Essentials of Weightlifting & Strength Training

First Edition

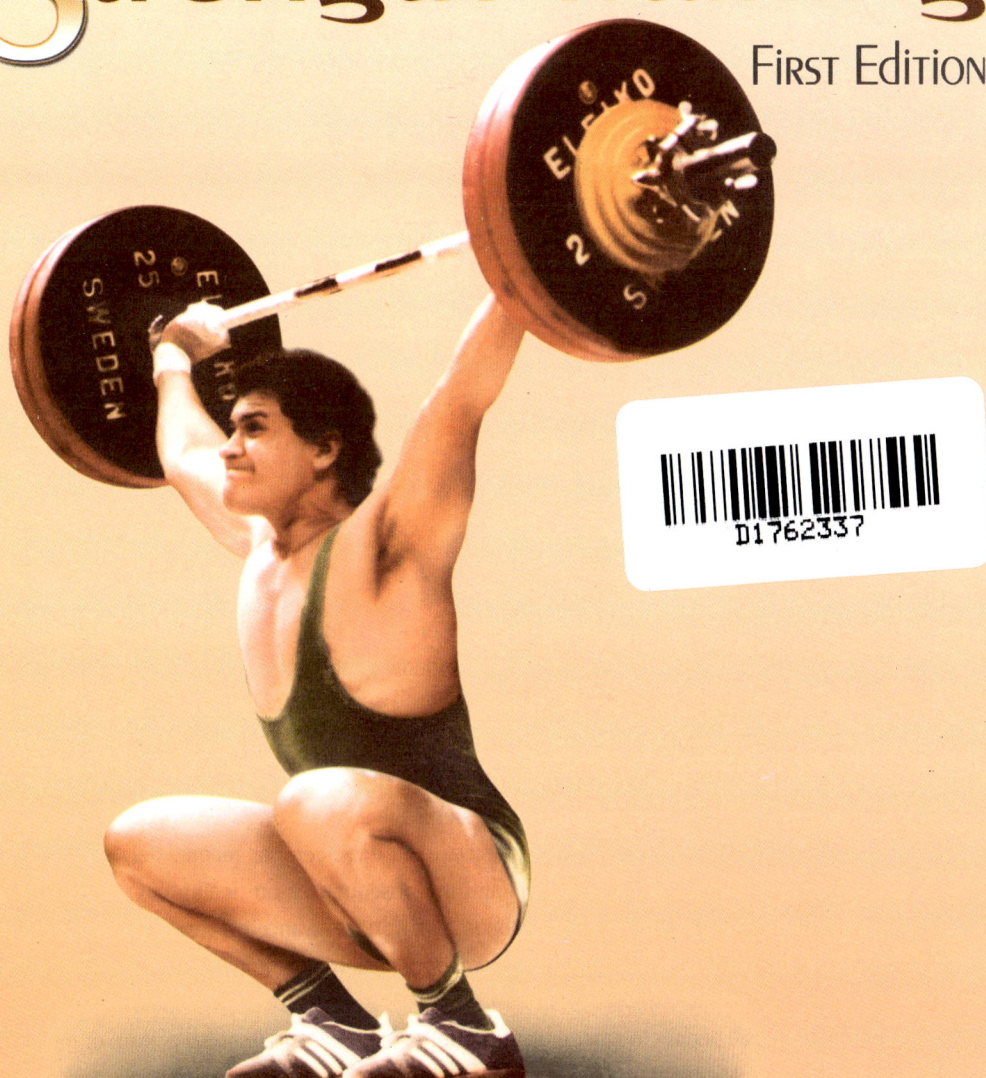

Mohamed F. El-Hewie, MD

SHAYMAA PUBLISHING CORPORATION
P.O. Box 501, Lodi,
New Jersey 07644-0501, U.S.A.

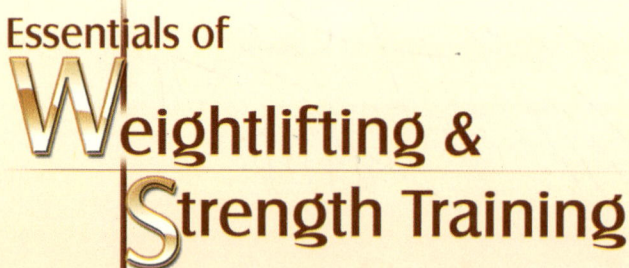

Essentials of Weightlifting & Strength Training

By **MOHAMED F. EL-HEWIE, MD**

Published by
SHAYMAA PUBLISHING CORPORATION
P.O. Box 501, Lodi,
New Jersey 07644-0501, U.S.A.

Copyright © 2003 by Mohamed F. El-Hewie, MD
World rights reserved. No part of this publication may be stored in a retrieval system, transmitted, or reproduced in any way, including but not limited to photocopy, photograph, magnetic, optic, or other record, without the prior agreement and written permission from the publisher.

Library of Congress Control Number : 2003090921
ISBN 0-9719581-0-6
Egyptian Deposit Number: 17423 / 2003.

1. Weightlifting– Textbook.
2. Strength Training—Manual.

First edition trade paperback printing October 2003
Printed in Alexandria, Egypt.

Includes descriptive and graphical analysis of physical exercises with drawings, photographs, charts, tables, and numerical presentation. The book bridges the gap between health, medical, and physical sciences in an effort to present the sport of Weightlifting in an academic form.

Disclaimer

The author presents his personal experience in Weightlifting and Strength Training in an educational and entertaining manner. The technical and medical analysis presented in this book represents the author's own views on the subject and does not represent peer review or institutional research work. The author, a physician and engineer, has relied solely on his own academic preparation to apply medical knowledge to physical exercise activity and its consequences on health and fitness. The author has utilized public information as well as professional academic information in his effort to advance his views. The author does not claim that the views presented in this book are flawless, since the entire domain of health and fitness is still evolving as our knowledge grows and expands.

Though the author is urging all people to contemplate strength training as an essential activity of modern living, the author spared no effort in explaining the limitation of human beings, in health and disease conditions. The author makes no warranty or representation, either expressed or implied, with respect to usefulness or safety of exercise or physical activity in conditions prohibited by medical advice. The author also does not intend to diagnose, treat, or prescribe medication with this publication.

Preface

This book is intended to serve as a compendium of those aspects of Weightlifting and Weight-Training that are essential to the development of physical strength. A prominent feature of this book is the in-depth coverage of scientific and medical aspects of a forgotten sport. The main theme of this book is the concept of **"progressive incremental resistance training"**. This is the basis of inducing physical adaptation to increasing activity. The book does not merely intend to explain execution of exercises or list commonly practiced exercises. In addition, this book elucidates the essence of developing **"healthy physical strength"**. This starts from the effects of exercise on genetic expression and ends by the cumulative effects of exercise over many years of life. Along these years, ill effects develop insidiously as a result of faulty exercise planning and execution. Many books tackle the subject of exercise description and plans of training. Yet, this book focuses on the balance among the various elements of physical strength such as endurance, flexibility, coordination, agility, and injury managements. The book offers expert advice on planning load volume and intensity of essential exercises, nutrition, and rest for the purpose of achieving breakthrough in strength development. These are presented in scientific context that aims for prevention of long term ill effects of inflexibility, unnecessary bodyweight gain, or increased vulnerability to preventable diseases.

The idea of writing a book about Weightlifting has haunted me since 1970s'. Yet, in those old days, the means of typing, drawing, and statistical analysis were quite discouraging in tackling such task of vast descriptive nature. Along thirty years, from the birth of the idea to deciding to proceed with writing and publication, many events have enriched my experience about the subject. Among these events was the exposure to men with great experience in international Weightlifting. The first coach, Ahmed Mutawa, who introduced me into Weightlifting, was the greatest impetus for my determination to lift for life. Unfortunately, he died from rheumatic heart disease in his thirties. The latter coach, Mohamed Al-Kassabany, was the greatest source of knowledge and motivation. His graduate study from East Germany, during the greatest strides in Weightlifting in 1960's, in addition to his paternal nurturing skills had greatly influenced my views. In addition, I am also grateful to the city of my birth, Alexandria Egypt, for the exposure it offered me to many Olympic gold medallists in Weightlifting. As a seaport, Alexandria has offered me unique exposure to international trends that lacked in the rest of the neighboring towns. I owe deep indebtedness to many teachers and professors who had shaped my academic acumen.

The book is organized into twenty chapters. Chapter 1: "Introduction", is a review on the role of Strength Training in health and fitness. Chapter 2: "Proper Lifting Techniques", presents the general rules of proper lifting. Chapter 3: "Fallacies and Their Critiques", discusses the common fallacies in the arena of exercising and nutrition. Chapter 4: "Weightlifting", presents Olympic Weightlifting to unfamiliar readers. Chapter 5: "Powerlifting", glances through the rising sport of Powerlifting in the western nations. Chapter 6: "Bodybuilding", discusses the role of Bodybuilding in developing muscular mass and strength. Chapter 7 : "Weight Training", presents the widely practiced sport of training with weight for general strengthening. Chapters 8 and 9 are detailed reviews of the mechanics of Olympic lifts and their assisting exercises. Chapter 10: "Endurance vs. Strength", offers the reader a review on the goal of any exercising activity. Chapter 11: "Axial Training vs. Peripheral Training", presents the author's personal bias in favor for axial training. Chapter 12: "Making Training Choices", is an effort to explore the many choices, others have made, in developing exercise strategy. Chapter 13: "Managing Load Volume & Intensity", details the planning of physical work to enhance strength and prevent overtraining. Chapter 14: "Health and Fitness", presents general issues of enhancing health by exercise and nutrition. Chapter 15: "Exercise and Preventable Diseases", reviews community trends in acquiring diseases and major risk factors. Chapter 16: "Exercise & Injuries", brings the reader to close understanding of exercise-related injuries. Chapter 17 : "Exercise and Science", presents the reader with abstract approach to scientific ideas that intertwine with all aspects of heath and fitness. Chapter 18: "Frequently Asked Questions", reviews common issues related to exercise and nutrition. Chapter 18 : "Training Women", discusses issues of specific concern to woman's fitness. Chapter 20: "Guidelines for Optimum Strength Training", sums all rules of exercise and the consequences of planning and performing.

Mohamed F. El-Hewie
Lodi, New Jersey, October 2003

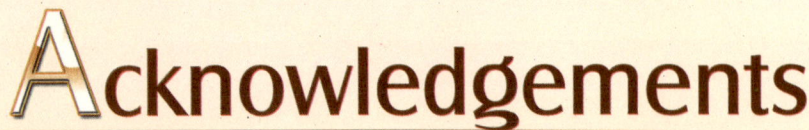
Acknowledgements

Statistical data:

I am indebted to the rich and generous information provided by many institutions. Among these are:

i. The **Center of Disease Control** of the USA for providing health statistics on American communities.

ii. The **World Health Organization** for providing health statistics on international communities.

iii. The **Olympic Museum of Lausanne,** Swiss for providing past Olympic records.

iv. The **International Weightlifting Federation** for providing statistics on world championships in Weightlifting.

v. The **Department of Agriculture** of USA for providing nutritional data on thousands of common food items.

Graphic work:

i. A very important contribution to the graphic work of this edition has been the invaluable work of my sister **Nadia F. El-Hewie,** who devoted many months in drawing and preparing photographs, charts, and tables.

ii. Cover design and photograph collection are credited to **Salah F. El-Hewie**. He has planned the entire layout of the graphic work and brought many capable graphic artists to carry out his plans.

iii. The painstaking artistic work was greatly enhanced by the contribution of the graphic engineers **Walid M. Fathy** and **Samah El-Fakahany.**

Book project management:

The chief burden of orchestrating this book project fell on the shoulders of my brother **Salah F. El-Hewie,** his wife, and two daughters. I am grateful for the tremendous effort undertaken by Salah and for his campaign of gathering information and photographs from many renowned Weightlifters and coaches and petitioning various capable and talented people for contribution to this book project. His meticulous editing, reviewing of the manuscript and graphics, and printing were instrumental in presenting this book in its current form.

Special thanks go to my 13-year and 10-year old nieces, **Shaymaa and Aliaa El-Hewie,** who managed the email and telephone communications between the different parties throughout the many months of printing and typesetting.

Graphic film production:

This was expedited by the sponsoring of **Al-Sawy F. Al-Sawy,** the chief executive manager of Graphic House Corporation, Alexandria, Egypt. His meticulous film production has saved many old photographs from getting wasted. His invaluable contribution and humble attitude had spared the author many daunting tasks of film preparation, touching, finishing, and production.

Book montage and color management:

The meticulous task of image composition, color choices, and figure adjustments were the work product of engineer **Sobhy A. Abul Fetouh.**

Book printing:

The combined effort of three printing firms from Alexandria, Egypt, has greatly expedited the production of this book and eliminated many formidable expenses. The three firms had sponsored and expedited the printing project of this book, despite their competitive work. Without such contribution from such very able printing companies, this book might have been delayed indefinitely. Thanks to these three managers for achieving such cooperation.

i. **Ashraf K. Said,** the manager and owner of Al-Mashreq printing company.

ii. **Abdel Fattah Al-Hadari,** the manager and owner of Al-Hadari printing company.

iii. **Ahmed M. Khamis,** the manager and owner of Al-Reyadah printing company.

Mohamed F. El-Hewie
Lodi, New Jersey, October 2003

Contents

1. INTRODUCTION   1

1.1 Recognition of a forgotten sport   1
1.1.1. Rapid expansion of urbanization   1
1.1.2. Increased access to medical knowledge   1
1.1.3. Increased affordability of strength training   1

1.2 Mystical thinking and sport   1
1.2.1. Mystical thinking among athletes   1
1.2.2. Mystical thinking among common people   2
1.2.3. Habits and healthy thinking   2
1.2.4. On the dynamics of human mind   2

1.3 Logical inference and sport   2
1.3.1. Logical inference and progress in sciences   3
1.3.2. The ultra-minute versus the gigantic universes   3
1.3.3. Similarities in health and physical sciences   3
1.3.4. Strength training and quality of ambulant living   3
1.3.5. The inevitability of human limitations   3
1.3.6. The dichotomy of physical and intellectual fitness   4

1.4 Role of herd conviction in sport   4
1.4.1. Constant and persistent modeling   4
1.4.2. Advent in communication   4
1.4.3. The proliferation of a forgotten sport   4
1.4.4. Passing habits between generations   5

1.5 Stigma about weightlifting   5
1.5.1. Class stigma of menial labor   5
1.5.2. Modern science discovers health in physical activity   5
1.5.3. Today's menial occupations   5
1.5.4. Growing need for exercising for good living   6
1.5.5. A sport of the tough and crude folks   6
1.5.6. Resistance training a new experiment   6
1.5.7 My personal experience with weightlifting   6
1.5.8. Surpassing others in the new sport   6
1.5.9. Getting involved in physical exercising   6

1.6 Social changes and sport   7
1.6.1. Epidemics of the past   7
1.6.2. Birth of new technological marvels   7
1.6.3. Military competition revolutionizes the sport of weightlifting   7
1.6.4. Contribution of the communist athletes to weightlifting   7
1.6.5. The rise and growth of the sport of bodybuilding   7
1.6.6. Proliferation of the sport of general weight training   8
1.6.7. Change in attitude towards physical training   8

1.6 State of knowledge   7
1.7.1. Proper resistance training leads to strength   8
1.7.2. Early education and systemic physical training   8
1.7.3. Education conveyed in play format   9
1.7.4. Children's demand for early training   9
1.7.5. The keys to proper planning of weightlifting program   9
1.7.6. The essence of the sport of weightlifting   9
1.7.7. Intermix of art and science   9
1.7.8. Lack of access to information   10
1.7.9. Causes of unpopularity of weightlifting   10

1.8 Discipline   10
1.8.1 The role of mental determination in weightlifting   10
1.8.2. The role of discipline in weightlifting   10
1.8.3. Access of information to the youth   11
1.8.4. Need for community-volunteer work by athletes   11
1.8.5. Scientific planning of resistance training   11
1.8.6 On the perplexing roots of discipline   12
1.8.7. On the rebellion of adult trainees against disciplinary rules   12
1.8.8. Discipline versus deprivation   12
1.8.9 On the compliance of trainees with planned schemes   12
1.8.10 On the nurturing of logical insight into one's own problems   13

1.9 Debates   13
1.9.1 Is Weightlifting an every day necessity?   13
1.9.2. How much weight training suffices for getting and staying fit?   13
1.9.3. How to avoid erroneously harmful training?   13
1.9.4. Search for ultimate role models   14
1.9.5. Weightlifting is a sport for everybody   14

1.10 Nutrition, exercise, and rest   14
1.10.1. Nutritional needs of athletes versus those for non-athletes   14
1.10.2. Natural exercises versus equipment-aided exercises   14
1.10.3. Making the best out of your rest time   15

1.11 Story of a little old lady   15
1.11.1. Setting priorities in a wise manner   15
1.11.2. Efficient selection of proper exercises   16
1.11.3. Implementing higher standards of training with plain common sense   16

1.12 Sound workout plan   16
1.12.1. Modest availability of space and equipment   16
1.12.2. Safety rules of proper progressive increase in resistance   16
1.12.3. Standards that achieve noticeable improvement   17

1.13 Basic rules   17
1.13.1. Essential exercises   17
1.13.2. Ancillary exercises   17

1.14 Exercise sequence   18
1.14.1. Essential exercises executed caudally   18
1.14.2. Ancillary exercises and mobility versus stability   18
1.14.3. Examples of improper sequence of executing exercises   18

1.15 Modesty and posture   18
1.15.1 Modest goal of staying physically fit   18
1.15.2. Essential muscles of posture   19

v

1.15.3.	Cumulative effect of posture enhancement 19	2.7.2.	The mysterious habit of yanking 34
1.15.4.	Benefits of healthy posture 19	2.7.3.	Yanking dissipates energy 34

1.16 Today's gym — 20
- 1.16.1. Role of health-club goers 20
- 1.16.2. Role of organizers of health-clubs 20

1.17 Proper equipments of resistance training — 20
- 1.17.1. Role of symmetry of motion 20
- 1.17.2. Use of simple and reliable equipments 20
- 1.17.3. Role of natural human movement 21

1.18 Serious daily habits — 21
- 1.18.1. Improper occupational activities 21
- 1.18.2. Improper lifting of a child from the floor 22
- 1.18.3. Improper lifting of a grocery bag 22
- 1.18.4. Improper bending on a sink 22
- 1.18.5. Sitting in couch 23
- 1.18.6. Alcohol consumption 23
- 1.18.7. Smoking 23

1.19 Highlights of chapter ONE — 24

2. PROPER LIFTING TECHNIQUES — 25

2.1 Lifting in everyday activity — 25
- 2.1.1. Lifting weights as a major cause of injuries 25
- 2.1.2. Who knows better about lifting? 25
- 2.1.3. Practical tricks of proper lifting 25
- 2.1.4. Knowledge versus Practice 26

2.2 Approaching lifting — 26
- 2.2.1. Centers of gravity of objects and humans 26
- 2.2.2. Vertical forces versus Horizontal forces 26
- 2.2.3. Standing very close to the object 26

2.3 Upper Body Posture — 27
- 2.3.1. Straight and upright posture 27
- 2.3.2. Shoulders elevation and chest thrusting 28
- 2.3.3. Demand for attention 28
- 2.3.4. Retracting the scapulae 29
- 2.3.5. Hardening the abdomen 29
- 2.3.6. Lifting Posture 29

2.4 Bend your knees — 30
- 2.4.1. Leaning versus squatting 30
- 2.4.2 Lifting instincts 30
- 2.4.3. Dreading knees bending 30
- 2.4.4. Use your knees as a probe in lifting 31
- 2.4.5. Wasting of knees and back muscles without exercise 31
- 2.4.6. Knees versus back injury 31

2.5 Habitual modeling — 31
- 2.5.1. Essence of proper lifting 31
- 2.5.2 Mastering the rituals of lifting 32
- 2.5.3. Learning through play 32

2.6 Shoulder versus arm pulling — 32
- 2.6.1. Role of the arms 32
- 2.6.2. Role of the Trapezius 33
- 2.6.3. Role of the Deltoid 33

2.7 Pulling versus yanking — 34
- 2.7.1. Knowing versus performing 34
- 2.7.2. The mysterious habit of yanking 34
- 2.7.3. Yanking dissipates energy 34
- 2.7.4. Timing of the lifting speed 35
- 2.7.5. How muscles adapt to resistance? 35
- 2.7.6. Normal course of training aftereffects 35
- 2.7.7. Yanking causes grave injuries 36
- 2.7.8. Perfecting lifting skills 36
- 2.7.9. Yanking versus adequate recruitment of muscle fibers 37

2.8 The approach phase — 37
- 2.8.1. Mental rituals during the approach phase 37
- 2.8.2. Physical attitudes during the approach phase 38

2.9 Initial phase — 38
- 2.9.1. Start position 38
- 2.9.2. Leverage of torque 39
- 2.9.3. Efficient recruitment of muscles 39

2.10 Equalization phase — 39
- 2.10.1. Essence of resistance and energy 39
- 2.10.2. Sequential hardening of muscles 40
- 2.10.3. Mid-foot arching 40
- 2.10.4. The stabilization of the ankles 40
- 2.10.5. The immense strength of the muscles of the knees 41
- 2.10.6. Hip position during lifting 41
- 2.10.7. The unique upright posture of lifters 41
- 2.10.8. The complex mechanics of the vertebral column 42
- 2.10.9. Leverage at the shoulder joints 42

2.11 Equalization phase — 43
- 2.11.1. Internal disturbance 43
- 2.11.2. External motion 43
- 2.11.3. Torques and forces 44
- 2.11.4. Synchronizing the Pull 44

2.12 Musculoskeletal back pain — 45
- 2.12.1. Prevalence 45
- 2.12.2. Nerve root syndrome 45
- 2.12.3. Muscular and fascial pain 45
- 2.12.4. Skeletal pain 45
- 2.12.5. Clinical presentation of lower back pain 46
- 2.12.6. Workup for back pain 46
- 2.12.7. Treatment of back pain 46
- 2.12.8. Spinoscopic examination 47

2.13 Highlights of chapter TWO — 48

3. FALLACIES AND THEIR CRITIQUES — 49

3.1 Aggressive marketing and health ethics — 49

3.2 Smoking and alcohol — 49

3.3 Sexual activity and training — 50

3.4 Deceptive information — 51

3.5 Fallacies on warming up — 51
- 3.5.1. Reasons for warming up 51
- 3.5.2. Physiology of warming up 52

3.6 Fallacies on warming up — 52
- 3.6.1. Purpose of the exercise 52

3.6.2.	Limitations of the exercise 52		4.2.8.	Brain control of muscle contraction 71	
3.6.3.	Function of lordotic back 53		4.2.9.	Speed of lifting 72	
3.6.4.	Power drive in the deadlift 54		4.2.10.	Repertoire of weightlifting exercises 73	
3.6.5.	Spinal disc herniation 54		4.2.11.	Load volume or "tonnage" 73	
3.6.6.	Overhand and underhand grips 55		4.2.12.	Exercise intensity 75	
			4.2.13.	Maximum lifts (1RM, one repetition of maximum) 75	
3.7	**Fallacies on Injuries and lifting**	**55**	4.2.14.	Recovery 76	

3.7 Fallacies on Injuries and lifting 55
- 3.7.1. Abdominal hernias 55
- 3.7.2. Knee injuries 56
- 3.7.3. Insidious deformities 57

3.8 Fallacies on sport versus exercise 57
- 3.8.1. Sport versus exercise 57

3.9 Fallacies on adaptation to technique 58
- 3.9.1. Adaptation to technique 58

3.10 Fallacies on weightlifting 58
- 3.10.1. Strength factor in weightlifting 58

3.11 Fallacies on weightlifting 59
- 3.11.1. Limitation of bodybuilding training 59

3.12 Fallacies on aerobics versus weight training 60
- 3.12.1. Aerobic fat burning 60
- 3.12.2. Planning load volume 60
- 3.12.3. Effective workout 60
- 3.12.4. Switching muscle fuels 60
- 3.12.5. Recuperation 61

3.13 Fallacies on nutrition and metabolism 61
- 3.13.1. Proper eating 61
- 3.13.2. Proper caloric intake 61
- 3.13.3. Metabolic factors 61
- 3.13.4 Old eating habits 61
- 3.13.5. Carbohydrate metabolism 62
- 3.13.6. Water balance 62
- 3.13.7. Nutrition and coronary artery diseases 62
- 3.13.8. Fat and protein diet 62

3.14 Muscular balance 63
- 3.14.1. Scapular balance 63
- 3.14.2. Stability 63
- 3.14.3. Agonists and antagonist muscles 63

3.15 Highlights of chapter THREE 64

4. WEIGHTLIFTING 65

4.1 Strength training in weightlifting 65
- 4.1.1. Evolution of weightlifting 65
- 4.1.2. Sport versus exercise 65
- 4.1.3. Constituents of weightlifting training 66
- 4.1.3.1. Pure strength exercises 66
- 4.1.3.2. Technique assisting exercises 67

4.2 Features of weightlifting training 67
- 4.2.1. General features 67
- 4.2.2. Daily training routine 68
- 4.2.3. Number of repetitions per sets 69
- 4.2.4. Number of exercises per session 69
- 4.2.5. Technique versus strength 69
- 4.2.6. Exercise sequence 70
- 4.2.7. Types of muscular contractions 70
- 4.2.8. Brain control of muscle contraction 71
- 4.2.9. Speed of lifting 72
- 4.2.10. Repertoire of weightlifting exercises 73
- 4.2.11. Load volume or "tonnage" 73
- 4.2.12. Exercise intensity 75
- 4.2.13. Maximum lifts (1RM, one repetition of maximum) 75
- 4.2.14. Recovery 76

4.3 Standard weightlifting training sessions 77
- 4.3.1. Standard training 77
- 4.3.2. Emphasis on the snatch technique 77
- 4.3.3. Emphasis on the clean and jerk technique 77
- 4.3.4. The snatch and the clean and jerk techniques 78
- 4.3.5. Reducing the volume for muscle recovery 78
- 4.3.6. Enhancing technical skills of the clean and jerk 78
- 4.3.7 Enhancing technical skills of the snatch 79

4.4 Training for competition 79

4.5 Assisting exercises of weightlifting 79
- 4.5.1. Squat 79
- 4.5.2. Major axial muscles of weightlifting 82
- 4.5.3. Power development and weightlifting training 83

4.6 International trends in weightlifting 84
- 4.6.1. Before World War II 84
- 4.6.2. After World War II 84
- 4.6.3. Olympic games of Atlanta 1996 86
- 4.6.4. Weightlifting in Egypt 1936 87

4.7 Highlights of chapter FOUR 88

5. POWERLIFTING 89

5.1 Basics of physical power 89
- 5.1.1. Training methods 89
- 5.1.2. Elements of physical power 90
- 5.1.3. Physical power of weightlifting 90

5.2 Powerlifting assisting exercises 90
- 5.2.1. Back Squat 91
- 5.2.1.1. Description of back squat 91
- 5.2.1.2. Variants of feet stance during back squat 92
- 5.2.1.3. Tweaking of squat technique 93
- 5.2.2. Front squat 94
- 5.2.2.1. Unique features of front squat 95
- 5.2.2.2. Description of front squat 95
- 5.2.3. Overhead squat 96
- 5.2.3.1. Description of overhead squat 97
- 5.2.4. Military clean 98
- 5.2.4.1. Real living emulation 98
- 5.2.4.2. Lifting styles 98
- 5.2.4.3. Description of military clean 99
- 5.2.5. Power clean 100
- 5.2.6. Hang clean 101
- 5.2.7. Military snatch 102
- 5.2.8. Power snatch 103
- 5.2.9. Deadlift 103
- 5.2.9.1. Description of the Ieadlift 103
- 5.2.9.2. Variants of the powerlifting deadlift 104
- 5.2.10. Bench press 104
- 5.2.10.1. Description of bench press 105

5.3	**Plans of powerlifting training**		**106**
5.3.1.	Parallel routine	106	
5.3.2.	Serial routine	106	
5.4	**Muscular imbalance**		**107**
5.5	**Power boosting modalities**		**109**
5.5.1.	Supersets	109	
5.5.2.	High intensity training	110	
5.5.3.	Slow motion training	110	
5.5.4.	Plyometrics	110	
5.5.5.	Calisthenics	111	
5.6	**Olympic weightlifting vs powerlifting**		**111**
5.6.1.	Lifting belt	111	
5.6.2.	Supportive clothing	112	
5.6.3.	Knee wraps	112	
5.6.4.	Squatting style	112	
5.6.5.	Power versus strength	113	
5.6.6.	Drug doping	113	
5.6.6.1.	False belief in drug enhancement	113	
5.6.6.2.	Mode of drug action	113	
5.6.7.	Mobility	113	
5.6.8.	Load volume	114	
5.6.9.	Longevity	114	
5.6.10.	Popularity	114	
5.7	**Highlights of chapter FIVE**		**115**

6. BODYBUILDING 117

6.1	**Essence of bodybuilding**		**117**
6.1.1.	New sport	117	
6.1.2.	New tools of fitness	117	
6.1.3.	New trends	118	
6.2	**Judging criteria**		**119**
6.2.1	Muscle mass	119	
6.2.2.	Muscular definition	119	
6.2.3.	Muscular proportion	119	
6.2.4.	Body shape	120	
6.2.5.	Posing performance	120	
6.3	**Bodybuilding diet**		**120**
6.3.1.	Body fat content	120	
6.3.2.	Dietary habits	120	
6.3.3.	Shedding calories by physical activities	122	
6.3.4.	Assisting medication	123	
6.3.5.	Bodybuilding model	123	
6.4	**Anabolic steroids**		**123**
6.4.1	Common drugs	123	
6.4.2.	Physiological effects	123	
6.4.3.	Psychological effects	124	
6.4.4.	Problems with illicit drug use	125	
6.5	**Back exercises**		**125**
6.5.1	Stiff-legged deadlift	125	
6.5.2.	Horizontal seated row	126	
6.5.3.	Bent-over row	126	
6.5.4.	Lever bent-over row	127	
6.5.5.	Chin-ups	127	
6.5.6.	Lateral cable pulldown	128	
6.5.7.	Dumbbell rowing	129	
6.5.8.	Lever rowing	129	
6.6	**Leg exercises**		**129**
6.6.1.	Squat	130	
6.6.2.	Calf raises	131	
6.6.3.	Cable hip adduction	132	
6.6.4.	Oblique leg press	132	
6.6.5.	Hack squat	133	
6.6.6.	Lying leg curls	133	
6.6.7.	Seated leg curls	134	
6.7	**Lower back exercises**		**134**
6.7.1.	Trunk twists	134	
6.7.2.	Lateral trunk bends	135	
6.7.3.	Hip extension from a bench	135	
6.8	**Abdominal exercises**		**136**
6.8.1.	Crunches	136	
6.8.2.	Incline sit-up	137	
6.8.3.	Leg raises	137	
6.9	**Weight training guidelines**		**138**
6.9.1.	Weekly training frequency	138	
6.9.2.	Symmetry rules	139	
6.9.3.	Range of motion rules	139	
6.9.4.	Returning from lay-off	139	
6.9.5.	Forced repetitions	139	
6.10	**Highlights of chapter SIX**		**140**

7. WEIGHT TRAINING 141

7.1	**Introduction**		**141**
7.2	**Strengthening elbow flexors**		**141**
7.2.1.	Applied anatomy of elbow	141	
7.2.2.	Brachial muscle	142	
7.2.2.1.	Barbell curls	142	
7.2.2.2.	One-hand cable curls	143	
7.2.2.3.	Dumbbell concentration curls	143	
7.2.2.4.	Cable curls	143	
7.2.3.	Biceps brachii muscle	144	
7.2.3.1.	Reverse barbell curls	144	
7.2.3.2.	One-hand dumbbell curls	145	
7.2.3.3.	Hammer dumbbell curls	145	
7.2.4.	Brachioradialis muscle	145	
7.2.5.	Wrist and finger extensors	146	
7.2.5.1.	Reverse wrist curls	146	
7.2.6.	Wrist and finger flexors	146	
7.2.6.1	Wrist curls	146	
7.3	**Strengthening elbow extensors**		**147**
7.3.1	Applied anatomy	147	
7.3.2.	Elbow extension exercises	148	
7.3.2.1.	Upright elbow extension	148	
7.3.2.2.	One-hand dumbbell elbow extension	148	
7.3.2.3.	Cable pushdown	149	
7.3.2.4.	Forearm kickback	149	
7.3.2.5.	Triceps dips	150	

7.4	**Strengthening the shoulders**	**150**
7.4.1.	Applied anatomy	150
7.4.2.	Shoulder elevation	151
7.4.2.1.	Shoulder shrugging	151
7.4.2.2.	One-hand dumbbell side bends	151
7.4.3.	Shoulder external rotation	152
7.4.3.1.	One-hand dumbbell rows	152
7.4.3.2.	Bent-over lateral arm raises	153
7.4.3.3.	Bent-over rows	153
7.4.3.4.	T-bar bent-over row	154
7.4.3.5.	Seated cable rows	154
7.4.4.	Shoulder internal rotation	155
7.4.4.1.	Barbell shoulder press	155
7.4.4.2.	Seated shoulder press	156
7.4.4.3.	One-hand shoulder dumbbell press	156
7.4.4.4.	Dumbbell front raises	157
7.4.4.5.	Cable front raises	157
7.4.4.6.	Dumbbell flyes	158
7.4.4.7.	Incline dumbbell flyes	158
7.4.4.8.	Inclined dumbbell press	159
7.4.4.9.	Cable flyes	159
7.4.4.10.	Deck flyes	159
7.4.4.11.	Pullover	160
7.4.4.12.	Bench press	160
7.4.4.13.	Inclined bench press	161
7.4.4.14.	Pushups	162
7.4.4.15.	Parallel bar dip	162
7.4.5.	Shoulder adduction and extension	163
7.4.5.1.	Chin-ups	163
7.4.5.2.	Cable pulldown	164
7.4.6.	Shoulder abduction	164
7.4.6.1.	Lateral arm raises	165
7.4.6.2.	Lateral deck raises	165
7.4.6.3.	Upright barbell arm rows	165
7.4.7.	Shoulder extension	166
7.4.8.	Shoulder flexion	166
7.5	**Strengthening the hips**	**166**
7.5.1.	Hip extension	167
7.5.1.1.	One-legged hip extension	167
7.5.1.2.	Goodmorning back extension purpose	168
7.5.1.3.	Horizontal back extension	168
7.5.1.4.	Dumbbell squat	168
7.5.1.5.	Inclined leg press	169
7.5.1.6.	Deadlift	169
7.5.1.7.	Back squat	169
7.5.1.8.	Front squat	170
7.5.2.	Hip flexion	170
7.5.2.1.	Horizontal leg raises	171
7.5.2.2.	Ladder vertical leg raises	171
7.5.2.3.	Parallel bar vertical leg raises	171
7.5.2.4.	Inclined sit-ups	172
7.5.2.5.	Vertical sit-ups	172
7.5.3.	Hip adduction	173
7.5.3.1.	Cable and machine hip adduction	173
7.5.4.	Hip abduction	173
7.5.4.1.	Floor and machine hip abduction	173
7.6	**Strengthening the knees**	**174**
7.6.1	Knee extension	174
7.6.1.1.	Back squat	174
7.6.1.2.	Front squat	174
7.6.1.3.	One-leg stepping on a block with weights	174
7.6.1.4.	Deadlift	174
7.6.1.5.	The clean and snatch	175
7.6.1.6.	Seated knee extension	175
7.6.2.	Knee flexion	175
7.6.2.1.	Leg curl	175
7.7	**Strengthening the ankle**	**176**
7.7.1.	Ankle flexion (dorsal flexion)	176
7.7.2.	Ankle extension (plantar flexion)	176
7.8	**Strengthening the abdominal muscles**	**177**
7.8.1.	Floor abdominal crunches	177
7.8.1.2.	Oblique bends	178
7.8.1.3.	Trunk rotation	178

8. THE SNATCH LIFT — 179

8.1	**Standard snatch technique**	**179**
8.1.1.	Preparation	179
8.1.2.	Induction of acceleration	179
8.1.3.	Induction of speed	179
8.1.4.	Induction of momentum	180
8.1.5.	Induction of weightlessness	180
8.1.6.	Overhead squatting	181
8.1.7.	Final ascent	181
8.1.8.	Barbell return to the floor	181
8.2	**Contest rules of the snatch lift**	**182**
8.3	**Training practice on the snatch lift**	**182**
8.4	**Specific features of the mechanism of execution of the snatch**	**183**
8.4.1.	Arm usage in transfer of forces	183
8.4.2.	Origin of lifting forces	184
8.4.3.	Momentum of head bouncing	184
8.5	**Learning the snatch lift**	**184**
8.5.1.	Discover your ability to perform formidable movements	184
8.5.2.	Individual variation in learning and objectivity	184
8.5.3	Learning with dummy objects	185
8.6	**Start position of the snatch**	**185**
8.6.1.	Analysis of the start position of the snatch	185
8.6.2.	Strengthening the start position of the snatch	186
8.7	**Phase of acceleration of the snatch**	**186**
8.7.1.	Analysis of the phase of acceleration of the snatch	186
8.7.2.	Strengthening the phase of acceleration of the snatch	187
8.8	**Phase of initiating momentum of the snatch**	**187**
8.8.1.	Analysis of the momentum initiation of the snatch	187
8.8.2.	Strengthening the phase of momentum initiation	188
8.9	**Phase of maximal speed of the snatch**	**188**
8.9.1.	Analysis of the phase of maximal speed of the snatch	188
8.9.2.	Strengthening the phase of maximal speed	189
8.10	**Phase of maximal momentum of the snatch**	**189**
8.10.1.	Analysis of the phase of maximal momentum of the snatch	189
8.10.2.	Strengthening the phase of maximal momentum	190

8.11	**Phase of shoulder abduction of the snatch**	**190**
8.11.1.	Analysis of the phase of shoulder abduction	190
8.11.2.	Strengthening the phase of shoulder abduction	191

8.12	**Phase of descent of the snatch**	**191**
8.12.1.	Analysis of the phase of descent of the snatch	191
8.12.2.	Strengthening the phase of descent of the snatch	192

8.13	**Phase of full squat snatch**	**192**
8.13.1.	Analysis of the phase of full squat snatch	192
8.13.2.	Strengthening the phase of full squat snatch	193

8.14	**Phase of full ascent of snatch**	**193**
8.14.1.	Analysis of the phase of ascent of the snatch	193
8.14.2.	Strengthening the phase of ascent of snatch	194

8.15	**Teaching the snatch lift**	**194**
8.15.1.	Framework of training for the snatch	194
8.15.2.	Heavy lifting versus fine movements	195
8.15.3.	Driving forces in multi-jointed machines	195
8.15.4.	Common mistakes in the execution of the snatch	195
8.15.5.	Landmarks of progress in the snatch	196
8.15.6.	Tweaking the snatch lift	196
8.15.7.	Assisting the snatch lift	197
8.15.8.	Proper sequence of the snatch in training sessions	197

8.16	**Highlights of Chapter EIGHT**	**197**

9. THE CLEAN & JERK — 199

9.1	**Standard technique of the clean**	**199**
9.1.1.	Preparation	199
9.1.2.	Induction of acceleration	199
9.1.3.	Induction of speed	200
9.1.4.	Induction of momentum	200
9.1.5.	Induction of weightlessness	201
9.1.6.	Descent under the bar	201
9.1.7.	Full squat clean	202
9.1.8.	Ascent from the clean squat	202
9.1.9.	Finalizing the clean	203

9.2	**Standard technique of the jerk**	**203**
9.2.1.	Preparation for the jerk lift	203
9.2.2.	Initiating the jerk lift	204
9.2.3.	Shoulder drive and leg lunging	204
9.2.4.	Stabilizing the jerk motion	205
9.2.5.	Recovering from the jerk motion	205
9.2.6.	Final jerk lift	206

9.3	**Contest rules of the clean and jerk lift**	**206**

9.4	**Training practice on the clean and jerk lift**	**207**
9.4.1.	Dissecting the motion of the clean and jerk	207
9.4.2.	Hang clean	207
9.4.3.	Hang pull	208
9.4.4.	High pull	208
9.4.5.	Push press	209
9.4.6.	Split jerk	209

9.5	**Proper lifting technique for the clean and jerk**	**207**
9.5.1.	Proper technique for the clean	210
9.5.2.	Proper technique for the jerk	210
9.5.3.	Training practice on the proper technique for the clean and jerk	212

9.6	**Pros and cons of explosive weight training**	**212**
9.6.1.	Risk factors	212
9.6.2.	Necessity of ballistic weight training	213

9.7	**Errors in the clean and jerk**	**214**
9.7.1.	The clean faults, causes and corrections	214
9.7.1.1.	Premature elevation of hips before raising bar	214
9.7.1.2.	Forward displacement of bar trajectory	214
9.7.1.3.	Backward displacement of bar trajectory	214
9.7.1.4.	Insufficient torso torque	214
9.7.1.5.	Insufficient full body extension	215
9.7.1.6.	Insufficient shoulder flexion	215
9.7.1.7.	Inadequate support of full body flexion	215
9.7.2.	The jerk faults, causes and corrections	215
9.7.2.1.	Insufficient leg drive	215
9.7.2.2.	Forward displacement during shoulder push	216
9.7.2.3.	Flawed leg split	216
9.7.2.4.	Backward displacement of bar during overhead arm extension	216
9.7.3.	General tips on technique	216

9.8	**Managing training load intensity and volume**	**217**

9.9	**Highlights of Chapter NINE**	**217**

10. ENDURANCE VERSUS STRENGTH — 219

10.1	**Physical endurance & strength**	**219**
10.1.1	Inherence and nurture	219
10.1.2.	Optimization of energy expenditure	219
10.1.3.	Optimization of energy expenditure in olympic weightlifters	221

10.2	**Ventilation, perfusion, and circulation**	**222**
10.2.1.	Gas exchange in rest and exercise	222
10.2.2.	Maximal oxygen consumption or VO2 max	223
10.2.3.	Mechanics of ventilation	223
10.2.4.	Circulation	223
10.2.5.	Metabolism	224
10.2.6.	Performance	225

10.3	**Running for endurance and strength**	**225**
10.3.1.	Burning fuel during activity	225
10.3.2.	Dynamic forces in running	226
10.3.3.	Muscle mass and disproportion in runners	226
10.3.4.	Muscle mass and flexibility issues in runners	227
10.3.5.	Muscular imbalance in runner	228
10.3.6.	Overweight and weakness in runners	228
10.3.7.	Lumbar deformities in runners	229
10.3.8.	Modern men's back	230
10.3.9.	Wasted leg muscles in runners	230
10.3.10.	Musculoskeletal stiffness	231
10.3.11.	Effect of regular and balanced activities on running	232

10.4	**Training for endurance and strength**	**232**
10.4.1.	Intermittent physical work	232
10.4.2.	Load volume and intensity in endurance and strength training	232

10.5	**Adaptation to exercise**	**233**
10.5.1.	Heart adaptation	233
10.5.2.	Skeletal muscle adaptation	234
10.5.3.	Increased maximal oxygen consumption	236

10.5.4.	Lactate threshold	237
10.5.6.	Efficiency of performance	237

10.6 Effects of age on strength and endurance — 238
- 10.6.1. Training volume and physical decline with age 238
- 10.6.2. Muscle mass reduction with age 238
- 10.6.3. Effects of age on training 238

10.7 Plyometrics — 240
- 10.7.1. General features 240
- 10.7.2. Plyometrics exercises 240

10.8 Highlights of Chapter TEN — 241

11. AXIAL TRAINING VERSUS PERIPHERAL TRAINING — 243

11.1 Axial training versus peripheral training — 243
- 11.1.1. Definitions 243
- 11.1.2. Difficulties with axial training 244
- 11.1.3. Popularity of peripheral training 245
- 11.1.4. Axial versus peripheral training 247

11.2 Effect of training emphasis on body composition — 248
- 11.2.1. Mineral depot 248
- 11.2.2. Rationing demands 248
- 11.2.3. Water content 249
- 11.2.4. Fat content 249
- 11.2.5. Protein content 250

11.3 Effect of training emphasis on cardiovascular function — 250
- 11.3.1. Heart and lung racing 250
- 11.3.2. Submaximal cardiac power output 251
- 11.3.3. Orchestrated central delivery 251

11.4 Effect of training emphasis on musculoskeletal functions — 251
- 11.4.1. Strength 251
- 11.4.2. Endurance 253
- 11.4.3. Flexibility 254

11.5 Effect of training emphasis on power output — 256
- 11.5.1. Involuntary control 257
- 11.5.2. Feedback regulation of axial muscles 257
- 11.5.3. Guiding the fire 257
- 11.5.4. Rationing your emotion 257

11.6 Effect of training emphasis on speed — 258
- 11.6.1. Mental will 258
- 11.6.2. Dynamics of moving mass 258
- 11.6.3. Muscular effects 259

11.7 Highlights of Chapter ELEVEN — 260

12. MAKING TRAINING CHOICES — 261

12.1 Setting goals — 261
- 12.1.1. Exposure and individual circumstances 261
- 12.1.2. Discovery conquest 261
- 12.1.3. Appearance and fitness 263
- 12.1.4. Power and strength 264

12.2 Age consideration — 265
- 12.2.1 Physiological consideration 265
- 12.2.2. Early start 265
- 12.2.3. Quest for power 265
- 12.2.4. Quest for height 266
  - 12.2.4.1. Hip flexors and abdominal muscles 266
  - 12.2.4.2. Exercising axial extensors 268
  - 12.2.4.3. Shoulder strengthening in children 269
  - 12.2.4.4. Whole performance and regional participation 270
- 12.2.5. Starting in late adolescence 270
- 12.2.6. Fundamentals versus details of workout 271
- 12.2.7. Starting in the twenties 272
- 12.2.8. Stimulating approaches 272
- 12.2.9. Permanent physical changes 273
- 12.2.10. Starting in the thirties 274

12.3 Fitness consideration — 274

12.4 Gender consideration — 276

12.5 Availability issues — 276

12.6 Bodyweight issues — 277

12.7 Muscular imbalance — 278
- 12.7.1. Shoulder and pelvis imbalance 278
- 12.7.2. Torso imbalance 279
- 12.7.3. Imbalance due to body disproportion 280
- 12.7.4. Imbalance due to weak arms and shoulders 281
- 12.7.5. Imbalance due to weak scapular muscles 282
- 12.7.6. Rectifying shoulder imbalance 282
- 12.7.7. Greatest weightlifting assets 283
- 12.7.8. Maximum strength with minimum muscle mass 284
- 12.7.9. Dealing with long limbed lifters 285
- 12.7.10. Weightlifting training, from start to end 286

13. MANAGING LOAD VOLUME AND INTENSITY — 291

13.1 Progressive strength training — 291
- 13.1.1. Source of information 291
- 13.1.2. Sets, repetition, intensity, and volume 291
- 13.1.4. Exercise intensity 292
- 13.1.5. Recuperative intervals 292
- 13.1.5. Periodization of load volume 292

13.2 Physical overtraining — 292
- 13.2.1. Causes of overtraining 292
- 13.2.2. Managing overtraining 293

13.3 Periodization of load intensity and volume — 294
- 13.3.1. Powerlifting periodization 294
- 13.3.2. Critique on the periodization of Powerlifting 294
- 13.3.2. Weightlifting periodization 294
  - 13.3.2.1. Number of daily lifts 294
  - 13.3.2.2. Monthly exercise-differentials 295

13.4 Details of a four-month period for weightlifting training — 294
- 13.4.1. First-month daily exercise-differentials 296
- 13.4.2. First-week daily exercise-differentials 297
- 13.4.3. Second-week daily exercise-differentials 298
- 13.4.5. Third-week daily exercise-differentials 299
- 13.4.6. Fourth-week daily exercise-differentials 300
- 13.4.7. Second-month daily exercise-differentials 302

13.4.8.	Fifth-week daily exercise-differentials	302		
13.4.9.	Sixth-week daily exercise-differentials	304		
13.4.10.	Seventh-week daily exercise-differentials	305		
13.4.11.	Eighth-week daily exercise-differentials	306		
13.4.12.	Third-month daily exercise-differentials	307		
13.4.13.	Ninth-week daily exercise-differentials	308		
13.4.14.	Tenth-week daily exercise-differentials	309		
13.4.15.	Eleventh-week daily exercise-differentials	310		
13.4.16.	Twelfth-week daily exercise-differentials	311		
13.4.17.	Pre-contest-month daily exercise-differentials	312		
13.4.18.	Thirteenth-week daily exercise-differentials	313		
13.4.19.	Fourteenth-week daily exercise-differentials	314		
13.4.20.	Fifteenth-week daily exercise-differentials	315		
13.4.21.	Sixteenth-week daily exercise-differentials	316		

13.5 Personal account with managing volume and intensity 316

13.6 Highlights of chapter THIRTEEN 324

14. HEALTH AND FITNESS 325

14.1 Role of exercise in health 325
- 14.1.1. Body systems of motion 325
- 14.1.2. Cellular adaptation to exercise 325
- 14.1.3. Physical appearance 327
- 14.1.3.1. Managing body Fat 327
- 14.1.3.2. Muscular machinery 327
- 14.1.4. Mobility 328
- 14.1.5. Gastrointestinal health 329

14.2 Flags of alarm 329
- 14.2.1. Headache 329
- 14.2.2. Constipation and indigestion 330
- 14.2.3. Muscle pain and stiffness 330

14.3 The pearls of fitness 331
- 14.3.1. Walking exercise 331
- 14.3.2. Optimum bodyweight 332
- 14.3.3. Aerobics 332
- 14.3.4. Caring for aching joints 334
- 14.3.5. Daily activities 334
- 14.3.6. Healthy diet 335

14.4 Source of information 335

14.5 Food and health 336
- 14.5.1. Macronutrients 337
- 14.5.2. Micronutrients 337

14.6 Food contents 340

Tables of foodstuff with high contents of protein, fat, carbohydrates, and vitamins 341

15. EXERCISE AND PREVENTABLE DISEASES 363

15.1 Prevetable causes of death in the USA 363
- 15.1.1. New challenges of urbanization 363
- 15.1.2. Health trends of modern American society 363

15.2 Prevalence of cardiovascular diseases 364

15.3 Heart diseases 364
- 15.3.1. Current state of knowledge 364
- 15.3.2. Heart attack 365
- 15.3.3. Heart failure 366
- 15.3.4. Cardiac arrest 366
- 15.3.5. Cardiac arrhythmia 367
- 15.3.6. Myocardial infarction 367
- 15.3.7. Rheumatic heart disease 367

15.4 Heart disease and cultural differences 368

15.5 Risk factors for heart diseases 369
- 15.5.1. Age 369
- 15.5.2. Gender 370
- 15.5.3. Alcohol 371
- 15.5.4. Heredity 371
- 15.5.5. Smoking 372
- 15.5.6. High blood pressure 372
- 15.5.7. Cholesterol 374
- 15.5.8. Overweight and obesity 375
- 15.5.8.1. Obesity 375
- 15.5.8.2. Overweight 376
- 15.5.8.3. Overweight and decline in health 376
- 15.5.8.4. Failure to reduce bodyweight 376
- 15.5.8.5. Obesity and overweight in children 376

15.6 Cost-effective and realistic prevention of heart diseases 377
- 15.6.1. Healthy Eating 377
- 15.6.2. Exercise 379

15.7 Cancer 380

15.8 Cerebrovascular disease 381

15.9 Autoimmune system 381

15.10 Diabetes Mellitus 382
- 15.10.1. Impact on public health 382
- 15.10.2. Glucose fuel 383
- 15.10.3. Insulin role 383
- 15.10.4. Preventive diet 383
- 15.10.5. Clinical manifestation 384

15.11 Highlights of chapter FIFTEEN 385

16. EXERCISE & INJURIES 391

16.1 Weaknesses and injury 391
- 16.1.1. Higher neural causes of muscular weakness 391
- 16.1.2. Lower neural causes of muscular weakness 391
- 16.1.3. Causes of peripheral muscular weakness 392

16.2 Group muscle weaknesses 392
- 16.2.1. Abdominal weakness 392
- 16.2.2. Hamstrings weakness 393
- 16.2.3. Supraspinatus weakness 393
- 16.2.4. Infraspinatus weakness 394
- 16.2.5. Weakness of spinal erectors 394
- 16.2.6. Quadriceps weakness 394

16.3	**Soft tissue injuries**	**395**
16.3.1.	Causes of injuries due to physical activity	395
16.3.2.	Alleviating physical injuries of soft tissues	395
16.3.3.	Ligament sprain 396	
16.3.4.	Muscle and tendon strain 396	
16.3.5.	Bursitis 396	
16.3.6.	Compartment syndrome 397	
16.3.7.	Soreness 397	
16.3.8.	Cramps 398	
16.3.9.	Role of exercise in injury management 398	

16.4	**Knee injuries**	**399**
16.4.1.	Meniscus injuries 399	
16.4.2.	Cruciate ligaments 400	
16.4.3.	Collateral ligaments 400	
16.4.4.	Arthritis 400	
16.4.5.	Tendon injuries 401	

16.5	**Injuries to the shoulder**	**402**
16.5.1.	Rotator cuff tear 402	
16.5.2.	Dislocation 402	
16.5.3.	Inflammation 402	
16.5.4.	Fracture 403	
16.5.5.	Adhesion 403	

16.6	**Back injuries**	**403**
16.6.1.	Causes of back injuries 403	
16.6.2.	Lower back pain 403	
16.6.3.	Herniated disc 404	
16.6.4.	Whiplash 404	
16.6.5.	Pinched neck nerves 404	

16.7	**Cortisone Injections**	**405**

16.8	**Highlights of chapter SIXTEEN**	**406**

17. EXERCISE & SCIENCE   407

17.1	**The entity of energy**	**407**
17.1.1	Disturbance versus life 407	
17.1.2	Space 407	
17.1.3	Distance 407	
17.1.4	Time 408	
17.1.5	Light 408	
17.1.6	Motion and rest 408	
17.1.7	Acceleration 408	
17.1.8	Force 409	
17.1.9	Inertia 410	
17.1.10	Momentum 410	
17.1.11	Gravity 411	
17.1.12	Charge 411	
17.1.13	Heat 411	
17.1.14	Energy disguises 412	

17.2	**The human organism**	**413**
17.2.1	Purposeful creature 413	
17.2.2	Wholesome nature 413	
17.2.3	Basic structure 413	
17.2.4	Muscles 414	
17.2.5	Regeneration 414	
17.2.6	Fat metabolism 415	
17.2.7	Carbon scavenging 416	
17.2.8	Nitrogen metabolism 416	
17.2.9	Biological energy 416	
17.2.10	Muscular energy 418	

17.3	**The cellular furnace of chemical fuel**	**419**
17.3.1.	The tricarboxylic acid cycle (TCA or the Krebs' cycle) 419	
17.3.2.	Electronic joggling 419	
17.3.3.	The enzymatic fuel guardian 421	
17.3.4.	Glucose transport 421	

17.4	**Power production by human body**	**422**
17.4.1.	Instinct 422	
17.4.2.	Human development 423	
17.4.3.	Strength training 424	
17.4.4.	Modern history of weightlifting 424	

17.5	**Energy flow in human body**	**425**
17.5.1.	Physiological changes due to exercise 425	
17.5.2.	Clinical changes due to exercise 426	
17.5.3.	Managing the flow of energy 426	

17.6	**Effects of exercise on the body**	**427**
17.6.1.	Digestion 427	
17.6.2.	Respiration 427	
17.6.3.	Cardiovascular 428	
17.6.4.	Immune defense 428	
17.6.5.	Kidneys 428	
17.6.6.	Bones 428	
17.6.7.	Mind 428	

17.7	**Managing chemical energy by live organisms**	**429**
17.7.1.	Energy in food intake 429	
17.7.2.	Energy flow within the body 429	
17.7.3.	Rest 431	
17.7.4.	Eating 431	
17.7.5.	Activity 432	
17.7.6.	Fasting 433	
17.7.7.	Warm-up 433	
17.7.8.	Vigorous activities 433	
17.7.9.	Warm-down 433	

17.8	**Highlights of chapter SEVENTEEN**	**434**

18. FREQUENTLY ASKED QUESTIONS   435

18.1	**Drug Use**	**435**
18.1.1.	Use of monoamine oxidase inhibitors 435	
18.1.2.	Anabolic steroids 435	

18.2	**Bodybuilding and self-image**	**436**

18.3	**Fat burning with diet and exercise**	**436**
18.3.1.	Daily caloric intake 436	
18.3.2.	Exercising for fat burning 437	
18.3.3.	Diet and muscle mass 437	

18.4	**Deadlift**	**438**	**19.4**	**Women's participation in sport versus men's participation** 462

- 18.4.1. Proper technique for deadlift 438
- 18.4.2. Variants of deadlift style 439
- 18.4.3. Definition of strength training 439
- 18.4.4. Essence of deadlifting 439
- 18.4.5. Sequence and percentage of deadlift 439
- 18.4.6. Deadlift and intensity of resistance 440
- 18.4.7. About pelvic circulation in deadlift 440
- 18.4.8. Deadlift and olympic weightlifting 440
- 18.4.9. Deadlift as an assisting exercise to weightlifting 441
- 18.4.10. Load volume of deadlift 441
- 18.4.11. Stiff-legged deadlifts and locked knees 441

18.5 Exercise and blood donation 442

18.6 Resistance training versus other types of workouts 442

18.7 Structuring workout sessions 443
- 18.7.1. Two-day split workout 443
- 18.7.2. Endurance versus weight training 444
- 18.7.3. Workout at home 444
- 18.7.4. Split day workout 445

18.8 Squat 445
- 18.8.1. Front squats and knee pain 445
- 18.8.2. Balancing knee extensors and flexors 446
- 18.8.3. Isolation versus compound exercises 446
- 18.8.4. Leg rxtensions and shear stresses 447
- 18.8.5. Leaning over during squat 448
- 18.8.6. Using waist belts during squats 448
- 18.8.7. Plateauing in squat 450
- 18.8.8. Squats and shoulder pain 450
- 18.8.9. Squat and deadlift rotation in workout 451
- 18.8.10. Squats and bench press synergy 451
- 18.8.11. Squatting with raised toes or heels 452
- 18.8.12. Rounded back during squatting 452

18.9 Learning the hang clean 453

18.10 Overhead dumbbell press 453

18.11 Personal trainers 454

18.12 Powerlifting versus bodybuilding 455

18.13 Shakiness during resistance training 455

19. TRAINING WOMEN 457

19.1 Long-term structured training for women 457
- 19.1.1. New trends 457
- 19.1.2. Development 457
- 19.1.3. brain and body mastery 457
- 19.1.4. Adaptation to long-term exercise 459

19.2 Women's view of strength training 460

19.3 Women's exercise and preventable diseases 460

19.4 Women's participation in sport versus men's participation 462

19.5 Women's view of strength training 465
- 19.5.1. Cardiovascular exercises 465
- 19.5.2. Axial back exercises 466
- 19.5.2.1. The clean lift 466
- 19.5.2.2. The snatch lift 467
- 19.5.2.3. The deadlift 468
- 19.5.2.4. Bend-over-and row (BOR) 468
- 19.5.2.5. Goodmorning exercise 468
- 19.5.2.6. Shoulder press and jerk 469
- 19.5.2.7. Seated back pushing 469
- 19.5.2.8. Seated trunk twisting 469
- 19.5.2.9. Back extension 470
- 19.5.3. Pelvic girdle exercises 470
- 19.5.3.1. Squat 470
- 19.5.3.2. Abdominal sit-ups 471
- 19.5.3.3. Leg lunges 471
- 19.5.3.4. Leg press 471
- 19.5.3.5. Leg extension and flexion 471
- 19.5.4. Shoulder girdle exercises 472
- 19.5.4.1. Bench press 472
- 19.5.4.2. Seated shoulder press 472
- 19.5.4.3. Cable rowing 473
- 19.5.4.4. Lateral push and pull 473
- 19.5.4.5. Shoulder shrug 473
- 19.5.5. Peripheral exercises 473

19.6 Highlights of chapter NINTEEN 473

20. GUIDELINES FOR OPTIMUM STRENGTH TRAINING 475

20.1 Nature of physical strength 475
- 20.1.1. Weight training versus endurance training 475
- 20.1.2. Essence of physical of strength 475
- 20.1.3. Developing strength 478

20.2 Fundamentals of strength training 478
- 20.2.1. Frequency 478
- 20.2.2. Gym 479
- 20.2.3. Program 479
- 20.2.4. Intensity of resistance 480
- 20.2.5. Goals 482
- 20.2.6. Lifestyle 482
- 20.2.7. Adjustment 482
- 20.2.8. Individualization 482
- 20.2.9. Documentation 483
- 20.2.10. Insight 483
- 20.2.11. Weight training guidelines 483

20.3 Effects of exercise 484
- 20.3.1. Mind and body 484
- 20.3.2. Adaptation to exercise 484
- 20.3.3. Immediate effects of strength exercise 485
- 20.3.4. Fat loss and weight training 486
- 20.3.5. Abdominal girth 486

20.3.6. Muscle fuel   487
20.3.7. Aerobic exercise   487
20.3.8. Overtraining   488

20.4 Training psychology   488

20.4.1. Drive and the psyche   489
20.4.2. Past experience   489
20.4.3. Present strategies   490
20.4.4. Assessing strategies   490
20.4.5. Workout anxiety   491
20.4.6. Workout counseling   491
20.4.7. Skillful workout   492
20.4.8. Training novice performers   492

20.5 Highlights of chapter TWENTY   496

Glossary   497

Index   509

Chapter 1 Introduction

1.1. RECOGNITION OF A FORGOTTEN SPORT

Weightlifting is becoming a well-structured field of knowledge that is forcing its way on modern everyday society. There are many reasons that make Weightlifting a superb method of resistance training and an adjunct to health and fitness, as follows.

1.1.1. RAPID EXPANSION OF URBANIZATION
Many people find it unbearable to endure the drastic weight-gain and muscular weakness as a result of diminished physical activity in today's urban and industrial communities. Yet, many others have succumbed to modern day diseases of obesity, hypertension, coronary artery disease, diabetes, and psychological stress. These maladies result, partially, from diminishing our metabolic ability to assimilate the food we consume, constructively. Most probably, such altered metabolism is a direct result of a decline in the activities of the many enzymatic complex, gene expression, and hormones that regulate every biochemical reaction in our cells. Alteration of the expression of our genetic moieties in response to lack of both constant and lengthy physical activity on daily basis, might explain the decline in our ability to maintain, proper body composition. The ultimate effect of urbanized life style is the loss of muscle mass, diminished strength, and improper function of many of our vital organs. In other words, urbanization becomes a synonym for stagnation and ill health. Weightlifting offers a natural stimulus to rejuvenate the functions and conditions of our cells, tissues, organs, and systems.

1.1.2. INCREASED ACCESS TO MEDICAL KNOWLEDGE
The new era of fast spread of information has contributed to the herd conviction regarding fitness as a "PLUS" to health. Other cultures have based its conviction on heroic figures. Some view smoking as a manly habit of strength and toughness that is associated with soldiers smoking in times of battles, leaders smoking in dealing with crises, and scientists smoking when discussing complex intelligent endeavors. The constant change in herd conviction is even apparent on the highest level of the social hierarchy. In the 1940's, it was acceptable to photograph a president of a nation wearing formal uniform while fishing in his leisure time. Forty years later, presidential candidates would strive to appear in a modest athletic style, jogging, working out, or wearing casual sports outfit. Today, we see increase in gym attendance of both young and old women that was unheard of few decades ago.

1.1.3. INCREASED AFFORDABILITY OF STRENGTH TRAINING
Strength training in the form of Weightlifting is becoming an affordable commodity on the personal level. The cost of buying a ticket to watch a baseball or a football game would suffice to pay the fees of an entire month in a modest health club. That, in addition to the added benefits of being in the center of the picture as a player, you are performing personal rituals, instead of being marginalized as a spectator in a frantic stadium. Closely meeting people and communicating with them in health clubs, away from the emotional drama of fanatic spectators, and the joy of using many amenities modern gyms provide; all make participation in health clubs a pleasant experience.

1.2. MYSTICAL THINKING AND SPORT

1.2.1. MYSTICAL THINKING AMONG ATHLETES
The mystic of what is a "plus" to health and what is not is still as vivid today as it was since the early times of our existence. Many athletes seek awkward ways to enhance their performance, even when it is evident that such ways are harmful to long-term health prospects. Anabolic steroids and many of the so called "energy boosting" supplements are among few in the jungle of relentless search for mystical strength. Apparently, the main enforcer of mystical thinking is the conviction of the greater society of the plausibility of such ideas. You would not step into any gym without observing the common trends of mystical believes, vividly apparent to the casual observer, as follows.
o You may notice the common practice of lifting weights to strengthen the part of the body that the person feels needs strengthening. For centuries, Weightlifters, farmers, factory workers, and household workers have long learned that performance of the whole body is the way to develop strength.

INTRODUCTION

- You may notice people showing up to training whenever they feel they want to train. Human intelligence forbids such irrational planning. Health and strength cannot be promoted without regular and long practices.
- You may notice people resorting to machine-exercises from beginning to end. Well, in real life, we use our brain to perform activities without machines lying around us. Thus, if exercise does not simulate real encounters of everyday activities then how would machine exercises alone foster fitness?
- You may notice personal trainers explaining to beginners how to exercise isolated muscles and demonstrating the genius in the science of anatomy. Yet, common people care less for anatomy. A reasonable person can intuitively sense the invaluable power of enhancing metabolism rather than enhancing few muscle fibers. Thus general activities and exercise can boost general health before getting distracted by anatomical details.

1.2.2. MYSTICAL THINKING AMONG COMMON PEOPLE
On the other extreme, many people attribute the gift of health to spiritual being and submit to a lifestyle of wishful expectation, praying without taking any substantial action to better their health. Most probably, the main reason for taking our health for granted, attributing it as given from higher authorities, is our constant observation of the mysterious ways our body and mind heal the so many traumatic scars. The alarming signs of adaptive trends among the common public are the overwhelming confusion with the diverse and ever-changing new discoveries and the indifference towards efforts of raising public awareness. Many people would not trust political or media campaigns and rather stick to their own vises, regardless of any truth in the former or serious flaws in the latter. Many further would trust their friends and relatives in trying new ideas of health and overlook the alien and remote voices of scientific authorities. Such mystical believes among the common people are being further enforced by the fast-food, tobacco, and health and fitness industries that aim at marketing their products rather than changing people's believes.

1.2.3. HABITS AND HEALTHY THINKING
The department of human behavior in our minds seems to be somewhat independent from the department of thinking. Many people describe habit changing as hard and needs constant or gradual effort to accomplish. Very few people can win the fight against ingrained bad habits. Smoking, overeating, using illicit drugs, and drinking are few among many destructive habits that are difficult to alter. The hypothesis of existence of biochemical causes of ingrained habits is constantly challenged on the basis of environmental and nurturing factors that may be causing both the biochemical changes and the habitual behavior, instead of being the effect of inherent disorders. The mysterious independence of behavior from thinking is vividly demonstrated in many areas of human behavior. Smokers, for example, might conceive the seriousness that smoking is causing them to lose muscle mass, sexual impotence, and respiratory failure, yet few smoker would even act seriously upon their conception of facts. The well-established proof that some habits are detrimental to health would undoubtedly skip the attention of mystical thinkers. Such curse of indifference to harmful behavior is costing nations enormous human resources, in caring for diseased smokers, lost work hours, and lost talents. The slow, but growing, awareness among the public about the cost incurred by letting people damage their health by destructive, yet preventable, habits is raising the debate on alternatives to protect the long term interests of the public.

1.2.4. ON THE DYNAMICS OF HUMAN MIND
Though we have made great strides in decoding the simplest rules that govern the physics and mechanics of material objects, we seem to be in the early stages of uncovering the dynamics of the human mind. Or, such dynamics might be so intriguing to yield themselves to simple abstract equations. The very early programming of the mind of infants and children may be more crucial for healthy mental development than the inherent genetic makeup of thinking or behavior. In many ancient societies, families were able to tolerate and love their children, even with extremes of behavioral problems, until developmental maturity rectifies many such behavioral difficulties. The value of warm, close, and loving environment in the early development of children may suppress many of the gene activities that present in the forms of depression, hyperactivity, overeating, smoking, or drinking. Without such tranquil and hopeful state of mind, health and fitness issues would not gain significant priorities in our daily plans.

1.3. LOGICAL INFERENCE AND SPORT

1.3.1. LOGICAL INFERENCE AND PROGRESS IN SCIENCES
It seems that omitting logical inference, when attending to our daily activities, is a norm of thinking, rather than an exception. That is evident in other human endeavors as with health habits. In astronomy, for example, mystical thinking had delayed our understanding of the extraterrestrial universe for thousands if not millions of years. Only when we deviated from our mystical perception of the universe when we began to conquer the new frontiers, fear free. Such new frontiers have brought us closer than we ever thought we would. With satellite communication, the skis are turned into new roads of lightening speeds of sharing and expressing ideas and dreams, with endless potential to better our living standards. Progress in these, apparently remote branches of sciences, has brought the human race closer in thinking and has greatly facilitated our understanding of health and disease issues.

Strength training is no exception in the history of illogical thinking. It has evolved rapidly during the last century for the same reasons that caused physics and science to excel. The need for strong and healthy soldiers to fight modern wars has thrust the creativity of military experts to figure out ways to promote strength through weight training. These efforts have culminated in rediscovering the old known methods of enhancing strength. Thus, **progressive regular weight training** has substituted old farming activities, with **strategic planning of intensity of lifting and volume of training** to prevent exhaustion and gradually build up physical strength, under the control of the training program.

1.3.2. THE ULTRA-MINUTE VERSUS THE GIGANTIC UNIVERSES

You would not engage in exercise without asking many questions about how food benefits our body, how drugs affect cells, how exercise alters body chemistry, or how body organs communicate with systems. In order to have any plausible answer, you would have to go as far as the stars, to understand the laws of the universe, and as deep as the atomic nucleus in order to realize the generality of the laws of physics to both the gigantic universe and the ultra minute world of nuclear particles. In nuclear sciences, similar deviation from mystical thinking had lead to the understanding of the atomic structure of matter. Such fresh air of thinking had sparked the light in a new era of nuclear and electronic marvels. Bridging the wide spectrum of knowledge has initiated a chain reaction of discoveries of antibiotics and many pharmaceutical agents that prolonged human lives and helped prevent and manag many diseases. Most of the unanswered questions about the molecular world of biological life are thought to have their secrets lying in the interactions of electrons of different atoms of the molecules of the body. The only successful attempt to describe such electronic world was made in the beginning of the last century in the form of describing particles as waves of energy. The wave theory has offered some explanation of how molecules might perform their activities, yet failed to account for the overwhelmingly complex molecular behaviors. No such theory has been yet devised to explain how few atoms could gather to form genes that control every feature of biological life.

1.3.3. SIMILARITIES IN HEALTH AND PHYSICAL SCIENCES

Without the daring adventure to conquer the ultra minute atomic universe, we would not have been able to step out into the unforgiving, immense, outer space. Mastering the fields of electrons and ions of the atoms, though crude and empirical, have helped us understand how our eyes see, ears hear, sensors transfer signals, and brain process information. The most amazing fact in all discoveries of atomic physics is that we never have seen any of the tiny particles themselves. Yet we have accepted the fact that they would not be seen within the limited scope of our human senses. Thus logical inference is our only alternative to explain the otherwise inexplicable observation. Sadly, it is very difficult to convey such logical consequences of introducing scientific wisdom into activities of large human population without many years of conviction, education, and raising public awareness. The most majority of people do not appreciate the need for exercise despite the fact exercise is proven fundamental to enhance and maintain health and prevent many diseases, both organic and psychological.

1.3.4. STRENGTH TRAINING AND QUALITY OF AMBULANT LIVING

Abstract logical inference has helped us master our affairs with great benefits. The evolution of human intelligence, that is strikingly evident in the scientific arena, is paralleled, though lagging, in the social arena. Recently we have witnessed the participation of women in Olympic Weightlifting, a sport that was thought to be too tough even for male trainees. Having gained some of their right for equality, women start rejoicing the freedom that comes with strength and health, of a relatively long, disease-free living. Many other segments of society are beginning to realize the importance of getting out and participate in some sort of activity in order to stay healthy. The principal difference between strength training and other activities is that strengthening stimulates the cellular chemistry and generates new building units for motion and growth. Running or walking increases energy expenditure but does little in growing new cellular protein or conditioning the cellular chemistry for vigorous energy production or balancing strength of various joints and muscles. That is because vigorous activity eliminates weak and fragile muscle fibers and induces reproduction of more effective fibers that suite the kind of activity you perform. The newly grown muscles enhance their neural control and participate effectively in the brain-to-muscle regulation, thus revitalizing the body to work more energetically. Less vigorous activities do not greatly alter muscle growth and can be attended with feeble muscle fibers. Promoting physical strength helps many people conquer new fields of employments, pursue their goals even at old age, and endure many traumatic life affairs with greater confidence.

1.3.5. THE INEVITABILITY OF HUMAN LIMITATIONS

Resistance training, apart from its beneficial health gains in warding off many diseases, bestows better quality of ambulant living. Sports that seem formidable to many people are rendered conquerable with proper resistance training. Understanding the physiology of exercise sheds light on the unexplored potential of human strength and health. Many preventable diseases can be avoided by eliminating their causes that lie in poor management of food consumption and energy expenditure. Exercise pushes the threshold of human limitation to higher levels, by bringing more insights into daily destructive behavior. Making exercising your daily relief goal eliminates ill habits that numb the mind, damage the lungs, or undermine the heart. What you gain from making exercise your daily goal are healthier joints that allow you to move freely, healthier lungs and hearts that ease your effort to perform many activities, and cheerful mind that is comforted by the achievement of sweating for good. Until clear cut limits are set for what is appropriate for certain age groups, I would like to stress that Weightlifters have pushed the envelop of physical performance beyond any expectation. Many new records are still being made and many formidable barriers have collapsed. The day when a 200 kg was thought the ultimate weight, man could lift bare-handedly, had passed by. New techniques of lifting have been invented, attesting to the persistence of man to master his or her affairs against all odds. Logical inference is what drives man to question the inevitability of the limitations he encounters, from weakness, aging, disease, failure, or even his inevitable demise. Of course, strength training would not enable you to do Biceps curls with a ton weight of steel, but will lead you to question the impossibility of such extreme power. Now, we know that humans have very close range of physical strength that does not match that of steel machinery. Yet strength training can lead us to perform activities that the best designed machine cannot perform.

1.3.6. THE DICHOTOMY OF PHYSICAL AND INTELLECTUAL FITNESS.
As with the dichotomy of understanding the minute structure of particles, which enabled us to master the extraterrestrial laws of planets and stars, is the dichotomy of bettering our physical fitness in order to better our mental health, and vise versa. The fact that many athletes score poorly on the intellectual scale of accomplishments is paralleled with the fact that many intellectuals fare poorly on the physical health scale. Adopting a scheme to introduce resistance training on your list of priorities is a smart way to better your body and mind. Not only because the body and mind are physically interdependent, but also because the mind has to learn through new activities and exposures to different and variable events of life. The greatest ideas in the human history have risen during playful activities. The laws of hydrodynamics were discovered in a swimming pond by observing water level rising when a new person dives into the water. The laws of gravitation were also discovered by observing objects maintaining motion even after external contacts have been ceased. The laws of flying were also discovered by watching birds mastering the forces of aerodynamics. The laws of electricity were discovered through playing with magnets. Thus the human mind seems to extrapolate natural events in order to learn their laws, rather than inventing laws anew, out of mere imagination.

1.4. ROLE OF HERD CONVICTION IN SPORT

1.4.1. CONSTANT AND PERSISTENT MODELING
It seems to me that the only way of swaying the herd conviction towards realistic healthy habits would be through constant and persistent demonstration of the benefits of practicing good planning of education, activity, and nutrition over long periods of time. In hoping to instill reality testing, of what is a **"plus"** and what is detrimental to one's health, mystical thinking has to be constantly challenged. Such effort of modifying herd conviction requires decades to gradually shift behavior towards constructive activities. The most productive application of habitual modeling is in the early years of life, when health habits can be condoned and overzealously practiced, when there are few regrets and setbacks to discourage continuation, when there is clear and material benefits from acting properly, and when there are adults who motivate the young to stay the course of disciplined living.

1.4.2. ADVENT IN COMMUNICATION
Fortunately, the advent in communication has contributed to sharing many stimulating concepts that would facilitate herd swaying in favor of recognition of the necessity to change one's lifestyle, for good. Today, we are closer to understand our inner personal identity and physical shortcomings than few generations ago. We are more aware of ways to alter our image when it interferes with our ability to enjoy good living. The major opposing forces to benefiting from advances in communication are the low socioeconomic status of many young people who have to struggle, just to afford living, apart from improving the quality of their living style. Many gyms do not allow youngsters to join for fear of accident liability. Moreover, membership fees and cost of transportation are burdensome to youngsters without strong social support. The openness on modern communication resources has brought people from very diverse cultures to agree on otherwise debatable issues. Before such global openness, many cultures were closed to outside ideas and athletes were viewed, as clowns by the rich and influential class of those cultures. I recall the days when the sons of the wealthy and influential people bragged about drinking milk in place of water, and eating butter and meat whenever they desire food. They were strong and chubby kids yet their future health was grim. The poor kids would settle for bread and grains and long hours of physical work, yet their physical energy was no match. Today, thanks to modern communication, we have better idea of what good food should be, and why activity is crucial to our health, as discussed in Chapter Fourteen.

1.4.3. THE PROLIFERATION OF A FORGOTTEN SPORT
The fact that the sport of "weight training" is proliferating exponentially in many communities is attributed to the concerted campaign of recognition of modern day health problems. Though such proliferation is directed toward commercial profit, it is nevertheless a positive step in the rebirth of a forgotten sport. The role of modern visual media

have raised our conscious awareness of **"PHYSIQUE"** and have propagated the most important idea we have learned over the years **that we can alter our physical image and enhance our sense of identity by exercise.** Weight training explores the vigorous potential of our body to overcome weakness and debility by intelligent and persistent planning of resistance training, and it is not a new invention. The rise of weight training is a logical consequence of displacing farmers and factory workers from physical labor and substituting man with machinery. The health clubs that are dispersed all over modern cities have gotten all their methods of training and fitness from farming and manufacturing industries. We always resort to our long history of struggle, from the remote past of the caveman, to modern urban living, whenever we stumble on perplexing problems. We did not forget that farmers used to work hard over half of the day and spent nights without electricity. We did not forget that old civilization were able to accomplish great projects with very primitive tools. Therefore, our past is what led us to reinvent weight training in order to maintain our species from demise.

1.4.4. PASSING HABITS BETWEEN GENERATIONS
The role of herd conviction is vital in instilling the habit of proper exercising and passing it from generation to generation. The reality of human development necessitates that newer generation have to rely on older generations for a good two decades, or so, before resuming independence from parents. Yet, the new generation would have to spend most of the remaining part of their life decompiling the early parental doctrine of growing up. The older ideas and habits pass relentlessly between generations and impede the spread of new ideas. Women used to play crucial role in passing old habits to children, and themselves, that is women, were denied most of the rights of equality with men. The long history of marginalizing the role of women still reek havoc in swaying half the population to gain equal access to fitness, as follows.
o   The most majority of women still believe that any thing to do with muscles has to belong to the man's world. Ironically, many laywomen even believe that muscles belong to man's anatomy of rugged appearance.
o   The association of muscles with locomotion mobility, internal mobility of fluids and intestinal contents, eyes mobility, and regulation of flow of vital circulation, seems to be an exclusive sort of knowledge that is accessible only to people with specific educational backgrounds.
o   From my personal experience, some women subordinate the necessity of muscles to the needs of good appearance. The simplest axiom of fitness that joints perform better with stronger and well-conditioned muscles has not yet conquered the territories of women's health society.

1.5. STIGMA ABOUT WEIGHTLIFTING

1.5.1. CLASS STIGMA OF MENIAL LABOR
The days when muscular development was viewed as a sign of a class of people performing menial jobs are about to fade into the remote past. Most probably, the early genuine message of glamorizing physical labor, portrayed in many religions, is gaining recognition anew. In some religions, a prophet would perform the same physical labor assigned to the least of his followers to demonstrate the heavenly doctrine of bringing equality among people and eradicate classes. Workers who toiled harder for earning living were viewed more honorable than others. From the medical point of view, laborers performing heavy physical activities fare better in health than people performing clerical jobs.

1.5.2. MODERN SCIENCE DISCOVERS HEALTH IN PHYSICAL ACTIVITY
To our surprise, modern science has consistently affirmed that physical labor bestowed unequivocal protection on our cardiovascular health. Heavy physical labor prevents deposition of atherosclerotic plaques into the arterial walls and helps preserve many organs from affliction with cardiovascular diseases. In addition, modern science has discovered the value of physical activities in maintaining healthy psychological development. Regular and continuous activities fulfill the respiratory requirements of cells allover the body and prevent cellular damage due to lack of nutrients or excess of metabolites[1, 2].

1.5.3. TODAY'S MENIAL OCCUPATIONS
On both sides of social classes, laborers and non-laborers, changes have occurred. Many menial occupations are now augmented with machinery that requires little labor to operate. Today, so many menial laborers are not as fit as compared to those few decades ago. Many laborers are overweight, have stiffed joints, frequent back and knee injuries, excessive smoking and drug addiction. Since menial laborers appreciate physical activities than other occupations, it seems that bettering the education of this segment of society would be more productive in bringing laborers to benefit from advances in information technology. Many laborers lack the knowledge of proper lifting technique or the course of action in dealing with over-exhaustion and injuries. Laborers are in more need to understand the side effects of smoking, alcohol, and drugs more than any other group in society, since the culture of peer pressure is a significant factor in substance usage.

---

[1] "Davidson's Principles and Practice of Medicine", C. Haslett, E.R. Chilvers, J.A.A. Hunter, and N.A. Boon, 18th edition, Churchill Livingstone, Edinburgh, UK, 1999. Pages 220, 245-247, and 530. ISBN 0443 059446.
[2] Exercise Physiology, energy, Nutrition, and Human Performance" by W.D. McArdle, F.I. Katch, and V.L. Katch, Lea & Febiger, Philadelphia, USA, 1991. Chapter 30 on Physical Activity, Health, and Aging. ISBN 0-8121-1351-9.

INTRODUCTION

1.5.4. GROWING NEED FOR EXERCISING FOR GOOD LIVING
Other non-laborers have resorted to fitness training for its added benefits of social acceptance and health and developed athletic muscular appearance. The alarming rate of mortality and morbidity that is associated with careers lacking physical activities has brought to the forefront the debate on the essential need for exercising for good living. Many of those who opt for office jobs content themselves with sedentary living, with sparse occasions of recreational activities. Such lifestyle will undoubtedly lead to ill health and costly medical care. Activity is a process that has to occupy most of our daily routines in order to prevent decline in health of organs and systems.

1.5.5. A SPORT OF THE TOUGH AND CRUDE FOLKS
Yet the stigma that Weightlifting is a sport of the tough and crude folks is still dominant in many cultures. It serves to justify, to many, that resistance training is exclusive to the strong. The reality is that every, and all people can gain from such superb tool of enhancing health. As we have mentioned, the historic roots of strength training stem from regular human occupation. It only takes gradual and regular exercising to go from A to Z in the field of strengthening. With many setbacks in between, Weightlifters learn to live with changing daily conditions in health. Also, building strong muscles is like building strong liver, heart, kidneys, and brain. These organs recognize no gender difference. All humans need strength to produce energy and to attend to their living needs.

1.5.6. RESISTANCE TRAINING A NEW EXPERIMENT
It is to the surprise of many that once they get started in such new realm of exercising they might surpass those who stuck to their old habits of rigid practice. Resistance training is an experiment that is conducted by the very diverse and individual humans, each of whom has his or her positive difference to add to the experiment and brings its conclusion into new heights. What new in strength training is the activation of the stem cells of the muscles to regenerate new and stronger muscle fibers. The stem cells listen to thousands of genes in order to differentiate into new cells. With such diverse and unique genetic makeup of each human being, strength development will vary among people. Some can develop strength faster and recuperate faster than others. Some others require individualized plans to produce results.

1.5.7. MY PERSONAL EXPERIENCE WITH WEIGHTLIFTING
On a personal level, I started learning Weightlifting at the age of sixteen, in 1966, when lifting weights was considered a clownish sport, practiced by factory laborers and street muggers. Few of my early peers had any elementary school education. I was among about eighty students selected from the class of honor students for my entire three years in high school. I never forget the worry of my mother who thought that having such privileged status of quality schooling should be protected by staying away from the class of illiterate Weightlifters. Yet, living those two diverse worlds was an enriching experience. My parents were the poorest of the poor, but they were there when I needed them. Many of my peers haven't had such blessing of guaranteed stability that is dearly needed in the early formative years in life. Since then Weightlifting became my passion and pursuit for happiness, for the rest of my life. I thought I was alone in appreciating such sport until the whole crowd of color TV, movie industry, and modern fitness awareness have recently discovered that forgotten sport of bumping iron.

1.5.8. SURPASSING OTHERS IN THE NEW SPORT
Among the few I have encouraged to change their training from Bodybuilding to Olympic Weightlifting is a fellow who has surpasses me and made it all the way to the Olympic games of Los Angeles 1984 and Barcelona 1988. More over I succeeded to convince him that sport and academic accomplishment could not be separated. He was able to join the law school and graduate as a lawyer, amidst his years of Olympic training. Unfortunately, when he deserted the academic spirit of logical thinking was when his bodyweight shot up and his injuries hampered his progress. Yet, above all, his entire life had been completely changed to better, with the inclusion of sport in his life. Sometimes, just being qualified to participate in the Olympics is the most an athlete can aspire to. So many others, I have thought would make good Olympic athletes, had fell short of their dreams. It is not a matter of luck that some people excel to the top and some do not. The combination of circumstances of financial, educational, familial, and personal conviction interplays in determining outcome.

1.5.9. GETTING INVOLVED IN PHYSICAL EXERCISING
As with the habit of getting immersed in academic disciplines, after realizing their potential to impact the whole society, is the habit of getting involved in exercising. You start appreciate the exaltation of getting stronger and healthier with proper planning. Your first lesson is learning the time course of events. Effective training requires certain number of sessions every week. Each training day, you are required to exercise for few hours. Recuperation also follows predictable course, according to the vigor and frequency of training. You will learn about the breaks between sets, the rest between sessions, and the effects of long rest on the body biology. Growth also follows predictable course and cannot happen in hours or days. The second lesson you will learn is how to plan strategic workout program by choosing few among many exercises, and how to order their sequence of execution. The third lesson will be getting content that you are in a process of evolution. Every day and every week of training, you are learning, discovering, and immensely understanding your inner body

biology. You would have to work in evolving better and wiser by modifying sleep, diet, and other activities to serve your body biology better.

1.6. SOCIAL CHANGES AND SPORT

1.6.1. EPIDEMICS OF THE PAST
In less than forty years since I starting lifting weights, the world has changed drastically. The epidemics of the past such as cholera, typhoid, malaria, tuberculosis, syphilis, and parasitic infections do not have the same eerie connotation as in the 1940's, and before. Man discovered ways to defeat bacteria and larger parasites. In the past, people have little to do to avoid affliction by air-borne, water-borne, or mosquito transmitted diseases. Today, most afflictions are caused by virus infection or inactivity. Most viral infections are preventable by behavioral changes, as well as most modern day diseases, such as hypertension, diabetes of adult onset, arteriolosclerosis, and cardiovascular disease. Even cancer could be avoided in many cases by enhancing our autoimmune systems. Exercise and education becomes paramount to modern living, because of the competing interests of manufacturing profiteers, public welfare, and political aspiration.

1.6.2. BIRTH OF NEW TECHNOLOGICAL MARVELS
In only few decades, people sensed the mysterious power of scientific accomplishments. I lived the conversion of the steam train into the diesel combustion engine. The train engineer, then tarred in black smog was now seated in a clean cabinet with colorful controls. Today, the train riders do not have to worry about rewashing their clothes after every ride on board or passing closer to the train. The invention of the television, the landing of man on the moon, the introduction of the internet were among few assuring hopes that would bring our planet together to work for common cause. There is definite proof that man became the master of the universe in just few centuries of rethinking the laws of nature and putting them to work to harness energy. We are now closer than ever to rectify many maladies that result from defects in the human genes, which should bring hope to many people with genetic disorders. As far as spreading health education and fitness awareness, it seems that economic improvements and availability of jobs are the most crucial factors in rendering the population aspiring to improve quality of life.

1.6.3. MILITARY COMPETITION REVOLUTIONIZES THE SPORT OF WEIGHTLIFTING
Ironically, achieving such advanced level of technical sophistication did not happen voluntarily. Without the two World Wars, national governments might have not recognized the immense benefits of scientific research. Competition for national security had thrust scientific research and development in many positive directions. Weightlifting was a major beneficial of such military competitions. Modern battles of the early part of the last century demanded heavy lifting of ammunitions and equipments for longer distances, hours, and across rugged terrains. Studying the nature of human physique to master such tedious physical labor has urged many military institutes to research resistance training for the sake of improving soldiers' ability to fight. The controlled military environment allowed testing and implementing new methods of enhancing fitness. The strict routines of eating, sleeping, and regular and coerced training have all eliminated procrastination of individuals and proved very effective in enhancing fitness.

1.6.4. CONTRIBUTION OF THE COMMUNIST ATHLETES TO WEIGHTLIFTING
During the cold war, 1945-1992, Weightlifters from the communist block have contributed significantly to advancing the sport to higher scientific levels, as follows and as discussed in Chapter Four[3].
o   They have excelled in optimizing the length of time a Weightlifter requires to progressively build strength, without regressing to fatigue and cardiovascular failure.
o   They also have perfected the sequence of executing exercises in a way that eliminate mechanical failure of major muscle groups, amidst training.
o   They also have succeeded in resolving the conflict of choice among the so many exercises that a weightlifter has to execute, to climb the hill to the peak of their performance. These three contributions to the sport of Weightlifting made the difference between scientific training and ad hoc training.

1.6.5. THE RISE AND GROWTH OF THE SPORT OF BODYBUILDING
In the western hemisphere, there was an intriguing world of personal freedom and economic prosperity. Western youth are concerned more with personal aspiration and the quick wealth and fame that are within reach in many western nations. Bodybuilding was blossoming as a new sport that enhances physical attraction and open new doors for young job-seekers. The endeavors of the early pioneers of Bodybuilding established the foundations of the sport and proved the feasibility of sculpturing human musculature, in many desirable shapes and with specific training methods. Many young people grew passion towards Bodybuilding because of its enhancement of appearance and strength, the freedom form supervised coaching, the so many artistic approaches to individualize one's own body, and the hope it offers of staying well.

---

[3] The Weightlifting Encyclopedia: A Guide to world Class Performance" by Arthur Drechsler, New York, USA, 1998. Chapter 6 on Putting It all Together: Developing the Training Plan. ISBN 0-9659179-2-4.

INTRODUCTION

Bodybuilding has developed in a vacuum that lacks any specific time frame to accomplish certain goals. That renders the sport a dangerous activity of building tissues that would impede, rather than enhance, many physiological functions, as follows and as discussed in Chapter Six.
- o Heavily built upper body, which lacks proportionate significance to the whole body motion, endangers the joints, particularly the knees.
- o Gaining excess muscular weight demands careful accounting of excess caloric intake that endangers the endocrine system. Building massive muscles, without due consideration of proper ranges of mobility of the many joints, leads to early onset of circulatory and respiratory problems due to restricted mobility.
- o The lack of proper sequence of executing exercises, in the sport of Bodybuilding, also renders the sport a crippling activity of stiffening tendons and damaging joints, with total disregard to the harmony of motion of properly functioning joints.

1.6.6. PROLIFERATION OF THE SPORT OF GENERAL WEIGHT TRAINING
As fitness has evolved in the last few decades, general resistance training becomes an alternative to Olympic Weightlifting and Bodybuilding. Today, weight training, as taught by most of fitness trainers, completely lacks the features of a sport, as follows and as discussed in Chapter Seven.
- o Neither the sequence of executing exercises is well thought of, nor is the number of exercises per session properly chosen.
- o Above all, it lacks the strategy of a concrete plan that adheres to physiological rules of enhancing functions, rather than arbitrarily focusing on strength of random muscles.
- o Such scheme of training offers a wider base to the so many people who had missed the opportunities to start training in the primes of their youth, when many complex issues were easily learnable.
- o It also offers a relaxed atmosphere of entertainment away from the strict disciplinary routine of systemic sports.
- o Since the wide majority of any population seems to have missed the opportunity of proper training, general weight training attracts many commercial businesses, seeking profit for its affluent clientele.
- o The health problems that face this wide segment of the population are easily preventable by active life style, way beyond walking to and from work.
- o The introduction of resistance training to common people is the wisest prescription physicians have to make to help their patients gain their independence from the costly health care system.

1.6.7. CHANGE IN ATTITUDE TOWARDS PHYSICAL TRAINING
Today, going to the gym become a sign of accomplishment, while in my early days it was considered a sign of recklessness and indifference towards academic glory that would ensure decent future. Such drastic change in people's attitude towards exercise proves that persistent persuasion works, over many years, in altering herd conviction.

1.7. STATE OF KNOWLEDGE

1.7.1. PROPER RESISTANCE TRAINING LEADS TO STRENGTH
The essentials rules that make the sport of Weightlifting a powerful aid in promoting health are well established. The simplest known axiom, on which Weightlifting is founded, is as follows.
"Consistent resistance to force leads to growth and strength, if performed properly and on long period of time".
That is very evident in the course of development of a newborn child. Persistent trials to kick, crawl, sit, stand, and finally walk and run are critical activities for growing up. After reaching that level of motor independence from the need of constant and immediate parental care, children develop strength of different parts of the body according to the sort of activities they engage in. Most children develop relatively strong legs compared to the upper limbs. This trend of differential strength, between upper and lower body, progresses unabated unless the person engage in specific activities that exercise the upper limbs. Thus, lower limbs that engage in walking and running get stronger, while the upper limbs that have little work to do get weaker. This is particularly noted in females.

Since most vital organs are located in the upper body (heart, lungs, and brain) and since the upper body gets minimal workout with regular daily activities as compared to the lower body, the result is that the respiratory muscles becomes disproportionately weak with respect to the bodyweight, and the upper body bone frame becomes disproportionately fragile with respect to the whole skeleton. Weak respiratory muscles and fragile upper body skeleton limit the individual capacity to lead active life, and predispose to inactivity.

1.7.2. EARLY EDUCATION AND SYSTEMIC PHYSICAL TRAINING
How do we forget the lessons of growing up? Many adults struggle with so many fitness problems that would have been avoided had they adhered to their past experience of growing up. The process of development and growth of childhood should not have been halted by an educational system that is heavily geared toward the sole process of literacy. The twelve years spent in basic education are mostly wasted in a system burdened with bureaucracies and self-service and less keen to

be trusted to manage those crucial years of educating children. Unfortunately, public education is not as profitable as gambling or tobacco industries, at least on the short run, and many politicians pander to the public sympathy towards education, with too many promises and too little deeds.

1.7.3. EDUCATION CONVEYED IN PLAY FORMAT
Even before the completion of childhood and early adolescence, a need to introduce a training program is the best way to bring the youth closely to understand the laws of nature. The mastery of athletic skills by a growing child lends assurance to the child's early experience of joyful play, which used to be his or her main occupation. Having neglected systemic physical exercises in the early years of primary and middle schools, children lose the proportionate fitness of body, limbs, and cardiovascular and pulmonary systems and become setup for many years of struggle to reverse such early life detour from proper training.

1.7.4. CHILDREN'S DEMAND FOR EARLY TRAINING
Other activities such as learning music, art, technical skills, and literacy should also be complemented with physical training. This can easily be argued on the basis of the anatomical fact that the heart, blood vessels, muscles, and bones constitute a great portion of the body, with their great demand for physical activities should be orderly prioritized. Many motor skills could not be acquired after the early years of adolescence because of the following:
o   Flexibility of pelvic and vertebral joints is progressively limited after puberty, in the absence of exercise.
o   Strengthening the major muscles groups (thighs, glutei, back erectors, and shoulders) is very difficult after late adolescence.
o   Endurance and ability to deal with vigorous stress decline sharply had regular exercise not started before the end of adolescence.
o   Balance and coordination are very difficult to acquire with taller and heavier bodies in the late adolescence.
o   Phobias from height, speed, vigorous activities set in by late adolescence.
o   Maximal reachable strength diminishes if exercise is not commenced around puberty or earlier.

1.7.5. THE KEYS TO PROPER PLANNING OF WEIGHTLIFTING PROGRAM
The knowledge accumulated about the proper strategy for planning resistance-training program encompasses multitude of basic rules that bridge the fields of physiology, kinesiology, and psychiatry. The early pioneers of Weightlifting relied on the stimulating milieu of regular and hard labor that is conducive to promoting strength. Competition brought insightful analysis and research that pushed the boundaries of human performance. The following issues promote proper planning for success in Weightlifting.
o   Nutrition is crucial to developing strength. Complex carbohydrates, vegetables, and proteins are paramount to building muscles and bones.
o   Building muscles and bones with aggressive Bodybuilding training could expedite the progress of the individual in Weightlifting, if (this is very important) running, flexibility, Calisthenics, and balanced whole body training are accounted for.
o   Building muscles with Weightlifting routines is also practical for people with good muscular mass and body proportions. Weightlifting routines are not the best choices to start with, for people with individual deficits such as narrow chest, weak shoulders and arms.
o   Combined routines of Bodybuilding and Weightlifting are favored by trainers in rush to get fast results. The fact is that young people require only few years to develop proportionate body ratios with Bodybuilding, combined with Calisthenics.
o   Destructives habits such as smoking, irregular and inappropriate sleep, alcohol and drug usage, and excessive sexual indulgence are significant obstacles to any progress in Weightlifting planning.

1.7.6. THE ESSENCE OF THE SPORT OF WEIGHTLIFTING
The essence of this sport is that muscular strength could be enhanced in parallel with joints' flexibility, whole-body coordination, cardiovascular, and pulmonary endurance, while maintaining maximum ratio of strength-to-bodyweight. Such optimization of positive functionalities and sparing overall body size is the ultimate goal of Weightlifting training, as follows.
o   Weightlifting is not a sport of strength alone. Many strong athletes bail out of Weightlifting because of lack of flexibility, synchrony of the technique, and improper balance.
o   It is not true that lifting maximum weight has nothing to do with the technique. A Weightlifter can lift heavy weight with much less effort and aftereffects than a much stronger non-Weightlifter.
o   Weightlifting emphasizes the three major muscle groups of the lower body, back, and shoulders. These are muscles that act on the axial region of the body. Peripheral limbs and muscles are trained in the interim of working out the axis.
o   Progressive increase in intensity of lifting and in volume of load is combined with structured rests and breaks, to progressively increase physical strength.

1.7.7. INTERMIX OF ART AND SCIENCE
The tools required to accomplish these goals are not only sound scientific backgrounds of anatomy, physiology, and kinesiology, but also practical experience on the performance and execution of wide spectrum of lifting techniques. Thus

both art and science intermix in delineating the strategy of planning robust resistance training program. This explains the new and constant breakthroughs of records and techniques thought of as remotely impossible to attain. Of course science alone cannot bring the basic elements of strong and determined individuals. Many accomplished Weightlifters are not well to do in science, yet most of them possessed the scientific mind without formal diplomas or education. As a matter of fact, curiosity, determined will, and little ingenuity have led many Weightlifters to the top.

1.7.8. LACK OF ACCESS TO INFORMATION
In environments totally alien to basic Weightlifting principles, the demanding standards of planning daily, monthly, and longer plans, have rendered the wealth of knowledge of the sport of Weightlifting less accessible to the masses of trainees and trainers. The following are examples of poorly informed trainees.
- Many trainees are still at the wrong belief that building big muscles enhances Weightlifting.
- Training certain regions of the body in some days and other regions in other days is widely practiced, and causes little to advance performance.
- The sequence of executing exercises is solely based on avoiding physical exertion rather than on integrating elements of mobility, coordination, and stability in proper order.
- Many still believe that the magic number of "TEN" repetitions per set is a mandate for success.
- Fitness machines are critical training tools. Most fitness machines create serious problems, from limiting the range of motion of joints, jeopardizing the mobility features of proper training, to seriously impairing the postural dynamics of coordination. There is no doubt that fitness machines can do more good in the hands of a knowledgeable trainer or trainee but they must not be the ultimate tool of training in public health clubs

1.7.9. CAUSES OF UNPOPULARITY OF WEIGHTLIFTING
The lack of wide access to proper training strategies has other underlying causes, as follows.
- The majority of academic curricula overlook Weightlifting as an eminent sport for enhancing public health. Other popular sports are promoted for the sake of their monetary return.
- The subject of Weightlifting has been left for ex-Bodybuilders and fitness trainers to promote to the public, with the result of serious flaws of portraying the sport to new comers. Many of the amateur fitness trainers have chosen this field as a short cut for earning income while having fun. Yet the subject is too complicated to be left to amateurs, and too unattractive monetarily to appeal to the prestigious universities that seek fast wealth with little resources.
- Health professionals are also overwhelmed with the fast paced progress of the medical sciences, have very little to do with structuring training for health and fitness. Physical therapy offers the minimal requirements for healing that keep people independent from the health system.

1.8. DISCIPLINE

1.8.1. THE ROLE OF MENTAL DETERMINATION IN WEIGHTLIFTING
Enduring the pain of enhancing physical strength is an uphill battle of internal struggle and temptation of lazy lifestyle, as follows.
- Weight training constitutes a struggle to understand what is occurring to the intriguing biological system in response to volitional activity.
- A practical understanding of the source and nature of the pain stimulus is required. You do not have to be a neurologist to train for Weightlifting, but you have to strive to understand the general concepts of what is serious and what is benign. Any part of the body that is not used to perform unaccustomed activity will protest in pain. You have to learn how to distinguish the different sources of pain that result from training.
- The complexity of the biological nature of the body and the mechanical aspect of Weightlifting leaves very little room for personal inclinations.
- The main drive for staying determined, even after setbacks, injuries, or even surgeries, is the realization that strength and fitness are paramount to freedom and happiness. The whole world won't deter strong and determined people.
- Your workout sessions are not mere physical sweating and hard labor but are fundamental biological obligation for nurturing your thought process. Exercise is as crucial to health, as sleeping and feeding.

1.8.2. THE ROLE OF DISCIPLINE IN WEIGHTLIFTING
Such desired discipline is not entirely new to us. We are familiar with the different phases of development from infancy, childhood, to adulthood, all of which require discipline to stay physically, mentally, and socially well. Though discipline is relative to the norms of different cultures, Weightlifting training requires strict observance of basic health rules in order to be able to master one's own health and fitness, voluntarily. Young trainees have long acquired their own identity and desire to rebel and experiment on their own, in order to reach their personal goals with their perceived reality. An older

and trusted figure might covey better insight to youngsters regarding the drawbacks of their naïve tackling of new challenges. As soon as the youngster senses that there is a complex and intricate world behind the superficial appearance of new issues, he or she may begin to appreciate patience and diligence in managing their health affairs, as follows.
- o A good night sleep or a day of relaxation may suffice relief of fatigue or anxiety better than any substance usage.
- o Slight modification of training might eliminate the boredom and stress of managing strength training.
- o Regular and persistent insertion of few exercises that specifically remedy one's individual deficits may add up to breakthrough in one's own level of fitness.
- o Determined search for and inquisition about a solution of a long burdensome issue may bring finality.
- o Skepticism towards common believes regarding limitations imposed by age, sex, or medical conditions may invigorate the mind to stay determined in working towards improving our condition.

1.8.3. ACCESS OF INFORMATION TO THE YOUTH
Access of information at early age can dramatically impact the society in guiding the youth to making better choices of disciplined practices, as follows.
- o Today, the famous and well-heard avenues of information propagation are commercial in nature, with main goals of making profit.
- o Most health and fitness information are geared towards prevention or management of diseases that target adults with lucrative resources who can afford to buy products.
- o Since the youth have little resources, particularly at the early age when starting new sports is very productive in making long term compliant and accomplished athletes, it follows that the youth need definite assistance from society if major changes in the trends of health and fitness are sought.
- o There is no doubt that developed nations enjoy unprecedented luxury of available fitness industries and clubs particularly in major cities. Yet, most commercialized fitness clubs offer gathering places for people with common goals, yet present formidable obstacles for the young. Those need role model, close personal guidance, and concrete plan to follow, rather than joining the crowd of confused population of health clubs.
- o Public health clubs offer access to the needy youth, just as venues to get them off the street for the sake of entertainment.
- o Proper access to information that is completely lacking in well-to-do societies, should focus on stimulating people to begin and continue structured sport for as long as they live. Since with the wide scale availability of basic preventive health standards, many people will live to advanced age than in the first half of the last century, thus encouraging people to engage in serious exercise will guarantee reduction on the drain of health resources in treating chronic preventable diseases such as diabetes, blood pressure, and cancer.

1.8.4. NEED FOR COMMUNITY VOLUNTEER WORK BY ATHLETES
It seems to me that community volunteer work, by accomplished athletes, could serve the purpose of providing access of information and guidance to the youth in this field of growing complexity of fitness knowledge, as follows.
- o What good is focusing on academic prosperity when the final outcome is drug addiction, alcoholism, and physically inactivity, even after graduating from prestigious universities?
- o Volunteer work of ex-athletes, with substantial accomplishments, with no conflict of interest of making profit by selling commercial products, might guide fitness industries to proper channels of benefiting both society and such industries, through stimulating the population to engage in invigorating exercise activities.
- o Many young, as well as adults, do not realize that it is possible for any individual to learn a new sport, and that passion and dedication to a beloved sport is very gratifying physically, psychologically, as well as intellectually.
- o Engaging in sport activities is not as hard as many people imagine. It only takes few months to get a sense of the required changes in the body to keep going. The predictable course of events of body adaptation and progressive improvements must be explained and emphasized repeatedly, in order to maintain participation in activities.
- o Explaining the required subsequent actions, to be taken when a setback is encountered, is assuring to beginners. When a herd of young beginners are taught about expected events and proper ways to manage them, adherence to training program becomes stronger. Many beginners were not taught that muscles and joints deteriorate without activities. When injuries happen, exercise is as important as ever, after the acute phase is managed. Having being injured should not be interpreted as a drawback to exercise, since all activities entail some risk.

1.8.5. SCIENTIFIC PLANNING OF RESISTANCE TRAINING
Resistance training is an enriching science of strategy planning, perseverance to accomplish enduring long-term goals, and practical experience in sensing what works and what do not, when health is at stake. It is the science and art, of play and fun that should be condoned, as equally as academic prosperity. The following supports this argument.
- o The individual has to accept stepwise approach. Things will get better in steps, the wiser the plan the larger the steps.
- o The general trend of the plan should be balance and simplicity. Overall balance cannot be attained with individual isolated exercises, no matter how tempting they are.
- o Apart from the general trend, an individualized component of the plan should deal with individual deficits. Thus, the plan may entail three or four general exercises that work out the whole body (each of them work out the whole body)

and one or two exercises that deal with individual isolated muscles or regions, such as chest, shoulder, arms, or abdomen. The individualized exercises lend more attention to distracting issues such as big belly, weak chest, overweight, and other concerns that may detour effective planning.
- o All individuals, beginners and advanced, have to devote most of their strength planning on back, pelvic, and shoulder strengthening, in that order of priorities. The rest of the body is trained in the interim, in addition to the individualized minor components. It is well known that distraction with "training isolated parts of the body" results in deformities of posture and premature decline in general strength. There are many people who can bench press over twice their bodyweight yet cannot perform back extension with even a 10th of that weight, or cannot squat with proportionate strength.
- o The main feature of scientific planning of resistance training is the realization of the concrete relationship between Intensity of individual exercises, Volume of accumulated exercises, and Predicted progress in strength. Intensity of physical activity is directly related to muscular growth in strength and size. Volume of accumulated physical activity is directly related to whole body adaptation to stimulus and the body's ability to evolve to higher state of strength. Predicted progress is based on tabulated tracks of other athletes with similar circumstances.

1.8.6. ON THE PERPLEXING ROOTS OF DISCIPLINE
Discipline is dearly needed virtue in this tough sport of health and fitness. But the roots of discipline are as perplexing as many other social traits. Teaching discipline to youth might be the most formidable task a mentor has to tackle. Using logical approach might fail with many defiant youths whose mind set serves finding their role among their peers, rather than contemplating a whole future awaiting them. The internal conflicts between primitive instincts and imposed demands for fitting in complex human society might tip towards urging desire for quick gratification, regardless of the consequences. It seems that there are earlier factors that play in the psyche of the young that may explain why some youngsters can adhere to tougher disciplines than others.

1.8.7. ON THE REBELLION OF ADULT TRAINEES AGAINST DISCIPLINARY RULES
Even with adults, barriers of rebellion work as in the case of youth rebellion. In many health clubs I have attended, many people do not show up for training until it is too late to reverse the deformities they have incurred, by not seeking knowledge earlier. The fact that physical development surpasses the rate of acquiring knowledge about health and fitness, in modern times, is attributed to the too many puzzling information that overwhelm people's mind. Many weigh the amount of effort needed to reverse ill effects versus the enjoyment of life they perceive, had they continued their prior activities. With the uncertainties about what best route to follow and the futility of such efforts, many people stick to what they know even if it does not lead to any progress.

1.8.8. DISCIPLINE VERSUS DEPRIVATION
The fact that should not be traded for personal gain or popularity is that **discipline is a sort of deprivation**, as follows.
- o We cannot eat what we wish, drink what we like, smoke in any capacity, exercise in any way we desire, without resorting to intelligent style of scientific strategy. As deprivation is relatively subjective issue, yet it defines certain norms of healthy behavior.
- o We should not expect to get rid of excess weight, which we have gained on many months or even years, by trying to reverse that excess in too short of a time period. There are many processes in the body that cannot be reversed on our own terms. The impact of excessive weight gain is widely manifested on many systems. A thorough understanding of the course of symptoms and signs associate with trials to reduce bodyweight is advised.
- o Many people have won the battle of weight reduction yet to face another battle of loss of bone mass, debility, lack of energy, or body deformities because of muscular imbalance. Resistance training benefits weight watchers by building the muscular machinery that is efficient in managing fat depot, better than just dieting.
- o Even if weight control is not your prime concern, you may appreciate the value of discipline and deprivation much better by exercising. That is because exercise is a practical learning of managing energy.

1.8.9. ON THE COMPLIANCE OF TRAINEES WITH PLANNED SCHEMES
The critical role of discipline is the compliance of trainees with a planned scheme, to accomplish the desired goals, as follows.
- o Sometimes boredom with frequent setbacks and lack of efficacy of a plan leads to incompliance.
- o Search for exit strategy of such unforeseen difficulties depends on prior experience, of confronting similar issues, and on making bold trials to experiment with new approaches to deal with individual shortcomings.
- o For example, trainees with weak lower body tend to avoid exercises that entail lifting from the floor, with subsequent aggravated weakness to the lower body and lengthy setback.
- o Likewise, trainees with weak upper body tends to avoid overhead lifting, to avoid embarrassment, with the result of worsening the function of the upper body.

- o Trainees with flexibility problems tend to favor military performance (stiffed legs without jumps or spring cushioning movements) to avoid imbalance.
- o Addressing individual deficits by adding exercises that remedy weak girdles, muscular imbalance, and limited range of motion should enhance performance on the long term and gains the confidence of the trainee in the rationale of a training plan.

1.8.10. ON THE NURTURING OF LOGICAL INSIGHT INTO ONE'S OWN PROBLEMS
Discipline, therefore, could be ingrained in one's daily routines when logical insight into the confronting problems is persistently sought and tested by regular exercise, as follows.
- o It would take just quick snap of mind to decide, in favor or against, performing certain exercises that might relieve the stress of a nagging problem, the trainee confronts.
- o As is the situation with other addictive rituals, nurturing a conscientious insight might be the only censor that sways the person toward the right course to fitness.
- o It might be said that just participating in structured training is a proof that the individual already possess reasonable insight to his or her inadequacies. Yet continuing the endeavor of training refines and expands that insight to other related world issues.
- o All living animals develop insight into the laws of nature by relentless activities, yet humans are privileged with intellectual development than the rest of creatures.

1.9. DEBATES

1.9.1. IS WEIGHTLIFTING AN EVERY DAY NECESSITY?
- o In many cultures physical training is not viewed as an every day necessity.
- o Yet, the new challenges of a constantly changing world, of new amenities and inventions, demand that we must take bold decisions to alter our life style in order to stay fit.
- o No health resources, of any magnitude, would cure or manage the consequences of inactivity of the majority of the population. The higher intake of calories and the minimal expenditure of energy by modern daily activities clog the blood vessels with excessive fat deposits, in the forms or arteriosclerotic plaques. Restricted and clogged circulation cause general deterioration of all body organs.
- o Since modern urbanization has reduced physical activities below minimal required levels, many people become baffled with what is essential and what is not. If people continue to believe that modern daily activities and modern eating habits are adequate enough for healthy living without regular vigorous exercises, the result might be gradual extinction of the human species, as was the case with the unfit dinosaurs.

1.9.2. HOW MUCH WEIGHT TRAINING SUFFICES FOR GETTING AND STAYING FIT?
What should workout consist of, to upset the vicious circuit of weakness and debility?
- o Definitely, walking to and from work, performing a strenuous job or demanding housework, is not sufficient as a substitute for systemic training.
- o Strenuous work duties induce deformities, stiffness, and imbalance, because neither is symmetry taken into consideration, nor is proper range of motion adhered to.
- o Dangers due injuries are very frequent in modern living. The weak and frail population has to deal with episodes of vigorous physical work such as lifting a child, shuffling snow, lifting a heavy bag of groceries, or opening a jammed door.
- o Vigorous weight training is not only intended to prepare the individual to competitive sports, but also to fare better in such everyday dangers. Therefore, weight training should be an everyday activity, in whatever type you choose to perform, as discussed in *Section 14.1.4* on Mobility and *Tip # 2,* thereof.

1.9.3. HOW TO AVOID ERRONEOUSLY HARMFUL TRAINING?
How could physical strength be promoted and not erroneously harmed by resistance training? The following offers some answers to this question.
- o The effort devoted to strength training is as beneficial as all efforts devoted to constructive activity. Strength training is a learning process that raises our level of awareness of the proper technique of movement, from walking, standing, running, sitting, or lying down.
- o Athletes perform every movement with much grace, for many years of life, compared to non-athletes. Refined motor skills aid in intelligent living. The first step to become an athlete is to start workout today and think about planning as you go. Think that athletes are not extraterrestrial aliens but rather people like you and me who started to work out earlier than the rest.
- o The vast majority of the population suffers from improper posture, weak limbs, chronic stiffness, and muscular imbalance, all of which would have been prevented with regular physical training.

INTRODUCTION

o You might be able to make up for missed opportunities of academic achievement, by reeducating yourself, but reversing the consequences of omitting exercise for many years is extremely difficult, if not impossible, and if not started soon.

1.9.4. SEARCH FOR ULTIMATE ROLE MODELS
Are there ultimate role models to strive for? The following argues the issue of seeking a role model in this context.
o As we grow up we alter our view of a role model according to how far we have accomplished in our pursuit of individual goals. There are many I have considered as icons at certain times who no longer rise to that level. When I was young I believed, like many young trainees, that big muscular men are icons. Now, I have developed a different scale for iconic merits, based on making choices in life that do well and do no harm.
o Big musculature would do a lot of harm, if not weighed against graceful mobility and decent intellectual achievement. Why would any sane person devote such time to get big without balancing his physique with intellectual knowledge?
o Definitely, building healthy physique is a plus. Yet, without ambition and dreams to better all aspects of life, strong physique does little to alleviate anxiety.
o Sport is an evolving field of activities and role models are also evolving. My advice is to keep open mind and to widen your scope of knowledge to be able to avoid pitfalls of different approaches of training.

1.9.5. WEIGHTLIFTING IS A SPORT FOR EVERYBODY
Is Weightlifting a sport for every body, or there are specific prerequisites in a person to become a Weightlifter?
o The zealous trend of Weightlifting coaches, that some people do not fit into the sport because they are too tall, have deformities, or slow learners, etc, stems from the narrow world of little ambition and exclusion of competitive sports.
o Many people will benefit from modern Weightlifting and do not have to compete in front of three Weightlifting judges. It suffices that they succeed to compete in front of the society at large with their new accomplishment.
o Weightlifting should be taught to all learning seekers, and should be introduced to non-seekers who do not have access to information. It is a sport for all vertebrate mammals with spinal body axis.

1.10. NUTRITION, EXERCISE, AND REST

The basic rule for promoting physical health is a triad of balanced nutrition, exercise, and rest. False promises of commercial health products that boost energy and exotic exercise equipments that substitute natural training are not within the realm of that balance.

1.10.1. NUTRITIONAL NEEDS OF ATHLETES VERSUS THOSE FOR NON-ATHLETES
A consensus on what is simple and affordable routine of nutrition is not out of reach.
o The nutritional aspect of this balance is mostly learned from parents, relatives, and friends. Eating habits are sometimes hard to change, particularly when rigid cultural taboos are in work.
o Healthy nutrition for strength training differs from the modest concept of weight-watchers, of assessing caloric and nutritional values of foodstuff.
o A Weightlifter must pick a nutritional regimen that, in addition of supplying the proper amount of calories and nutritional requirements for anabolic processes, must also produce minimal strain on the digestive tract. Many non-athletes tolerate carrying around heavily loaded large intestine for many years of their lives. The predominance of distended bellies, asthenic limbs, and deformed postures among modern human population are direct results of imbalanced habits. An athlete would be hampered with a full belly.
o Nutrition that keeps the guts within reasonable size, does not impede respiration, venous return, or circulation in vital organs, is critical to athletic success. The rule of thumb is that food or regimen that leads to infrequent bowel movement; dark colored or malodorous stool should be avoided. Food of animal origin and fatty meals fall into this category as discussed in *Section 14.3.6* on Healthy diet.
o Shortening the transit time of the digested food, through the colon, permits unobstructed venous return, vigorous respiration, and efficient channeling of blood to working muscles during ambulance. Simply, athletic nutrition should reduce the main function of the large intestine, of putrefaction of undigested food, to a level that minimizes the pressure on abdominal organs.
o In all Weightlifting exercises, diaphragmatic excursion during vigorous breathing requires empty guts to allow full inflation of the lungs during inspiration. The habit of maintaining constantly deflated guts, with minimal residues of undigested food, may be the healthiest habit gained from physical training.
o Reducing the physical pressure on the kidneys, with light guts, would decrease the chances of developing hypertension due to ischemic kidneys. Reducing the putrefaction in the large intestine would help avert colon irritation and many other maladies that result from restricting the smooth flow of blood in the major venous channels.

1.10.2. NATURAL EXERCISES VERSUS EQUIPMENT-AIDED EXERCISES
The second element of the balance is exercise. Here, all the confusion begins about what constitute a proper exercise plan. Whom would you trust as guidance for planning your exercise? The following shed some light on this issue.

- o Natural exercise cannot be substitute by daily work activity, equipment-aided exercises, or by electrical stimulating devices. During daily activity, we repeatedly use the same groups of muscles to perform the intended work.
- o In contrast, during systemic training, we survey the weak muscle groups and the stiffened joints and aims at restoring strength and flexibility, where they are compromised. Moreover, systemic exercise refines the motor and sensory skill of the intricate nervous system
- o Equipment aided exercises are supposed to supplement but not substitute freestyle lifting. Seated exercises and restricted motions, of many aiding equipments, undoubtedly restrict joints mobility and precludes many muscle groups from developing natural strength and responsiveness to stimulation. Equipment aided training is a curse for healthy capable people. It is a deceiving habit that will steal from you the vigor of getting fit and staying healthy for many years after. The pros and cons of aided exercises are discussed in Chapter Seven, on Weight Training issues.
- o Free lifting integrates the coordination of muscle sensors, with the extrapyramidal nervous system, to modulate skeletal muscles in such a way that strength and mobility are optimized. Free lifting is not easy, but when practiced regularly, for few months, stamina and endurance will ensue. Freestyle lifting is elaborately discussed in Chapters Four, Eight, Nine, Eleven, Twelve, and Thirteen.

1.10.3. MAKING THE BEST OUT OF YOUR REST TIME

The third element of the balance is rest. Rest by avoiding exercise, avoiding exertion in daily activities, and sleep, is a two-edged weapon, as follows.
- o The sleep part of the balance has been drastically impacted, in the modern times, with the invention of electricity and television. It became very hard to convince people that regular and adequate sleep is as important as dedicated exercise and nutrition.
- o Excessive sleep, over ten hours, reduces muscular tone of the paravertebral region, to dangerously low levels. With lowered tone, fewer muscular fibers perform the whole task of movement. This results in muscular strain and injuries to lower back, after long hours of sleep.
- o Also, inadequate sleep, less than six hours, increases the sympathetic activity and renders the cardiovascular and respiratory systems over-sensitive to any physical effort. This precludes the trainee from completing adequate exercise session.
- o The other eight hours of work, or home-related activities, significantly determine your achievement in the world of fitness. A factory worker can surpass any athlete, if carefully plans his eight hours of tedious work. A simple example is to try to equally use both hands alternatively during the eight-hour workday. The long history of achievements of factory workers in Weightlifting attests to the effect of long day of activity on fitness.
- o Another healthy habit to practice, on-job activity, is the bending of knees, slowly and carefully, each time a weight has to be lifted. The best habit of all, in this context, is to try to constantly memorize and execute the proper technique, when faced with a task of lifting.
- o The remaining eight hours of the day should be utilized on the basis of the activities of the other sixteen hours. The crucial index of "fitness to exercise" is the heart rate and force of beats. An exhausted person feels the pounding of hyperactive heart, out of proportion to physical effort. Fever is another sign that should be watched before attempting to exercise. Of course clear consciousness is of utmost importance in any physical activity. Any medication such as alcohol, antihistaminic medication, hypnotics, or any drug that impair consciousness should be cleared off the body, at least a full twenty four hours prior to exercise.
- o The experience accumulated over the past 100 years, of documenting Olympic athletes, points to the fact that about two hours of vigorous physical exercise maximally enhances the performance of an athlete. Some programs favor a day of complete rest off vigorous training, plus another day or two of double shifts of workout, each week. That is an eight to seven workouts per week, with a day off. Of course, many self-taught athletes would not be able to plan such heavy schedule without erring on the side of straining the heart to failure. Scientific training is thus founded on the fact that graduation of the magnitude, duration, and frequency of application of resistance, on many months, is the key to enhancing fitness. That defines **"progressive incremental resistance training"**.

1.11. STORY OF A LITTLE OLD LADY

1.11.1. SETTING PRIORITIES IN A WISE MANNER

I like to cite a brief story, I have witnessed, that coveys lessons on how to plan a robust training program using plain common sense. In a busy health club in New York, during the rush hours, when it is hard to even find a space to stretch your arms without hitting somebody, there came an old black lady with a thirty-pound barbell in her hands, looking for a spot in front of a mirror. When she got to the end of the room, she pushed away few plates, to clear an area around her, and started working out, by lifting the bar from the floor to her shoulders and then pushing it overhead. That is exactly what all Weightlifting trainers advise their trainees to do. Full range of axial motion is common sense, scientific strengthening, and it promotes health effectively.

1.11.2. EFFICIENT SELECTION OF PROPER EXERCISES
She repeated that for few sets, and then moved to the Smith machine, added two forty-five pound plates, lied on her back on the floor, under the suspended barbell, and started pushing the weight upwards and lowering it with her feet. She used the bar hook to hang the bar at the end of each set. The former, upright lifting, is a great challenge to the sympathetic nervous system, that has to work overzealously to maintain blood flow to the upper body during standing. The latter, Smith machine, lying down is a great challenge to the heart compliance with excessive venous return. Thus, that lady simply challenged two major and vital body systems, heart and brain, within few minutes from starting exercise.

1.11.3. IMPLEMENTING HIGHER STANDARDS OF TRAINING WITH PLAIN COMMON SENSE
She was sweating heavily, more than the other big and tough guys around her. Neither of them had lifted any weight from the floor. Everybody else was using benches and machines. Such a story shows how a person, without any past experience, can use simple common sense in making their workout a very powerful tool of promoting health. No single person in that health club had benefited from his or her workout better than that little old lady. She had implemented all fundamentals of scientific training just by relying on her own instincts, as follows.
- o She wasted no time in distraction by isolated muscles.
- o Trained the muscular groups that deserve highest priorities to maintain proper posture.
- o Resorted to extremes of exercises that require perfect coordination, mobility, strength, and, most importantly, demand excellent cardiopulmonary performance to endure vigorous strain, in recumbent versus upright postures.
- o Pacing a training plan, the way that lady has done of speechless seriousness and dedication, reveals the strong will of a determined person.

1.12. SOUND WORKOUT PLAN

1.12.1. MODEST AVAILABILITY OF SPACE AND EQUIPMENT
A sound workout plan could be defined as follows:
- o A plan that requires modest availability of space and equipment. The common practice of commercial health clubs of crowing the gym floor with all kinds of shinning fitness equipments is only intended to attract unwary new members, yet do not serve the purpose of simplifying training.
- o Simplicity of the training area is crucial in focusing attention on planning, without the distraction of accessory equipments. The oldest model of a training area is that of a platform, a barbell set, a ceil-and-wall ladder, and a parallel bar pair. The rest of equipments should be totally isolated in separate rooms from the main working place.
- o With bars weighing 10 to 20 kg (22 to 45 lbs), you can almost perform most of the ancillary exercises, without the need for aiding equipments.
- o Vertical and horizontal ladders are essential for pulling exercise of the pectoral girdle, while parallel bars are essential for the pushing exercises of the pectoral girdle.
- o The rest of modern equipment is useful in supplementing freestyle exercises, for the sake of strengthening of particular groups of isolated muscles.
- o Heavy reliance on equipments could lead to serious imbalance by overriding the natural mechanisms of motion. For example, heavy use of chest machines can lead to imbalanced of the pectoral girdle that requires a wide range of mobility to accomplish its function. Pectoral muscles can be heavily trained, in parallel with balanced freestyle lifting, without upsetting the shoulder balance.

1.12.2. SAFETY RULES OF PROPER PROGRESSIVE INCREASE IN RESISTANCE
Proper training plans adhere to safety rules of performing exercises in the proper sequence of increasing difficulty, as follows.
- o Many beginners, and even advanced athletes, underestimate the invaluable benefit gained from starting a workout set with a bare bar, that does not have plates on it. On daily basis you will see people start their resistance training with a weight that is very close to the maximum they could lift.
- o With systemic professional training, trainees will learn to content themselves with progressive increase of resistance.
- o Exercises that do not involve weights precede those that require weight. Exercises that require full and vigorous power to execute are only performed with fully warmed up body.
- o Developing the sense of how injuries occur, what tissues would be harmed, and what course of management of an injury would follow is a sought goal of systemic training. This is discussed in Chapter Sixteen.
- o Safety consideration not only prevents injuries but also aids in avoiding setbacks and in understanding the nature of each muscle group in the body. Exercises that seem apparently unsafe discourage people from performing crucial activities such as the Snatch and the Clean and Jerk. Without these whole body activities, some muscles waste away very fast and require constant training to stay fit. Some other muscles can be developed fast and can aid significantly in perfecting newly learned techniques.

- o   The resilient groups of muscles that demand special consideration in training are those that are constantly overlooked in training. Examples of such resilient muscle groups are the Biceps, Serratus anterior, Rhomboids, and paraspinal muscles. All of which work on erecting the upper body and keep the shoulders in proper posture, when arms transfer force to the vertebral axis.

1.12.3. STANDARDS THAT ACHIEVE NOTICEABLE IMPROVEMENT
Proper training plans adhere to specific technical training standards that lead to noticeable improvement in health within reasonable time, as follows.
- o   Training standards have been evolving over a documented history of a hundred years.
- o   The drive for that evolution was the competition for strength, with least body weight. Age and height of the competitors are still not accounted for in judging competitors. Gender, however, has lately been addressed by a criterion for judging competitions. Women have participated in international and Olympic Weightlifting.
- o   The normal course of evolution started by the idea that getting big and strong is a desired goal of training.
- o   Then the idea that speed and agility could tip the balance, in favor of little athletes, has approximated the training standards to healthier levels.
- o   The latest development was a natural extrapolation of our growing knowledge about physical performance. Such knowledge has been, mostly empirically gained from many tales of successes and failures, of countless number of Weightlifters. From those who stuck to the habit of heavy lifting every time they train, those who developed their own rituals from spirit, nutrition, to relaxation, to those who dug deeper into the analysis of the dynamics of the lifting technique.
- o   Today, the basic tenet of modern Weightlifting is the simultaneous inclusion of the three fundamental regions of the body, in most exercises, in such a way that maintains both nervous responsiveness and muscular effectiveness in a harmonious balance. The three regions are the thighs, torso and shoulders.
- o   Training that entails random exercises of isolated parts of the body will fail in balancing strength, coordination, and mobility, apart from the development of disproportionate physique.

1.13. BASIC RULES

1.13.1. ESSENTIAL EXERCISES
The theme of this book revolves about basic rules that aim at averting the frustration of many trainees with the tedious task of planning workout programs, as follows.
- o   Trainees are confronted with many exercises to choose from, and many individual problems that require lengthy and appropriate planning to resolve. To simplify matters, optimum training is attained by focusing on two phases of workout.
- o   The first phase is **"essential exercises"**. That is equivalent to a combination of warm-up and the minimally required amount of physical work essential for staying fit.
- o   Essential exercises can be executed in less than half-hour, in a space that is two-arm span wide, be it your bedroom, office, kitchen or bathroom.
- o   You do not need membership to any fitness club to get fit. Thus keeping the idea of getting fit on the top of your conscience is, most probably, the first habit you have to master to reach your goals.
- o   Essential workout is the common denominator between all levels of training. Whether you have never worked out before, or you are on the top of advanced athleticism, essential workout should consist of three exercise portions: an exercise or more for each of the legs, torso, and shoulders.

1.13.2. ANCILLARY EXERCISES
The second phase of training is the **"ancillary exercises"**. This has the following features:
- o   This is ancillary in the sense that it is meant to advance fitness, beyond the common average, to that of higher athletic performance.
- o   Ancillary exercising requires a strategy of perfecting the details of individual exercises, the details of daily and long-term inclusion of these exercises in workout, in addition to developing the skill of assessing progress on shorter and long runs.
- o   They involve external resistance, in the form of lifting barbells, dumbbells, or lifting one's bodyweight, as in chin-up and parallel bar dip exercises. Again, no external resistance should be added before adequate muscular and ligamentous warm-up preparation has been completed.
- o   Ancillary exercises require higher skill, such as knowledge of how to perform exercises that target certain anatomical structures or physiological functions. Examples of exercises that demand higher skill are Squat, Clean and Jerk, or treadmill exercises. Though anybody can perform those exercises, by mimicking other athletes, there is a definite advantage in learning how to dissect the motion into its basic elements. This aids in the remedying specific individual deficiencies, excelling in particular exercises, and averting chronic injuries.
- o   The simplest example is that of the treadmill runners, in which chronic shoulder deformity is incurred by habitual hunching of the chest cage while treading. Treading without paying attention to exercises that retract the scapulas and

INTRODUCTION

lift the shoulders will aggravate hunching, reduce the breathing capacity, and restrict the venous return in the upper arms leading to weaker arms.
- o Ancillary exercises are intended to advance rather than to maintain physical fitness. Thus, a well-planned scheme must be in work to gradually increase resistance without compromising proper lifting technique.
- o It is futile to try to muscle with resistance if your technique of execution violates the norms of anatomical and physiological performance. For example, trying to squat a weight that exceeds your ability to maintain straight back could cause more harm than good. Or, trying to complete a set of ten-repetitions on a shoulder exercise, while feeling pain within the shoulder, might derail you for many months of serious tendonitis or osteochondritis.

1.14. EXERCISE SEQUENCE

1.14.1. ESSENTIAL EXERCISES EXECUTED CAUDALLY
- o The sequence by which exercises are to be performed is not an arbitrary proposition, or is a personal preference.
- o Essential exercises are executed caudally. This means that shoulders are exercised first, then the torso, and finally the legs. In this order, the trainee increases the participation of body regions, as he or she proceeds from the head downwards, to the foot. Increased participation of the parts of the upper body, as the warm-up proceeds from head to feet, corresponds to increased resistance to gravity, as viewed by an observer at the sole of feet.
- o The beginning of this phase of workout entails more mobility exercises, since the shoulders support light and free limbs. The ending of this phase entails more stability exercises, since the feet support heavier and more fixed limbs.
- o Mobility exercises, which begin this phase of workout, ought to entail higher number of repetitions per set (five to ten), while stability exercise, which end this phase, ought to entail fewer repetitions per set, say one to five.
- o The product of the number of "repetitions per set" by the weight of body region involved, amounts to a certain level of workout that the heart can tolerate per each set. This level is quantified as **load volume**.

1.14.2. ANCILLARY EXERCISES AND MOBILITY VERSUS STABILITY
The sequence of performing exercises in the ancillary phase of workout follows these different rules.
- o High mobility exercises, of ancillary training, involve wider range of joints and have to precede high stability exercises, regardless of the caudad (from the head to the legs) or cephalad (from the legs to the head) sequence.
- o Low resistance exercises precede high resistance exercises. Thus, the Clean and Snatch precede the Deadlift and Squat.
- o Finally, exercises that involve higher number of joints precede those involving lesser number of joints.
- o The dominant trend in all this is to allow monotonous gradient of recruitment of muscle fibers by the extrapyramidal [4] nervous system.
- o In simple layman's words, this trend gives sufficient time for the preparation of the nervous system to reach its highest level of muscular responsiveness. The nervous system cannot recruit muscle fibers that are depleted from CP-ATP [5] fuel supply, fast enough to perform vigorous activities.

1.14.3. EXAMPLES OF IMPROPER SEQUENCE OF EXECUTING EXERCISES
Examples of executing exercises in improper order are numerous, as follows.
- o Many trainees start by exercising their legs, by either warming up the legs heavily or even omitting the warm-up all together. This habit exposes the upper body to sudden stress, before appropriate levels of muscular tone and perfusion are achieved. It traumatizes the shoulder and the back leading to long- term problems of stiffness and loss of full range of motion.
- o Many trainees start heavy shoulder training (ancillary shoulder training) without executing essential workout of the torso and legs. This trend precipitates back injuries, both in the upper back muscles, which transfer the forces from the upper arms to the axial column, and the lower back, which stands the bouncing and jolting of the upper remote parts of the body.
- o Advanced athletes are more vulnerable to injuries than cautious beginners. Overconfidence and forgetfulness of the serious consequences of improper lifting technique are the worst enemies of advanced trainees. Moreover, the sense of egoistic eternity that drive advanced athletes to higher levels of accomplishments is, in many times, challenged by the reality of aging, fatigue, or other irregularities in health.

1.15. MODESTY AND POSTURE

1.15.1 MODEST GOAL OF STAYING PHYSICALLY FIT
Essential workout means exactly that.

---

[4] The extrapyramidal system integrates function of three brain structures: cerebrum, basal ganglia, and midbrain. It just integrates associated movements, posture, and autonomic functions. Its inhibitory and facilitatory functions define physical performance. Source "Correlative Neurology & Functional neurology" 16th edition, by Joseph G. Chusid, California, USA, 1976. Page 16. ISBN 0-87041-015-6.

[5] CP-ATP refers to a molecular shuttle, in muscle cells, that comprises of Creating Phosphate and Adenosine Triphosphate molecules. These are "high energy" carriers that supply immediate energy to the actin-myosin protein to generate kinetic energy. It thus circumvents the slow availability of energy from glucose burning, or glycolysis.

INTRODUCTION

- o The minimum workout you would need to stay physically fit and able to endure unexpected extremes of stress.
- o That modest goal is a mere reminder of the different systems of the body to stay viable.
- o Albeit its modesty, essential workout bestows longevity on many vital body functions, which would otherwise decline insidiously over time.
- o Famous exercises such as those for Biceps, Triceps, chest, abdominal exercises are not essential.
- o You can break your heart running and laboring to attend training sessions, yet miss what is essential in enhancing your fitness, effectively and hassle-free.
- o Again, essential workout can be accomplished in twenty to thirty minutes. It involves exercises for the torso, legs, and shoulders, without getting into detailed muscular isolation.

1.15.2. ESSENTIAL MUSCLES OF POSTURE

- o Essential exercises deal with the bulkiest and most needed groups of muscles, all of which are working on the posture, rather than the extremities.
- o You do not need huge biceps, or chest or abdomen to have athletic posture unless you have balanced shoulders, torso, and legs muscles. That is because all vertebrate mammals main posture by spinal axis and four limbs.
- o Balancing the strength of major muscles helps you carry your head and have open chest cage that does not hamper the breathing of the lungs and the beating of the heart.
- o While you work hard to build up and maintain your proper posture, you then can insert few exercises to work out peripheral and assisting muscles.
- o Think like a civil engineer. Before worrying about the windows and the decoration, dedicate most of your time balancing the frame of your skeleton.
- o You might sit next to a person with arm biceps as big as your waist size, yet what matter is the balance of your frame of posture. Proper posture is an index of balanced and intelligent activities.

1.15.3. CUMULATIVE EFFECT OF POSTURE ENHANCEMENT

- o Few minutes of shoulder training, everyday, have cumulative effects that outmatch many activities in enhancing your feeling of vibrant health.

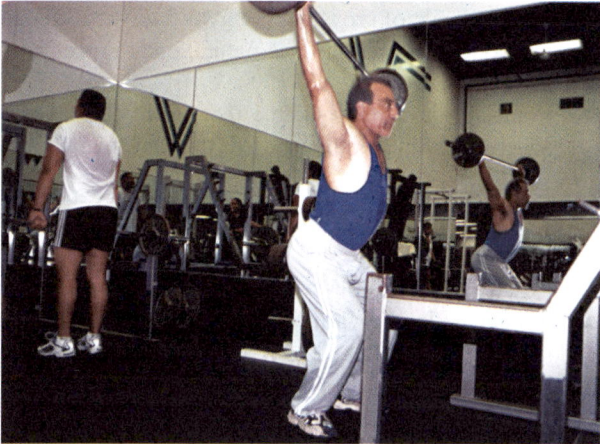

Figure 1.1. A trainee is shrugging 40 kg barbell from the racks behind another trainee executing Overhead Press and Squat with the same weight. Notice the body proportions of the trainee using the rack. Also notice the straps around his wrists and the stiffed knees.

- o The shoulders carry the arms and transmit forces to the region of the vertebral columns that spans the distance from the base of the skull to the top of the pelvis.
- o Strengthening the shoulder balance eases all activities that involve the use of hands and arms. The very basic activities such as eating, showering, writing, or dressing could be performed easier with stronger shoulders and will improve the minute to minute feeling of well being.
- o Strengthening the shoulders supports the vertebral column in carrying the skull and brain, without easy fatigability, for long hours.
- o Strengthening the shoulders enhances maintaining the chest cage hanging below the clavicles, instead of collapsing on the lungs and hearts causing fatigue, shortness of breath, and whole body weakness.

1.15.4. BENEFITS OF HEALTHY POSTURE

- o Similarly, few minutes of torso exercises, everyday, enhance your personal appearance beyond any gain from other modern medical treatment modalities.
- o The so many people with stiff, weak, and injury-prone torso attest to the increase demand to educate people about torso exercises.
- o So many people have their occupation altered due to susceptible lower back that is easily helped by modest workout.
- o The benefit of maintaining strong and healthy shoulders and torso are multifaceted. From positive self-esteem, feeling of better body image, to enjoying the privilege of having many occupations to choose from, to the luxury of enjoying many entertainment activities without restriction.
- o Also feeling strong and well helps in pursuing your goals in whatever avenue you choose.

1 INTRODUCTION

1.16. TODAY'S GYM

1.16.1. ROLE OF HEALTH-CLUB GOERS
o   Weight training, as practiced in many health clubs in major cities, is in state of chaos. Such dismal state of affairs also reflects the reality of the current educational system.
o   Many health-clubs goers aim at mediocre goals, of either enhancing their physique or controlling their bodyweight. Going to the gym just to accomplish little goals could do more harm than good.
o   When science and art are implemented in weight training, the whole lifestyle is impacted in many positive ways. For example, a trainee who spends most of his time to develop strong chest can incur serious back and knee injuries, if he forgets the need for whole body training and warm-up. That is because strengthening the chest requires support of the vertebral column and legs, as spines bridge the pelvic and the pectoral girdles.
o   Also, normal movement during the daily activities requires a balance between the two girdles.

1.16.2. ROLE OF ORGANIZERS OF HEALTH-CLUBS
o   Health clubs have to cater to such disinterested population that seeks quick gratification.
o   Many ambitious and innovative ideas have shaped some aspects of today's gym. Aerobics and yoga are the best examples that prove that it is possible to create good tutors and many faithful followers, when a new concept is well articulated to the public.
o   Today's weight training lacks such appeal as well as clear execution strategy that invigorate wide public acclaim. Health clubs would not walk the long path of educating their members on how to become athletes.
o   Clubs contribute to the mediocrity of resistance training by diverting resources away from research.
o   The epidemic of crowding the gym floor with equipments, and leaving little room for freestyle training, is perplexing. Freestyle exercises advance natural body movements, while machine-aided exercises topple the natural balance of the body.
o   Ironically, it is very possible that health clubs, with little informed research, can equally profit and in the same time adhere to the moderate standards of proper Weightlifting, rather than reinventing a crippling sport, *Figure 1.1*.

1.17. PROPER EQUIPMENTS OF RESISTANCE TRAINING

1.17.1. ROLE OF SYMMETRY OF MOTION
o   Symmetry in Weightlifting refers to evenness on both sides of the body around a vertical line.
o   Symmetry is observed in many movements that enhance human performance.
o   Asymmetric exercises, such as one-hand exercises and Calisthenics, should not be performed without first strengthening the major symmetrical muscle groups around the vertebral column, pelvis, and shoulders.
o   Asymmetrical movements generate shearing forces across the vertical line of symmetry and can lead to strain, sprain, dislocation, and disc bulging. .
o   Asymmetrical movements may also involve lifting heavier on one side of the body than the other, such as lifting a barbell that is not adequately lubricated at the carrying cylinders. This is the case with newly introduced polygonal barbells.
o   In the year 2001, a well-known chain of health clubs in USA replaces all the round plates of barbells by multi-sided polygonal plates. These have two gripping holes near their periphery and patent information engraved on them, *Figure 1.2*. Such unwise decision to replace round plates with polygonal ones is a live proof of the poorly informed management of health clubs.

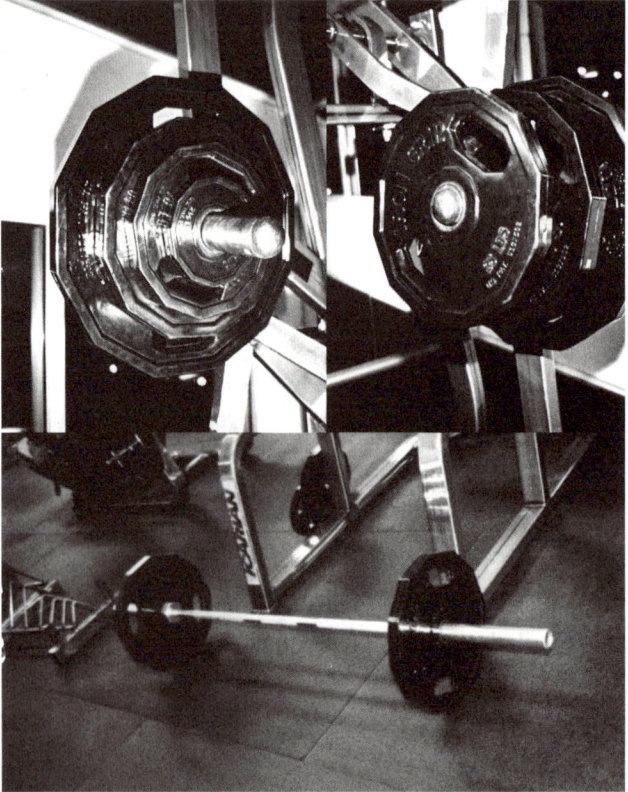

Figure 1.2. Polygonal plates, patented by the USA patent authorities, now replace round plates in many health clubs, in complete defiance to international trends of progress in standardizing fitness training.

1.17.2. USE OF SIMPLE AND RELIABLE EQUIPMENTS
o   Polygonal barbell plates cause injuries to the wrists, shoulders, back, knees, and ankles, because they lack circular symmetry, *Figure 1.2*.

- o With their poor freedom of revolving, polygonal plates impede the angular movement of the whole body.
- o Pulling a barbell, with polygonal plates, from the floor is dangerous to the lower back, since the bar would not follow the natural trajectory of normal human motion.
- o A 12-sided polygonal plate, weighing 20 kg, has maximum diameter of 45 cm, a minimum diameter of 43 cm, and 12 facets on its periphery, each is 12 cm long.
- o When lifting from the floor, a barbell loaded with polygonal plates and without adequate lubrication, horizontal shifts from the vertical plane of fall line may cause serious shearing forces.
- o That is because the polygonal plates are stuck, in place, on a twelve centimeters long flat facet and are not free to follow the imposed horizontal shift. When trying to lower the bar by hands, at the end of the lift, the whole barbell rolls on the pointed tips of the polygon, to rest on the flat facets.
- o One side might roll forwards, while the other backwards, ending in an unsightly setting and may rub against the shins, wounding them.
- o Also using polygonal plated barbells, in other exercises, traumatizes all moving joints since it lacks free revolution of the plates on the carrying cylinders.

1.17.3. ROLE OF NATURAL HUMAN MOVEMENT
Modern barbells are loaded with weight plates that can revolve freely on well-lubricating rolling balls, inside the plate carrier cylinder. These serve the following purposes.
- o Free revolving of weight plates allows for free hand extension and flexion at the wrist.
- o When such natural hand movement is prevented by high friction, between the weight plates and the bar held in the hands of the lifter, this results in forcible shearing stress at the wrists, shoulders, back, pelvis, knees, and ankles.
- o Shearing forces cause long- term inflammation of these joints because they, the shearing forces, run across the fall line of lifting at oblique angles.
- o If the lifts involve the lower back, as in seated Shoulder Press, the shearing stress at the shoulder joints is magnified many times at the lower back, due to the long arm of force between the shoulder and lumbar region.
- o If the lift is executed in standing position, as in Hang Clean or standing Shoulder Press, the greater magnification of shear stress occurs at the knees, resulting in premature wear and tear of menisci and cartilages of the knee joint.
- o Although most dumbbells are rigid structures, they are often held by one hand. That frees the shoulder from the restricted tie of both hands, on a barbell. Thus with dumbbells one can stiffen the wrist joint and allow the elbow and shoulder to move freely with minimal traumatic shear stress.
- o From the above discussion, it is apparent that judging the quality of fitness equipments is solely based on their compliance with natural human motion.
- o With the growing stream of invention of new fitness equipments and designers, whose credentials are questionable, it is wiser to adhere to the use of fewer numbers of simple and reliable equipments.

1.18. SERIOUS DAILY HABITS

1.18.1. IMPROPER OCCUPATIONAL ACTIVITIES
Improper lifting at workplaces is pervasive in industrial occupations. In most situations, emphasis is directed to preventing acute and serious injuries. Many workmen find themselves performing heavy work with inadequate equipments and for long hours, as follows.
- o Truck drivers spend many hours sitting, thus lose full range of motion of the legs and back due to weakening of muscles and shortening of tendons.
- o Physical work after long hours of sitting, without warm up, predisposes to injuries.
- o Bending the back, instead of squatting and extending the back, is common, due to weak thighs. This predisposes to bulging of the spinal disc, or disc herniation.
- o Lifting weights with bent elbows causes the upper back to cave in and leads to hunching of the upper back, after few years of poor technique.
- o Asymmetrical lifting is another flaw in the procedure of lifting. Lifting heavy weight with one hand or while standing on one foot cause shearing and twisting torques that traumatize the vertebral, shoulder, and pelvic structures, *Figure 1.3*.

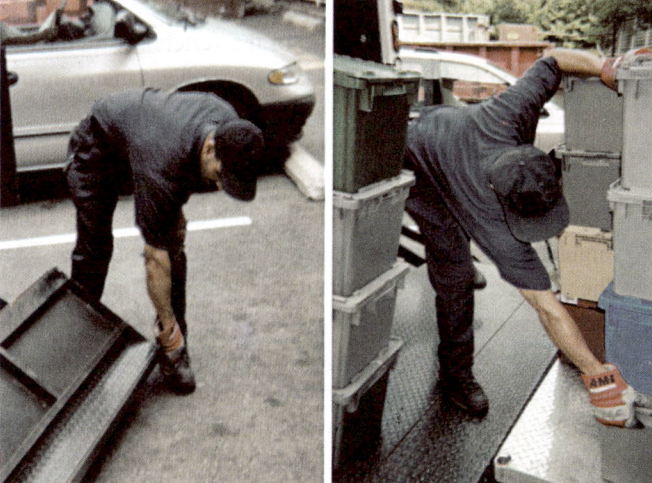

Figure 1.3. Asymmetric lifting by standing on one foot, while bending, could cause serious lower body paralysis.

1.18.2. IMPROPER LIFTING OF A CHILD FROM THE FLOOR
Lifting a child from the floor, without standing evenly on both feet and bending the knees, may cause serious back injury, as follows.
o   This is most common is tall and thin parents.
o   Lifting a child without bending the knees would increase the magnitude of torque on the lower back muscles. The torque is calculated as the product of the weight held by hands and the horizontal distance between the arms and the lower back.
o   Lifting a child without proper warm-up of the muscles of the back is very common when an adult tries to lift while sitting, getting off bed, consuming alcohol, when the neuromuscular integrity is compromised, or when not paying attention to the proper technique of lifting.
o   Injuries due to improper lifting of a child can be severely aggravating, from few weeks of low back pain, shoulder pain, neck pain, to many years of back pain and weakness..
o   Physiotherapy might offer some help in relieving the pain and inflammation of a torn muscle or herniated disc, but exercise is the role of thumb for long-term health prospect.
o   The smart way of exercise, in this particular case, is not to lift before few seconds of warming up your back, knees, and shoulders prior to lifting. This should raise the tone and enhance the circulation in the working muscles.
o   The second advice is to lift your child as frequent as possible, to develop the strength and endurance of repeating the same labor, when you have to. Above all, little children are not supposed to exert themselves for longer times, since they have no way of knowing the limits of their hearts, and carrying them by parents is beneficial for both the child and the parent.

1.18.3. IMPROPER LIFTING OF A GROCERY BAG
Lifting a grocery bag by one hand, after long period of relaxed sitting, is dangerous, as follows.
o   This is another common way of injuring the lower back, neck and shoulder.
o   Since lifting groceries is not the most desirable task in our daily activity, the lack of motivation to tackle such task with proper lifting technique contributes to the increased rate of injuries.
o   Other situations that might also contribute to injuries are poor weather conditions, high heels, smoking, over filled stomach, or improperly loaded grocery bags. Amazingly, injuries that occur during such situations might surpass, in severity, those incurred during training.
o   Developing the habit of proper lifting, when psychological elements are in play, could only be acquired through lengthy routine of resistance training.
o   Supposedly, such length of time and devoted commitment to such specialized training might raise the unconscious order of priorities to the degree that psychological detraction would not impair motor skills.
o   Thus planned training could be considered an investment in countless number of benefits that characterize intelligent living and an addition to the repertoire of personal refinement.

1.18.4. IMPROPER BENDING ON A SINK
Bending on a sink to reach a faucet early in the morning, soon after getting off bed, is a common cause of back injury, as follows.
o   After a night sleep, the muscles of the vertebral column are in their lowest level of tone. Few minutes of leg pedaling, while still in bed, would dramatically prevent many injuries to the lower back that would otherwise cause annoying inconvenience.
o   A simple test to avert lower back injuries, after long hours of sleep, is to slowly bend your back, by leaning forwards, and try to sense any tightness, spasm, or any unusual feeling in the lower back region.
o   If that was the case, you should immediately stop all bending activities and start warming up your back. This stimulates the muscle units and reduces the spasm of those few fibers that have to deal with the entire bending stresses.
o   The simplest routine of warming up your back, prior to bending, in addition to leg pedaling while in bed, is by moving your arms and legs as if you are walking still. That is, the left arms moves forwards with the right leg, and both alternate with opposite limbs. That would generate a twisting movement along the longitudinal axis of the vertebral column and stimulate the spinal and lateral back muscles.
o   Next, is the exercise that brings the knee closer to the chin by flexing the thigh on the abdomen, the chest on the abdomen, and the head on the chest. That will stimulate the spinal muscles, by stretching.
o   Of course, the safest posture to protect your back, while bending on a sink, is to harden your back in a straight posture, bend your knees slightly, and harden your abdominal muscles. The first and third tricks are meant to stabilize the vertebra posteriorly and to reduce the dragging forces of the guts anteriorly.

o   Bending the knees would provide a cushioning shock absorber and protects the back muscles from sudden contraction.

1.18.5. SITTING IN COUCH
Couches are found in almost every modern home and are related to spinal injuries as follows.
- o   With its low level and comfortable soft cushioning, a couch plays a role in incurring disc herniation, by allowing the back to curve in exaggerated round form.
- o   Getting up from a low couch, by excessive forward leaning, exacerbates the back convexity and thrusts the spinal disks backwards and laterally.
- o   Crossing legs while seated in a couch causes lower back, neck and shoulder injuries. Crossing legs throws one's bodyweight towards one side, while the head is thrown towards opposite side. Thus the lower back is curved laterally into one direction while the neck is curved into the opposite direction.

1.18.6. ALCOHOL CONSUMPTION
Apart from the heated debate on alcohol consumption and its role in a vast spectrum of social mishaps, consumption of alcohol plays a major role in injuries to bones, joints, muscles, tendons, and nerves, as follows.
- o   Alcohol has direct numbing effect on the sensory and motor control of muscles, as well as on the central control of motion and stability.
- o   Yet the crucial issue that skipped many advocates for moderate consumption of alcohols is that humans have to confront so many struggles, to better their lives, and that each such struggle requires clear consciousness, not only for few short hours but for extended number of years.
- o   Resistance training is one of such activities that require drug-free body and mind. Building healthy and fit physique is a serious business that requires concerted and persistent effort, to adhere to dynamic strategy.
- o   Systemic training is harsh, even on those who never drink alcohol, since it differs from academic work in that it requires both the planning and the performance.

1.18.7. SMOKING
Smoking has been the focus of concern of preventive health authorities, probably since the triumphant success of antibiotics and vaccination in eradicating or diminishing the epidemics of the past. The following issues relate to smoking and health.
- o   Unfortunately, the problem with battling smoking lies within battling the will of the masses that are cynical toward the consequences of such destructive practice.
- o   No progress could be made in fitness planning without strong self-esteem. With every cigarette lit, the smoker senses the relentless dragging forces of his or her act of indulgence in a purposeless ordeal.
- o   The elation of the exotic odor of tobacco and the joy of being in a company of peers of smokers are short lived. Sooner, the smoker has to face the consequences of indulgence.
- o   There would be constant decline in his or her ability to perform so many demanding physical activities, constant worsening in his or her ability to digest or enjoy food, and constant and persistent decline in the desire to tackle complex issues. Loss of self-esteem undermines any planning of building strength by training.
- o   Of course, had the person had the determination to comply with a serious plan of resistance training, it would be fairly assumed that he or she would be able to gather strength and bail out of such course of declining quality of life of smokers.
- o   Resistance training puts to test the actual changes smoking afflicts on the body. A smoker feels diminished strength when trying to resist the weight every passing day with smoking. As the inhaled carbon monoxide competes with hemoglobin for oxygen, active tissues suffer most of impaired respiration.
- o   Moreover, the vasoconstricting effect of nicotine diminishes the blood supply to those tissues. Thus, not only the respiratory complications that manifest vividly with training, but also the very early alteration on active tissues that demonstrate themselves early in the development of pathological changes due to smoking.
- o   Such early signs might skip those who do not engage in fitness training, as is the case with most smokers. Another effect of smoking on training is the lack of adaptation of the respiratory mechanisms to vigorous exercise.
- o   At the peak of muscular contraction, both heart rate and respiratory rate increase in proportion to the severity of contraction. This requires adequate hydration of the air passages to stand the increased evaporation of water and dryness of mucus.
- o   Smokers suffer from inconvenient throat and tracheal dryness with exertion. That forces the smoker to stop exercising and abandon his or her fitness planning, most probably to resort to smoking that is the main culprit in his or her misery.

INTRODUCTION

1.19. HIGHLIGHTS OF CHAPTER ONE

1. The basic rule for promoting physical health is a triad of balanced nutrition, exercise, and rest.

2. Many people will benefit from practicing modern Weightlifting and do not have to compete in front of three Weightlifting judges.

3. The fact that should not be traded for personal gain or popularity is that discipline is a sort of deprivation.

4. Health professionals are overwhelmed with the fast paced progress of the medical sciences, have very little to do with structuring training for health and fitness.

5. Physical therapy offers the minimal requirements for healing that keep people independent from the health system.

6. The essence of this sport is that muscular strength could be enhanced in parallel with joints' flexibility, whole-body coordination, cardiovascular, and pulmonary endurance, while maintaining maximum ratio of strength-to-bodyweight.

7. The simplest axiom on which Weightlifting is founded is that **"consistent resistance of force leads to growth and strength if performed properly and on long period of time"**.

8. The lack of proper sequence of executing exercises, in the sport of Bodybuilding, renders the sport a crippling activity of stiffening tendons and damaging joints with total disregard to the harmony of motion of properly functioning joints.

9. Weightlifting explores the great potential of our body to overcome weakness and debility by intelligent and persistent planning of resistance training.

10. Many people attribute the gift of health to spiritual being and submit to a lifestyle of wishful expectation.

11. You can break your heart running and laboring to attend training sessions yet miss what is essential and what is not. Essential workout can be accomplished in twenty to thirty minutes. It involves exercises for the torso, legs, and shoulders without getting distracted by detailed muscular isolation.

12. Strengthening the shoulder balance eases all activities that involve the use of the hands and arm, supports the vertebral column in carrying the skull and brain, without easy fatigability for long hours, enhances maintaining the chest cage hanging below the clavicles instead of collapsing on the lungs and hearts causing fatigue, shortness of breath, and whole body weakness.

13. Bending the back, instead of squatting and extending the back, is common among all people and is due to weakened thighs. This predisposes to bulging of the spinal disc and results in sciatica (pinching of the sciatic nerve), weakness, pain, and or lower body paralysis.

14. The safest posture to protect your back while bending on a sink is to harden your back in a straight posture. Bend your knees slightly, and harden your abdominal muscles. Bending the knees would provide a cushioning shock absorber and protects the back muscles from sudden contraction.

15. Smokers suffer from inconvenient throat and tracheal dryness with exertion. That forces the smoker to stop exercising and abandon his or her fitness planning. He or she will, most probably, resort to smoking, the main culprit in his or her misery, instead of exercise.

Chapter 2 Proper Lifting Techniques

2.1. LIFTING IN EVERYDAY ACTIVITY

2.1.1. LIFTING WEIGHTS AS A MAJOR CAUSE OF INJURIES
Lifting weights is a process we encounter in everyday life. Lifting a child from the floor, grocery bags, household appliances, books, even lifting our own body, while sitting, standing, or leaning, is always the major cause of injuries to joints and muscles. How many people have you known experienced back injuries by just sitting or leaning improperly? Injuries due to lifting are caused by the following:

o Entirely **new lifting position, or heavy weight** that has not been lifted before.
o Inattention or **distraction by other stimuli**, such as talking, other affairs in the surroundings, or other personal concerns.
o **Improper technique,** or lack of practicing of lifting. The technique of lifting cannot be taught by posters or lectures alone. **Practice** and constant tweaking of the technique are essential to perform correct lifting.
o Lifting when **not ready** to perform physical activities, such as after getting off bed, under the effect of drugs, when having dizziness spells, or when not feeling good.

2.1.2. WHO KNOWS BETTER ABOUT LIFTING?
I used to think that those who deal a lot with lifting would know better about proper lifting than others, yet I observed the following.

o I found, from my medical practice in rural farming towns, that **farmers** do not know better than urban inhabitants. Farmers depend on practice and strength with very little understanding of proper techniques. Many farmers start the new farming season without gradual exercise, after six months or so of relatively inactive living. Many incur lower back injuries during that transition from long hours of inactivity to vigorous activity.
o **Engineering students** may know more about the laws of mechanics but practice none of what they learn on the gym floor. So are the **medical students** and doctors who are notorious in breaching what they teach, and being taught.
o **Bodybuilders** and weight trainers are not any better. Many Bodybuilders lift for many years with flawed techniques. Hunching the upper back, bending the elbows while lifting, driving up the barbell with the back instead of the lower limbs, are among many mistakes Bodybuilders make.
o The **National Safety Council** distributes posters explaining safe techniques of lifting, with serious flaws in their explanation. A sketch of a person squatting to lift a box, next to him an advice to bend knees and drive the weight upwards with the knees not the back. While that sounds reasonable logic, lowering the hips below the knees is very dangerous in lifting unless the person is well trained. If you follow the advice of the National Safety Council without thrusting your chest and straightening your elbows you might fall, with the box on the top of you. Because deep squatting drags the vertebral column downwards and bent elbows cause the chest to cave in.
o Athletes are not immune to improper lifting. The worst injuries happen to over-confident athletes, when they overlook the basics of their trade.

2.1.3. PRACTICAL TRICKS OF PROPER LIFTING
Very simple tricks distinguish proper lifting from traumatic lifting, as follows.

o **Bending your knees** while leaning on a sink is a trick that prevents serious lower back injuries. Knee bending relaxes the Hamstrings and permits the pelvis to tilt forwards and the lower back to remain straightly extended.
o **Thrusting the chest** forwards and upwards, like "soldier's stance", transmits the forces of the weight to the middle and upper back, instead of the upper back alone.
o Keeping the **elbows straight** when lifting from the floor, and using shoulder shrugging, utilizes the biggest muscles such as the Trapezius, instead of the small muscles such as the Biceps.
o **Hardening your abdomen** prior to lifting or bending will prevent pooling of blood in the guts and redistributing it to the spinal nerves and muscles.

2. PROPER LIFTING TECHNIQUES

- o You cannot lift weight with buttocks falling below the knee level, unless you have well-toned and stretchable thighs. You have **to lift the hips gradually and slowly** from above the knee level upwards.
- o Your back should **never yield to hunching** (rounding or bulging backwards). You better drop the weight if you feel that your back is about to buckle, in order to avoid injury.

2.1.4. KNOWLEDGE VERSUS PRACTICE
Understanding the basics of proper lifting can help you make your living less troublesome, as follows.
- o Knowledge of the basic rules of proper lifting does not substitute practical training.
- o Proper lifting requires the nervous system to **synchronize muscle units** to produce specific levels of power. Such neural synchrony requires time and practice in order to build substantial neuromuscular control.
- o Proper lifting requires conditioned **reflexes of muscle spindles and tendon sensing organs**, in order to be well tuned and ready to respond on time. This requires gradual and regular lifting, not just thinking and learning.
- o Lifting any weight requires **cardiovascular and pulmonary** responses. These develop with practice. Remember that motion requires life and life does not come cheap. Demands put on the heart, lungs, and cells due to lifting have to be met by practice and not by mere conviction.

2.2. APPROACHING LIFTING

2.2.1. CENTERS OF GRAVITY OF OBJECTS AND HUMANS
- o Approach the object you are about to lift very closely. Each material object has a **"center of gravity"**. Try to figure out visually, before attempting to lift, a point where that object would balance itself around, if hung upwards from that point. Having roughly estimated the point or center of gravity, now move closer to that point of the object, such that it lies as close as possible to your feet.
- o In Weightlifting, all barbells and dumbbells can be centered over the front of the feet.
- o You then have to figure out your own center of gravity. Why? Bringing the centers of gravity of your body and the object closer to a vertical line eliminates unnecessary torques. Torques, in this case, are forces that tend to rotate or twist your body to either bring you closer to the object or cause the object to fall. These forces are generated by the pull of gravity on the centers of the body and object. Torques are generated by displacing these forces apart from the vertical line of gravity.

2.2.2. VERTICAL FORCES VERSUS HORIZONTAL FORCES
- o The force of gravity of the earth is directed in simple **vertical lines**. When we try to lift properly, we try to reduce all force to mere resistance, against the pull of the gravity. Thus we have to bring all forces closer, on one vertical line, not only to exert the minimum effort in lifting, but also to avoid forces that are directed in horizontal directions.

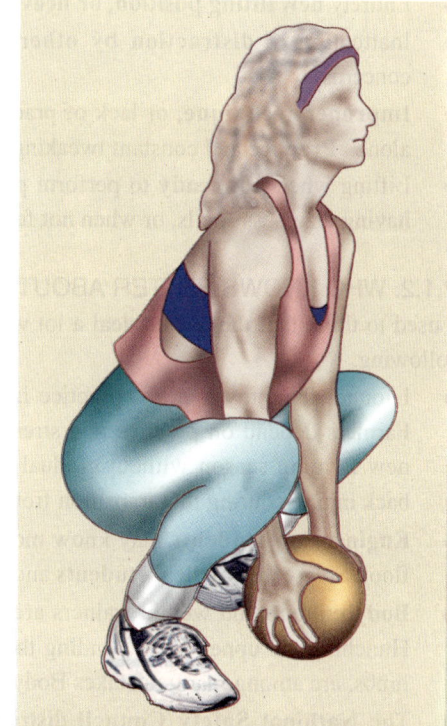

Figure 2.1. Stand very close to the object you are about to lift. Maintain straight back and elbows and bend your knees. The chest must be thrust forwards and upwars.

- o Horizontal forces are not very friendly to human anatomy. We spend years to grow up vertically and little time to develop musculoskeletal support for horizontal shearing forces.
- o Your center of gravity falls on the **front third of your feet** while standing. If you are sitting, your center of gravity falls on the ischial tuberosities, the bones we sit on. If you are kneeling, the center of gravity falls on the kneecaps. If you are lying on your back, the center of gravity that matters is that of the working part of the body.

2.2.3. STANDING VERY CLOSE TO THE OBJECT
- o Now, approximate the center of gravity of the **object,** you intend to lift, to the vertical plane of your own center of gravity. This minimizes the shearing forces on the back, *Figure 2.1.*
- o **Barbells** have a space under them where you can advance your feet under and to the font of the bar. When you bend to lift the bar, the bar may be felt stuck against the shins. This is the right start position for lifting. When lifting begins, the knees will extend and the bar should not rub the shins.
- o Lifting heavy objects in **workplace** might pose a danger of falling and injuring the toes. Objects that are hard to grip, heavier than usual, or never been lifted before in workplaces, require extreme consideration of other safety rules before any attempt to perform proper lifting technique.

o Remember that proper lifting techniques are prescribed to lifting objects that are familiar to us and that have to be lifted **regularly and repeatedly** in order to accomplish certain goals. This is not the case for newly encountered heavy industrial objects in the workplace. You should not risk placing any part of your body under or close to newly encountered heavy objects before you have assistance by others. Know the stability of the object, have good grip on the object, and have mechanical tools that aid in case of accidental falls.

Table 2.1. Comparison between lordotic versus kyphotic postures, during lifting.

Lordotic back[1]	Kyphotic back[2]
1. The Lordotic posture is unequivocally the safer and more efficient way to lift weights. It helps prevent injuries by using the erector muscles that reduces shear forces, *Figures 2.1 and 2.3*.	1. Exacerbate shear forces on the interspinous ligaments and may causes sudden disc herniation, during flexing the spine and lifting with knees straight, *Figure 2.4*.
2. Overextending the spinal axis increases the compression of the spines, due to the contraction of the erector spinae muscles, in order to safeguard against transient virtual forces and prevent dangerous flexion. The erector spinae are activated enough to generate torque that far exceeds the static torque generated by lifting.	2. Untrained people lift weights by rounding their backs because of weakness of back erectors. Rounding the back activates stretch reflex, and hence increases muscular tone. This still not sufficient even to support unloaded back. The increased prevalence of back pain and injuries may be attributed to relying on the passive posterior ligaments, and the thoracolumbar fascia, to support the back spine.
3. The intervertebral joints are also located lateral to the spines, one on each side, and posterior to the spinal cord. Thus the spinal erectors are located posterior to the joints. The spinal erectors have multiple origins, insertions, and directions, which make them powerful and respond vigorously to strength training.	3. Weak muscles can be strengthened with strength training, and can help eliminate functional back kyphosis. Untrained workers do not bend over and round their backs instinctively, when lifting, but do so out of disinterest in performing tedious jobs. Children maintain perfect lordotic back instinctively, even with their relatively heavy head and light lower body weight, *Figure 2.2*.
4. Muscles are contractile tissues that comply with the voluntary control of the individual. Also, muscles are rich in blood supply and can grow newer and stronger fibers, by hyperplasia and hypertrophy. Ligaments only react to stretch, not to nervous control. Ligaments can restore elastic energy but cannot generate contractile force. They have poor blood supply and heal slowly, with fibrosis. Previously injured ligaments are less elastic and thus incapable of withstanding heavy forces without tearing.	4. Stretching the muscles beyond their ability to pull the spines weakens the contraction of the spinal erectors, of kyphotic back. This creates anterior shear forces on the unsupported spines. The net shear results from the sum of the upper bodyweight and the external weight. Kyphosis displaces the line of action of weights forwards, thus deforms the spinal discs.
5. Experienced Weightlifters can lift twice their body weight in the exercise of Goodmorning and Deadlift. This cannot be achieved without contractile muscles, and not ligaments. Balance between the Iliopsoas and spinal erectors can maintain horizontal pelvic platform, on which L5 can gain stable support during heavy lifting, instead of depending on unpredictable recoil forces.	5. Kyphosis may prevent the 5th lumbar vertebra (L5) from sliding forwards, by stretching the posterior ligaments, as long as the stretch forces in these ligaments are high enough to maintain balance. But heavy lifting requires active muscles, to deal with external forces under the control of the nervous system not on the recoil tendency of ligaments.

2.3. UPPER BODY POSTURE

2.3.1. STRAIGHT AND UPRIGHT POSTURE

Before descending to grab the object, you should prepare the upper body for proper posturing, as follows.

o **Thrust your chest upwards and forwards** by straightening your back and sucking your belly inwards. This will lend some **free excursion** to the diaphragm, in case that excess inhalation is required. Thrusting the chest forwards and upwards puts the back in proper **extension** that fits lifting. It also brings shoulder plates closer, and evenly **distributes the forces** on the middle back. Thrust chest also elevates the ribs of the chest cage and increases **chest volume**. The increased chest volume creates suction pressure (negative pressure) and aids in **returning venous blood** from the lower body to the chest. The enhanced venous return enhances **arterial flow** out of the chest, to vital exercise organs.

o The **straight back (or better lordotic back)** will guarantee balanced blood flow to the front and back of the spinal cord along its course in the spinal canal. Lordotic back is a concave back, since the lower back dips forwards, between the two banks of back erectors, on both sides. It relieves the vertebral discs from imbalanced load and prevents disc

---

[1] Lordotic back refers to backward bending or concave, or arched in lower back, where the spines advance in a forward curve, in the middle of the lower back.
[2] Kyphosis refers to forward bending, or hunching, or rounding of the upper back, where the spines retreat in a backward convex curve.

bulging[3] (herniated disc). Straight back and thrust chest bring the shoulders and arms vertical on the center of gravity and help transmit forces, from the arms to the vertebral column, without caving in the chest or buckling the back.
o The debate over lordotic versus kyphotic back is summarized in **Table 2.1**.

2.3.2. SHOULDERS ELEVATION AND CHEST THRUSTING

o Now, shrug your shoulders upwards and backwards. As you advance in training, you will master this trick of **retracting the scapulas** and keeping the arms at a distance, on the sides of your body.

o This posture elevates the collarbones upwards and allows for free return of venous blood from the arms. Now, the arms are in a state of readiness to **grab, pull, or push**.

o Skipping this posture results in strangulation of blood vessels of the **upper arms**, by the lowered collarbones, and subsequent loss of grip and or consciousness during maximum lifting.

o Scapulas are the two backbones - known as the shoulder plates- located behind the chest cage, one on each side. When the scapulae are retracted they are stuck tight to the chest cage and closer to the vertebral column. In this position, the scapulas lift the lateral ends of the collarbones upwards and allow **tight transfer of forces along the arms-shoulders-vertebral link**.

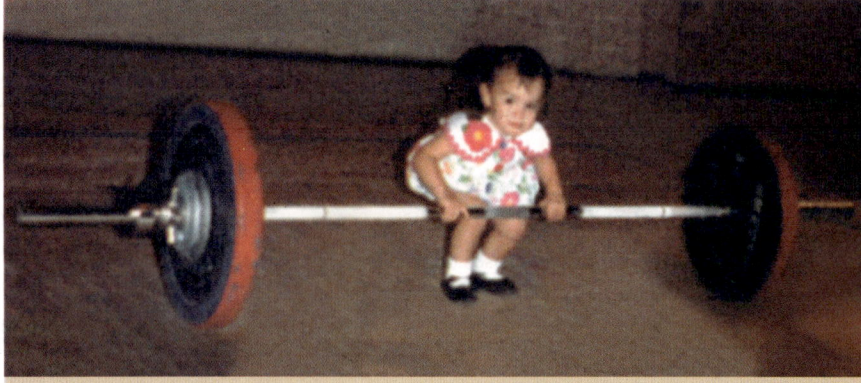

Figure 2.2. A 22-months old toddler emulating the start position. Perfect knee bending, straight back, and symmetric grips. Her bent elbows are attributed to the great height of the barbell.

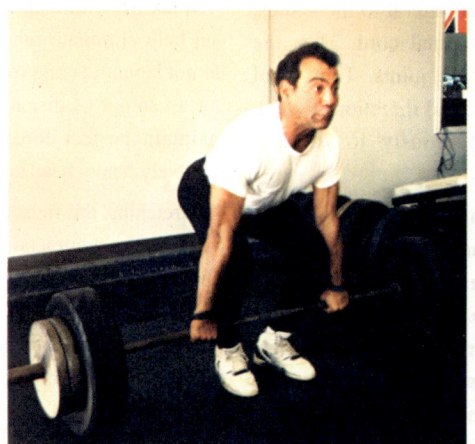
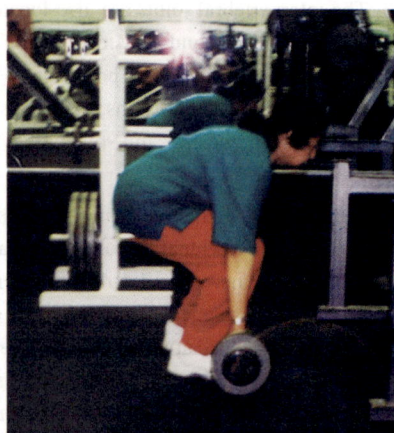

Figure 2.3. Start Position. Hyper-extended back. Thrust chest. Straight elbows. Bar close to shins.

Figure 2.4. Inexperienced lifter. Scapulas are not retracted. Back buckles in.

2.3.3. DEMAND FOR ATTENTION

o The **"attentive posture"** of hyper-extended back, thrust chest, and retracted shoulder plates is an awkward posture; so many people find it demanding.

o It is the most practiced posture by military personnel and athletes.

o This posture enables the **chest cage** to move freely and puts the **arms** in the proper position to deal with aggressive tasks. Remember that the arms of mammals are not directly attached to the vertebral column, but rather to the scapula and the clavicle. Four-legged animals do not have to bother with this posture, since their chest cage is hanging downwards, from the vertebral column.

o Assuming the attentive posture for lifting requires practice to utilize the proper mechanisms of transferring forces, from the **major axial muscles to the limbs**. People with no lifting experience tend to rely on limb muscles to lift objects. This traumatizes the joints that link the limbs to the vertebral axis. Regular working out of the major axial muscles builds sound musculoskeletal frame.

o Though attention is a **voluntary activity** that controls posture and senses, it affects involuntary processes such as circulation, respiration, and neural control. The chain of reactions that occurs during resisting forces depends greatly on attentive posture, in order to complete successful rounds of lifting and lowering weights without dizziness, imbalance, or falls.

o Many exercises could not be performed without extreme emphasis on attentive posture. The Front Squat, Overhead Squat, the Snatch, and the Goodmorning, all require serious attention to execute safely and properly.

---

[3] Disc bulging refers to "herniated spinal disc" In this pathological condition, the gelatinous core of the spinal disc, called "nucleus pulposus", escapes from the fibrous sheath of the disc and might disrupt surrounding nerves.

2.3.4. RETRACTING THE SCAPULAE [4]

The basis for retracting the scapulae before starting lifting lies is in the anatomy of the shoulder girdle, as follows.
- o A basic principle of muscular contraction is to pre-activate the muscle before committing it to full contraction. This is the pre-stretch **muscle spindle reflex**.
- o Thus hardening the muscles around the scapulae, before starting any physical effort, stimulates the **central neurons** that regulate muscular contraction.
- o The neurons, in turn, determine which muscle fibers to stimulate and regulate in the immediate events. This is the process of **muscular synchronization**.
- o The **feedback** (back and forth communication between the neurons and the muscle fibers) impacts the flow of blood to the muscles in concern and briefs the higher nervous centers to prepare the heart, lung, and the entire system for the event.
- o For a layman, retracted scapulas amounts for the appearance of arms hanging vertically, relaxed, and separated from the body by few inches, as if they are hanging from the two sides of a "T", **Figure 2.3**.

2.3.5. HARDENING THE ABDOMEN

Sucking in your abdomen is a good habit that ensures the following:
- o Spasm or higher tone in the abdominal wall squeezes the major abdominal veins, the inferior vena cava, and helps the **returning venous blood** from the lower limbs. This is rhythmic squeeze that is regulated by the brain, and not constant gripping.
- o Increases your cardiac output by preventing pooling of blood and fluids in the **abdominal organs**.
- o Reduces the drag force of the guts, on the diaphragm, and promotes **vigorous breathing**, when need calls for it.
- o Supports the abdominal wall and prevents the guts from escaping outside the **abdominal cavity,** causing hernia.
- o Balances the back extension, with abdominal hardening. This permits free **circulation in the spinal cord** and averts lower body weakness. Recall that venous congestion raises both the pressure of the cerebrospinal fluid and spinal venous pressure, and impairs the functions of the spinal nerves that supply the lower body and the rest of the body below the head level.

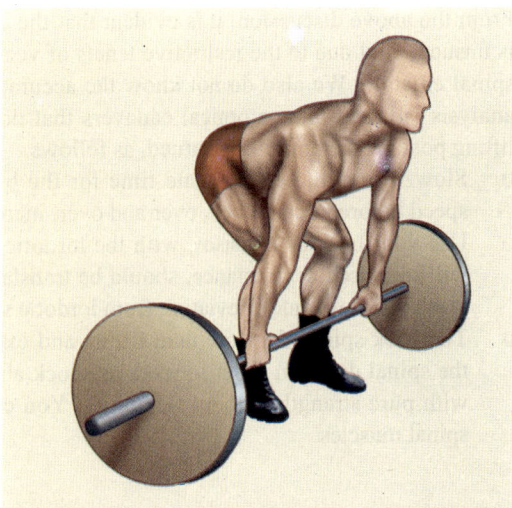

Figure 2.5. Inexperienced Bodybuilder. High hips during lifting cause back injuries.

2.3.6. LIFTING POSTURE

Bipedal animals require exquisite dynamic control and static stabilization of the body axis during motion, on the narrow platform of two feet. The effort to understand how lifting forces originate and interact, in order to maintain such graceful and strong performance of lifting, has progressed on many fronts. One such front is the assumption that there exists two motor units that support the spinal axis from within and from without, during lifting.[5] The outer motor unit is undisputable entity. Yet, the inner motor unit is a questionable factor, in lifting posture, as follows.
- o The inner motor unit is thought to stiffen the spinal vertebras from inside the body. This is thought of as a preparatory stiffener of the axial skeleton. It encompasses the inner walls of the abdominal cavity [6] and the ceiling and floor of the abdominal cavity. These are the diaphragm and pelvic floor musculature.
- o The outer unit extends the vertebras from outside. It encompasses the outer abdominal muscles (external and internal abdominal oblique muscles), back erectors (Erector spinae and Latissimus dorsi), hip muscles (Gluteus maximus, Hamstrings, Adductors, and Iliopsoas).

The two motor units are believed to work in concert to stabilize the axial vertebras. The flaws with this assumption of inner stiffening and outer mobilization are as follows.
- o The inner abdominal wall muscles are activated prior to any leg or shoulder movement in order to regulate gas and fluid circulation, in preparation for the frantic chaos of blood pooling by muscles and heart acceleration during lifting. This early activation may be of no mechanical significance in stabilization, other than preventing vessels form kinking and nerves from pinching, by equalizing pending fluid perturbation.
- o The pulling forces, on lumbar spines, by contracting abdominal walls cannot contribute to lordotic posture, unless such forces squeeze the major abdominal structures. The resulted increase in intra-abdominal pressure, through the

---

[4] Retraction of the scapula refers to bringing the shoulder blades together, in the back of the chest. This throws the shoulders backwards and advances the chest forwards.

[5] For related discussion, refer to the book titled "The spinal engine" by Serge Gracovetsky, Springer-Varlag. New York, USA. 1988.

[6] The inner abdominal walls are supported by the Transversus abdominis and deep Multifidus transversospinal muscles that span two to four vertebras.

PROPER LIFTING TECHNIQUES

synergistic action of the abdominal walls and the thoracolumbar fascia, cannot exceed vascular blood pressure. Also, mechanical forces work maximally along vertical plane, where major muscles exert their forces, while the abdominal muscles exert extension perpendicular to that plane.

- o The increased intra-abdominal pressure flexes the spines, while the abdominal contraction extends them. Thus abdominal forces serve internal purposes, not external support of spines, since they originate and end, from and into, the spines.
- o The contraction of back musculature may create internal hydraulic pressure within the investing fascia. This does not aid in the erection of the spine, from a flexed position, yet aids in the sliding of ligaments and tendons on bones. Spinal erection requires direct action along tendons of active muscles.
- o Many people suffer from back pain, due to an imbalance between the inner and outer units, during long hours of inactivity. Inactivity causes relaxation of the two motor units thus leads to venous congestion that weakens the spinal erectors. Many heavy weight lifters have huge bellies, with weak abdominal musculature; yet can lift very heavy weight. Thus abdominal musculature suffices in preventing visceral hernias, not spinal stiffness. The claim that the movement created by the outer motor unit depends on the segmental stiffness created by the inner motor unit, through preventing spines from buckling, is therefore flawed.

From the above discussion, it is evident that the effort of understanding the mechanical spinal balance of bipedal mammals is unsuccessful due to the restrictive tenets of vector analysis. We do not know how strong are the too many branches of the spinal erectors. We also do not know the accurate three-dimensional measurements of their insertions and directions. Our analysis is based on anatomical cadavers that do not move and are dried in preservatives. Yet, the practical approach to lifting posture is empirically learned, as follows.

- o Slow lifting allows adequate time for the brain to control muscular support. Speed progresses with training. Never speed before you practice, over and over, incrementally, until you know your bounds.
- o Use your back as a sensor, with the lordotic posture as a baseline. Any deviation from lordotic baseline, against your willful muscular resistance, should be translated into an increase in the magnitude of external force. Only training will teach you how much deviation from lordotic spine should you tolerate.
- o The back spines do more than lifting and extending. They dampen vibration by the cushioning gelatinous material of the spinal discs. In order to work as shock absorbers, the spinal axis requires flexibility training. You cannot lift safely with pure strength without flexibility. You cannot maintain safe lifting posture with tired, spastic, painful, or relaxed spinal muscles.

2.4. BEND YOUR KNEES

2.4.1. LEANING VERSUS SQUATTING

- o Do not start by leaning forwards to approach the object with stiffed knees. This is a universal mistake, committed by almost all people across cultural lines. Common people prefer leaning forwards, to bending knees, because it uses the most conditioned muscles of the buttocks, the Glutei.
- o Proper lifting aims at **balancing different muscle** groups to prevent chronic muscular wasting. Thus we will focus on sparking more life into the thighs, torso, and shoulder muscles.
- o Bending your knees will **bring your shoulders vertically,** over the object, and the center of pulling will fall on the line of the centers of gravity.
- o Bending your knees will also force the **back to incline,** rather than to remain horizontal. Inclined back drastically reduces shearing forces and diverts most of the muscular pull to the lifting process.

2.4.2. LIFTING INSTINCTS

In *Figure 2.2,* a twenty-two month old toddler is mimicking a forty-four year old lifter, *Figure 2.3,* as follows.
- o Perfectly bending her knees.
- o Holding the bar at the middle.
- o Keeping the bar above her feet.
- o Her back is perfectly straight and slanting, with almost 45 degrees angle with the ground.

This is the first time this toddler ever saw a barbell, yet she was able to approach the bar from the right direction and position herself as adults do, with no trouble. Older people do not have such keen ability to emulate others. All beginners, I have encounters, have to be taught and reminded, repeatedly, to perform the above steps. They execute one step just to miss the other steps. Many sessions would pass-by until an adolescent learns what that toddler emulated in few seconds. As people grow older, it seems that instinct are overshadowed by other concerns and learning becomes harder.

2.4.3. DREADING KNEES BENDING

- o Many people dread bending their knees, particularly women, having demanding jobs and housework.

- o If bending your knees are troubling that means you should forgo lifting until you take care of this issue. Hurting the knees while lifting is less serious than hurting the back.
- o Use your knees as a probe to figure out if you should continue the task of lifting or forgo lifting altogether.
- o When you get used to bend your knees, while lifting, they will get stronger if you work them out every day or every other day, for a while. If you lift once every few weeks you are definitely at high risk of knee and back injuries. Knees and back do not fare well without exercise.

2.4.4. USE YOUR KNEES AS A PROBE IN LIFTING
- o But, why should you bend your knees and not your back? The back has the vertebral column, which host one of the most privileged structures of our body, the spinal cord, and though it can bend slightly at each vertebra, it should be kept as straight as possible.
- o The spinal cord is as thick as the index finger, carries millions of nerves and few blood vessels, and it does not stand the extremes of kinking or compression.
- o The back also has the shock absorbers, the "intervertebral discs", which act to dampen jolting vibration. Imbalanced bending results in herniating those discs, with grave consequences.
- o Also, the back muscles, though strong, are not as flexible and ready to perform as the thigh muscles. The back muscles do not possess great range of motion, or great blood supply, are short and branch very often, into many insertions and from many origins.

2.4.5. WASTING OF KNEES AND BACK MUSCLES WITHOUT EXERCISE
- o The back joints permit bending, by cumulative minimal angulation, at each joint along the vertebral column. Neglecting exercises of any region of the vertebral column leads to wasting of muscles, weakness of tendons and ligaments, and consequent limited range of motion of that region.
- o The back has to be strengthened by mostly isometric exercises. These entail very little or no bending between joints. On the other hand, knees require mostly isotonic exercises. These entail bending of knees during resisting. Isometric exercises are complex and require experience. They constitute the basic tools in yoga.
- o Exercising the back is frightening to most people, and is erroneously performed by most Bodybuilders, Powerlifters, and weight trainers. Most of them overlook the fact that any exercise, of the lower or upper body, has to be balanced with exercising the linking joints of the back.
- o The back muscles are mostly tendinous, as they perform isometric stabilization and endure enormous forces. The knee muscles are very fleshy. Both knee and back muscles have multiple pinnation and many points of origin and insertion. These enable them to exert forces in many directions and at high power.
- o Knees are easier to exercise than the back, since there are only two knees, while there are twenty-four intervertebral joints on each side of the spines, forty-eight total. The knees are specialized in bending, by maximal angulation in a single joint. The bones are long and strong, their joints are well-adapted to articulate, by specialized cartilages, menisci, and wide range of motion, and are supported with strong muscles, in almost all direction of the knee range of motion.
- o Neglecting back and knee exercises render the person incapable of performing many activities. Few weeks without leg and back exercises negatively impact fitness and set a vicious circuit of weakness, instability, injury, and stiffness. The best method of breaking out of that vicious circuit is progressive resistance exercising. This is executed without weight, and with one's own bodyweight, for higher repetitions and full range of motion, until circulation and nervous control reach robust levels.

2.4.6. KNEES VERSUS BACK INJURY
- o It would take the knees over forty years of life before they start showing signs of ailment due to constant wear and tear. Earlier knee injuries result from improper use, overweight, lax muscles, or accidents.
- o In contrast, a single improper action can severely injure the back at any age. The probability of improper use of the back is higher than that of the knees. Because most of us use the knees in many activities and have acquire better knowledge of how to avoid injuring them.
- o Most back injuries due to improper lifting are avoidable, by adequate warm-up, gradual and progressive intensifying of resistance, and proper technique.
- o Acute soreness due to heavy training could predispose to severe injury if the person does not learn how to alleviate soreness, with regular and gradual activity. Running is magical cure for acute back soreness after training. Even ten minutes of jogging or running, after stressful training, would relieve the inflammation of the lower back structures.
- o Regular Weightlifting has proven to bring the back and knees to exceptional strength and adequate range of motion.

2.5. HABITUAL MODELING

2.5.1. ESSENCE OF PROPER LIFTING
- o Now, although you did not yet start lifting, I can assure you that, if you can initiate the three previous steps, every time you intend to lift anything, that your are a pro Weightlifter, regardless of how much weight you can lift.

PROPER LIFTING TECHNIQUES

- o Comprehending the risk involved in lifting is a real sign of your appreciation of the complexity of the body, and the laws of nature.
- o In order to reach that level of awareness, whether you are a trainer or a trainee, you need to adhere to the rituals of proper lifting, in order to avoid any surprising mishap.
- o Any time you squat, or bend your back, or move something with your hands, you will have plenty of information about your fitness that should guide your training. Stiff or weak knees should alert you to either excess weight issue, general condition affecting your well being, or need for lower body exercising. Shaky or weak back should alert you to real need to start moving, and to increase exercising time and intensity.
- o As with all energy issues, proper lifting is promoted with immediate commitment to exercise and regular and frequent exercising. The more you perform, the deeper the level of engagement of the nervous system, and the richer the skills you acquire.

2.5.2. MASTERING THE RITUALS OF LIFTING

- o **"Stand close to the weight. Keep your chest thrust forwards and upwards, shoulders elevated and thrown backwards, and scapulae retracted. Bend your knees. Maintain straight back. Tighten your abdomen"**. I repeated this slogan thousands of times, to my fellow trainees and to myself, and it works as a perfect reminder and stimulating ritual.
- o Like all activities, actions start from the brain. Thinking precedes acting. Thinking about the plan of lifting is a serious business in Weightlifting. Coaches implore their trainees to think about the phases of execution of a technique, rather than thinking about how heavy the weight might be. Thinking about the phases of lifting technique imposes the higher command of the brain on the nervous system, that might, otherwise, fall into chaos of hesitation, poor timing of recruitment, and distraction with trivial circumferential details.
- o The will of the mind to master muscular power cannot be exaggerated. Many lifters loose self-esteem when they overlook the significance of meditation during performance. Many others put their minds to work with ease, and iron-will, by memorizing certain rituals of concentration and harmony.

2.5.3. LEARNING THROUGH PLAY

- o There will be thousands of objects to lift during the entire life of a human being, but learning this simple technique of performing that ominous task has never been taught in learning institutions, or family setting.
- o This resulted in very lucrative business for chiropractors and physicians, attending to injuries of the back, shoulders, knees, and arms.
- o Early life activities deepen the individual's awareness, for the need of regular activities to stay fit. Late starters stumble upon argumentative reasoning, on the duration of exercise, the sequence of execution, or even the utility of sweating for resistance training.
- o Playful activities ingrain memories of active living, exploring, new experiences, adaptation to failures and successes, and understanding our limitation and potential. Play in itself should be a goal, not just a mean to some gain. All the wealth in the world might secure us shelter, food, and social status, but play is a tool of learning the essence of existence.

2.6. SHOULDER VERSUS ARM PULLING

2.6.1. ROLE OF THE ARMS
- o Hold the weight and never think about lifting the weight from the floor by bending the elbows, or using your Biceps, before your knees comes closer to full extension, *Figures 2.6* thru *2.8*.
- o The Biceps are not the muscles of first choice to lift heavy weights. They are third in priority. Biceps remains in isometric contraction, to stabilize the shoulder joints, until the weight is driven into motion by the strong leg drive.

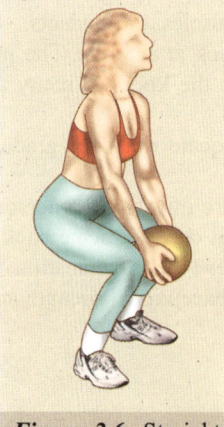

Figure 2.6. Straight arms. As long as the legs are still extending.

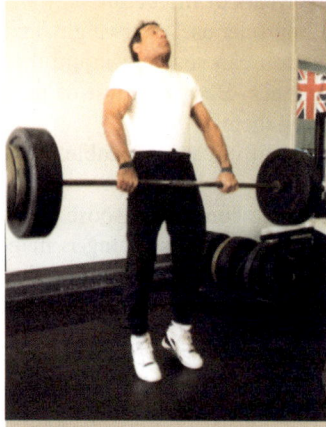

Figure 2.7. Fully extended legs. The rams will begin bending.

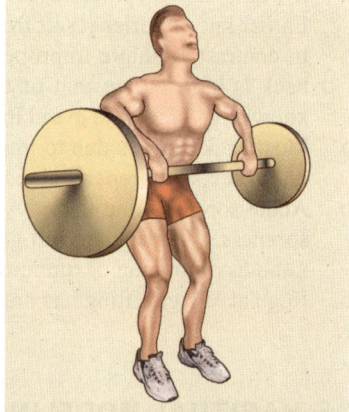

Figure 2.8. Faulty technique. Both elbows and knees are bending.

PROPER LIFTING TECHNIQUES 2

o The very first muscles that should engage in any movement of an object are the Trapezius. The leg drive cannot commence before the Trapezius stabilize the scapulas and transfer the sense of resistance from the arms, through the scapulas and vertebral column, to the legs.
o The isometric contraction of the Biceps, without any shortening, stimulates the stretch reflex, and renders the muscle stronger, when elbow flexion commences, as the weight is passing over the upper portion of the thighs.

2.6.2. ROLE OF THE TRAPEZIUS
Trapezius is a superior puller, compared to the Biceps. The fibers of the Trapezius run in many directions and span a vast space, from origin to insertion, *Figure 2.9*. Because of its location behind the neck, it escapes the attention of lay folks and is, always, ignored during lifting by lay folks. Weightlifters work out the Trapezius in, almost, every exercise, *Figure 2.10*. That is because the Trapezius performs the following essential Pulls.
o Shrugs the shoulders, when the bar is maximally driven upwards, above the upper mid-thighs, by the leg drive.
o Retracts the scapulas, when the bar is moved upwards, below the upper mid-thighs during the Deadlift phase.
o Elevates the shoulders and retracts the scapulas, when the bar is moved below the level of the breasts.
o Rotates the scapulas, when the bar is pressed, jerked, or snatched, overhead.
o Distributes the forces of pull along the upper thoracic vertebras and cervical vertebras, in a pattern that can induce or prevent hunching of the thoracic vertebras.

Most people tend to erroneously believe that muscles that are closer to the handgrips are reliable movers. The fact is that peripheral muscles only act like claws or hooks that grip objects. The real movers are the axial muscles, such as the Trapezius. This is farther explained as follows.

o In *Figure 2.9*, a Bodybuilder, masses the Trapezius and the shoulders, while neglected the lower back erectors. His lower back is not in good proportion to the upper body. This disproportion predisposes the athlete to frequent muscular injuries.
o In *Figure 2.10*, a Weightlifter expresses hypertrophied Trapezius, yet the size of his shoulders is in good proportion to his bodyweight. He has minimal probability of back injury.
o In *Figure 2.11*, the designers of George Washington Bridge, in New York, opted to use pulling cables from the vertical structure to the terminals of the bridge, in order to balance the vertical forces on the bridge. The cables transmit the forces from the horizontal bridge to the vertical structures. This is exactly the role of the Trapezius. The Trapezius transmits forces from the ends of the scapulas to the vertebral axis.

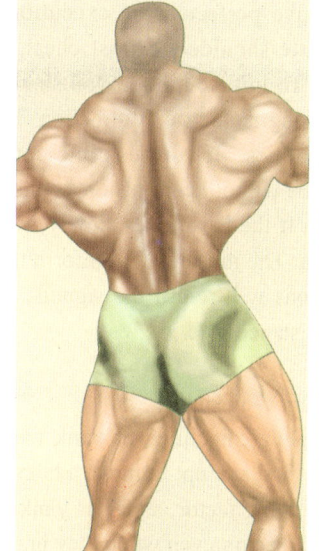

Figure 2.9. Disproportionate muscular hypertrophy in a Bodybuilder.

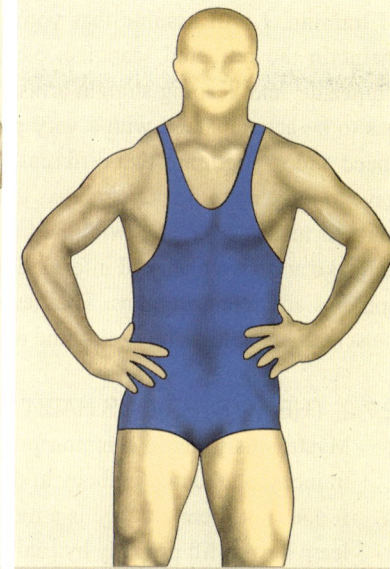

Figure 2.10. The Trapezius muscle is hypertrophied in Weightlifters in proportion to strength.

2.6.3. ROLE OF THE DELTOID
Second, in pulling order, is the Deltoid. The Deltoid is not as bulkier as the Trapezius. By virtue of its middle location, along the pulling line, its size suits its function. The relatively small size of the Deltoid imposes these two limitations on the lifting technique:

o You should not let the bar trajectory moves away from your body, particularly during the Deltoid pull. This is the phase of shoulder abduction of arms, when the bar is moving over the torso. Many lifters let the bar rubs against their cloths, in order to minimize Deltoid stress.
o Lay people tend to lift by flexing the shoulders, by moving the upper arms forwards, instead of abducting them laterally by moving the upper

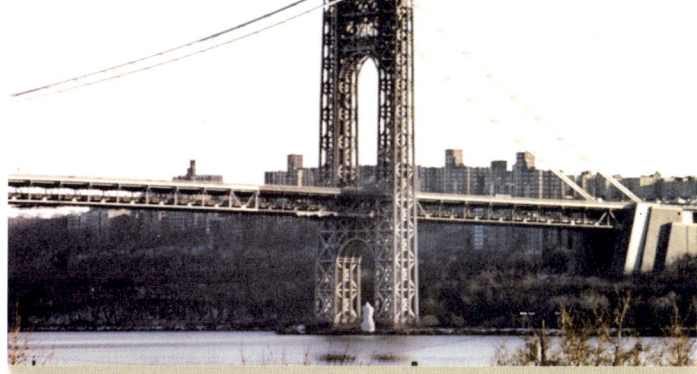

Figure 2.11. In civil design, a bridge is suspended by cables to vertical columns. The body anatomy follows similar design rules. The arms transmit forces to the vertebral axis through the Trapezius muscle. These keep the shoulders elevated, and suspended from the vertebral axis.

arms to the sides, laterally. Abduction of arms forces the bar trajectory to follow the body profile, brings the centers of gravity closer. Flexion of arms moves the centers of gravity apart, makes the weight heavier.

2 PROPER LIFTING TECHNIQUES

These Deltoid features limit the maximal transmission of forces from the arms to the back. Without proper trajectory of the heavy bar, the shoulders would shut off and fail to lift the weight. Thus the smaller Deltoid, with respect to the larger Trapezius, works as a safety valve to prevent back injuries.

The wrists begin to generate torque only after the shoulder abduction is over, when the bar approaches the shoulder level. From this sequence of pulling, it is clear that the peripheral portions of the limb act as rigid levers that convey the resistance to the body. The proximal (closer to the vertebral axis) portions act as dynamic pullers. So, keep your arms straight at the elbows, when initiate the very early lifting movement. If the Trapezius muscles are healthy and strong then you will have better control on the pull of weights, over the torso region.

2.7. PULLING VERSUS YANKING

2.7.1. KNOWING VERSUS PERFORMING
I am very sure that, it is easier to read and understand the rituals of proper lifting than to apply them when performing. Every Weightlifter struggles with memorizing these rituals, yet misses on few of them during performance. When all rituals of proper lifting are executed fully, during a lift, they give the feeling of being on the top of your game, at that particular moment. But there will be more incidents of skipping and missing of proper rules of lifting, as an inherent nature of training. I will assume that you have perfected the execution of the rituals, not just understand them, as follows: maintain the retracted scapulae, elevate shoulders, thrust chest, keep straight and inclined back, while hardening the Trapezius, and keeping straight arms. To initiate motion you should now proceed slowly to test the weight. The slow pull has to be accompanied with a very strong isometric contraction. Before you move on, make sure that you remember that speed and strength are two different entities. If you rush into convulsive yanking of the weight from the floor, then you have to remember the next trial has to be without convulsion, without yanking, and with total mastery of your focused mind on your muscular contact with the bar. If the bar moves slowly, your muscles will communicate better with their neurons, and take and give plenty of information. The muscles will inform the neurons about the magnitude of resistance, via muscle spindles and tendon organs. The neurons will return the signals, with responsive command, in order to recruit sufficient muscle fibers to team up against the resistance.

2.7.2. THE MYSTERIOUS HABIT OF YANKING
o   Mysteriously, most common people are inclined to yank weights during lifting. You will see many inexperienced trainees jolt their entire body in the first attempt to move a heavy weight.
o   It does not seem that age is a modifying factor, as far as yanking of new weight is concerned. Common people do not learn how to lift properly by trial and error, even when they practice for many years of their life.
o   Indulged athletes, in contrast, learn by trial and error, in addition to exposure to the experience of their trainers. That is attributed to the fact that athletes perform sport as a goal in itself, and dig deeper into its intricate details.
o   Explaining to people the proper technique of overcoming the inertia of material objects is a very frustrating experience. Only lengthy training would approximate the practical meaning of the laws of nature to beginners. Hopefully, as training progresses, a trainee would learn that forces do no impart their effect instantaneously.
o   A college graduate might digest the concept of resistance, taught in many disciplines, faster than folks with lesser education. Yet, learning how to tame resistance for our own good requires a lot of work.
o   Resistance is a universal concept. For example, if you drill a hole in a tank full of water, the water would not leak all together, instantaneously, but rather on a long time. That is proportional to the size of the hole, the viscosity of the fluid, and the head of fluid level. The resistance to fluid flow is applicable to other forms of flow: flow of electrons, flow of electromagnetic waves, and flow of force on matter.

2.7.3. YANKING DISSIPATES ENERGY
o   Trained lifters learn that yanking weights dissipates their energy, and leaves the barbell dead in its place.
o   Slow pulling allows many natural processes to complete their normal course.
o   If the weight is light, your body will maintain the prior posture. The sensors of the Trapezius convey the information to the entire spinal array, along the back, and the spinals muscles increase or decrease recruitment of its fibers, to support the extra load.
o   If the elbows are still kept straight, until the knees are fully extended, that will prevent the confusion of communication between the working muscles (Trapezius) and the postural muscles (Spinal erectors).

o Slow pulling allows you to fully contract the thigh muscles, Glutei, back muscles, and the Trapezius, in order to convey force to the barbell, along iron-grid of levers of hardened muscles on bones.

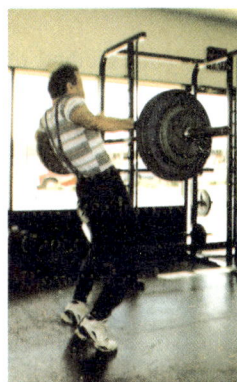
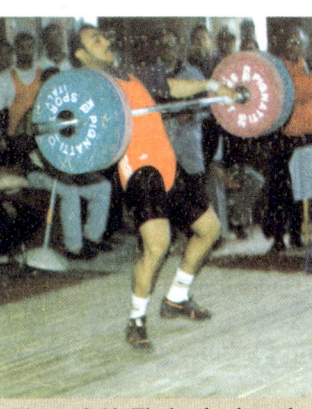
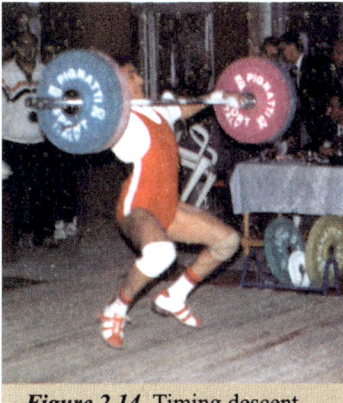
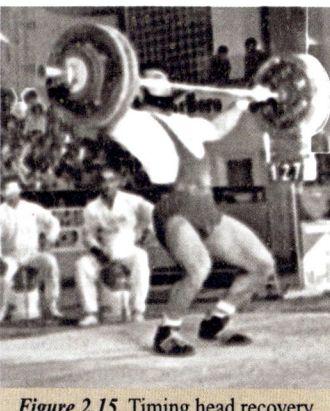

Figure 2.12. Timing shoulder abduction.   *Figure 2.13.* Timing backward bouncing.   *Figure 2.14.* Timing descent.   *Figure 2.15.* Timing head recovery.

2.7.4. TIMING OF THE LIFTING SPEED
o You can then proceed to the phase of speedy displacement of the barbell as follows, *Figures 2.12* thru *2.15*.
o The Trapezius contracts, farther more, to shrug the shoulders. All the four lifters, in these figures, shrug the Trapezius, abduct the arms, hop on the feet balls, and throw their heads backwards, in order to move the center of gravity of the body backwards.
o The Deltoids contract and shorten to abduct the arms.
o The Biceps contract, not only to bend the elbow, but also to support the shoulder balls in their sockets, by the long heads of the Biceps.
o The spinal muscle pulls the 24 spines, of the 24 vertebras, of the lumber, thoracic, and cervical regions, in addition to the skull. Only one lifter, *Figure 2.15,* is wearing a waist belt. This show how confident Weightlifters are, about the strength of their back.
o Maintaining vertebral alignment is a fundamental tenet of proper lifting and can only be achieved, during the initial phase of lifting, by slow and strong displacement of the barbell. Weightlifters are trained to react timely to the possibility of encountering any vertebral misalignment, before they proceed with the Pull.

2.7.5. HOW MUSCLES ADAPT TO RESISTANCE?
o Long before the weight departs the floor, a solidly tightened back will alert the lifter of what is lying ahead, and whether the lift has to be aborted, to avoid a crippling injury.
o The best virtue a Weightlifter has to learn is not to be charismatic or self-defiant. Know the nature of force. Let your grips loose, and release the barbell, whenever alarming strains arise. Training teaches you what is alarming and what is not.
o Adaptation to resistance cannot happen with casual training. Many, if not all, modern Weightlifting authorities agree on one thing that is lifting from the floor to overhead has to be performed at least daily. Everyday, to the end of life, adaptation to lifting will keep evolving. Your hesitation will wax and wane according to your involvement in training. The longer the interruption of training, the greater is the hesitation in tackling lifting.
o Lifting from other than the floor, such as Bench Press, Cable Rowing, and arm exercises, will not transfer to adaptation in whole range lifting. The same could be said about gymnastics, wrestling, and other sports. You have to perform the pattern of sport you intend to master. That is because you are refining the neuromuscular adaptation, not just muscular strength.
o Assisting exercises add fine touch, but also may work against you. A hugely developed shoulder, when done by dumbbells, will not have the same range of motion as when done in sport related activities. So, next time you should not wonder when you see people squatting, deadlifting, or bench-pressing extremely heavy weights, yet cannot lift proper Clean or Snatch. Heavy and slow training works out some muscles, yet heavy and fast training works out different muscles. The former are slow twitchers while the latter are fast twitchers. Each belongs to different motor neural family.

2.7.6. NORMAL COURSE OF TRAINING AFTEREFFECTS
o It all starts with the early sore and painful muscles after performing new activities. Soreness decreases within days, as tolerance to similar activities increases.

2 PROPER LIFTING TECHNIQUES

- o   Training then proceeds with gradual increase in strength of resistance and quicker recovery. The range of motion adapts to the new activities in a slow fashion.
- o   When the level of conditioning peaks, soreness goes unnoticed and the lifter experiences fatigue more than soreness. Thus adaptation becomes more generalized as fitness progresses. Local soreness indicates local weakness, shortening of ligaments or tendons, or poor conditioning of circulation and innervation.
- o   Advance trainees put deep faith in thorough warm-up as an effective way to prevent soreness. Your method of warm- up will grow wiser as you find your way around strength training. The following are some tips on warming up that might deepen you faith in its effectiveness.

   i. Any time you warm-up you should never forget squatting for at least a dozen of times. Even if it is your Bench Press day, squatting means a lot to the sympathetic activity, since the nervous system has to regulate blood flow during the taxing changes of posture in squatting and standing.
   ii. At least a dozen repetitions of bending the torso on the legs (Goodmorning exercise) will prepare the back erectors to vigorous activities.
   iii. Warming up, without weights, until inducing perspiration will guarantee you sore-free workout. To get that far in sweating means that you have to reduce pauses and side talks.
   iv. Your touch with ground is your gauge to fitness. If you can stand on your feet balls and control your weight gracefully for few seconds that indicates your preparedness to begin strength training. Calf muscles, when warmed up thoroughly, will test the harmony of the cardiovascular, pulmonary, and nervous system. Remember that ballet dancers could sense any gain in Bodyweight just by feeling the difficulty of hopping on the feet balls. That is because the lower legs are very tight compartments, where circulation is scant and muscles perform mostly postural activities. Thus feeling good on your feet balls means good circulation in that compromised part of the body.

2.7.7. YANKING CAUSES GRAVE INJURIES
- o   Yanking during lifting a barbell, pulling a child by the arm, or during opening a jammed door can result in grave injury to the spinal cord, shoulder, or leg joints.
- o   Yanking adds an extra dynamic force of resistance that might exceed the maximum limit of ligaments, tendons, bones, and cartilages.
- o   Yanking creates ischemic injuries, avulsions, or even fractures, or causes complete loss of balance.
- o   Sometimes you see Weightlifters scream, pull, snatch, jerk, or strain, while lifting, yet you never see them yanking the weight.
- o   Vigorous activities are timed in such manner that synergy is the outcome, rather than chaos. Weightlifters spend many years in lengthy experimentation with timing the speed of lifting until they can automate perfect execution of lifting.
- o   When the barbell is dead still on the floor, the only way to lift is to proceed very slowly, by imparting force on the bar. The duration of such slow pull varies, from very brief to a protracted second (1/60th of a minute). Variation in the duration of Pull depends on your ability to recruit sufficient muscle fibers and muscle groups, to generate force adequate to energize the barbell into motion. If your most effort falls short of the threshold required for inducing motion, then the slow pulling allows for room to terminate the task of lifting. Yanking will deprive the mind from the opportunity to decide on bailing out, without risking injury.

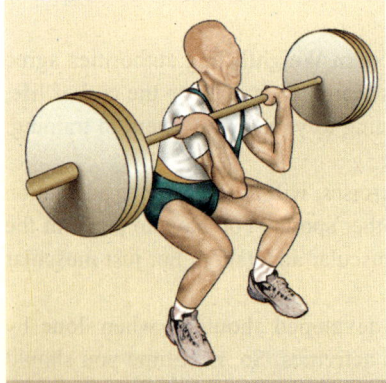 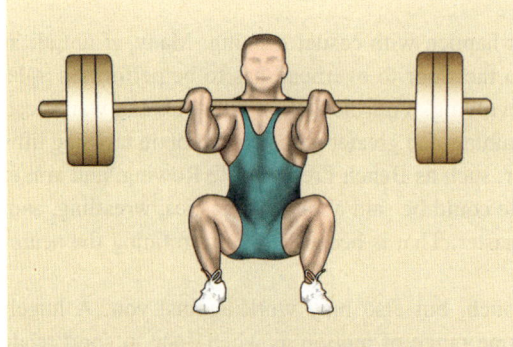 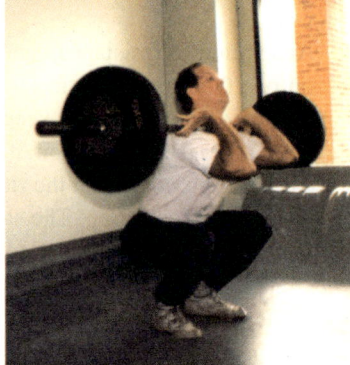

Figure 2.16. Shoulders failed to flex and elbows failed to flip and elevate. This might cause injury to wrists and elbows.

Figure 2.17. Strong shoulder flexion creates a flat platform for racking the bar on the shoulders and demands flexibility of the shoulders and the back.

Figure 2.18. Shoulder flexion requires flexible wrists and back that requires regular practice.

2.7.8. PERFECTING LIFTING SKILLS
- o   **Reciting the plan of execution.** Weightlifters learn to amplify the few seconds, prior to lifting, into a detailed plan of execution. When you lift you are on your own, under the mercy of your own ability to quickly make determination on

what to do next. When you develop confidence in the reliability of the laws of lifting, you would not worry about failure. Because most failures in Weightlifting are due to overwhelming fear of performing under a heavy weight.
- **Lifting rituals.** At the peak of your training, you will master these rituals of lifting.
  i. The centers of gravity of the barbell and of your bodyweight have to come very close to one vertical line.
  ii. Extend the knees before executing maximal pulling, because bent knees stand in the way of vertical ascent.
  iii. As the barbell approaches the thighs, during ascent, its center of gravity departs significantly from the center of gravity of the body and the lifter has to hyper-extend his or her body, hop on both feet balls in order to bring the centers of gravity into a vertical line.
  iv. As the barbell approaches the chest, in the Clean lift, the shoulders are abducted, by spreading uppers arms laterally.
  v. As the barbell approaches the shoulders, in the Clean lift, the shoulders are flexed, by flipping the elbows forwards under the barbell.
  vi. In order to support a heavy bar on the shoulders you have to thrusting the chest forwards and upwards, in order to create a horizontal flat bed to rack the bar on the shoulders, *Figures 2.16* thru *2.18*. You should never support the bar on your wrist and elbows. The forearm is not adapted to heavy compression. The bar should seat on the shoulders and the upper end of the sternum.
  vii. As the bar moves overhead, the head has to pass under the bar, as soon as the bar is elevated above the level of the eyebrows. Passing the head forwards under the bar aligns the centers of gravity and maintains balance with minimal shoulder strain.
  viii. **Voluntary and involuntary actions.** While you may well understand the difference between a perfect bar trajectory and a lousy one, your performance has little to do with your understanding. Your performance depends mostly on practicing and striving to execute theoretical proposals of technical lifting. Even if you are advanced lifter, fears and hesitation may sneak into your mind and cause old, dormant habits to dominate acquired ones.
  ix. **Individual variation.** The lessons learned from a hundred years of Weightlifting should top all lessons learned from all other sports combined. There is great potential of overcoming weakness, with patient and planned Weightlifting training for months. Also, strength training is affordable as long as we are in the company of air and gravity. Lifting weights at young age might contribute to better compliance of various ligaments, to execute extremes of motion. Many years of neglecting exercise could result in irreparable shortening of ligaments and deprives the trainee from the wide range of flexibility, needed to maintain extreme posture during lifting. Yet, the most debated issue of neglecting exercise is the extent of decline with age in efficacy of the nervous system. That orchestrates the proprioreception performance. Whether there is a specific age limit for developing and acquiring higher skill of motor harmony, or the accumulation of problems, caused by neglecting exercise, are too difficult to remedy, depends on individual circumstances.

2.7.9. YANKING VERSUS ADEQUATE RECRUITMENT OF MUSCLE FIBERS

- Lifting proceeds very slowly from the beginning, by imparting force on the weight to just equalize its inertia.
- That proceeds by adding more force of pulling; yet keep in mind a very serious possibility of aborting the lift at any sense of unfamiliar feeling. Aborting a lift in progress by a trained Weightlifter is executed very decisively and swiftly. In contrast to beginners, trained lifters would seek no second opinion to opt out a risky lift.
- Yanking allows no such time for probing the risk ahead. It could cause disc herniation or joint dislocation, even before getting any feeling of the heaviness of weight.
- Slow, progressive lift allows recruitment of additional muscle fibers, circulatory blood flow, and host of biological activities essential for the task of generating physical force.
- Try to gently yank a stationary car on flat surface with its transmission put in neutral. You will see that your effort is wasted in shaking the part of the car in the immediate contact with your body, with very little effect on the entire car. It takes not just a swift short notice to move objects but a persistent calculated effort.
- If you do not yank the weight then you would have to put up with the agony of lengthy muscular spasm during the slow procedure. This is the normal course of building strength. Fortunately, today's agony will, very soon, become a thing of the past and you will be proud of being more knowledgeable about fitness.
- The slowly pulled ligaments and the painfully spastic muscles will adapt to forces of resistance, by seeking more blood supply, modifying the firing schemes of their sensing nervous elements, and evolving to new and strong structures that will last for a while long.

2.8. THE APPROACH PHASE

2.8.1. MENTAL RITUALS DURING THE APPROACH PHASE

- Trainers spend many months, or even years, in refining the attitude of their trainees towards approaching a lift. Lifting can turn to be a devastating undertaking without proper approaching rules.
- Beginners have to learn to focus utterly on lifting and overcome any distracting thought. Shyness, fear of exposure to the public, or overconfidence undermines the balance and the harmony of lifting and may result in serious bodily injury or loss of self-confidence, due to failure.

PROPER LIFTING TECHNIQUES

- o This is the most intense moment the athlete might experience. The fear stems from concerns that one's strength might betray him, his will may crumple, or his preparation is no match for the occasion.
- o The process of approaching a heavy lift is a ritual process that involves all previously acquired habits, sense of inner tranquility, and ability to master the entire body in concerting effort. Memories from previous experience tide the mind over these critical moments of decision-making. Individual variation in focusing and optimizing every bit of energy, in order to achieve efficient performance, is very diverse.
- o The dynamics of this meditative focusing aims at manipulating the autonomic nervous system. Thus a focused athlete can learn to lower his heart rate, relax all muscles, and suppress all secondary, reflexes in preparation for a big storm of calculated actions and emotions.

2.8.2. PHYSICAL ATTITUDES DURING THE APPROACH PHASE

- o Most, if not all lifters, start the initial phase by hopping on the front part of their feet. Lifters start by standing on the feet balls, lifting the heels, and pretending to adjust their standing position. This stimulates the lower leg muscles, the entire system of equilibrium, and arousal for the task ahead.
- o They relax and shake their arms and shoulders to allow all possible perfusing capillaries to nurture the arm muscles. Thus tense lower legs and relaxed upper limbs will reverse the gravitational gradient on the circulation. Gentle shaking of limbs and torso, alarms the lifter about any spastic muscle that defies shaking, by its spastic state. He thus has to force his mind to further relax such annoyed muscle. Though we know that muscular relaxation is not under voluntary control of the individual, there are many learned tricks of inducing muscular relaxation, such as breathing deeply and slowly. Many people, for example, learn how to dilate or constrict their pupils with meditative techniques.
- o Most, if not all lifters, will squat to the bar gripping position with a very standardized approach: knees bending, lower back lordosis, upper back vertical, neck and head on vertical line with the heels, shoulders falling behind the front of chest cage, well-retracted scapulae, and arms hanging loosely and freely, with minimal spasm, landing vertically on the bar.

2.9. INITIAL PHASE

2.9.1. START POSITION

In the initial phase of lifting, the lifter has to assume a starting position that recruits the major muscles in proper sequence. The upper body will contract by isometric mode, thus hardening the elbows, shoulders, and spines, without shortening of muscles. The lower body will contract by isotonic contraction. Thus the knees and hips are bent, in order to be extended by shortening of contracting muscles. This position utilizes the relatively strong muscles of the lower body to overcome the inertia of the weight and initiate displacement of the barbell from the dead point. This serves to unfold the semi-seated body into straight, upright posture.

The physical appearance of a **"pyramidal start-position"** is enhanced by performing active positioning of the musculoskeletal joints, as follows.
- o Balance your scapulas such that they are closer, together, in the back.
- o Balance your shoulders such that they are evenly horizontal and thrown backwards, behind the chest.
- o Thrust your chest forwards such that your upper back remains as close to flat and straight posture as possible.
- o Your arms should hang loose and vertical on the bar.
- o Force your lower back to arch inwards in a concave posture. This is done by the combined actions of back erectors and hip flexors (Iliopsoas). To feel that your back is correctly positioned in lordotic form, you must have your belly stuck tightly to the thighs.

These balancing tasks align the lines of forces from the vertebral column, through the scapulas, to the arms, in such a way as to eliminate losses.

With the upper body stretched and the lower body bent, at the knees and hips, lifting will be initiated by the Glutei and Quadriceps. The entire body will pass through a sequence of hardening of joints, between the pelvis and shoulder, in order to transferred forces to the barbell and to the floor, simultaneously. Every subsequent phase in the process of lifting depends on this early posture. Lax joints or muscles negatively impact the simultaneity of transfer of force and might topple the entire effort of lifting, to failure. This might strain specific joints of the body, precipitate tear, rupture, dislocation, sublaxation, or even fracture. The sequence of contracting muscles proceeds as follows.

  i. **Control of contraction.** The muscles that carry bodyweight are contracted mostly by the effect of that weight, and slightly by voluntary actions. The upper body muscles can be contracted, after being aligned, by pulling on the bar, while still maintaining alignment. Of course, maximal contraction of muscles cannot be accomplished voluntarily without pulling or pushing against external objects. We cannot force muscles to contract maximally by mental determination without external resistance. Thus when we start pulling the weight, during lifting, muscles show hidden forces, by feedback process between the muscle sensors and the neurons. All what we can do is to decide on global issues, such as how far or how fast the barbell will travel. If the body developed prior memory of the strength required to execute our higher wishes, mental commands could then be executed to the fullest extent of the body's ability.

ii. **Pre-stretching.** Most well trained Weightlifters overdo deep squatting, prior to assuming the start position. Some would squat until the ischial tuberosity (the bone we sit on) seats on the Achilles tendon (the back of the ankle), for few seconds, before assuming final position for lifting. The purpose of deep squatting is stretching the Quadriceps, the Glutei, and the back erectors. Stretch puts these groups of muscle on highest alert to initiate lifting. Trying to assume the start position without the pre-stretching rituals surprises the motor memory of the lifter, and causes hesitation during the early probing phase of lifting.

iii. **Movers.** The first groups consist of the bulkiest muscles of the body. Their anatomical fiber grouping are multi-pinnate, having very wide origin, and act on long bones to produce maximum torque. This group extends the hips and the knees and drives the barbell from dead rest, to maximal displacement.

iv. **Stabilizers.** Next, in hierarchy, are the Trapezium, Rhomboids, and Deltoids. This group of muscles will kick in with peak power after the barbell clears the knee and becomes ready for maximum speedy displacement. Initially this group was the stretchers when the first group was doing the moving. The stabilizers are less bulky than the movers, act for shorter distances, and have fewer pinnas. This group only shrugs the shoulder, retract the scapula, and flex the arms, and benefits largely from the preceding drive of the first group.

v. **Weightlessness.** Third, in hierarchy, are the Biceps, Triceps, and Calves. They are least in pinnation, mostly longitudinal in direction, act on long bones and two joints, and weakest of the three groups. This group operates during the weightlessness phase by fixing joints or contracting at high speed to lead the barbell to final destination.

2.9.2. LEVERAGE OF TORQUE

o Training entails understanding the mechanics of gravity. The untrained hardens the muscles in the close proximity to the barbell, such as those of the hands and arms, and omits the remote muscle such as the Glutei and Quadriceps.

o The simple fact of mechanics, that skips common people, is that **"a weight held in the arms generates a reaction at the knees, or at the feet, equals to that weight plus a torque, or a couple, that depends on the displacement of the weight from the knee, or the feet, respectively."**

o Thus the feet carry the highest burden in lifting, the knees are next, while the arms are least in carrying the burden. Arms carry the weight but they do not have to lift the bodyweight or support the maximally produced torque.

o Leverage means that individual muscles have to team up, in harmonious fashion of contraction, in order to maintain motion of the whole bodyweight. The moving bodyweight pivots around joints and creates angular and linear momentums. Thus momentum is a cumulative memory of the sum of forces generated by all isolated muscles on the mass of moving objects. Muscles that contract out of harmony diminish the net momentum.

o Momentum refers to the amount of motion. It thus correlates with the mass of the moving weight and the speed of that mass. Because speed has to have specific direction, therefore we refer to momentum in straight lines as linear momentum, whereas that in curved directions as angular momentum.

o Leverage is generated by the added effects of the contracting muscles on the long, solid bones. Leverage is so crucial to lifting. If you use isolated muscles to lift weights you run into the problem of straining ligaments, tendons, and muscles. Whole body performance is the essence of lifting by proper leverage, since whole body is capable of generating maximum momentum.

2.9.3. EFFICIENT RECRUITMENT OF MUSCLES

o Training aims at mastering efficient motor recruitment skill. Farmers incur many serious back injuries, even after many generations of skillful farming. Fatigue, stress for making living, variation of seasons, and sparse irregular labor may explain the high prevalence of injury among farmers.

o Weightlifting sport differs from farming, and other physical labor, in its purposeful and playful learning trends. This stimulates curiosity to discover the mechanics of motion. Other than making profit from lifting weights, athletes are driven with mysterious believes of doing well to themselves, by promoting strong physique. Even injured lifters would wish to return to their glorious days of top performance.

o The skill of synchronizing muscular recruitment, during lifting, demonstrates the vitality of a fit and healthy body to perform exceptionally, when trained to do so. Focusing on mastering muscular recruitment, and suppressing the distraction of circumferential thoughts, cannot be exaggerated. Many people lack such ability of devotion to playful activities that require mental concentration.

2.10. EQUALIZATION PHASE

2.10.1. ESSENCE OF RESISTANCE AND ENERGY

o The goal of the initial phase was to **prepare the person** to the state of vigorous exertion, optimize the performance of anatomical configuration of the human body, and orchestrate the musculoskeletal recruitment process.

PROPER LIFTING TECHNIQUES

- o The final product of the initial phase is the **"pyramidal start-position"**. From that position, the person is apt to exert internal forces to equalize external resistance in the most efficient manner.
- o The essence of resistance is **regulation and control** of flow of all kinds of energy. Resistance regulates the flow of electrons in wires, nerves, and all materials. Resistance to energy flow makes it possible to invent electronic devices, made biological life a possibility, and lent materials different physical properties.
- o Because resistance is the language of energy, **resistance training** is a vehicle of transforming energy into health. It seems that all forms of biological life possess the instinct of active pursuit of overcoming resistance. Such pursuit separates life from death. It also colors health with different shades of a wide spectrum of feelings, from feeble and ill to robust and vibrant.
- o The matter is the ultimate maker of resistance. As we have learned after many centuries of accumulated knowledge, matter and energy are two forms of a single being. The resistance is generated when these two entities interact with each other. Inertia, of material objects, requires energy to translate objects into different states, of displacement or speed. Particles in materials require energy to allow their electrons to stream in electric currents. Underground fluid requires energy to permeate through soil pores.

2.10.2. SEQUENTIAL HARDENING OF MUSCLES

In order to overcome the inertia of an object, the lifter proceeds from the **"start-position"** of the initial phase, to a well thought of process of sequential hardening of muscles. The purpose of the sequential hardening is not only to equalize the weight of the barbell, without any significant upward translation, but also to ignite a process of firing along many nerve endings and neurons that will bring the memories of prior experiences to replay the lifting. In this phase, six major groups of joints maximize their muscular stability (with minimal sensible mobility) to its fullest, in a sequential manner, as follows.

- o Muscles are hardened in cycles of **feedback regulation,** between the sensors of the handgrips and the proprioreceptors of the feet stance.
- o The arms pull on the handgrips and transmit forces to scapular muscles.
- o The scapular muscles pull on the vertebral column and skull and thus trigger the proprioreceptors along the axial joints. The scapular muscles also pull on the chest cage and clavicles and thus trigger respiratory and circulatory responses.
- o The vertebral axis transmits forces to the legs through the pelvis. The legs react by resisting forces and transmitting signals from the feet stance.
- o The feedback circuit is reversed and amplified, with more muscular recruitment and more muscular power generation, until the motion proceeds in lifting. The number of feedback circuiting depends on the reserve of muscular recruitments and the amount of resistance encountered.
- o The lower back is the center of the circuit. Yet, all parts along the pathway of the circuit have to check in, with their potential to participate in subsequent circuiting, until the goal of resisting external forces is achieved.
- o As far as the lifter is concerned, sequential hardening of muscles is learned with very little explanation about its dynamics. Weightlifters learn that they cannot harden their entire body simultaneously. You cannot perform total convulsive muscular spasm to lift weights. The sequential contraction and relaxation limits hardening of muscles to required directions, without compromising perfusion of the rest of the body.

2.10.3. MID-FOOT ARCHING

- o The mid-foot arch allows free blood flow during heavy lifting. This arch is maintained in part by the intrinsic muscles of sole, and in part by the peroneal, tibial, and toes muscles. Toes have to have blood supply during lifting, through the feet arch.
- o Now, the entire bodyweight is distributed on the heels (80%) and the metatarsal heads or feet balls (20%).
- o In all sports involving performing while standing, arching the middle of the feet indicates alertness of the performer. Even in sports such as skiing, where feet are heavily guarded in hard boots, arching and throwing the bodyweight of the feet balls allow better control of the mechanics of motion.
- o The outstanding features of the human feet will be put to test in the following events of lifting. No other animal can demonstrate such ability to balance the entire body, in addition to lifting up to three times its weight, plus the added momentum of the high speed lifting. No other animal can balance itself, on two feet, on a straight line, and perform so gracefully and strongly, as humans.

2.10.4. THE STABILIZATION OF THE ANKLES

- o The ankles are stabilized by large and small muscles, in the back, front, and deep in between, of the tibia and fibula. The large muscles are the Gastrocnemius, Soleus, and anterior Tibialis. These perform powerful actions. The small muscles of the toes and the peroneal muscles perform fine stabilization of the ankle, through supporting the toes and the sole.
- o Stable ankles even the entire bodyweight on the articulating surfaces. Unevenly stressed ankle locks off and impedes the performance of graceful lifting technique.

PROPER LIFTING TECHNIQUES

o All forces of lifting affect the ankles more than any other joints in the body. These forces are the Bodyweight, the weight of barbell, and the virtual weights arising from the motion of these material weights.

2.10.5. THE IMMENSE STRENGTH OF THE MUSCLES OF THE KNEES

o The optimum knee angle to equalize resistance depends on both the length of the femur (the thigh bone) and the range of motion of the hip joints. The three variables manage to keep the back straight and inclined, above the horizontal line. Knee angle over 90 degrees between tibia and femur, is appropriate for this phase of lifting.

o The massive Quadriceps in front, the Hamstrings in the back, and the lateral ligaments on the sides stabilize the knee joint. Stable knees evenly distribute weight on their articulating condyles. Unevenly loaded knees impede the technique of motion of upward drive or downward flexion.

o The knees are hinge joints that are well suited for bending and should be relied upon in all lifting from the floor level. Substituting the bending of knees, by that of the hips, contributes to the stiffness and wasting of the muscles around the knees and the growth and strength of the muscles around the hips. This imbalance of muscular form leads to unsightly body appearance of bulky buttocks, at the middle of the body, with thin and weak limbs. After many years of improper lifting, by bending the hips instead of the knees, the majority of the population loses the precious freedom of unrestricted ambulance. Early aging has its root in such sedentary living.

o Weightlifting is the only sport that has, single handedly, explored the immense capabilities of the muscles of the knee to perform the extremes of motion. Ordinary walking, aggressive running, wrestling, and many other motor activities would not rise to the level of Weightlifting training, in developing and conditioning all groups of fibers around the knee joints. These groups run in many directions, to different lengths, and are inserted into tendons along wider areas and shapes. Conditioning such formation of muscular pinnation is unique to Weightlifting.

2.10.6. HIP POSITION DURING LIFTING

o Lay folks, along with many animals such as horses, cows, and camels, rely heavily on the muscles of the buttocks during lifting. Weightlifters have revolutionized the skill of lifting, by delegating upward driving forces to the knees. In developed countries, the invention of seated toilets has contributed to the wasting of the muscles of the knees. Natives of undeveloped countries maintain highly flexible knees, until late ages.

o The use of the hip joints during lifting is indicative of the level of training of a lifter. Well-trained lifters keep the hip joints half way between the floor level and the head level during the equalization phase. Untrained lifters elevate the hips prematurely. This throws the back into horizontal position; the head and shoulders are distanced away from the center of gravity of the weight. Getting untrained lifters to maintain the mid-position of the hips, between the head and feet, requires a lot of building of proximal muscles of the pectoral and pelvis girdles.

o Equalization of resistance commences by gradually intensifying the contraction of the Glutei muscles, while the rest of the body is stretched at constant tone to support the transfer of forces to the barbell. Thus the Glutei initiate equalization, while the rest of the muscles react by more supportive fixation, without any lax motion. As with all joints, the Glutei are counteracted by the opposing muscles, Iliopsoas. Balancing the strength of both groups, Glutei and Iliopsoas, is vital in maintaining the hip balance with minimal trauma to the articulating surface of the joint.

o The fact that the gluteal muscles, in humans, maintain the unique upright posture signifies the role of these muscles in locomotion and lifting. The rapid wasting of the Glutei results from avoiding lifting from the floor. Many trainees underscore the significance of the Glutei in locomotion, because their role does not manifest itself before lengthy training and understanding of the mechanics of locomotion.

2.10.7. THE UNIQUE UPRIGHT POSTURE OF LIFTERS

After few years of training, Weightlifters develop a characteristic shape of pelvic bones, as follows.

o The sacrum becomes heavier and more convex, the ilium rough, heavier, and stout. A Weightlifter could keep his trousers on, without the need for waist belt or suspensors, due to the well convex sacrum.

o The gluteal muscles waste away with avoiding lifting from the floor, long inactivity, and in alcoholics and heavy smokers. The loss of convexity of the sacrum is manifested by the frequent falling of the trousers below the waist line and predisposes to higher frequency of back and knee injuries. Wasted Glutei in alcoholics explain the straight form of sacrum, the less roomy pelvic cavity, the bulging of the belly outside the pelvic cavity, and wasted muscles above and below the Glutei.

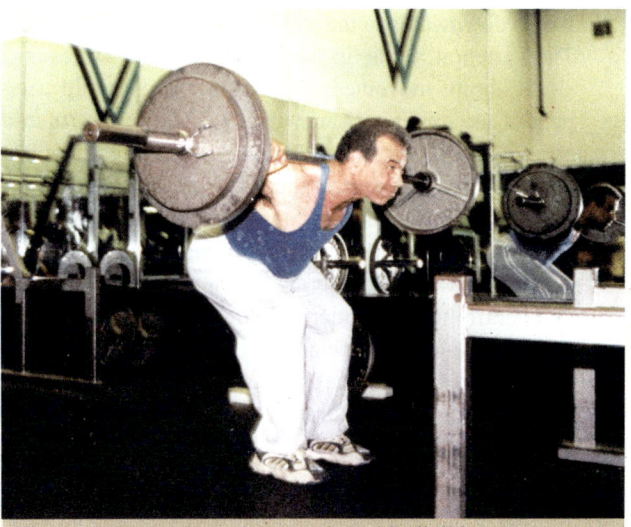

Figure 2.19. Goodmorning exercise with slightly bent knees.

2. PROPER LIFTING TECHNIQUES

- o The action of the Glutei, on the back of the hip joint, is counteracted, on the front of the joint, by the iliofemoral ligament, the strongest ligament in the entire body. This ligament is responsible for keeping the torso attached to the legs in the most vigorous activities we undertake. Thus lifting from the floor accomplishes the most basic benefit of health and fitness, of strengthening the link between the upper body and the lower body.
- o Strong upper-to-lower body link enhances the performance of the proprioreception nervous system and the cardiovascular system, and conditions the person to tackle the most demanding tasks that require whole-body strength, *Figures 2.19* and *2.20*.

2.10.8. THE COMPLEX MECHANICS OF THE VERTEBRAL COLUMN

Coaches should persistently emphasize to their trainees the complex mechanics of the vertebral column, as follows.

- o In all vertebrates, the vertebral column hosts bundles of millions of nerve fibers, to and from the brain and the whole body. Different groups, of these millions of nerves, enter and exit the vertebral column at few holes along the sides of the column, to reach their destinations.
- o The fact that forces are transferred along the back of the vertebral column is crucial in lifting. The joints of articulation are located behind the spinal cord bundles and are supported by many muscles and ligaments, along the back of the vertebral column.
- o The front of the vertebral column contains the chunky bodies of the vertebras and the intervertebral discs, but contains no joints. The front of the vertebral column acts merely as a shock absorber cushion. The two sides of the vertebral columns (between the front and the back) contain the exit and entrance holes, and the whole traffic of nerves, in and out of the spinal cord, *Figure 2.21*.

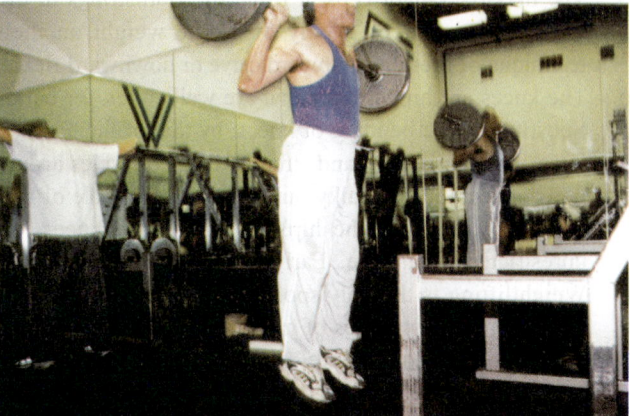

Figure 2.20. Jumping after bending is an outstanding exercise that works out the linking joints between the upper and the lower body parts, with emphasis on the fast twitching muscle fibers. Notice the poor guy in the back, warming up for squatting with completely skewed posture.

- o During lifting, the vertebral column has to be kept concave (arched inwards or lordotic), when viewed from the back. Bending any of the vertebral joints (rounding or hunching) increases the pressure inside the intervertebral disc that is formed of gelatinous substance enclosed in fibrous sheath and may predispose to spinal disc herniation.
- o Inside the vertebral canal are located the vascular channels that supply the spinal cord on its front and back surfaces. Bending the back during lifting disturbs the blood flow to the spinal cord by stretching the vessels on the back surface while kinking those on the front.
- o Straining during strenuous lifting aggravates the congestion in the front surface of the spinal cord during bending, because of the kinked vessels. The resulted disturbance of blood flow to the spinal cord, during lifting with bent back, could abort transfer of information signals along the central nervous lines and lead to failure of lifting, falls, or injuries. Keep in mind that the spinal cord, like the eyes, is an extension of the brain.
- o Keeping straight or lordotic back is half the task. The other half of the task is to keep the back inclined, as close to vertical as possible. The more vertical the back is, the less are the shearing forces across the vertebral column. Shearing forces are hostile horizontal forces that tend to dislocate the joints, strain ligaments, deform discs, and kink the vital blood vessels on the spinal cord. Vertical forces are well handled by the vertebral joints. These joints transfer forces downwards to the pelvic girdle, and upwards to the pectoral girdles.
- o The vertebral joints, in the vast population, are overwhelmingly unconditioned, even to common daily activities. A slight abrupt movement of the upper body could trigger inconvenient back discomfort, for many days. Injuries and pain of the spines consume huge medical resources in developed nations. As with the knee muscles, Weightlifting has exploited the vertebral column to the highest level of stress, with ingenuity and perseverance. The mechanics of articulation of the vertebral column are perfected with training. The potential of exceeding all expectation of strength, with minimal increase of bodyweight, has been relentlessly pursued. Today's top Weightlifters can, bare-handedly, lift three times their bodyweight from the floor to overhead, at unprecedented speed and grace.
- o If the back fares well, during the equalization phase, the lifter gains confidence in his or her ability to move the weight and control its destination. Distressed back impacts other vital organs, in a negative manner, causing clumsy or failed lifting technique. During lifting, the difference between distressed back of a well-trained lifter and a beginner is that the former may gradually intensify the distress, yet to bail out prior to incurring trauma. A beginner might zap through a traumatic effort before realizing the consequences of traumatizing the back.

2.10.9. LEVERAGE AT THE SHOULDER JOINTS

At the shoulders, a "T" formation of muscles and bones convey forces, back and forth, between the vertebral column and the upper limbs, as follows.

o All activities performed by the arms involve the shoulder muscles. Even with the complete elimination of the action of the shoulder muscles on the arms (such as resting the elbows on a table during typing), the shoulders affect the posture of upper body. When not conditioned by exercise, weak shoulders convey the feeling of fatigue and lack of energy.
o Unconditioned shoulders might cause a person to spend longer hours in sleep, after a regular day of activities. Strong shoulders enhance the blood flow to the brains, through maintaining unrestricted carotid and vertebral vessels. They also enhance limb circulation, through maintaining the passage of the limbs major vessels, under the clavicles.
o During the equalization phase, the shoulders act as mere stretchers, until the bar has cleared the knee joints. When lifting from the floor, the shoulders are located mid-way between the weight and the brain. By virtue of their location, they only maintain posture of the upper body and delegate the process of equalization to the lower muscles. The proper posture is that of forwardly thrust chest, retracted scapulas, and straight upper back and neck. This posture guarantees adequate respiration and circulation to the whole body.

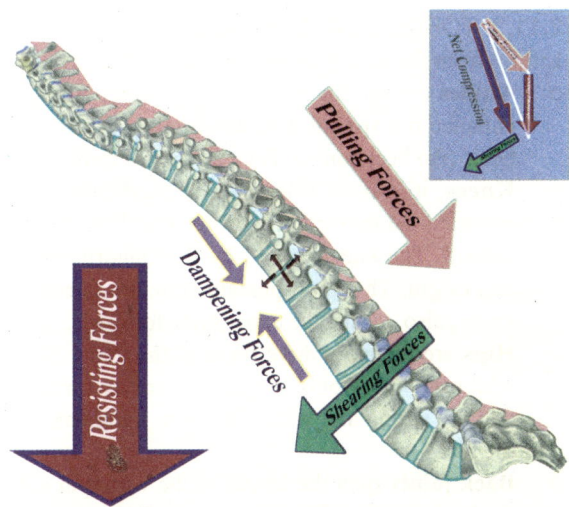

Figure 2.21. The mechanics of vertebras. Intervertebral joints lie on the back. Spinal tunnel lies in the middle. Discs that perform cushioning lie on the front. Spinals nerves exit and enter from the sides.

o The rationale behind limiting the relative motion of the shoulder, upper limbs, and scapulas, during the equalization phase, and even till the barbell clears the knees, is partially explained above in terms of physiological effect on the lifter. In mechanical terms, if two remote parts of the body were accelerating simultaneously, in different directions and with different forces, it would be very difficult to predict the net outcome of motion. Most probably than not, simultaneous forces, in different directions and at different locations, result in clumsy technique. Simplification of motion, to a driving force by the lower body accompanied by tensile force by the upper body, enhances lifting performance by focusing the mind of the lifter on two isolated, yet consecutive tasks.

2.11. THE PHASE OF EXTERNAL MOTION

2.11.1. INTERNAL DISTURBANCE

Only a portion of the force imparted on the object is utilized in setting the particles of that object into **apparent external motion**. The other portion of the force upsets the internal particles of the object. While the object remains apparently motionless, its particles are set into **internal motion**. All material objects inhere such basic internal reaction to external disturbance. Different states of matter manifest such internal reactions in different manners, as follows.
o **Gases** manifest dramatic internal effects in reaction to forces, by virtue of their weak inter-particular bonds.
o **Liquids** are slower than gases in expressing internal responses to forces.
o **Solids** have stronger inter-particular bonds and are the slowest, of the three states, to respond to forces. A considerable portion of the energy required to move solid objects is consumed as heat due to the fore-mentioned strong inter-particular forces.

When equalization forces (exerted by the lifter) surpass the internal forces (the inertia of material objects), the object would not still move arbitrarily. There is another force that has to be overcome to bring the object to a weightless state.

2.11.2. EXTERNAL MOTION

As the lifter maintains exerting force beyond that point of inertia equalization, the object moves according to the laws of conservation of motion. The apparent motion is thus the result of the upward **vertical pull** minus the gravitational **downward pull**, as follows.
o At the bottom, where the barbell rests on the floor, the barbell commences motion from **zero velocity**.
o Every passing moment, the velocity increases by an infinitesimal, in proportion to the elapsed time and the exerted force.
o The summation of these infinitesimal increments of the velocity of the barbell reaches certain levels where it matches the velocity of contraction of the muscles of the lifters.
o When this happens, the lifter will be able to guide the barbell to its final destination, be that the shoulders as in the Clean, or overhead as in the Snatch.

A well-trained Weightlifter learns how to **time the moment** where his pull matches the sum of the gravitational pull and the pull due the acquired acceleration.

2.11.3. TORQUES AND FORCES

Lifting from the floor follows a trajectory that is determined by seven major joints, as follows.
o **Ankles** control the entire body posture. Ankles transfer the weight from the heels to the front of the feet in order to enhance the **spring and cushioning** effect. This is achieved by the pull of the calves on the calcaneus bone of the heels (the heel bones). Thus the ankles torque the whole body forwards.
o **Knees,** in trained lifters, are strengthened beyond the limits that many people might believe could happen. Knees generate the upward drive force that lifts the body, the barbell, and stands the upward acceleration of both body and barbell. The knees extend by the Quadriceps, which are multi-pinnate; each pinna has different direction, insertion, and origin. The multi-pinnate structure is rich in blood supply and in the width of origin of pulling forces. Thus the knees, also, torque the upper body forwards.
o **Hips** are the main drive force of the torso. They differ from the knees in that they torque the entire torso backwards, while the knees only torque the femurs forwards. As with the knees, the hips are supported by multi-pinnate Glutei that are strong and wide. The front ligaments of the hip joints are the strongest in the body and prevent dislocation of the hip.
o **Back joints** span the length of the vertebral column. These joints generate the extension of the back by the action of the back erectors. They play as stabilizing joints rather than as mobilizing.
o **Shoulder** joints are critical in both controlling the trajectory of the barbell, as well as the free flow of blood and air through the neck inlet. The shoulders protect the passage of blood vessels under the clavicles to the arms, elevate chest cage to allow open trachea and vessels passages through the neck. The shoulders stabilize the pull, while the legs are moving the body, and complete the pull when the legs finish their task. The shoulders torque the arms, with the bar, to higher levels.
o **Elbows** play two roles. They stabilize the upward pull and end the pull by bending the forearms on the upper arms, to rack the bar on the shoulders or above.
o **Wrists** also play two roles. They extend during the phase of lifting below the shoulders and flex above the level of the shoulders.

The major torques are maximal around the hips, knees, and ankles. Torques have to be minimized at the wrists since hand tendons cannot endure excessive forces. Torques are generated when forces act away from the vertical line of the centers of gravity. Torques tend to bring the centers of gravity closer.

Advanced Weightlifting comprises mastering the maximization of torque of the body joints, while keeping the barbell moving under vertical forces with minimal bar torque. Remember that torques are forces that act in curved direction around pivots.

2.11.4. SYNCHRONIZING THE PULL

o As the barbell is gaining speed upwards, below the level of the kneecaps, it is not prudent to exert the most burst of power by yanking the barbell. Below the level of the kneecaps, the barbell is too slow to yield to the strongest pull, and it is wiser to maintain **slow and strong** advancing, at least up to the level of the kneecaps. Strong and slow pull cannot be perfected without solid hardening of the body, from the hips upwards. As long as the shoulders are kept behind thrust chest, in the "T" **posture** with the vertebral axis, then slow and strong Pull can proceed steadily.
o Having passed the kneecaps, the course of ascent is free for the ultimate speed. This is accomplished by the forward **thrust of the hips and the extension of the back.**
o The final burst of power comes from the **shoulder muscles** that generate vertical pull. This elevates the bar to the top of the thighs, by the shrugging of the upper fibers of the Trapezius. Simultaneously, the Glutei and spinal erectors generate a torque at the hip joint. That throws the upper body backwards around the hip joint.
o Portion of the vertical Pull is generated by the **calf muscles,** particularly at the end of the shoulder shrugging. This happens when the lifter elevates the heels off the floor, to add extra displacement to the barbell above the upper thigh. A similar portion of the torque is generated by the calves that throw the entire body backwards, around the feet balls.
o Having extended the entire body and hopped on the feet balls, the shoulder kicks in, with **abduction of the arms** to slide the bar from the top of the thighs to the breast level. Standing on the feet balls, with heavy barbell held in both hands, cannot last for long. Thus shoulders abduction has to proceed very instantaneously, and is immediately followed by elbow elevation (**shoulder flexion,** in the Clean lift). This occurs in the same time of **dipping with knees and hips** to lower the body under the barbell. In the Snatch lift, the shoulder abduction is followed by immediate extension of elbows and wrists to place the bar overhead.
o Timing the Pull, therefore, has to start, below the kneecaps, with **slow isotonic contraction** of the lower body and **strong isometric contraction** of the upper body.
o Above the kneecaps, a torque with the head and hips (as two terminal weights on the vertebral axis) **speeds lifting** quite bit. As the bar approaches the upper thighs, a trained lifter will **waste no time in performing the final Pull.** This is the stage of weightlessness, as the upward Pull generates sufficient acceleration to counteract the gravitational Pull.

2.12. MUSCULOSKELETAL BACK PAIN

Back injury is also discussed in details in Chapter Sixteen, on Exercise and Injuries.

2.12.1. PREVALENCE
Musculoskeletal low back pain is one of the most common complaints among adults and is encountered more frequently with lifting. Lower back pain is not a common complaint in children and, when present, is more likely to be due to factors other than musculoskeletal causes, such as meningitis or neoplasm. Lifting causes lower back pain through its effects on the nerve root, muscles, tendons, ligaments, joints, and bones. Most causes of lower back pain are not life threatening; however, significant morbidity is associated with chronic lower back pain. Also, most cases of back pain treated in the emergency department are not true emergencies, but rather apprehension on the side of a patient unfamiliar with spinal issues. A significant number of patients with low back pain are unable to return to their normal daily routines or function in a productive work environment, due to excessively unstable spinal structures.

2.12.2. NERVE ROOT SYNDROME
Weak spinal structures, such as the spinal discs, deform under shear stresses, produce anatomical impingement on nerve root. This is characterized by sharp, localized radicular pain that may be accompanied by abnormal skin sensation, or paresthesia. Impinged nerve root can be diagnosed by stretching the root, while raising the leg of the opposite side. This straight leg-raising test causes substantial pain on the side of impingement. Minor anatomical deformities due to lifting may cause irritation of the nerve root. This produces dull, poorly localized pain, without paresthesia or radiation of pain.

Structural deformities that cause nerve root impingements are:
o **Herniated spinal discs** are produced either by forceful shearing imbalance or by discs degeneration. The thinned or torn sheath of the disc allows the nucleus pulposus to protrude out of the central cavity of the disc, against an adjacent nerve root. The most common locations for herniation are the lower back discs. The lowest disc at L5/S1 is involved more than the discs at L4/L5 and L3/L4. Massive herniation of disc material into the spinal canal, at the cauda equina, compresses the caudal sac. This presents as bilateral sciatica, with lower extremity, bowel, or bladder dysfunction, or paralysis. It may require immediate decompression surgery to prevent permanent neurological damage.
o **Spinal stenosis** is the narrowing of the disc space, due to aging. The narrowed intervertebral space limits the range of motion of the vertebral column and produces inflammation and nerve root impingement, with slightest trauma and without disc herniation. Radiographic studies show evidence of degenerative joint disease. Patients with this disease process often complain of progressive pain, down the lateral aspect of the leg, during ambulation (pseudo-claudication). This sort of pain is caused by neurologic compression, rather than the circulatory compromise in claudication. The stoop test helps distinguish true claudication from pseudo-claudication. Patients with true claudication sit down to rest when pain occurs, while patients with pseudoclaudication[7] attempt to keep walking by stooping or flexing the spine to relieve the stretch on the sciatic nerve.
o **Spinal degeneration** due to aging is the proliferation of degenerative changes in the nucleus pulposus, its annular sheath, and surrounding structures (spinal canal or foramina). With prolonged standing or walking, proliferation causes root impingement, instability due to pseudo-spondylolisthesis[8], and morning stiffness.

2.12.3. MUSCULAR AND FASCIAL PAIN
Pain originating from muscular and fascial sources is felt over localized areas, restricted to a peripheral nerve. It is characterized by tenderness, loss of range of motion in the involved muscle groups. Stretching the affected muscle group may relieve the pain. When generalized stiffness, fatigue, and muscle ache and tenderness are encountered Fibromyalgia may be suspected. Soft tissue pain, during the lifting years, is attributed to lingering recuperation from intense lifting or overtraining. A day or two of rest, hot sauna, massage, sleep, and proper nutrition may expedite recovery and increase subsequent body strength. However, soft tissue pain due to autoimmune inflammatory condition may require analgesic medication to relieve the inflammation.

2.12.4. SKELETAL PAIN
Pain due to bone and joint afflictions are rare in Weightlifting. The following are the main causes of skeletal pain.
o **Infection** of the bones of the spines causes osteomyelitis. This is a serious process that requires immediate attention in order to avoid chronic side effects. Clinical findings are nonspecific, and the patient may be afebrile on presentation. Classic presentation includes pain on palpation of the vertebral body, elevated sedimentation rate, and complaints of pain, out of proportion to physical findings. Patients particularly at risk for development of osteomyelitis include

---
[7] Pseudoclaudication differs from claudication in that limping is not caused by vascular factors in the pseudo limping, as in the true limping.
[8] Pseudo-spondylolisthesis refers to degeneration or deficient development of the structures of the vertebra.

patients who have undergone recent back surgery, intravenous drug users, patients with immunosuppression, and those with a history of chronic pelvic inflammatory disease.
- o **Inflammation** of the joint ligaments such as in the sacroiliac joints. This pain presents over the sacroiliac joints, radiates to the anterior and posterior thighs, and is worse at night or by prolonged sitting or standing. Sacroiliitis usually presents with pain over the involved joints and no peripheral neurologic findings.
- o **Malignant tumors** of the spine can be primary or metastatic. Most primary spinal tumors are found in patients younger than 30-year of age and usually involve the posterior vertebral elements. Metastatic tumors are found mostly in patients older than 50-year of age.

2.12.5. CLINICAL PRESENTATION OF LOWER BACK PAIN

Patients most often complain of pain in the lumbosacral area (lower back). Pain starts at a sudden, during lifting and may last few days to weeks. The pain is gradual with degenerative causes, over days or months, and progressively worsens. The pain is exacerbated by movement or by prolonged sitting or standing. Lifting or moving furniture can precipitate the pain. Infectious causes may produce systemic symptoms such as fever, weight loss, dysuria, cough, and bowel or bladder problems. Infection causes pain by inflammation. Chronic steroids may predispose to infection or compression fractures by demineralization of bone. Also, anticoagulants may result in bleeding or hematoma that causes pain by compression

On physical examination, a patient with back pain has limited range of motion and, or neurologic deficits in peripheral motor function, sensation, and deep tendon reflexes. Straight leg testing, with the patient lying on his or her back, reveals nerve root impingement. Abdominal examination must exclude intra-abdominal pathology. Rectal examination is carried out on men older than 50 years to assess prostate size and exclude prostatitis. It is also performed on any patient who may have cauda equina syndrome, to assess rectal tone and perineal sensation. Also, rectal exam is performed on younger males who are febrile and have urinary complaints. Pelvic examination is performed, if necessary, on females complaining of menstrual abnormalities or vaginal discharge.

Classic presentation includes numbness in a dermatomal distribution (skin areas supplied by specific sensory nerves) corresponding to the level of disc involved, with findings of motor weakness and reflex loss. Herniated discs have different presentations depending on the location, *Table 2.2*.

Table 2.2. Locations of herniated spinal discs and their symptoms.

Location of disc hernia	Radiation of pain	Motor weakness	Sensory loss	Reflex loss
L3/L4	Front of the leg	Knee extension	About the knee	Loss of knee-jerk reflex
L4/L5	Side of the leg	Foot dorsiflexion	Web of the big toe	No reflexes lost
L5/S1	Back of the leg	Foot plantar flexion	Back of calf and lateral foot	Loss of ankle jerk

2.12.6. WORKUP FOR BACK PAIN

Urinalysis is performed to exclude systemic diseases, other than musculoskeletal or an exacerbation of chronic back pain. Complete blood count (CBC) and erythrocyte sedimentation rate (ESR) are performed if the patient is febrile or may have an epidural or spinal abscess or osteomyelitis. ESR has moderate specificity; sensitivity is relatively high in cases of abscess.

Lumbosacral spine series are expensive and expose the gonads to more radiation than a chest x-ray, but most have little value in directing therapy, particularly among patients younger than the age of fifties. Malignant involvement of vertebral bodies can be evident on plain film when as little as 30% of the vertebral body has been replaced. Other indications that suggest the need for radiographic imaging include chronic steroid use and acute onset of pain in older or very young patients.

CT scan and MRI are generally considered the studies of choice for more precise imaging of the vertebrae, paraspinal soft tissues, discs, or spinal cord. Myelography, followed by CT scan, is often used to enhance diagnostic imaging. Ultrasound may be useful if the differential diagnosis includes appendicitis, a pathologic pelvic process, or abdominal aneurysm. True emergencies that necessitate imaging include a history of malignancy, new evidence of nerve entrapment, back pain associated with paralysis or gross muscle weakness, bowel or bladder function loss, and an epidural hematoma or abscess is suspected

2.12.7. TREATMENT OF BACK PAIN

Traumatic injury requires full spinal precautions. Non-traumatic injuries are made more comfortable by supporting the lower extremities with a pillow or blanket. New neurologic deficits, accompanied by bowel or bladder dysfunction, may be caused by cauda equina syndrome, which mandates emergency imaging and consultation.

Conservative therapy is the mainstay of treatment, as even those with true sciatica generally respond with fast recovery. Ultimately, only few patients with sciatica or with true disc herniation require surgery. Conservative therapy traditionally includes the following:
- **Bed rest**, once the cornerstone of treatment, is no longer widely employed. Even brief bed rest is not necessary except in patients with true sciatica. In this case, the supine position decreases pressure on the spinal cord itself. Early return to work on light duty or restricted activity seems to lead to better long-term outcomes.
- Use of **hot or cold compresses** has never been proven scientifically to speed symptom resolution, but some patients may experience brief relief. Gentle flexion/extension exercises are helpful. Spinal traction is ineffective.
- Pharmacological therapy involves both **anti-inflammatory** medication and **muscle relaxants**. Narcotics may be employed initially to gain relief, but their chronic use is associated with increased functional impairment. Steroids, while highly recommended by some practitioners, lack prospective confirmation of their value. Many physicians feel a single burst or short course of oral steroids can be beneficial, particularly in those with a significant degree of inflammation. Epidural steroid injection may also bring significant short-term relief, but this treatment is not without adverse effects and has not been shown to provide lasting benefit. Unless the patient is allergic to the medicine or it is otherwise contraindicated, severe lower back pain in patients admitted to the emergency department can be improved significantly with a combination of the following NSAIDs (non steroid anti-inflammatory drugs) and muscle relaxants.
    i. Ibuprofen (Ibuprin, Advil, Motrin) and Naproxen (Anaprox, Naprelan, and Naprosyn) treats mild to moderate pain by inhibiting inflammatory reactions and pain. It decreases prostaglandin synthesis.
    ii. Flurbiprofen (Ansaid) acts as analgesic, antipyretic, and anti-inflammatory. It also decreases prostaglandin synthesis.
    iii. Ketoprofen (Oruvail, Orudis, Actron) relieves mild to moderate pain and inflammation.
    iv. Cyclobenzaprine (Flexeril) is skeletal muscle relaxant that acts centrally and reduces motor activity of tonic somatic origins. It influences both alpha and gamma motor neurons.
    v. Acetaminophen (Tylenol, Panadol, Aspirin Free Anacin) and Acetaminophen and codeine (Tylenol #3) this is the drug of choice for pain in patients with documented hypersensitivity to aspirin or NSAIDs, with upper GI disease, or who are taking oral anticoagulants.
    vi. Hydrocodone bitartrate and acetaminophen (Vicodin ES) is a drug combination indicated for the relief of moderate to severe pain.

In patients without true sciatica or nerve root findings, follow-up is managed by the patient's private physician. If these findings are present, follow-up by an orthopedist or neurosurgeon is preferred. Short-term physical therapy with gentle exercises may be of some benefit. Outpatient therapy generally consists of a combination of muscle relaxants and NSAIDs. In certain cases, a short course of prednisone may also be helpful. Prognosis is quite good for most patients presenting with mechanical back pain. Few of all patients with lower back pain have long-term problems.

Patient education centers on prevention. This includes promoting weight loss where indicated, performing back strengthening exercises, teaching proper lifting technique, increasing overall physical conditioning. Back belts, which are commonly worn in occupations with heavy lifting, have not been proven to prevent back injury.

2.12.8. SPINOSCOPIC EXAMINATION
This modern diagnostic, non-invasive tool assesses the performance of the back by using a computerized setup of video cameras, skin motion detectors, and electrodes to monitor the motion of body curves and muscular activity, under incremental increase in load. The computerized spinoscopic examination specifies the degree of normality of spinal function, estimates an individual's spinal capacity in a simulated work environment, and records changes in condition. This automated analysis guarantees uniformity of evaluation, facilitates patient's follow-up over time, helps tailor treatments and predict outcomes. Thus a clinician with a Spinoscope can perform the task of a skilful training coach who is able to pinpoint anatomical and functional weakness and plan remedial exercises for correcting deficits.

Spinoscopic examination provides the following data:
- During resisting incremental load, the Spinoscope captures skin displacements of the body motion of the trunk and pelvis, by skin motion monitors. **The displacements of skin markers** are averaged during a dynamic movement and can provide information on the range of motion of the hips and trunk.
- The differentials of the skin displacements provide the **velocity and acceleration** of the body segments under loaded movements.
- Surface electrodes capture the electric muscular activity over Multifidus transversospinal muscles and can assess increase of **electrical activity** of the paraspinal muscles. This aids in differentiating chronic lower back pain from the normal.
- Isometric and isokinetic responses of the body motion arc, in response to resistance, are also assessed from skin **displacement analysis under load**.

PROPER LIFTING TECHNIQUES

The captured data provides the following diagnostic information.
- o Asymmetric patterns of motion are detected from the analysis of motion skin markers. Data collected during asymmetrical movements have some correlation with the presence of pathology and pain, especially torsional injuries.
- o The lumbosacral angle, the angle between the T12/L1 disc and the L5/S1 disc, is measured from the analysis of skin markers, placed over the spine. This permits assessing the degree of dynamic back lordosis.
- o The differentials of the skin displacements, over the longitudinal axis, facilitate assessing inter-segmental mobility of the spines. There are significant differences between the normal and injured spinal mobility.
- o The pattern of coordination between the pelvis and spines, during resistance of force, can be compared to those of control groups, or to previous patterns of the same person, in order to evaluate changes in condition. Lower back pain alters the following patterns:
    i. Voluntary **changes in coordination in order to avoid pain** results in abnormal responses to resistance during motion.
    ii. Incremental resistance determines the **threshold for abnormal motion**. Identical load patterns exclude subjective interference.
    iii. **Excessive muscle action** at particular segments can be pinpointed and help localize site of injury or weakness.

2.13. HIGHLIGHTS OF CHAPTER TWO

1. Bending your knees while leaning on a sink prevents serious lower back injuries.

2. If bending your knees are troubling that means you should forgo lifting until you take care of this issue.

3. Approximate the center of gravity of the object you intend to lift to the vertical plane of center of gravity of your body.

4. Proper lifting aligns all force to resist the pull of the gravity. This minimizes the shearing forces on the back.

5. Knees and back do not fare well without exercise

6. When approaching the weight, stand close to the weight. Thrust your chest upwards. Slightly elevate shoulders. Retract scapulae. Bend the knees. Maintain straight back. Tighten your abdomen.

7. Forces do no impart their effect instantaneously. Yanking the barbell dissipates your energy and leaves the barbell dead in its place

8. During Weightlifting, focus utterly on lifting and overcome any distracting thought.

9. A weight held in the arms generates reaction at the knees, equals the weight plus a torque that depends on the displacement of the weight from the knees.

10. The essence of resistance is the regulation and the control of flow of all kinds of energy.

11. Freestyle lifting strengthens the link between the upper body and the lower body, by strengthening the Glutei, Iliopsoas muscles, and the iliofemoral ligaments

12. Remember that motion requires life and life does not come cheap. Demands put on the heart, lungs, and cells due to lifting have to be met by practice and not by mere conviction.

13. You should not risk placing any part of your body under or close to a newly encountered heavy objects before you have assistance by others. Know the stability of the object, have good grip on the object, and have mechanical tools that aid in case of accidental falls

Chapter 3
Fallacies and Their Critiques

3.1. AGGRESSIVE MARKETING AND HEALTH ETHICS

The advent of cybernetics has brought to the forefront the issue of unethical practice of misinformation in the field of health and fitness. The diverse specialization in that field has complicated the debate about the ethical standards of the profession, as follows.

o **Deceptive marketing:** Many self-proclaimed professionals have tarnished the reputation of the health care profession by spreading fraudulent information and marketing health supplements that serve no purpose other than cheating the public. Such unethical misinformation spreads skepticism and confusion about the proper approach to healthy living. Unwary citizens are dismayed with the pushy trickeries of "aggressive marketing" that distastefully intruded on a humane profession.

o **Consumer protection:** The lack of peer review on the advertisement on radio, television, and Internet leads to an uproar of spread of deceptive information. It is doubtful that the government will, in any time soon, effectively curtail the wide spread of deceptive health industries. As for consumer protection agencies, they cannot compete with affluent profiteers of deceptive health products. Therefore, the best protection for the consumer seems to reside in the education and awareness of the public.

This chapter discusses some of the common mischievous practices of concern to health and fitness.

3.2. SMOKING AND ALCOHOL

Advertisement on smoking and alcohol is a vivid example of the deliberate propagation of deceptive information. Smoking and alcohol are the principal culprits in stealing a major segment of the population away from healthy and fit living. The following factors interplay into this dilemma.

o **Advocacy:** Pro-smoking advocates have vested interests in marketing products, regardless of any health complications. Many media outlets launch vicious attacks on anti-smoking advocates, accusing them of trying to rip us of our personal freedom, beginning with the privilege to smoke. They capitulate to the wide spread of unhealthy habits, condone obesity as a personal choice, and mock health advocacy for disease prevention as an intrusion on freedom.

o **Educators:** Educational authorities seem to have given up on the effort of informing the public about healthy choices. They contribute to increasing the acceptance of dangerous habits by embracing moderation, instead of advocating the benefits of complete abstinence from alcohol.

o **Religious institutions:** Even some churches have contributed to such pervasive habits of drinking by making alcohol part of their communion. The fact that alcohol is the single factor that has devastated many people's health precludes its association with goodness.

o **Enforcing ignorance:** The insidious advertisement for alcoholic beverages in association with high quality food services is another trick to encourage alcoholic consumption and to equate it by essential food requirement. The misconception of alcohol as a booster to digestion is so pervasive that it demonstrates the ignorance of the public about the harmful effects of alcohol. Many people even discount beer from alcoholic beverages, and many others discount moderate consumption of alcoholic beverages from the toxic effects of alcohol. The fact is that alcohol is not only inessential to healthy living but also an infamous culprit in slipping down a slippery slope of sick living.

o **Scientific fallacies:** The new trend of praising alcohol for its benefits on reducing myocardial infarction, lowering low-density lipoproteins, and its antioxidant benefits is another chapter in deceiving the public. Most of the scientific articles that track the effect of alcohol on the prevention or reduction of the incidence of myocardial infarction demonstrate the vanity of modern scientific research. The apparent cause of reporting realistic epidemiological facts regarding a specific group of moderate and regular alcohol consumers, does not justify the vanity of tedious statistical analysis to enforce a bad habit. If alcohol consumption has any benefits at all, would not it be prudent to weigh these benefits against the destruction it brings on society?

3. FALLACIES AND THEIR CRITIQUES

- o **Effects on training:** Even the slightest consumption of alcohol would skew the best fitness program in the world. Robust fitness planning requires long-term clearness of conscience in order to concentrate on the workout and to assess the very insidious development in motor skill and performance. Any chemical dependence deprives the trainee from the objectivity to make proper decisions when difficulties arise. In resistance training, there is constant stream of difficulties that arise every workout, with every move of weight or bend of a joint or beat of heart. Enhancing sound plans of health and fitness is harder than reconstructing a city, since you have to perform all the task of the many departments of utility, planning, and financing. Such undertaking is no joke, *Figure 3.1*.
- o **Human vulnerability:** The damning facts about the vulnerability of human addiction are manifested in various behavioral trends, as follows.

  i. Most alcoholics have, unintentionally, slipped away from moderation.
  ii. Most heavy smokers cannot quit, even after developing very apparent health problems as a result of smoking.
  iii. Many acquaintances of television, Internet, or radio would not resort to change the channel or the site when harmful information is distastefully promoted.
  iv. The epidemic of obesity, overweight, diabetes, high blood pressure, and ischemic heart disease afflicts the rich and the poor, the high and the low social classes, and the educated and the not so well educated. It is mainly due to poor habits and human vulnerability to lean towards easy and naïve choices in life of overeating and inactivity.

Profiteers of smoking and alcohol products prey on such human vulnerability to addiction and inaction.

3.3. SEXUAL ACTIVITY AND TRAINING

- o **Sexual priority:** Young athletes have to factor sexual activity into planning for training. Strained understanding of sexuality can incur heavy toll on the future of youth. Taming sexual activity to its proper significance into the whole future of a young trainee is a demanding task. The fact is that youth training is a partial aspect of the integrated learning process that has to be aided with understanding the ultimate goal of learning.

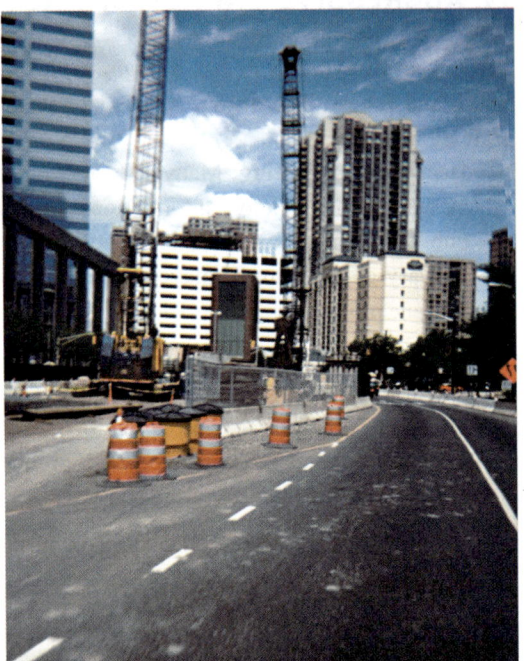

Figure 3.1. Building a city is much easier than building healthy body. To plan a fitness program you alone have to perform all the tasks of planning, developing, and laboring. You will need clear and healthy mind to accomplish your plan, in one life chance.

- o **Unplanned birth:** A serious consequence of unplanned sexual activity is the birth of a child. The economic needs for raising a child are significant burden on young people with little resources. This raises the issues of abortion versus adoption as an alternative solution of family planning. Either option results in serious consequences on the living and the newborn. The trauma of abortion deprives the woman of moral integrity that is dearly needed for peaceful conscience. The very instinct of revering the life of a newborn is fundamental for the innate integrity of the person's mind. Adoption is equally shattering to the healthy mind. It does not make any sense to plan for health and fitness, if the individual does not revere the lives of his or her own offspring. Whether the individual could compartmentalize such disparity of concerns and succeed in planning healthy living is doubtful.
- o **Social enforcers:** The approach of advising youth with practicing safe sex overlooks the drain of mental energy involved in social distractions and failures associated with short term gratifying activities. It is very important to explain to the young the enormous potential they possess to enjoy better life with wise planning and patience. The fear of homosexuality among the youth makes the conviction of abstinence from heterosexual sex a dislikable alternative. Though homosexuality is not the destiny of abstinence, it detracts many insecure youth to seek a fit into the mainstream of heterosexual peers. Such detraction in itself contributes to other aspects of behavior of trying to please others instead of focusing on real personal goals. The issue of sexuality could be brought to the right order in the personal concerns by advancing other skills and motivations in the life of the young. The hypocritical treatment of the media to homosexuality, as norm of life, should be appreciated in terms of the political and public influence on the media. The media and other health organization have chosen less confrontational approach to the issue of homosexuality due to realistic existence in society. Yet, in the field of health and fitness a sound scientific approach have to be followed to deal with health issues.

- **Self-esteem:** Teaching the young to develop their independent personality, without yielding to the pressure of others who try to attract them to a shallow world of sexual obsession and isolation, is a good way to advance healthy sexual identity. Resistance training demands physical strength that is a culmination of whole set of healthy practices. Understanding the biological aspect of human body is crucial to fitness training and the issue of sexuality has to fall along the lines of enhancing biological functions rather than tampering with the well being of a healthy individual.

3.4. DECEPTIVE INFORMATION

Whether it is deliberate deception or unconscious ignorance, the fact that there are abundant examples of misuse of the media through active and organized campaign of deception and fraud. Most of these fraudulent schemes are legally evasive; yet breach all rules of ethics. These are few examples of fraudulent health products.
- "**Holly water** for sale": A radio health program advertises for holly water that cures all diseases by virtue of its unique quantum magnetic fields. The host claims to be a physician practicing in Washington State and claims to discover the secret of quantum magnetism of a brand of water that cures all diseases.
- "**Oil that cures** many maladies": Another program sells the oil of Oregano as a cure for every ailment under the sun. Claiming that guaranteed potency Oregano oil has ability to destroy many different kinds of microorganisms including bacteria, fungus, virus and parasites and that it promotes a healthy immune system.
- False hopes for **fat burning** by enzymatic therapy that claims to be a remarkably effective weight loss aid, with a sensible diet and regular exercise, and accelerates the loss of body fat, while maintaining muscle tissue integrity. The therapy claims to be an improve form of DHEA (testosterone precursor) that is clinically proven safe and effective and clinically proven to burn fat and promote weight loss. The catch here is that sensible diet and exercise will do the job without the product itself.
- "The **Ultimate Aid For Low Carbohydrate Dieters**": claims that it helps inhibit carbohydrate digestion and absorption and helps maintain healthy glucose levels. Thus, you can eat all you want and still lose weight!
- "The **Ultimate Body Sculpting System For Lean Muscular Look**": claims to be designed for athletes, fitness enthusiasts, and anyone else who wants to dramatically improve their body composition (lean body mass to fat ratio). It also claims to benefit healthy body composition; increased growth hormone; reduced body fat; increased lean body mass; optimized metabolism; increased stamina; increased muscular performance. All are vague and convoluted issues that are hard to substantiate.
- "Help Reduce **Unsightly Cellulite**": claims to help rid you of embarrassing cellulite and to effectively prevent and relieve cellulite from bunching up on the thighs and hips and reduce unsightly fatty deposits under skin.
- "Increase **Testosterone and Promote Muscle Strength**": claims to increase free testosterone, enhance recovery, promote tissue repair.
- "Just In Time For Summer **Fuel For Exercise**- Calcium Pyruvate": claims to help you achieve optimum health and fitness, increase energy and stamina, and may assist weight loss.
- An amino acid, a derivative of Glycine, claims to improve overall performance and endurance, to enhance oxygen utilization, to reduce lactic acid buildup, to improve muscle recovery after strenuous exercise, and to significantly improve physical and mental performance.
- "**Magnetic mattresses** for sale": claims that it cures arthritis.
- "**Human growth hormone for sale**": claims the potential to reversing aging and building muscles.
- Secret for a diet that will **revolutionize health** is supported by irrelevant biochemical facts and scientific references in order to prey on the vulnerability of common people.

Others pitch in with their own experience without adequate qualifications and find strong promoters to sponsor their rising star, as long as they are skilled in marketing their tricks. Also, celebrity writers propagate such fraudulent ideas by relying on their fame.

3.5. FALLACIES ON WARMING UP

3.5.1. REASONS FOR WARMING UP
Misconception: *"Warm-up causes rise in temperature and increase in the ability of the muscle to contract forcefully"* (see footnote3, page 53).

Critique:
- Muscles do not contract forcefully by mere use or by rise in temperature but rather by preparation of the nervous system to **recruit** appropriate number of different muscle fibers, for different warm-up tasks. Unconditioned people, for example, might suffer from sense of cold and dizziness during warm-up and may not be able to proceed with core exercises, for which they warmed up.
- Fuel burning in the healthy biological tissue is not similar to burning fires. The temperature does not rise abruptly in healthy muscle. The feeling of warmth is due to more heat generation, rather than to temperature rise. Heat and temperature are different things. When you put your hand on a metal surface, and then on a wooden surface, in the same room temperature, the metal feels cooler than the wood, yet both have the same temperature. The metal conducts

your hand's heat quicker and gives you the feeling of cold.
- o During warm-up, the body temperature rises due to thermal as well as mental factors. This regulation originates in the hypothalamus, which affects voluntary cerebral function and involuntary peripheral vascular flow.[1] Thus, improved performance with warm-up is mainly nervous in origin and not merely local.
- o Only during sickness that the cellular respiratory chain is impaired. Sick tissues fail to use the chemical energy of ATP molecules to generate kinetic energy. Instead they generate thermal energy that causes fever. Thus fever is a sign of sickness. When the person has fever, neither muscles nor heart could sustain resistance training.

3.5.2. PHYSIOLOGY OF WARMING UP
Misconception: *"Warming up pumps fresh, oxygenated blood to the muscles, raise the blood pressure, increases the heart rate, and helps eliminate the waste products of exercise"*.

Critique:
- o Rising blood pressure is caused by constriction of blood vessels and increased vascular resistance. This does not serve to perfuse working muscles. The rise in blood pressure during exercise serves to perfuse the vital organs that lack skeletal muscles[1].
- o Exercise causes sudden pooling of blood into active muscles and deprives vital organs from blood, unless blood pressure rises. The blood flow to muscles increases, instead, because of **sympathetic vasodilatation** in the muscle. Thus warm-up increases the autonomic **nervous stimulation** and more blood capillaries are opened to perfuse the tissue.
- o The **pooling of blood** in working muscles is what provides for the excess oxygen and energy requirements, and not the increased blood pressure or the heart rate. **Increased heart rate** lowers the oxygen level, due to speedy transit of blood through the lungs and less time to exchange oxygen. Only when cardiac output increases and lung perfusion increases when blood oxygen level increases.
- o **Waste products** are not best eliminated during warming up. They pile up and stimulate the sympathetic flow. This activates more blood vessels to dilate (in selective tissues) and more closed ones to open, so as to get ready for pending vigorous exercise.

3.6. FALLACIES ON DEADLIFT

3.6.1. PURPOSE OF THE EXERCISE
The Deadlift, as its name indicates, is a lift that is short of a full lift. In the Deadlif, the barbell does not reach the shoulder level and the lift "dies" before the arms can sustain further elevation of the weight. Deadlifting is best defined as the exercise that strengthens axial muscles and ligaments that oppose gravity. These are the thighs, Glutei, Spinal erector, and Trapezius in that order. Thus, it is not an exercise for the lower back solely as is the situation of Goodmorning exercise, relatively speaking. After few months of Deadlifting, the lifter develops the following characteristic features of axial hypertrophy.
- o The Trapezius becomes apparent on the sides of a muscular neck.
- o The vertebral column sinks between enlarged spinal erectors.
- o The Glutei thicken and form tight buttocks.
- o The thighs enlarge noticeably in the front of the upper legs, if the technique is executed correctly as discussed in *Section 5.2.9* on Deadlift.
- o The skeletal curvature expresses the antigravity, lordotic lower back.

3.6.2. LIMITATIONS OF THE EXERCISE
The Deadlift movement is also characterized by the unique feature of **concentric contraction**. It commences with maximum contraction of the thighs from initially relaxed and flexed knees. This is in contrast to squatting from a rack, where contraction gradually starts from fully extended knees and reaches maximum at full Squat. In this respect, Deadlifting mimics natural driving movement of the axial muscles, from the feet upwards. Yet, this advantage is undermined by the limited range of motion and slow contraction of muscles, as follows.
- o If the Deadlift is not followed by overhead exercise, then the spinal muscles shorten, become strongly stiff, the back loses its flexibility, and frequent injuries are bound to occur. The worst enemy to the integrity of the lower back is immobility, since it causes stiffness. Deadlifting, in Bodybuilding training, is the wrong recipe for strong lower back. In this sport, Deadlifting aggravates stiffness due to the lengthy recovery of few days after such traumatic exercise. In Olympic Weightlifting, very high mobility and wide range of motion of the lower back is practiced in the Snatch and

---

[1] "Samson Wright's Applied Physiology" by Cyril A. Keele and Eric Neil, Oxford University Press, London, UK, 1971. Pages 133, 139, 246, 337, and 339. ISBN 0 19 263321 X

Clean and Jerk. Here, the Deadlift have to be gauged to a certain percentage of the maximum Clean lift. The best remedy to lower back stiffening after the Deadlift is, therefore, mobility in the form of running. Running generates waves of massaging vibration along the spinal structures and thus facilitates relief of inflammation.
- The second worst enemy to the integrity of the lower back is bulking too much mass on the upper peripherals. Looking muscular in the upper half of the body and neglecting the lower body is a costly mistake. If you have gone that way, it is better to start sooner by increasing the volume of lower body training to avoid future crippling injuries. In the Deadlift or heavy Squat days, at least ten minutes of running, at the end of the training session, is very healthy in preventing knee swelling and overnight discomfort. Few sets of Squat, even at low intensity, increase the volume of load on the legs and enhance their growth.
- However, such doctrine of lifting heavier, and rectifying inflexibility and imbalance by more heavy lifting of different variety of exercises, overlooks the dual nature of neuromuscular regulation. Aggressive voluntary exercises are operated by pyramidal neural tract. They lack the fine control of involuntary postural regulation by the extra-pyramidal neural system. You should test your progress in postural balance to avoid inflecting serious problems with regulation of muscular tone such as Parkinsonism or highly spastic muscular tone. This may manifest in decline in ability to perform fine motion such as writing, typing, performing fine hand operations, or inability to behave in docile manner.[2]

The following are examples of common fallacies about Deadlift.

3.6.3. FUNCTION OF LORDOTIC BACK
Misconception: *"Deadlifting with bent back is dangerous because the lower back initiates moving the barbell instead of the lower body."* [3]

Critique:
- The reason that during the Deadlift the back has to slant, with an acute angle with the vertical plane, is to reduce the shearing forces on the intervertebral joints and to transfer the vertical drive of the lower limbs to the bar, with less horizontal losses. The lower back is stressed in either case, since it links the upper and lower parts of the body. The most important thing in the Deadlift is maintaining muscular contraction of the entire back, along the vertebral column, in exaggerated extension, in order to keep the vertebrae on straight line, whether leaning forward or not.

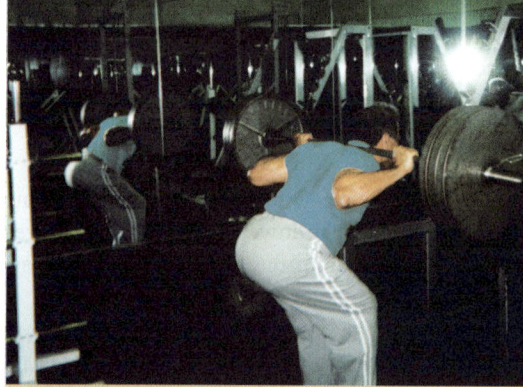
Figure 3.2. Goodmorning with heavy weight, 315 lbs.

- You would not be able to keep straight or hyper-extended lower back if you do not retract your shoulder plates behind your chest. That is because the Deadlift involves forces that transmit from the vertebral column to the arms, passing by the scapular bridge, in the interim. Retracting the two scapulas guarantees that forces will flow from the thoracic part (behind the chest) of the vertebral column, as well as from the cervical part (behind the neck) of the vertebral column to the arms, through the Trapezius muscles. The Deadlift has to start with the scapulae retracted fully and the chest cage thrust forwards in front of the shoulders (when viewed from the side view of the lifter). This guarantees that the arms efficiently transfer forces from the vertebral axis to the barbell, without obstructing the thoracic outlet, strangulating the blood flow to the arms and terminating the resistance. The major traffic of blood vessels occurs under and above the collarbones. These have to be kept elevated during any lifting. Lax scapulas present as caved in chest and cause hunching the thoracic portion of the vertebral column, as well as the lower back.

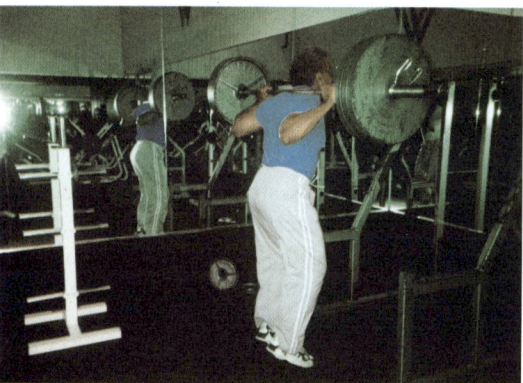
Figure 3.3. Jumping from Goodmorning.
Bending the back forwards in the Goodmorning exercise is not dangerous even with 140 kg barbell (315 lbs), even with jumping on the toes. The danger is in loosening the back muscles while resisting weight. Keeping straight tight back and moving with caution and relying on past experience are keys for strong and healthy back.

- The main danger lies in buckling in of the intervertebral joints. This may cause bulging of spinal discs or dislocating the intervertebral joints. But mere bending of the back, with tightly extended posture, is well tolerated, *Figures 3.2* and *3.3*.

---
[2] "Samson Wright's Applied Physiology" by Cyril A. Keele and Eric Neil, Oxford University Press, London, UK, 1971. Pages 288 thru 303, on muscle tone and regulation of posture.. ISBN 0 19 263321 X.
[3] "The new encyclopedia of modern bodybuilding" by Arnold Schwarzenegger with Bill Dobbins,Simon & Schuster, New York 1999.

3 FALLACIES AND THEIR CRITIQUES

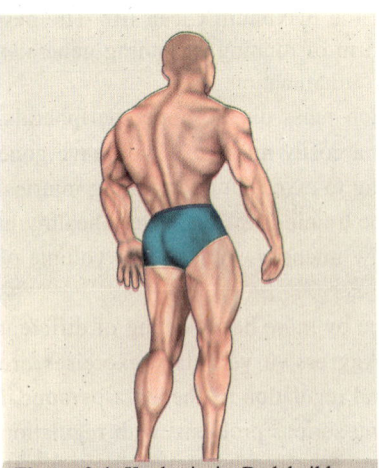
Figure 3.4. Kyphosis in Bodybuilders (hunching of the upper back) results from avoiding freestyle lifting for many years, and building imbalanced, massive upper body muscles.

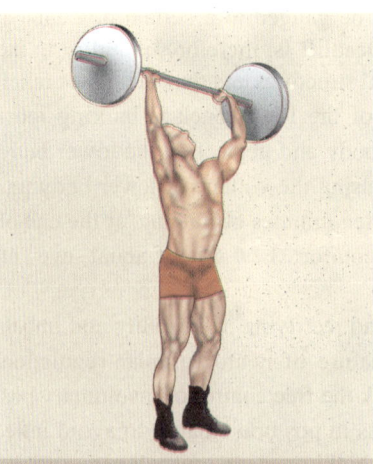
Figure 3.5. Hunching disturbs the forces of balance. The lower lumbar vertebras are too stiff to extend backwards enough to maintain balance. The shoulders are also too fixed to tolerate overhead lifting. Elbows have limited range of motion.

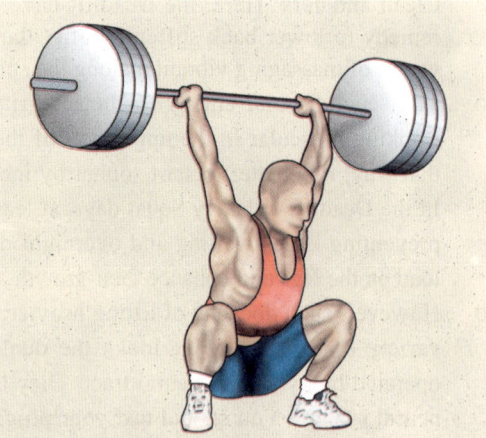
Figure 3.6. A Weightlifter is very comfortable with overhead lifting, in a Squatting position with fully flexible and strong lower back and shoulders. This shows exquisitely balanced vertebral column that allows the lifter to push a heavy weight above his head.

3.6.4. POWER DRIVE IN THE DEADLIFT
Misconception: *"Deadlift with the head kept up and the back kept straight, causes the Glutei, leg muscles, and lower back to generate maximal upward drive force on the bar."*

Critique:
o Neither the head nor the back posture causes maximal upward drive. The main drivers are the Glutei and the Quadriceps. The lower back acts like a lever that transmits the drive upwards along the vertebral column. From the vertebral column, the forces spread to the arms via the scapulas, by means of the Trapezius, Rhombi, back erectors, and front vertebral muscles of the neck.
o To maximized upward drive, you ought to spread the shoulders sideways in "T" shape formation with the vertebral axis and thrust the chest upwards and forwards. This will make the arms feel like making solid conduit with the body axis. Keeping your head up, without first thrusting your chest forwards, is a bad habit that results in upper back hunching and neck injuries.
o Neglecting the "T" angulation, between shoulders and the vertebral column, is responsible for deforming the upper thoracic curvature and enhances the hunching of the back. That is very noticeable in Bodybuilders, *Figures 3.4* and *3.5*. In Bodybuilding, the stiffened shoulders are due to bulky Deltoid muscles, shortened tendons, and stiffed ligaments. With meticulous planning a trainee can maintain such coordination that keep forces in balance and enhances performance, *Figure 3.6*.
o Keeping the back straight without hardened scapulas is useless, since forces will cause buckling of the upper chest. Overextended back (arched forward or lordotic) is very fundamental to heavy lifting, because forces travel along the back surface of the vertebral axis through the spinal joints, ligaments, and muscles. There are no erecting muscles anywhere else but in the back of the vertebral axis. Overextending the back ensures that the forces transmitted downwards the vertebral axis are balanced by the reacting forces transmitted upwards through the spinal joints. With straight back, the muscular strength is barley balancing the external forces. Yet with overextended back the over tightened spinal erectors exceed the external forces in strength and are able to accommodate virtual forces (forces that might unexpectedly appear due to sudden motion). Also, see *Section 2.3* on Upper Body Posture.

3.6.5. SPINAL DISC HERNIATION
Misconception: *"During Deadlift the spinal discs are simultaneously compresses on the front more than the back. Keeping the head up and the back straight distributes the stress and reduces the chance of injury."*

Critique:
o The purpose of proper back posture during lifting is not to distribute the stress on the intervertebral discs, but rather to reduce them to minimal. This is best achieved by overextending the back and not by keeping it straight or keeping the head up. Overextending remove all stresses from the discs and transmits them along the articulating joints, which are located on a plane behind discs. As I have mentioned before, the intervertebral discs are not involved in steady lifting. They serve as shock absorbers during relative movement between the vertebras, *Figure 3.7.*
o The pivotal points, in the center of the surface of articulation of these joints, align well with the central axis of the

spinal cord. Since the spinal cord is about an index finger thick, it bends evenly along its entire length when the vertebral joints bend. This even bending reduces the pull on the spinal cord, during bending the torso, and consequently leaves the existing and entering nerve trunks undisturbed.

o Remember that you should not try to overextend your back in the way I have described unless you have advanced in Weightlifting and that you understand the significance of essential warm-up, progressive graduation of resistance, and the whole analysis of proper training, *Figures 3.8* thru *3.10*. Overextending ligaments that lack flexibility, habitual conditioning, and warm-up may cause serious injury.

3.6.6. OVERHAND AND UNDERHAND GRIPS
Misconception: *"Deadlifts grips with an overhand grip and an underhand grip"*.

Critique:
o Asymmetric bar gripping, with overhand and underhand grips, is a dangerous practice. Asymmetry affects the anchoring of the humerus heads on the joints of the shoulders. Thus one arm is rotated more than the other and the shoulder rotators contract unevenly on each side, conveying twisting forces to the upper spinal region.

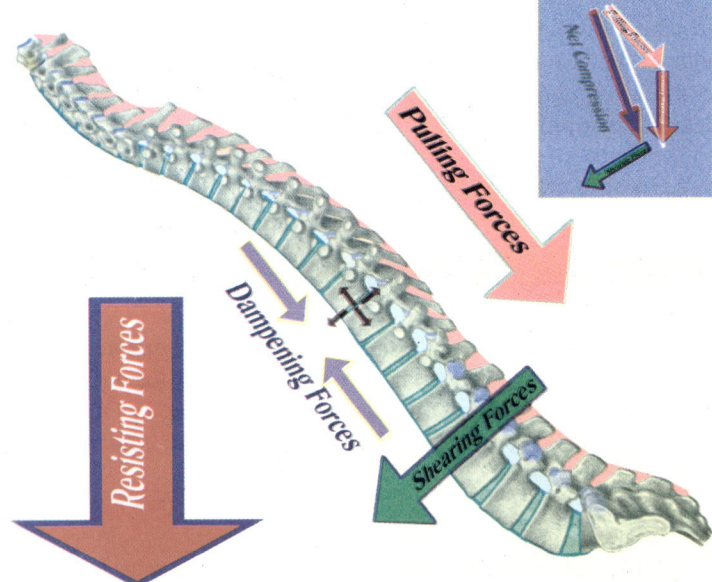

Figure 3.7. Spinal discs and spinal joints. Forces transmit along the back of the vertebral columns. Cushioning occurs along the front of the column.

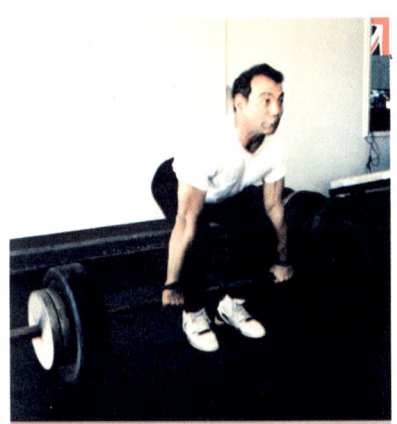

Figure 3.8. Overextended back, adequate chest thrust, and proper angle with vertical, while lifting heavy weights, ensures adequate safeguard against virtual forces.

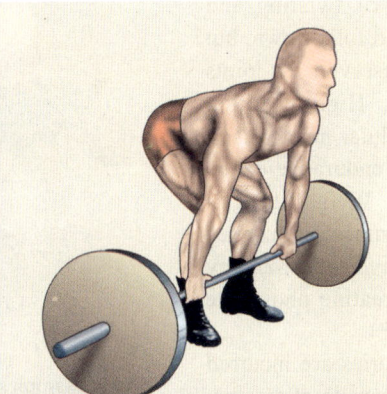

Figure 3.9. Maintaining straight back puts the vertebral joints in insecure misalignment position and could cause serious injury on sudden motion.

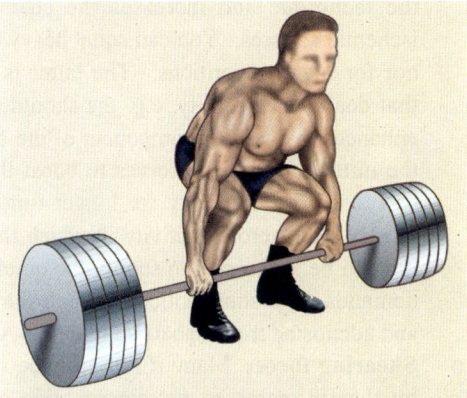

Figure 3.10. Notice the loss of hyper-extended lower back, hunching of upper back, and caving in of the chest, in a Bodybuilder.

o This is apart of the uneven loading of the articulating surface of the upper arm, the humerus, which could cause traumatic arthritic changes. When you deal with heavy weight you better grip the bar symmetrically and do not reinvent unnecessary styles. You could alternate the symmetrical grips if you are targeting a specific anatomical structure.

o With either handgrip, you should remember to balance your shoulder muscles. Whatever muscles you have tightened will shorten and undermine your shoulder mobility, unless you perform stretching exercises with the same load volume and duration in reversing tightening. Simply put, whatever you have labored to tighten must be equally stretched.

3.7. FALLACIES ON INJURIES AND LIFTING

3.7.1. ABDOMINAL HERNIAS
Misconception: *"Males have a congenital weakness in the lower abdominal wall that gets torn on heavy lifting when breathing is withheld and abdominal pressure is raised too high. A tear in the abdominal wall is called a hernia"*[3]

3 FALLACIES AND THEIR CRITIQUES

Critique:
Both males and females can have congenital or acquired defects in the abdominal walls. [4] Hernia is the protrusion of abdominal contents through these defects. Thus both males and females can have hernia. Hernias do not occur frequently in athletes during training. Hernias occur in people with feeble muscular abdomen or congenital defects but not in all males. Also, no **tear** occurs in hernia but rather imbalance in muscular contraction that allows the abdominal viscera to extrude through defects in the abdominal wall. Regular exercise may prevent hernia by strengthening muscles and regulating bowel movement.

3.7.2. KNEE INJURIES
Misconception: *"Injuries to the knee occur during heavy Squats due to stress of bending, bouncing at the bottom, or squatting bellow parallel."*

Critique:
The idea that **heavy Squats** stress bent knees has deterred many people from even contemplating lower body exercise. Heavy Squats do not cause knee injuries as long as the anatomical and physiological rules that govern the knee structures and function are upheld. The best example is seen in Olympic Weightlifters squatting deep, fast, bounce and recover beautifully as demonstrated in *Figures 12.33, 12.34, 12.48, 12.50-51,* Chapter Twelve. The following are the main causes of knee injury.

The following are the main causes of knees injury.
- **Irregular squatting** schedules allow the knee muscles to waste faster, the ligaments to shorten and stiffen, and the proprioreceptors of motion to become sluggish. Regular daily leg exercise is essential for developing not only bulky muscles but also responsive neuromuscular balancing ability. Regular leg training enhances the readiness of the lower body.
- **Highly repetitive squatting.** The lower limbs serve stability function and strengthening them with heavier resistance is superior to repetitive low resistance. Squatting ten times per set is gruesome, wears the cartilages, worsens the technique and increases the chance of twisting and ischemic stresses. You can squat heavy and fully down, but not for many repetitions. The latter is reserved for joints that deal with mobility, e.g. the shoulders. High repetition enhances the aerobic component of the cellular metabolism, the mitochondria, and serves to boost the endurance of the cell to carry on activity for longer times. Weightlifting is mostly an anaerobic activity in which the muscles enzymes have to be stimulated to supply the quick and robust energy demands on a short notice, through the creatine phosphate and adenosine triphosphate shuttle (CP-ATP).

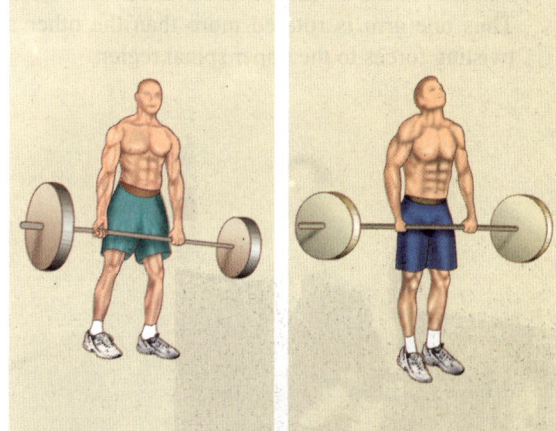

Figure 3.11   *Figure 3.12*
Two examples of partial overloading exercise that do more damage than good. Both trainees show poorly trained lower body, yet they shrug heavy weights from a rack support, for short distance. The only result of this famous exercise is stiffness of all the extensors and trauma to the knee in the standing position. After few months of such traumatic training, trainees suffer from frequent knee and back injuries and reduced ability to perform agile movements. Shrugging should only complement full range of freestyle lifting from the floor, to overhead. You should stop that damn exercise if you notice limited flexibility of the back, shoulder, or knees.

- **Shearing forces.** Many if not all knee injuries are incurred by shearing stresses, not compressing or tensile stress that obey anatomical rules. Many injuries occur during walking, running, or using the knees in the wrong sequence of exercises, when their readiness is inadequate.
- **Momentum.** Developing huge upper body on narrow "lower base stance" predisposes the knees to injury if the upper body is stopped suddenly during walking or running. As when a person tries to avoid colliding with an object. The probability of faring better in this situation is higher with proper body proportions.
- **Partial loading** of the knee articulating surfaces, with extremes of weight resistance, is another major cause of knee injuries. Partial overloading encompasses short-range exercises with heavy loads, without constantly assessing the consequences on the knee performance, as follows.
    i. Excessively heavy Deadlift without equally exercising the upper body and without assessing flexibility or agility. If **deadlifting** to that extreme limits knee flexibility or reduces agility drive, it should direct your attention to a traumatic damage of a partial area of the knee.
    ii. Another example is performing **Half Squat** from a rack. Loading a barbell with excessive weights and dipping for

---
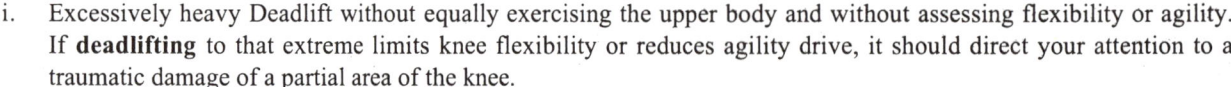
[4] "Bailey & Love's Short Practice of Surgery" by A. J. Harding Rains and H. David Ritchie, H. K. Lewis & Co., London, UK. 1975. Page 1059.

few inches in the Squat is a serious traumatic exercise. It crushes the cartilage, deforms the menisci, and causes quick and chronic knee injury.

iii. **Leg press** machine with twenty plates or more is a sadistic, partial overloading, of the anterior third of the knee surface. It deforms and wears the knee cartilages and the renders the trainee to life-long disability.

iv. **Shrugging a heavy bar** from the rack, without incorporating the exercise in a whole program of evaluation of knee performance. Shrugging 300- or 800-pound barbell from a rack might be a priding subject to brag about with friends, but it does not put you on the right path to health and fitness, *Figure 3.11* and *3.12.*

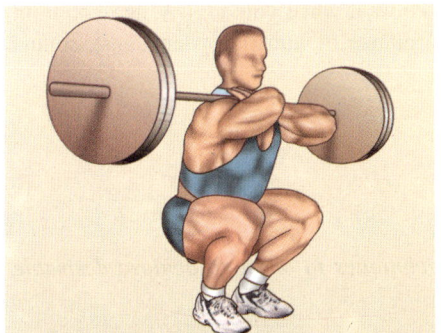
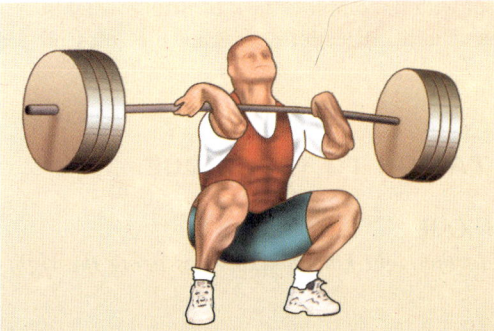
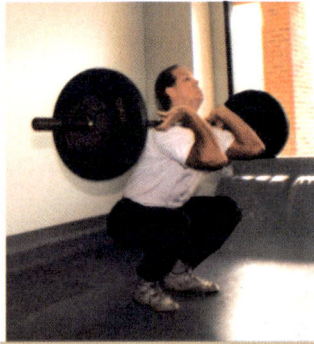

Figure 3.13   *Figure 3.14*   *Figure 3.15*

Figure 3.13. Due to loss of flexibility of his shoulder joints, a Bodybuilder has to cross forearms and put the palms on the top of the bar, instead of under the bar. This demonstrates the severe stiffness in the forearm extensors that prevents the wrist from extending and carrying the bar in hand grip under the bar.

Figure 3.14 and 3.15. Weightlifters demonstrate fully flexed shoulders and elbows, with fully thrust chest and hyper-extended lower back.

3.7.3. INSIDIOUS DEFORMITIES
Misconception: *"Bodybuilders do not suffer training-related injury beyond muscle strain or sprain."*

Critique:
Bodybuilders incur more injuries and deformities than any other sport because of the lack of professional standards of training, self-medication, and unclear goals. An example of lack of intelligent standards of Bodybuilding training is the sequence of routine of training. Bodybuilders work out the chest, then the back, then indulge in the most stressful exercise of Deadlifting, for three sets, of four to ten repetitions each.
Tackling the Deadlift with unconditioned pelvic muscles traumatizes the back severely and sets the process of weak stiffened back, *Figures 3.9* and *3.10*. Deadlifting has to follow freestyle lifting from the floor, either the Clean or the Snatch, until the freely lifted weight comes closer to the weight intended for Deadlifting. Thus the thigh muscles and the Glutei experience a gradual increase in resistance, instead of the abrupt heavy Deadlift after upper body training.

Also, shortening of ligaments and tendons in Bodybuilding is pervasive and life-long problem. Bodybuilders cannot flex the shoulders in Front Squat due to seriously imbalanced scapular muscles, *Figure 3.13*. Buckling of the upper thoracic vertebras is exclusive to Bodybuilding training due to lack of floor lifting with proper technique, *Figure 3.4*. Insidious and permanent deformities render trainees unfit to many sport activities and lead to short longevity in fitness. The shallow definition of injury as an acute and distressing pain is misleading. Long term stiffness and progressive loss of range of motion of joints are incurred due to insidious injuries. These undermine fitness and thwart planning for competitive sports.

3.8. FALLACIES ON SPORT VERSUS EXERCISE

3.8.1. SPORT VERSUS EXERCISE
Misconception: *"Bodybuilding is a sport of form while Weightlifting is a sport of measurement."*

Critique:
"Form" refers to the quality of performance, as an indication of fitness. Body shape, per se, does not amount for good form, unless it engages in skillful motor skill. Bodybuilding, the way it is advertised in popular circulation, defies all principles of fitness, by virtue of its untoward effects on the mobility of joints, the heart performance, the endocrine system, the mental state of obsessed worriers, and indulgence in self-medication. The invaluable experimentation with Bodybuilding in the last half-century can be put to its best use by integrating Bodybuilding methods of enhancing muscles into performance-

oriented planning. This should aim at follow-up assessment of changes in ligaments, muscles, joints, and cardiopulmonary functions, as training proceeds. Performance-oriented planning is a synonymous to scientific sport and is the main theme of this book.

The term "scientific sport" is coined by the author to refer to the integration of multiple disciplines of science in the planning exercise program that enhances health. In Weightlifting, the process of integration started by common people experimenting with lifting weights. This is followed by the efforts of some engineers who founded guidelines for efficient lifting techniques. Along these efforts, experienced retired lifters and fitness educators were experimenting with alteration in the style of lifting with young beginner lifters. With some state support, the sport benefited from the efforts of medical experts in experimenting with the intensity and load of training that can promote performance. The integration of all such efforts were not possible without the genuine belief of those involved in Weightlifting that they have to depend on multiple scientific disciplines in order to deal with the ominous task of lifting weights. You know it when you do it. When you train to lift weights your thoughts expand in all directions, seeking the roles on performance of nutrition, sleep, rest, sexual activity, and amount of training.

3.9. FALLACIES ON ADAPTATION TO TECHNIQUE

3.9.1. ADAPTATION TO TECHNIQUE
Misconception: *"You have to do the right kind of exercises using the right techniques in order to achieve desirable adaptation of the nervous system"*

Critique:
The nervous system controls muscular contraction, as the digestive system controls the muscular nutrition, and the cardiac system controls the muscular perfusion. These systems adapt, not to right exercises or right techniques, but to right planning of long-term workout. Adaptation does not depend on the right technique and right exercises alone, but on a plan that incorporate these two, along with previously learned rules of enhancing integral aspects of fitness. Mobility, flexibility, strength, coordination, and endurance are few functions that require body adaptation to enhance fitness.

You could perform the best technique of execution; yet err on the imbalance of body proportions, joints mobility, or catabolic induction by overtraining. The fact that many trainees believe that they become experts in health and fitness, as soon as they build few big muscles, shows the over-simplicity of the followers of this sport. The shortest way to achieve the adaptation you wish to have is through persistent and regular exercise. Yet, achieving adaptation of invaluable impact on your health and fitness demands lengthy thinking and strategic planning. Any person can hold two dumbbells and perform improper exercises, yet develop big muscles anyway. Yet, to develop healthy adaptation you need to keep your mind open to new discoveries and learn how change with the tide of progressive evolution in learning.

3.10. FALLACIES ON WEIGHTLIFTING

3.10.1. STRENGTH FACTOR IN WEIGHTLIFTING
Misconception: *"Weightlifters are most concerned with ultimate strength. They do a lot of Bodybuilding training and work on balanced development of all the muscle groups."*

Critique:
Strength alone has failed many athletes to become accomplished Weightlifters. I witnessed the strongest athletes frustrated by the demanding nature of the high performance of Weightlifting. Weightlifting requires healthy joints, tendons, and nervous coordination, in addition to strength. Weightlifters perform very agile dynamic skill that requires split-second cooperation of the cardiopulmonary and neuromuscular systems. Such performance requires maximal efficacy when the laws of mechanics are put to immediate test. Strength training is a partial component of Weightlifting and is developed through exercises that emulate Weightlifting freestyle. Emulation of skillful motion ingrains habitual performance and induces the mind to perform by automatic reflex, with very little burdensome thinking and hesitation. Developing balanced group of muscles is also a partial requirement. The other requirements of Weightlifting are:

o   Flexible tendons and ligaments without impeded range of motion,
o   Smooth articulation of joints that permit non traumatic bending and extending,
o   Cardiovascular system that tolerate vigorous gradients of cardiac outputs, and
o   Neuromuscular system that is developed to perform complex balance.

Bodybuilding, on the other hand, is a static training that is executed in a state of mental vegetation and can disturb all vital mechanical functions of the locomotive and cardiopulmonary systems. Bodybuilding is not a standardized sport and its mentors are poorly equipped to lay its basic scientific health guidelines. It is not structured for disciplining and enriching youth personality but for immediate gratification of building firm and big body. The strides made in experimenting with muscular development, in Bodybuilding, can be of great help to other sports if integrated with skillful performance.

3.11. FALLACIES ON FITNESS

3.11.1. LIMITATION OF BODYBUILDING TRAINING
Misconception: *"Bodybuilding training is one of the best methods of achieving physical fitness"*

Critique:
Isolation exercising. Fitness does not start with big muscles, yet may ends with it. Bodybuilders mass bulky muscles that defeat the purpose of fitness. Does today's Bodybuilding enhance this early stage of fitness adaptation? The answer is no. Bodybuilding violates the very essence of fitness that is large heart-size to body-size ratio is the optimum index to fitness. The downfall of Bodybuilding sport is "isolation" exercising. When a muscle is trained in isolation, the entire cardiac output is used to train that particular muscle. Whereas, when the whole body performs in natural motion, there is too little heart pumping capacity with respect to the wildly developed massive system. Thus enhancing the cardiovascular system should guide Bodybuilding training.

Dynamics of circulation. Building massive muscular body disturbs the hemodynamics considerably. That is because the heart does not have the ability to hypertrophy indefinitely, as do skeletal muscles, and in the same time maintains healthy pulsation and contraction in a massive body-size. Any person who is not fit, his right heart would not tolerate such extra load of blood flow and could suffer from sudden irregularity in pulsation. That might force the entire body to cease any physical activity. When we exercise, the very first event takes place in the beating heart, in the form of increased hemodynamics. Therefore, muscular building has to be planned to serve the goal of maintaining healthy heart. The heart of a fit person acquires enough strength and elasticity to tolerate the excessive hemodynamics of exercise. When exercise is properly planned, the heart muscle enlarges, tolerates more transitions in its state, and develops rich circulation to adapt of exercise vigor. In addition, the heart will adapt to nervous and hormonal controls to deal with the havoc of physical stress. In aerobics, Weightlifting, wrestling, gymnastics, swimming, running, golfing, or football, the entire body is used simultaneously, allowing higher ratio of heart-to-body performance.

Dynamics of respiration. Also during exercise, signals from the pressure and the chemical sensors, along the major blood vessels, regulate hemodynamics. These nervous and hormonal signals affect the control centers of respiration and circulation. If the person were fit, the central nervous system would have been adapted, sometimes ago, to respond to the changes as a result of exercise. It will send the right signals to the lungs to open new blood vessels, allow more breathing capacity, and reach the optimum gas exchange rate, of carbon dioxide and oxygen. On the other hand, if the person is not fit, breathing becomes difficult, either fast and inefficient or slow and labored. In that case, the unfit person has to stop exercising to catch breath. Does Bodybuilding enhance this pulmonary function at best? The answer is: slightly, but not on the long run, because of the isolation nature of exercising individual muscles.

Dynamics of perfusion. Pumping of the blood by the heart, and filtering it by the lungs, is followed by the flow of blood from the left side of the heart to the whole body. If the person were fit, the left heart would tolerate the exuberant amounts of blood return and should be able to pump it to the systemic circulation to reach all parts of the body, including the heart muscles themselves, through the coronary arteries. Unfit persons feel abnormal sensation on the left side of the chest, left shoulder, face, or extremities. Because, in this case, the left heart is unable to handle that extra task of receiving and delivering the extra blood, returning from exercising muscles. The features of the heart that impose the healthy or ailing feeling reside in the strength of the heart muscles, the harmonious regulation of its contractility and impulsivity, and the conditions of the four valves that regulate the blood flow through the heart. Thus, in cardiac terms, fitness is best described as conditioning the heart to be free from violations, such as flowing of blood in the wrong direction due to leaky valves (regurgitation), or hesitating to proceed in the right direction due to irregular heart rhythm (turbulence), or slowing the flow due to weak heart walls (congestion). These violations negatively impact the entire health, particularly the brain, the heart, the lungs, and the kidneys, which are vital to vigorous short-term activity.

Dynamics of innervation. Fit performance relies on the nervous control of all muscular activities and blood flow. The significance of refining the motor nervous system by exercise warrants serious consideration. As with acquisition of new skills, the brain adapts to learning by devoting specific areas to specific skills. Learning two languages, for example, is proved to require more than one brain area to process different languages. The complexity of such brain adaptation depends largely on the age of acquiring new learning skills. Thus, Bodybuilding should be used as an adjunct to enhancing fitness as a remedial solution to individual deficiencies. Building optimum mass of musculature is essential to healthy nervous system. Since muscles are the fastest furnaces of fuel, they drive the energy expenditure of the body towards anabolic state,

3 FALLACIES AND THEIR CRITIQUES

which enhances the performance of all body systems, and the nervous system in particular. Nobody should trade the mobility, agility, flexibility, and coordination for the arbitrary and subjective art of Bodybuilding. As the brain adapts to new learning of skills, the peripheral innervation also adapts by refining recruitment function of different muscle fibers and muscle groups to enhance performance beyond primitive ordinary levels. The lesson learned from Bodybuilding is that pushing aerobic muscular activity to higher level of resistance greatly enhances muscular growth. This lesson should be applied to enhancing the components of multi-joint complex exercises that enhance full range of motion.

3.12. FALLACIES ON AEROBICS VERSUS WEIGHT TRAINING

3.12.1. AEROBIC FAT BURNING
Misconception: *"Resistance training significantly increases your metabolic rate at which your body burns fat. That is why weight training is superior to aerobic exercise for people who want to lose fat."*

Critique:
The metabolic rate of burning fat is maximum in aerobic exercises (as in birds and long distance runners) and minimal in anaerobic exercises (such as in weight training). The best fat burner ever is aerobics. Aerobic activities such as dancing, skiing, running, swimming, walking, rowing and bicycling have immense benefits on cardiovascular and mental well being, as well as on weight control. Aerobic folks know how to generate virtual forces by accelerating and decelerating body parts, with their kinetic energy converted to muscular tension. Resistance does not have to be rigid objects as barbells and dumbbells or weight machines.

Weight training is vigorous, bursting muscular activity that relies on the creatine Phosphate as a fast source to generate ATP. It builds muscle mass but is not nearly as healthy, and heart protective, as aerobic exercise. Yet, strong muscles make you more attractive and make it easier for you to maintain an ideal weight.

Fat tissue is not an inactive tissue, it is very active manufacturing hormones, responding to hormones, delivering and depositing fats. It is a rich source of energy and causes health problems when it interferes with vital biological functions such as circulation. Yet, we cannot live without fat since it is the precursor of most hormones and it enters in the membranes of all cells. Exercise guarantees that fat does not stand in the way of getting nutrients to cells. Like driving your car on abandoned country roads, you may find vegetations growing in the middle of the road and blocking your access to the other end of it. Fat deposits on the arterial walls cause similar blocking of blood flow. The core of the problem of excess fat is excess intake of calories and immobility. If you are fat and start by weight training alone you may become less mobile and get fatter and fatter.

3.12.2. PLANNING LOAD VOLUME
Misconception: *"Brief and intense workouts are highly effective and take less than four hours a week. Working out more is not better."*

Critique:
The intensity of workout must evolve as the plan of training unfolds. It depends on the age of the person, his or her goals, and previous history of advanced training. False promises of magic formulas, of briefness and shortness, do not accomplish goals. Many people require longer training hours to alter long incurred problems of excess or less bodyweight or deformities. There are many instances when a person is encouraged to work out more than once a day, with due attention to the volume of load to avoid over-training. This is discussed in details in Chapter Thirteen, Managing Load Volume and Intensity.

3.12.3. EFFECTIVE WORKOUT
Misconception: *"Workouts with weights only three days a week and aerobic training three days a week, on alternating days, is very effective."*

Critique:
This is very arbitrary plan and has no foundation whatsoever. Weight training should be preceded and followed by aerobic exercises, in the same session, to avoid stiffness and inflammation. Planning weight training should not be based on the method of exercising, but rather on the goals one wants to achieve. Also, training for bodyweight control should integrate aerobic and resistance, in coherent manner, to accomplish solid results. Aerobics enhances endurance while resistance training enhances strength; both are needed for long compliance with exercise plan. Yet, endurance and strength are very difficult to maximize, simultaneously. Thus you cannot adhere to strict rules of alternative days if you do not see progress.

3.12.4. SWITCHING MUSCLE FUELS
Misconception: *"Effective weight training helps burn fat and taps into the energy of dormant fat and use it to fuel the growth of muscle"*

FALLACIES AND THEIR CRITIQUES

Critique:
Fat storage is not tapped into by weight training since it requires aerobic conditions. Only sustained physical activity taps into fat depots, via hormonal activation of lipase enzymes and stimulation of fat cells to hydrolyze natural fat and release fatty acids. The liver can metabolize the glycerol portion of the released fat, while the muscles utilize the fatty acids. Many weight trainees cannot burn fat if they cannot control their dietary intakes. Thus, the energy of weight training does not come from fat energy, in the first place. Weight training only conditions the body to perform better and stronger, but it is up to the individual to use such improved performance and alter his or her eating habits.

3.12.5. RECUPERATION
Misconception: *"It is important to give your muscles time to recover from exercise stress. If you work out again before the muscles have had time to rebuild, you will short-circuit the recovery process."*

Critique:
This does not mean that you cancel your workout because of soreness or even injuries. A wise plan of workout should account for predicting sore muscles and working different ones on different sessions. Even injuries could be handled with training uninjured parts, unless general rest is required, as in major injuries. Most soreness is relieved by warm-up and exercises rather than by rest and immobility. Also, the level of recovery form stress increases as training advances. You should gain more insight on what constitutes normal recovery period, from advanced trainers, books, or other sorts of informative media.

3.13. FALLACIES ON NUTRITION AND METABOLISM

3.13.1. PROPER EATING
Misconception: *"Eating is not the key to fat loss. You need plenty of good quality nutrition to build a healthy body"*

Critique:
Unfortunately, in developed nations, eating is the key for fat loss. People consume more calories than expending energy. Building healthy body does not require plenty of food. This depends on individual needs. Good quality nutrition may be obtained by eliminating bad food rather than by adding more good food. Thus cutting the caloric intake might fulfill the condition of good nutrition. Excessive weight gain has to be dealt with disciplined eating habits, with no illusion about the danger of excessive caloric intake.

3.13.2. PROPER CALORIC INTAKE
Misconception: *"Animals that graze constantly, but in far lesser amounts have low body fat and lean muscles. We should graze, not binge. Eat more often than you do now in order to transform your body and feel better"*

Critique:
Eating every few hours stimulates the satiety center and renders the individual addicted to constant eating and subsequent weight gain. Human gastrointestinal tract takes over six hours to digest and absorb a meal, and over twelve hours to eliminate the remains of a meal. Some food may remain in the esophagus or the stomach even after two hours of its ingestion. Also, frequent eating necessitates frequent oral hygienic measures; otherwise the teeth will suffer from accumulation of food remains. If we eat every two hours then floss and brush as often, there will be no plenty of time left to enjoy our healthy living. The advice, of credible health authorities, of eating five servings of fruits and vegetables daily has very solid health foundation. Since fruits and vegetables consist largely of water, have balanced solute composition, contain fibers and vitamins, and contain no cholesterol, they serve all the purposes of healthy nutrition. They do not increase bodyweight or accelerate dental decay. They do not upset digestion. They balance vitamin needs. And, finally they sustain healthy cardiovascular system, as discussed in *Section 14.3.6* on Healthy Diet

3.13.3. METABOLIC FACTORS
Misconception: *"When you eat every few hours, you'll have more energy, less hunger pangs and cravings, you'll be creating a "metabolic environment" that supports healthy fat loss and muscle gains."*

Critique:
Eating every few hours suppresses fat loss since the body will have easier source of energy of food intake. Muscle gain occurs only by exercise not by eating more frequently than necessary. Emphasis on metabolic magic that burns fat and builds muscles is unrealistic. Many people are deceived with the argument that frequent eating causes fat loss and end up in notorious obesity that is difficult to control.

3.13.4. OLD EATING HABITS
Misconception: *"About 8,000 years ago, the Egyptians learned to farm and shifted over to consuming more carbohydrates,*

3. FALLACIES AND THEIR CRITIQUES

primarily in the from of grains. They actually became an obese society with widespread heart disease, stunted growth, and malnutrition." [5]

Critique:
There is no way to rely on statistics of 8000 years ago. We cannot even trust the statistics of few decades ago. Grains are not pure carbohydrates and Egyptians had other diseases of the temperate Africa other than nutritional problems. Also, there is no valid epidemiological data about any ancient life of that remote past. Just few centuries ago, epidemics were widespread all over the world. One does not have to dig in the remote past to justify absurd views. In the old farming society and with poverty, obesity was not the main culprit in causing illness.

3.13.5. CARBOHYDRATE METABOLISM
Misconception: *"Eating a high carbohydrate diet over a long period of time causes" insulin resistant" and develops adult-onset diabetes, which can lead to obesity and heart disease. It also stimulates the appetite and cause mood swings".*

Critique:
Total caloric intake is more important than eating specific food ingredient. Even excess protein or fat would lead to obesity, adult-onset diabetes, and cardiovascular disease. Diabetes does not cause obesity, yet obesity is a major cause of diabetes. The high insulin level, in insulin-resistant states, does not cause more obesity, since the body is resisting its effect, but causes muscle wasting, since no immediate source of glucose becomes available. Insulin is an anabolic hormone. When the cells receptors resist binding with insulin, they do not uptake glucose and thus cannot synthesize enough pyruvate. This is the entry substrate for fat synthesis from carbohydrates. Insulin resistance is thought to be caused by these three culprits: abnormal antagonists to insulin in circulation, abnormal insulin molecules, or defective cellular receptors to insulin.

3.13.6. WATER BALANCE
Misconception: *"The best ways to get rid of water retention is to drink more water, not less. Water retention is just another aspect of your body's survival mechanism."*

Critique:
This is a moronic idea. Water retention cannot be treated with more water. Water retention refers to kidney troubles in filtering excess body water. This might be due to effects of medication on the kidneys. Some diseases cause secretion of an antidiuretic hormone that leads to water retention. Also, low blood protein causes water retention due to low osmotic pressure of the blood plasma. Liver disease cause water retention by both increased portal hypertension and reduced blood proteins. Heart failure causes water retention by failure to circulate fluids. Thus, water retention has to be dealt with clinically with professional care.

3.13.7. NUTRITION AND CORONARY ARTERY DISEASES
Misconception: *"Symptoms of coronary heart diseases could be reversed by diligent lipolytic diet, nutritional supplements and chelation therapy."* [6]

Critique:
Any diligently compliant patient will do well without having to experiment with unproven treatment modalities. Diligently compliant patients can overcome many difficulties by mere exercises without the need for absurd diet that will undoubtedly worsen their conditions. Also, chelation therapy, nutritional supplements and lipolytic diet are the "rip off" tools of many commercial practices. Offering medical solution to every human malady is impractical. Exercise and low caloric intake resolve and improve coronary problems that do not require prescription medications. Chelation is a questionable and risky practice that offers false hopes. Heart patients do not have such healthy liver that can metabolize the heavy fat and protein diet that is prescribed by advocates of low carbohydrate diets. Middle class patients cannot afford the exuberant expenses of extensive and unnecessary laboratory tests that cost a fortune in unproven therapeutic modalities.

3.13.8. FAT AND PROTEIN DIET
Misconception: *" Stopping your cravings through abstinence, rather than moderation, could be accomplished by high fat and protein diet".*

Critique:
Abstinence could be accomplished without further food intake but rather discipline. Abstinence is the remedy of many diseases that result from excessive indulgence and not following lethal diet of high fat and protein that can lead to cancer and cardiovascular diseases. Abstinence could be enforced by indulgence in exercise activities and spending longer times away from food sources. Our closest relatives, the chimpanzees, do not develop cancer colon, since they do not consume

---
[5] "Body-for-life : 12 weeks to mental and physical strength" by Bill Phillips with Michael D'Orso, 1st edition. HarperCollins Publishers, New York, 1999.
[6] "Dr. Atkin's New Diet Revolution" by R.C. Atkin, Avon Books, New York, USA. 1999. ISBN 0-380-80368-2.

meat. Since the body can synthesize most aminoacids and fatty acids from carbohydrates, with the help of vitamins and minerals, it is apparent that humans need few essential animal byproducts to live healthy. These are the essential aminoacids, essential fatty acids, and vitamin B_{12}. Other than that, vegetables are the safest form of food source for humans.

I personally doubt if fat and protein from animal sources are of any value to human health, other than in minute amounts. You do not have to be an expert to notice the difference is composition of vegetables and animal products. Fruits and vegetables have loose structures since they do not have the high-pressure circulation system as animals. Such loose composition of plants contains plenty of fluids and less of packed fats and proteins. Food from animal sources such as meat, cheese, eggs, and fish have very condensed structures and thus contains highly packed fats and proteins, with less water. Also, fats from plants are mostly long chains of unsaturated fatty acids attached to glycerol. These are easily hydrolyzed by the human cells and used to fuel exercise. On the other hand, animal fats contain high percentage of saturated fatty acids and cholesterol. Cholesterol is only synthesized by animals and cannot be used as energy fuel. Cholesterol structure contains four aromatic rings, which stay together during its metabolism to bile or sterol, but never into pyruvate for fuelling Tricarboxylic acid cycle[7].

3.14. MUSCULAR BALANCE

3.14.1. SCAPULAR BALANCE
o   Weight training emphasizes on strengthening muscles with repetitive lifting with very little focus on posture.
o   Bodybuilders neglect the upper and middle back muscles that help keep the shoulders elevated and chest thrust forwards. The upper and middle back muscles are the scapula retractors, the shoulder extensors and external rotators, such as Infraspinatus, Teres minor, and rear Deltoid. Not only sufficient strengthening of these muscles is required but adequate posture and proportionate strength is needed to prevent caving in of the chest. Heavy training of pectoral and Deltoid muscles adds good look to the upper body but pulls the clavicles forwards and causes caving of the upper chest.
o   Weightlifting depends entirely of scapular strength and mobility. Stability of the scapulas is demonstrated while lifting from the floor or overhead. Balanced musculature around the scapulas allows them to rotate around the shoulder and maintain proper posture. Winging, caving in, or shaking while lifting are signs of imbalance.

3.14.2. STABILITY
In multi-jointed creatures, stability is implemented by some joints during the mobility of other joints. Thus not all joints move simultaneously, otherwise, forces of motion would oppose each other and render the motion purposeless. During lifting, the upper body implements stability during the leg drive phase of lifting from the floor. The lower body implements stability during upper body extension and flexion, in the late phases of lifting. The back implements stability more than any other region of the body by virtue of its situation in the middle of leverage. Stability is also implemented while walking, standing, or sitting by the parts of the body that do not require mobility.

Nervous feedback information flows between the brain and the stabilizing muscles to determine the degree stability required and to refine postural tone. Sensors from the limbs, back, neck, and special sensations pool their inputs to local and central neurons that master stability and balance. Stability under high resistance is only possible by training the muscle sensors and ligament ganglia to identify tolerable levels of resistance. Thus stability evolves with training through promoting nervous control and strengthening muscular effectors.

3.14.3. AGONISTS AND ANTAGONIST MUSCLES
Misconception: *"The abdominals are strengthened when one exercises the back, just as the Biceps are strengthened when one exercises the Triceps."*

Critique:
This is an old and wrong belief. Muscles cannot be strengthened unless they resist force that tries to separate their origin from their insertion. Back exercises do not affect abdominal strength since they do not intend to spread the chest cage away, or towards, the pelvis against resistance. Abdominal exercises require bending of the chest cage towards the pelvis against a sort of force. Be that gravity or pushing against objects. The Triceps pulls on a joint as a first-degree lever, with

---

[7] TCA, or tricarboxylic, also called citric acid cycle, or Krebs cycle. It refers to a series of aerobic oxidative enzymatic reactions in aerobic organisms involving metabolism of acetyl Co-A and producing high-energy phosphate compounds, which serve as the main source of cellular energy. It was discovered by the British biochemist Sir Hams Adolf Krebs, in 1936.

FALLACIES AND THEIR CRITIQUES

the pivot lying between force and resistance. Thus the Biceps is not exercised during Triceps training, except to stabilize the shoulder by its long head. Also, the Triceps are not exercised during Biceps training, since the Biceps pull on the forearms between the joint and the resistance without any need for triceps support, other than to stabilize the shoulder. The same could be said about Quadriceps and Hamstrings. While squatting works out Quadriceps, Hamstrings only stabilize the pelvis in the interim.

3.15. HIGHLIGHTS OF CHAPTER THREE

1. Robust fitness planning requires long-term clearness of conscience to concentrate on the workout and to assess the very insidious development in motor skill and performance. Chemical dependence deprives the trainee from the objectivity to make proper decisions when difficulties arise. In resistance training, there is constant stream of difficulties that arise every workout, with every move of weight, or bend of a joint, or beat of heart.

2. The trauma of abortion deprives the woman of moral integrity that is dearly needed for peaceful conscience. The very instinct of revering the life of a newborn is fundamental for the innate integrity of the person's mind. Whether the individual could compartmentalize such disparity of concern and succeed in planning healthy living is doubtful. It is very important to explain to the young the enormous potential they possess to enjoy better life with wise planning and patience.

3. Though homosexuality is not the destiny of abstinence, it detracts many insecure youth to seek a fit into the mainstream of heterosexual peers. Such detraction in itself contributes to other aspects of behavior of trying to please others instead of focusing on real personal goals. Teaching the young to develop their independent personality without yielding to the pressure of others who try to attract them to a shallow world of sexual obsession and isolation is a good way to advance healthy sexual identity.

4. Deadlifting is best defined as the exercise that strengthens axial muscles and ligaments that oppose gravity in the vertical direction. With overextended back, the over-tightened spinal erectors exceed the external forces in strength and are able to withstand virtual forces. Overextended back is very fundamental to heavy lifting. Forces travel along the back surface of the vertebral axis, along the spinal joints, ligaments, and muscles.

5. Deadlifting is best defined as the exercise that strengthens axial muscles and ligaments that oppose gravity in the vertical direction. With overextended back, the over-tightened spinal erectors exceed the external forces in strength and are able to withstand virtual forces. Overextended back is very fundamental to heavy lifting. Forces travel along the back surface of the vertebral axis, along the spinal joints, ligaments, and muscles.

6. Remember that you should not try to overextend your back in the way I have described; unless you have advanced in Weightlifting and that you understand the significance of essential warm-up, progressive graduation of resistance, and the whole analysis of proper training. Overextending ligaments that lack flexibility, habitual conditioning, and warm-up may cause serious injury.

7. Heavy Squats do not cause knee injuries as long as the anatomical and physiological rules that govern the knee structures and function are upheld. Irregular squatting schedules allow the knee muscles to waste faster, the ligaments to shorten and stiffen, and the proprioceptors to become sluggish.

8. An example of partial loading is excessive heavy Deadlifting without equally exercising the upper body and without assessing flexibility or agility.

9. Bodybuilding, the way it is advertised in popular circulation, defies all principles of fitness by virtue of its untoward effects on the mobility of joints, the heart performance, the endocrine system, the mental state of obsessed worriers, and indulgence in self-medication. Bodybuilding is a static training that is executed in a state of mental vegetation and can disturb all vital mechanical functions of the locomotive and cardiopulmonary systems.

Chapter 4 Weightlifting

4.1. STRENGTH TRAINING IN WEIGHTLIFTING

4.1.1. EVOLUTION OF WEIGHTLIFTING

Strength training exercises greatly focus on enhancing the strength and development of the major groups of muscles. Weightlifting is unique in its hundred years history of persistent experimentation with the following elements of strength training.
o   Combinations of diverse **exercises** of global nature.
o   **Sequence** of execution of such exercises.
o   **Amount of time** spent in working out, on daily, weekly, and annual basis.
o   Variation of **intensity** of resistance that leads to building up of strength rather than exhaustion.
o   Variation of **volume** (cumulative intensity over time) that allows replenishment of body reserves and growth.
o   **Individualization** of exercises that can remedy various physical deficits of various individuals.

The chronological evolution of Weightlifting is briefly summarized as follows, *Table 4.1.*

Table 4.1. Changes in weight classes and contested lifts in Weightlifting during the last century.

Bodyweight divisions				Contested lifts (Years)	
Bodyweight divisions until 1992	*Years held*	*From 1996-now*		*Contested Lifts*	*Years held*
Flyweight	52 kg	1972-1992	54 kg	One-handed Snatch	1896-1924
Bantamweight	56 kg	1948-1992	59 kg	One-handed Clean and Jerk	1896-1924
Featherweight	60 kg	1920-1992	64 kg	Two-handed Clean and Press	1928-1972
Lightweight	67.5 kg	1920-1992	70 kg	Two-handed Clean and Jerk	1896-now
Middleweight	75 kg	1920-1992	76 kg	Two-handed Snatch	1928-now
Light Heavyweight	82.5 kg	1920-1992	83 kg		
Middle Heavyweight	90 kg	1952-1992	91 kg		
Class of 100 kg	100kg	1980-1992	99 kg		
Heavyweight	110 kg	1972-1992	108 kg		
Superheavyweight	Over 110 kg	1896-1992	Over 108		

o   In 1896 Olympic games in Athens, Greece, Weightlifting was contested in one- and two-handed lifts.
o   During the turmoil of World War I, Weightlifting was included in 1912 and 1916 games.
o   In 1920 Olympic games in Antwerp, Belgium, competition were held in five bodyweight divisions contesting in three different lifts.
o   In 1924 Olympic games in Paris, France, the contesting lifts increased by two. These were the two-handed Snatch and the two-handed Clean and Press.
o   In the Olympic games of 1928, the one-handed lifts were eliminated and the two-handed lifts were contested.
o   In 1972 Munich Olympic Games, East Germany, the two-handed Clean and Press was contested for the last time.
o   The bodyweight divisions have changed too, as well as the method of awarding medals.
o   In 1964 Tokyo games, Japan, the technical rules were changed to allow the bar to touch the thighs during the lift. Thus, the upper body does not have to work hard to maintain the bar away from the body during ascent.
o   The efficiency of lifting technique evolved from the **spring method** of descending under the bar to the **deep Squat** style of retrieving the bar. Accompanying this evolution, the relative importance of the muscles of the upper extremities in the technique of lifting diminished. Those of the lower extremities increased, *Figures 4.1* thru *4.3.*

4.1.2. SPORT VERSUS EXERCISE

The obvious differences between Weightlifting experience and the other modalities of strength training such as **Bodybuilding, Powerlifting, and general weight training** are:
o   Weightlifting strengthening-exercise religiously observes the need to maintain optimally lean body with **minimal**

weight increase. Enhancing strength while observing lean bodyweight is in congruence with modern scientific guidelines of health and fitness. In young age, beginner athletes mostly have no slightest clue of the consequences of increasing body mass, even if it is pure lean muscles. In all animal species, maintaining higher **cardiac index** positively impacts the health and longevity of an individual within that species. The cardiac index is the quotient of the cardiac output by the square of body height.

o Weightlifting strengthening is no nonsense, **simple and pragmatic,** approach to getting things done in short time and with definite results. Very little hypothetical disputes surround this sort of strength training. Substantial gains materialize within few weeks, in the form of progressively increased ability to lift heavier and heavier weights, with progressive speedier recovery. Bodybuilding training is very deceptive, since it builds individual muscles with little or no monitoring criteria to avoid stiffness, imbalance, or incoordination. Powerlifting training borrows most of its exercises from the Weightlifting, yet lacks integrated total performance of the body.

o Weightlifting training has **definite time** frame to enhance strength, **definite sequence** of execution of exercises to avoid injuries, and **definite requirement** of progressive, continuous, and regular practice to build strength. Also, Weightlifting strength training would not fail a trainee by causing long-term injury, due to faulty anatomical or physiological approach.

o Advancing in Weightlifting training is a **reliable index** of progressive development in integrated muscular, nervous, cardiovascular, and pulmonary performance. Such advancing is quantified by assessing the level of **endurance**, the **power** of lifting, the **speed** of performance, and the **flexibility** to perform high quality technique.

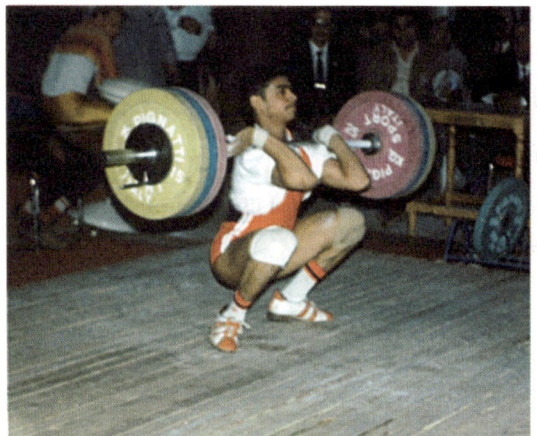

Figure 4.1. Deep Squat in the Clean lift in 1995, Egypt was thought formidable in 1950's.

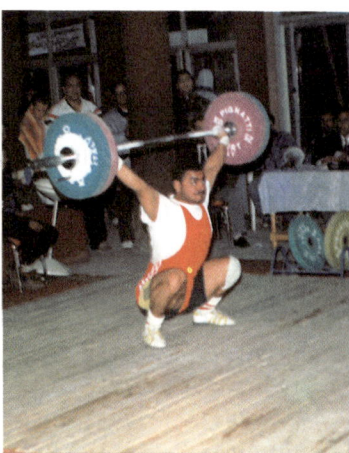

Figure 4.2. Deep Squat in the Snatch lift in 1995, Egypt, also thought formidable in 1950's.

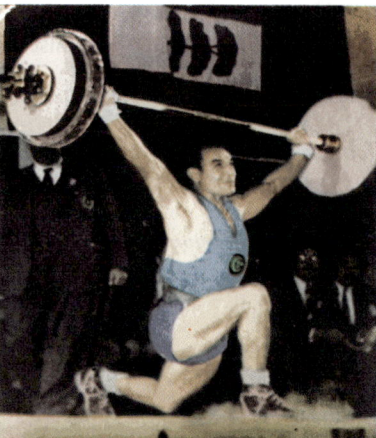

Figure 4.3. Mahgoob, of Egypt, in leg lunge in the Snatch lift, year 1951, Paris, France. Also, see Figure 4.17.

4.1.3. CONSTITUENTS OF WEIGHTLIFTING TRAINING

4.1.3.1. Pure strength exercises

These constitute about **one fifth (20%) or more** of the standard Weightlifting training schemes. In Powerlifting, this increases to 100%, which leaves no room for advancing other skills. Almost all Weightlifting authorities agree on one thing, that strength training is no substitute to real performance of ballistic lifting. You can have all the strength you wish yet fail to concert its timing during performance. The fundamental strength exercises that constitute about 90% of all strength exercises, in Weightlifting, are:

o **Deadlifts and Pulls.** The distinctive limitation to the Deadlift is that the weight being lifted should NOT exceed 180% of the maximal of a classical full range lift. Thus, if a trainee's maximum Clean lift is 100 kg his or her Deadlift should not exceed 180 kg. Powerlifters and many new comers to Weightlifting notoriously violate this basic empirical rule. The Deadlift could cause serious knee and hip injuries when it is left to hike to the maximal power of the trainee. Any trainee could Deadlift way above his maximal Clean. Since it is partial range exercise, it has to be curtailed if the wholesome fitness is of prime concern.

o **Squat.** The Squat is also curtailed with an upper ceiling of about 140% of the maximal Clean Lift. Heavier than that immensely hardens the ligaments of the lower limbs and traumatizes the articulating surfaces of the knees and hips. This shortens the longevity of the Weightlifter in competitive sport. As you can see, Weightlifting training puts less emphasis on extremes of power of isolated limbs. Excessive Squatting and Deadlifting undermines the upper body mobility and hinders the technique of floor-to-overhead lifting. A fit Weightlifter is a whole-body performer and not just a powerful athlete with less resourceful repertoire of skills. The Deadlift and Squat constitute as high as 40% of the entire workout volume.

- o **Press.** Overhead Shoulder Press targets the balancing muscles of the scapulas and therefore strengthens the upper body. Front Shoulder Press strengthens the suspending muscles of the chest cage as well as the shoulder muscles. Back Shoulder Press strengthens the upper Trapezius in addition to the shoulder muscles. No press is possible without active Serratus anterior muscles. These muscles that run on the sides of the chest originate from the ribs and wind behind the chest cage to pull the medial border of the scapulas, laterally and forwards.
- o **Goodmorning.** Bending over with weights on the back of the shoulders, with slightly bent knees, strengthens the Hamstrings. The entire back is kept extended and hardened with no buckling in. Extending the hips with explosive jumps strengthens the Glutei as well.

The other 10% are the chest, abdominal, and arm exercises.

4.1.3.2. Technique assisting exercises
These constitute the rest of Weightlifting training **(80%)** and are intended to enhance the Clean and Snatch lifts, as follows.

- o **Clean and Snatch pulls**, from the floor or from the hang, *Figure 4.4*. These target shoulder elevation. They beautifully enlarge the Trapezius, neck muscles, and upper back axial muscles. The Pulls differ from Deadlifting in distributing the weight on wider span of the thoracic vertebras, due to the rotation of the scapulas around the shoulder joints. The Pulls intend to strengthen the lower phases of lifting. They strengthen the chain of links during moving the weight above the kneecaps until it passes the pubic area.

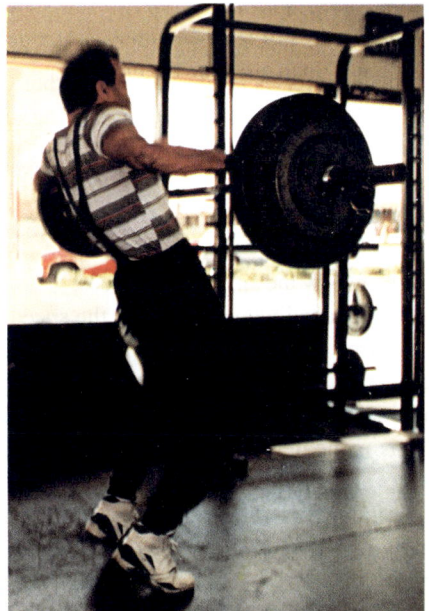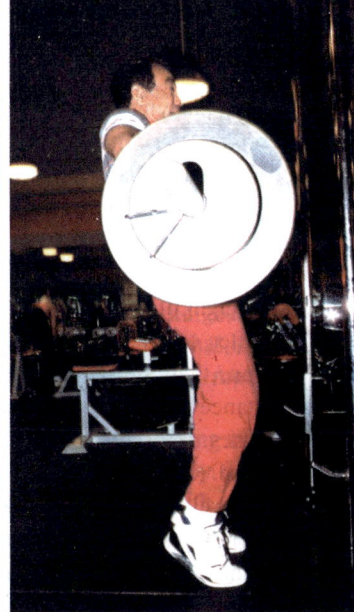

Figure 4.4. Clean pull (left) and Snatch pull (right) put great emphasis on strengthening scapular muscles.

- o **Clean and Snatch from the hang.** These are performed with variant percentage of isometric upper body contraction, speed and height of lift, and eccentric contraction. Lifting from the hang, or from above the knee level, strengthens the upper body. The Clean from the hang targets shoulder flexors and abductors, particularly during the process of dipping under the bar, in Squat position. This is a formidable flexibility and strength exercise that demands high flexibility of the lower back, shoulders, and Hamstrings. The Snatch from the hang strengthens the scapular balance in the widely abducted and elevated arms posture. It requires high flexibility of the upper back and shoulders.

- o **Jerk** from behind and front of the neck, with leg lunges, overhead descent Squat, or power pressing, is paramount to preventing buckling in of the upper back. As the weight is jerked upwards, the shoulder plates rotate sideways (laterally), the upper back hyper-extends, and the chest cage thrusts upwards and forwards. Only humans can perform such upright lifting overhead, on straight vertical posture. Jerking while descending, in squatting motion, is multi-girdle, complex balancing exercise. Power Jerking with strong leg drive is multipurpose exercise of power, balance, and flexibility facets. Recall that Jerking cannot be substituted with static Press. The former is ballistic and fast twitching, whereas the latter is slow twitching.

- o **Power Clean and Snatch,** with various handgrips, start from the floor and end on the shoulders in the Clean lift, or overhead in the Snatch. These are fundamental, full-fledged, strengthening exercises of the whole body. In addition to the whole body strengthening, the Clean lift targets the shoulder flexors and chest elevators. The chest cage and the collarbones support the weight in front of the vertebral columns during back extension. The Snatch lift targets the shoulder abductors and the scapular balancing muscles.

4.2. FEATURES OF WEIGHTLIFTING TRAINING

4.2.1. GENERAL FEATURES
Weightlifting training sessions have both fixed and variable features. The **fixed features** regard the sequence of executing exercises, the duration of a session, the number of sessions per week, and the annual load curve trends. The **variable features** regard the insertion or exclusion of accessory exercises to remedy individual deficits. These features make Weightlifting training an easy-to-master art and science. The most difficult feature of Weightlifting strength training is the

execution of the technique that requires few years of learning. The following are general features of Weightlifting training.
- Weightlifting training sessions last about ninety minutes and could be performed twice daily, but less than ten sessions per week.
- Training sessions starts with about fifteen minutes of warm-up. Some advanced Weightlifters use weights in most of their warm-up time.
- Core exercises often consist of six groups; each group consists of four to eight sets, each set consists of one to six repetitions. The interval between each set ranges from two to five minutes depending of the fitness condition of the trainee, the intensity of the training, and the temperature of the training room. Longer intervals could lead to poor technique or injuries.
- The six exercise groups have constant sequence. The first three exercises are classical, full range or quasi-full range lifts that start from the floor. These exercises might focus on either Clean and its strengthening alike, the Snatch and its strengthening alike, or a mix of the Clean and the strengthening alike of the Snatch, or vice versa. The other three exercises are a combination of shoulder, legs, and back strengthening exercises, as follows.
    i. The Deadlifts always ranks **first in sequence** in this group, and fourth in sequence in the entire session.
    ii. The shoulder Jerk follows Deadlift in sequence.
    iii. The Legs are **last**.
  Abdominal and peripheral exercises follow the six core exercises.
- The weight of a lift is increased or reduced judging by both the speed of lifting and the body posture during lifting. If the lifter can perform proper control over the speed of lifting along the trajectory, without showing regression in motion, then subsequent set, in that particular exercise, should progressively increase. Incremental increase in resistance promotes coordinated strength. Regression in the bar motion, particularly below or above the shoulder indicates excessive loading. This mandates either reducing the weight of the barbell or terminating that particular exercise. Regression is judged by:
    i. Lax elbow during overhead lifting.
    ii. Uneven shoulder elevation.
    iii. Shaking legs, arms, or torso.
    iv. Extremely congested face.
- The annual distribution of load volume consists of periods of strengthening, periods of restful recovery, and periods of emphasis on the competitive lifts.

4.2.2. DAILY TRAINING ROUTINE

Planning daily workouts has to account for past accomplishments, future goals, and the current condition of the trainee. The following are the main issues in planning daily Weightlifting routines.

- **Quick evaluation:** Under normal conditions *(defined as absence of known serious health conditions or prior surreptitious destructive behavior)* quick assessment is undertaken for the rate, regularity, and force of the heart beating, the presence or absence of murmur, rate of respiration, and bodyweight. In young beginners, evaluation of absence or presence of wheezes, cough, odor of the breath, and body temperature is important to exclude asthma, respiratory disorders, diabetic ketosis, and rheumatic diseases, respectively.
- **Warm-up** consists of preparation of cardiovascular, neuromuscular, and musculoskeletal *(heart, muscles, joints, and nervous system)*. General warm-up without weights lasts for about fifteen minutes. Special warm-up of the shoulder and pelvic girdles, the back and knees is carried out with light weights and lasts for shorter duration.
- **Core exercises** consist of one or both standard Weightlifting lifts, one or both strengthening exercises of Weightlifting lifts, Squat, and Jerk, as follows:
    i. Number of exercises: 5 to 7 (average 6).
    ii. Total number of sets: 25 to 35 (average 28).
    iii. Number of repetition per set: 1 to 5 (average 3).
  For example, if one intends to perform six different kinds of exercises, each exercise is executed in five sets, each set consists of three repetitions. This forms a standard 30-set session.
- **Individualized finishing exercises** targets neglected or weak body regions.
    i. This includes exercises for abdominal muscles, chin-ups, dips, arm exercises, and Bench Presses.
    ii. The choice of the number of exercises and the intensity of resistance depend on the resources of the trainee, such as availability to train longer and multiple sessions per day.
    iii. Muscles that seem to defy strengthening efforts have to be worked out more frequently.
- International lifters may work out more than once each day. Most lifters reserve a day off, every week. The duration of daily workout ranges from four to six hours, split into two or three training sessions per day. This redundant range of energy expenditure depends on the bodyweight and mobility of the trainee.

4.2.3. NUMBER OF REPETITIONS PER SETS
Repetitive lifting of a weight, without letting off hand gripping, is common strengthening practice. Repetitive lifting is not allowed in competition since, in this case, only the best single lift that counts. The number of repeating lifts varies, as follows.

High repetition: This varies from six and up.
o High repetition increases the muscle **size and strength** but strains the exercised muscles to the extent of interfering with acquiring higher technical skill of simultaneously employing many joints.
o High repetition with weights less than 60% of maximum **consumes the immediate fuel** that sustains muscular action and renders the neuromuscular control temporarily dysfunctional. Any effort to perform highly coordinated technique, after high repetition of contraction, could predispose to failure and injury to the joint, tendon, cartilage, or the whole body.
o The main goal of repetitive lifting of light weight is to benefit from the enhanced endurance of working a weak or resilient muscle or muscles. It is very effective way to enhance **vascularity, size, and tone** or sense of strength, in an otherwise lax muscle.
o It suits individual weak muscles such as the chest, arms, or abdomen. It is also suitable for purposeful **sculpturing** of specific body region.
o Athletes from other sports acquire strength and skillful technique by performing strengthening exercises that **simulate** the sport they practice. Since most fine **motor skills cannot be reciprocated** among different sports, repetitive lifting wont enhance skills of a particular sport but rather enhances a weak link or region.

Medium repetition: This is very common practice in all strengthening modalities.
o Repetitive lifting from three to five times, with weights over 60% of maximum, both **strengthens and bulks** major muscle groups.
o It is commonly used in the Bench Press, Squat, Pulls, and Deadlifts when a **breakthrough of a plateau** is desirable.
o It could cause overtraining due to the high intensity and long duration of **expending energy**.
o All **machine exercises** could be performed with medium repetitions since the technique of lifting is not very crucial.
o Exercises that do not involve high speed and do not span both shoulder and pelvic girdles could be repeated, up to six times per set.

Low repetition: *This is practiced mainly in Weightlifting.*
o Weightlifters have long abandoned the decimal ritual of repetitions. Repetitions of one to three lifts per set of technically challenging exercises are the dominant rule in Weightlifting.
o These involve the floor-to-overhead exercises such as the Snatch and Clean and Jerk. The heavier the weight, the less is the number of repetitions.
o Weights that are less that 60% of the maximum of certain exercises are not very beneficial for acquiring strength. These are judiciously used in warm-up, rehabilitation, or recovery from long inactivity.

4.2.4. NUMBER OF EXERCISES PER SESSION
Weightlifting sessions consist of four to eight different core exercises. A month or two prior to a contest, the numbers of sets per daily sessions is reduced from six or eight, to four or five. The repetition of lifts per each set and the weight of the lift are determined by the intended load volume. Each training session comprises of an average of fifteen minutes of warming up, fifty minutes of core exercises, and about twenty minutes of accessory exercises. Such definitive time frame of the three segments, number of sets, exercises, and weight percentage, makes Weightlifting planning less cumbersome, than planning endlessly protracted Bodybuilding training. The latter sort of training leaves the trainee with too much worries regarding inability to adhere to ambitious, yet self-defeating planning.

The different daily exercises may be related to either enhancing technical skill or promoting strength. At least one core exercise has to emphasize **Weightlifting style**, either in the form of classic-, military-, or power-style. Also, at least one core exercise has to emphasize strengthening of the **legs, back, and shoulders**. This is entirely different from Bodybuilding or Powerlifting where those three diverse regions are not combined in single training sessions. The remaining core exercises may either enhance the Weightlifting style, executed earlier in the session, or the one that was not executed, or both.

4.2.5. TECHNIQUE VERSUS STRENGTH
In clear distinction from Bodybuilding, Powerlifting, and general weight training, Weightlifting exercises are performed to enhance both the technique and the strength.

Strength. Lifting *higher, heavier, and more frequently* enhances **strength** but stiffens the ligaments and partially **loads** the joints. This is practiced most by beginners, when individual deficits need to be rectified, and up to two to three months away from the competition date. Prior to competition, strengthening exercises average about one fourth the total number of sets per session. During off-season, strengthening rises to almost three fourth the total number of sets.

Technique. Technique enhancement is accomplished by *squatting as deep as needed to retrieve the bar, lifting heavier, faster, and for lesser repetitions*. This permits the lifter to concentrate on refining the trajectory of the moving weight, figuring out which muscles need more enhancements, in order to remedy deficits, and develop robust neuromuscular coordination. Two to three months prior to the date of competition, the number of sets of exercise that emphasizes refinement of skill increases to 75% of the total sets. These exercises should simulate real competition, in terms of the load and preparation time. The barbell weight should start from 75% of the maximum and increases to exceed the maximum, if the condition of the trainee permits and his or her performance promises successful trials. No attempt should be made to emphasize on the technique if the trainee has missed three or more workout sessions. Irregular training routine undermines progressive skill acquisition and requires emphasizing on strength, until the level of fitness catches up with the previous rate of progress.

4.2.6. EXERCISE SEQUENCE

The sequence by which exercises are executed is learned from many decades of experience and follows specific rules.
- Exercises that require intricate technique and multi-joint involvement are executed earlier in the core segment of a training session (after warm-up). This encompasses the Clean and Jerk and the Snatch.
- Exercises that strengthen a particular phase of the lifting process should follow the classical lift they intend to strengthen.
    i. The **Deadlifts and Pulls** are executed after the classical lifts since they strengthen the lower phases of the lift.
    ii. The **Presses and Jerks** are executed after Deadlifts since they follow the normal sequence of floor-to-top strengthening.
    iii. **Back Squat** is always left to the end of the core Weightlifting segment. The back Squat is the most important strength exercise and is usually executed every workout day during the strengthening season. The maximal weights are repeated from one to three times and preferably with a pause at the bottom. Regular and wise squatting develops the ability to squat deeply with pausing without knee damage or injury. Lighter weights are used in explosive jump and fast squatting. The best back Squat record of heavyweight weightlifters is 380 kg (837 lbs) with a Clean and Jerk of 260 kg (573 lbs). Front Squats are less frequently performed with respect to the back Squat as it requires longer recovery time and strains the chest. The best Front Squat for heavyweight weightlifters is 300 kg for three reps.
- Exercises that involve less number of joints and low speed are left to the end. This encompasses the Squat, the abdominals, Chin-ups, Bench Presses, and Dips.
    i. **Starting with large muscles.** Amateur trainers believe that starting training session by exercising the larger muscle groups guarantees completion of the most demanding exercises and avails the trainee for the remaining portions of the daily program. This is not the case in Weightlifting training.
    ii. **Learning discipline.** Weightlifting discipline is a learning process in which a trainee cannot impose his or her wishes in defiance to basic requirements of a well-established training regimen. Yet, it is not, by any means, a sadistic approach of workout. After few weeks, the trainee will start to gain confidence in the rational of training major axial muscles, in progressive incremental intensity of resistance.
    iii. **Starting with isolated muscles.** Starting by exercising isolated muscles interferes with the harmonious integration of the functions of the nervous, muscular, articular, cardiovascular, and pulmonary systems. A strained muscle, amidst the chain links of skillful motion predisposes to injuries by shifting the burden of lifting onto otherwise unstrained joints, ligaments, or tendons.

4.2.7. TYPES OF MUSCULAR CONTRACTIONS
- **Multi-joint dynamics.** During freestyle lifting, different parts of the body perform different types of muscular contractions. That is because the human body folds and unfolds around multiple joints in order to lift weights in the shortest possible trajectory.
    i. **Movers of joints.** In the early phase of the lift, below the knees, the lower half of the body performs **isotonic contraction** (concentric contraction) by extending the joints and maintaining uniform muscular tone in order to mobilize the weight.
    ii. **Stabilizers of joints.** During that phase, the upper body performs **isometric contraction** by fixing the joints and hardening the muscles in order to stabilize the body.
    iii. **Transition between contractions.** The transition from one type of contraction to the other involves **isokinetic contraction** (uniform velocity of motion with varying degree of contraction).
    iv. **Shifting contractions.** Above the knee level, lifting proceeds by reversing the orders of contractions, to isotonic in the upper body and isometric in the lower body. Isotonic contraction serves joint mobility while isometric contraction serves joint stability. Now having got this jargon off my chest, I would like assure the reader that

such arcane terminology does not invent new phenomena other than what we usually do during everyday activities.

　　v. **Reverse contraction** (negative contraction or eccentric contraction) takes place when resisting force while elongating the muscle. Negative contraction occurs when lowering the weight proceeds slowly. Reverse pulling are performed in strength training. Resisting the free fall of the bodyweight during squatting, the free fall of the barbell during the Press, the free fall of the bodyweight during Chin-ups, are examples of reverse contractions.

- **Enhancing the different types of contractions**
    i. **Isometric contraction** is enhanced by particular exercises, once or twice weekly.
        a. Less than eighth of the weekly total sets of exercises are devoted for isometric strengthening.
        b. These exercises involve longer duration of hardening muscles without shortening. The Clean and Snatch from the hang are examples of isometric exercises, when performed with slow and protracted pull.
        c. Each set encompasses three to five *repetitions*. Pure isometric exercises are uncommon.
        d. This sort of training is performed to hasten recovery from injuries, after long interruption of training, or stressing resiliently weak muscle group. Increasing the duration of joint fixation, during lifting, serves the purpose of isometric training.

    ii. **Isotonic contraction, or concentric contraction** is enhanced by plenty of exercises.
        a. It constitutes over three quarters of the weekly total sets of Weightlifting training.
        b. These exercises involve concentric contraction that shortens muscles and bends joints while maintaining uniform muscle tone. All normal lifting with continuous motion involve isotonic contraction.
        c. Powerlifting is very deficient in isotonic-dominant exercises since the three basic lifts (Squat, Deadlift, and Bench Press) leave little range of motion to maintain isotonic contraction. Most of the Powerlifting contractions are isometric-dominant.

    iii. **Reverse contraction, or eccentric contraction, or negative contraction** is performed in heavy loads exceeding 75% of the maximum.
        a. It constitutes less than fifth of the weekly total sets of exercises.
        b. These exercises involve eccentric contraction in the form of lengthening of the muscle while resisting lowering of weights. Lowering your body slowly in the chin-ups workouts the Biceps, in the parallel bars dips the Triceps, and in the Clean the Biceps and the Trapezius.
        c. This is very effective method of stimulating muscle growth and strength. Eccentric exercises should not be performed prior to contests since they require long recovery time in order to return muscle tone to comfortable levels.
        d. It should be emphasized that the different types of muscular contraction could be incorporated as a modification of the basic exercises. For example, the Clean lift could be modified to **"Clean from the Hang"** with slow Pull. The pull is protracted for five to ten seconds duration with back extension and fixed elbows, along the distance from the kneecaps to the upper thigh. The reverse contraction could be performed by slowly lowering the weight from the shoulders to the floor on a period of five to ten seconds.

4.2.8. BRAIN CONTROL OF MUSCLE CONTRACTION

- **Cortex.** The primary motor cortex is the brain center that controls voluntary muscles and is located in the vicinity of the anterior central sulcus of the cortex. Control is conducted by firing of electrical signals by the neurons of this brain area. These signals are transmitted downwards the nerve fibers to reach remote locations.

    i. **Signals.** Firing occurs as bunches of signals of frequencies ranging from 15- to 33-pulse per second (frequency varies with fiber recruitment). Regular training should affect the firing frequency and amplitude profile of the brain signals that distinguish trained from untrained individuals.
    ii. **Activity of cortex.** Thus voluntary control of muscle contraction originates in the brain cortex and lasts for the entire duration of muscular action. The higher cortical signals reach the motoneurons in the spinal cord, the anterior horn cells or AHC. From the AHC, lower motor signals spread through the final common pathways, the peripheral nerves, to reach peripheral muscles.

- **Transmission.** Electrical firing from higher brain centers reaches the different muscles at intervals that depend on the distance of the muscle from the cortex. The interval between the firing of the brain cortex and that of the motor unit ranges from 12 to 53 milliseconds, shorter at the neck and longer at the sacrum.
- **Gated control.** The motoneurons of the spinal cord act like transistors or controllable-gated source of signals. On its own, motor neurons are capable of exciting peripheral muscles, as is the case of upper motor neuron lesions. Yet, upper motor control from the brain initiates, sustains, and grades the voluntary action beyond mere spastic activities. The ability of trained athletes to influence muscular activity, from utter silence prior to lifting to maximal contraction during lifting, takes place in the motoneurons. These are affected by diverse inputs, as follows.

i. Inputs from the **cerebellum, other motor neurons, and from afferents of muscle spindle** enter the motoneurons of the spinal cord and regulate the fine control and recruitments of muscle fibers during contraction. Thus, highly skilled and graceful movements by athletes are affected by cerebellar control as well as general muscular conditioning.
ii. Inputs from the **brain stem** convey signals on respiration, circulation, and arousal and modify motor outputs from the brain and cerebellum. Integrating these vital processes with muscular activities is promoted with regular and continuous training.
iii. Inputs from the **special sensory organs** (eyes, ears, and nose) covey both reflex signals from the midbrain and voluntary signals from the brain to the motor area and modify their motor output. Visual, auditory, and olfactory signals from the workout environment affect the performance of trainees.
iv. It is very important for strength trainees to understand the dual status of muscular regulation, during **REST** and **MOVEMENT**. During voluntary movement, voluntary control of muscles originates from the cerebrum, propagates through the pyramidal neural tract, reaches the terminal muscle via the alpha-motoneurons through the peripheral motor nerve, and ends on *muscle fibers*. It is modulated by the sensory nerve of muscle spindles. During rest, involuntary control of muscle tone originates from many areas in the brain and brain stem, propagates through the extra-pyramidal neural tract, reaches muscles via the gamma-motoneurons through the motor peripheral nerve, and ends on *muscle spindles*. Muscle tone regulation by the extra-pyramidal system modulates voluntary control and distinguishes spastic from relaxed toned muscle. Thus, a well-relaxed muscular system during rest interval will undoubtedly perform powerfully, and in compliance with one's will, when movement is initiated.

4.2.9. SPEED OF LIFTING

Over the years, Weightlifters have gained knowledge of how to enhance strength. By trial and error, most of the complicated rules of mechanics were well mastered.

o **No yanking rule. Yanking an object** at rest in order to induce motion is an inefficient way of lifting. Initiating motion efficiently requires strong and steady contact with the object and slowly advancing the contact as the object complies. This rule of "no yanking" stems from the limit imposed on accelerating massive objects by their inertial resistance to change state of motion.

o **Equal reaction rule.** As soon as the object moves smoothly, that is at uniform velocity or closer to uniform, no time should be wasted to let the motion die. This rule stems from the reaction of objects to forces acting on them. If the force diminishes, so does the reaction.

o **Generation and control of speed.** Weightlifters develop well-adapted proprioreceptors -the sensors of pressure, vibration, and speed- and motor coordination to implement these two rules. This elucidates the important relationship between the speed of lifting and the strength of the athlete. Untrained lifters exhaust by attempting to speed the barbell when the *laws of mechanics do not permit* such change of state. A special feature of Weightlifting is that the generated *quantity of motion or momentum* is substantially higher than other strength training modalities. The momentum is a measure of the speed of a moving object and its mass, conjunctly.

o **Graceless lifting.** Meddling with graceless lifting is not condoned in Weightlifting training. Clumsy technique predisposes to long-term problems, ranging from acute rupture of tendons, trauma to the joint cartilage or bone. Graceless lifting is characterized by:
  i. Lifts that advance in speed then suddenly regress without the control of the lifter.
  ii. Favoring one side of the body over the other.
  iii. Bouncing noticeably away from the vertical fall line.
  iv. Departure from the normal pattern of the bar trajectory.

o **Timing energy expenditure** according to productive acceleration of the barbell is the basic goal of training. For example, you can stand on a gigantic bridge across a vast space and induce the bridge to vibrate by specific jumping pattern, though you might not know exactly which pattern would cause the most effect on the bridge until you conduct a thorough experiment. Timing of acceleration occurs partly in the inner ears, which are equipped with three semicircular tunnels of fluids, in three perpendicular planes, with acceleration sensor in each tunnel. Thus, the ears can coordinate the three Cartesian components of acceleration of the body in the three dimensional space. Training refines this anatomical and physiological function and leads the trainee to master speed and strength relationship in amazing grace.

o **Explosive lifting.** The high momentum in Weightlifting increases the threshold of firing of the tendon ganglia such that these would not shut not off the motor neural unit before heavier forces are encountered. The familiar examples of tiny Weightlifters lifting about three times their bodyweight attests to this sort of adaptation. The upper limit on the **speed of lifting** maximal weights by humans has compelling explanation, as follows.
  i. Firstly, the living muscle fibers contract by circuits of neural networks that require intervals of the order of microseconds to **transmit stimulating signals.** Living muscle fibers do not cross-communicate without nerves.

ii. Secondly, living muscles have a safety mechanism to **shut off muscular contraction** if acceleration exceeds previously tolerated maximum. The tendon ganglion fires the shut off signals, while the muscle spindles fire the stimulating signals to recruit additional units. This safety mechanism forces the lifter, with acquired learning, to test the yielding of weight to motion prior to incrementally increasing the force of pulling or pushing.

iii. Thirdly, all substances have maximal **tolerance to deformation.** Organic substances might vary in this property among species. Yet, there still exits a characteristic threshold of deformation to tendons, muscles, cartilages, and bone.

iv. The Snatch lift requires between 3 to 4.5 seconds, with the maximum speed not exceeding 1.8 meter/sec. Of course, there is no such thing as minimal speed of lifting maximum weight. Since lifting signifies force, which is the **change of the quantity of motion,** the change of motion peaks during maximal force of lifting.

4.2.10. REPERTOIRE OF WEIGHTLIFTING EXERCISES

The most commonly practiced strength training exercises are listed in *Table 4.2*.

Table 4.2. Exercises commonly performed in Weightlifting training.

Core Weightlifting Exercises	Accessory Weightlifting Exercises
The Clean group:	**The Pull group:**
o Classical Clean and Jerk.	o Deadlift with variable handgrips.
o Clean from the Hang, with Squat.	o Pull from the hang, with variable handgrips.
o Military Clean.	o Pull from the hang, with jump.
o Clean from the Hang, with isometric Pull and rapid dipping.	o Shrugging, with isometric arm contraction.
o Clean with wide handgrip.	**The leg group:**
o Clean with eccentric contraction (negative contraction) during slow lowering of the weight to the floor.	o Front Squat.
	o Back Squat.
The Snatch group:	o Squat, with barbell held overhead.
o Classical Snatch.	o Squat, with jump.
o Snatch from the Hang, with Squat.	o One leg stepping, with weight.
o Military Snatch.	o Leg lunges, performed once in a while as a change of pace.
o Snatch from the Hang, with isometric Pull.	**The back group:**
o Snatch, with narrow handgrip.	o Goodmorning. This is executed with slightly bent knees.
The Jerk and Press group:	o Goodmorning, with jump.
o Classical Jerk from the rack.	o Hyperextension exercises. These are performed to stretch sore or overtrained back.
o Shoulder Press, with variable handgrip.	
o Shoulder Press or Jerk, with full Squat.	

Balanced combinations of these exercises constitute Weightlifting training. These are the basic ingredients of the sport of Weightlifting. Exercises are included in training sessions according to some common **guidelines**, as follows.

i. Of course, Weightlifters never execute all these exercises each training session, or regularly in cycles.
ii. The choice of exercise is personal and depends on required individual needs.
iii. Many of theses exercises are seldom performed by many Weightlifters whereas others are commonly shared among them.
iv. Exercises that strengthen certain anatomical parts are usually not duplicated in the same session. Thus, the front Squat or the back Squat falls in different sessions. Also, the Goodmorning or Deadlift falls in different sessions.
v. Unless the trainee aims at targeting specific weak links in his or her lifting sequence, there is no need for duplicating assisting exercises that serve similar anatomical region.
vi. Substituting exercises for other exercises reduces boredom; enhances unforeseen elements of motion, and works out unforeseen assisting anatomical elements.

4.2.11. LOAD VOLUME OR "TONNAGE"

o **Buildup versus exhaustion.** Due to the redundancy of the standards of strength training, efforts are made to tailor such standards to individual needs. Naturally, a layman would rightfully believe that exercise could lead to *exhaustion and even irreversible lethal injuries*. The most dreaded injuries are the internal ones and those that show very little if any alarming signs.

i. Injuries to the heart valves could remain concealed for years before being diagnosed.
ii. Injuries to the knee and hip joints could be confused for seasonal ailments till disabling level of pain are reached.

iii. Insidious chronic injuries to ligaments and tendons affect the musculoskeletal posture of the entire body and creep stealthily on the unwary trainee over many months of imbalanced training.

- **Cumulative effects.** Finding a reasonable measure of the **cumulative effects** of lifting weights enhances our ability to avoid the pitfalls of exercise and guess ways to breakthrough plateaus. The **volume,** or the total weight of certain lifts, is used to gauge the *volume of exercise load*.
    i. The volume of a daily training session is defined as the product of the barbell weight, the number of sets, and the number of repetitions of certain exercises.
    ii. Since there is no consensus on the specific exercises to incorporate in the formula, the volume is a relative index to different individuals.
    iii. Issues such as joint imbalance due to neglecting certain aspects of training, improper sleep cycle, use of recreational or illicit chemical enhancer interfere with the interpretation of the volume index.

- **Energy expenditure.** There must be some accurate way of estimating the **energy expenditure** of vigorous exercises, yet that would be time consuming since full account of the motion of the weight has to be considered. The fact that constant new records are still being made signifies that human limits are far from being reached. Thus, realistic volume assessment does not have to be very accurate. Roughly estimated, Weightlifters average, in cumulative total of Weightlifting exercises, as follows.

    i. Annual   600 to 3000 tons
    ii. Monthly   50 to 300 tons
    iii. Weekly   10 to 60 tons

- **Pre-contest volume.** As an empirical index, the volume is tailored to personal conditions and preparation to contests. The average volume for a trainee is roughly estimated by few months of observation and tracking. Average volume is a reliable index, particularly, when fitness and health seem to wane as a result of overload. Conveniently, training programs assign different **levels of volume** of light, intermediate, or heavy, in order to assess overloading problems. **Prior to contests**, the monthly volume is distributed in ascending order, from one week to another.
    i. The week prior to the contest accounts for a high portion of volume, that is less than 40% of the monthly volume. **The last week** prior to the contest, however, starts with heavier daily volumes and ends with lightest volume, just at the day prior to the contest date. That takes into account that the weekly volume is still the heaviest of that month and that the total number of exercise groups are less than five. The exercises of the last week are purely similar to real contest lifts. The number of repetitions also does not exceed two per set.
    ii. **Four weeks** prior to the contest, the volume starts from low, about 1/8 monthly volume, and gradually increases to maximum by the last week, about 2/5 monthly volume. *Increasing the volume,* gradually to a maximum at the contest date, will foster responsiveness and total fitness to peaking levels. The low weekly volume, thirty days before contest, allows for refining the technique and enhancing total body recuperation.

- **Evolutionary changes.** In the last century, evolutionary changes had led to drastic increase in the maximum endurable volume of load by Weightlifters, as follows:
    i. The *age of new beginners* has greatly dropped to early adolescence. This has led to the appearance of outstanding Weightlifters by the peak age of strength, 18- to 25-year of age.
    ii. The lifting style has advanced from foolishness, to craziness, to ultimate madness. Until the late 1950's, Weightlifting was dominated by *springing the legs while pulling*. This emulates movements by large animals, such as camels and horses, of getting up by kicking front legs forwards and body upwards. That was the proper style for stiff-legged, old athletes. Looking back, lunging the legs while lifting sounds like a foolish way that violates all rules of mechanics. Most probably, camels and horses perform the lunging of the fore limbs, because the forelimbs in all mammals are weaker than the rear limbs and have to be spread wide, unbent, to be able to commence further extending.
    iii. By 1960's, **deep squatting** under the barbell was then thought to be utter craziness. Balancing a human lifter, with weights exceeding twice his bodyweight, on two feet was thought formidable.
    iv. By 1990's, **squatting during Jerking** was introduced by few lifters at the top of class. Due to its enormous strain on the shoulders and back, we do not know if that latest evolution in technique would ever prevail
    v. The advent in the learning process, also, led to simplification of daily planning and focusing on the major aspects of **strength and performance**. Today, Weightlifters execute very few exercises and many weekly sessions.
    vi. The most influential changes are of course, the **social ones**. Larger and larger pools of diverse nationalities of Weightlifters have stimulated the evolution of the sport. Lifters from the communist nations had revived a dead sport by virtue of their limited access to luxurious living. Lifters from socialist nations have contributed by early start and dedicated supervised training. Affluent small nations have coupled western technological advances, dedication to socializing sports, and the relatively slow pace of living, to further revive Weightlifting.

vii. On the subject of **anabolic steroids** usage by the soviet lifters, some believe that western pharmaceutical technology should offer the western athletes more advantage and that the soviet advances in Weightlifting are attributed to the limited alternatives of social engagements. The Romanian scandal of usage of drugs in recent competitions, as well as other eastern bloc athletes, does not justify the loss of competitiveness of American lifters. This decline had long started before wide-scale testing for enhancing drugs.

4.2.12. EXERCISE INTENSITY

This refers to the **average lift weight**. Intensity may refer to specific exercises, or to training sessions of certain interval, *Figure 4.5*. Exercise intensity is the main impetus of all strengthening activities. Intense resistance to forces promotes physical strength when planned according to scientific guidelines. The rest of our venture, in managing exercise intensity, is to minimize damage to health while enhancing strength, as follows.

- **Relative to bodyweight.** In order to increase strength, intensity of resistance has to increase as bodyweight increases. The relationship between resistance and bodyweight cannot be a linear one, though. As the bodyweight increases, higher intensity is required to achieve balanced strength. This is based on the maximum lift for each exercise, keeping in mind the maintenance of well-balanced performance. The main reason for the nonlinear relationship between intensity and bodyweight is the change in leverage, of muscle pull on bones, due to the nonlinear height and bodyweight relationship.
- **Prior to competition,** exercise intensity has to be reduced to allow replenishment of body reserves. However, reduction in intensity has to adhere to common guidelines in order to avoid muscular wasting. Longer periods of **lower exercise**

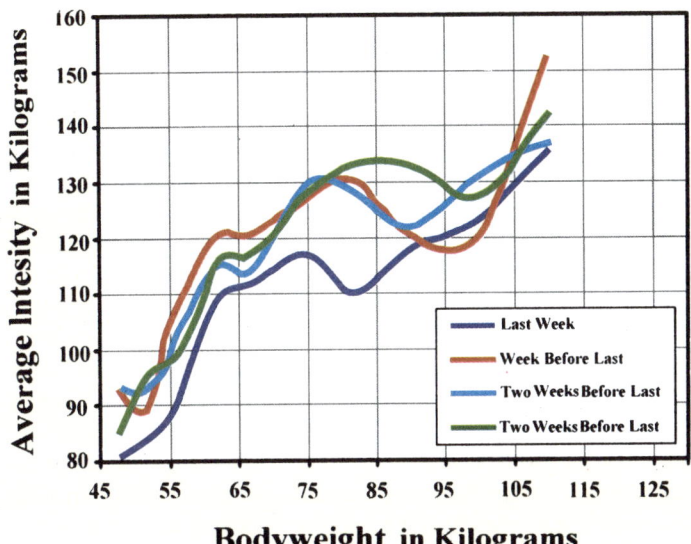

Figure 4.5. Exercise intensity of ten olympic weight classes prior to a contest

intensity, of 20% or more from average intensity, could lead to decline in strength and performance. One has to opt for higher exercise intensity rather than volume, during the **final weeks prior** to contest. This ensures robust neuromuscular coordination rather than depletion of vital body resources. In a nutshell, the following practices would lead to substantial enhancement of both strength and technique:

  i. Exercise intensity: 75% of maximum lift
  ii. Sets per exercise group: 5 to 6
  iii. Repetitions per set: 1 to 3
  iv. Exercise groups per session: 2 to 3 (core classical lifts).
  v. Sessions per week: 5
  vi. Total intense lifts / week: 180 (lifts of 75% 1RM) = 6 sets x 2 reps x 3 exercises x 5 days.
  vii. The three exercise groups are picked from this short list: Classical Snatch, Classical Clean and Jerk, Squat, or Shoulder Press

- **Redundancy in planning**. Of course, a trainee might find him- or herself in more or less different condition that necessitates adjustments to these general rules, which above all are quite redundant.
  i. Today, international Weightlifters practice up to 120 times of **maximum lifts** each month, within the context of monthly exercise volumes of about 100 ton.
  ii. During training, most Weightlifters do not exceed what they can lift in **competitions**. The top heavyweight can lift 210 kg in the Snatch and 260 kg in the Clean and Jerk during peak competition, while his training would not exceed 200 kg and 245 kg, respectively.
  iii. **Heavy lifters** require more training sessions per week and higher intensity of load. A heavyweight lifter uses average training weight of 190 kg in the pulls and Squats with 170 kg as the first set, followed by 50 kg jumps, until the maximum weight is reached.

4.2.13. MAXIMUM LIFTS (1RM, ONE REPETITION OF MAXIMUM)

This is defined as 90% of what a trainee could lift in his or her best condition. As the lifter advances in lifting, his maximum lift keeps increasing until certain plateau is reached. The most lift that constitutes 100% of maximum is only tried few times prior to competition, or when the lifter exhibits continuous increase in strength from one week to another week. Surprisingly, all people, athletes and non-athletes, are limited as of the most they could lift. Unless significant changes take place in their habits, maximum limits are formidable to overcome. Weightlifting addresses this hurdle by intense exercising according to the following rules.

- o In Weightlifting, one **1/3** of the monthly volume consists mainly of the **maximal of classical lifts**.
- o Another **1/3** of monthly volume consists of the major **assisting exercises,** such as the Pulls and the Squats.
- o The remaining **1/3** encompasses all remaining **assisting exercises**.

This gives you an idea about how trying is to just maintain previously achieved strength. Beating old records with few kilograms is a double accomplishment of both reaching and breaching old records. Maximum limits imposed on the ability of animals to generate force are multifaceted. The following is an effort to enumerate the main factors contributing to plateauing of strength to fixed maximal value.

- o The driving force for movement resides in the *heart*, since plants do not have such organ. A *heart* that fails to comply with the demands of movements limits such effort. The heart might fail to beat faster, stronger, in tandem with cellular demands, or leaks. All these heart difficulties, which are not under the full control of the individual, limit strength. Rest, nutrition, sleeping habits, drugs, smoking, alcohol, and diseases affect the performance of the heart and thus affect maximal physical strength.
- o A *nervous system* that is not conditioned or equipped to synchronize well-coordinated muscular activities imposes limits. The nervous system of trained individuals has the memory of dealing with recruitment and synchrony of needed muscle fibers, the ability to recover timely, and the potential for improvement in performance.
- o *General conditions* that interfere with both delivery of nutrients and removal of by-products impose limits. These generally depend on the socioeconomic and educational status of the individual. People with limited access to information become isolated from learning healthy ways of bettering their style of living.
- o The *genetic* factor is quite compelling but remains vague, in large populations. There are people born with natural strength that surpasses the average norms of population. I did not believe in miraculous strength until I witnessed by my own eyes a Sudanese national with average bodyweight who was able to resist the weight of an empty van, with his chest and arms, laying on his back, while the rear wheel of the van moved slowly, in reverse, over his chest. In that show, the so-called Sudanese Hercules was able to lift an average donkey, hung with a rope around its belly, with the jaws of the man clenching the rope. Such natural strength is a myth.
- o Biochemistry offers little explanation of the cellular physiology of strength. The *muscle cell* fuels kinetic energy by high-energy transport molecules, CP and ATP. The amount of these molecules in muscle cells, in addition to the amount of muscle fiber protein "myoactin"[1] determine the rate of energy production. Aside from the catalysts of the release of energy from ATP and the contraction of myoactin, the formation of these strength moieties holds part of the secret for physical strength. Synthesis of ATP and muscle protein requires great cycling of the cellular furnace, the tricarboxylic acid cycle or TCA cycle. This biochemical cycle uses acetyl Coenzyme-A and the final byproducts of all foodstuffs. The TCA cycle generates ATP and many substrates that enter in protein synthesis. The TCA cycle is operated by few enzymes and catalysts that determine its cycling efficiency. The most important factors that we can affect are the availability of vitamins and minerals for efficient cycling of energy through the TCA cycle. Vitamin B complex and calcium play major role in the cleavage the carbon skeleton of foodstuff and transport of electrons in the TCA cycle. Thiamin deficiency (vitamin B_1), for example, can cause serious loss of muscular strength and neural deficits.

4.2.14. RECOVERY

Unused muscles atrophy despite the availability of ample nutrients. Conversely, exercise stimulates muscular growth, even in states of whole body catabolism, such as in malnutrition, fasting, or over training.[2]

- o Exercising **THREE** days per week maintains strength.
- o Exercising **FIVE** to **SIX** days per week increases strength.
- o Exercising **EVERYDAY** and for **LONGER DURATION** maximizes strength.
- o **One week** without exercise causes about 15% loss of previously acquired exercise strength.
- o **Three weeks of rest** causes about 50% loss of previously acquired exercise strength.
- o **One year of rest** causes over 55% loss of previously acquired exercise strength.

With eight workouts per week, one should keep in mind proper volume, intensity, balance between strength and mobility, and meticulously monitoring body response. You should not venture in haphazard, intense frequent training. This sort of overtraining defeats the purpose of scientific planning of strength training. The latter takes into account the body adaptation to the volume and intensity of resistance and tweaks many factors in order to prevent exhaustion and foster strength.

---

[1] Myoactin comprises of actin and myosin protein. It exists in muscles in the form of fibrils that slide to produce muscle contraction in the presence of calcium ions and adenosine triphosphate molecules.

[2] "Harrison's Principles of Internal Medicine", by Thorn, et al. McGraw-Hill. 1977. Page 364.

4.3. STANDARD WEIGHTLIFTING TRAINING SESSIONS

4.3.1. STANDARD TRAINING
To illustrate how to manipulate Weightlifting training sessions during different periods of the annual load curve, the following are examples of standard training sessions.
- o **Warm-up.** Each session starts with warm-up. Warm-up for ten minutes without weight or with light weights simulating the subsequent weight exercise.
- o **Core exercises** are performed in sets that comprise of repetitive execution of the same exercise in the same manner without a break. The percentage of maximal load in each lift determines the intensity of resistance. Core Weightlifting exercises have specific common features. These are mostly **floor-to-overhead** lifts such as the Clean and Snatch. Many lifters perform the Snatch every workout day. The Clean and the Jerk are better executed as a whole to maintain **shoulder to pelvic balanced** proportion. **Shoulder presses** are not widely practiced today as in the past, prior to 1972.
- o **Finishing.** Each session may end with accessory exercises such as chin-ups, dips, abdominal sit-ups, or running. These serve individual enhancement of areas of deficit. Running or brisk walking are very effective in reducing or preventing acute episodes of inflammation, hours after exercise, particularly, in old and advanced lifters. At least ten minutes of running may ease night sleep after heavy training.
- o Many lifters reserve **separate workout** days for the Clean and Jerk or the Snatch. Each whole lift, of the Clean or Snatch, is followed by its assisting exercises from the floor, from the hang, or while standing on a raised surface. Thus on the Clean and Jerk session, for example, the classical lift is executed in a group of four to eight sets. This is then followed by the Clean Pull, or Clean Deadlift, or Clean from the hang, for another group of four to six sets. Alternatively, the latter group may be substituted by the Snatch Pull, Snatch Deadlift, or Snatch from the hang.

4.3.2. EMPHASIS ON THE SNATCH TECHNIQUE
This prototype session focuses mainly on the Snatch lift and its assisting exercise, the Deadlift or Pull, **Table 4.3**.
- o Core exercises emphasize the technique and strength of the Snatch lift.
- o Two basic strengthening exercises, for the legs and back, are routinely added.
- o The simplicity of the session contributes greatly to refinement of the complex technique of the Snatch.
- o This session may be supplemented by another session, in the same day that targets peripheral muscles or assisting exercises that strengthen major muscles.
- o The sequence of exercises is logical and proceeds from whole body workout (in the Snatch) to partial strengthening (in the Squats).

Table 4.3. Standard Weightlifting training session emphasizing on the Snatch lift

Exercises	Number of sets	Number of sets x (% Projected 1RM x Number of repetitions)			
		1st subset	2nd subset	3rd subset	4th subset
Snatch	8	2(60% x 3)	2(70% x 3)	2(80% x 2)	2(90% x 2)
Pull for Snatch	6	2(80% x 3)	2(100% x 3)	2(120% x 3)	
Goodmorning	4	2(50% x 6)	2(70% x 6)		
Squat	6	2(80% x 3)	2(90% x 3)	2(100% x 3)	
Total	24				

4.3.3. EMPHASIS ON THE CLEAN AND JERK TECHNIQUE
This prototype session focuses of the extra strength needed for the heaviest lift, the Clean and Jerk, **Table 4.4.**
- o Here the trainee starts with the Snatch. This is lighter than the Clean and is used to add extra warm-up and strength to the axial muscles.
- o With the Snatch preceding the Clean, it is possible to start with 70% of the maximum in the Clean.
- o The Shoulder Press serves shoulder strengthening which is very fundamental to the Clean. One has to remember that Shoulder Press is not a substitute to overhead Jerk. The latter is ballistic and entails different neural responses and different virtual forces.
- o The Pulls and Deadlifts are replaced with the Goodmorning and the Snatch. Both serve strengthening the axial major muscles as well as the Hamstrings.

Table 4.4. Standard Weightlifting training session emphasizing on the Clean and Jerk lift

Exercises	Number of sets	Number of sets x (% Projected 1RM x Number of repetitions)		
		1st subset	2nd subset	3rd subset
Snatch	6	2(60% x 3)	2(70% x 3)	2(80% x 2)
Clean and Jerk	6	2(70% x 3)	2(80% x 3)	2(90% x 2)
Seated Press	4	2(60% x 4)	2(80% x 4)	
Goodmorning	4	2(50% x 6)	1(70% x 6)	1(80% x 6)
Squat	6	2(60% x 3)	2(70% x 3)	2(80% x 3)
Total	26			

4.3.4. THE SNATCH AND THE CLEAN AND JERK TECHNIQUES
This prototype session focuses on the classical lifts, in addition to the routine of leg and back exercises, **Table 4.5**.
o   The Clean and Jerk is a combination of lower and upper body workout with emphasis on the axial muscles.
o   Lifting from the Hang reduces the lower body drive and strengthens the upper back muscles.
o   Hanging the bar at the knee level or the mid-thighs and pulling very slowly (5-6 seconds) to the shoulders enhances isometric contraction. Speeding occurs closer to the shoulders.
o   The Snatch from the hang strengthens the upper back muscles.
o   The Press has been substituted by the Snatch from the Hang to strengthen the upper back and shoulders.
o   Even with such heavy session, the Goodmorning is a very useful exercise.

Table 4.5. Standard Weightlifting training session emphasizing on both the Clean and Jerk and the Snatch lifts

Exercises	Number of sets	Number of sets x (% Projected 1RM x Number of repetitions)			
		1st subset	2nd subset	3rd subset	4th subset
Clean and Jerk	8	2(60% x 3)	2(70% x 3)	2(80% x 2)	2(90% x 1)
Isometric Clean from the Hang	4	2(80% x 5)	2(90% x 5)		
Snatch from the Hang	8	2(60% x 3)	2(70% x 3)	2(80% x 2)	2(90% x 1)
Goodmorning	4	2(50% x 6)	2(70% x 6)		
Squat with slow descent	4	2(100% x 1)	2(120% x 1)		
Total	28				

4.3.5. REDUCING THE VOLUME FOR MUSCLE RECOVERY
This prototype session is a restful workout of fewer sets, lighter load, and basic exercises, **Table 4.6**.
o   The weight of the barbell is kept as low as 70% of the maximum to enhance speed and coordination.
o   Both the Clean and Snatch work out the major axial muscles.
o   The seated Shoulder Press allows resting of the legs while working out the upper body.
o   The Squat is kept light, rather than being completely omitted.
o   The low volume of this session allows recovery and replenishment of body reserves.

Table 4.6. Standard Weightlifting training session of low volume for active recovery

Exercises	Number of sets	Number of sets x (% Projected 1RM x Number of repetitions)	
		1st subset	2nd subset
Classical Clean	6	2(60% x 3)	4(70% x 2)
Classical Snatch	6	4(60% x 3)	2(70% x 2)
Seated Press	4	4(60% x 3)	
Squat	4	4(60% x 3)	
Total	20		

4.3.6. ENHANCING TECHNICAL SKILLS OF THE CLEAN AND JERK
This prototype session addresses the special needs of strong shoulder elevators and flexors in the extremes of squatting and overhead extension, **Table 4.7**.
o   All phases of the Clean and Jerk are individually and collectively worked out by encompassing the different lifts of each phase.
o   The common critique on splitting the Clean from the Jerk is that splitting reduces whole body strength. Yet splitting might enhance technique and reduce overtraining. It is all up to your preference.
o   The front Squat is easier in this session since the shoulders are already worked out and stimulated in the range of motion required for full shoulder flexion.
o   The inclined Press targets the upper chest and shoulders that are heavily involved in the Clean and Jerk.
o   The entire session focuses mostly on the upper body, with the lower body being worked out in the interim of strengthening the Clean and Jerk.

Table 4.7. Standard Weightlifting training session of technique enhancement for the Clean and Jerk

Exercises	Number of sets	Number of sets x (% Projected 1RM x Number of repetitions)		
		1st subset	2nd subset	3rd subset
Clean	7	1(50% x 3)	2(60% x 2)	4(70% x 1)
Clean Pull	4	1(60% x 2)	1(70% x 2)	2(80% x 1)
Jerk from the rack	6	2(60% x 2)	2(70% x 2)	2(80% x 1)
Front Squat	5	2(70% x 3)	3(80% x 3)	
Press inclined bench	4	2(60% x 3)	2(70% x 3)	
Total	26			

4.3.7. ENHANCING TECHNICAL SKILLS OF THE SNATCH

This prototype session focuses on the strengthening of the different working muscles of the Snatch, **Table 4.8**.
- o All phases of the Snatch are being worked out, with the upper back being strengthened in the hyperextension posture.
- o The Squat is inserted here since the Snatch lifts are all lighter than maximal limits and the volume of the session is moderate.
- o Squat has to be left to the end since the other three exercises are technically complex and require high flexibility.
- o The chest and the front of shoulders are not strained here and could be worked out in another session in the same day.
- o This is a classical session of teaching the Snatch to beginners or refining that for the advanced lifters.

Table 4.8. Standard Weightlifting training session for technique enhancement of the Snatch

Exercises	Number of sets	Number of sets x (% Projected 1RM x Number of repetitions)		
		1st subset	2nd subset	3rd subset
Snatch	6	2(50% x 2)	2(60% x 2)	2(70% x 1)
Snatch Pull from the hang	4	2(80% x 2)	1(90% x 2)	1(100% x 2)
Snatch from the hang	6	2(50% x 2)	2(60% x 2)	2(70% x 2)
Squat	4	1(70% x 3)	2(90% x 2)	2(70% x 1)
Total	20			

4.4. TRAINING FOR COMPETITION

Modern competitive Weightlifting requires dedication to training, in the form six to eight training sessions per week. Training sessions can be held twice daily, each session lasts 90 minutes, with one day off each week. Detailed discussions on training periods, session managements, and load volume-intensity are presented in Chapter Thirteen.
- o **Weekly sessions.** This can take the form of morning training sessions for fives days and evening training sessions for two to three days each week. Some sessions may have to be cancelled if signs of overtraining develop.
- o **Session duration.** Continuous workout might not exceed a total of two hours per session.
- o **Load curve.** A training cycle, of few months duration, **starts** with heavier volume at low intensity and ends with low volume and high intensity. Heavy volume is achieved by increasing the number of sets per exercise groups. Low volume with high intensity is achieved by few sets of heavier lifts.
- o **Daily volume.** Daily, the trainee performs less than forty sets of a balanced combination of the Clean and Jerk, the Snatch, and assisting exercises. Each set consists of one to five repetitions. Exercise groups usually range from four to eight groups each training day.
- o **Average loads.** The intensity level should not drop below 60%, with average intensity of about 80% of the maximum.
- o **Preparing for competition.** The maximum attempts of lifting should be reduced during the early months prior to the contest to allow for general buildup of strength and to prevent trauma due to weakness or poor conditioning.
- o **Frequency of maximal lifts.** Thus, a trainee could try to reach the maximum of the Clean and Jerk, or the Snatch, three to five times per months and increase the attempts as the contest approaches.
- o **Daily regimen.** Usually the morning sessions are assigned to the classical technical lifts. The evening sessions are designated for the assisting exercises to remedy individual deficient aspects of training.
- o **Approaching contest.** As the contest date approaches, the volume drops and the intensity increases. One month prior to the contest date, the maximum lifting attempts climb to the top, to reach 20 or so, for each lift.
- o The week or so prior to the competition, three sessions per week are considered reasonable with avoidance of all strenuous activities.

4.5. ASSISTING EXERCISES OF WEIGHTLIFTING

4.5.1. SQUAT

The illusion that heavy squatting enhances maximal lifting is very deceptive. Squat strengthens the knees but does little to synchronize driving force during real lifting. Therefore, squatting has to be gauged within the framework of advancing performance.
- o **Leg drive.** Weightlifting training requires strong and flexible legs for both the Snatch and the Clean and Jerk. The legs are the main drive force in freestyle lifting. The three muscles that generate the upward drive force and torques around the leg joints are:

i. ***Quadriceps***. The Quadriceps are the front muscles of the thigh. They are stretched prior to shortening, by bending the knees and lowering the hips to the horizontal level of the knee. Pre-stretching enhances recruitment of the different pinnas of the Quadriceps.
ii. ***Glutei***. The glutei are the muscles of the buttocks. They extend the hips and differ in their action from the Hamstrings in their oblique directions, their action on the femurs as well as the upper back of the pelvis, and their explosive Jerky contraction. The Glutei are pre-stretched by bending the hips in the start position. The stretch reflex is well known to generate as much muscular force of contraction as the muscle spindles are elongated, by stretching.[3]
iii. ***Hamstrings***. The Hamstrings reside behind the upper legs. These are main hip extensors when the knees are straightened and fixed. They are pre-stretched by the lifter leaning forwards, with almost-straight knees, to begin the over-knee acceleration of the bar.

o **Limitation of leg drive**. The Clean and Jerk in particular depends on the strength of the legs. Naïve propositions, of solely enhancing leg strength by squatting in order to promote the Clean and Jerk, are flawed because of the following.
  i. The **recovery** period after squatting impacts subsequent workouts. This has to be balanced for their negative effects on technique enhancement.
  ii. Increase in the number of repetitions per set over three repetitions, for six sets or more, will strengthen the legs though might interfere with **legs' flexibility**.
  iii. The legs generate the most **powerful driving** force in Weightlifting over a relatively small range of motion at the knee, hip and ankle joints. That is because of the multiple origins, directions of action, and sizes of the muscles of the thighs and glutei. Yet, this power depends on the conditions of the heart and lungs. These two are affected by the upper body status during lifting, as well as the protracted aftereffects of squatting effort.
  iv. Even with awesome strong legs, Squat depends on the **scapular balance**. Strong shoulders and back permit vigorous respiration and circulation to supply enough oxygen and blood to the legs.
  v. The 1970's, legendary Vasily Alexeyev (soviet superheavy weight class) was one the opponents of heavy squatting. His strength stemmed from his well relaxed and rested; yet heavily trained muscles. Alexeyev body contours defied any athletic appearance. He believed that results in Weightlifting are not dependent on high results in the Squat, *Table 4.9*.

Table 4.9. Examples of Squat records and Clean and Jerk of superheavy Weightlifters

Weightlifter	Country	Bodyweight	Year	Clean, kg	Back Squat, kg	Front Squat, kg
Aslanbek Yenaldiev	Soviet	Superheavyweight	1992	245	455	
Leonid Taranenko	Soviet	Superheavyweight (147.5 kg)	1988	266	380	300
Antonio Krastev	Bulgaria	Superheavyweight (172.5kg)	1987	255	390	310
Vasily Alexeyev	Soviet	Superheavyweight	1972	256	270	
Mark Henry	USA	Superheavyweight (181 kg)		220	432	325
Paul Anderson	USA	Superheavyweight (150 kg)	1952	220	454	
Anatoly Pisarenko	Soviet	Superheavyweight		262.5	290	

o **Changes in the role of leg drive.** The current literature on Weightlifting portrays the current trends in training. However, changes in trends happen insidiously as well as acutely, as follows.
  i. Jerking heavy weight with deep squatting, instead of leg springing, was introduced in the 1990's.
  ii. Pulling the bar on the back of the shoulders, after passing the head under and in front of the bar, was also introduced in competitions.
  iii. Reducing the number of exercises per session, and increasing the number of workout sessions per week, was learned since the 1950's.
  iv. Although Squats, Bench Press, and Deadlift are the most important assistance exercise, many believe that the future of Weightlifting will bring major changes, with sole reliance on the classic **Clean and Jerk** (Clean, Hang Cleans, Hang Pulls, High Pulls, Push Press, Split Jerk), **Font Squat, Snatch** (Hang Snatch, Overhead Squat, Press under with quick drop), *Table 4.10*.

---

[3] Stretching a muscle induces reflex stimulation through a circuit of sensory nerve fibers, spinal motoneurons, and motor nerve fibers. The delay between stretching and stimulation is about 0.5 to 0.9 millisecond. Stronger stretching induces stronger stimulation. This is segmental reflex within the same muscle. In addition, extensor stretching induces flexor inhibition. This is inter-segmental reflex between muscles and their antagonists. "Best & Taylor's Physiological Basis of Medical Practice" 9th edition, by John R. Brobeck. The Williams & Wilkins Company. Baltimore, 1973. Pages 9-72 to 9-74.

v. Enhancing the Clean and Jerk or the Snatch might rely completely on **more training of the same kind,** with different intensity and load volume.

Table 4.10. Examples of the relative association of strength in assisting exercises and strength in whole lifting of superheavy Weightlifters (All weights are in kilograms). Source: http://www.iat.uni-leipzig.de/weight/htm and personal files.

Name	Country	Bodyweight	Snatch	Clean & Jerk	Back Squat	Bench Press	Deadlift
Antonio Krastev (1981-87)	Bul	172	216	260	390	210	345
Evgeni Popov	Bul	152	200	242.5	365	220	365
Serge Reding	Blr	133	182.5	235	400	240	350
Sergei Alexeev	Rus	147	175	235	420	220	330
Andrei Mustrikov	Rus	114	177.5	232.5	360	230	362.5
Shane Hamman	US	164	187.5	230	457.5	250	332.5
Ken Patera	US	150	175.5	229	372.5	255	355
Mark Henry	US	181	180	220	432.5	240	410
Bruce Wilhelm	US	148	182.5	220	362.5	255	360
Taito Haara	Fin	132	175	217.5	405	227.5	362.5
Jerome Hannan	US	154	175	217.5	362.5	227.5	362.5
Viktor Naleiken	Ukr	131	167.5	212.5	410	232.5	370
Andrew Kerr (1973–75)	GB	136	155	200	357.5	250	382.5
Jon Cole	US	123	155	195	408.5	276.5	400
Thomas Magee	Can	127	147.5	195	390	260	367.5
Lars Noren	Swe	140	145	191	422.5	250	406
G Badenhorst	RSA	140	140	177.5	450	250	402.5
Bill Kazamaier	US	145	130	170	420	300	402.5
Don Reinhoudt	US	157	117.5	167.5	425	275	402.5

GB : Great Britain, BUL : Bulgaria, Rus : Russia, Blr : Belarussia, Fin : Finland, Swe : Sweden, RSA. South Africa.

o **Methods of Developing Leg Strength**
  i. *Submaximal training*. It is well known that one does not have to train with maximal resistance, all the time, in order to strengthen the legs. One can make significant improvement employing primarily small (up to 70%) and medium (up to 80%) weights. This loading should be combined, on occasions, with large and maximal weights. However, maximal weights should make up only about 16% of the total load in Squats.
  ii. *Preparatory training*. It has also been known that noticeable improvement in Squat results can be achieved, after only six weeks of training. By chiefly utilizing small and medium weights for Squat, one can preserve a good "functional state", a necessary condition for systematic training. This moderate stressing of the legs is designed for the preparatory stage. The six-week training cycle of squatting is divided into two stages. Each stage consists of three weeks. In the first stage, the **volume rises** with a relatively constant average weight of the barbell, in the range of 70% and 80% of the best back Squat. The high volume serves whole body conditioning by enhancing energy production. In the second stage, the volume decreases while the **intensity increases** in the range 80% to 105%. The low volume in the second stage fosters active rest, while the high intensity fosters muscle growth by eliminating weak and fragile fibers. During the six weeks, Squats are performed three times per week, with no more frequency than every other day.
  iii. *Peaking of volume*. The preparatory training cycle of the legs begins with increasing the barbell weight every other session, but adhering to the limit of below 80% of current maximal weight. The other alternating sessions remain at the same barbell weight and volume of training, in regard to the number of sets and repetitions of weight. This medium intensity and high volume stage is an activation process of the subsequent anabolic stage. It lasts for three weeks and comprises of twelve Squat sessions, of about five sets per session, and three or four reps per set. The net total of lifts in this stage ranges from 180 to 240 Squat lifts of less than 80% 1RM.
  iv. *Peaking of intensity*. After three weeks of high volume Squat preparation, the barbell weight is progressively increased by 5% incremental increase each session. That starts by adding 5% barbell weight to the end of the previous stage of 80% of 1RM. This is accompanied by progressive decrease in number of repetitions and increase in the number of single-repetition sets. Within five sessions, in the stage, intensity peaks from 80% to about 105%. Yet, subsequent drop in intensity, during the remaining seven sessions of the three-week segment, and the progressive increase in barbell weight during each session accounts for average intensity in the range below 85%, but above 80%. The total volume of twelve sessions, of six sets per session, with average two reps per set, amounts to 144 lifts. One fourth of these lifts have intensity below 90% 1RM and about one tenth exceeds 90% 1RM. The percentages are mere estimates that serve as a guide in preventing overtraining.

v. ***Whole body and leg load volumes.*** The Squat cycle intertwines with whole body training. Squatting volume reserves slightly over 20% of whole body volume and should be kept around 80% intensity. Thus the six-week preparation, of 240 lifts of high volume and 144 lifts of high intensity in Squatting, will total about 1800 lifts in all exercises. This averages 300 lifts per week, or 50 lifts per session, in six-session week. On the average, the maximum intensity in Back Squat should exceed 130% of the maximum of Clean and Jerk. If one's Squat results are substantially below this figure, the volume of Squats should be increased to 30% of the general volume of loading, instead of 20%.

vi. ***Mobility.*** This requires greater recovery system beside anaerobic exercises of Weightlifting. Running, sprints, jumps, and sport games enhance the aerobic components of leg structures, other than muscles mass. Bear in mind that adequate nutrition and rest, during the 24-hour of the day, are crucial for exercise to yield any positive outcome. If overtraining is suspected, rest and relaxation must be contemplated for few days and load volume must be reduced. Rest and nutrition help restore the extra-pyramidal nervous regulation to normal and reduces muscular spasm and poor recruitment.

4.5.2. MAJOR AXIAL MUSCLES OF WEIGHTLIFTING

o **Extensors.** The extensors of the legs and trunk are the major lifting muscles in the body, as follows.
   i. The muscles most important, in lifting from the floor, are undoubtedly the **Quadriceps**, *Figures 4.6* thru *4.8*. The Quadriceps torque the femurs around the knees in order to lift the body, loaded with weight.
   ii. The **Hamstring** muscles are stretched during the initial acceleration, during the lifting from the floor to the kneecaps. Stretch stimulates the muscle spindle reflex to recruit more fibers and increases the magnitude and duration of firing. This Hamstring effect kicks in the final acceleration from the kneecaps to full extension of the body on raised heels. Here, the Hamstrings extend the hips, thus translating the Quadriceps drive to the torso.
   iii. The **Glutei** differ from the Hamstrings in their action on the upper femur. By their oblique direction behind the hips, the glutei stabilize the hips during both the upward extension of the body as well as during the descent.
   iv. The **back erectors** work as a lever, transmitting the forces of the lower body to the upper body. Their action is mainly isometric, strong contraction with little bending of the joints.

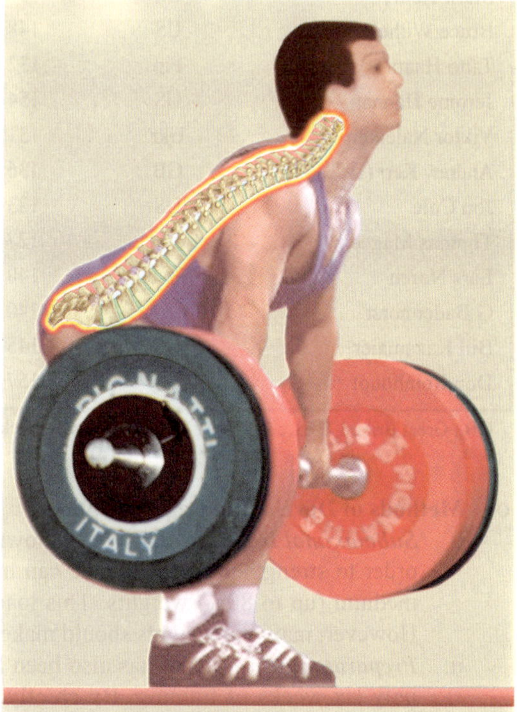

o **Scapular muscles**. These transmit the forces from the vertebral axis to the arms. Scapular muscles are paramount to lifting in maintaining the chest cage widely patent (open), under the heavy load on the upper limbs. Their support of the upper skeletal configuration permits the heart and lung to perform their vital functions, and protect the freedom of passage of the major vessels to the arms and brain, as follows, *Figure 4.9*.

Figure 4.6. The leg drive and lordotic back posture are fundamental to lifting.

   i. The scapulas do not articulate with the vertebral column and rely entirely on muscular pulling for transmission of forces. This configuration permits the scapulas to move freely, in many directions, and give the arms greater range of mobility
   ii. The scapulas are triangular in shape. They move as a result of the muscular pulling on their three edges and two surfaces. The scapulas also play crucial role in supporting the chest cage during lifting. The way the scapulas manipulate the balances of forces on their edges and surfaces is through their attachments to the clavicles, arms, chest, and vertebral axis.

o **Shoulder muscles**. The **Deltoids** are the major shoulder muscles that abduct and flex the shoulder, as follows.
   i. The Deltoids are crucial to front Squat, upper pulling, and Snatch.
   ii. Strong Deltoids are not a substitute to strong front vertebral neck muscles. These pull the chest cage upwards during the loading of the front chest. This explains why strengthening the Deltoids, in isolation, is not a substitute for performing the Clean and front Squat.

o **Methods of developing back strength**
   Pulls. Pulling weights from the floor to full body extension, with straight arms, brings the barbell to the top of the thighs. Further pulling takes place by three actions that serve to move the shoulder plates beyond their isometric fixed state at the beginning of the lift. The three actions are as follows.

i. Back hyperextension is enhanced by the balance of the Erector spinae and Hamstrings, on the back, and Iliopsoas on the front.
ii. Shoulder shrugging is produced by the upper Trapezius. Pulling, while jumping forwards in the middle of the pull, is practiced by some lifters, in order to jolt the Trapezius with excessive impulsive force.
iii. Arms abduction is generated by the Deltoids and Supraspinatus.

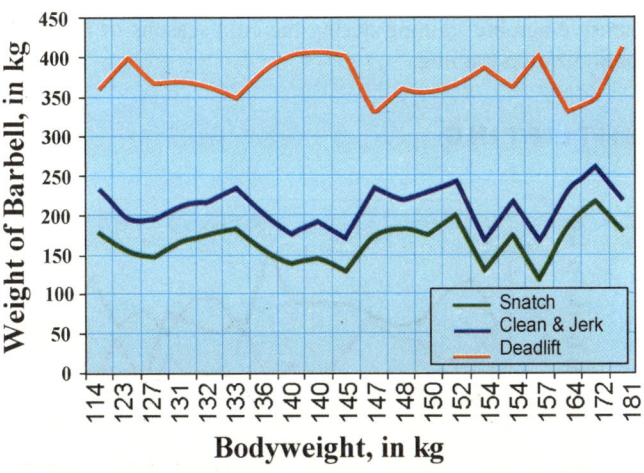

Figure 4.7. Superheavy Weightlifters Deadlift less than double the maximum Clean lift. Yet the Deadlift curve shows a trend of hindering the Snatch and Clean lifting. The more the weight lifted in Deadlift the less weight lifted in Clean and Jerk and Snatch. Compiled from *Table 4.10*.

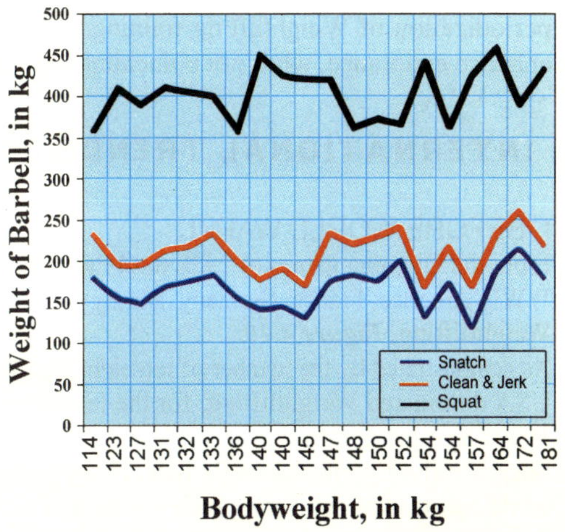

Figure 4.8. Weightlifters Squat more than they Deadlift. The reverse of peaking and dipping of the three curves demonstrate the same hindrance effect of the Squat on the Clean and Snatch. Compiled from *Table 4.10*.

Pulling accelerate one's ability to move heavy weights within few weeks. It is the most effective way of strengthening back erectors and scapular muscles. Executing Pulling in various stages, of progressive increase in the height of the pull, facilitates dissecting the motion into its simple and easy-to-learn technique. Advanced lifters maintain balanced chain of muscular links by regular and progressive pulling from the floor. This always has to be balanced by performing overhead pushing, even in a few numbers of sets, in order to balance scapular forces.

Goodmorning. This strengthens the Hamstrings and Glutei by isotonic contraction and the back erectors by isometric contraction. Goodmorning has to be performed with slightly bent knees and hyper-extended back. Many Weightlifters can perform the Goodmorning with weights that exceeds their maximum in the Clean lift. Goodmorning is also executed with jumping while extending the hips. Military Goodmorning with stiffed knees is not encouraged since it might cause Hamstring tear. Also, it is a fallacy to believe that Goodmorning strengthens the abdominal muscles.

4.5.3. POWER DEVELOPMENT AND WEIGHTLIFTING TRAINING
Developing power by Weightlifting training is subjected to theoretical as well as practical guessing, as follows.

Theory: Some analysts claim that power gained by Weightlifting training is not transferable to other athletic activities, such as jumping. Thus, Weightlifting training is presumed as distinct and separate skills, with distinct and separate abilities from those experienced in different sports. These views are based on the assumption that muscular power is controlled by brain motor-programs that determine muscular explosive movements. Thus weigh training that approximates sporting movements only affects the brain programs and may develop transferable power. Weightlifting differs from weight training of sporting activity in these respects.
o The velocity in Weightlifting peaks in the middle of lifting in opposition to that of weight training of sporting activity, which peaks at the end of motion, such as sprinting vigorously at the end of a race.
o The velocity dips with increasing resistance to the limbs, in Weightlifting, while in sporting activity maintaining higher velocity by means of powerful effort is the desired goal.
o Postural alignment adapts to Weightlifting differently from that in weight training of sporting activities. Weightlifting gears towards balancing vertical forces while sporting activities require many directions of balance.
o Developing general power using non-specific exercises improve physiological hypertrophy and strength not skill.
o Power movements are better trained in a pattern specific to that practiced by sport activity since abilities are non-transferable and are subjected to specific movement patterns for their selected use

Practice: The claim that Weightlifting training has a pattern that is non-transferable to other sports activities omits the following issues.
o Different individuals have different brain capacities of motor programming. Some athletes excel in more than one sport with exceptional accomplishments.

4 WEIGHTLIFTING

- o The claim that velocity-force relationship in Weightlifting affects power development in a way that differs from that of other sports activities, that do not involve the dampening effect of lifting, is not substantiated with concrete proof. Strengthening coordinated major axial muscles is a plus to developing power that suits any sport.
- o The only deterrent to gaining transferable power between Weightlifting and other sports is over training. This leaves little stamina to perform other activities beside Weightlifting.
- o Serial cross training is well proven to enhance skill. For example, a trainee can greatly benefit from training on swimming during the months of summer, with reduced load volume in strength training, when he or she return to full periodization of Weightlifting training. In addition, extensive aerobic training during the cold seasons of the year can enhance endurance, when not coinciding with ongoing periodization training.

4.6. INTERNATIONAL TRENDS IN WEIGHTLIFTING

4.6.1. BEFORE WORLD WAR II
- o From the Olympic games of 1920 until the beginning of WWII, America, France, Germany, and Egypt, dominated Weightlifting, *Figure 4.10*.
- o As demonstrated by the number of top eight Weightlifters, USA dominated Weightlifting, for the last time, in the 1932 Olympic games.
- o Surprisingly, Egypt, then a British colony and a third world nation, was competing with France and Germany, second to USA.
- o In 1936, Germany dominated the Olympic Weightlifting while the other three nations started declining until the present time.
- o Taking into consideration the relative population of the four nations, USA ranked last in terms of its relative contribution to the top eight positions of Weightlifting. Moreover, the noticeable decline of the USA participation in higher ranking continued a steep downhill course until this day.

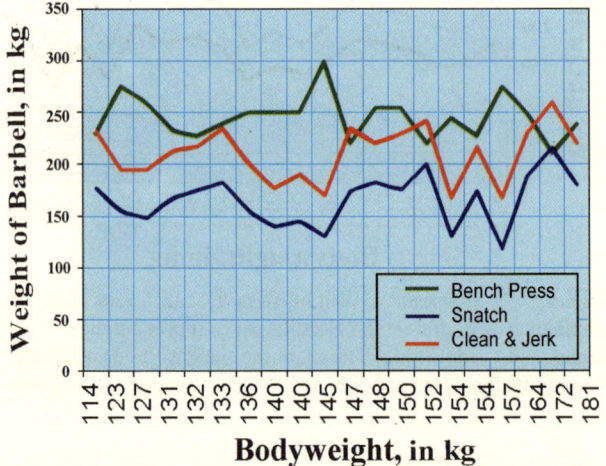

Figure 4.9. Weightlifters Bench Press less than they Deadlift but more than they Clean. Again the hindrance effect of the Bench Press is evident from the reverse of peaking and dipping of the corresponding curves. Compiled from *Table 4.10*.

4.6.2. AFTER WORLD WAR II
A new era of communist dominance has commenced, with dramatic revolution of the sport of Weightlifting. The Soviet, since 1956 until 1990, has never ceased to break all previous records. The Soviets were followed by East Germany, Bulgaria, and Poland as the four giants of Weightlifting of modern times. Only late during 1980's, when a new breed of nations had excelled into the front. China, Japan, Koreas, Greece, and Turkey are showing a trend that monopoly is a fallacy in Weightlifting. It must be noticed that, these later years, accomplishing top ranks in Weightlifting is tremendously difficult task.

- o **Human limit of strength**
  The most important observation from these international trends of climbing and declining of nations and the constant uphill stampede of records are:
  i. **Research**, on the national scale, was the major impetus for uncovering the human potential of developing strength without gaining excess weight. Without the aggressive experimentation on all aspects of strength training, it would be impossible to discover the optimum training methodology that we know today.
  ii. **Military** competitions through a breed of military officers, keen on exploring the unknown, coincided with the first man in space in 1961. Strength training became the focus of promoting strength among soldiers.
  iii. Human limits of lifting heavy weight may still be in state of constant **evolution**. The potential of the cardiopulmonary function to endure such new challenges of strenuous exercise demonstrates the evolution process. The enhancement of human ligaments, tendons, muscles, and bone by exercise, enables Weightlifters to lift over three times bodyweight and at high speed. This is another sign of evolving sport.
  iv. Though unpopular and almost overlooked by news reporters, health professionals, and sports fans, strides in Weightlifting are planting the **seeds of future revolution** in strength training.

- o **Western trends**
  Western countries are enjoying affluent economic state that influenced athletic education and practice in all levels. Most the gyms in USA are geared to general fitness for profit. **Gyms** stock the training floors with shining machines to impress unwary clients. General weight training is the dominant form of resistance training in western nations. This comprises of working out individual muscle groups, using aiding machines for training, and splitting the training days for upper body and lower body sessions. Such simplistic and misleading methods of training are so pervasive in the ailing athletes of western nations.

Also, in western nations, the **school system** is more dismal than the fitness industry. Teachers worry about litigious fears, physical safety, and the demands of intolerable cost of living than the future of the new generation they are supposed to prepare for future challenges. The **government of** western nations is a product of the popcorn culture of entertainment, self-serving, and mainstream popular alliance. **Role models** are also lacking in nations that fared poorly in health training of the vast populace.

i. The American model had shifted toward the physical attractiveness of big and strong.
ii. The best top American Weightlifters left no trace of motivation of others. Few youth know or hear of
iii. Weightlifting training. Most believe that Powerlifting is synonymous to Weightlifting.
iv. The entire concept of perfect performance is lacking in the norms of American culture.
v Most believe that a role model Weightlifter should earn higher in Hollywood or get better contract with entertaining agents.

In most western nations, the **public** is divided into two parties, as far as sport is concerned. A party that is entertained, has the power to buy game' tickets, food, and drinks to watch frenzy of clowns of athletes. That party would also consume the national health resources by ailing hearts, joints, and minds. The other party of entertaining athletes that gamble with their future to excel in sport, with very little emphasis in excelling in academic or social skills. Most of such entertaining sports end in life threatening injuries.

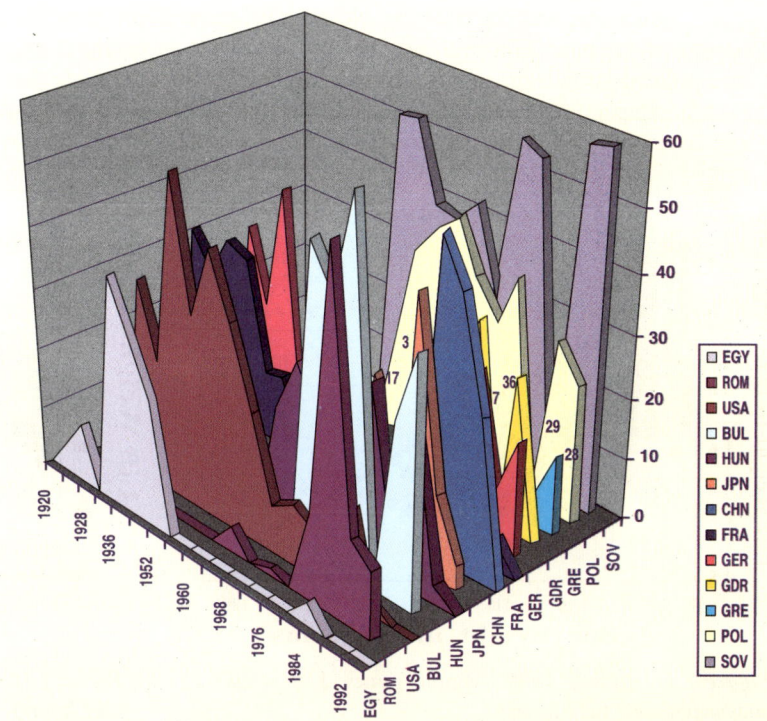

Figure 4.10. Number of top eight ranking Olympic lifters in the Olympic games since 1920 for different nations

The **media** is as guilty as the other players in marginalizing Weightlifting as a viable health and fitness tool. The louder and powerful media form the public perception of strength training. Armed with an arsenal of impressive bodily photography, phony medical supplements, and marketing experts, many fitness magazines and media have contributed to the apathy of today's youthful athletes. This left the fitness literature jammed with erroneous methods of training. Bodybuilders pioneer the fitness of ignorance, building huge muscles, disregarding health issues of healthy bodyweight, flexibility, and coordination.[4] The competitions of the fitness industry for profit have resulted in a public that believes that sport is exclusive to privileged few.

o **State support**
The fact that communist and socialist nations are dominating Weightlifting sheds light on the impact of state support for promoting sports that promote public health. It might be said that in socials settings, athletes are coerced by lack of alternative opportunities, or might be recruited by governments. Under any system, Olympic athletes have to consume most of their resources to get to the top and are subject to severe personal sacrifices in pursuing these goals. Even in western nations, most athletes who do not participate in a popular sport have not benefited financially, on a large scale. When injured prematurely, many end up underemployed, in dismal living situations.

o **Local trends**
Getting started in strength training without proper coaching or adequate knowledge about the different disciplines involved in health and fitness, leads the majority of people to make short cuts in exercise. The most common practice in improvised weight training is working out muscles that are easily visualized or felt. **Exercising individual groups of muscles** is pervasive in all cultures and countries that lack active physical education campaigns. Even well educated people in many cultures do not bother to advance their knowledge about exercise planning. As if that sort of play does not deserve keen intellectual effort. Such practice consumes many years of training without leading to the desired

---
[4] "The new encyclopedia of modern bodybuilding" by Arnold Schwarzenegger with Bill Dobbins, Simon & Schuster, New York 1999 and "Body-for-life: 12 weeks to mental and physical strength" by Bill Phillips with Michael D'Orso, 1st edition. Harper Collins Publishers, New York, 1999.

goals. Mainly, because there are too many muscles, and there are endless ways of training them. If you know how to train the Biceps in five of six different ways, each in a handful of sets, each set in a handful of repetitions, how many years would it take you to get your Biceps the way you want them to be?

In addition, designating alternate workout sessions for specific body parts undermines muscular balance. With **split body training,** you would need a sophisticated computational program to analyze your proportions, your balance, speed, flexibility, and coordination. No such program is yet domesticated. Bumping iron without learning from the lessons of the past leads to injury. History is always an essential impetus to the evolution of the human brain. The accumulated knowledge in physical training enforces the principle that "lean and mean is better than big and mean". That is simply translated to the fact that active whole body workout takes away the size and promotes strength, whereas isolated exercises may enlarge scattered muscles, yet prejudice whole body fitness.

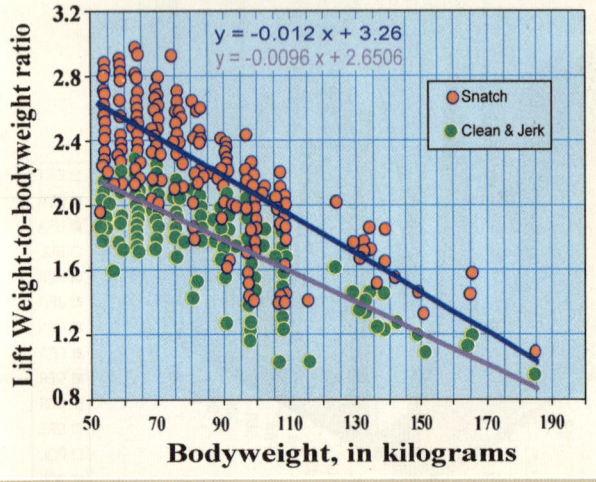 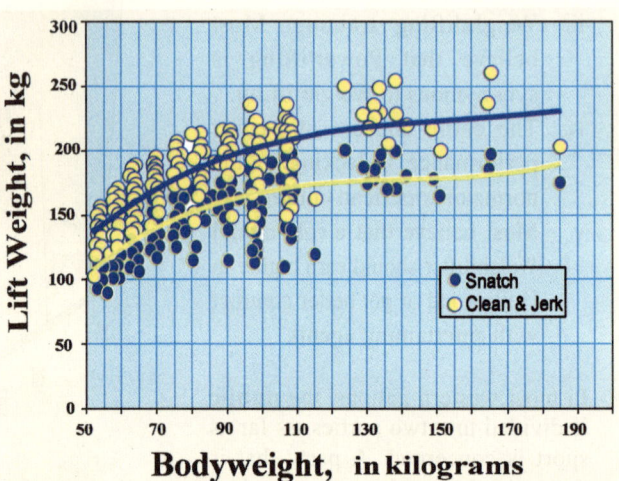

Figure 4.11. Atlanta 1996 Olympic games. Lift weight-to-bodyweight ratio (217 lifters).

Figure 4.12. Atlanta 1996 Olympic games. Lift weighs in kg (217 lifters).

4.6.3. OLYMPIC GAMES OF ATLANTA 1996

In the 1990 Olympic games in Atlanta, USA, the trends of developing strength in relation to the bodyweight proves the old principle of the superiority of leanness and mobility over mass and immobility, *Figures 4.11* and *4.12*. From these tables, the ratio of lift-weight to bodyweight relative strength (RS) decreases as the bodyweight (BW) increases according to the equations:

    Clean and Jerk: RS   = 3.26 - 0.0120 x **BW** (kg).
    Snatch: RS   = 2.65 - 0.0096 x **BW** (kg).

If one has to use these equations to estimate the maximum work done by the top Olympic Weightlifters, one has to borrow the weight-to-height relationship from epidemiological data. The average American male population exhibits bodyweight-to-height relation according to the equation:

                        BW (kg) = 0.88 x **Height** (cm) – 74.

Multiplying the lift per bodyweight ratio by the height yields the average work done per each kilogram of the lifter (WDKG). This gives

    Clean and Jerk: WDKG = 0.0006 **BW** (kg) + 3.9047 (meters)
    Snatch: WDKG = 0.0007 **BW** (kg) + 3.1804 (meters)

The average work done per each kilogram of the lifter is the vertical distance to which a kilogram of body can lift an equal weight. From this crude analysis, we can make the following observations.

o   These are guiding relationships of the work done per kilogram of the lifter's weight of top Olympic athletes of Atlanta 1996.
o   The main limitation of increasing the relative work is due to the increase in the height of the lifter. This explains why stocky, short lifters made historical records because the bodyweight was the only factor under consideration.
o   There exists a maximum on the amount of work that can be done by top human Olympic lifters.
o   If there were any fairness in the Olympic games, this formula would be the best judge to athletic performance.
o   The 7.23 meters landmark represents the maximum work done in the two Olympic lifts per kilogram of bodyweight.
o   The most work done per body weight was in the 85 kg class, where 8.47 meters were exceeded.
o   The 70 kg and 100 kg Olympic weight classes were able to reach the 8.25 meters of relative work.
o   Under 70 kg and above 85 kg Olympic weight classes, the relative work done diminishes.
o   If there is such a thing as optimum weight, 85 kg average height person accomplishes the most relative work done.

It should be emphasized strongly that we have made the following approximations when derived the above equations:
    i.   We borrowed the weight-height ratios of average American adult male population to deduce an approximate figure for the heights of the Olympic Weightlifters.

ii. Many of the heavy weight lifters do not adhere to that representation. Because the Olympic committees and the Weightlifting organizing authorities do not record heights of the competitors, we have resorted to that method to analyze the performance of different top lifters. Borrowing epidemiological data of one population and using it in another population is a well-practiced method to analyze data retrospectively, when the researches lacks specific data.
iii. An example of the inaccuracy is a weightlifter that weighs 180 kg, according to our height-weight formula; he is supposed to be 289 cm tall (9.62 feet), which is an impossible height for Weightlifters.
iv. We assumed that the lifting distance equals to the height of the lifter. While Weightlifters lift above their heads, they dip under the weight at lower distances. Thus, the height was taken as the average distance that approximates the phase of the lift. Keeping in mind that the plates of the barbell position the bar at 22 cm elevation above ground, which makes our assumption more realistic.

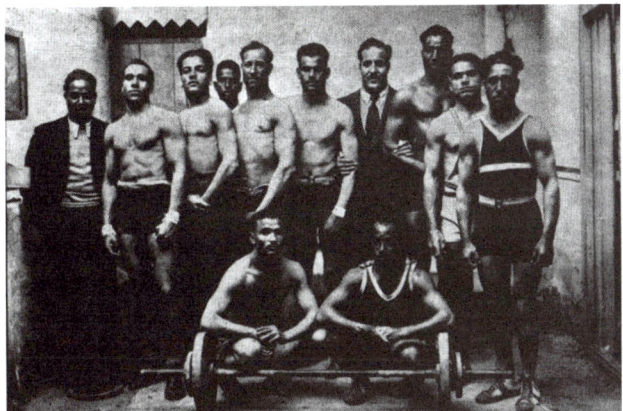

Figure 4.13. The 1928 Olympic gold medallist Mr. El-Sayed Mohammed Nosseir, in a suite and tie, with athletes of local club. The gyms of that era were as simple as a wooden platform and a locally machined barbell, 1936 in Egypt.

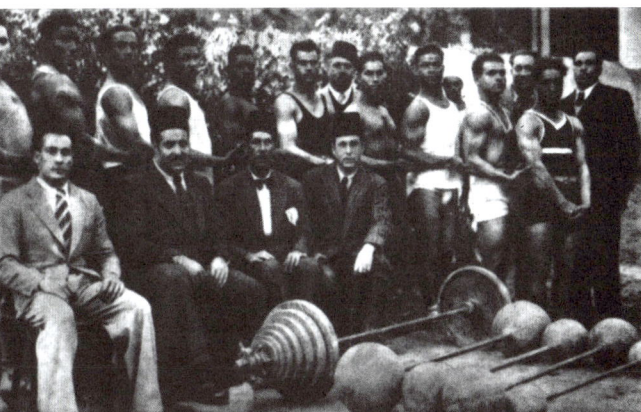

*Figure 4.14 El-Sayed Mohammed Nosseir, (seated second from left) Egy*pt, Weightlifting gold medallist of the Olympic games 1928, Amsterdam, class 82.5 kg (Press 100, Snatch 112.5, Jerk 142.5) is celebrated as an national icons by the locals of a south Egyptian town, in 1936.

4.6.4. WEIGHTLIFTING IN EGYPT 1936

In 1936, Weightlifting was in its infancy. Public gyms were very scarce and in very dismal state. The Olympic gold medallist El-Sayed Mohammed Nosseir lifted only 100 kg in the Press, 112.5 kg in the Snatch, and 142.5 in the Clean and Jerk in the weight class of 82.5 kg. Today, these records are 180 kg in the Snatch and 210 kg in the Clean and Jerk, while the Press is cancelled. Such modest level of lifting is attainable today with few months of training. Yet in 1936, Mr. Nosseir

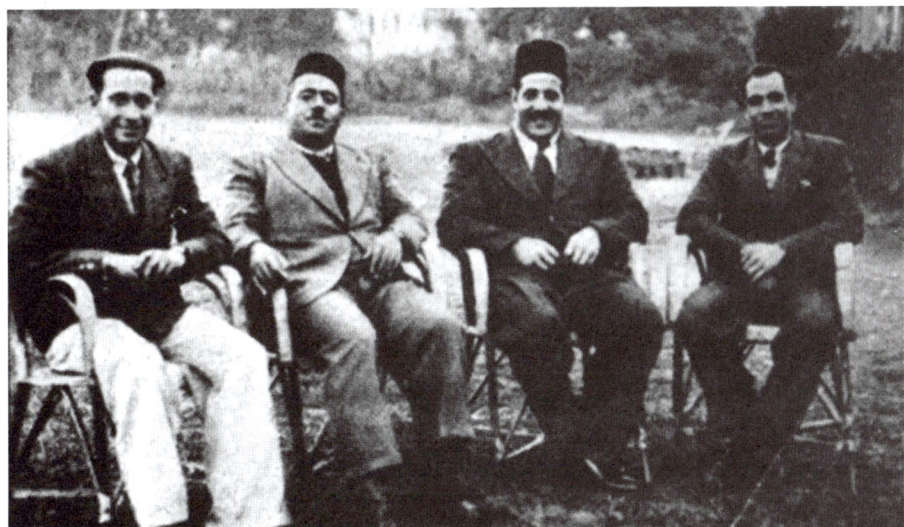

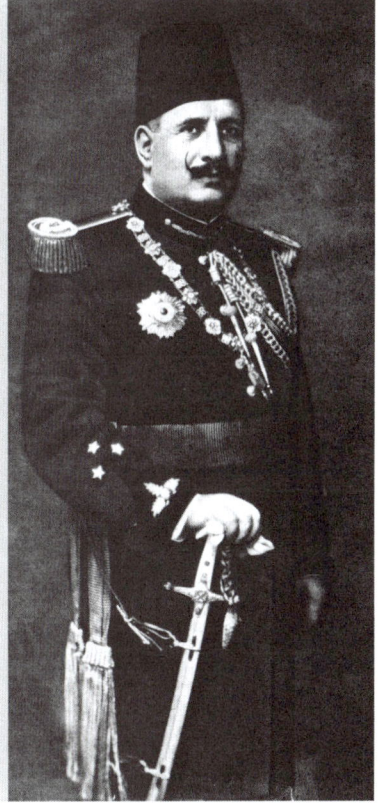

Figure 4.15. Seated (above): Al-Sayed Noussir (afandi) (third from left), Special welcome for a national Weightlifting hero by the high class of the town, Egypt 1936.

Figure 4.16. Standing (to the right) King Fouad had died from dental infection. In 1936, antibiotics were not yet discovered. His obituary was published in "Al Lataif Al Musawara", Vol. XXII, Cairo, June 1936: " as follows: "In last April 28, 1936 Egypt was shocked with the loss of its dearest great king, Fouad the First. This had brought deep sadness which was only relieved with the arrival of the young beloved prince, his greatness Farouk the First, who had renewed hope to the noble royal family and the sad nation."

was treated as a hero with prestige and access to power throughout his entire life, and all over the nation, *Figures 4.13* thru *4.15*. The king of Egypt died in 1936 from dental infection that is treatable today with antibiotics, *Figure 4.16*. These were discovered in 1942. Half a century later, the earlier champions of Weightlifting are still active in campaigning for the sport, *Figure 4.17*. The three people in the last figure traveled from far and remote areas of Egypt to attend a Weightlifting contest, in which they are viewed as role models and icons of the old and glorious days of the nation.

4.7. HIGHLIGHTS OF CHAPTER FOUR

1. Weights that are less that 60% of the maximum, of certain exercises, are not very beneficial for acquiring strength. Intense resistance is the main impetus to all strengthening activities. Intense resistance of force promotes physical strength when planned according to scientific guidelines.

2. Weightlifting training has definite time frame to enhance strength, definite sequence of execution of exercises to avoid injuries, and definite requirement of progressive, continuous, and regular practice to build strength. Also, Weightlifting strength training would not fail a trainee with long-term injury, due to faulty anatomical or physiological approach.

3. Weightlifting training sessions last about ninety minutes and could be performed twice daily, but less than ten sessions per week. Training sessions starts with about fifteen minutes of warm-up. Some advanced Weightlifters use weights in most of their warm-up time.

4. Core exercises often consist of six groups; each group consists of four to eight set, each sets consists of one to six repetitions. The interval between each set ranges from two to five minutes depending of the fitness condition of the trainee, the intensity of the training, and the temperature of the training room. Longer intervals could lead to poor technique or injuries.

5. The annual distribution of load volume consists of periods of strengthening, periods of restful recovery, and periods of emphasis on the competitive lifts.

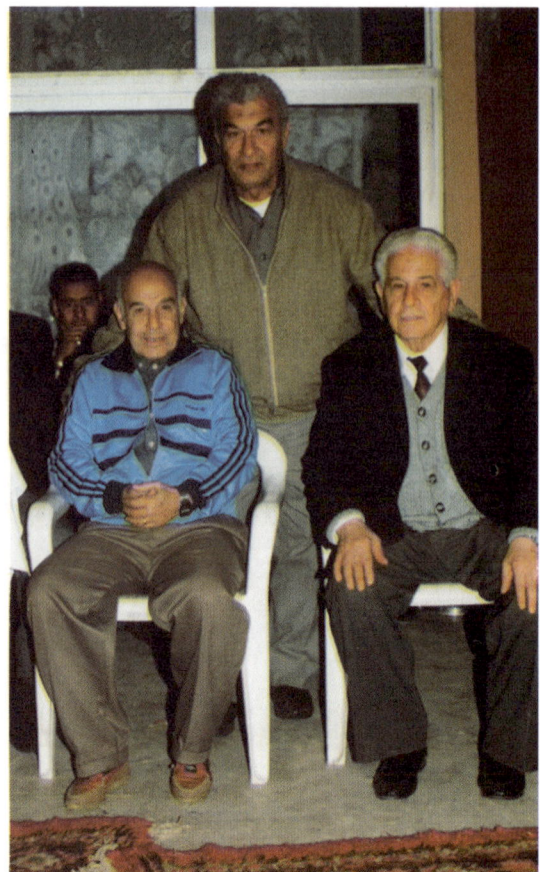

Figure 4.17. Mahmoud Fayad (dressed in a suit and tie) is a Weightlifting gold medallist of the Olympic games of 1948, class 64 kg (Press 92.5, Snatch 105, Jerk 135 kg). Mr. Mahgoob is seated on the left and photographed lifting in 1951 in Paris, Figure 4.3. Standing in the middle, Mr. El-Kassabay, who has pioneered modern scientific Weightlifting in Egypt. The author is one of his students. The style of lifting and routine of workout were major deterrents of that era. Most Weightlifters prior to 1942 died at very young age, due to the epidemics of infectious diseases, such as tuberculosis, typhoid, and cholera. Photo taken in 1995.

Chapter 5
Powerlifting

5.1. BASICS OF PHYSICAL POWER

5.1.1. TRAINING METHODS

The development of physical power by structured training is learned from a long history of human evolution. This relies on the different aspects of energy to enhance physical power as follows.

o **Plyometrics** emulate wild life activity of jumping, climbing, and sprinting. It utilizes the inertial energy of the body to promote power by altering the speed and acceleration of body motion. This sort of activity engages major muscle groups in coordinated complex movements. Their disadvantages lie in the need for spacious training room and complex training education, in addition to the high prevalence of injuries due to the dynamic nature of Plyometrics. Plyometrics help develop the power of either the pelvic or the shoulder girdle, but not both, since the girdle that generates momentum is the one that develops strength. Runners and jumpers, for example, develop awesome lower leg muscles while gymnasts develop strong shoulders and arms.

o **Machine aided training** utilizes different machine designs to strengthen different parts of the body. This method of training offers many people the hope of overcoming individual deficits and of strengthening and balancing weak and neglected muscle groups and joints. In the hands of mathematically and anatomically minded people, this method offers enormous potential of enhancing physical strength. The major disadvantages are the temptation of complete reliance on machines that may seriously cause muscular imbalance. Also, there is a lack of monitoring criteria to assess the proper direction of training, since a sitting person has limited awareness of his or her ability to function in real conditions.

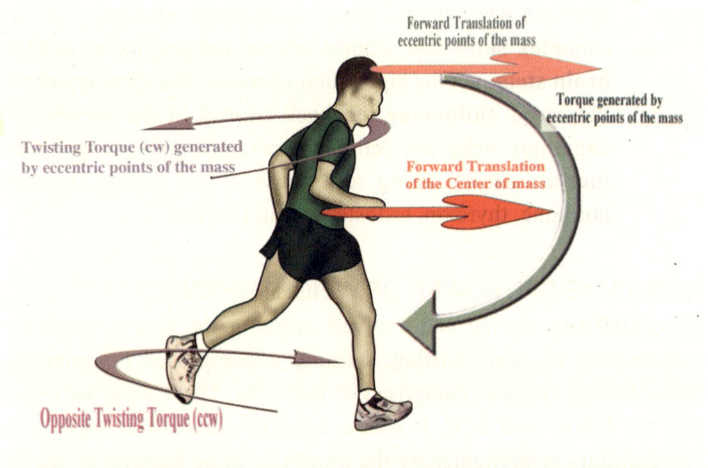

o **Freestyle lifting** utilizes weights of barbells and dumbbells to further enhance the inertial energy of Plyometrics and increase physical power, in short time and beyond conventional standards. This method of training emulates normal activities and reveals the unlimited potential of humans to develop physical power. It is basically founded on the principle: "train the way you intend to fight". The clear disadvantages of freestyle lifting are the need to understand the course of progressive resistance training, overtraining, the relationship between intensity and load volume, over many weeks of training. In addition, weight training entails a tedious learning process of lifting techniques.

Figure 5.1. As the center of mass moves (translates) it creates both translation and torques at the off-center points. Torques are balanced with muscular contractions that work to maintain dynamic balance. Back erectors counteract torques that tend to cause fall. Torques that tend to swing the body towards the sides are counteracted with hip abductors and collateral back muscles.

The different methods of enhancing physical power share this common concept:
Massive bodies tend to revolve around the center of the mass when the initiating force is applied off-center. Physical power is developed when muscles resist such revolution of body parts in order to maintain balance, **Figure 5.1.**
Altering the timing, direction, magnitude, and site of action of force application promotes endless skills of managing physical power. Few of the acquired skills dominate individual performance and shape his or her characteristic identity as an athlete. The above three methods of training complement each other in many ways and should be integrated in any training program.

5.1.2. ELEMENTS OF PHYSICAL POWER

To quantify the components of power development of each method the following elements of human power are considered.

- Power of muscular contraction **(dynamic elements):** This is the critical component of biological power. The muscles are the powerhouses of converting chemical energy into kinetic energy. By virtue of their biological living capabilities, they adapt to activities by growing new dynamic elements, tweaking their biochemical reactions in response to stimulation, and most importantly, altering their reaction to neural signals in response to activities, as follows.
    i. Hypertrophy and increase of density and tensile property of the connective tissue, tendons, and ligaments.
    ii. Type of muscle fibers used in activity, fast- and slow- twitchers.
    iii. Groups of muscles used according to their leverage power and points of insertion into bones.
    iv. Type of muscular contraction used to enhance posture versus enhancing movement, isometric versus isotonic contractions.
- Power of bone support **(static elements):**
    i. Bone grows in density and strength to support the pull of ligaments, the pressure of excessive virtual forces, and the shearing forces of twisting torques.
    ii. Bone responds to hormonal control by regulating the balance of calcium and phosphate ions in the blood. All cells require inorganic phosphates to synthesize ATP molecules from ADP, during glycolysis. Also, all cells require calcium ions to operate many essential biological reactions. Calcium release during muscular contraction activates various stages of the TCA cycle and the conversion of Pyruvate into acetyl CoA, for aerobic energy production.
- Power of synchronization of actions **(optimization elements):**
    i. Lower neural changes occur in the motoneurons of the **spinal cord**. These changes affect the firing rate and synchrony of firing of the motoneurons. They serve increase recruitment of motor units and increase muscular coordination.
    ii. Higher neural changes occur in the **brain** in the form of integration of visual, auditory, equilibrium, proprioception, sensory, and motor stimuli. These changes take place in the cerebrum, cerebellum, and brain stem and serve control of actions of lower neurons.
    iii. Complex skills that require intense integration of mechanical functions rely on the autonomic functions of the **brain stem**, not the higher brain centers. The changes affect the heart, lungs, vascular, and central nervous system.
    iv. Increased **endocrine** feedback control of the metabolism of vigorous physical work. This affects the mood, cognition, behavior, cellular respiration, protein synthesis, and management of energy expenditure. The shift in fuel utilization during rest, activity, and fasting is under the control of insulin, glucagon, adrenaline, growth hormone, thyroxin, testosterone, and cortisol.

5.1.3. PHYSICAL POWER OF WEIGHTLIFTING

Weightlifting started and evolved utilizing the above-mentioned three methods of training. Apart from competitive presentation of Weightlifting, training encompasses Plyometrics, aided training, and freestyle lifting. Until 1920's, Weightlifting contests comprised of four lifts. These were the one-hand Snatch, the Clean and Press, the two-hand Snatch, and the Clean and Jerk. It was a sport of blue-collar hard laborers and tough folks. Part of the training routine of Weightlifters is strengthening the groups of large muscles of the thighs, back, and shoulders. This strengthening segment of Weightlifting has evolved, over the years, to **Powerlifting**. Another part of Weightlifting training is building the assisting muscles that enhance the technique of Olympic lifts. The assisting muscles of importance in Weightlifting are arms, abdomen, and chest. This refining segment of Weightlifting has also evolved, over the years, to **Bodybuilding**. The evolution of the new sports was arbitrary, since there is no reason for assuming that an athlete can perform one sport and not the others. Few people have appreciated the benefits of enhancing performance by all available means of sound training, rather than getting distracted by the propaganda of advocates of one sport or the other.

Powerlifting has offered great temptation because of the following.
- Its attractive and stimulating name that connotes "Power". Many people confuse Powerlifting for all weight-training activities.
- The simple routine of three lifts. Squat, Deadlift, and Bench Press.
- This new sport has relieved many beginners from the formidable task of finding a Weightlifting coach that can commit himself, for at least three years, teaching the Olympic technique of lifting. Training a Weightlifter is a daunting task that requires close interpersonal relationship in order to bend old habits, to adapt to systemic vigorous training.
- Powerlifting eliminated the hurdle of simultaneous use of the pelvic and shoulder girdles. This requires tedious training to balance the head, hip, and feet during high-speed resisting motion. Such simplicity of using one girdle at a time encouraged many beginners to dream of getting strong and enjoy the excitement of competitive strength sport. During the Squat and Deadlift, Powerlifters concentrate on the lower body motion while stabilizing the upper body. During the Bench Press, the upper body moves while the lower body is kept stable. With this simple technique, people

can powerlift as long as they live with no need to worry about complex technique, demanding flexible joints, and robust balance.

5.2. POWERLIFTING ASSISTING EXERCISES

Training to build up physical power and remedy individual deficits takes the form of many months of regular training efforts, of at least three times per week, for a minimum of on hour duration per training session. The following exercises are performed during this process, prior to the phase of competition.

5.2.1. BACK SQUAT

5.2.1.1. Description Of Back Squat

Anybody can put a bar behind the shoulders and perform Squat. Yet, progressing in Squat and easing its burden requires understanding certain tweaking techniques to enhance physiological and anatomical functions. The following is a description of the different steps of Back Squat.

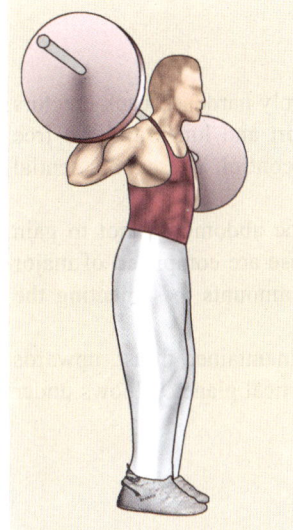

Figure 5.2. Start position for Back Squat.

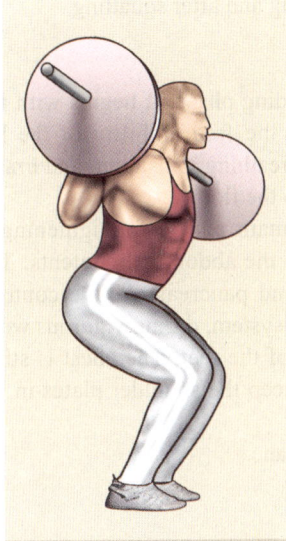

Figure 5.3. Initiating Back Squat.

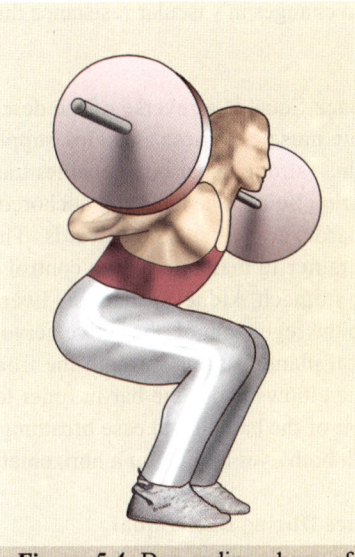

Figure 5.4. Descending phase of squatting.

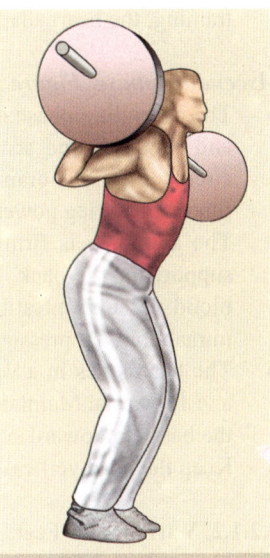

Figure 5.5. Ascending phase of Back Squat.

Start position, Figure 5.2.
- The barbell is placed on a rack at the height of the shoulders.
- Stand facing the racked barbell. Hold the bar with a handgrip, slightly wider than the shoulder-width.
- Step forwards to place both feet in a vertical plane under the barbell. Dip by bending knees and hips. Pass your head, under the racked bar, to the front of the bar.
- Now, the bar is placed across the back of the shoulders and Trapezius, on the spines of the shoulder plates.
- Place the feet about shoulder-width apart, with the toes slightly pointed out to the sides.
- Thrust the chest forwards. Keep the back tight and curved inwards in lordotic posture. Keep abdomen firm and gut sucked in. With the tar loaded on the back of shoulders, move away from the support knobs, before squatting.
- Keep the center of the bar in a vertical plan on the lower back and on the middle of both feet.
- Do not let the bar fall freely on the back of the shoulders. Push upwards with both hands to keep shoulders tight and force the shoulder plates to stick to the chest cage (by contracting the Serratus anterior). The hand's push on the bar pulls the collarbones upwards and eases circulation to the arms and head.

Initiating Squat, Figure 5.3.
- Squatting is initiated by lowering the hips backwards and downwards, by bending the knee and the ankles. If hips do not move backwards then the person would be forced to lift the heels and move the knees forwards. Pushing the hips backwards, while maintaining upward thrust of the chest, forces the lower back to arch inwards (concaved lower back).
- Progression of the Squat requires two actions: (1) increasing the forward and upward thrust of the chest and (2) increasing the lordosis of the lower back in order to maintain vertical torso.

- o The trickiest technique, in this initial negative contraction of the lower body, is maintaining firm isometric contraction of the shoulders and arms. Solid support of the bar, on the arms, shoulders, and scapulas, evenly distributes the weight along the upper vertebral spines, as well as to the back of the skull. Lax arms puts the weight on narrow point on the center of the upper back and create a callus of keratinized dead tissue.
- o Shakes and tremors may result from lax lower back or shoulders, which impair blood flow through the spinal arteries or the neck arteries (carotid), respectively. Lax muscles not only cause direct mechanical kinking of the underlying vital organs, but also impair sympathetic control of blood flow and contribute to circulatory disturbances. These are the main causes of tremors.

Descending phase, Figure 5.4.
- o The descent phase of squatting comprises of resisting force while the thigh muscles are elongating. This sort of eccentric contraction causes more soreness and increase in muscle mass than the ascending phase of Squat.
- o The heels should never lose good contact with the floor. In addition, the arches of the feet (between the heel and base of toes) should be kept high and firm to avoid flat footing while lifting heavy weight.
- o During Squat, the largest muscles of the body contract maximally and, therefore, trap voluminous portion of the whole blood in the lower body. These muscles are the Quadriceps, the Glutei, the Hamstrings, the Iliopsoas, and the back erectors. The trapped blood causes significant reduction on circulation. Trained athletes, learn to effectively relax the lower body muscles prior to initiating Squat to help endure serious circulatory compromise during squatting. With training, the heart adapts to changes in vascular resistance during and after squatting.

Ascending phase, Figure 5.5.
- o The ascending phase of Back Squat is a reverse of the descending phase. It begins with firmly hardened back erectors and shoulder and scapular muscles. These muscles support the free mobility of the heart and lungs and the free circulation to the brain. Thus, strong upper body enables the breathing, pulsation, and brain control. These are essential functions for leg power during Squat. The heels are anchored to the floor.
- o The abdomen is firmly hardened and sucked inwards. The main reason for tightening the abdomen is not to gain support for the back, but rather to maintain active control on the abdominal contents. These are comprised of major blood vessels, intestines, stomach, kidneys, bladder, liver, and pancreas. Active control amounts to subjecting the intraabdominal pressure to the regulation of the active nervous system, during vigorous work.
- o The bar moves in a vertical plane, passing through the front of the feet. The chest is still maintained thrust, upwards and forwards. Maintain the elbows under the bar in order to keep the shoulder plates in vertical planes. Elbows under the bar help upward support of the barbell and ease breathing.
- o Keep the head vertical with both eyes looking in a horizontal plane.

5.2.1.2. Variants Of Feet Stance During Back Squat
Feet stance during Back Squat depends on the group of muscles that are intended for strengthening as well as on the height of the lifter. Feet stance varies from standard shoulder-width, slightly narrower or wider, or significantly wide stance. The following is a short description of the common feet stances encountered in Powerlifting.

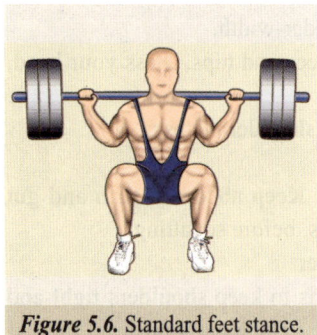
Figure 5.6. Standard feet stance.

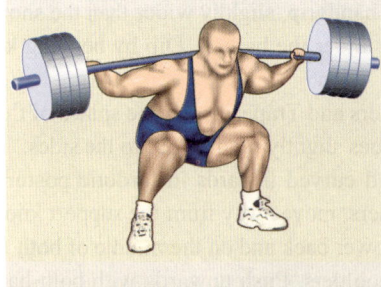
Figure 5.7. Feet stance of an overweight lifter.

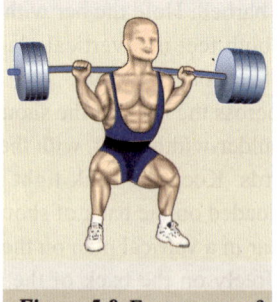
Figure 5.8. Feet stance of a short lifter.

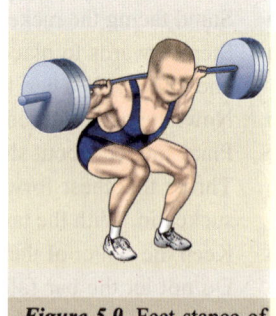
Figure 5.9. Feet stance of a tall lifter.

Standard shoulder-width stance provides the following benefits and limitations, *Figure 5.6.*
- o Normal leg stance adheres to anatomical function of the joints. It evens the loads on the joints and permits deep and safe Squat.
- o It aids in developing flexibility and full range of motion.
- o It requires long and regular training, since symmetric muscles require constant strengthening in order to remain symmetric.
- o The long travel distance makes it daunting, in fatigue conditions.

Widely separated feet have the following pros and cons, *Figure 5.7*.
o   Shorten the abductors and extensors and elongate the hip adductors. Shortened muscle may remain contracted if not stretched.
o   Overload lateral knee condyles and ease the stress of medial structures, particularly if a medial meniscus was injured.
o   Impair deep Squat since the knee cannot fully bend when twisted in this stance.

Overweight athletes have specific limitations regarding feet stance, *Figure 5.7*.
o   Body overweight imposes inflexibility on the shoulders, back, pelvis, and knees. Inflexibility interferes with standard feet stance.
o   Wide gripping of the bar, during Squat, weakens shoulder support and limits the shoulder mobility.
o   Wide stance and half squatting limit the hip mobility and overload partial surfaces of the hips and knees. Both heavy bodyweight and lifting are detrimental to knees and hips.
o   Bulging abdomen undermines circulation to lower limbs and back.
o   Both bulging abdomen and throwing the elbows backwards hampers breathing efforts.

Short-limbed athletes exhibits highest leverage forces and can lift much heavier than others, of the same bodyweight, *Figure 5.8*.
o   Short bones of the legs amplify the strength of the Glutei and Quadriceps and shorten squatting descent.
o   Back erectors exert relatively less work to support the weight and transfer forces to the legs.
o   Short arms and strong shoulders easily support the weight of the bar in the vertical plane and ease breathing.

Long-limbed athletes encounter different leverage issues, *Figure 5.9*.
o   Long legs are easily injured with poor alignment than short and chubby legs. Athlete resort to strengthen muscles and maintain vertical posture of legs in order to enhance knee and hip stability.
o   Strengthening the back extensors and shoulders aid in supporting the weight while descending, on closely separated feet.
o   Tall lifters are in more need for regular training and proper nutrition in order to maintain active control of joints.

5.2.1.3. Tweaking Of Squat Technique
o   The "**fall-line**" is the vertical line in a vertical plane that passes through the bar, the middle line between the thighs and the feet. The further the head and hip from that vertical plane, the harder it is on the back to recuperate after exercise. Deviation from the fall line amounts to creating unnecessary torque on the back, hips, knees, and ankles.

o   The weight of the barbell is supported by the spines of the two shoulder plates (**scapulas**). Each shoulder plate is snuggly pulled onto the chest cage by many muscles, in all directions. Therefore, just putting the barbell on the back of the shoulders would work out many muscles around the shoulder girdle. Even before commencing any squatting, shoulder balance takes place the moment you load weight on your back, as follows.
   i.   The Trapezius pulls the outer edges of the scapulas upwards and pushes the scapula towards the chest, when arms are lowered below the shoulders.
   ii. The Latissimus dorsi pushes the lower edge of the scapula towards the chest.
   iii. The Rhomboid muscles pull the medial edge of the scapulas to the center of the back (medially).
   iv. The Levator muscles elevate the medial edge of the scapulas.
   v.   The Scapular muscles (Supraspinatus, Infraspinatus, Subscapularis) transfer forces to and from arms and scapulas.
   vi. The Serratus anchors the medial border of the scapula to the chest.

o   Prior to squatting, try to get a sense on how the **six groups of muscles** stabilize the barbell on the upper back, as follows.
   i.   Pushing on the bar with both hands, in the upward direction, activates the Trapezius pull towards the back of the head and the Serratus pull towards the sides of the chest.
   ii. Thrusting the chest cage, forwards and upwards, activates the Trapezius pull to the middle of the back and Serratus pull on the sides of the chest.
   iii. Keeping the elbows closer to the sides of the chest requires the scapulas to be pulled closer in the back, by the lower Trapezius fibers and Rhomboids, and anchored by Serratus pull to the chest.
   iv. Moving the elbows backwards and away from the chest requires rotation of the scapulas away from the chest cage and causes the chest to cave in.

o   No squatting is safe or easy without arching in the lower back (**concave lower back**). This is done by moving the upper body backwards and the lower back forwards, at the waist level. The spinal erectors support the vertebral column and thus remove the pressure from the spinal discs (intervertebral discs). Tight and firm spinal erectors convey the weight of the barbell to the lower legs and eliminate the annoying firing of the back, had it been lax. The concave and well-supported back permits free circulation to the spinal cord, both in front and back surfaces.

- Prior to squatting, keep both **knees unlocked**, by slightly bending them. Keep the arches of the feet tight by standing on the heels and the balls of the feet, instead on laying the soles of feet flat on the floor of the shoes. Slightly bent knees activate the stretch reflex of Quadriceps and Glutei. These enhance muscular control of the knees. Unlocked knees are more supported than straight knees by the stretched Quadriceps and Hamstrings. Also, active knee-control fosters the floating of the heavy weight on the inner knee fluid, thus distributes the weight evenly on the articular surfaces.

- The "**start position**" is completed by adjusting the stance, knees, shoulder plates, chest, arms, lower back, and head in such a way as to provide maximal support to the weight, maximal breathing ability, and maximal joint stability. The next step is to further tighten the back erectors to commence descending with weight. All movements below and above the lower back could not be initiated without tight **back erectors**. That is because all movements around the ankles, knees and hips have to be linked to movements around the neck, shoulders, and spines, through the back erectors.

- With tight back erectors, descending takes place by rotating the femur, from vertical to horizontal position. This pushes the knees to the front and the hips to the back of the fall-line. Descent must proceed with both heels anchored to the floor and the upper body as close as possible to the vertical plane. **Descending** occurs by eccentric contraction (negative contraction) and must proceed slower than ascending. That is because, during descent, both the weights of the barbell and body, and their acceleration, are directed downwards, against muscular resistance. Free fall or fast descending, are prohibited as they may tear tendons and avulse their attachments to bones.

- Fast **ascending** is tolerated by advanced lifters since it occurs under the control of muscular contraction, with upward acceleration and downward weight pulls. Fast ascending, even with high jump, is practiced by advanced Weightlifters. Since descending activates stretch reflexes it, therefore, greatly increases ascending force.

- Squatting all away down to the heels, and bouncing upwards and downwards, is not encouraged, for beginners, without a coach. **Full squatting** with bouncing is practiced by Weightlifters to enhance flexibility of the thigh muscles. Even frog jumping, in full Squat, is well known to enhance the development of thighs in advanced training setting. You can start practicing deep Squat and deep bouncing with no weight and with gradual stretching of the knees. Trying to bend inflexible knees trigger acute pain that might induce severe heart pounding. When bending succeeds in overcoming inflexibility then your heart will remain quite during deep squatting. Only then, you can proceed with increasing external weights. Troubling full Squat may be attributed to conflicting flexion and extension reflexes. Deep squatting by advanced lifters activates the extension reflex and inhibits the flexion reflex around the knees such that the Quadriceps would not be resisted by spastic Hamstrings.

- It might take a beginner two years before learning not to let the **pelvis** tilts downwards while squatting deeply. In untrained people, the pelvis tilts after the thighs dip below horizontal plane. Tilting pelvis rotates the buttocks downwards and drags the vertebral columns in a convex curve at the lower back. This leads to the drop of the chest on the thighs with probable injury of the back. Trained lifters maintain solid back erectors and Iliopsoas such that the abdomen is stuck tight to the thighs and the lower back is kept tightly concave, on horizontal pelvis.

- The simple way to evaluate the **balance** of Iliopsoas (hip flexor) and back erectors is to compare overhead lifts to shoulder level lifts. Overhead lifts require greater hip flexors to maintain hip stability. For example, the duration and weight used with a stand-alone torso, during seated upper exercises, are good index to balanced hip flexors and back extensors. People with imbalance pelvis cannot exercise for long, while seated without board-supported back.

- As long as the lifter learn the trick of maintained **non-fluttered tight back erectors** he or she will not have difficulty ascending and descending, until the thighs fatigue. Shaky back erectors distract the mind from performing any movement with the weight and give the sense of complete apprehension towards squatting. It is very dangerous to attempt squatting with shaky back erectors, as in situation of returning to exercise after long interruption, convalescence from illness, fever, lack of warm-up, distraction in the environment, or overtraining.

- **Ascending** begins with movements above and below the lower back that acts as a leverage link. The head, chest, and arms push upwards, and slightly backwards, and the thighs and Glutei push upwards and forwards.

5.2.2. FRONT SQUAT

Front Squat and Back Squat do not refer to strengthening of the front or the back of the thighs. Both front and Back Squat equally works out the Quadriceps. The only difference between them is that the Front Squat is performed with weights loaded in front of the vertebral column. It requires the scapulas (shoulder plates) to move away from the chest cage. Front Squat mainly strengthens the thrust of the chest and elevation of shoulders during squatting. Weak shoulder elevation causes the collarbones (the clavicles) to drop on the underlying blood vessels supplying the rams. This causes sudden weakness and numbness of arms during lifting heavy weights. Thus, Front Squat mainly strengthens the groups of muscles that balance rotated shoulder plates and flexed shoulders. These muscles are the Deltoids, the Serratus, the Trapezius, the long head of Biceps, and the back erectors. Front Squat is, therefore, a measure of flexibility of the shoulders and back erectors and thrust of the chest.

5.2.2.1. Unique features of Front Squat
o The **group of muscles** that supports the weight of the bar on the front of the shoulders is uniquely strengthened by Front Squat.
  i. The shoulder flexors elevate the upper arm in a forward plane, forcing the scapulas to depart the chest cage. These muscles are: the Deltoid as prime flexor, long head of Biceps as stabilizer, Pectoralis minor as stabilizer, Serratus anterior as scapula rotator, and Trapezius as shoulder elevator.
  ii. The anterior vertebral muscles, the Scalenes and Sternomastoids pull the chest cage upwards and backwards and transfer the forces to the back erectors. Thus, font Squat greatly enlarges the neck muscles.
  iii. Holding the bar with a grip larger that the shoulder-width, while flexing the shoulders, is formidable to many bodybuilders and Powerlifters. This position requires strong lateral rotation of the upper arms with strong pulls of the Infraspinatus and Serratus anterior, in addition to strong Biceps long head anchorage.[1]
o Since the weight of the bar is racked on the chest, as well as the collarbones, it creates **downward torque** on the upper half of the body that tends to throw the body forwards. To reduce the magnitude of this torque, the bar has to be seated deeply at the root of the neck, right on the top of the sternum (front bone of the chest). This brings the bar closer to the vertebral column. Developing such neck support to heavy weights requires many years of training to allow the muscles of the shoulders to elevate the bar away from the air passages and the major blood vessels. Young beginners may endure such annoying discomfort at the neck for few weeks before developing tolerance to heavy weights. Old beginners are required to develop shoulder muscles to tolerate the snuggly-racked bar at the base of the neck.
o Any **upper back hunching** or weak shoulder elevation makes Front Squat troublesome. The net difference between Front and Back squatting is the downward torque of the Front Squat. That has to be opposed by the upward torque of the shoulder flexors, chest elevators, and upper back erectors.
o The Front Squat tests the elasticity of the carotid **arteries and veins** and may cause dizziness and collapse. It requires sufficient shoulder and chest elevation in order to remove the weight of the bar from squeezing the neck vessels.
o While the shoulder and chest elevators are tightly contracted in the Front Squat, the lower body is skimped of substantial **blood supply** that feeds the upper body. This increases the burden of the Front Squat on the entire performance.
o As Back Squat has its main impetus in hardening the lower back, Front Squat has its impetus in **tightening the shoulder** and chest elevation. In Front Squat the lower back is unconsciously hardened by the downward torque of the bar and the upward resistance.
o What eases proceeding with the Front Squat are two movements. As the hips are descending backwards and downwards, the elbows are elevated upwards and forwards. These two movements maintain the bar in the vertical plane of the fall line.

5.2.2.2. Description of Front Squat

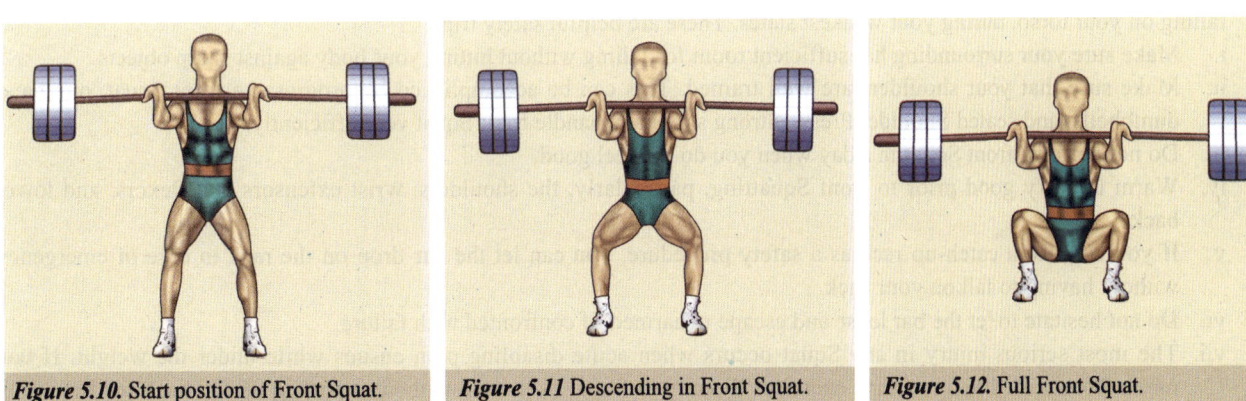

Figure 5.10. Start position of Front Squat.   *Figure 5.11* Descending in Front Squat.   *Figure 5.12.* Full Front Squat.

Start position, Figure 5.10.
o This is similar to that of Back Squat, with the only difference of racking the bar across the chest and the front of the shoulders.

---

[1] Strengthening muscles in isolation does not enhance Front Squat, which is an axial exercise that relies on pelvic and shoulder girdles. This multi-girdle coordination requires super-segmental regulation of flexion-extension reflexes. Simply stated, many major muscles have to "**give and take**" in order for the CNS to sustain control on front squatting with weight.

POWERLIFTING

- The bar is gripped as in the Clean, with both palms facing upwards when the bar is racked on the shoulders, and not the arms.
- The arms should never carry the weight away from the shoulders otherwise sever wrist injury ensues due to overstretching digital and wrist tendons.
- Thrust chest, hardened abdomen, and erected lower back, all help rack the bar above the shoulders and secure it in place by the bulk of hardened Deltoid, in front of the bar.
- The feet are placed as in the Clean stance, slightly wider than shoulder-width, with toes slightly pointed to the sides.

Descent phase, Figure 5.11.
- Descending starts with additional arching in the lower back, elevating the elbows upwards, and moving the hips backwards and downwards.
- As descending proceeds, both tight back and thrust chest prevent falling of the bar, from behind the Deltoid's blocking bulge.
- Descending forces the lower back to lose concavity. This is further aggravated by the forward torque generated by weight loaded in front of the shoulders. If the squatter were young or long-trained, he or she would be able to maintain lower back concavity. Untrained squatters need to work their way to gain such control on lower back flexibility. This is accomplished by regular training for months and years.
- Leaning forwards is not well tolerated in front squatting. If the bar slides over the arms, from its secure location on the shoulders, it should be allowed to fall freely to the floor and quickly released by the squatter.
- If you have to release the bar, and have no helper or catch-up rack, then let the bar fall forwards and push yourself away, backwards. Remember to avoid hitting your head against any surrounding object. You might fall on your buttocks with no or little discomfort. If you do not act quickly enough, the bar might fall in your lap and force you to fall on your back. In this ugly fall, your knees are still bent and the barbell is over your belly, while lying down. A standard barbell has over twenty-centimeter radius plates that is sufficient to bridge the bar over your belly and prevent internal injury. Thus, you would most probably recover from backward fall with few elbow bruises and knee strains, but nothing major.

Full Squat, Figure 5.12.
- Full squatting with heavy weight is not encouraged unless the athlete is advanced in Weightlifting. It carries the serious risk of collapsing under the bar. At least six months of training are required for a young beginner to develop shoulder and back control, during deep Front Squat.
- Squatting to depth, where thighs are parallel to the floor-is safe. Yet, you have to remember to release the barbell without hesitation if things go wrong. That happens if either the back erectors shut off or the thrust chest caves in. A quick backward kick with the buttocks generates sufficient torque to throw the bar away from the knees, while being released.
- A standard Olympic barbell has plates of sufficiently large diameter to prevent crushing the chest had the barbell falls on the chest, in case of falling on your back with barbell on the top of you.
- The most important safety rule in front Squat is planning an exit strategy before getting entangled under a heavy bar falling on your torso, during your weakest states. These are helpful safety trips.
    i. Make sure your surrounding has sufficient room for falling without hitting your body against sharp objects.
    ii. Make sure that your shoulders are well trained. This can be accomplished by progressive front Squat, one-hand dumbbells, and seated Shoulder Press. Strong shoulders handle front Squat very efficiently.
    iii. Do not perform front Squat in a day when you do not feel good.
    iv. Warm up very good prior to front Squatting, particularly, the shoulders, wrist extensors and flexors, and lower back.
    v. If you can use a catch-up rack as a safety procedure, you can let the bar drop on the rack in case of emergency without having to fall on your back.
    vi. Do not hesitate to let the bar loose and escape unharmed, if confronted with failure.
    vii. The most serious injury in any Squat occurs when acute disabling pain ensues while under the weight. If you move from seated and machine exercises directly to Squat exercises, without warming up the back for flexibility and strength, you may be heading for troubles. Acutely spastic spinal muscle can incapacitates you entirely and undermines you ability to bail out of dangerously heavy barbell. Remember that acute spinal pain during lifting is a life-threatening occurrence and must be prevented by all means, such as gradual increase in resistance, thorough warm-up, proper technique, and serious mindedness.

5.2.3. OVERHEAD SQUAT
The Overhead Squat is a highly coordinated exercise of the shoulders and legs. It simultaneously enhances the stability of the legs and the mobility of the shoulders, in one complex exercise. The following are some special features of Overhead Squat.

- o It differs from the Back Squat in that the overhead weight is transferred to the upper vertebral column through the **arms and scapulas.** Squatting with both arms elevated overhead is a challenge to muscular balance. It is the most difficult exercise to Powerlifters and Bodybuilders since it requires great shoulder mobility and balance, in a two-girdle exercise.
- o While Back Squat commences with hardening of the lower back and Front Squat commences with hardening the shoulder and thrusting the chest, overhead Squat commences with locking the **upper Trapezius muscles** and excessively forward thrusting the chest. The upper Trapezius stabilizes the outer edges of the scapulas. Thrusting the chest stabilizes the medial borders of the scapulas through the Serratus anterior muscle.
- o Squatting with overhead weight is frightening to old, novice trainees. As soon as the trainee masters the trick of hardening the **Trapezius and thrusting the chest**, the trainee will soon learn to keep the arms straight and firm while focusing on the squatting and hardening the lower back.
- o The skill of performing complex balance at the shoulder and pelvis is easily gained with **persistent training**. The muscles of the shoulders have to learn to maintain the overhead weight in the vertical plane of fall line, while the lower limbs perform the reposition of the knees, hips, and curvature of the lower back.
- o Narrow grips of the bar test the strength of the Supraspinatus and its ability to anchor the humeral ball when the long head of the Biceps is becoming less tense.

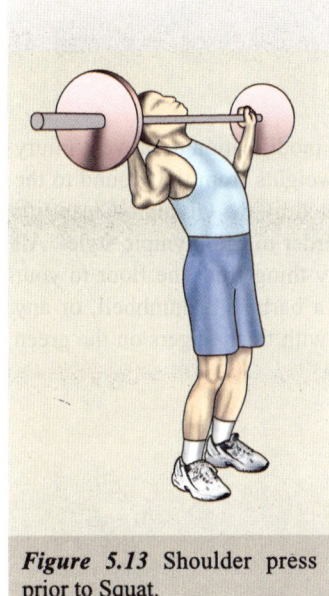

Figure 5.13 Shoulder press prior to Squat.

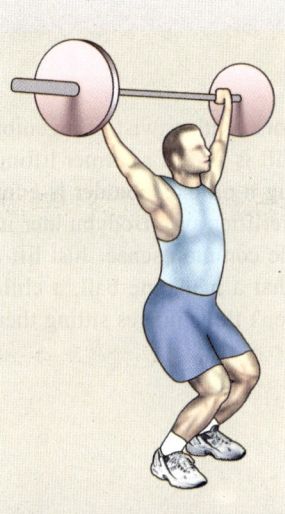

Figure 5.14 Squatting while shoulder pressing.

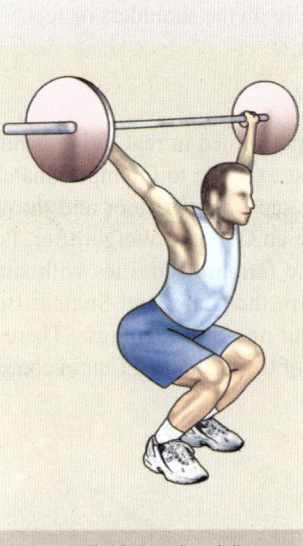

Figure 5.15 Overhead Squat.

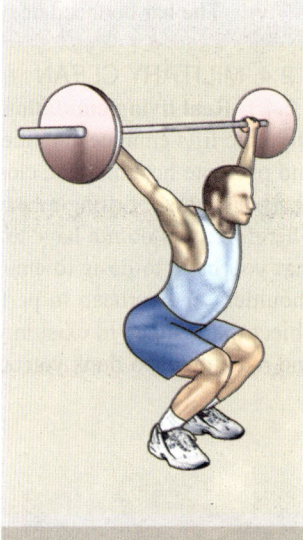

Figure 5.16 Ascending in overhead Squat.

5.2.3.1. Description of Overhead Squat
Start Position, Figure 5.13.
- o Shoulder Press prior to Overhead Squat helps prevent shoulder injury and is performed as warm-up, or as full-fledged strengthening exercise. Thus, instead of just performing Overhead Squat, you can Shoulder Press and then Squat, while the bar is clearing the face region.
- o While the bar moves upwards, the head clears the way by tilting backwards.
- o The chest is thrust and the knees are ready to bend.
- o When the bar passes the level of the eyebrows, the head advances forwards under the bar, which is felt as being moving backwards.
- o Descending is possible when the head moves forwards, the hips move backwards and downwards, and the knees bend.

Squatting and pressing, Figure 5.14.
- o As the bar clear the head, by Shoulder Pressing upwards and dipping downwards, squatting becomes smooth by balancing the bar with the front head mass and the rear pelvic mass.
- o The locking of the upper Trapezius and rear Deltoid fibers and hardening the back erectors allow the mind to focus on the eccentric contraction of the lower body.
- o The quick descent has to be halted by contracting the Glutei and thighs at the desired braking point.
- o If the squatter never experienced utilizing the shoulder, back, and lower limbs in such single complex coordination, it might take few weeks of training to master the overhead descent.

Descending phase, Figure 5.15.
- o The depth of overhead squatting depends on the flexibility of the shoulders, back, knees, and hips. Weightlifters can Squat full, and even step forwards by shuffling the feet, while balancing the overhead weight.
- o Pointing the knees outwards, to the sides, brings the hips forwards and reduces the acute concavity of the lower back.
- o Overhead Squat can proceed with ascending, without lowering the bar to the chest or the back of the shoulders. Alternatively, the trainee may opt to lower the bar during ascending from Squat and elevate the bar during descending.

Ascending phase, Figure 5.16.
o   Ascending can follow a short pause after descending or commences immediately after reaching the lowest descent.
o   Ascending is helped by locked shoulders, thrust chest, and concavely hardened lower back.
o   Push the buttocks forwards and upwards and thrust the chest upwards while ascending.
o   Any laxity or hesitation in the elbows will be amplified many folds, as felt by the shoulders and back. This may cause failure to ascend or stress to the shoulders, elbows, and wrists.
o   Aborting squatting or ascending should be executed promptly by releasing the bar and escaping the nearest exit. If the bar lies vertically in front of the feet, it is then feasible to escape backwards, by the body. Release the bar loose, by straightening the wrists and letting the bar drop freely to the floor.
o   If the bar falls in a vertical plan behind the feet, let the bar drop behind the body by thrusting the buttocks forwards and loosening the grip. In either case, you might avoid falling by deciding quickly on aborting the Squat if things do not look good, as in the following conditions:
    i.   The elbows or shoulders relaxed unexpectedly.
    ii. The overhead bar bounced excessively to the front or to the back.
    iii. The heels left the ground and messed up the stance.
    iv. The back erectors shut off unexpectedly.
    v.   Sudden acute feeling has risen along the back.
    vi. The bar bounced unevenly on the shoulders or feet.

5.2.4. MILITARY CLEAN
5.2.4.1. Real living emulation
Olympic lifts emulate activities performed in real living conditions, with a twist of ingenious modification to prevent injury and promote health. The closest example to Olympic Snatch lift is that of a farmer lifting weights from the ground to the back of a horse. Lifting a heavy sac from the floor and throwing it on the shoulder is emulated by the Olympic Clean lift. Therefore, you do not have to be an Olympic Weightlifter, Powerlifter, or a Bodybuilder in order to lift Olympic style. All that you have to do is to emulate farming activities with simple common sense. Just lift any thing from the floor to your shoulders or overhead to perform the Clean and Snatch. Be that a medicine ball, a child, a barbell, a dumbbell, or any object that happen to exist in your near surroundings. There aren't three judges sitting there with their fingers on the green and red buttons to flunk you out of the health and fitness contest.

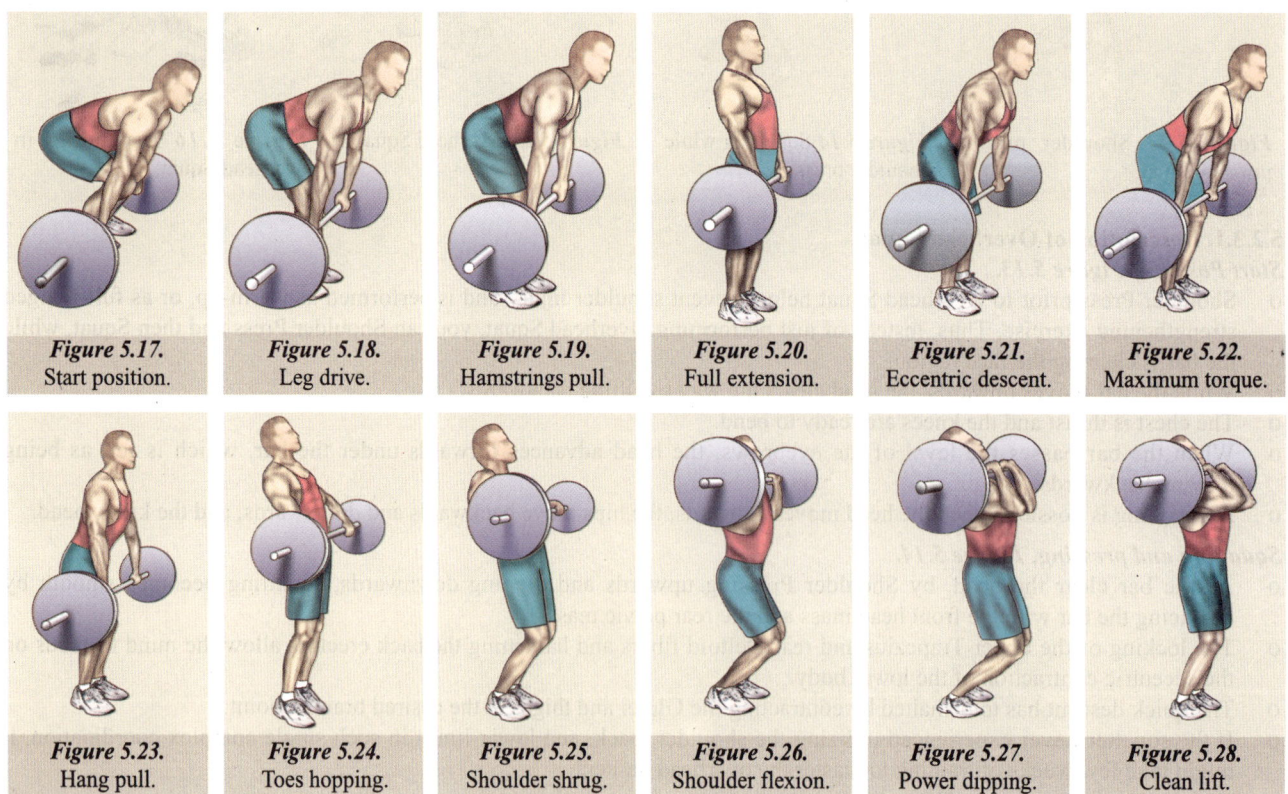

Figure 5.17. Start position. *Figure 5.18.* Leg drive. *Figure 5.19.* Hamstrings pull. *Figure 5.20.* Full extension. *Figure 5.21.* Eccentric descent. *Figure 5.22.* Maximum torque.

Figure 5.23. Hang pull. *Figure 5.24.* Toes hopping. *Figure 5.25.* Shoulder shrug. *Figure 5.26.* Shoulder flexion. *Figure 5.27.* Power dipping. *Figure 5.28.* Clean lift.

5.2.4.2. Lifting styles
The Olympic Clean and Snatch are practiced in different training styles, to promote different components of performance, for different body conditions, as follows.

POWERLIFTING

The **"Military"** style of lifting
o   This is an oversimplified, stiff, and stable version and suits beginners, overtrained athletes, recuperating conditions, or people with resilient muscular imbalance due to weakness or stiffness.
o   The military Clean is simple, weight room exercise that develops strength of major muscles, in one efficient style.
o   When performed improperly, Military Clean has the potential for back injury and reinforcement of improper technique. Proper technique enhances muscular balance.
o   Military Olympic lifts are stiff, stable, and entail high pull without dipping. When the bar is elevated above the kneecaps, the body remains extended and the shoulders perform high pull.
o   The Clean amounts to lifting the barbell from the floor and racking it on the shoulders. Military Clean is performed as the Power Clean without the dip under the bar, when the bar passes over the chest.
o   The Military Clean suits conditions of sore and uncoordinated body. It is performed to strengthen major axial muscles when highly coordinated exercises are burdensome.
o   Military Clean is intended to strengthen the following.
    i.   The major body extensors: the thighs, Glutei, back erectors, and Trapezius.
    ii. The shoulder movers: Deltoid back fibers, Latissimus dorsi, Supraspinatus, upper Trapezius, and long head of Biceps.
    iii. The scapulas' movers: the Rhombi, Levator scapulae, Trapezius, and Serratus anterior.

The **"Power"** style of lifting requires an advanced level of muscular responsiveness to impulsive Jerky forces at the knees, hips, back, and neck. The "power feature" stems from the ability to lift faster and stronger with some degree of bending knees and hips in order to shorten the vertical distance of pulling.

5.2.4.3. Description of Military Clean

In this style of the Clean, you bring the barbell from the floor all away to the shoulder level, without attempting to ease the lift by descending to meet the bar halfway down. It is performed as follows, *Figures 5.17* thru *5.24* and *5.28*.
o   Stand at the barbell with both feet advancing under the bar. The big toes should be seen **in front of the bar** (if bare footed) while the bar covers the front third of the feet, as seen from above, *Figure 5.17*.
o   Keep the feet separated with a distance of at least one-foot apart, and no more than shoulder-width. Sometimes you might like to entertain closely stuck feet, or slightly separated feet, during the Clean, to test your balance.
o   Prior to descending to grip the bar, practice the **chest thrusting** and shoulder backward throwing. Advanced lifters remember that trick in their younger years and leave the shoulder thrust to the moment of lifting. The main purpose of chest thrusting is to stimulate the upper back, position the scapula and shoulders in lifting position, elevate the diaphragm upwards, and tighten abdominal muscles.
o   You can descend anyway you want to grip the bar. The best habit is to **descend by bending the knees** and hips in the same time and maintaining the torso as vertical as possible, with the arms hanging loose over the bar.
o   Hold the bar with at least a **shoulder-width grip** with both palms facing backwards. If you prefer the thumb-hook grip as many Weightlifters do, it is up to you and to the length of your thumbs to enhance this secure gripping.
o   Remember that you are not going to lift the barbell with the strength of the Biceps. The arms only work as stabilizers for most of the lifting, all the way up to the chest level. Thus, **keep the arms straight** at the elbows and relatively relaxed until lifting starts. The Clean feels bit easier if you remember not to bend the elbows until the entire body is vertically straight and the bar elevated above the middle of the thighs. Bending the elbows earlier causes the chest cage to retreat and the scapulas to wing away from the chest. This makes the Clean harder, if not formidable.
o   Capable lifters commence the Clean with the **hips kept slightly above the knees level**. This start position puts the back in a pyramidal slope as vertical as possible and helps the chest thrust.
o   **Upward drive** of the weight originates from the concentric contraction of thighs and Glutei. The **thighs** produce torque around the knees in proportion to the length of the femur and the strength of the thighs. The **Glutei** produce torque around the hips in proportion to the length of the torso and the strength of the Glutei. The torque produced by the Glutei is only effective as long as the back erectors stay contracted and transmit the torque to the shoulders.
o   As soon as the weight of the barbell is **equalized, and the barbell commences moving** upwards, any slack in the stabilizing muscles of the upper body can lead to failure of lifting. The bar proceeds upwards, slowly and strongly controlled, until it passes over the kneecaps, *Figure 5.18*.
o   Above the kneecaps, the Glutei and back erectors contract vigorously to produce the final torque at the hips. This thrusts the hips forwards and helps move the bar uniformly, in a weightless state.
o   After the leg drive ends, upper body drive begins. When your body is fully extended, lean backwards and hop on your feed balls. Your arms are still firmly straight. As your heads bounces backwards, start shrugging the shoulders, *Figures 5.17* thru *5.24*.
o   Your training will help you time the shoulder shrug and swiftly proceed with shoulder abduction, *Figure 5.25*. From here, the strength of your shoulders and arms will determine how much abduction can you generate, at the shoulders. When no further shoulder abduction is possible, you have to engage the front Deltoids, in ballistic shoulder flexion, in order to pull the bar to the shoulders, *Figures 5.26* thru *5.28*.
o   Your entire training in Weightlifting will emphasize on how to promptly utilize the shoulder muscles. You will learn to generate momentum by the masses of head and pelvis and the velocities of rotation on the ankles, knees, hips, and shoulders. While you generating momentum, you will master muscular recruitments in the various phases of joint

mobility.
- Moving the bar on the torso, from the level of the lower abdomen to the upper chest, demonstrates the difference between novice and skilled lifters, *Figures 5.20* thru *5.25*. **Novices use Biceps**, Deltoid, and Trapezius to meddle with a formidable situation, when a heavy barbell is positioned below the shoulder and above the thighs. Such inexperienced meddling makes the lightest weights extremely heavy. Since the shoulder balls are only half spheres, therefore, reaching maximum range of motion, when the weight still below the shoulder level blocks further lifting with the shoulders.
- **Skilled lifters thrust chest** to bring the vertebral column and the bar closer. This increases the range of motion of the shoulders and helps further abduct the arms, using upper and back fibers of Deltoids. Shoulder abduction, by moving arms to the sides, is followed by shoulder flexion, by moving elbows forwards and upwards. Thus, skilled lifters make use of the scapular rotation to amplify shoulder rotation. If scapular rotation is not utilized then the shoulder rotation is a problematically limiting factor in lifting
- While the bar is approaching the shoulder level, the skilled lifter recruits the front fibers of the Deltoid in elevating the humerus under the bar and racking it on the shoulders.
- Instead of lowering the hips and knees to reach the bar below the chest, in attempt to rack it on the chest, the **Military Clean intends to protract the Deltoid upward pull** and augment it with slight hopping on the feet ball.
- When the bar is racked on the shoulders, the **elbows should be elevated** in the front, as high as the level of the shoulders, *Figure 5.28*. If that is not feasible, a wider grip should be attempted later in the next attempt. Novices tend to bend the wrist to rack the bar on the shoulder or let the bar sit on the handgrip with straight wrist, which traumatizes the hand flexors and causes sore wrist.
- Having racked the bar on the shoulders, you have many options to manage the rest of the Military Clean. You can lower the bar to the floor and repeat the exercise. You can perform Shoulder Press, then lower the bar to the back of the shoulders and perform Goodmorning or Squat. Alternatively, you can leave the bar racked on the shoulders and perform Front Squat.

5.2.5. POWER CLEAN

The Power Clean is a basic strength training exercise of major muscles. Proper technique can be learned and memorized in few months. Training emphasizes on synchronizing joint movements, maintaining centers of moving weights in vertical lines, and abandoning ill habits of premature bending of elbows, lax stabilizing joints, or yanking the weights below the knees. It is performed as follows, *Figures 5.17, 5.18,* and *5.22* thru *5.28*.

- The Power Clean does not begin with the starting stance at the barbell. There is certain preparatory work you have to consider prior to beginning this exercise.
    i. In addition to warming up general body and particular joints, the athlete has to reach the bar with **focused mind** and vivid imagination of the pending phases of lifting. Lifting Power Clean depends heavily on mental presence, since each phase of lifting demands implementation of specific rules.
    ii. Before proceeding with your workout, make sure that the bar is well lubricated and freely rotating within the loading cylinders, to avoid any wrist injury. Even lifting platform, securing collars or locks, and sufficient clearance from other people are basic requirements of freestyle lifting.
    iii. Your nightmare may lay in a new encounter to the gym that never saw freestyle lifting. People who do not know what you are doing may attempt to grab a plate or a collar in your vicinity while you pulling the explosive phase. A crowded gym should alert you to those who may dart "out of the blue" in your vicinity and during lifting.
    iv. Another contributing factor is that many people in the gym are either trying to mind their own affairs, by avoiding eye contacts with others, or shy from others and not paying attention to freestyle lifting. That requires larger travel distances than machine-aided exercises.
- The **stance** begins with feet placed a shoulder-width apart and the front third of the feet advanced under the bar. Keep the bar close to shins of the lower legs. The knees are bent, hips lowered, and arms land straight to grip the bar, slightly at a span wider than a shoulder-width. The knees stay inside the arms and above, and slightly in front, of the bar. Thus, it seems that the knees are blocking the way of the bar when it commences upward motion, *Figure 5.17*. You have the option of standing with very closely separated feet if you are working on your balance, or working on stretching the structures at the hips.
- The back retains a concave posture (arching in), by **tightening the back erectors and thrusting the chest forwards**. The concave lower back maintains shoulders in the vertical plane above the bar and prevents the pelvis from tilting downwards. If you want practice stretching the pelvic structures, you can force the buttocks to sit on the heels while tightening both lower back and abdomen. The pelvis is kept in balanced position with the back erectors opposed by hip flexors (Iliopsoas). If the pelvis keeps tilting downwards against your will, you might have to strengthen the Iliopsoas, with weights, during the crunches on declined benches. Strong Iliopsoas pulls the lower back towards the femurs during full Squat.
- The **heels stay stuck** to the floor until the bar is elevated to a level above the thighs. The heels only depart the floor when the bar is elevated above the kneecaps. Recall that the feet are not dumb flat parts of the body. While you're standing, you're distributing your weight on the heels and the balls of the feet, the heads of metatarsal bones. The space between the heels and the feet balls is kept elevated from the floor, to allow blood flow to the "poor tissues" of the feet. Although modern sport shoes account for such needs, it helps to learn managing your affairs when things do not meet your demands.

- o The **role of the arms** in the Clean and Snatch lifts opposes the belief of lay people. Arms do not generate lifting drive. They only complete the drive generated by axial muscles Weightlifters do not solely rely on arm strength to lift heavy weights. Prior to lifting, the arms are kept straight and relaxed. During below-groin lifting, the arms remain straight and firm. Arms contracted isometrically during that time to allow the transfer of the lower body drive to the bar, through the back extensors and scapulas, *Figure 5.18.*
- o **Upward movement** of the bar commences by extending the knees and hips in steady slow and strong motion, while lower back maintains lordotic posture. Maintaining all upper body muscles firm, without lax motions, allows raising the shoulders with the bar hanging in the arm grips. The bar is kept close to the body by retaining straight elbows, lordotic back, and thrust chest. Heels are stuck firmly to the floor. The center of mass of the body is moving backwards, behind the vertical plane at the heels, in order to balance the weight of the bar in front, *Figure 5.22* and *5.23.*
- o Above the kneecaps, the bar moves faster with the aid of the final and forward thrust of the hips, the full extension of the knees, the sustained stabilization of fixed and firm upper body, and straight solid elbows.
- o When the knees and hips finish **full extension**, further upward pull on the bar comes from shrugging the shoulders and hopping on the feet balls, *Figure 5.24.* With advanced training, the lifter will learn to elevate the heels without elevating the whole feet. Yet, some top Olympic lifters jump off the ground during this process. This combination of actions requires backward bouncing of the head and upper body. Backward upper bouncing occurs during the forward thrusting of the hips. Thus an upward force is generated, in addition to a torque, that brings the bar weight close to the vertical plane of the fall line.
- o After the Trapezius exhausts shrugging the shoulders, the Deltoids kick in to **abduct the upper arms** and exert further pull on the ascending bar, *Figure 5.25.* The timing of recruiting the Deltoids is critical in facilitating the Power Clean. Any hesitation in the timing of the actions of the shoulders may lead to failure to lift.
- o The Deltoids cannot abduct the arms above the shoulder level without rotating the scapulas. Below the shoulder level, the front of the Deltoid could be quickly recruited to **elevate the elbows under the bar** (by shoulder flexion) and rack the bar on the front of the shoulders. This is aided by simultaneous dipping with the knees and hips, during exerting the final pull, *Figure 5.26* thru *5.28.*
- o The successive sequence of shoulder shrugging, abduction, and flexion serves the purpose of bringing the **bar very close to the chest** during the weakest range of motion of the shoulders. The elevated elbows throw the bar in the groove between the Deltoid and the clavicles. Most athletes have enough flexibility at the wrists and can tolerate overextending the wrist while with bar seated on the shoulders. Others, with stiff wrist flexors, opt to open their handgrips and let the bar seat on the tips of the fingers.
- o With the bar racked on the front of the shoulders, the back is kept firmly extended, shoulders tightly flexed, and the hips and knees are straightened. From here, this posture aids complete upward lift or repeat the Clean from the floor.
- o The bar is slowly lowered, by lowering the elbows to release the bar from the "shoulder seat". The bar slides downwards over the front of the chest, under control of the arms, until it reaches the top of the thighs. The hips and knees then bend as the bar slides on the thighs. Squat down, with the bar held in both hands, and maintain lordotic back posture. The bar is then lowered, close to the shins, and placed on the floor. The body should be in the same position as at the beginning of the lift.
- o Lowering the bar can be more dangerous than elevating it. Many lifters opt to drop the weight on rubber floors. Before the invention of rubber floors, we used to drop the weight on wooden floors and take care of the floor repair afterwards. Poor alignment of the back, during lowering the bar, can cause devastating disc injury. In addition, underestimating the danger of eccentric contraction of muscles without serious attention on the lifter's part contributes to back injuries.

5.2.6. HANG CLEAN

The Hang Clean strengthens the upper phases of the Clean lift. It is not an exercise that should be performed in isolation of the whole Clean training. That is because the hang Clean only strengthens a partial phase of the lift. The other phases of the Clean lift are very important and should not be omitted from training plan.
- o The bar is held by both hands, in standing position, with a shoulder-wide grip. Equipped gyms provide stands of various heights to support the bar. The **start position** takes the form of slightly bent knees, forwardly thrust chest, retracted scapulas, shoulders fall behind the chest, firmly concaved lower back, and straight arms holding the bar above the kneecaps, *Figure 5.20.*
- o The initial lifting of the Hang Clean is extremely difficult for untrained folks. During early initiation of lift from the hang, neither the arms initiate the lifting, nor does the shoulders shrugging kick in. Before the bar commences upward movements, the upper body has to **bend forwards,** *Figure 5.21.* This brings the head in a vertical plan in front of the toes and moves the hips backwards, behind the vertical fall line *Figure 5.22.*
- o Novices start lifting with heads lying vertically on the bar. Vertical descent with hips and knees reduces the momentum generated by bouncing the head and body on the feet balls.
- o The forward leaning brings the bar in a vertical plane with the back fibers of the Deltoids, and the middle fibers of the Trapezius. Lifting starts with slight knee extension that further **throws the head forwards**. Then hips and lower back extension follows, while the upper body still retains solid firm contraction. These few movements by big muscles set the bar in motion *Figure 5.23.*

POWERLIFTING

- o While the body is assuming full extension, the head and the upper body will be moving across the vertical plane of the fall, line, from the front to the back. **Shoulder shrugging** commences after full body extension is reached. Shoulder shrugging brings the bar to a level above the thighs, *Figure 5.24*.
- o While the head and upper body are crossing the vertical plane, the heels are elevated to amplify the torque of the upper body around the footballs. In the same time, the shoulders abduct the arms to bring the bar closer to the body and elevate the bar further to the chest level *Figure 5.25*.
- o . The catch-up and the lowering phases are the same as the Power Clean, *Figures 5.26* thru *5.28*.

5.2.7. MILITARY SNATCH

The Military Snatch is stiff and stable form of the Snatch. It entails a high pull without dipping by the hips or knee. The barbell is lifted from the floor to an arm-stretch overhead, without being racked at the shoulders. The bar is held with a grip wider than the shoulder width. It is then lifted from the floor and thrown above and behind the head, with straight arms. The following is a description of the military Snatch.

- o The starting stance is the same as in the Military Clean, Power Clean, and Power Snatch, *Figure 5.29*.
- o In the start position, the hips descend to the horizontal level of the knees.
- o The handgrips are wider than shoulder-width. This forces the chest to come closer to the bar than in the Clean. The arms are stretched straight at the elbows, all the way until the entire body is upright and extended with the bar elevated above the thighs *Figures 5.29* thru *5.34*.
- o The chest is thrust forwards and the shoulders placed behind the chest. This ensures well-retracted scapulas.
- o The back erectors should remain tight and maintain lordotic lower back.
- o As any lifting from the floor, lifting starts with further hardening the back extensors. This allows movements above and below the waist to link together, in an upward unison, *Figures 5.29* thru *5.32*.
- o With the lower back kept firm, the thighs and Glutei drive the body upwards while the upper body remains in isometric contraction (firm with no shortening of muscles or bending of joints) to stabilize the weights that is hanging down in both hands, *Figure 5.30*.
- o When the bar is elevated above the kneecaps, the upper body starts to bounce backwards while the hips are pushed forwards. The two masses, the head and pelvis, move in counter directions by the actions of the thighs and Glutei, *Figures 5.32* thru *5.34*.
- o Shoulder shrugging comes to play when the body is overextended, the bar reaches above the thighs and very close to the body, and the head moves behind the vertical fall line, *Figure 5.34*.
- o Arms abduction follows shoulder shrugging and elevates the bar from below the level of umbilicus to an arms-stretch overhead. Without dipping with the hips and knees, the Deltoids, long head of Biceps, Supraspinatus, and Serratus anterior work very hard to move the weight overhead, *Figure 5.38*. Skip *Figures 5.35* thru *5.37*, when doing Military Snatch.

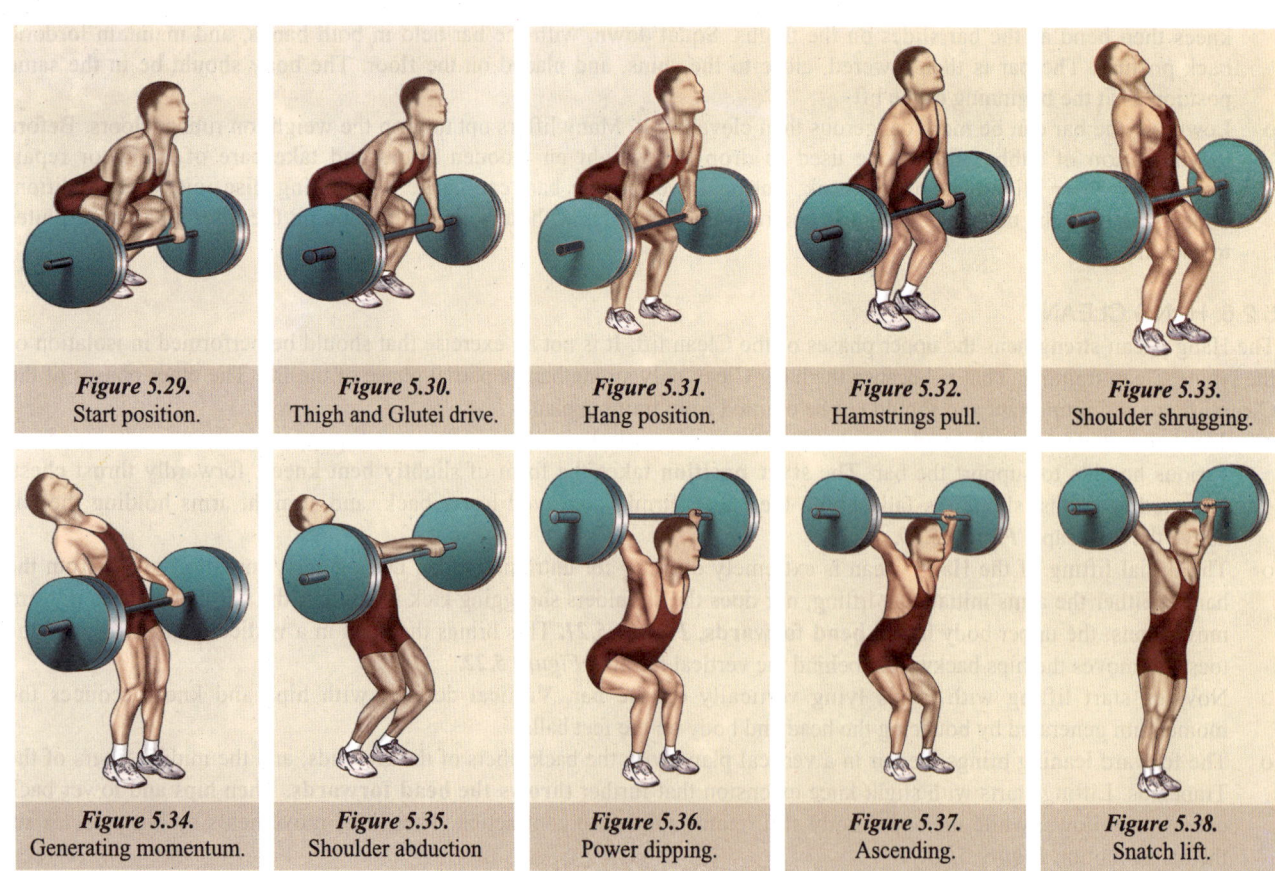

Figure 5.29. Start position.

Figure 5.30. Thigh and Glutei drive.

Figure 5.31. Hang position.

Figure 5.32. Hamstrings pull.

Figure 5.33. Shoulder shrugging.

Figure 5.34. Generating momentum.

Figure 5.35. Shoulder abduction.

Figure 5.36. Power dipping.

Figure 5.37. Ascending.

Figure 5.38. Snatch lift.

5.2.8. POWER SNATCH

This differs from the Military Snatch in the upper phase of the pull. The lifter has to dip with the knees and hips to shorten the distance of upward pull. Dipping starts as the bar reaches the breast level. At this level, the upper and back fibers of the Deltoid guide the barbell upwards and behind the shoulders, as follows.

o   The bar is pulled up to the breast level as in the Military Snatch, *Figures 5.29* thru *5.34*.
o   With the center of the body falling behind the fall line, the lifter abducts both shoulders to bring the bar from below the chest to shoulder level, *Figure 5.35*.
o   From the shoulder level, throw the bar backwards and upwards and dive with your head and body forwards and downwards. This is done by dipping with bending knees and hips on anchored heels, *Figure 5.36*. The danger in this stage lies in the loss of attention, or poor timing of head attack, or excessive throwing of the bar backwards and upwards. Injuries to the chin, nose, or forefront occur with such mistiming. With practice, such skill is easily gained.
o   You should not use custom-manufactured barbells that have rough indentation. These cut the skin as sharp razor blades. Professionally manufactured bars have smooth indentation and are friendly to human skin.
o   The quick dip of the hips is opposed by quick extension of the arms under the bar. These opposing movements prevent substantial drop of the bar, while the body moves from above and behind the bar to under and in front, *Figure 5.37*.
o   After the bar is secured in extended hands above the shoulders with the head advanced across the fall line and the hip retreated behind the fall line, ascent starts with hardening the Trapezius and back extensors and extending the hips and knees, *Figures 5.36 thru 5.38*.

5.2.9. DEADLIFT

The Deadlift is a simple exercise that entails lifting weights from the floor to the level of mid-thighs. Therefore, Deadlift is a partial strengthening exercise. Heavy deadlifting is a measure of whole body strength, not fitness or performance. Performing this exercise without including exercises of whole range of motion, in total planning, is a serious mistake.

5.2.9.1. Description of the Deadlift
The following are the features of the Deadlift exercise.

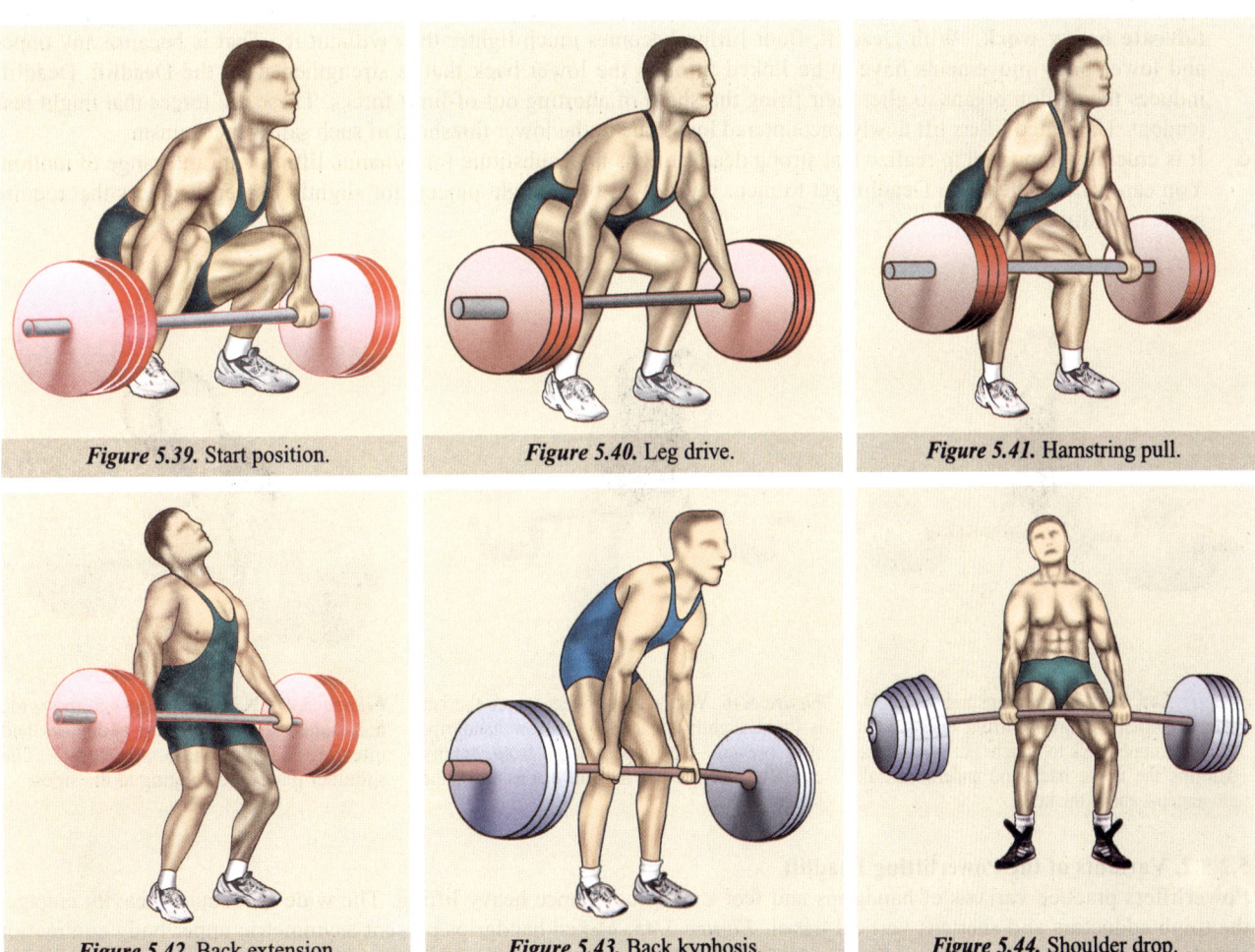

Figure 5.39. Start position.   *Figure 5.40.* Leg drive.   *Figure 5.41.* Hamstring pull.

Figure 5.42. Back extension.   *Figure 5.43.* Back kyphosis.   *Figure 5.44.* Shoulder drop.

o   The Deadlift could be performed in many ways, with one common rule, that is the **back muscles** have to be kept sufficiently contracted to support lordotic back, without any wiggling, *Figures 5.39* thru *5.42*.

5 POWERLIFTING

- Lifting with slightly bent knees adds more shearing stress on the back and requires exquisite hardening of the back to avoid sudden slipping of the spinal disk. The stiff-legged Deadlift is known as the **"Romanian Deadlift"**. It is only practiced with beginners and women interested in fast tightening of the back muscles. Its major drawback is that any lapse of attention could lead to grave injury.
- Lifting with **bent knees,** with hips lowered to the knee level, puts the back in optimal lifting position. This pyramidal posture brings the back extensors closer to vertical plane. The shoulders are positioned vertically on the bar. The chest is thrust upwards and forwards, *Figure 5.39.*
- Keeping the **knees inside the arms** prevents shortening of the hip abductors and evenly spreads the load on the entire surface of the knees. Wide feet stance shortens the distance of elevation and eases lifting but predisposes to chronic arthritis of the knees and hips. Wide stance directs forces obliquely on the hips, knees, and ankles, thus limiting the loading surface to oblique directions, *Figure 5.45.*
- Handgrips that are narrower than shoulder-width pull the scapulas forwards and concentrate the weight on convex (hunched) upper back. With a **shoulder-wide grip**, the scapulas can remain retracted to the chest cage and balance the distribution of pulling forces along the upper back. Thus, lifting heavier for shorter distances prejudices the integrity of the shoulder posture and causes long term deformed shoulders, *Figures 5.43* and *5.44.*
- Holding the bar with mixed handgrips, one palm facing backwards and the other facing forwards, undermines the shoulder balance. Such asymmetric grips load one shoulder ball in one way, while the other ball is loaded in a different way. The arm, with the palm facing forwards, has shortened Infraspinatus and laterally displaced tendon of the long head of Biceps, *Figures 5.45* thru *5.47.*
- The Deadlift is performed by pure upper body isometric contraction and pure isotonic contraction of the lower limbs. If not balanced by exercises of full range of motion of the shoulders then serious **shoulder immobility** develops.
- The Deadlift should be aborted, not when the back buckles, but when encountering any sense of **pending buckling**. Even if you succeed in lifting a heavy load, after allowing the back concavity to be lost, you are subjecting your back to unnecessary risk. That is not just the ordinary risks that athletes usually take, but rather a risk that could leave you paralyzed for very little gain. You might be able to lift heavier weights in the future if you work on strengthening your back, *Figures 5.43* and *5.44.*
- Apart from its strengthening effects of the body extensors, the Deadlift mainly increases the whole body ability to **tolerate heavy work**. With Deadlift, floor lifting becomes much lighter than without it. That is because any upper and lower body movements have to be linked through the lower back that is strengthened by the Deadlift. Deadlift induces the tendon organs to alter their firing threshold of aborting out-of-limit forces. These are forces that might tear tendons. Untrained lifters lift newly encountered loads due to the lower threshold of such safety mechanism.
- It is crucially important to realize that strong deadlifting is no a substitute for dynamic lifting with full range of motion. You can lift very heavy in Deadlift yet to incur injuries on lifting light objects for slightly longer distances that require some mobility of joints.

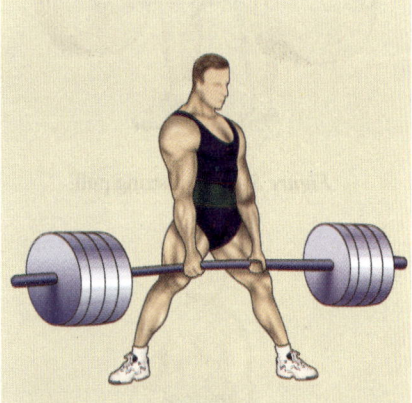

Figure 5.45. Narrow handgrips and wide feet-stance shorten the upward lifting distance but force the upper back to hunch. Such technique deforms the upper back and undermines all movements above the head.

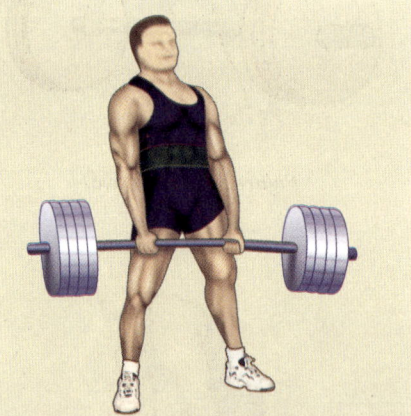

Figure 5.46. With narrower feet-stance the bar is lifted slightly higher. The narrow handgrips still prevent the upper back from totally extending, in spite of the full extension of the lower back.

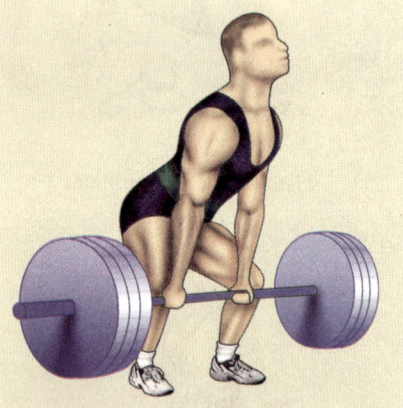

Figure 5.47. Narrow handgrips and wide feet-stance shorten the hip abductors and interferes with chest thrusting. The shoulder plates are winging to the sides.

5.2.9.2. Variants of the Powerlifting Deadlift
Powerlifters practice variants of handgrips and feet stance to enhance heavy lifting. The wide feet stance heavily engages the thigh adductors and shortens vertical travel, *Figure 5.45.* Mixed handgrips present asymmetric upper body contraction and thus offers stimulating feeling, *Figures 5.45* and *5.47.*

5.2.10. BENCH PRESS
The Press while lying on a bench is the most famous exercise in the entire world of modern weight training. It gained such worldwide fame because of the following.

POWERLIFTING

o   Bench Press works out one of the most cherish part of the body, the chest-that hosts the heart and lungs. Developing strong chest embodies athletic achievements.
o   Easy to perform exercise. It can be performed without warm-up, when tired, injured, or bored. It requires least amount of coordination.
o   Progress is quit fast for all people even those with relative weakness of the back. Thus, it gives the sense of accomplishment with least amount of effort.
o   It does not require sophisticated coaching and it offers the option of finding many partners, since many people perform this exercise.

The Bench Press is a shoulder exercise. That is true. Remember you cannot train the chest if you do not have shoulders. The chest works out because of the direction of force that requires the Pectoralis major to resist, in the front of the shoulder. Thus, in order to balance the shoulder muscles, the Bench Press has to be part of whole shoulder training. That includes inclined and declined Bench Presses, seated Shoulder Press, Bent-over and row, Chin-up, and Dips. The Bench Press could be enhanced by progressive increase in load, as well as by assisting exercises such the one-hand dumbbell exercises. Dumbbell exercises work out all directions of the shoulder movements.

5.2.10.1. Description of Bench Press
Although performing Bench Press is very simple, yet some trainees make bizarre mistakes in its execution. The following is brief description of the exercise.
o   Lay on your back on the designated bench. Your eye should be positioned vertically under the bar. This allows the bar to move away from the rack when held in both hands and elevated off the rack. This way the bar will not be hitting the supporting parts of the rack.
o   Hold the bar with both palms facing upwards. You should see your knuckles under the bar. Do not invent reverse handgrips. These are not feasibl anatomical movements. Make sure that your handgrips are evenly positioned on the bar from its middle, or ends.

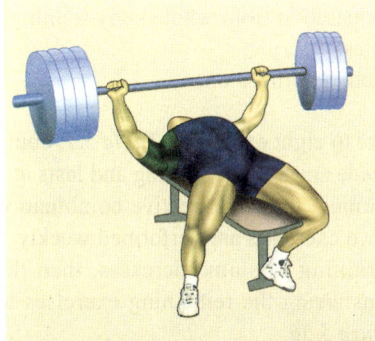

Figure 5.48. Acutely concaved lower back and abducted thighs aid in shortening the travel distance of the bar and support the body on hard solid girdles.

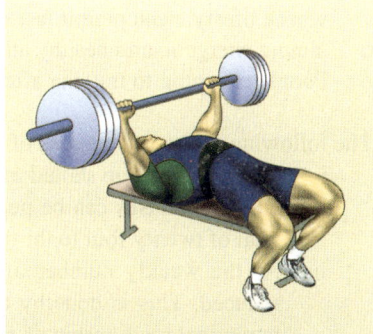

Figure 5.49. Ideal position of shoulder-wide handgrips, and similar width feet stance.

o   Before you start lifting, ensure that both feet are well supported on the ground. Also, ensure that the barbell is evenly loaded. This is your last minute checkup routine.
o   Your shoulder plates, buttocks, and feet support lifting the bar from the rack. It is better to arch your lower back away from the bench. This lordotic back will ensure your active protection of the spinal discs.
o   As you prepare the arms and shoulders to move the bar from the rack, thrust the chest upwards, tighten the shoulder plates against the bench, and arch your lower back.
o   One of the bizarre mistakes, some lifter make, is going into frantic convulsion prior to lifting heavy weight. Save your energy for muscular work. If you concentrate on lifting you would not need excessive excitation to lift.
o   As the bar is lifted from the rack, it must move forwards, few inches, in order to move freely. Now, you support the weight of the bar on shoulder plates, buttocks, and feet.
o   The direction of your elbows, during descent and ascent, determines which muscles resist the weight. Elbows directed to the outside, away from your body, mostly work out shoulder adductors. These are the Pectoralis major, Subscapularis, and long head of Biceps. Elbows directed downwards, with respect to your vertebral axis, or close to the sides of the body, mostly work out the shoulder flexors. These are the front Deltoid, Pectoralis minor, and upper fibers of the Pectoralis major.

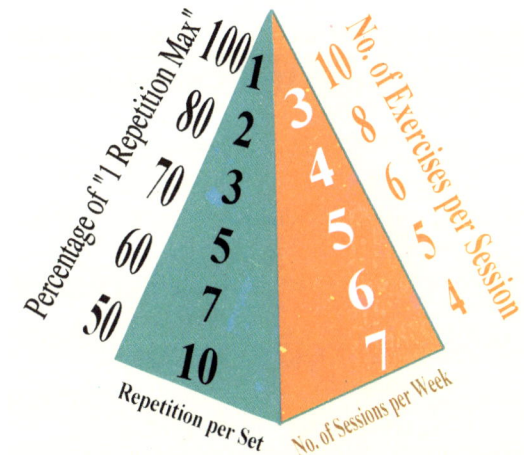

Figure 5.50. The pyramidal relationships between Number of repetitions per sets, Number of sessions per week, Number of exercises per session, Average percentage of maximal weight.

o   Slow descent operates by eccentric contraction. This is used to enhance hypertrophy. Fast ascent operates by concentric contraction. This fosters strength.
o   The bar may be lowered on a wide range, between the junctions of the second rib with the sternum to the xiphisternal joint (the lowest point of the sternum, just over the stomach). Usually, people lower the bar slightly above the level of nipples.

5 POWERLIFTING

o Many people prefer pausing in the bottom before commencing ascent. This serves stretching ligaments and muscle spindles that reset the stretch reflex to higher thresholds and enhance muscular strength in short duration.

5.3. PLANS OF POWERLIFTING TRAINING

Powerlifting is a newly invented sport with subjective planning strategies. In order to avoid long-term deformities, the following routines integrate full range of motion and balanced muscular performance. The **"parallel routine"** comprises of exercises that work out all major muscles in each session. The **"serial routine"** comprises of split-session exercises for specific muscle groups.

5.3.1. PARALLEL ROUTINE
This approach intends to work out different parts of the body in each session. It is a full-body training. It suits people with the following conditions:
o Beginners aiming at muscular balance without prejudice to specific body parts.
o People with resourceful circumstances that can afford to train for over an hour, exclusive time on the gym floor, and whose lifestyle can permit fast recuperation from whole body training.
o Young energetic and healthy athletes.
o People returning to training after long intermission.

The following four combinations of five to eight exercises, *Table 5.1*, could be performed, in parallel routine, as follows.
  i. General warm-up should precede any weight training and lasts at least ten minutes.
  ii. **Eight exercises** can be performed, in the respective combinations, *Table 5.1*, in consecutive training sessions. A total of twenty four to thirty two exercises are performed weekly.
  iii. As the weekly number of **training sessions** increases, then the number of exercises, per combination, may be reduced. This is done by transferring the remaining exercises to the following training session, according to the pyramidal relationship of *Figure 5.50*.
  iv. Each exercise should be performed, at least, in three sets, and no more than eight sets, with an average of five sets.
  v. Each set of exercise should be performed, at least, once (one repetition), and no more than ten times (repetitions), with an average of five repetitions.
  vi. The number of repetitions should decrease with **increasing the weight**, to a single repetition for the maximal weight (1RM).
  vii. The weights should increase, from at least 50% of the maximal weight (1RM) at the first set of each exercise, by **incremental increases** with each successive set. Maximum weight averages anywhere from 70% of 1RM to 100%, depending on the planed load volume.

Table 5.1. Parallel routine of strength training. The four combinations are performed in four consecutive training sessions. The four sessions are repeated in cycles. Each session encompasses **whole body** training.

	Combination No. 1	Combination No. 2	Combination No. 3	Combination No. 4	Anatomy
1	Lateral Pull-down, OR Bent Over Row	Chin-up, OR Pull Over (on flat bench)	Cable Rowing OR Goodmorning	Clean Pulls, OR Deadlift	Back
2	Military Clean	Power Clean	Power Snatch	Military Snatch	Whole Body
3	Bench Press OR Decline Bench Press		Inclined Bench Press	Dumbbell Flyes Press, OR Dips	Chest
4		Seated Back Press, OR Seated Front Press	One Hand Press		Shoulder
5	Calf Raise, OR Leg Raise (on bench)	Front Squat	Back Squat	Overhead Squat, OR Back Squat	Legs
6	Lying Triceps Press	Biceps Curls	One Hand Biceps	Standing Triceps Press	Arms
7	Crunches		Sit-ups	Lateral Waist Tilting	Waist

5.3.2. SERIAL ROUTINE
This approach emphasizes one major part of the body in split-sessions. It suits people in the following categories.
o Those that need to gain excessive muscular mass, without regard to technical skills of performing complex coordinated movements.
o People with special need to develop particular parts of the body to meet other sports' needs.
o Very advanced athletes that can perform high intensity training and recuperate fast.
o Old athletes with limited cardiovascular reserves. Those cannot endure parallel routines.
o Rehabilitation of injured body parts that require extra amounts of load volume to build up strength.

Table 5.2. Serial routine of strength training. Four combinations of eight exercises are performed in four consecutive training sessions. The four sessions are repeated in cycles. Each session encompasses training of a **specific region of the body.**

	Chest Workout	Back Workout	Shoulders & Arms Workout	Legs Workout
1	Power Clean, OR Goodmorning	Chin-up, OR Pull Over on flat bench	Military Clean, OR Snatch Pulls	Military Snatch
2	Bench Press	Power Snatch, OR Cable Rowing	Shoulder Press	Goodmorning, OR Deadlift
3	Incline Flyes	Deadlift Standing Shoulder Press	Triceps Press	Back Squat, OR Front Squat
4	Dips	Front Squat	Barbell Curl	Decline Bench Press
5	Back Squat, OR Leg Raises		Back Squat , OR Leg Raises	Lateral Waist Tilting
6	Crunches	Crunches	Crunches	Crunches

Serial training could be made complete with little addition of general exercises. These are added to the core exercises for the purpose of priming of the region of interest, as follows.
- o After warming up, an exercise of the whole body is performed. This works out the major muscles of the thighs, back erectors, shoulders. This exercise can be Power or Military, Clean or Snatch.
- o Since all exercises affect the torso, a lower back exercise is performed every session in the form of Goodmorning, or Pulls from the floor. The abdomen is worked out every session.
- o The region of concern, in a particular session, receives three different core exercises. These regions are the chest, the back, the legs, or the shoulders.
- o Exercises start with at least 50% of maximal load (1RM) on the first set. That is executed from three to ten repetitions.
- o Successive sets involve incremental increase in weight and decrease in the number of repetitions.

5.4. MUSCULAR IMBALANCE

Imbalance of muscular coordination is encountered in all unfamiliar activities and has the following features:
- o Muscular imbalance becomes burdensome when it **interferes with regular** activities or when it assumes a course of relentless decline in strength and mobility. In these situations, muscular imbalance starts to raise concern as a pressing health issue.
- o Muscular imbalance affects **all people**, in one form or another. It results from favoring activities and disregarding balanced development of the musculoskeletal system. Various occupations that require daily repetitive tasks, for many years, mold the body in permanent form. Favored exercises that emulate daily work activity compound muscular imbalance.
- o Imbalance can be **purely functional.** That demonstrates itself only during certain activities in the form of limited range of motion, inflexibility of joints, pain or discomfort on trying to push the limits, or loss of strength at certain range of motion, such as:
    - i. Inability to **touch certain parts of your back** with one hand but not the other, due to tight shoulder muscles.
    - ii. Inability to perform **Front Squat** with elevated elbows due to weak Serratus anterior, Supraspinatus, and Deltoid.
    - iii. Inability to perform **seated Shoulder Press** without back-stand support due to weak Iliopsoas, Serratus anterior, and back extensors.
    - iv. Inability to perform **Overhead Squatting** due to weak Iliopsoas, Serratus anterior, upper Trapezius, and back extensors.
    - v. Inability to perform the **upper phase of the Clean,** without swinging the bar away from your chest, due to weak shoulder abductors.
    - vi. Inability to perform full **Back Squat,** without raising your heels or leaning forwards, due to weak back extensors and Iliopsoas.
    - vii. Inability to **Back-Squat** with thrust chest and vertical back, without tilting your head upwards and backwards, due to weak back extensors, Iliopsoas, and Serratus anterior.
- o Muscular imbalance can be easily observed as **change in the posture** of walking, standing, sitting, or lying down. Imbalanced activities cause shortening and tightening of some groups of muscles, while weaken other muscle groups. The loss of balanced strength, flexibility, and endurance of the muscular elements of a joint deform the composition and integrity of the bone, cartilage, tendons, ligaments, and bursa surrounding the joint, as follows.
    - i. Drooping of arms in people with **wasted shoulder muscles**. Weak shoulders show in drooping of the arms over the chest and belly, with no or little gap separating the arms from the torso, while standing relaxed.
    - ii. Wasting of arms, shoulders, and chest are very common in women. This predisposes to shoulder dislocation, sublaxation, and arthritis.
    - iii. Loss of lower **back curvature** (normal concavity) due to weak back erectors and Iliopsoas.
    - iv. **Rounded upper back** due to weak back erectors and forward translation of the shoulders. This deformity

POWERLIFTING

predisposes to tendonitis, arthritis, bursitis, or tears of the rotator cuff muscles of the shoulder joint, *Figure 5.51*.
  v. **Exaggerated neck curvature,** in compensation for rounded upper back. This deformity predisposes to cervical and thoracic dysfunction and entrapments of the brachial nerve plexus.
  vi. **Bulging belly** due to weak abdominal support and weak breathing muscles.
  vii. **Wasting of buttocks and thighs** due to lack of activity of the lower body. The hip flexors (Iliopsoas and Rectus femoris) and erector spinae muscles become tight and short, while the abdominal muscles and Gluteus maximus are weakened.
  viii. Swayback with anterior pelvic tilt, **increased lumbar lordosis**. This deformity predispose to lower back pain, discomfort or dull ache in the buttocks during Squat.

o Muscular imbalance is very **difficult to prevent, recognize in timely fashion, or rectify** in the majority of cases. Due to the long course and insidious development of muscular balance, it escapes recognition by many people. Those accommodate muscular imbalance as a sort of "identity characteristics" instead of trying to rectify its causes.

o Weight training resolves some problematic aspects of muscular imbalance. By developing new and strong muscle fibers, strength training can alleviate, if not rectify, imbalance. The Olympic lifts require great deal of muscular balance. Both the Snatch and the Clean and Jerk require great deal of shoulder mobility, in the upward and backward directions. Weightlifters neglect the chest to greater extent compared to Powerlifters. Each strengthening activity offers unique gain. Olympic lifts develop the fast twitching muscles fibers and thus enhance functional balance. Powerlifting enhances slow twitching muscle fibers thus fosters postural balance.

o Powerlifting consists of the three lifts: Deadlift, Squat, and Bench Press. These three lifts work out legs, back and chest and favor wide range of body types. Almost anyone, long limbed or short limbed, can aspire to be competitive in Powerlifting, for many years of his or her life. Muscular balance could be maintained if the Powerlifter realizes the limitation of the three lifts. The three lifts lack the following **component of muscular balance**.

  i. The three lifts are performed with the shoulder plates entirely seated on the back of the chest. There is no **shoulder abduction** in Powerlifting exercises. Also, there is no shoulder flexion except during Bench Press with narrow grip. There is no overhead elevation. These could be corrected by Plyometrics exercises without weights or with lightweight that involve shoulder abduction, flexion, and overhead elevation. Few sets of Power Snatch, Power Clean, or Shoulder Press, with variable grips, could easily remedy these shortcomings. These remedial exercises should be done in equal proportion to the core Powerlifting exercises in order to avoid **permanent shoulder freezing**.

  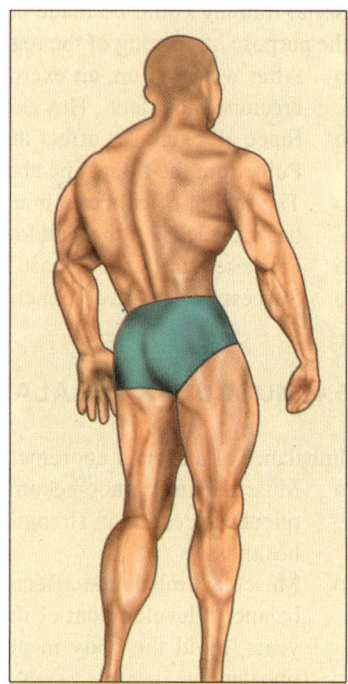

  Figure 5.51. Bencher's chest: The shoulders and chest are rounded forwards. The arms are internally turned. The Pectorals, Deltoids, and scapular muscles are hugely developed but with forward translation.
  The tight muscles are: upper Trapezius, Sternocleidomastoid, the Pectoralis, and Levator scapulae.
  The weakened muscles are: Rhomboids, deep neck flexors, and erector spinal muscles.
  Curves: increased cervical curve, increased thoracic kyphosis, and lost lower back lordosis.

  ii. The Deadlift ceases at full body extension without an effort to shrug shoulders, extend back erectors, or abduct shoulders. Thus, the shoulder structures perform **pure isometric contraction,** without any dynamic motion. Bizarre stances of feet, such as widely spread feet, severely traumatize the knee and hips. Trauma develops due to adding horizontal forces and pointing the load on narrow area of the articulating surfaces. The lateral condyles of the knees carry the entire load, and the heads of the femur are exposed to enormous shear stress. These shortcomings could be avoided by standing in neutral position, where the legs fall vertically below the hips. The limited range of pull of the Deadlift could be compensated with few light sets of Power Clean form the hang and from the floor.

  iii. The Squat **with wide feet-stance** does the same damage to the knees as the Deadlift with wide feet stance. These, partially and discriminately, traumatize the lateral knee condyles, menisci, and hip joints. Squatting to parallel shortens and stiffens the knee ligaments and joints and prevents the strengthening of the lower back in fully squatted position. Building stronger thigh muscles is wiser than damaging the knees with oblique bending. Full squatting could be practiced with lighter weights prior to loading heavier weights.

  iv. The Bench Press strengthens the front of the shoulder, the Deadlift the upper aspect of the shoulder. There is a need to strengthen the back and the lower aspects of the shoulder with exercises such as rowing and chin-ups.

  v. The three lifts lack enhancement of normal **human posture**. The Squat involves leaning forwards, the Deadlift does not involve thrusting the chest forwards with elevated shoulders, and the Bench Press is performed in lying down position. These could be remedied by performing Front Squat, seated or standing Shoulder Press, and overhead Press and Squat, *Figure 5.52*. The easiest postural exercises are the Power Snatch and Clean and Jerk.

These work out the vertebral column, when the head and hip move backwards and forwards, across the vertical plane at the feet balls.
- o Efforts to rectify muscular imbalance may succeed or fail to achieve desired goals according to the following contributing factors.
    - i. **Awareness** of the presence of the problem, the need for solution, and the available treatment options.
    - ii. The **duration and severity** of the imbalance. Bony deformities are not good candidates for conservative correction, though great benefits can be gained from efforts to improve muscular imbalance and foster better living conditions with a chronic problem.
    - iii. **Stretching** with safe techniques, and for long term, ameliorate many imbalance conditions. Yoga training can reverse long incurred imbalanced if practiced long enough, at least six months or so.
    - iv. **Strength training** requires good understanding of the functional and physical anatomy of muscles and joints. Few weeks of progressive strength training can develop active muscles that antagonize short and tight muscles. Activating weak muscles may greatly increase strength on a wide range of motion.
    - v. **Aggressive modalities** such as chiropractic manipulation, use of ice or heat after traumatic exercises, ultrasound, and electrical muscle stimulation may tide extreme cases over critical periods, but not for long term correction. Aggressive approaches induce more insults to biological structures and worsen scarring.
    - vi. **Nutrition** may play a significant role in those with borderline nutritional status and those require boosting energy to sustain persistent training. Nutritional elements that deserve some consideration are vitamins from vegetables and fruits. Most of the vitamins that regulate the metabolism of carbohydrate, fat, and protein occur in natural food.

5.5. POWER BOOSTING MODALITIES

5.5.1. SUPERSETS

Supersets are common modalities of stimulating strength and growth, in relatively short times. From my own experience, supersetting holds the secrets of developing fast strength for accomplished lifters. It is very effective strength training modalities during strength-development season. It is counterproductive during technique-enhancement season. It has these common features.

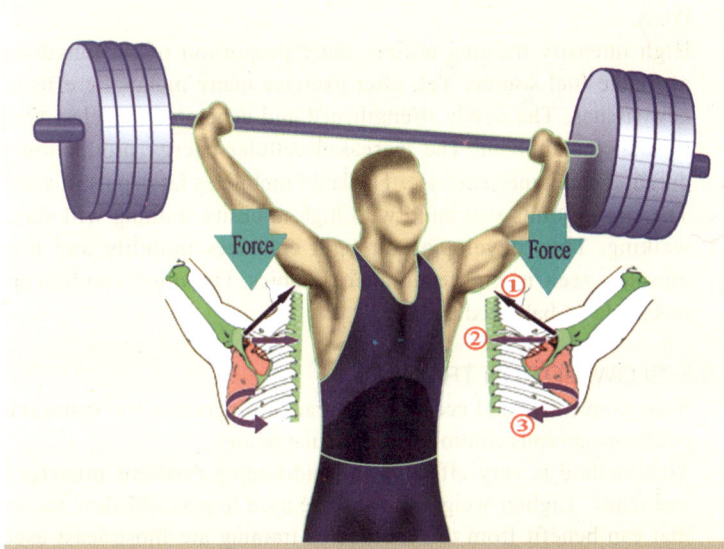

Figure 5.52. Overhead shoulder exercises: Weightlifting strongly balances these scapular muscles:
- o The scapular elevators: upper Trapezius, circle 1,
- o The scapular retractors: middle Trapezius, circle 2, Serratus anterior, circle 3, and Rhomboids,
- o Upper arm extensors: rear Deltoid, Infraspinatus, Teres minor, Triceps long head, and Latissimus dorsi, and
- o Upper arm external rotators: Infraspinatus, Teres minor, and rear Deltoid.

These muscles thrust the chest upwards, transmit forces to upper and middle back, evenly, and stabilize the shoulder during overhead lifting.

- o This modality is most probably introduced by motivated and energetic athletes. It is a primitive way of catching up with the many exercises, many muscles, and limited amount of time available for training.
- o Exercising **more than one muscle, in consecutive sets**, instead of performing consecutive sets of one exercise. The groups of muscles involved in consecutive sets may be related in action, or in priority of strengthening.
- o You can exercise the **Biceps,** for example, with two of three different exercises in consecutive sets. Thus, you can perform Biceps curls, dumbbells curls, and chin-ups, in supersets, in order to enhance Biceps size and strength.
- o Similarly, you can exercise the **thighs** with two or three different exercises, in supersets of Back Squat, leg extension, and power Clean, in order to enhance Quadriceps size and strength.
- o You can exercise **shoulder, back, and thighs** in supersets of standing Shoulder Press, Goodmorning, and Front Squat, in order to enhance whole body strength, in short time.
- o You can perform **Bench Press**, flyes with dumbbells, and pullover, in supersets to enhance chest development.
- o You can exercise the **extensors and their counterparts, the flexors**, in consecutive sets to enhance joint stability. The back erectors are exercised with the Iliopsoas in supersets, of Goodmorning and crunches, to stabilize the pelvis. The

Bench Press can be performed in supersets with the bent-over row to stabilize the shoulder. The Biceps with the triceps to strengthen the elbows.
- o Because two or three exercises are intertwined together, **break intervals** have to be reduced to avoid cooling down during active training and to maintain neuromuscular coordination. Thus, either exercise intensity has to be reduced, to avoid overtraining, or the athlete has to be well trained to endure stressful training.
- o Supersets can be a portion of a standard training routine or can constitute the whole routine. The number of repetitions should not exceed ten, with an average of three to six repetitions per set. The number of exercises in consecutive sets should not exceed three, to avoid neuromuscular incoordination.

5.5.2. HIGH INTENSITY TRAINING

High intensity resistance knock down the weak and fragile muscle fibers and activates the muscle cells to re-grow newer and stronger fibers. It also induces systemic hormonal changes in order to integrate all organs in performing activity. Both cellular and systemic adaptation of the body to intense training culminates in fostering physical strength.
- o In order to enhance muscular strength beyond normal training activities you have to adhere to these simple rules. Increase the weight of the barbell over **60% of 1RM**. Perform one to five lifts, average three lifts, each set. Repeat the set for at least three times. Take twenty seconds to three minutes **break intervals** between sets.
- o With adequate rest between training sessions, and proper nutrition, high intensity training enhances **muscular strength.** This is more effective than training with weights that could be repeatedly lifted over five times per set.
- o The **maximal weight** of the barbell that could be lifted for at least once, with good technique, should steadily increase over few weeks. Factors that interfere with gaining strength are aging, overtraining, lack of rest, or poor nutrition.
- o High intensity training has to fit within well-structured **load volume chart** to avoid server overtraining. It also could be performed on separate muscle groups or separate functional skills, on partial basis of whole training. Thus, you can perform high intensity on the power Clean, plus low or medium intensity on other exercises in the same session. Alternatively, you can cut down the total number of exercises per session and focus on three or four high intensity exercises. The fundamental exercises that promote power are the Power Clean, the Deadlift, the Squat, and the Bench Press.
- o High intensity training utilizes more proportion of carbohydrates than fat due to the nature of immediate need of available fuel source. Yet, after exercise many metabolic effects remain active to replenish reserves and regenerate new tissues. The newly strengthened and generated muscles, tendons, bones, and ligaments will be of great assets to cellular metabolism. The increased cellular energy production facilitates future intensity training, as well as long duration endurance exercise. The latter mobilizes fat depots in very efficient manner.
- o The strong joints you build with high intensity training will stabilized your posture during running, jogging, or brisk walking. Thus developing strength enhances mobility and prevents tightening, weakening, or wasting of major muscles, seen in high endurance aerobics. Optimum combination of high intensity and long duration endurance is reachable by balanced training.

5.5.3. SLOW MOTION TRAINING

- o Slow concentric and eccentric contraction increases the **isometric component,** during the isotonic contraction. This enhances nervous control over muscular action.
- o This method is very effective in conditioning **resilient muscles** that require constant stimulation to develop strength and mass. Lighter weights have to be used to perform slow motion, in both directions of lifting. The parts of the body that can benefit from this method of training are those least used in daily activities in full range strengthening. The muscles of the calves, forearms, lower back, thighs, chest, shoulder-extensors, -elevators, and -flexors, Biceps, and hip flexors, are good candidates for isometric slow motion training.
- o Slow motion training cannot be performed in the last month, prior to competition, since it undermines muscle flexibility and coordination during complex motion. Slow motion induces tissue congestion and edema thus interferes with neuromuscular coordination and recuperation from training.
- o Its main application is stimulating muscles that are lagging behind general body development. It is practiced only on casual basis, since it leads to accumulation of fluids within the active muscles, causing soreness and tightness.
- o The following exercises may be performed slowly in both directions of lifting: Calf Raising, Back Extension, Bench Press, Cable Rowing, Shoulder Shrugging, Shoulder Press, and Biceps Curls.

5.5.4. PLYOMETRICS

Plyometrics are exercises that utilize the body inertial energy to generate resistance and strengthen muscles.
- o Because the entire bodyweight is utilized in generating resisting forces, the athletes should have **well-conditioned limbs** to withstand such excessive forces. Gradual strengthening exercises by weight training, in combination with progressive Plyometrics exercises, should help limbs stand excessive impulses.
- o Powerlifters, Weightlifters, and beginners who intend to use Plyometrics may utilize these exercises as **assisting** to weight training. Cross training enhances the discovery of points of weakness, overweight issues, lack of endurance

issues, or inflexibility problems. Well-trained thighs, lower back, and shoulders can be put to real test during Plyometrics.
- o Plyometric exercises are unique in working out muscles that propel the bodyweight into airborne state and ensure solid **structural and functional integrity**. These might have other invaluable effects on the psychological and endocrine system due to their invigorating and entertaining nature.
- o Cardiovascular development advances at the same rate as **musculoskeletal development.** This is in contrast to Bodybuilding and "weight training", where muscles and bones development surpasses cardiovascular development. This renders the athlete "out of breath" when performing endurance activities.
- o The unique feature of Plyometrics is the heavy workout of the **lower legs**, below the knees, which is the main gauge of feeling and controlling walking, standing, jogging, and running. The lower legs are poorest in blood supply since the arteries of the lower limbs flow in tight and narrow compartments. That makes the lower limbs a constant source of pain and discomfort of arthritis and peripheral arterial disease. Plyometrics enhance the blood circulation to the lower legs and make people with arthritic knees enjoy active running and jumping for many years. Even swollen arthritic knees develop great stability and flexibility after gradual and progressive Plyometrics exercises.
- o Exercises of common use in strength training are:
    - i. **Platform depth jump** is performed by jumping from a higher level (box) to lower level (platform). Landing on the lower level is cushioned by the springing action of feet, knees, and hips. The muscles around these joints can work out hard by imposing greater cushioning resistance, instead of falling freely with lax body collapsing to the ground. This parallels eccentric contraction during squatting, yet with an impulsive component.
    - ii. **Vertical depth jump** is a modification of the previous exercises. At the end of the depth-jump, the person performs subsequent vertical jump. This stretches the body in the air by trying to reach highest vertical level. This involves both eccentric contraction (negative contraction during landing) and concentric contraction (during jumping vertically).
    - iii. **Depth push-up** is performed with straight body, close to horizontal, with feet kept on an object above the head level, and hands put to two raised blocks or boxes or hand-held bars. This is an old and famous exercise is performed on two-sided wooden triangle or lower parallel bars. The upper body performs push-ups by bending and extending the elbows. The advantage of raising the feet above horizontal and lowering the upper body below the surface of the side boxes, or bars, is adding more resistance and range of motion to the Pectoral and Deltoid muscles.

5.5.5. CALISTHENICS

Calisthenics differ from Plyometrics in the theme of exercise. These focus of creating artistic flavor to exercising. As with Plyometrics, Calisthenics generate greater inertial energy and require greater joint flexibility and strength to avoid injuries. The assisting component of Calisthenics is simpler from dedicated performance. It is incorporated in public gyms' aerobics with different levels of complexity. The main goal of Calisthenics is relaxing nervous control of muscles in performing graceful and complex motions.

5.6. OLYMPIC WEIGHTLIFTING VS POWERLIFTING

5.6.1. LIFTING BELT

Most weight trainees do not understand the function of lifting belts. Many of the world's best Weightlifters compete without a belt. The benefits of developing natural torso are multifold, as follows.
- o Belts do not aid the spinal erectors in extending the trunk. Sufficient intraabdominal pressure, produced by abdominal strength and strong spinal erectors can be developed by structured training and without belts. Continued belt use retards muscular development if it is tightened for long times, or has a bigger width that limits bending.
- o Belts are used as **warning devices**. These pinch at the edges, when buckling of the lower back ensues during lifting. The pinch alarms the lifter to release the weight in order to avoid injury. Confident lifters trust their own senses. If backstretch becomes extreme, confident lifters rely on their humble compliance to yield and dump the weight.
- o Belts restrict the **range of motion** specially when they are wide and tough. Restricted back motion limits flexibility and stretch and predisposes to stiffness, weakness, and injury. Though large and polished leather belts look sexy to outsiders, they are not serving human needs as they are perceived to be.
- o Belts prevent many **back injuries** in many industries that require physical activities or lengthy hours of idle sitting and inactivity. For lay folks, belts are the most practical way to circumvent injury, herniation, or even overeating. In this case, a waist belt acts as a stimulant to the skin to remind the person with the events at the waist level of the body, such as distending belly or buckling lower back. Belts also keep the back warm and improve sensation. That is not the case for motivated athletes who strive for strength, flexibility, and ability to perform without the drag of noncompliant, retarded waist.
- o Tight **belts impede circulation** and lead to damming of returned blood in the lower body. The back muscles suffer more from congestion and poor circulation from tight belts, than without them. The desired increased intra-abdominal

pressure is one that is pulsating in synergy with respiration and heart beating. Abdominal pressure is beneficial only when it enhances pumping blood and blowing air, not when it applies all times, needed or not.
- o Powerlifters ought to refrain from imitation of practices seen in **commercial advertisement** when these defy scientific wisdom. If lifting the heaviest weight gets you a trophy, you should weigh such gain against the cost of crippling injury. That may not seem as acute or dramatic as you might expect, but rather insidious crushing of cartilages and bones and scarring of tendons and ligaments.

5.6.2. SUPPORTIVE CLOTHING
Lifting suits serve few purposes such as:
- o Suspending the testicles during vigorous training to prevent contusion and internal bleeding.
- o Preventing the exposure of the lower back during bending, by uniting the lower and upper halves of a suit at the waist. Standing for few minutes sweating with exposed lower back undermines the performance of strength athletes, particularly in cold or ventilated environment.
- o Appearance that is appropriate for a sport of bride and passion. Above all, athletes do not design their own suits and, most probably, they are tempted by the attractive choices made by designers.

5.6.3. KNEE WRAPS
Knee wraps are commonly used by old athletes and those with many years of training.
- o Wraps are never intended for use by young lifters with healthy joints. If the cartilages and menisci of the knees are elastic and whole, then no significant tear or wear would cause swelling, pain, or discomfort.
- o Training the young to develop strong muscles around the knees, without incurring internal knee injury, is a real struggle. Many young lifters want to get strong fast and train enthusiastically. Imposing rigorous standards of volume, intensity, and technique is not feasible in many cases when institutional support is lacking.
- o Although the knees are surrounded by tendons and ligaments in all directions, there are still some gaps between these structures, where the synovial sac of the knee is not well supported. When the inside of knee is swollen, by inflammatory fluids, the knee capsule press through the unsupported weak spots. These are located around the patellar tendon, behind the knee, and above the patella.
- o Knee wraps support the weak spots to contain the knee capsule under pressure and keep inflamed structure apart, within the knee. Wraps also keep knees warm and press against skin, thus reducing throbbing pain due to inflammation.
- o Olympic lifting technique does not allow use of thick, heavy-duty wraps, because the bulk of material behind the knee, during full Squat, can cause injury. Powerlifters only Squat to parallel with heavy weights that cause crushing injuries to the cartilages and menisci. Their use of heavy-duty wraps is justifiable.
- o It is important to keep in mind that top athletes in any sport should not be the ultimate models to follow. Since sports are evolving, it is wiser to think rationally and prevent injuries due to passionate bias towards favored icons.
- o Also, training without knee wraps does strengthen the body's own connective tissue. Wraps only serve the purpose of supporting weaker spots in the body design, of ligament and tendons. Wraps are not facts of life but rather helpful aids for the old and injured athletes.

5.6.4. SQUATTING STYLE
The style of squatting used by Powerlifters is intended for lifting as much weight as possible.
- o Powerlifting Squat depends on forward lean of the torso, low bar placement on the back, wide feet stance, and descent to parallel depth.
- o These deviations from standard Squat shorten the distance of travel. It utilizes much leverage in order to minimize the work of descending and ascending, during squatting. No wonder why some Powerlifters squat up to four times their bodyweight.
- o The leverage gain from shortening the distance of travel in Powerlifting Squat amounts to avoiding the bowing of tendons around the pulleys, such as the Quadriceps tendon at the knees or the Glutei tendons at the hip.
- o Long-term training, with short travel distances, stiffens the tendons, ligaments, and muscles.
- o The extremely heavy weights that excite the young and healthy athlete are not great achievements, as it apparently seems to be. Heavy lifting, in partial range of motion, predisposes to pathological changes.
- o Heavy lifting is a function carried out by voluntary muscles. The injured structures such as cartilages, bones, and ligaments are coerced to support beyond their limit to irreversible damage. Young athletes are sport overzealous individuals with less appreciation of future consequences of living with injuries.
- o Weightlifter's style of Back Squat is much better for overall athletic development. Yet, it limits the amount of weight that can be handled. Even if a Weightlifter could squat with excessively heavy weights, the rational of balancing performance of the whole body deters Weightlifters from enhancing a single partial exercise to the extent of irreversible damage.
- o Weightlifters strive to lift heavy weights in full range of motion, and some have lifted triple their bodyweight in the Clean and Jerk lift.

5.6.5. POWER VERSUS STRENGTH
Powerlifting is indeed a sport of power, as follows.
- o   Although lifting heavy weights slows the speed of motion, it imposes enormous demands on the heart, lungs, and vascular system that amounts to the ultimate power of human performance. Weightlifters execute higher dynamic motion, but much less isometric contraction than Powerlifters do.
- o   Isometric contraction of muscles, during Powerlifting, makes the estimate of the measurable power output- force x velocity- an artifact, since it ignores the physiological dynamics of longer duration under high potential energy.
- o   Olympic lifting is only popular in countries where there are infrastructure of Olympic trainers, facilities, and educational resources to support the teaching of the sport. Powerlifting, on the other hand, has spread in countries with fast pace lifestyle, where young people have to depend on themselves to secure housing, jobs, and education with little governmental or social support. Olympic training for competition is impractical in such fast pace countries.
- o   The issue of superiority of Olympic lifting in developing explosiveness, and Powerlifting in developing power, is absurd. That is because neither explosiveness nor power is an independent feature of strength. Weightlifters train for strength and speed to execute competitive lifts. Powerlifters, on the other hand, worry less about speed and live within the constraints of time limitation enjoying very invigorating sport.
- o   Integrating the good of both Olympic and Powerlifting is a wise choice. Performing cycles of the Clean and Jerks, Snatch, or Overhead Squat, prior to Powerlifting, ensures balanced musculoskeletal system.
- o   To maximize strength of muscles, joint movements have to be performed at specific speeds in order to increase neural activation of the motor unit. This activation enhances synchronization of recruitments of the elements of motor units, promotes motor memory to resistance activity, and alters the contractile properties of muscle. It also alters the muscle tensile connective tissues.

5.6.6. DRUG DOPING

5.6.6.1. False belief in drug enhancement
Drugs that enhance physical performance are plaguing most sports activity of modern times.
- o   The overwhelming and naïve trust of athletes in manufactured substances that claim to boost nature to new horizons is incomprehensible. The myth that a pill or injection substitutes structured efforts, in improving nutrition, exercise, and recuperation, has long been associated with human belief in unknown powers.
- o   Resorting to drugs to enhance performance is a distraction from the main purpose of sport. Sport serves the purpose of educating the mind with realistic insights about complex human transactions. Insights such as the need for strength and wellness to perform mental function. This need makes the association between the body and the mind clearer than ever. Insights such as the consequence of picking proper food, and consuming proper amounts of it, on the wellness of the person. This could better be appreciated by testing physical fitness in sport. Insights such as comprehending the role of science in human activities put the person in unison with his environment.
- o   Drugs circumvent such nurturing aspect of sport and lead the person to making poor choices. The young and ambitious athlete that wants to fit into a team, and gains the admiration of overzealous coach, may opt make every effort to excel in sport against all axioms of wisdom. The young may justify the demanding pressure to excel as a motivating stimulus to achieve great goals.
- o   Many pretend to understand the mechanism of action and the long-term effects of used drugs. The sheer facts about drug users are that they do not realized the vulnerability of the body to intrusive behavior. They do not realize the limitation of science that makes even the most knowledgeable physician retreats from interfering in questionable conditions. They do not realize the greed of the unscrupulous drug manufacturers whose main aim is to profit at any cost.
- o   Powerlifter are at highest risk of drug doping by virtue of their inclination to a sport that is knowingly promote the ultimate power, despite skimping mobility, coordination, and flexibility.

5.6.6.2. Mode of drug action
- o   Supplying sufficient muscle **fuel** such as creatine. Creatine is available in diet rich in protein and is made in the body. There is doubt that creatine supplements differ from any normal protein diet.
- o   Affecting **hormones** that regulate protein synthesis. No authority could claim that hormonal manipulation is safe or predictable. The sensors triggered by drugs change their threshold of response to stimulus and require higher and continuous supply of drugs to achieve the same effects. This could not be met without accurate measurements and monitoring. The feedback mechanism of the body hormonal control is difficult to predict with administering illicit drugs. While the drug might help build muscles, it may suppress or aggravate other endocrine or immune functions.
- o   **Stimulating** the nervous system to increase arousal and aggressiveness. This method alters mood and neuromuscular system and may impair judgment and ability to avoid serious injuries.

5.6.7. MOBILITY
Powerlifting offers the luxury of easy and slow motion activity that suits many people with busy minds.

POWERLIFTING

- o The need for attending ballistic barbells in Weightlifting, moving within hair-thin distances closer to the body, is eliminated. Thus, a Powerlifter can enjoy music, read a book, or wander through his inner thoughts between sets of strength training.
- o The downfalls of performing activities, lying down on benches, are loss of control of mobile impulses and wasting essential mechanisms of dynamic movements. This could be compensated by limiting the duration of lying down, during exercise.
- o Since the technique of dynamic movement is not paramount to Powerlifting, most Powerlifters do not see the value of coordinating heavy, full range of motion lifting.
- o Strengthening alone does not make Weightlifters lift more, since the strong muscles could completely be rendered useless by inflexible joint, stiff tendon, or imbalanced performance. Under high-speed resistance, some of the strongest Weightlifters fail to dip in Squat, stretch shoulder overhead, or balance head with back, hip, and feet.
- o Powerlifts are performed with shoulder plates fully seated on the chest. Thus, the ligament, tendons, and muscles are merely strengthened and tightened in that restrictive position. In addition, to the tendency to squat to parallel thighs without fully squatting, both the pelvis and the shoulder girdles are subjected to tightening and shortening of muscles.
- o Overhead training, with various handgrips on barbell, helps flex and elongate the tight shoulder structures. Overhead exercises such as Shoulder Press, Jerk, and Snatch, force the scapulas to move away from the chest cage and rotate around the lateral ends of the collarbones. In this position, the forces transmitted from the arms through the scapulas will affect the middle back region and enhance the muscles that counteract kyphosis (hunch back).

5.6.8. LOAD VOLUME

Powerlifting offers another great advantage of high intensity training. Thus, a large load volume could be easily attained in short time. In fact, Powerlifting training could be supplemented with few minutes of aerobic exercises (such as running) to accomplish well-rounded training sessions in less than hour duration. The Deadlift, Squat, and Bench Press target groups of large muscles and eliminate the boredom of dealing with sculpturing exercises. That requires many hours of training.

Competitive Weightlifters train seven to eight times weekly, spread over five or six days. They perform the Snatch and/ or Clean and Jerk related movements, back and/or Front Squats, Snatch and/or Clean Pulls, Deadlift, or Goodmornings, in a plan of balancing joints. Their goal is to achieve full range lifting. The major challenge of Olympic training is balancing the proportions of these exercises to maximize performance, not mere strength of different body regions. Weightlifters exercise with weight over 60% of maximal (1RM), for a minimum of four exercises, each consists of five to sex sets of one to three repetitions. This amounts to over 100 lifts at over 60% 1RM every training session.

In both sports, overtraining is easily reached, particularly in the untrained, undertrained, very young, elderly, and people with conditions that impair recuperation. These occur during catching cold, fever, anemia, poor nutrition, or demanding lifestyle. Both sports, too, require the athlete to use the large muscles of the body in "bursts" that tremendously enhance strength. If taught and trained properly, these are very safe to perform. In the early stages of training, increased strength gains contribute to maximum power output. As potential strength-gains diminish, then other velocity-oriented means contribute to maximum power output. Progressive increase in load volume of training is paramount to increase power and strength in the young athletes, over periods of months. Old beginners and old athletes require slower rate of progressive increase in load volume to avoid ill effects of overtraining.

5.6.9. LONGEVITY

Performing regular and vigorous physical activities, for the longest years of life, depends mainly on individual circumstances of appreciating sport. Many competitive athletes abandon sport entirely after retiring. Many others exercise for the rest of their lives. Little twists of fate contribute to leading athletes to triumph or to quit altogether. Deeply ingrained knowledge, of the value of exercise in health and longevity, plays in that fate. From my own experience, an Olympic lifter was persuaded to convert from Bodybuilding to Weightlifting. There, he surpassed all of us and reached the top Olympic team. As soon as his Olympic years were over, he entirely quitted at the age of thirty-five and never came back to the gym. Injuries, dedication, strict weight control, and many years spent in climbing to the top add up to the burnout of top athletes. Those start lifting early in life. Another crucial factor in abandoning exercise prematurely, in the competitive sport, is the immense aura of glorifying top winners and abandoning losers. Losers that were, one day, glorified winners retreat to oblivion to avoid embarrassment. Also, zealous trainers discourage athletes on the downside of the competitive accomplishment curve from participating even as role models for new comers.

5.6.10. POPULARITY

The unpopular status of Weightlifting can be summarized as follows.
- o In USA Olympic Weightlifting is a dead sport, very rarely practiced in public gyms, very scarce coaching infrastructure, no available equipments or setups for freestyle lifting, and no funding of any sort.
- o Olympic lifts such as Clean and Jerk and Snatch seldom ring a bell to lay people and are confused for Powerlifting.
- o Weightlifting has less recognition and reward than Powerlifting with its invigorating name.

- o Gyms do not carry bumper plates, many switched to polygonal plates, and not all gyms condone tossing barbells on the floor.
- o Olympic lifts are dangerous if not performed under the tutelage of an experienced coach, particularly with young motivated athletes.
- o Olympic Weightlifting is hardly covered by public media or during reasonable viewing hours.
- o The Hollywood portrayal of weight training as a method of becoming big, muscular, and tough influences the majority of beginners for seeking muscular size, at any cost. Many people believe that getting big and muscular amounts for becoming healthy. Many young athletes would not bother practicing Weightlifting since it does not offer impressive appearance of well-defined huge muscles.
- o Most trainer act as cheerleaders promoting popular exercises such as Biceps curls, Bench Press, etc. They disregard whole body exercises such as the Clean and Snatch. People do not have to compete in Olympics to perform whole body exercise that produce benefits in short time.

5.7. HIGHLIGHTS OF CHAPTER FIVE

1. Massive bodies tend to revolve around the center of the mass when the initiating force is applied off-center. Plyometrics utilizes the inertial energy of the body to promote power by altering the speed and acceleration of motion. Plyometrics engages major muscle groups in coordinated complex movements.

2. The three methods of training, Bodybuilding, Powerlifting, and Weightlifting complement each other in many ways and should be integrated in any training program. Bear in mind that there are no authoritative boundaries between these modalities of strength training. In addition, the impressive naming of these sports should not discourage you from practicing and implementing their best strategies. The aura of "Olympic lifting" repels many people from attempting to practice the Snatch or Clean and jerk. Think that farmers are more "Olympic" than many people believe.

3. The Olympic lifts emulate activities performed in real living conditions, with a twist of ingenious modification to prevent injury and promote health. The closest example to Olympic lifting is that of a farmer working in the field. Lifting a heavy sac from the floor and throwing it on the top of a truck is emulated by the Olympic Snatch lift. Lifting a heavy sac from the floor and throwing it on the shoulder is emulated by the Olympic Clean lift.

4. Weightlifters strive to lift heavy weights in full range of motion and some have lifted triple their bodyweight in the Clean and Jerk lift. Freestyle lifting utilizes weights of barbells and dumbbells to further enhance the inertial energy of Plyometrics and gain the advantage of increasing physical power beyond conventional standards, in shorter training times. The advantages of this method of training are that it emulates normal human activities and reveals the unlimited potential of humans to develop physical power

5. Machine aided training utilizes different machine designs to strengthen particular parts of the. The advantage of this training is the hope it offers to many people to overcome individual deficits and strengthening and balancing weak and neglected muscle groups and joints. In the hands of mathematically and anatomically minded athlete, this method offers enormous potential of enhancing human power.

6. The extremely heavy weights that excite the young and healthy athlete are not great achievements, as it apparently seems to be. Heavy lifting in partial range of motion predisposes to pathological changes. Heavy lifting is a function carried out by voluntary muscles. The injured structures such as cartilages, bones, and ligaments are not voluntary and are coerced to support beyond their limit to irreversible damage. Young athletes are ardent sport overzealous individuals with less appreciation of future consequences of living with injuries.

7. Descending occurs by eccentric contraction (negative contraction) and must proceed slower than ascending. That is because, during descent, both the weights of the barbell and body, and their acceleration, are directed downwards, against muscular resistance. Free fall, or fast descending, is prohibited as they may tear tendons and avulse their attachments to bones. The most serious injury incurred during Squat occurs when acute disabling pain ensues while under the weight. If you move between seated and machine exercises directly to Squat exercises, without warming up the back for flexibility and strength, you may be heading for troubles. Acutely spastic spinal muscle can incapacitates you entirely and undermines you ability to bail out a dangerously heavy lift.

8. Fast ascending is tolerated since it occurs under the control of muscular contraction, with upward acceleration and downward weight pulls. Fast ascending, even with high jump, is practiced by advanced Weightlifters. Since descending activates stretch reflexes it, therefore, greatly increases ascending force.

POWERLIFTING

9. As long as the lifter learn the trick of maintained non-fluttered tight back erectors he or she will not have difficulty ascending and descending, until the thighs fatigue. Shaky back erectors distract the mind from performing any movement with the weight and give the sense of complete apprehension towards squatting. It is very dangerous to attempt squatting with shaky back erectors, as in situation of returning to exercises after long interruption, convalescence from illness, fever, lack of warm-up, distraction in the environment, or overtraining.

10. Resorting to drugs to enhance performance is a distraction from the main purpose of sport. Sport serves the purpose of educating the mind with realistic insights about complex human transactions. Insights such as the need for strength and wellness to perform mental function. This need makes the association between the body and the mind clearer than ever. Insights such as the consequence of picking proper food, and consuming proper amounts of it, on the wellness of the person. This could better be appreciated by testing physical fitness in sport. Insights such as comprehending the role of science in human activities put the person in unison with his environment.

11. Overhead exercises such as Shoulder Press, jerk, and snatch force the scapulas to move away from the chest cage and rotate around the lateral ends of the collarbones. In this position, the forces transmitted from the arms through the scapulas will affect the middle back region and enhance the muscles that counteract kyphosis (hunch back).

12. Most trainer act as cheerleaders promoting popular exercises such as Biceps curls, Bench Press, etc. They disregard whole body exercises such as the Clean and Snatch. People do not have to compete in Olympics to perform whole body exercise that produce benefits in short time.

13. It is important to keep in mind that top athletes in any sport should not be the ultimate model to follow since sports are evolving it is wiser to think rationally and prevent injuries due to passionate bias towards favored icons. Also training without knee wraps does strengthen the body's own connective tissue since wraps only serve the purpose of supporting weaker spots in the body design of ligament and tendons. Wraps are not facts of life but rather helpful aids for the old and injured athletes.

Chapter 6 Bodybuilding

6.1. ESSENCE OF BODYBUILDING

6.1.1. NEW SPORT
o The last half-century has witnessed proliferation of resistance training in building strong muscular physique. Bodybuilding has emerged as **an new sport,** in its own rights, due to the long hours required to build up strong muscles and the interference of the building process with other activities.

o The elements of fatigue, loss of flexibility, and protracted soreness, due to acute and prolonged resistance training, preclude Bodybuilders from performing parallel sports like activities. That requires full range of motion, speed, and coordination.

o The rise of the new sport of Bodybuilding is attributed, mostly, to its **accessibility to all people**. Anybody can start, from somewhere along the path of Bodybuilding, and labor to accomplish his or her perceived goals, without the coercion of a coach, team, or any higher authority.

o Such easy accessibility is not without drawbacks. Almost all those involved in Bodybuilding have limited understanding of the long-term consequences of building large muscles that hinders mobility. Many Bodybuilders incur chronic deformities because of the dominance of mainstream trends of **large and strong** physique, rather than fit and healthy individual. The constant discouragement of performing aerobic, running, and global exercises, other than isolated training, costs many Bodybuilders their fitness and graceful outlook.

o The new sport has also alerted its followers to the value of **good nutrition**. Almost, everybody, practices Bodybuilding for few months, and interacts with other fellows, will learn something new about nutrition. The concept of estimating caloric contents of food intake became popular, thanks to Bodybuilding advertisement.

o The new sport arrived, right on time, with the global proliferation of urbanization and industrialization. Modern lifestyle has resulted in the wide prevalence of modern day diseases of overweight, cardiovascular diseases, high blood pressure, diabetes, cancer, and psychological disorders. Public health clubs of Bodybuilding promote self-esteem of young people as well as older adults who have slipped away from healthy living style. Many young people use gyms as gathering places of nurturing and learning other **social interactions,** by way of Bodybuilding.

6.1.2. NEW TOOLS OF FITNESS
o The positive gains from such devoted process of body enhancing and its predicted outcome, over few months and years, renders Bodybuilding a great tool of shaping the future of many athletes. Bodybuilding premises a concrete approach of enhancing physique for those lacking **physical strength**. The key for benefiting from such great tool is patience and determination, not genetics or myth.

o The critique on the lack of **transferability of skills,** from Bodybuilding exercises to real sport skills, should not undermine the benefit gained by empowering skilled athletes with strong muscles. Those are not mere addition, of inert musculature, but rather enhancement of body hormonal system, metabolism, morale, and sense of accomplishment. Most importantly, individuals can build up strong physique during certain period and then work on sports enhancement in a different period. The limitation of building massive musculature has to be weighed against the gain of enhancing balanced musculoskeletal system.

o The critique, on the **lack of cohesiveness** of training isolated muscles and on the undesired outcome of bulking masses of muscles of improper proportions that disfigure motor skill, could be easily rebutted by introducing slight modification in Bodybuilding routines. Many Bodybuilders are getting into the habit of running, as a way to reduce fat. Encouragement of aerobics and running for mobility gain can make the difference in acquiring cohesiveness. This is another way of enhancing coordination. Bodybuilders dread aerobics because of the fear of overtraining.

o Training isolated parts of the body, in separate sessions with heavy load volume or intensity, achieves large and strong muscles. Great stimulation of long-neglected muscles takes place during exercising individual muscles. That is because the entire cardiac output is diverted towards working out such isolated muscles. That enables the athlete to enhance his or her weak spots. However, isolated training also seriously undermines the ability of muscles to perform synchronized motions. Synchrony requires proper recruitment when multiple joints are engaged in concerted activity. **Isolated training** suppresses the responsiveness of the nervous system, during complex activities.

- Bodybuilders resort to either **shape or size** of muscles or the **maximal strength** of muscle groups as a guide to training. Both guiding criteria are not perfect in planning proper strength training. Though the size and shape of muscles may relate to strength and performance, they do not predict actual deficits, unless more realistic index of performance is used. In addition, maximal strength of individual muscle groups overlooks the relative importance of muscle groups in, relation to performance.
    i. As an example, a Bodybuilder with large and strong arms and shoulder may fail to properly contract the back stabilizers of the scapulas, while lifting heavy dumbbells, resulting in pinching the long thoracic nerve and paralyzing the Serratus anterior muscle. This injury manifests as **winging of scapula**. Habitual lifting from the floor would have prevented this injury by developing roomy musculoskeletal structures.
    ii. Another example is that the ratio of strength of Biceps muscle to that of the Triceps has little to do with performance since each muscle performs **different leverage action**. The Triceps pulls on a lever where the pivot center lies between the pulling force and the resistance. The Biceps pulls on a lever where the pivot center is on one side of the muscle and the resistance is on the other side of the pulling force. Thus, the Triceps can perform vigorous and fast pull for longer travel than the Biceps, even though their shape and size may indicate proper ratios. In addition, the extension reflex that regulates Triceps action differs from the flexor reflex of the Biceps.
    iii. In addition, the forearm flexors differ from the extensors in their **configuration of performance**. The forearm flexors work synergistically with finger flexors during griping the bar. The forearm extensors contract against two forces: the weight of the barbell and the clinching forces of the flexors. The forearm flexors might not give away, on time, to allow the extensors to bring the wrist to extended position. Many Bodybuilders injure their wrist during lifting due to the imbalance between the forearm flexors and extensors. That is unrelated to shape or to maximal strength of the forearm. Regular lifting from the floor conditions the forearm extensors for heavy physical work.

- Most critiques are rightfully directed towards **deficient axial strengthening** in Bodybuilding. The "mirror obsession" distracts Bodybuilders from seeing what is needed to be balanced while enforces the impressive progress in front-view appearance. The side-view and the back view are insufficiently emphasized by mirror viewing.
    i. The **dynamic view** of performance is very hard to appreciate without elaborate understanding of mechanics. All novice Weightlifters do not understand gravitational forces when objects are set in motion. Generated torques, momenta, and elimination of unnecessary components of forces are completely alien to novice lifters. All novice lifters tend to move weights at a distance from their bodies. They bend their elbows prior to stabilizing the shoulder plates and shrugging the shoulders.
    ii. The dynamic view could be easily enhanced by slight modification in Bodybuilding routine by enforcing the value of dynamic exercises of multiple joints. This can be accomplished with low intensity lifting. A Bodybuilder that could bench press twice his bodyweight should try to perform complex exercises. Multi-joint exercises such as Power Snatch, Power Clean, Jump Squat, or Overhead Squat can help discover weak dynamic links in his or her buildup.

6.1.3. NEW TRENDS

- Bodybuilders have utilized the common experience of their times, that **resistance training develops muscles** when practiced regularly and beyond normal limits. Those limits were rationalized as normal in relation to one's current condition of fitness, rather than to one's potential to enhance strength. It was observed that long and regular resistance training increases tolerance to heavy physical labor[1].
- While Weightlifters were busy, setting rules of fairness in judging strength of athletes based on bodyweight and strict rules of lifting, Bodybuilders were busy modifying the regimen of preparation for contests. By doing away with technical limitations and bodyweight restraints, Bodybuilders maintained the volume of training load, by **increasing repetitions and reducing intensity**. Thus, in Bodybuilding, the same volume of physical work was maintained, or even exceeded, by utilizing the biological ability of the human body to perform better, at slower rate.
- Repeating resistance strokes, over three times per set, was proven effective in enlarging muscle mass and strength. The critique on poor efficiency of recruitment, by repetitive low intensity resistance training, points to the reduced strength of sizable muscles due to lack of nervous control adaptation. Such adaptation is easily acquired if no long-term deformities have been developed. Many Bodybuilders were able to acquire new skills and excel beyond normal

---

[1] Brief exercise training may alter the gene expression for the enzyme nitric oxide synthase of vascular endothelium, which forms nitric oxide gas and may be part of the vascular adaptation seen after training. Exercise causes shear stress by the frictional force of blood flowing through arteries. Nitric oxide may contribute to spectacular exercise performance. Source: Medical Science, Sports Exercise 1995 Aug; 27(8): 1125-34. Also, produced nitric oxide is a short-lived gas that penetrates membrane and regulates the function of other cells. Source: The Nobel Prize in Physiology or Medicine 1998.

average when their training encompassed flexibility and endurance routines. In addition, acquiring new explosive movements requires enhancing fast twitching muscles. Those are controlled by different motoneurons and neural reflexes and are developed by ballistic activities.
o   Though doing away with technical barriers and Weightlifting restraints had led to new discoveries of manipulating human body, it created serious structural problems of neglecting **axial framework of strengthening**. All Bodybuilders suffer, during complex dynamic motion from supporting the huge muscles they labored to develop, without properly enhanced linking muscles.

6.2. JUDGING CRITERIA

As Bodybuilding is evolving, new criteria are also evolving for judging muscular development. Current judging criteria put more emphasis on muscular shape than on performance. Muscular performance is to less extent accounted for, during demonstration of body motion during contest posing. Voluntarily contraction of muscles during posing does not account for strength against resistance. Resisting external forces is completely different from resisting imaginary forces, since muscular recruitment is not under the direct control of the voluntary mind.

6.2.1. MUSCLE MASS
o   Strong muscles must develop sizable mass compared to weak muscles. Yet, strength has also neural component, beside the size of the muscle.
o   In addition, general strength is based on optimum proportion of the strength of working muscles of specific activities. Thus, Wrestlers, Weightlifters, and Powerlifters present significantly different configuration of muscular strength.
o   Bodybuilders develop muscular mass that performs no specific skill, other than local resisting motions of isolated muscles.
o   Enhancing muscular mass is a fundamental goal in Bodybuilding. Mass is then complemented with other qualities in order to accomplish functional musculoskeletal system.
o   In today's urban and industrial society, the general population has adapted to inactivity with loss of muscle mass and deposition of more fat than those of earlier generation. Proper exercise and sound eating habits cannot reverse the modern trends of inactivity without careful accounting for energy expenditure and food intake. Many hours of weekly and daily activities are required to stop the decline in wasting of human body and deforming of musculoskeletal system.
o   Focusing on muscular mass without planning long term, healthy lifestyle, defeats the purpose of the new sport of Bodybuilding. Those who start Bodybuilding training today should plan for life long participation in sport, since alternative lifestyles outside the gym environment is mostly sedentary in nature. To achieve this goal diverse and cross training should complement bulking muscles. In addition, gaining excess bodyweight during training years might be very difficult to reverse after quitting workout. In addition, it is desirable to work out all life long. The majority of athletes give up training all together as early as their thirties and forties.

6.2.2. MUSCULAR DEFINITION
o   Muscular definition refers to the appearance of striations and sharp contours of anatomical boundaries of muscles. It is maximal in skinny people and those with very low subcutaneous fat.
o   Muscular definition demonstrates the skill of the Bodybuilder in training as well as nutritional discretion. It exposes anatomical knowledge of trainees in picking exercises and their physiological knowledge of mastering the proportions of protein, fat, carbohydrates, and water in their body.
o   Of course, good definition without adequate muscular mass does little to promote Bodybuilding.
o   Muscular definition is a reliable gauge of long-term adherence to disciplinary regimen. As long as energy expenditure outpaces energy intake, muscular definition holds fast.

6.2.3. MUSCULAR PROPORTION
o   This is the most debated issue in Bodybuilding. All Bodybuilders agree on the ambiguity and arbitrariness in judging good from bad proportion.
o   Visual assessment of proportion is very subjective. There are no standardized rules for resolving disputed judgments.
o   A Bodybuilder that worked very hard to develop extraordinary muscular mass and definition may be defaulted for improper proportion of some part of the body or another. Thus, the hard work is not always rewarded with higher recognition.
o   Even if advances in measurement of muscular size and proportion are made, the best muscular proportion might never amount to greater muscular performance in other sports. That is because muscles work with internal processes, mostly, unrelated to external proportions. Your right shoulder, for example, might have the same proportion as your left shoulder, yet the right shoulder, in many right-handed people, performs more effectively than the left shoulder.

6.2.4. BODY SHAPE
- Although muscular proportion accounts for proper relative measurements of muscles, it does not amount for overall shape.
- Hunchback, bowlegs, scoliosis, and other abnormal curvatures distort the shape of a Bodybuilder despite proper proportions.
- Balanced anatomical training adds endless shapes to muscles, other than proportion and definitions. Esthetics is another subjective criterion of judging Bodybuilding. Esthetics is relative to various cultural norms.
- The ratios between shoulders, breasts, waist, and hips constitute fundamental characteristics of judging physical body shape and psychological perception of what is attractive and what is not.
- Variations in body shape are dictated by differences in the size, shape, and proportion of muscle, fat, and bone. The distribution of body fat portrays complex images of the lifestyle of a person, from inactivity, sexuality, eating and elimination, personal hygiene, sleeping pattern, and participation in social interaction. Judging beauty based on fat distribution over the body is like reading a book about the personal activities of the individual. A greater than normal fat content can increase the likelihood one's body shape will vary from the norm.
- Muscular impressions of a body also portray complex images about the activity, robust mobility, intelligence in mastering his or her destiny, through controlling body composition, and social participation in constructive activities.

6.2.5. POSING PERFORMANCE
- The effort of a Bodybuilder to display his or her skillful art of enhancing physical health is demonstrated by visual presentation, on stage.
- Bodybuilders demonstrate various posing performances to display muscular assets and ability to execute impressive movements that show harmonious musculoskeletal performance.
- The conditions of the skin are major factors in demonstrating healthy physique. The skin color, grooming, consistency, and tone convey much information on the health, habits, and personality of the Bodybuilder.
- Other personality attributes also affect judging in Bodybuilding contest. Facial expressions and poise reveal convincing information about the athletic attributes of the trainee.

6.3. BODYBUILDING DIET

Where the sport of Bodybuilding is practiced there is, usually, little or no difficulty in obtaining the proper ingredients of healthy diet. Those who can afford the luxury of enhancing their physique, building clubs and gyms, and manufacturing machines for training should be least to worry about proper dieting. The essence of healthy nutrition is frequent meals, of proper mix of nutrients, and of minimal amounts sufficient to maintain proper energy balance. Exotic supplements and drugs only add flavor to the ambience of social belonging without any significant contribution to enhancing health and fitness.

6.3.1. BODY FAT CONTENT
- The relative absence of subcutaneous fat can enhance the appearance of muscular development by revealing the size, shape, and striations of the underlying muscles. It is no secret, that Bodybuilders work on fat reduction, only short time before competition. This episodic, strict dietary regimen makes it difficult to maintain long-lived and stable bodyweight and body composition.
- The body fat in competitive Bodybuilders, during the off-season, ranges from 9% to 16% and drops as low as 5% on the competition day. This is measured by hydrostatic weighing. Cutting down fat content is planned during the last three months prior to contest. Fat reduction is achieved by frequent weighing in order to assess progress and adjust diet, dietary restraints, and aerobic activity (in the form of cycling, running, and walking two to five hours daily).
- Dietary fat is reduced if progress in cutting body fat content is not adequate, two to three months prior to contest.
- If, after cutting down dietary fat, body fat content remains high then a reduction in total caloric intake is warranted, one to two months prior to contest.
- Eliminating low caloric roughage, eating six to eight smaller meals daily, and eliminating foods known to produce intestinal gases reduce intestinal volume.
- Extracellular and subcutaneous fluids are reduced by reducing sodium intake and increasing bland water intake.

6.3.2. DIETARY HABITS
- Most competitors progressively restricted their diets two to four months before competition.
- Beginning two to three days before the competition, fluid restriction and dehydration practices are common among athletes with weight problems.
    i. Competitive Bodybuilders consume between 2000 to 4000 kcal per day, with an average of less than 30 kcal/kg bodyweight/day (one kilo calorie is equivalent to a Calorie, the latter is used for food content of calories).
    ii. Daily protein intake varies from 150 to 250 grams constituting about 30% of daily caloric intake.
    iii. Daily carbohydrate intake ranges from 200 to 400 grams constituting about 50% of daily caloric intake.
    iv. Daily fat intake varies from 20 to 60 grams constituting about 20% of daily caloric intake.

o   Three to four weeks prior to contest, Bodybuilders may lower caloric intake by 10% in order to induce fat reduction without undermining strength. This may amount to a loss of few pounds of lean bodyweight, and double that of fat.
o   The most popular source of protein is white chicken meat, lean fish, egg whites, and canned tuna packed in water.
o   All basic nutrients meet or exceed the RDA (recommended daily allowance), except calcium (75%) and zinc (71%). In addition, nutrition supplements are used by, nearly, all Bodybuilding competitors.
o   The high intake of carbohydrate stimulates Insulin secretion by the pancreas. Insulin is a hormone that activates specific receptors on the cellular membranes of fat, muscle, and liver cells. Insulin facilitates and increases the transport of glucose to muscle and liver cells. It can also increase Lipoprotein Lipase action and thus enhances the synthesis and storage of triglycerides in fat cells. Cutting down on carbohydrate and fat intake enhances utilization of stored fat in energy production. This is done by lowering the secretion of Insulin and increasing that of Glucagon.
o   Exercise increases the muscle's sensitivity to Insulin, predominately, during the 4 to 6 hours after exercise. During this time, muscle glycogen synthesis has been shown to be greater with ingestion of simple, as compared with complex, carbohydrates. After six hours from exercise cessation, muscle glycogen can be re-synthesized near pre-exercise levels, within 24 hours, equivalently with either carbohydrate form. After 24 hours, muscle glycogen can increase very gradually, succeeding normal levels, over the next few days. The effect of exercise on metabolism might take place through the endocrine secretion of the hormones Adrenalin, Growth hormone, Testosterone, Cortisol, Glucagon, and Thyroxin.

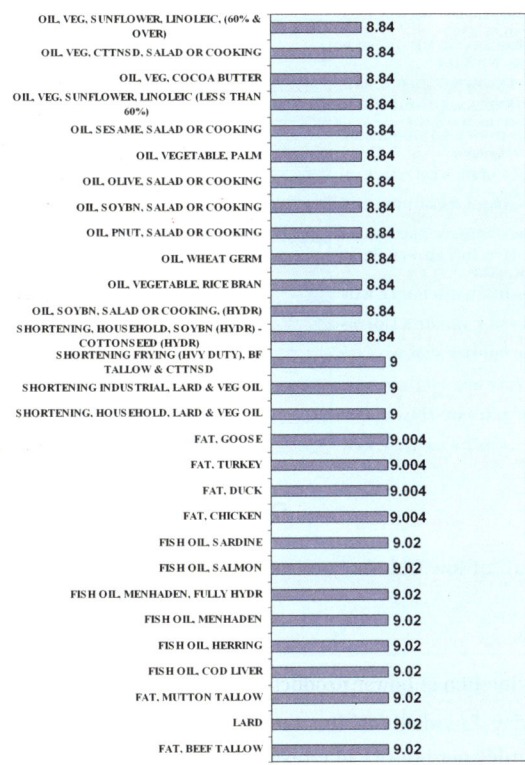

Figure 6.1. Foodstuff of high caloric contents over eight Calories/gram.[2]

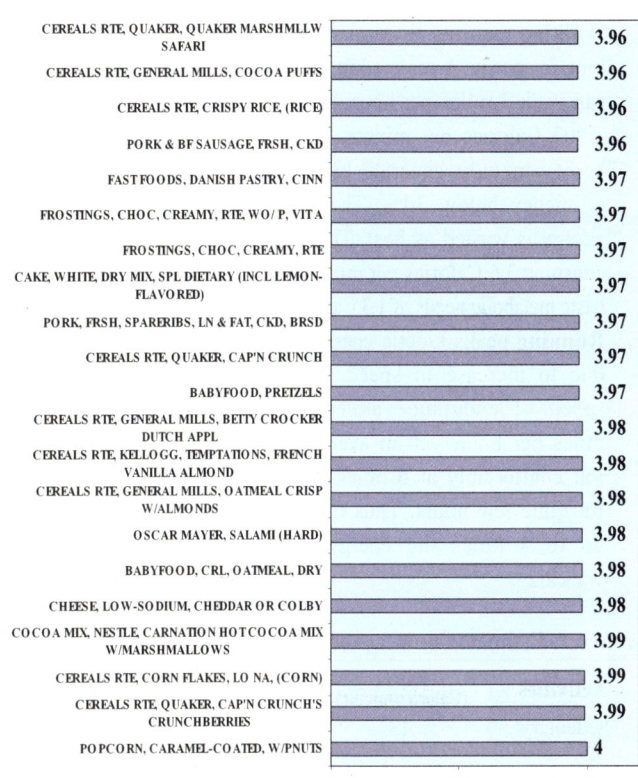

Figure 6.2. Foodstuff of medium caloric contents below four Calories/gram.[2]

o   The selection of food items is crucial to controlling caloric intake and limiting the exertion of fat reducing activities. *Figures 6.1* thru *6.3* show the caloric contents of common foodstuff. In addition, see Chapter Fourteen for Tables of Foot Contents
o   **Oils and animal fat** provide over **EIGHT** Calories per gram, *Figure 6.1*. Examples of high caloric content food items are: beef tallow fat, lard, fish oil, fat from chicken, duck, turkey, and vegetable oil.
o   **Diary products, cereal, lean meat, and cakes** provide medium caloric contents, below **FOUR** Calories per gram, *Figure 6.2*. Examples of such food items are: popcorn, cereals, cheddar cheese, pretzels, white cake, chocolate creamy frostings, and pork and beef sausage.
o   **Vegetables** provide less than **ONE** Calories per gram of intake, *Figure 6.3*. Examples of these low caloric contents food items are: lettuce, spinach, squash, cabbage, and cucumber.

---

[2] **Source:** http://www.nal.usda.gov/fnic/foodcomp/

6 BODYBUILDING

6.3.3. SHEDDING CALORIES BY PHYSICAL ACTIVITIES

Although caloric content of foodstuff is the principal criterion in assessing the effect of food intake on energy balance, yet there are other important aspects of different food items that affect health and fitness. Animal proteins, for example, cause more digestive problems than vegetables, because of the low fiber and the high nitrogen content of animal protein. In addition, fat disturbs the digestive system more than fruits and vegetables, because of poor emulsification and the low water content of fats. Therefore, the assumption that caloric contents of food determine the amount of activity needed to shed the calories of certain amount of food intake is purely hypothetical. A high protein or high fat diet will undoubtedly hinder performance and undermine your ability to shed the high calories from food intake. The hypothetical relationship, between intake of calories and the duration of physical work needed to burn these calories, can be roughly estimate as follows, *Table 6.1*.

o **Sedentary living** requires the basic metabolic needs to sustain biological function such as respiration, circulation, and metabolism. An adult male weighing 70 kg would require 1880 Calories per day for basic needs. Thus, minute rate of caloric need falls in the order of 1.3 Calories per minute.

o **Walking** requires physical work to produce kinetic energy. A male adult weighing 70 kg can walk 3 miles per hour, which consumes 0.902 Calories per minute. Yet, the human body can only generate kinetic energy at efficiency below 30%. The other 70% of energy is wasted as heat. Thus walking can consume 3.6 Calories per minute, in excess to basic metabolic needs of 1.3 Calories per minute.

o **Running** peaks kinetic energy consumption due to increase in speed. The maximum speed of endurance athletes reaches 13 miles per hour, yet an average person can run comfortably at 6 miles per hour speed for quite few hours. Thus running can burn up to 4 times the energy consumed in walking.

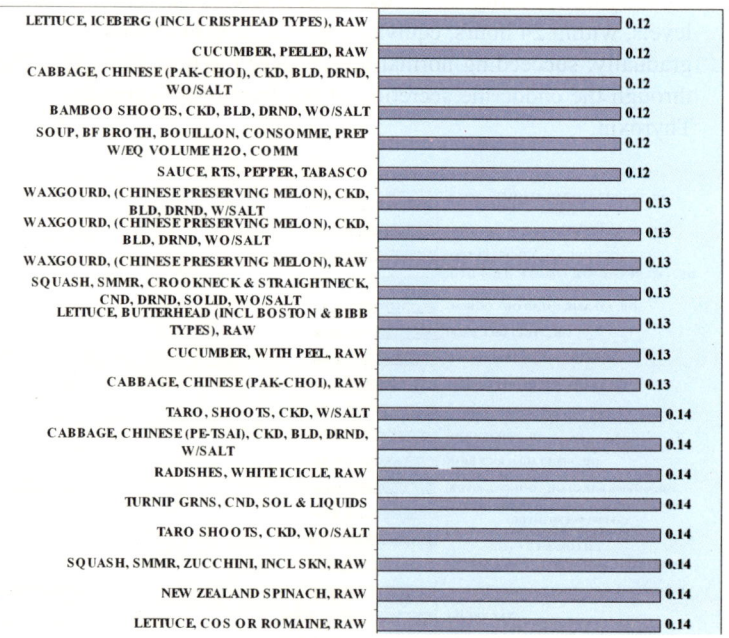

Figure 6.3. Foodstuff of low Caloric content, below 0.15 Calories/gram.

Table 6.1. Estimated power production for five sorts of physical activities.

Activities	Power (Calories/minute)	Empirical estimation of power production
Sedentary,	13	Basal metabolic rate = 1880 Calories/day. Divide by 24 hrs, then by 60 min.
Walking	~4.9	A person weighing 70 kg can walk 3 miles per hour (134 cm/sec). Multiply 1/2 the mass by the square of the speed, to get energy per second. Multiply by 60, for a minute rate. Divide by 4.1868 E+10 to get food Calories per minute. This yields 0.902 Calories. With efficiency of 25%, we get 3.6 Calories as kinetic energy/minute. Add to basic metabolic rate of 1.3 Cal/min to get 4.9 Cal/min.
Bicycling	~8	Assume that bicycling yields less than double the 3.6 Cal/min for walking and add the basal metabolic rate.
Swimming	~11	With heat loss and movements, a rate of 11 cal/min is suggested based on the following data. Water thermal conductivity at 20 °C is, k = 0.0014386 cal/sec.cm. °C (For reference see footnote[3]) Body surface area for an average person is, A= 12000 sq.cm. Difference between body and water temperature is, T-To = 17 °C. Proposed distance for temperature gradient = 1 cm. (entirely hypothetical) Heat flux in 1 minute (Cal) = kA(T-To)/(x-xo) 60= 17.61 Cal. (17608 cal).
Running	~20	The best marathon runner has speed less than 13 miles per hour. That is more than 16 times the power production from brisk walking. An average person can run at 6 miles per hour for quite few hours. That is 4 times power production in walking. Thus, 20 Calories/minute is suggested.

---

[3] "Heat Transfer", by J.P. Holman, second edition, McGraw-Hill, New York (1968).

- o **Cycling** utilizes the lower body more effectively and enhances anaerobic power production due to resistance workout. It is estimated to burn the average of the two activities, walking and running.
- o **Swimming** shed calories at lower rate than running since floatation reduces resistance. The main factor in shedding calories during swimming is the heat loss from the body to the water. Water conducts heat at much greater rate than air. For example, at 50°F the air has thermal conductivity of 0.0143 Btu/hr.ft. °F, whereas that for water is 0.388 Btu/hr.ft. °F. Thus, the water conducts heat at a rate 27 times that of air. In a swimming pool of 68 °F temperature, the difference between the body temperature and water temperature determines the rate of heat loss. The body can lower skin temperature to reduce hypothermia but within certain limits, say 86 °F (30 °C). In addition, water motion determines the gradient temperature at the skin. This is a great unknown in the estimation of heat loss during swimming. My assumption of 1 cm distance for temperature gradient is completely subjective. The last factor is the skin surface area that dissipates heat to the water. This is taken as 1.2 square meter for an adult male. An estimate of 11 Calories per minute of energy consumption is a mere guess.

6.3.4. ASSISTING MEDICATION
- o Many Bodybuilders believe that nutritional supplements are necessary for optimal progress. Many claims made for commercially marketed supplements for Bodybuilding are not supported by scientific research.
- o Probably, all Bodybuilders self-administer medications such as anabolic steroids, HCG, laxatives, and diuretic.
- o Bodybuilders and Weightlifters have used androgenic enhancers to increase muscular size and to remain competitive. Some athletes simultaneously use different anabolic steroids, commonly referred to as "stacking". That is adding the effects of combined medication. Anabolic stacking begins with a low dosage of particular compounds and then increases the dosage, until a peak intake is reached. After peaking, dosages and compounds are gradually reduced, or "tapered". A cycle usually lasts 6 to 16 weeks and may be repeated throughout the athlete's career.

6.3.5. BODYBUILDING MODEL
In order to reach top achievements, in Bodybuilding, trainees follow general rules, in training, dieting, and monitoring progress. These rules can be summarized as follows.
- o Planning to win contests is an impetus to training. Winning Bodybuilding competitions is a reward for serious planning and training.
- o Optimum weight of a Bodybuilder falls in the range 220 to 230 lbs. This is compared to 185 to 200 lbs for Weightlifters. Top Bodybuilders can lower their body fat to approximately 4%.
- o Weight training is performed approximately five days a week. Workouts usually begin an hour after the completion of a meal. Strength training is reduced, few days before the contest, in effort to restore muscle growth in size.
- o Meals were usually spaced approximately 2.5 to 3 hours apart. Eating less, more often, reduces abdominal circumference by shortening intestinal transit time and reducing intestinal volume. In addition, foods suspected of causing gas are eliminated. Foods containing salt are discontinued, two days before the contest, in effort to deplete subcutaneous water.
- o Tap water is replaced by distilled water two days before the contest to ensure reduced intake of unwanted minerals.
- o An adequate amount of dietary fat is needed, not only for digestive gains but also for essential nutrition. The proportions of fat, carbohydrates, and protein are subject to modification. That depends upon body composition and overtraining status.

6.4. ANABOLIC STEROIDS

6.4.1. COMMON DRUGS
Table 6.2 lists commonly, though illicitly, used anabolic steroids by many Bodybuilders.
The main therapeutic usage of these medications is intended for bone marrow activation in the treatment of aplastic anemia, cancer, and osteoporosis. They mainly work on the growing cells and enhance synthesis of protein.

Table 6.2. Anabolic androgenic steroids commonly, though illicitly, used by Bodybuilders.

Generic Name	Trade Name	Common usage
Oxymetholone	Anadrol 50	Treat aplastic anemic
Oxandrolone	Anavar	Treat osteoporosis
Nandrolone Decanoate	Deca-Durabolin	Treat anemia due to low Erythropoietin
Nandrolone Phenpropionate	Anabolin-I.M.	Antineoplastic
Ethylestrenol	Maxibolin	Treat refractory anemia and osteoporosis
Testosterone Propionate	Testex	Androgen replacement and cancer treatment
Testosterone Enanthate	Andryl	Androgen replacement and cancer treatment
Testosterone Cypionate	Depo-testosterone	Androgen replacement and cancer treatment
Stanozolol	Winstrol	Prophylactic to angioedema

6.4.2. PHYSIOLOGICAL EFFECTS
The long-term effects of illicit anabolic steroid usage depend mostly on the health condition of the individual. The type of drug, dose, frequency of use, age, and concurrent drug use, all play a role in modifying long-term effects. All effects might be fully reversible within several months after cessation. Yet, idiosyncrasy, due to drug reaction, might also bring unexpected results. These effects, mostly, impact the liver, serum lipids, reproductive system, psyche and behavior, glucose

---
[4] Source: http://www.fda.gov. Product: ANABOLIC STEROIDS.

metabolism, cerebrovascular accidents, prostatic changes, and immune function. From this wide range of side effects of anabolic steroids, one can see their ominous affliction on health, as follows.

- **Cardiovascular disturbances**
  i. Disturbance in **glucose metabolism** affects neural regulation of the cardiovascular system. Hyperinsulinism and decreased glucose tolerance develop because of alteration of cellular receptors to Insulin.
  ii. Disturbance in **fat metabolism** causes changes in lipoprotein fraction, through the effects of anabolic steroids on liver and fat cells. The increased breakdown of neutral fats causes increased blood level of triglycerides.
  iii. Disturbance in **liver synthesis** of clotting factors causes increased blood concentration of several clotting factors. These have serious effect on clogging of brain and coronary arteries.
  iv. Hypertensive and myocardial changes, caused by anabolic steroids, may be attributed to disturbances in fat and carbohydrate metabolism.
- **Liver disturbance**
  i. Disturbance of fat metabolism induces cholestasis in the liver bile ducts. This produces obstructive **jaundice**
  ii. Disturbance in liver functions, by anabolic steroids, affects the integrity of **blood capillaries**. This produces a condition of subdermal rupture of tiny blood vessels, known as Peliosis hepatis.
  iii. Disturbance in the protein and nucleic acid synthesis of liver cell produce **hepatocellular hyperplasia and adenomas**
- **Disturbance in reproductive system**
  i. Exogenous androgens, of anabolic steroids, suppress the pituitary production of gonadotrophic hormones. These are necessary for gonadal growth and synthesis of endogenous androgens. With prolonged use of anabolic steroids, gonads atrophy and their size and function diminish.
  ii. Disturbance in liver functions decreases sex hormone-binding globulin, which is responsible for transferring hormones from their glands, through circulation, and to remote targets.
  iii. Disturbance in secondary sexual characters due to decline in endogenous androgen. **Gynecomastia** is enlargement of male breast due, in part, to hormonal disturbances. **Deepening of voice** and **increased baldness** are other side effects of anabolic steroids.
- **Disturbance in female reproductive system**
  i. Exogenous androgens suppress the pituitary function and thus decreases FSH, TSH, and LH. These hormonal changes induce menstrual abnormalities, shrinkage of the breasts, deepening of the voice, increased libido, acne, body hair, clitoris size, and male pattern baldness.
  ii. Liver disturbances, due to anabolic steroids, decreased sex hormone-binding globulin and thyroid-binding proteins. These reduce total level of these hormones in the blood.
- **Anabolic effects**
  i. Anabolic steroids can increase strength and muscle mass when accompanied by adequate protein, calories, and strength training. Thus, both intake of food and exercise are important for benefiting from anabolic steroids. These gains are not long lasting. Few months in illicit use of external hormones suppress the endocrine system and require total dependence on external supplement of hormones. External dosage is very difficult to regulate to body needs. In addition, external hormones may trigger insensitivity of the body cells to the antigenic structure of external hormones.
  ii. The hypothesis that short use of anabolic steroids might not permanently afflict the endocrine feedback control is not substantiated.
  iii. Intense training stimulates cells to the convert chemical energy contained in food intake into useful biological molecules of high energy. This process of cellular energy production produces the many ingredients needed for amino acid synthesis. Anabolic steroids are hormones that affects cellular uptake of glucose, fat degradation, and fuel consumption. With exercise and food intake, protein synthesis proceeds at greater rate with anabolic steroids.
  iv. Human body can synthesize nonessential amino acids from the carbon atoms of carbohydrates and fats, combined with the nitrogen obtained from metabolized aminoacids. Thus, there is no need for excess protein intake to build muscle mass.
  v. Anabolic steroids may play a physiological role in the regulation of fatty acid oxidation in liver and fast twitch muscle mitochondria, even in the absence of intense physical training.
  vi. Anabolic steroids depress endogenous secretion of testosterone, since external testosterone elevates serum testosterone level throughout usage. Serum testosterone abruptly decreases below normal levels after cessation of usage of anabolic steroids. The recovery of endocrine system from external suppression depends on the duration of usage and the health of the person.

6.4.3. PSYCHOLOGICAL EFFECTS

Though anabolic steroids are not classified as psychoactive compounds, these have very strong influence on sexual desire and aggressive behavior. Patients treated with therapeutic routines of testosterone attest to the strong effect of medication in stimulating thinking and mood aspects of the brain activity. The fact that a human embryo differentiates into a male fetus under the effect of intrauterine testosterone secretion also proves the role of this hormone on growing stem cells. The effects of this medication on normal people, that have normal endocrine balance, are uncertain. Reports of mood changes, aggressive behavior, and altered somatic perceptions with medication are among those uncertain side effects, as follows.

- o Behavioral changes due to anabolic steroid use present in violent acts and psychotic episodes of manic behavior.
- o Thought changes present in the form of bizarre ideas and unreal perception similar to brief schizophrenic episodes.
- o Mood changes occur in the form of labile feelings and expressions.
- o Disturbance is transient and may relate to special drugs and individual health condition.

6.4.4. PROBLEMS WITH ILLICIT DRUG USE

- o The lack of regulatory authority on illicit drugs contributes to the lack of standards of the contents, dosage, and length of usage of uncertain chemical substances. Thus, illicit drug users are under the mercy of unscrupulous drug manufacturers.
- o The conservative views of sports authorities support the rationale that practicing sports should not be a mean of aggressive and ignorant self-destruction. Since we know little about the long-term effects of many essential drugs, we have very limited resources to perform accurate and protracted research on recreational and nonessential drugs.
- o Athletes, on the other hand, have entertained the short-term gains of strength and mass due to anabolic steroids but they lack any resources to document pre- and post-effects of illicit medication. This is compounded by natural denial of side effects that might develop insidiously. Testosterone, in particular, affects thought process and lights many areas in the brain that deal with sexual desire and aggression. It is thus no surprise that one can use illicit drugs and misperceive their ill effects.
- o In addition, due to the effect of androgens on the hypothalamus and the impairment of feedback through hypothalamus-pituitary-endocrine gland axis, one should not doubt the ominous effect of anabolic steroids on the personality and the immune status of the individual. The other ominous effects of anabolic androgens on cellular metabolism of aminoacids raise more suspicion on their role on carcinogenesis and antibody synthesis. Both processes require activation of specific genes in the translation and transcription phases of amino acid synthesis.

6.5. BACK EXERCISES

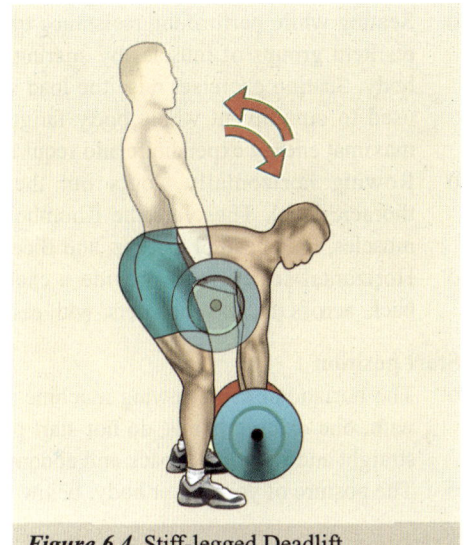

Figure 6.4. Stiff-legged Deadlift

Bodybuilding exercises emphasize anatomical regions of the body. Slow motion exercises work out the slow twitching muscle fibers. These exercises are the principal tool of enhancing strength for non-athletes, as well as athletes. Most exercises are performed in sets of four or more. Each set is performed up to ten times, without a break, other than transient change in speed or a pause.

6.5.1. STIFF-LEGGED DEADLIFT

Lifting weight from the floor to midthigh level with straight knees is called "stiff-legged Deadlift". The Deadlift portion is attributed to the incomplete lift, short of the shoulder level.

Purpose
- o The main **Purpose** of stiff-legged Deadlift is strengthening the **Hamstrings** by isotonic contraction, by shortening the muscle fibers while resisting force, in addition to strengthening the scapular and back muscles by isometric contraction. Thus, stiff-legged Deadlift enhances pelvic extension and upper body stability.
- o Stiff-legged Deadlift differs from standard Deadlift in that the latter requires bending knees. This reduces the tension on the Hamstrings and shifts the burden to the glutei and lower back.
- o The lower back functions as a transfer lever. It contracts isometrically through the entire duration of the exercise.
- o Although there are many exercises for Hamstrings strengthening, such as Goodmorning, yet stiff-legged Deadlift engages shoulder and pelvic muscles in one exercise, thus increases effectiveness.

Start position
- o The height of the plates on the barbell determines the range of motion of the Hamstrings. Standard plates weigh 45 lb (20 kg), with 22.5 cm radius, and allow 90 degree bending, at the hip. Using smaller plates (10 and 15 kg) helps bending further when lowering the barbell to the ground.
- o Standing on an elevated platform with both feet, while the barbell's plates are standing on lower ground, allow excessive bending.
- o Before pulling any weights from the floor, you should approach the barbell as you do with the Clean lift. Stand with feet placed at shoulder width apart, handgrips slightly wider than shoulder width. Your feet have to advance under the barbell in the first lift. This reduces forward torque by approximating the centers of gravity to vertical plane, *Figure 6.4.*

Execution
- o The first floor lift may require bending knees and hips, as if you are Deadlifting to full upright position. Initiating stiff-legged Deadlift in the first trial requires confident, experienced, and fully warmed up lifter. This simply means that

stiff-legged Deadlift is not for beginners and not for those returning from long intermission of physical training. It requires highly toned back muscles.
- From the beginning to the end of this exercise, your lower back has to be kept concave (arched in), not just straight.
- Keep your arms straight and hardened, at the elbows. This is a risky and dangerous exercise because the lower back has to resist a torque with a lever width of the torso's length and a force of the sum of the barbell weight plus the upper bodyweight. Though this torque is not extreme, it performs under the mercy of fully stretched Hamstrings, by way of stiff-legged posture.
- With fully thrust chest, stable scapulas, and raised shoulders, bend the hips, as in Goodmorning, in order to lower the barbell until the plates are just an inch or so above the ground. Slight bending of knees safeguards against rupturing the Hamstrings.
- Do not round the lower back at any stage, even if you enjoy the stretching action of bent lower back. It is much better and safer to force the hips to bend, rather than rounding the lower back. As time passes, the hips will gain more range of motion as well as the lower back.
- You should not excuse your self by lifting heavier weights with rounded back. Proper technique with straight back will lead to progressive improvement, while poor technique predisposes to injury.
- Stiff-legged Deadlift could be executed in repetition from three to ten per set but never until fatigue. Fatigue while performing risky exercises should be seriously discouraged.

6.5.2. HORIZONTAL SEATED ROW

Horizontal pulling of a loaded cable, while seated, is called "Horizontal seated row". Rowing describes the action of moving the arms back and forth, while maintaining slow and steady body motion.

Purpose
- Seating while performing resistance training is intended to enhance resilient groups of muscles by sparing the work done by the lower body. Seating exercises raise the load volume of training. These are used to circumvent whole body fatigue, when the trainee reaches maximal energy expenditure and requires a break in load.
- Rowing horizontally works out the scapulae retractors at the thoracic level. These are the Rhomboids, middle Trapezius, Teres muscles, long head of Triceps, and Biceps.
- Horizontal seated rows provide a chance to sculpture great upper back, across the two shoulders, with easy and convenient exercise.

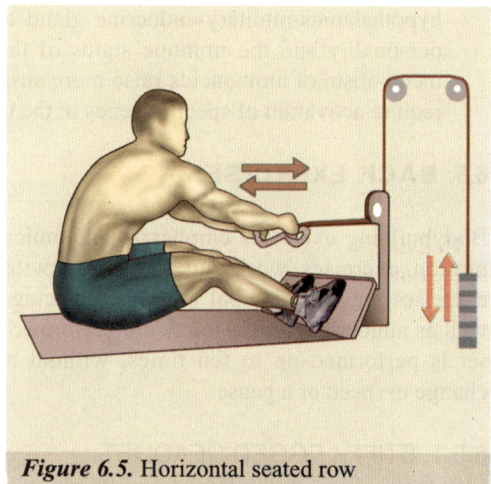

Figure 6.5. Horizontal seated row

Start position
- The horizontal cable rowing machine provides a seat, cable handle, and feet support. After holding the cable handle with, one or both hands, do not start pulling unless your lower body is well supported at the feet and hips. Maintain straight and tight lower back and abdomen and slightly bent knees, *Figure 6.5.*
- The posture of your lower body, below the shoulder, will determine which muscle groups will work out hard.

Execution
- Before initiating the pull, ensure that your chest cage is thrust forwards and upwards. That indicates that your vertebras are correctly aligned. Maintain chest thrust throughout pulling.
- Pulling may end at waist level, upper abdomen level, or breast level. Each level corresponds to different muscle groups. I prefer the upper levels of pulling in order to eliminate the action of Latissimus dorsi. These can be worked out by many other exercises.
- If you bounce your back backwards and forwards, you also work out the back erectors. This shifts the pulling burden to multiple muscle groups.
- This exercise can be performed in sets from three to eight, with repetitions from three to ten per set, and with progressive weight increase.

6.5.3. BENT-OVER ROW

Standing on a hard surface and bending the upper body to horizontal level, while pulling weight upwards by both hands, is called "Bent-over rows", *Figure 6.6.* It differs from stiff-legged Deadlift in that, in the bent-over row, the torso remains horizontal while the arms moves upwards and downwards, with weights. It differs from horizontal cable rows in its great demands to balance the body and weight on only two feet, rather than sitting.

Purpose
- Strengthening the retractors of the scapulas in addition working out the lower back and Hamstrings with isometric contraction.
- Rising, while rowing upwards, alters the contraction of the lower body to concentric contraction.

- o Bending torso to above horizontal level strengthens the upper fibers of Trapezius and the back fibers of Deltoid.
- o Bending torso to horizontal level strengthens middle fibers of Trapezius plus Teres major and minor.
- o Rowing to lower abdomen, from the floor, strengthens the Latissimus dorsi.

Start position
- o Bend knees slightly and bend over bar with hardened and arched in lower back. Arching of lower back in is judged by upward thrust chest and sucked in belly.
- o Hold the bar with overhand grip with width that varies according to your goal of targeting specific fibers. Wide handgrips shorten travel and feel easier due to pre-stretch reflex. Narrow handgrips increase travel and enhance range of motion.

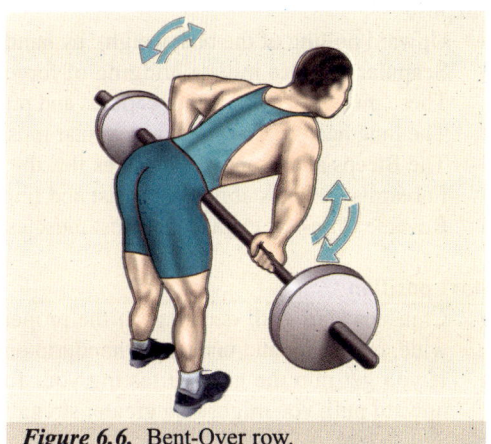

Figure 6.6. Bent-Over row.

Execution
- o With securely stable feet stance and hard and alert lower back, slowly pull the bar upwards without yanking.
- o Depending on your goals, the bar may be pulled towards waist, chest, or shoulder. Of course, the best technique would be pulling upwards to the chest since the other two options are often enhanced in other exercises, such as shoulder shrugging and chin-ups.
- o Performing Bend-over and row with inclined torso, on regular basis, accomplishes very little in enhancing back muscles. You have to diversify the angle of bending of torso, the width of handgrip, and the direction of rowing.
- o Strength of scapular retractors is gained by few repetitions of progressively increasing weight, for four to sex sets. Muscular definition and bulking are achieved by repetitions over five times per set.
- o The exercise comprises of upwards pulling and lowering the barbell by both hands, without too much back bouncing. This two-way stroke is a single repetition. A set consists of three to ten repetitions.

6.5.4. LEVER BENT-OVER ROW
Upward pulling on one end of a loaded lever that is anchored to the floor at the other end is called "Lever bent-over row". The anchorage of the lever adds a horizontal component to the vertical resistance that forces the entire body to perform constant backward pulling, in addition to rowing, *Figure 6.7*.

Purpose
- o Has the same purpose of freestyle Bend-over row.
- o Resisting against lever supported at one end works the lower scapular muscles harder.

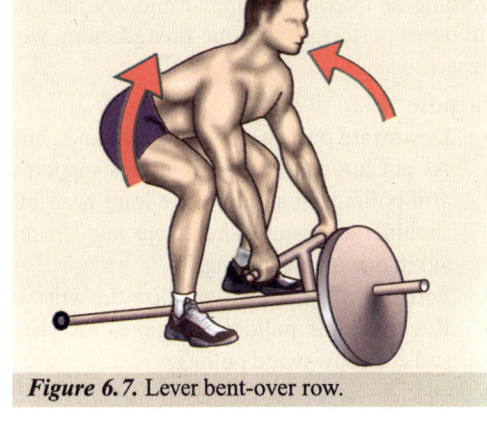

Start position
- o Bend knees slightly and bend over bar (fixed at one end at a corner) or lever handle with hardened and arched in lower back.

Figure 6.7. Lever bent-over row.

- o Hold the bar with overhand grip with width that varies according to your goal of targeting specific fibers.
- o Holding a bar in the middle increases the range of motion to its maximum.

Execution
- o With securely stable feet stance and hard and alert lower back, slowly pull bar upwards without yanking.
- o Depending on your goals, the bar may be pulled towards waist, chest, or shoulder. Choosing to pull on the central bar gives you more mobility and strength than a bar with "T" cross handle.

6.5.5. CHIN-UPS
Holding an overhead object, by both hands, and pulling your bodyweight upwards is called "Chin-ups". The Chin-up feature describes elevating your chins to high level during pulling your body upwards. This exercise is the mainstay of strengthening shoulder extension and elbow flexion, *Figures 6.8* and *6.9*.

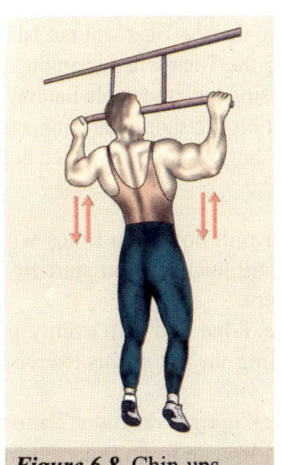 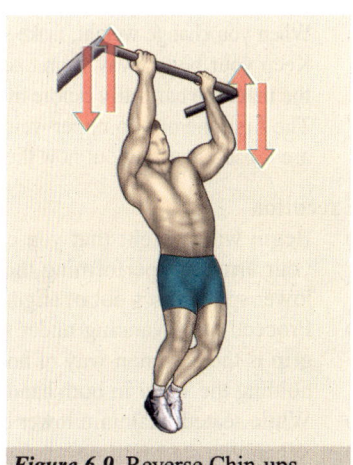

Figure 6.8. Chin-ups.   *Figure 6.9.* Reverse Chin-ups.

BODYBUILDING

Purpose
o Upward pulling of the bodyweight, by hands, strengthens the upper body.
o Scapular muscles initiate bridging of forces on the chest cage in order to avoid caving in on the vital chest structures. These muscles stabilize the scapulas and pull the upper arms to extend the shoulders.
o The long head of Triceps aids scapular muscles in shoulder extension.
o The Biceps and Brachialis muscles flex the elbows and aid in upward pulling.
o Forearms flexors stabilize the wrist and fingers during elbow flexion.
o Reverse Chin-ups engage the chest muscles in shoulder extension and ease upward pulling.

Start position
o Chin-ups start with deciding on the proper handgrip, width, and direction. You have the options of narrow, medium, wide, overhand, and underhand handgrip on the Chin-up bar.
o If you get into the habit of testing your finger grips, by slightly opening and closing your hand grip before initiating upward pull, you might gain greater strength in hand gripping. This spares your the time of performing wrist curls.

Execution
o As usual, before initiating the Pull, ensure that your chest cage is thrust forwards and upwards. This brings the fibers of the scapular muscles into proper anatomical directions that prevent kyphosis.
o If your arms cannot generate enough power to elevate your bodyweight, you are not alone. You may execute few repetitions, even one is good, but increase the number of sets. You can cheat by performing leg drive to help your muscles initiate the shortening.
o If your muscles are in a bad shape, you should begin with an aiding machine that gives you some help in elevation. These work by pushing your bodyweight upwards at the heels, or knees, by specially designed platform.
o As you advance in training, your bodyweight will be able to initiate the pulling of Chin-ups by slow and strong Biceps and Latissimus dorsi contraction.
o The exercise proceeds by elevating and lowering your bodyweight for one to ten times in a set, and repeating that set from three to eight times.

6.5.6. LATERAL CABLE PULLDOWN

Holding an overhead loaded cable, by both hands, and pulling the cable downwards is called "cable pulldown". Cable pulldown performs the same strengthening work of Chin-ups but offers the advantage of grading resistance in incremental steps.

Purpose
o Downward pulling of weight, by hands, strengthens the upper body.
o As in Chin-ups, scapular muscles support chest cage from caving in during arm pulling. In addition, the long head of triceps aids scapular muscles in shoulder extension. The Biceps and Brachialis muscles flex the elbows and aid in downward pulling.
o Forearms flexors, also, stabilize the wrist and fingers during elbow flexion.
o Reverse cable pulldown engages the chest muscles in shoulder extension and ease downward pulling.

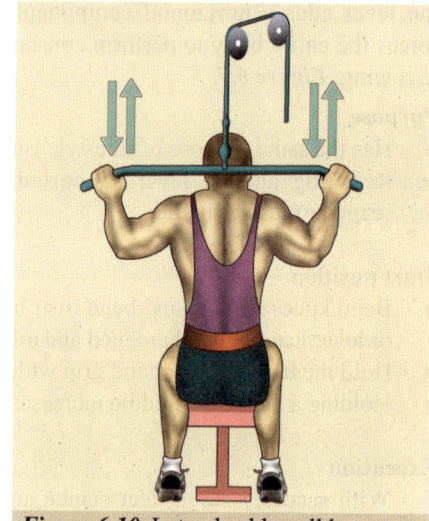

Figure 6.10. Lateral cable pulldown.

Start position
o Cable pulldown starts with deciding on the proper handgrip, width, and direction. The presence of the T-bar limits your options of handgrips.
o You will be seated, upright vertically under the T-bar.
Remember that some machines lack balancing support of the T-bar weight. When you change weight, make sure that the T-bar will not fall loose on your head. Keep your body away from under the T-bar when changing weight and inspect the machine carefully before messing with the cable loading.
o The first one or two upper weight blocks should be connected permanently to the cable to balance the T-bar weight. If these are loose, then find out how the T-bar would be balanced before changing weights.

Execution
o Begin with weight that you can pull down ten times without bouncing your head or torso. This guarantees that only your arms are performing the pulldown. If you start by heavy weight and proceed by yanking, you might pull your lower spinal discs out of alignment.
o Proceed by advancing under the T-bar and grip evenly by both hands around the middle of the bar. Usually overhand grip is the common way of holding the bar in this exercise. Now proceed by sitting, with both arms stretched overhead, holding the T-bar in both hands.
o While seated, maintain lower back upright erection. Thrust your chest. Tighten your abdominal muscles.
o When you start pulling, you will initiate force from the front of your elbows that is the Biceps insertion point. You will

see the Biceps harden and bulge when pulling starts. If you cannot start by bending the elbows, and have to yank the weight by upper back pulling, then make sure you have warmed up your back thoroughly. Otherwise, you might have to terminate your workout if spinal strain ensues unexpectedly.
o Proceed by pulling the T-bar downwards to the root of the neck, in the front, or the nape of the neck, behind the shoulders, *Figure 6.10.* Of course, you can pull lower, even to the belly button, if you desire. This works out the Triceps to greater range of motion.
o You can even pause or proceed by letting the T-bar ascent under your control. If you let the cable loose it might snap cut. Also slow ascent enhances eccentric contraction of the muscles of the arms and scapulas.

6.5.7. DUMBBELL ROWING
Purpose
o Dumbbell rowing are superior exercises in strengthening desired muscles. The unrestricted movement of one hand gripping fosters neural control of scapular muscles. Thus, greater number of muscle fibers and muscle groups engage in resistance.
o Rowing strengthens scapular retractors and shoulder adductors. These muscles waste quickly with inactivity.

Start position
o One-handed dumbbell rowing can be executed by bending the hips, slightly bending the knees, and rowing without the support of a bench.
o It can also be executed by kneeling over a bench, with one knee, and hanging the working arm downwards, on the side of the standing knee.
o The dumbbell can be lifted prior to bending or kneeling or after assuming those positions, *Figure 6.11.*

Execution

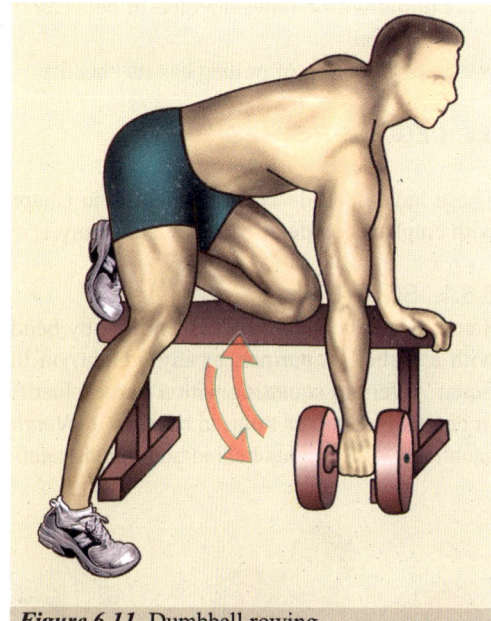

Figure 6.11. Dumbbell rowing.

o Pulling a dumbbell, in any manner, from the floor while bending will strengthen scapula retractors. Yet, the best beneficial posture is to maintain the torso horizontal by bending the hip at 90-degree angle with the spines. Maintaining horizontal torso works out the middle and low scapular muscles.
o If you raise the torso above horizontal, you will be strengthening the upper scapular muscles. These are already manageable by many other exercises such as the Clean, Snatch, Deadlift, or Shoulder Shrugs.
o Pulling with elbows pointed in three different directions works out three different muscle groups.
   i. Pulling with elbows moving close to the side of the body works out Latissimus dorsi and long head of Triceps.
   ii. Pulling with elbows pointed away from body works out the back fibers of the Deltoids and the upper retractors of the scapula.
   iii. Pulling with elbows in between previous directions works out lower retractors of the scapulas.
o Torso should be kept stationary while arms and scapulas are performing the rowing. Only during heavy pulling, torso should bounce to assist in breaking the slow motion.

6.5.8. LEVER ROWING
Purpose
o Horizontal pulling on loaded levers works out retractors of scapulas, extensors, and adductors of shoulders.
o Since there are hinges and solid levers, you have very limited control on the trajectory of pulling. These are very localizing exercises that target specific muscle fibers.
o All lever machines are condemned for their limited range of motion, concealing asymmetrical dynamics, and very localizing action. These drawbacks might be pluses to someone who uses these machines to complement wholesome workout regimen.

Start position
o These machines make start position simple since they have torso support, seat, lever handles, and fixed trajectory of motion.
o Sit on machine seat, abut your chest against vertical board pad, and hold the lever handles with both hands, or one hand if you intend to perform one hand rowing, *Figure 6.12.*

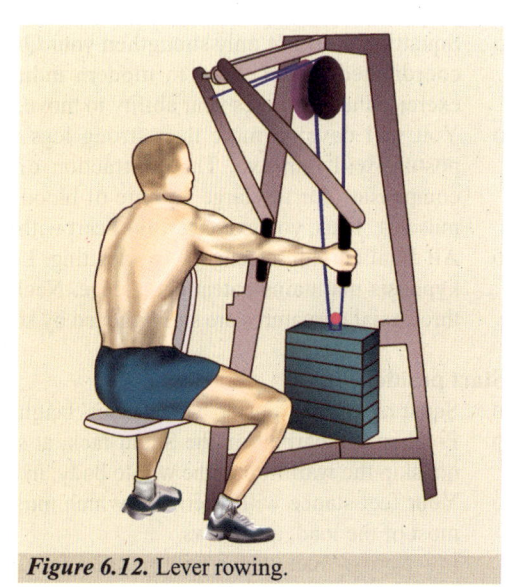

Figure 6.12. Lever rowing.

Execution
- As with any arm pulling, you should start the first pull slowly with hardened lower back and abdomen and without yanking. Sudden pulling of heavy weight is risky.
- With your chest and belly abutting vertical support and your feet evenly stuck to the ground, pull lever handle backwards.
- You have few options when pulling. Pulling with elbows falling in vertical planes, to the sides of the body, strengthen the shoulder extensors, mainly the Latissimus dorsi.
- Pulling with elbows directed away from the body, in a horizontal plane, strengthens the shoulder transverse adductors. These are the middle scapular retractors.
- Pulling with elbows directed in between the previous planes, obliquely, enhances two motions, shoulder adduction and extension.
- Each direction of pulling has its benefits

6.6. LEG EXERCISES

These have been described in details in Chapter Five. In this section, I will touch lightly on general exercises for the leg with emphasis on detailed applied anatomy.

6.6.1. SQUAT

Standing on the floor and descending, by bending both knees and hips, is called "Squat". "Back Squat" refers to squatting with a barbell, a partner, or any weight, on the back of the shoulders, during descending, *Figures 6.13* and *6.14*. "Front Squat" refers to squatting with a barbell loaded on the front of shoulders and held by both hands. Front Squat is discussed in details in Chapter Four, in relation to Weightlifting, and Chapter Five, in relation to Powerlifting. Squat can also involve squatting with weights held in both hands, such as dumbbells *Figure 6.15*.

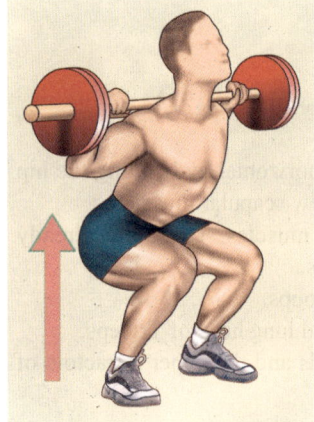
Figure 6.13. Back Squat with neutral feet stance.

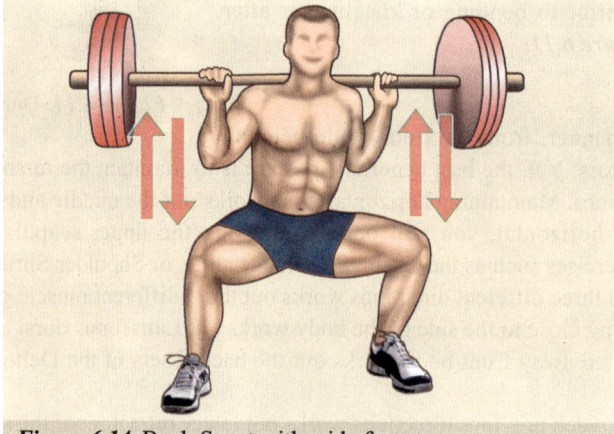
Figure 6.14. Back Squat with wide feet stance.

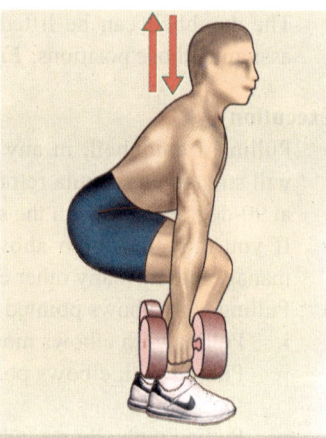
Figure 6.15. Squat with dumbbells

Purpose
- Squatting does not only strengthen your Quadriceps but also engages the shoulders, lower back, and pelvic muscles in coordinated action. Prior to modern industrialization, squatting was a common practice in everyday life. It is an exercise that promotes your ability to move, run, and lift heavy objects.
- You will develop more than strong legs with squatting. Your tolerance to weights will increase and your general posture will improve. The contraction of the large muscles of the thighs will make your heart race in order to compensate for the large volume of blood that is trapped in the contracted Quadriceps, glutei, Hamstrings, and back muscles. Thus, you exercise your heart with squatting.
- All axial curvatures engage in squatting. Low back lordosis prevents spinal discs from dislocation. Upper back normal kyphosis maintains patent chest cage. Neck concavity balances the head on the neck and prevents forward fall. These three axial curvatures are strengthened by squatting, with and without weight.

Start position
- Squat racks are adjustable to athletes' heights and some of them have safety cross bars to catch falling barbells.
- Position the barbell on the Squat rack, at shoulder height. Before you move to the next step, make sure that you did not skip the warm-up of the whole body, in addition to the special stretching of the legs, back, and shoulders.
- Your feet stance will determine which muscles will do the work and which part of your knee and hip joints will carry most of the load, as follows.
  i. Narrow feet stance with parallel feet aligns the Quadriceps tendon with the middle fibers of the Quadriceps and stretches the hip abductors.

ii. Neutral or normal feet stance evens the load on the hips and knees.
   iii. Wide feet stance throws most of the weight on the lateral knee compartment and stretches the hip adductors.
   Thus, you have to manipulate your feet-stance to custom sculpture your own body
o After you decide on which feet-stance you going to use, advance one foot under and to the front of the racked barbell. The other foot will help you remain in balance. Now pass your head under the bar by bending your knees in order to place the bar over the back of your shoulders. If you intend to do Front Squat then skip this move.
o Before off loading the barbell from the rack, make sure that your body is centered in the middle of barbell, your chest cage is thrust, your abdomen is sucked in, and your lower back is arched in.
o Load off the bar from the rack to your shoulders using both hands. The upward lift originates from the thighs. The vertebral column must maintain lordotic curve during and after off-loading. This guarantees stable scapulas while performing Squat. With proper squatting style, your body frame will adapt to unconscious and automatic proper posture if unusual circumstances ensue.

Execution
o Having loaded off the barbell from the rack you need to move away from the supporting rack knobs in order to start squatting. With heavy weight, you need to move slowly and cautiously to avoid twisting your lower back. If one side of the barbell collides with the side of the rack, you might suffer acute twisting force, unless you move very slowly.
o Before starting the Squat, perform the rituals of aligning and balancing your joints, as follows.
   i. Thrust the chest cage upwards and forwards.
   ii. Elevate the shoulders to make "T" crossing with the axial column.
   iii. Arch in your lower back to form concave curvature, not just flat or straight back.
   iv. Slightly bend the knees and throw most of your bodyweight on the feet balls.
   You will use the heels as sensors to your balance and land on them for support, if balance is undermined. In other words, the middle of your soles will work like shock absorbers by varying the tension in the arches of the feet.
o Since you are about to embark on the most strenuous venture that your body is designed to endure, therefore, you will need extra blood pumping capacity. You will use your belly to pump extra blood back to your heart. Your belly should resume higher tone, contract and relax, massaging the major abdominal vessels and augmenting blood passage from lower limbs to chest. So, do not let your belly hang loose, but rather breathe with it, by exhaling and inhaling when running out of breath.
o You can now Squat slowly and ascend slowly. Your speed in both directions will vary according to your progress, confidence, and robust fitness. Early in training life, try to content yourself with humble learning, one step at a time, slow and right technique better than charismatic and risky performance.

6.6.2. CALF RAISES
Standing on a hard floor, or on the edge of a hard step, and elevating the heels upwards, is called "Calf Raise". It can be done with weight or without weights, *Figure 6.16* and *6.17*. Calf raises can also be performed while seated and loading weights on the thighs. Seated calf raises emphasize Soleus strengthening alone, since the Gastrocnemius is not stretched during knee flexion. Calf raises are also performed on the laying down leg press machine. Here you can call them "calf press", if you wish.

Purpose
o Calf raises strengthens the ankle joint by exercising the Gastrocnemius, Soleus, and the feet evertors.
o Ankle strengthening serves both postural as well as dynamic activities. The Soleus muscle is a main postural effector while the Gastrocnemius responds more to vigorous stimuli, such as sprinting.

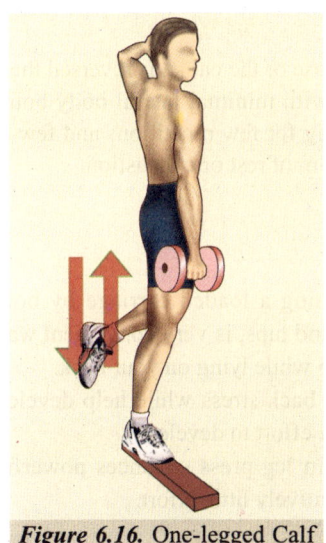

Figure 6.16. One-legged Calf Raises.

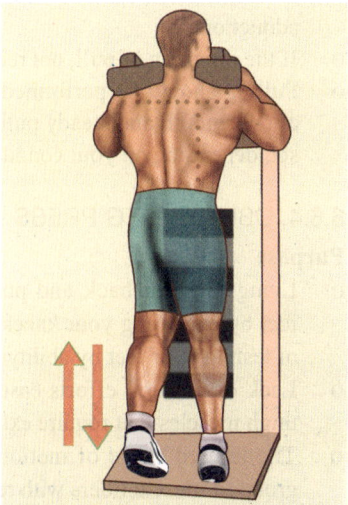

Figure 6.17. Two legged Calf Raises.

o The greatest benefit of calf strengthening is enhancing peripheral circulation in a part of the body that is often subjected to arterial insufficiency and venous congestion.

Start position
o Whether you hold the weight in your hands, on the shoulders, or on the thighs, the start position in leg raises entails vertical elevation of the heels under resistance.
o Mere hopping on the toes would strengthen the calf muscles beautifully. Yet, added weight enlarges the muscle mass, not just endurance, as in the case of aerobics.

Execution
- Raising the heels against weight can proceed either slowly or fast. In the latter case, the person must be young and well trained to avoid avulsion of the Achilles tendon.
- Raising the heels also can be performed with the toes directed inwards, forwards, or to the sides. This serves strengthening the direction of the ankle movement that is suspected as a weak link in motion.
- The vertical travel distance depends greatly on the flexibility of the ankle, the strength of the calf muscles, and the fitness condition of the trainee.

6.6.3. CABLE HIP ADDUCTION

Cable hip adduction is performed while standing on one leg and supported by holding hand-held stand. The unsupported leg pulls a loaded cable, horizontally and from the side to the middle, by ankle attachment, *Figure 6.18*. Hip adduction can also be strengthened by seated machine exercise, with both thighs pushing on loaded pads form the sides inwards, to the middle. Sumo Deadlift also strengthens and stretches the hip adductors with much heavier weights.

Purpose
- Strengthening and stretching the hip adductors with weights facilitates stable walking, running, sprinting, and lifting. The hip adductors are located at the inner upper aspect of the thighs and often become short and weak with inactivity.
- Cable hip adduction strengthens thigh adductors besides, the lateral spinal muscles.

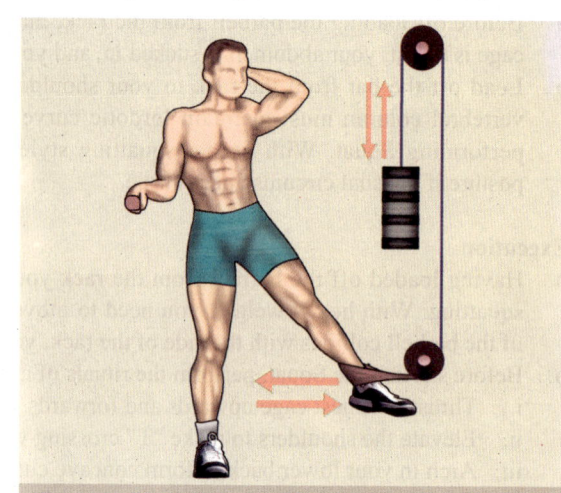

Figure 6.18. Cable hip adduction.

Start position
- Cable hip adduction requires thorough warm-up of the lateral spines in order to avoid ligamentous sprains.
- Because one leg is performing pulling of resisting cable while the other is supporting the body, additional upper body support is needed. That is done by holding to a close-by hand held stand or fixed handle.

Execution of cable hip adduction
- Cable adduction by the legs is executed by attaching the handle of the low, and horizontally moving, cable to the ankle of the unsupported leg, of a standing person. The unsupported leg should be able to pull the cable away from the machine, from outside to the middle, relative to the standing person. Thus, the inner upper thigh muscles perform adduction.
- If the direction of pull, not release of the cable, is reversed then the hip abductors will be worked out.
- Pulling should be performed with minimal lateral body bouncing or yanking. Thus, a light weight should be used to allow smooth and steady pulling for few repetitions and few sets. Weight should be increased every set, or every other set, depending on your condition, of rest or exhaustion.

6.6.4. OBLIQUE LEG PRESS
Purpose
- Lying on your back and pushing a loaded carriage by both feet by extending your knees and hips, is very convenient way of testing your feet by ability to while lying on your back.
- Lack of postural efforts eases back stress while help develop thigh muscles that require extra effort to develop.
- The limited range of motion in leg press enhances powerful group of muscle fibers with relatively little effort.

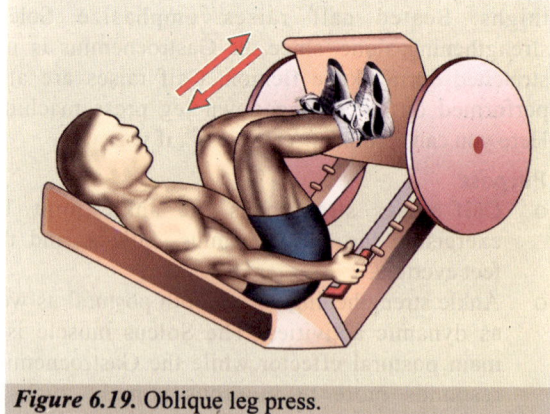

Figure 6.19. Oblique leg press.

Start position
- Before getting under the loaded sliding carriage, make sure that the safety knobs and sliding surfaces are in operable conditions.
- While moving your body under the carriage, do not hold onto the carriage or yank it. The carriage can slide accidentally by jerky movement and causes injury.
- Lie on your back on the lower fixed back support. This is mostly a padded board that is oblique to the ground surface.
- With the carriage racked at the top of the sliding rails, raise your feet to abut against flat metal surface of the carriage. Here is your feet stance on the moving carriage that can take various forms. You can put your feet close together, few inches apart, or widely separated. You can also change the angle of the feet with the longitudinal mid-body plane, by raising or lowering your feet contact with the carriage.

o   Hold the two control arms that will release the carriage when you load the weight on your feet. You will not rotate the control arms before you are ready to lift the carriage with both feet, *Figure 6.19*.
o   To get ready for lifting arch your low back on the oblique board such that your weight falls on the back of the hips and the back of the shoulder plates.

Execution
o   Start with weight that you can lift few times with smooth and comfortable motion. Then increase the weight every set, or every other set. As usual, a set consists of one to ten repetitions, each comprises of upward pressing and lowering of the loaded carriage.
o   As your body hardens against the back support, slowly push the carriage upwards, with both feet.
o   When the knees are straight and you feel that your back is securely supported, rotate the control arms outwards to free the sliding path of the carriage. Now the carriage can be lowered downwards the oblique rails by bending your knees by negative contraction of the thighs and glutei.
o   You can lower the carriage until the thighs stick to the abdomen. Shorter travel of the carriage limit tendon and ligament stretch and can undermine flexibility of the lower body.
o   At the lower end of the leg press, you may want to pause for stretch or proceed with reversing the motion. Upward pushing is called the "press" motion since to urge the weight to go away, upwards. This is the concentric contraction phase.
o   If you like to torture yourself by combining the leg press with other assisting leg exercises, in one session, you should have a second look into the rationale of unnecessarily wearing the delicate structures of the legs, in brief duration. This assisting exercise is better executed during fatigue conditions when standard Squat is more tiring.

6.6.5. HACK SQUAT
Purpose
o   Similar to lying leg press but with different back and chest configuration.
o   Different body inclinations alter your positional sense of leg exercises. Leg pressing with hack sled machine gives different sensation for Quadriceps activities. The other two leg exercises of Squat and Leg Press challenge the equilibrium apparatus of the inner ears in all three directions of motion. Thus, each exercise feels different according to the input of the vestibular ear sensors on the brain control of the leg motion.
o   Neither Hack Squat nor Leg Press is a substitute for upright standard squat.

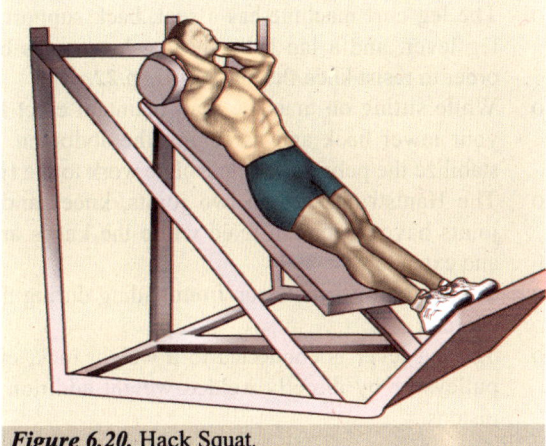
Figure 6.20. Hack Squat.

Start position
o   Lie on your back on the sliding carriage of the Hack machine. Your start position begins with bent knees and hips. Your feet stand on the inclined and fixed feet support of the machine, *Figure 6.20*.
o   Place the support shoulder pads on your shoulders while your hands hold the extended support bars. Since you are pushing with your shoulders upwards, maintain thrust chest cage and hardened belly, even if you are lying against a board.
o   Your lower back should be arching above the carriage bed, with your buttocks and upper back touching the bed firmly.

Execution
o   With firm upper body and back, straighten your legs by extending your hips and knees. This will move the loaded carriage far away from your feet.
o   Resistance results from a load of plates attached to the sides of the moving carriage, while sliding downwards and upwards by bending knees and kips.

6.6.6. LYING LEG CURLS
Purpose
o   Flexing the lower legs at the knees against resistance from behind the ankles, while the thighs remains stable, works out the Hamstrings.
o   Since the Quadriceps is shut off, by lying down, the antagonist to the Hamstrings is the posterior cruciate ligament (PCL). This unique exercise stretches the ligament PCL more than any other exercise.

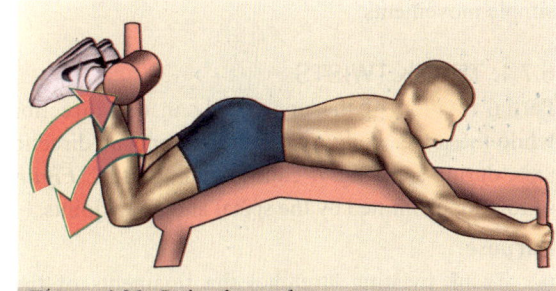
Figure 6.21. Lying leg curls.

BODYBUILDING

Start position
- Lie face down on the special machine and anchor your ankles under the padded lever, *Figure 6.21*.
- The hip joints have to be kept extended with the torso and thighs abutting the bench surface.

Execution
- While maintaining fixed upper body, by holding the support handles of the machine, and tightening the buttocks to maintain straight hips, bend your knees to raise the loaded lever upwards.
- Resistance results from weights attached to a pivoted leverage assembly that moves the weight upwards when ankles are pushed against the padded lever.

6.6.7. SEATED LEG CURLS

Purpose
- Bending knees against resistance, at the back of the ankles, works out the Hamstrings, in addition to the cruciate ligaments.
- Since the bodyweight is eliminated from the affecting the Quadriceps, by the sitting position, the Quadriceps is not antagonizing the Hamstrings in the leg curls. The posterior cruciate ligaments resist the posterior translation of the tibias over the femur, by the action of the Hamstrings.
- Thus curling the legs while seated differs from the Goodmorning, in the elimination of the action of the Quadriceps, though both exercises work out the Hamstrings.

Start position
- The leg curl machine has a seat, back support (optional), padded leg lever, and a lap belt. The leg lever goes behind the ankle in order to resist knee flexion, *Figure 6.22*.
- While sitting on machine seat, maintain erect torso by arching in your lower back and hardening the abdomen. These two actions stabilize the pelvis and help isolate work to the Hamstrings.
- The Hamstrings act on two joints, knees and hips, and the hip joints have to remain fixed while the knees are curling (bending and extending).
- The lap belt prevents you from sliding during the **execution** of the exercise.
- The leg lever is connected to a weight rack, either by cables and pulleys or by directly welded weight addition rod. Hydraulic machines are connected to resisting air compression pistons.

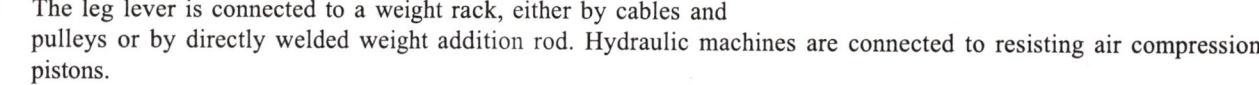

Figure 6.22. Seated leg curls.

Execution
- Leg curling starts by pushing against the padded leg lever with the back of the ankles, while the upper body is kept steady.
- No yanking is allowed during leg curls in order to avoid tearing the Hamstrings.
- Bending the knees, from the straight leg position to perpendicular tibia on femur constitutes the concentric contraction phase.
- Straightening the knees constitute the eccentric contraction phase.
- Both phases could be performed with different speeds to induce muscular hypertrophy or endurance.

6.7. LOWER BACK EXERCISES

Bodybuilding exercises for the lower back differ in specificity from those for Powerlifting, in regard to isolating the targeted muscles by simple movements.

6.7.1. TRUNK TWISTS

Partial rotation of the upper body in one direction, during standing, while the lower body rotates in the opposite direction around a vertical axis, during standing, is called "trunk twists", *Figure 6.23*. The degree of rotation is limited by the spinal and sacral joints.

Purpose
- Trunk twisting stretches the ligaments of the spinal joints and transverse processes along the vertebral joints.

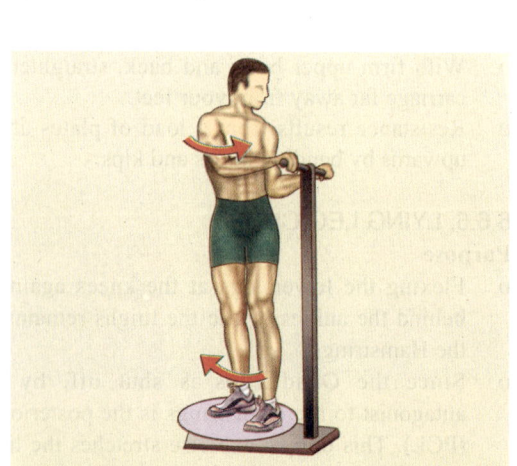

Figure 6.23. Trunk twists.

o   It is a fundamental exercise for spinal mobility and strength. It prevents shortening and calcification of ligaments thus prevents "vertebral freezing". This is a major cause of spinal injuries.
o   It must be performed along with back bending exercises of the spinal erectors, in order to add strength to mobility.
o   The strengthening and toning of the abdominal oblique and transverse muscles is also an added benefit from this exercise. Yet, these muscles can be better strengthened without such serious twisting. Abdominal muscles require high repetition that is beyond the limits of twisting of spinal joints.

Start position
o   If the machine for trunk twisting were available, it would help ease eye and ear stress during the rotatory motion of twisting. In addition, rotating discs enhance momentum generation. Holding onto the support handle prevents falling.
o   The low back should be positioned vertical, with the head lying on a vertical line passing through the heels.

Execution
o   Trunk twists are executed by moving the lower body in one rotatory direction and the upper body in the opposite direction, utilizing the hand held support as an initiating point.
o   Maximal rotation is reached when the face is looking in a direction opposite to the direction of the toes. Close to 180-degree angle is reachable by people with flexible neck, back, hips, knees, and ankles.
o   Twisting is reversed after maximum rotation. Maximum twisting after reversal constitutes one cycle. This is repeated from few cycles up to ten or more but not exceeding fatigue limit.
o   This exercise cannot be used for serious weight reduction since it involves asymmetric spinal joints.

6.7.2. LATERAL TRUNK BENDS
Standing on a hard floor and bending the upper body to the side is called "lateral trunk bends". It can be executed with or without weights, with arms in any position, from the sides of the body to overhead position, *Figure 6.24.*

Purpose
o   Like trunk twists, lateral bends stretch the ligaments of the spinal joints and transverse processes along the vertebral joints. It is also a fundamental exercise for spinal mobility and strength and must be performed along with back bending exercises of the spinal erectors.
o   The added hand held weight of dumbbell, or a plate, enhances the strength of lateral spinal erectors and abdominal oblique muscles.

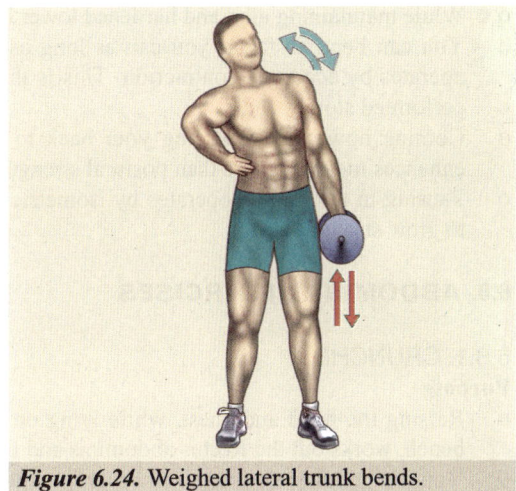
Figure 6.24. Weighed lateral trunk bends.

Start position
o   Lateral bends should start without weights, with both sides of the truck warmed up with progressive vigor, for few repetitions. The feet stance is preferably wider then the shoulder span.
o   The most common mistake is the hunching of the upper back while bending to the side. Thrust your chest forwards and upwards and maintain low back lordosis, even if you are not bending forwards.
o   Before adding weights, ensure that your lower back is ready to bend and resist. Thus any annoying discomfort in the low back might alert you for either the need for more warm up, or for complete cessation of activity of that region, for the time being.

Execution
o   Bend your upper body, from the waist up, to one side such that the hand on the bent side reaches downwards, below the knee level. Remember that bending to the side means that your head remains in the vertical plane that passes through both feet and shoulders. Thus, your head should not move to the front of that plane.
o   After reaching planned maximal bend, remember to remain tight and cautious. Do not talk while bending and do not pause for long. In addition, do not attempt to reach beyond you limits of bending, particularly with heavy weights.
o   Reverse the bending to the other side and repeat that cycle for up to ten repetitions, if you can. After a short break, less than 2.5 minutes perform another set. Total number of sets should exceed three. Preferably, you should progressively increase the weight, if you feel that you can.

6.7.3. HIP EXTENSION FROM A BENCH
The back extension bench allows the person to anchor both feet under a support bad while the upper half of the body projects outside

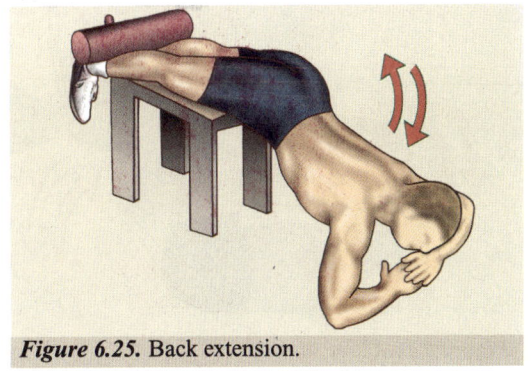
Figure 6.25. Back extension.

the opposite side of the bench. If your front thighs face the bench then your projected upper body can bend downwards, to the floor, and then return to horizontal level, by reversing the motion. This is called "back extension", *Figure 6.25*. If the back of your thighs face the bench then your projected upper body can move backwards to horizontal level and returns upwards. That is called "abdominal sit-ups".

Purpose
o   Extending the back, with and without weights, from low level to horizontal, strengthens the Hamstrings and Glutei by concentric contraction while the back performs isometric contraction.
o   The reverse, lowering from horizontal level to low level, operates by eccentric of the Hamstrings and glutei.
o   The greatest benefit of back extension by downward lowering of the body is the stretching, rather than compressing of the spinal joints. Thus, the spinal muscles work out by contraction, while the spinal joints are saved from the irritation of compression.

Start position
o   Place the front of your thighs on a flat bench or the specially designed bench for back extension. Anchor your feet under the provided pad support or let a partner hold the back of your, while you perform the exercise.
o   You can perform the exercise without weights or with plates or barbell placed on the back of your shoulders or held in front of your chest by both hands.
o   The weight of your upper body, plus the extra weight, makes the resisting force. The speed of bending also adds virtual forces.

Execution
o   While maintaining alert and hardened lower back, lower your projected torso downwards by bending at the hips.
o   You can bend as far as you can as long as your Hamstrings can tolerate stretch. Remember that lowering the back operates by eccentric contraction. This is the kind of contraction that can enhance your strength and muscles mass if performed slowly.
o   Coming upwards, by raising your back to horizontal, operates by concentric contraction. This kind of contraction enhances mobility more than postural strength.
o   Pausing in the middle operates by isometric contraction. This can induce intense soreness and stimulate weak muscles to grow strong.

6.8. ABDOMINAL EXERCISES

6.8.1. CRUNCHES
Purpose
o   Raising the head and chest, while lying on the back, and maintaining buttocks and lower back stuck to the floor or bench, works out the Rectus abdominis and front muscles of the neck.
o   You are bending your torso to bring the chest cage towards the lower half of your belly, not the thighs, *Figure 6.26*. Thus, you will not get up by using the Iliopsoas.
o   The oblique abdominal muscles can either work out by performing sit-ups on the side of the torso or on a chair, *Figure 6.27*.

Start position
o   Lie on your back on a flat bench or on the floor. Both hands are kept behind head or on the chest, with or without weight.
o   Both legs are bent at knees and hips or kept straight. Feet can be supported under feet support in specially designed crunch boards, or by letting a partner hold them while you raising your upper torso.
o   You can superset crunches with hip flexion by raising both head and chest and legs while maintaining lower back abutting the floor.

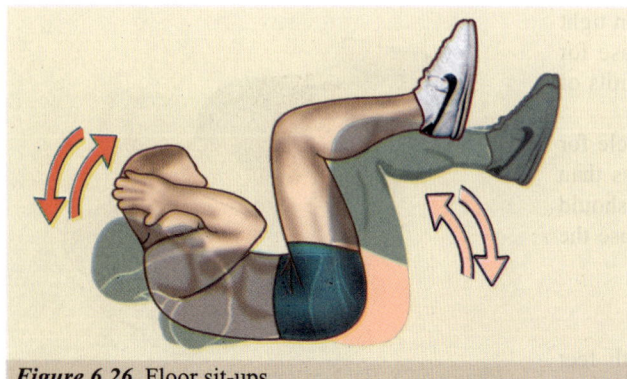

Figure 6.26. Floor sit-ups.

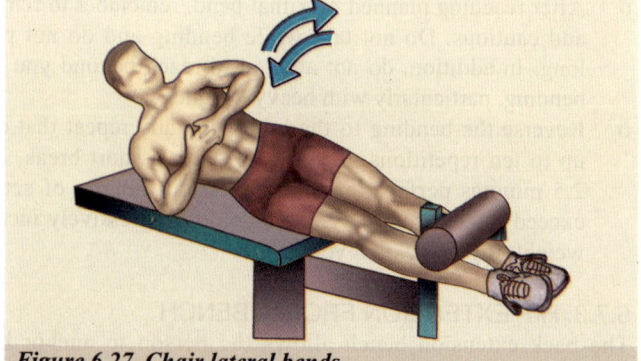

Figure 6.27. Chair lateral bends.

Execution
o   Start exercise by hardening your abdomen, thrusting your chest and supporting your head.
o   Raise your head and chest from horizontal. Your range of motion will not be great since the Rectus abdominis only maintain flat belly. It works mostly by isometric contraction to maintain postural flat abdomen.
o   You can also perform isometric contraction by slightly elevating the head and chest, without apparent raising, and then relaxing them back.
o   Remember that flat belly requires more than strong muscles. It requires less distention of guts and proper transit of contents. These all depend on dietary habits and aerobic activities. The strong abdominal muscles only contract when you want then to do so. Yet, high tone requires habitual low abdominal pressure and more general mobility than just executing few sets of exercises.
o   Reverse the motion after a short or no pause, at the end of raising. As with other exercises, you need to repeat that set from three to ten times or more.

6.8.2. INCLINE SIT-UP
Purpose
o   Lying on your back on inclined bench or board, with you head down the incline, and raising your head and chest, while the lower back is sticking to the bench, works out the Rectus abdominis. This flexes the chest lower border to the upper border of the pelvis, in the front. Raising the torso from the bench works out
o   the Iliopsoas while the Rectus abdominis experiences isometric contraction, *Figures 6.28 and 6.29.*
    Neck flexors and front vertebral muscles
o   are also worked out.

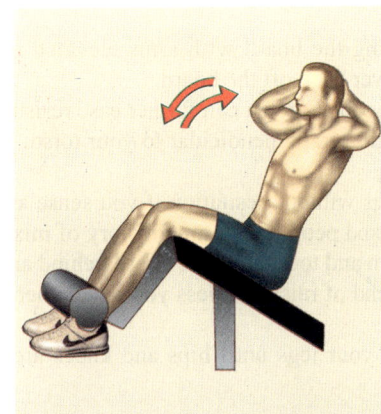 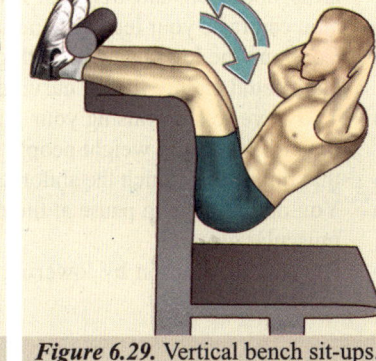

Figure 6.28. Inclined bench sit-ups.   *Figure 6.29.* Vertical bench sit-ups.

Start position.
o   Lie on your back, on inclined bench, designed with feet hooks to pull the bodyweight upwards during raising. The head is placed downhill. Both hands are held behind head or held together in front of the body.
o   Hook both feet under designated feet support while bending hips and knees.
o   You can use weight plate in both hands and place the plate on your chest or behind the head. The closer the plate to the thighs the easier is the raising. Behind the head plates are the most difficult to raise since the collar bones would squeeze the arteries to the upper arms and make the weight feels terribly heavy.
o   Without weights, you could perform more sets and reach greater range of motion, in addition to promoting your endurance.

Execution
o   Start **Execution** by hardening the feet hook to the feet support in order to prevent sliding and falling of the bench. Next, arch your lower back upwards and tighten your abdominal muscles before raising from the bench.
o   If you use weight, you should begin with light weights and progressively increase weights from one set to the other.
o   Raising can include multi-purpose movements. Raising the neck, chest, lower back from bench, while bending the hips and anchoring the feet under hook, will work out neck, abdominal Rectus muscle, and hip flexors.
o   You could add extra movement by raising pelvis and slightly extending the knees in order to make your chin touches knees. Thus, you come to complete elevation away from the board.
o   Reverse the motion after a short or no pause at the end of raising. As with other exercises, you need to repeat that motion from three to ten times or more, and for three sets or more.

6.8.3. LEG RAISES
Purpose
o   Leg raises works out the muscles in front of the hip joints (hip flexors), the Iliopsoas. Its functional value is more important than its anatomical outlook.
o   You need hip flexors every time you perform back extension. Thus when you sit, stand, walk, run, laugh, scream, talk, or perform any vigorous activities such as coughing, sneezing, or moving bowels, you have to extend you back to permit spinal nerves to travel freely along the spinal cord.
o   Hip flexors prevent the back from bouncing backwards and thus enhance erect, upright posture.

Start position
o   Lie on your back on incline board or bench, *Figure 6.30.* You can start on horizontal bench in order to try the exercise. Then increase the angle of inclination, in order to increase the difficulty of resistance. Lying supine on your back and raising your legs works out the anterior (front) muscles of the hip joints. Yet, if you also raise your pelvis from the

board you can work out the abdominal muscles. This modification requires strong arms and well-conditioned back muscles and is very difficult for heavy or weak trainees.
- o You can also begin without any added weight to your lower body or you can fix light dumbbells or other weights to your ankles.
- o If you want to further reduce resistance you can bend your knees in order to minimize the torque of the lower body around the hip joints. Thus, addition of extra weights to the lower body or keeping straight knees intensify the torque. You can also do without weights; yet increase the speed of raising to generate more momentum by the moving lower body.
- o Hold the fixed sides of the board or bench with both hands, with arms elevated above shoulders. Make sure you are not grasping loose board that would move and break apart when pulling commences.
- o Leg raises are also performed on vertical stands with elbow support, *Figure 6.31*.
- o Ladder leg raises are beneficial in stretching the upper body while the lower body performs the exercise, *Figure 6.32*.

Execution
- o While lying on your back, holding the board with arms elevated over shoulders, start execution by hardening your arms, abdomen, and arch your lower back off the board.
- o You can raise your legs by bending hips or you can further ease resistance by bending knees too.
- o Continue the leg raising until thighs are perpendicular to your torso. You can exceed this point if you are sure that your back could endure further curving.
- o You have to stop raising your legs without hesitation if you sense any stretching pain, strain, or unusual feeling at the lower back. Light weight people and people with long history of mixed training could perform hip flexion to the extent that thighs may touch the abdomen and toes touch the board behind and above the head.
- o You do not have to pause at the end of raising unless you have other thoughts in mind, such as stretching or fatiguing a muscular group.
- o Reverse the motion by lowering your legs until hips and knees are straight again. This is just one repetition of few more to come.

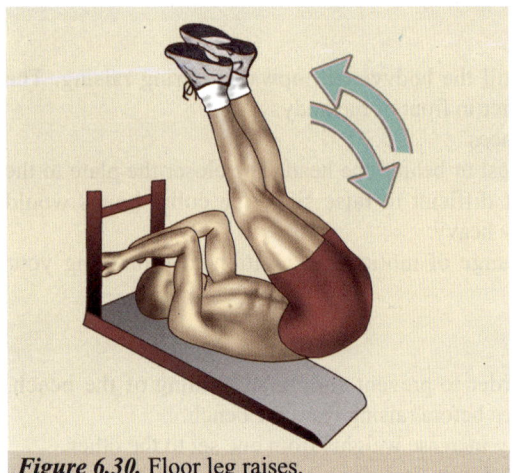

Figure 6.30. Floor leg raises.

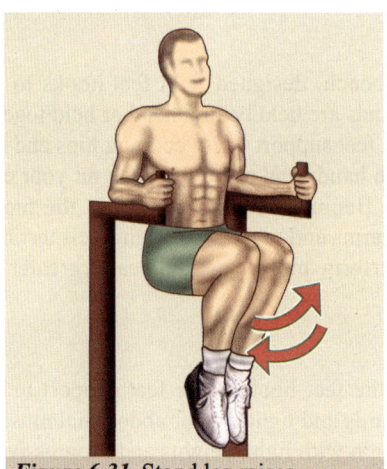

Figure 6.31. Stand leg raises.

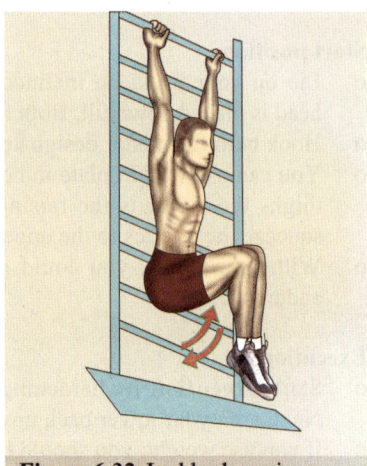

Figure 6.32. Ladder leg raises

6.9. WEIGHT TRAINING GUIDELINES

6.9.1. WEEKLY TRAINING FREQUENCY
- o The proper number of training sessions per week depends on many factors. The most important factor being the heart condition of regular pulse, normal beating force, and comfortable response to physical vigorous activity. All factors that interfere with the performance of the heart have to be taken into consideration when deciding on training. Lack of sleep, medication, overtraining, or diseases can afflict the dynamics of the heart and necessitate longer intermission between training sessions.
- o Beginners, young or old, have to start with three sessions per week, equally spaced. This allows time for recovery and adaptation.
- o When the trainees show signs of adaptation, in the form of quick physical recovery and passionate interest in more training, the number of session may increase up to 6 sessions/week.
- o When the trainee reaches the level of competitiveness and plans for future competition, sessions may be further increased to include two or three double-sessions per day, per week.
- o Few weeks prior to competition, weekly sessions should be reduced, depending on individual adaptation to stress and recovery, but not less than three sessions/week.
- o The most important factor is the cumulative volume of load over few weeks. The frequency of training is intended to find an optimum level of sustaining buildup of muscles without fluctuating between loss and gain.

6.9.2. SYMMETRY RULES
- All people suffer from postural asymmetry, in one form or another. For example, right-handed people have stronger right arm and shoulder. Many people have one leg stronger than the other. The purpose of training is to maintain postural asymmetry minimal.
- Training with barbells does not eliminate asymmetry, since other groups of muscles may conceal asymmetry by uneven synergy. Barbells eliminate the actions of many adducting muscles since the bar obviate adducting resistance.
- Dumbbells, when used in one-hand exercises, aggravate asymmetric problems vividly and help in locating the weak muscles that cause them.
- Strengthening the weaker muscles, with few extra repetitions over the other side, alleviates asymmetry.
- Thorough warm-up helps weaker side catch up with stronger side.
- Universal machines with rigid moving bars and levers are notorious in aggravating asymmetry, since the lifter adheres to the machine trajectory regardless of which muscle he or she is using to perform that exercise.

6.9.3. RANGE OF MOTION RULES
- The range of motion of a joint is served by various groups of muscles. Performing exercises with limited range of motion, for long time, jeopardizes the integrity of the joint. The neglected muscles waste and the ligaments around the joint shorten and stiffen.
- Full range of motion is not as dangerous as people think. You just have to learn not to exceed anatomical limitation. There is a difference between full range of motion and exaggerated range of motion.
- Full Squat, with buttocks seating on the back of the heels, is widely practiced in Weightlifting, while it is dreaded in other sports.
- Full lowering of the barbell on the shoulder, during Shoulder Press, is not as dangerous to the cuff rotators as many Bodybuilders claim.
- Hyperextension of the back during Deadlift, Squat, and Goodmorning is not serious practice, as Powerlifters claim.
- Serious injuries due to exceeding limits of motion results from:
  i. Sudden or quick alteration in habit without gradual conditioning in strength and duration.
  ii. Trying to increase the range of motion of a joint that is badly frozen, due to long-term poor training.
  iii. Exceeding normal anatomical limits and incurring injuries to structures.
  iv. Fast and uncalculated motion that result in generating unforeseen virtual forces.
- Enhancing the range of motion of some joints affects those of other joints. Hyper-flexible back, for example, allows greater range of motion of overhead exercises and front Squat.

6.9.4. RETURNING FROM LAY-OFF
- The length of duration of lay-off affects adaptation to re-acquiring higher levels of fitness.
- The nature of activities during lay-off, also, impacts adaptation to fitness training.
- Lengthy inactivity, excessive alteration in body weight, or loss of muscle mass complicate re-acquiring prior fitness level.
- The wisest approach to undo ill effects of lay-off is to prolong warming up time or even to content yourself with aerobic and Plyometric exercises for few workout sessions before engaging in resistance training by weights.
- Soreness can be reduced to minimum by gradual and protracted light exercises with high repetitions of full range of motion exercises. Sweating during warm-up enhances local metabolism of working muscles and reduces after-exercise soreness.
- Adequate rest and proper nutrition also hasten recuperation. Light balanced meals are easy to prepare without the need for fancy nutritional supplements.
- Perform exercises that have global nature such as Squat, Goodmorning, Bench Press, Shoulder Press, Clean and Snatch. You can perform these exercises with just a 45 lb (20 kg) bar without any added weights to it. Just execute the motion for few sets and few repetitions in order to get the feeling of stimulation of resistance.

6.9.5. FORCED REPETITIONS
- Forced repetitions are not objectionable if the trainee could maintain proper technique. The habit of persisting to push beyond limits is dear to athletes.
- Forced repetitions are commonly practiced to stimulate resilient muscles to gain extra strength. The excess production of lactic acid, due to excessive work, makes extra repetitions feel as hard as increasing the force of resistance with less repetition. Yet, excessive lactic acid accumulation undermines the technique by impairing neural control.
- The other gains of forced repetition are the enhancement of aerobic elements of the cells. These mitochondrial elements are increased in number when aerobic respiration is forced to take place during excessive work. Performance of the right arm in many right-handed people is an example of how forced repetitions alter the function of muscles. Repeatedly working the right arm makes it stronger than the left arm.
- Of course forced repetitions have to be restricted to isolated muscles, such as the Biceps, Triceps, Latissimus dorsi, and so on. You should not exceed normal repetition in exercises that involve multi-joints, complex technique, or high speed.

- o It is unwise to perform excessive repetitions with heavy weight on a limited range of motion. Performing Shoulder Press or Bench Press with heavy weight, for a short range of travel, causes joints to lose flexibility and induces ligaments to remain short and stiff, in addition, it traumatizes partial strained area of the working joints.
- o Forced repetition could play positive role in increasing flexibility of a joint that has long suffered from neglect. Excessive repetition on Goodmorning exercises, forearm curls, and abdominal exercises, with light resistance could bring these exercising regions to better figures of strength and flexibility.

6.10. HIGHLIGHTS OF CHAPTER SIX

1. The critique on the lack of **transferability of skills,** from Bodybuilding exercises to real sport skills, should not undermine the benefit gained by empowering skilled athletes with strong muscles. Those are not mere addition, of inert musculature, but rather enhancement of body hormonal system, metabolism, morale, and sense of accomplishment. Most importantly, individuals can build up strong physique during certain period and then work on sports enhancement in a different period. The limitation of building massive musculature has to be weighed against the gain of enhancing the musculoskeletal system.

2. The critique on the **lack of cohesiveness** of training isolated muscles and on the undesired outcome of bulking masses of muscles of improper proportions that disfigure motor skill could be minimized by slight modification in Bodybuilding routines. Many Bodybuilders are getting into the habit of running, as a way to reduce fat. Encouragement of aerobics and running for mobility gain can make the difference in acquiring cohesiveness.

3. Training isolated parts of the body, in separate sessions with heavy load volume or intensity, achieves large and strong muscles. Great stimulation of long-neglected muscles takes place during exercising individual muscles. That is because the entire cardiac output is diverted towards working out isolated muscles. That enables the athlete to enhance his or her weak spots. However, isolated training also seriously undermines the ability of muscles to perform synchronized motions. Synchrony requires proper recruitment when multiple joints are engaged in concerted activity. **Isolated training** suppresses the responsiveness of the nervous system, during complex activities.

4. Bodybuilders have utilized the common experience of their times. That **resistance training develops muscles** when practiced regularly and beyond normal limits. Those limits were rationalized as normal in relation to one's current condition of fitness, rather than to one's potential to enhance strength. It was observed that long and regular resistance training leads to higher ability of tolerating resistance.

5. Though doing away with technical barriers and Weightlifting restraints has led to new discoveries of manipulating human body, it created serious structural problems of neglecting **axial framework of strengthening**. All Bodybuilders suffer, during complex dynamic motions from supporting the huge muscles; they labored to develop, without properly enhanced linking muscles.

6. In today's urban and industrial society, the general population has adapted to inactivity with **loss of muscle mass** and deposition of more fat than those of earlier generation. Proper exercise and sound eating habits cannot reverse the modern trends of inactivity without careful accounting for energy expenditure and food intake. Many hours of weekly and daily activities are required to stop the decline in wasting of human body and deforming of musculoskeletal system.

7. I have my own doubts if abdominal exercises would flatten your belly. It might give you strong abdominal muscles, but flat belly requires more than strong muscles. It requires less distention of guts and proper transit of contents. These all depend on dietary habits and aerobic activities.

8. The most important factor is **the cumulative volume of load** over few weeks. The frequency of training is intended to find an optimum level of sustaining buildup of muscles without fluctuating between loss and gain.

9. The range of motion of a joint is served by various groups of muscles. Performing exercises with limited range of motion for long time jeopardizes the integrity of the joint. The neglected muscles waste and the ligaments around the joint shorten and stiffen.

10. The wisest approach to undo ill effects of lay-off is to prolong **warming up time or even to content yourself with aerobic and Plyometric** exercises for few workout sessions before engaging in resistance training by weights.

11. It is unwise to perform excessive repetitions with heavy weight on a **limited range of motion.** Performing shoulder press or Bench Press with heavy weight for a short range of travel causes joints to lose flexibility and induces ligaments to remain short and stiff, in addition, it also traumatizes partial strained area of the working joints.

Chapter 7
Weight Training

7.1. INTRODUCTION

Weight training exercises are founded on the following simple rules of bone and muscle leverage.

o   When a muscle contracts it generates force along the line between its origin from one bone to its insertion on another bone.
o   If one of those two bones is kept fixed to an external object such as ground, bench, or a machine support then the other bone can be moved by the muscular force, around the nearby joint.
o   If the mobile bone is resisted from free moving by external force such as barbell, dumbbell, medicine ball, or weight loaded cable then the muscle has to generate more force in order to sustain motion.
o   When the muscular force equals the external resisting force then the joint does not move. This sort of muscular contraction is referred to as "isometric contraction" since the two bones maintain fixed static state.
o   If the muscular force exceeds the external resisting force then the joint moves in the direction of muscular shortening by concentric contraction (isotonic). The concentric feature arises from shortening of the muscle fibers towards the middle "center" of the muscle.
o   Finally, if the muscle generates force that is less than the external resistance, but sufficient to allow control, then the joint moves in the direction of the external resistance (negative contraction) and the muscle elongates by eccentric contraction. Thus, the muscle fibers elongate away from the middle "center" of the muscle.

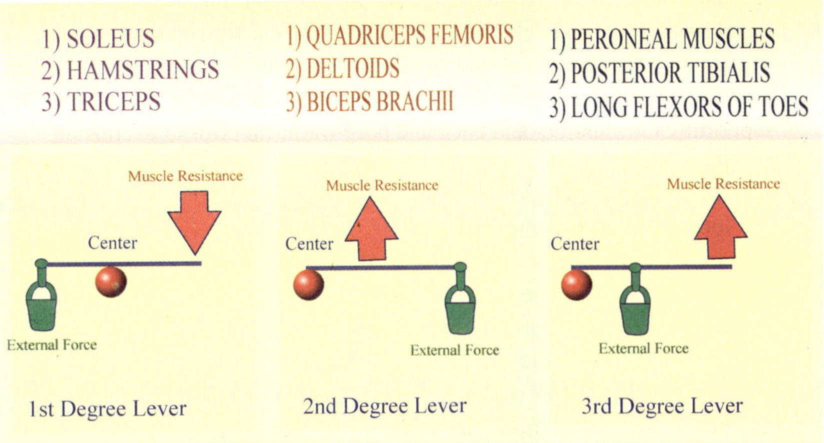

Figure 7.1. The three types of levers configuration.

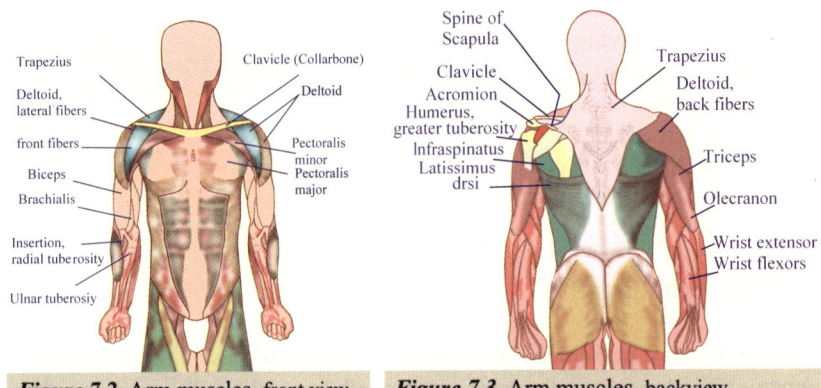

Figure 7.2. Arm muscles, front view. **Figure 7.3.** Arm muscles, backview.

7.2. STRENGTHENING ELBOW FLEXORS

7.2.1. APPLIED ANATOMY OF ELBOW

The elbow flexors are the muscles that bring the forearm towards the upper arm[1] against a force of resistance that tries to separate them apart. The force has to be applied on the palm of the hand or the front of the forearm. Flexion is achieved by a 2nd degree lever, where the insertion of the muscles on the forearm lies between the elbow joint and the point of force

---
[1] Upper arm refers to region between shoulder and elbow. Upper limb refers to the whole arm.

application, - the hand. This muscle-to-bone arrangement implies inherent relative weakness of the flexors since the lever-arm of resistance is much smaller than the lever-arm of force, *Figure 7.1.* The 2nd degree lever arrangements imposes minimal compression or tension, on the upper arm. The resistance and force are parallel and opposite in direction, comprising a couple that tends to separate the scapula away from the chest cage by way of the long and short heads of the Biceps. This couple of forces makes flexor training strenuous to the upper back.

The elbow is flexed by the combined actions of the following five muscles: Biceps, Brachialis, Brachioradialis, common wrist flexors, and common wrist extensors, *Figures 7.2* and *7.3*. In order to exercise the elbow flexors, the following peripheral and axial muscles participate in muscular balance during resistance training:
o **Peripheral muscles:** The forearm muscles control the hand gripping. The Triceps and Biceps transmit the forces to the scapulas, the Deltoid, Pectoralis, Teres, and scapular muscles stabilize the shoulder joints.
o **Axial muscles:** The Trapezius and Latissimus dorsi convey the scapular forces to the spinal axis.
o **Muscular balance**: All forces applied to the elbow flexors are balanced by forces at the shoulders and spinal axis. Shoulder or back pain or discomfort, during exercising the elbow flexors, stems from weakness of the muscles supporting the shoulder and back and poor warm-up prior to exercising.

7.2.2. BRACHIAL MUSCLE

This is located in front and above the elbow, sandwiched between the Biceps and the humerus bone, -the bone of the upper arm-, *Figure 7.2*. It originates from the upper arm, bridges the elbow, and ends in the forearm. This is a pure elbow flexor since it originates from the front surface of the lower half of the humerus and inserts into the ulna, the medial bone of the forearm. The Brachial muscle flexes the elbow by pulling the ulna to the humerus. The fibers of the Brachial muscle are shorter than those of the Biceps, with a wide difference between the length of the shortest and the longest fibers due to its wide origin from the lower two thirds of the front of the humerus. The Brachialis is exercised by:

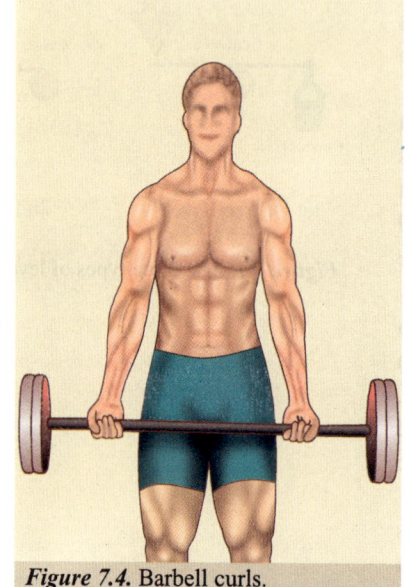

Figure 7.4. Barbell curls.

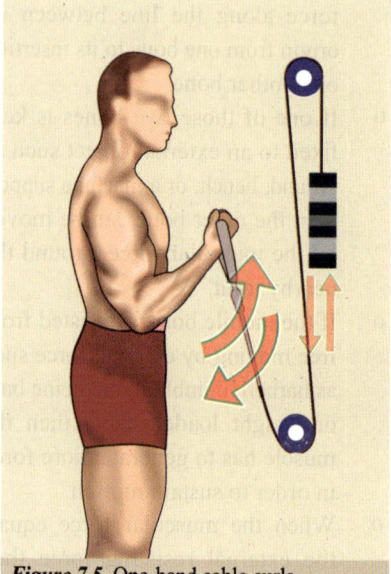

Figure 7.5. One-hand cable curls.

1. Barbell curls.
2. One-hand cable curls.
3. Dumbbell concentration curls.
4. Cable curls.

7.2.2.1. Barbell Curls
Purpose
The barbell curls, in *Figure 7.4,* work out the Brachial muscle more than the Biceps since the forearm is supinated and the humerus and ulna fall on the same plane of elbow rotation. The underhand grip on the bar puts most of the weight on the little, ring, and middle fingers, which transmit forces to the ulna. The common wrist flexors assist the Brachial muscle in flexion while the long head of Biceps stabilizes the shoulder and assist in elbow flexion by pulling the radius -the lateral bone of the forearm- towards the humerus.

Execution
o Arm barbell curls are performed while standing, by holding a bar with underhand grips, with palms facing forwards.
o Lift the barbell by bending the elbows to bring the barbell from the initial location, at the upper thighs upwards to the level of the chest.
o If the entire body or the upper body bounces back and forth during bending of the elbows then the Brachial muscle will contract by two modes, isometric contraction followed by concentric contraction.
o Pure concentric contraction requires very stable body while the forearms raise the barbell upwards.
o Lowering the barbell very slowly enhances eccentric contraction and causes fast growth of the muscle, within weeks.
o The common mistake in performing barbell curls is hunching the upper back. Keeping upright back, elevated shoulders, retracted scapulas, and thrust chest, all benefit the working muscles by facilitating circulation and respiration and prevents developments of deformities of the, all shoulder girdle.

7.2.2.2. One-hand cable curls
Purpose
The One-hand curls, in *Figure 7.5,* impose more tension on the short head of the Biceps but still exercise mostly the Brachialis. You should resort to one-hand exercises in order to stimulate growth and strength of muscles that lag behind, in both. One-hand exercises require less cardiac output and oxygen consumption than whole body exercises, in addition to their effective enhancement of the mind-over-body control, through stimulating neuromuscular control of the particularly emphasized muscle. One-hand exercises are awesome ways to enhance body parts beyond all norms, as seen in Bodybuilders and elite Weightlifters.

Execution
- One-hand exercises are asymmetric since they put more stress on one side of the body than the other side. They should be performed after thorough warm-up.
- Slowly increase the weight, in progressive steps, from set to subsequent set, and with frequent alternation between the two sides of the body. Starting one-hand exercises with heavy weight and high repetition can undoubtedly cause spinal injury. This strains one side of the spinal erectors more than the other side and thus destabilizes the spinal joints.
- Upward pulling should proceed slowly and without yanking. This is not a ballistic exercise. Therefore, you should not try to pull in haste.
- Downward lowering of the weight should also proceed very slowly in order to enhance eccentric contraction.
- If you bounce your entire body then you are fatiguing the shoulders and back, in addition to the upper arm muscles. Focused elbow bending, with stable body, fosters local growth of muscle, in size and strength. Yanking stresses the supporting tissues of the muscles, such as the ligaments, tendons, and elastic fibrous tissue.

7.2.2.3. Dumbbell Concentration Curls
Purpose
Concentration curls, in *Figure 7.6,* bring the coracoid process, - the origin of the short head of biceps at the shoulder-, into a straight line with the Biceps line of action. This posture relaxes the tension on the Biceps and forces the Brachial muscle to resist the most. The noticeable bulging of the Biceps during concentrated curls is due to the short distance between its origin and insertion, by way of leaning down with the upper body. The bulging Biceps is less stretched in this position. This one-hand elbow flexion exercise is unique in enlarging the muscles around the cubital fossa, -front pit of the elbow joint. This a rhomboid shaped pit is formed by the borders of the Biceps, Brachialis, Brachioradialis, and radial flexor muscles of the wrist, *Figure 7.2.*

Execution
- While seating on a bench, or leaning forwards with the torso, hold a light dumbbell with underhand grip. The arm that holds the weight should fall vertically downwards with straight elbow.
- If you can bend the elbow without moving it from the vertical line of the upper arm then you do not need to support the elbow from behind. The basic idea is to maintain vertical upper arm.
- You might have to support the elbow with the other free hand or by abutting it against the inner side of the thigh.
- Lift the dumbbell while the palm maintains facing forwards. If you twist your hand you will be engaging more of the Biceps action.
- The main benefit of this exercise stems from slow upwards and downwards motion. It is mainly designed for hypertrophy of the muscles in the front of the elbow.

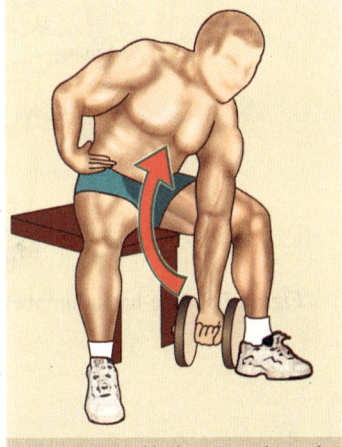 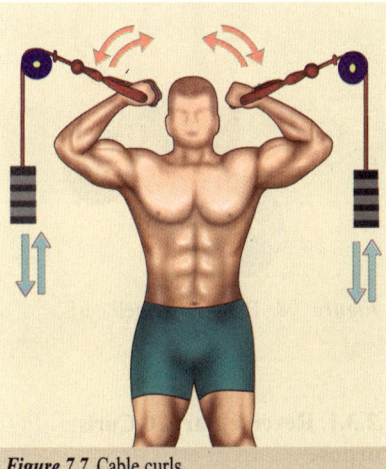

Figure 7.6. Dumbbell concentration curls.   *Figure 7.7.* Cable curls.

7.2.2.4. Cable Curls
Purpose
Bilateral curls by cables*, Figure 7.7,* accomplish the same effect of concentration curls but with proper shoulder and back alignment. The elevated shoulders work out the long head of Biceps by isometric contraction since they stabilize the shoulder elevation for the length of the exercise. In this elevated shoulder posture, the Supraspinatus along with the Trapezius abduct the shoulders and stabilize the scapulas during curling. This is a symmetric upper arm exercise that also enhances chest and shoulder posture.

WEIGHT TRAINING

Execution

o Adjust the level of the cable final pulley in order to exercise the muscles you wish to target. A pulley at the shoulder level will mainly strengthen the upper arms muscles. Lowering the pulley would stretch the Deltoid and the Supraspinatus, in addition to the upper arm. Raising the pulley above the shoulder level would limit the range of motion of the elbows at full flexion.

o Slow initiation of pulling and slow release of cable is the essence of this exercise. As with concentrated curls, this exercise is meant to enhance size and strength of the upper arm muscles, not the speed of pulling.

7.2.3. BICEPS BRACHII MUSCLE

The Biceps brachii bridges both the shoulder and elbow joints by two heads, without any attachments to the bone of the upper arm, *Figure 7.2.* It flexes either joint when the other joint is kept fixed. It has two bellies, or heads, a short and a long head. The tendon of long head of Biceps travels in the groove between the two tuberosities of the humerus. These are two bulging surfaces on the bone of the upper arm, in front and to the side of the shoulder. The tendon reaches the upper margin of the glenoid cavity, the socket of the shoulder ball over the head of the humerus, and attaches to the supra-glenoid tubercle. The short head of Biceps originates from the coracoid process, which is a bony projection from the scapula above the shoulder ball, lateral to the clavicles. Both long and short heads are inserted into the radius bone of the forearm by the common Biceps tendon.

The Biceps brings the radius towards the humerus. The insertion into the radius makes the Biceps a major forearm supinator that rotates the forearm laterally to bring the palms facing forwards. The Biceps takes advantage of the leverage support of the humerus by pulling the forearm towards the shoulder without being inserted or originated from the humerus. It thus acts as a linking tensile structure, between the elbow and the vertebral axis, through the shoulder and across the humerus. The Biceps brachii is exercised by:

1. Reverse barbell curls.
2. One-hand dumbbell curls.
3. One-hand dumbbell hammer curls.

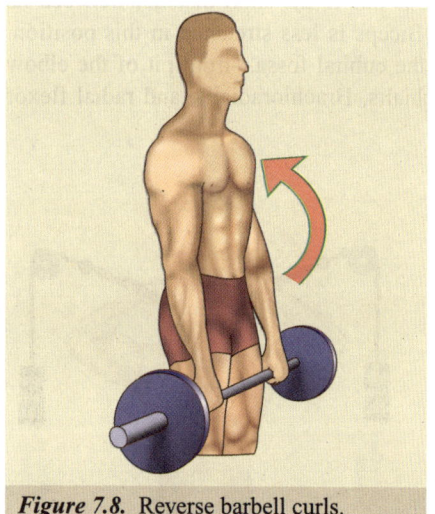

Figure 7.8. Reverse barbell curls.

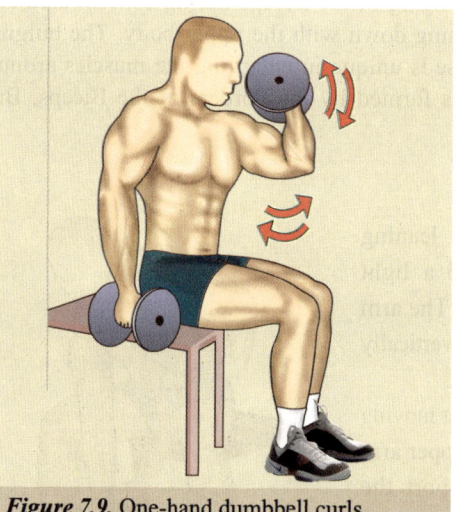

Figure 7.9. One-hand dumbbell curls.

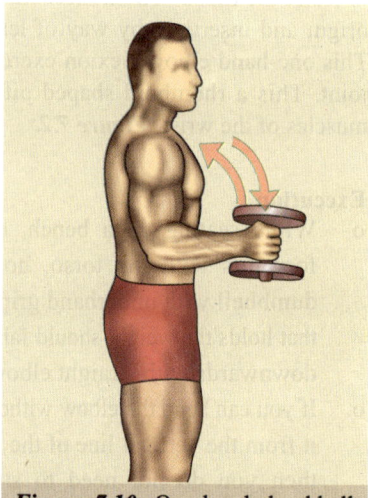

Figure 7.10. One-hand dumbbell hammer curls.

7.2.3.1. Reverse Barbell Curls

Purpose

The reverse curls, *Figure 7.8,* are performed with the forearms in prone position, with palms facing backwards with overhand grip on the bar. This brings the radius and the humerus on the plane of elbow rotation and minimizes the effect of Brachialis. The overhand grip puts most of the weight on the thumb and index finger, which transmit forces to the radius. The wrist extensors and the Brachioradialis assist the Biceps in elbow flexion. The particular sensation of intense muscle tone with reverse curls stems from the effort of the Biceps action to supinate the forearms against the resistance of the limiting bar between the two hands.

Execution

o If you haven't performed reverse curls before, then you should start with very light weight. You will need to perform this exercise for the rest of you life, if you want to maintain wrist-elbow-shoulder strength. You will often need to warm up with this exercise before any lifting from the floor. That is because reverse curls rotate the two forearm bones around the wrist and elbow joints thus warm up the pronation and supination of the forearm. These are fundamental function of the human forearm.

- o Hold the barbell with shoulder-width handgrips. Narrower width causes upper back kyphosis. Greater width of handgrips impairs elbow flexion.
- o Lift the barbell by bending the elbows while maintaining steady body posture. Sometimes you might have to slightly lean forwards to initiate muscular contraction.
- o The worst mistake you would ever make, in reverse curls, is letting your wrist go soft while lifting. This would overstretch the finger tendons on the back of the wrist and might cause inconvenient inflammation, in the form of cystic swellings along the tendons on the back of the hands. Remember to maintain the wrist in neutral position. That means that you should maintain the hand and the forearm on straight line. When you warm up sufficiently, then you can play with wrist extension and flexion during reverse curling.
- o Again, lift slowly and lower the weight slowly in order to enhance the size and strength of muscles. If you perform ballistic motion, you take the risk of injuring your back and shoulder. Ballistic reverse curls are safely performed during the Clean from the floor since the full range of motion here does not surprise the back or shoulder muscles.

7.2.3.2. One-Hand Dumbbell Curls
Purpose
This exercise works out the short head of the Biceps with the Brachialis, *Figure 7.9*, by flexing the elbow and shoulder consecutively. Both the Brachial muscle and the Biceps bring the ulna to the humerus by flexing the elbow. The Biceps brings the humerus to the coracoid process by flexing the shoulder. Care must be taken to avoid upper back hunching during elevating the upper arm. A hardened abdomen and upright lower back facilitate upper bodywork through preventing blood pooling in the lower body. This is achieved through sympathetic activity during the alerted upright posture.

Execution
- o One-hand dumbbell curls are the oldest known weight training exercises that are well perceived even to people who have never practiced weight training. There isn't any simpler motion than moving both arms with weights, held in each hand, for the sake of strengthening the arms.
- o You can perform the exercise seating or standing. You can also alternate hand motion and change the direction of the hand.
- o Hold two dumbbells, one in each hand. With one arm kept straight hanging downwards, bend the elbow of the other arm. Keep the upper arm vertical until the elbow is fully bent. Then raise the upper arm of the bent elbow by flexing the shoulder. The entire arm motion should be kept in an anterior-posterior plane. Thus, the hand should not bounce to the side or the middle, relative to the body.
- o When the working arm reaches the level where the upper arm becomes horizontal, then you can either pause to enhance the short head of Biceps or slowly reverse the motion, lower the elbow, and extend the forearm.
- o After reaching the lowest downward point, repeat the same action on the other arm, while the lowered arm take a stretching break.

7.2.3.3. Hammer Dumbbell Curls
Purpose
Curling the arms, with the wrist in mid position between supination and pronation can equally strengthen both the Biceps and the Brachial muscles, *Figure 7.10*. The posture of the forearm maintains equal pull on the radius and ulna during elbow flexion. The one-hand feature eases the effort of lifting and permits greater enhancement of load volume on this essential part of the body. It must be emphasized that variation in forearm postures fosters strengthening of the forearm tendons and bone support of these tendons. That is why Weightlifters and Bodybuilders can develop strong handgrips and wrist movers by varying the lifting posture with both hands.

Execution
- o Like dumbbell curls, hummer dumbbell curls start from the side of the thighs, move forwards and upwards, and end at the shoulder level. Then the motion is slowly reversed.
- o Two dumbbells, one in each hand, alternate in ascending and descending, with only one arm working at any particular moment. If only one dumbbell is used then care must be taken to prevent straining the spinal axis with asymmetric lifting by one arm. Thus, the lower back and legs should be sufficiently warmed up.

7.2.4. BRACHIORADIALIS MUSCLE
The Brachioradialis does not duplicate the action of either the Brachial muscle, which draws its origin from the upper arm similar to Brachioradialis, or the Biceps, which inserts into the radius also similar to Brachioradialis, *Figure 7.2*. It differs from both muscles in its insertion on the distal end of the radius. Thus, the Brachioradialis muscle acts as elbow flexor and forearm supinator, but with point of action located far distally from the center of the body, on the radius. The farther insertion of the muscle on the forearm makes the lever-arm of resistance closer to the lever-arm of force. This muscle draws the radius to the humerus through pulling the far end of the radius.

Reverse barbell curls strengthen the Brachioradialis, *Figure 7.8*. Weightlifters circumvent the multiplicity of these exercises by the performing the power or military Clean lift from the floor, which includes the reverse barbell curls in addition to shoulder shrugging, shoulder flexion, and back and leg extension.

7.2.5. WRIST AND FINGER EXTENSORS

This group of muscles shares common origin at the lateral epicondyle of the humerus. This is the bulging part of bone at the upper and outer side of the elbow, *Figure 7.2*. They extend the wrist and fingers during lifting any object with overhand grip. This sort of extension is called "dorsiflexion", since the dorsum of the hand is bent on the forearm.

Wrist extensors are strained by repetitive wrist curling, as in the common condition of **"tennis elbow"**, and become inflamed and painful. These muscles are strengthened along with the other elbow flexors with the **reverse curls** of *Figure 7.8*.

7.2.5.1. Reverse Wrist Curls
Purpose
Reverse wrist curls, *Figure 7.11*, eliminate the elbow flexion and focuses on the wrist and finger extension. This is done by resting the elbows on a stable object such as thighs or a bench. The old tool of a wooden or metal rod, with a rope attached to a weight and to the middle of the horizontal rod, is still a perfect wrist-curling tool. Strengthening the elbow, wrists, and fingers extensors is paramount to any lifting. After few years of training, the tendons and bony structures of the elbows, forearms, and hand will develop sizable dimensions as a result of strengthening of tendons, muscle growth, and enlarging of the bone. Untrained people suffer from weakness of those structures and experience acute pain when lifting unaccustomed objects. Though the forearm extensors cannot be strengthened indefinitely, due to the limited room of the forearms, lifters learn how to use the shoulder muscles in bringing the weight close to the body during lifting. This lifting technique minimizes the displacement of the bar away from the center of masses and thus reduces the torque on the forearm extensors. You can easily tell whether the person has advanced in Weightlifting by the magnitude of displacement of the bar from the body, while lifting for power.

Execution
o You can perform reverse wrist curls standing, seating, or squatting. You can also curl with forearm hanging downwards or kept horizontal by flexing the elbow. You can also support the forearms on your thighs while seating, on a bench, or keep them up by contracting the Biceps.
o Hold a light barbell with overhand grip. The knuckles of your hands will be facing forwards and upwards, during the exercise.
o Curling in reverse proceeds by slowly lowering the hand as far as the finger tendons can tolerate the tension and then elevating the hand as far as the wrist can tolerate the dorsiflexion. The forearms should stay immobile. The only rotating parts are the hands that move around the wrist joints.

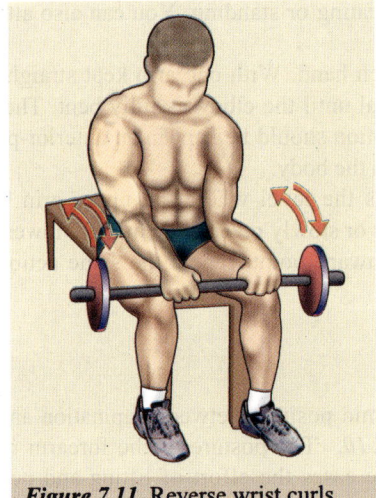 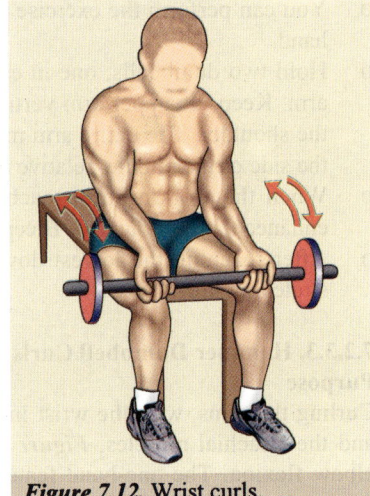

Figure 7.11. Reverse wrist curls.   *Figure 7.12.* Wrist curls.

o If you are using the horizontal rod with attached rope in its middle then you can alternate spinning the rod with both hands. Here, spinning proceeds by bringing the back of the fingers upwards in order to work out the wrist extensors.
o Remember that reverse curling entails crossing of the ulna and radius. The radius bone crosses from the outside of the arm, at the elbow, to the middle plane of the body at the wrist, while the ulna crosses from the middle to the outside. This forearm posture causes great soreness afterwards and might interfere with subsequent exercises that require fine hand motion.

7.2.6. WRIST AND FINGER FLEXORS
This group of muscles drives its origin from the medial epicondyle of the humerus, which is the bulging part of the bone of the upper arm at the upper, inner side of the elbow. These flex the wrist and fingers. These can be strengthened along with the elbow flexors as in *Figures 7.4* thru *7.7, 7.9* and *7.10*. Pure isolation of the wrist flexors is done by **wrist curls**, *Figure 7.12*, with the elbows supported on a fixed object.

7.2.6.1. Wrist Curls
Purpose
Exercising the forearm flexors is important to lifters and non-lifters. Non-lifters with weak wrist tendons, muscles, and bony structures easily experience "carpel tunnel syndrome" with repetitive finger flexion. Training promotes the growth of these structures and allows better tunneling of the flexor tendons through their long and tortuous course, from the wrist to

the distal phalanxes of the fingers. Weightlifters depend on strong wrist and forearm flexors during Front Squat, Jerk, Press, and Snatch lifts. Strengthening the wrist flexors and extensors builds stronger handgrip and enhances the body response to the handheld weights. Warming up with wrist extension and flexion with light weights may make the difference between success and failure in Weightlifting that is heavily dependent on those wrist functions.

If you keep the balance of the wrist flexors and extensors on the top of your mind, you will find many ways to strengthen these vital muscles. You can accomplish this task amidst many general exercises without the need to worry about including such long list of exercises in your routine. The Chin-ups are the best example for strengthening the wrist flexors. Here, you can exercise the wrist, fingers, and forearm flexors by loosening and tightening your hand gripping on the bar while pulling or lowering your body or while hanging down the Chin-up bar. The Bench Press and Pushups are other examples where you can exercise the wrist and finger flexors by bending and straightening the wrist while the elbows are extended.

Execution
o   As with reverse curling, you can perform wrist curls standing, seating, or squatting. You can also curl with forearm hanging downwards or kept horizontal by flexing the elbow. You can also support the forearms on your thighs while seating, on a bench, or keep them up by Biceps contraction *Figure 7.12*.
o   Hold a light barbell with underhand grip. The knuckles of your hands will be facing downwards and backwards, during the exercise.
o   Wrist curling proceeds by slowly lowering the hand as far as the wrist tendons can tolerate the tension and then elevating the hand as far as the wrist can tolerate flexion. The forearms should stay immobile, too. The only rotating parts are the hands that move around the wrist joints.
o   If you are using the horizontal rod with attached rope in its middle then your handgrip is the reverse of the previous exercise. You will be placing the rod on the top of your palms.
o   Wrist curling entails no crossing of the ulna and radius. The ulna carries most of the weight while the radius maintains balance.

7.3. STRENGTHENING ELBOW EXTENSORS

7.3.1. APPLIED ANATOMY
o   The elbow extensors are a group of muscles that pull the forearm away from the upper arm against a force of resistance that tries to push the forearms towards the upper arm. The force must be applied at the palm of the hand or along the back surface of the forearm.
o   The elbow extensors are the Triceps and Anconeus muscles, *Figures 7.13* and *14*. The Triceps differs from the Biceps in that it drives a wide origin from the humerus, has multiple pinnation and wide insertion into a broad tendon, and its fibers run in many directions. The Triceps has three heads and one common tendon that are inserted into the olecranon process. This is the tip of the back of the elbow and the proximal end of the ulna.

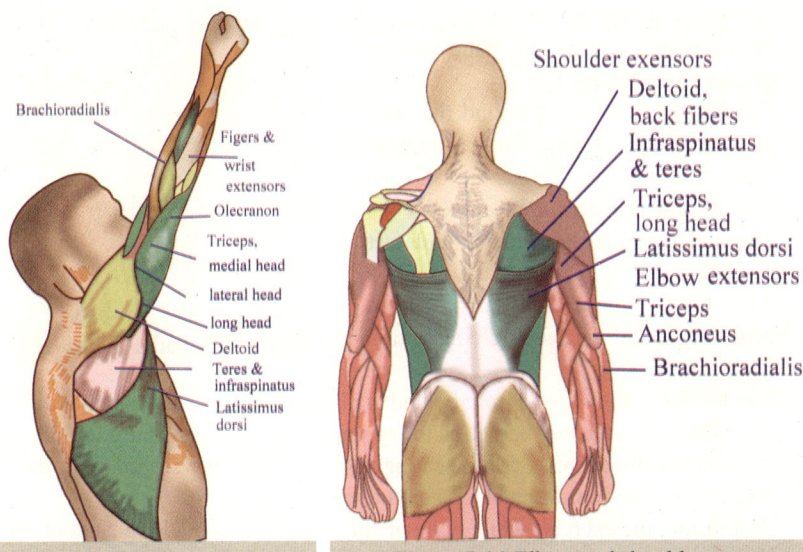

Figure 7.13. Elbow extensors.   *Figure 7.14*. Elbow and shoulder extensors.

o   The **long head of the Triceps** originates from the infra-glenoid tubercle, under the shoulder cavity. It pulls the Triceps tendon medially (thus acts as shoulder adductor) and upwards (thus acts as elbow and shoulder extensor). It can be trained separately from the other two heads if the elbow kept fixed, extended or flexed, while the upper arm is adducted (brought from the side towards the body) against force that tries to pull it away from the body, to the side.
o   **The lateral head** of the Triceps originates from upper back of the humerus. It is inserted into the common Triceps tendon. This head pulls the tendon laterally thus antagonizes the medial pull of the long head during shoulder adduction. The lateral head also pulls the common tendon upwards thus extends the elbow. If the lateral head is weak, the long head will pull the common tendon obliquely on the olecranon, thus causing friction and inflammation of the elbow joint.
o   **The medial head** has a vast origin in the lower part of the back of the humerus. It is inserted on the two sides of the Triceps common tendon. The fibers of the medial head pull the Triceps tendon upwards, laterally, and medially.
o   The Triceps resists the forces applied to the forearm by a 1st degree lever arrangement, *Figure 7.1*. Intense and long training of the Triceps enlarges the bony and soft tissues of the olecranon process and its attached structures. This

muscle-to-bone leverage arrangement imposes double compression on the upper arm, since the resistance and force are parallel and directed upwards (from elbow towards shoulders). The compressed bone adapts to training by thickening and strengthening.

7.3.2. ELBOW EXTENSION EXERCISES

Elbow extension works out the Triceps along with other forearm and shoulder muscles. The following are common Triceps strengthening exercises that utilize elbow extension:

1. Upright elbow extension.
2. One-hand dumbbell elbow extension.
3. Cable pushdown.
4. Forearm kickback.
5. Triceps dips.

7.3.2.1. Upright Elbow Extension

Purpose

Upright elbow extensions is unique in enlarging and strengthening the Triceps with progressively increasing resistance. You can develop awesome Triceps mass with lightweights and progressively increasing your minimal baseline as you progress. You cannot do that in parallel bar dips or Pushups, without cumbersome modification.

Execution

o Upright elbow extension, *Figure 7.15,* is usually performed while standing or seating using a barbell with overhand grips. Overhand, here, refers to placing the palm of the hand on the top of the bar when it was on the floor. During the overhead posture, the hand will be placed under the bar.
o The barbell is lowered behind the head with minimal, if any, body or upper arm movement.
o The elbow is better kept close to the ears and vertically over the shoulder, if possible.
o The lowering of the barbell can proceed slowly if eccentric contraction is desired.

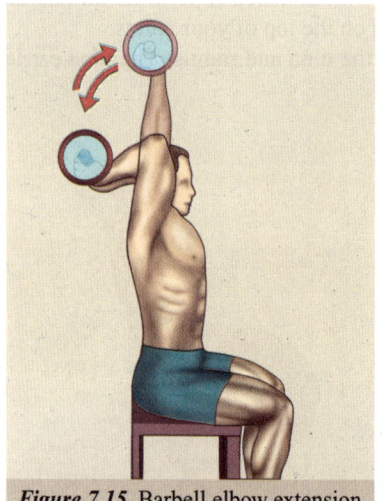 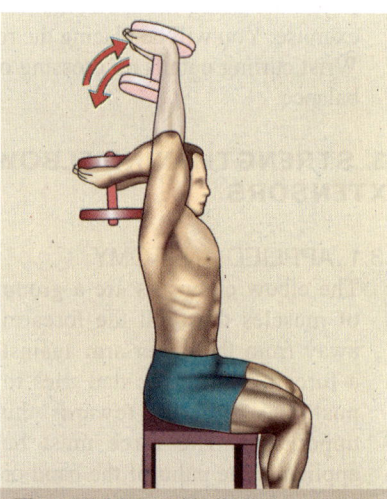

Figure 7.15. Barbell elbow extension. *Figure 7.16.* Dumbbell elbow extension.

o The barbell is then raised from behind the head to full arm extension with the elbows still kept closer to the ears.
o The advantage of using barbell is the symmetrical loading of the shoulder structures.
o Performing the exercise while seating rests the legs, but strains both the Iliopsoas and spinal erectors. These muscles balance the pelvis and spinal axis on the seat.
o Performing the exercise while lying on the back relaxes the long head of the Triceps and the upper Deltoids.
o Keeping the elbows close to the ears increases the isometric tension in the long head of Triceps, by way of shoulder adduction, and works the lateral and medial heads of the Triceps harder then the long head.
o Widely separated elbows put most of the resistance on the long head of the Triceps. The long head of the Triceps is easily exercised in many activities such as Cable rowing, Bend-over rowing, Chin-ups, Deadlift, Clean, and Snatch.

7.3.2.2. One-Hand Dumbbell Elbow Extension

Purpose

o Elbow extension by dumbbells offers more control and manipulation of the muscle recruitment. It requires maximal balance between the long and lateral head of Triceps and the various fiber groups of the Deltoid muscle. Here, there is no limiting bar, as in the case of the barbell extension. Thus, the adducting muscles of the shoulder are activated by overhead dumbbell workout.
o One should resort to one-hand dumbbell exercises when muscular imbalance is suspected to be caused by specific individual muscles. Alternatively, when growth and strength are desired with maximal cardiac and respiratory efforts dedicated to such intense partial exercises.
o One-hand exercises are very nurturing to the body when complementing a wholesome axial training routine but not when comprising the main routine of training. In the latter case, you cannot balance the equation of proportion of size, strength, flexibility, and coordination with training scattered parts of the body.

Execution
- In *Figure 7.16*, the upper arms should be kept upright, the elbow close to the ears.
- The hand that grips the dumbbell should not cross the central plane between the right and left sides[2] of the body. This can be achieved by lowering the weight to touch the shoulder plate from behind and on the side of the extending elbow.
- One-hand dumbbell extension should proceed slowly, upwards as well as downwards, in order to enhance eccentric and concentric contraction.
- Full range of extension and flexion will ensure steady stretching of the tendons and ligaments and thus prevent freezing of elbows. You should lower the weight to touch the body, even if you have to use lightweight.

7.3.2.3. Cable Pushdown
Purpose:
Pushing a loaded cable downwards against upward force of resistance is called **"pushdown"**, *Figures 7.17* and *7.18*. This offers easy approach to Triceps strengthening. Thus, if you are weak in the parallel bar dips then you can work your way towards strengthening the Triceps by progressive increase in resistance with cable pushdowns. These machines are widely used in gyms and require little preparation to get started. The low location of the elbows, beside the waist, requires minimal scapular balance, compared to the upright elbow extensions. This is a disadvantage for people who avoid over shoulder lifting since the scapular muscles lose their ability to coordinate lifting the shoulder with weights held in hand. Pushdown exercises are recommended in states of fatigue or overtraining as a substitute of over shoulder upright elbow extension. The overhand grip strengthens the wrist flexors, *Figure 7.17*, while the underhand grip strengthens the wrist extensors, *Figure 7.18*.

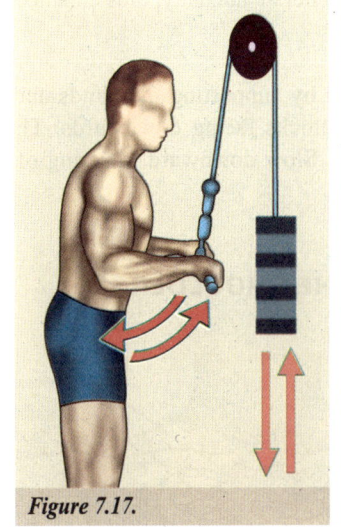
Figure 7.17.

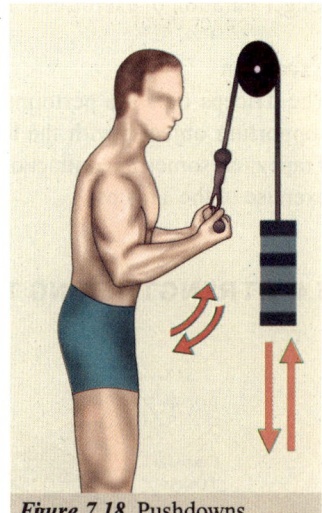
Figure 7.18. Pushdowns.

Execution
- Remember that you are working on the Triceps. Thus, maintain good body stability and only move the forearms around the elbows. The upper arms should be kept as still as possible.
- Also, remember to thrust your chest and maintain lordotic back. Since this exercise emphasizes arm strengthening, the back and chest are supported by isometric contraction and can incur significant strain by just standing still.
- Downward pushing and upward return should proceed as slowly as possible.

7.3.2.4. Forearm Kickback
Purpose
Forearm kickback is performed while standing and leaning forwards, *Figure 7.19*. The horizontal posture of the humerus forces the long head of the Triceps to contract isometrically, during the whole duration of exercise. Consequently, the lateral head has to counteract the contraction of the long head, thus leaving the medial head of the Triceps to kick the forearm backwards. Forearm kickback quickly enlarges the lateral and long head of the Triceps by the isometric contraction that imposes intense inner tissue pressure.

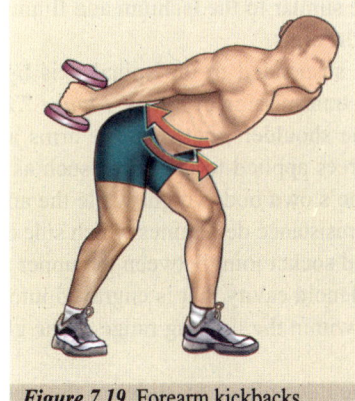
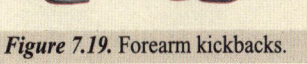
Figure 7.19. Forearm kickbacks.

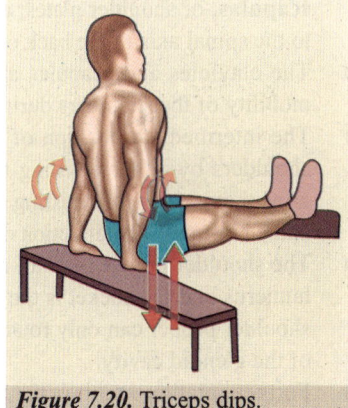
Figure 7.20. Triceps dips.

Execution
- You can perform forearm kickbacks with or without weights. You can also stand with feet placed a shoulder width apart or advance the foot on the opposite side of the working arm. Uneven stance twists the spinal axis and might cause back injury if the spines are not sufficiently warmed up and the duration of the exercise was protracted.
- You should bend both knees in order to relax the spines. You also should bend the torso to horizontal level in order to stretch the back erectors.

---
[2] The central plane between the right and left sides of the body is called "coronal plane". It divides the body into front and back portions.

o   With the elbow elevated backwards and upwards, keep the elbow close to the side of the body.
o   Kickbacks are then performed with the rotation of the forearm on the elbow while the upper arm is kept still in horizontal level. The forearm can be extended to fully straightened arm and the returned back downwards.
o   Slow and steady kicking and returning enhance strength and size. Ballistic motion can traumatize the elbow and the Triceps tendon.

7.3.2.5. Triceps Dips
Purpose
Triceps dips involve elbow extension. They differ from parallel bar dips in reducing the action of the chest muscles and putting less than the whole bodyweight on the Triceps, *Figures 7.20*. They are easier than the parallel bar dips and allow longer duration of exercises at moderate intensity, thus enhance size over strength.

Execution
The Triceps dips are performed by supporting the hands and heels on raised objects and lowering body in between the supporting objects, with the buttocks facing downwards. The upward push requires Triceps concentric contraction and Trapezius isometric contraction. Slow downward lowering of the body can be greatly utilized as an eccentric contraction exercise of the Triceps.

7.4. STRENGTHENING THE SHOULDERS

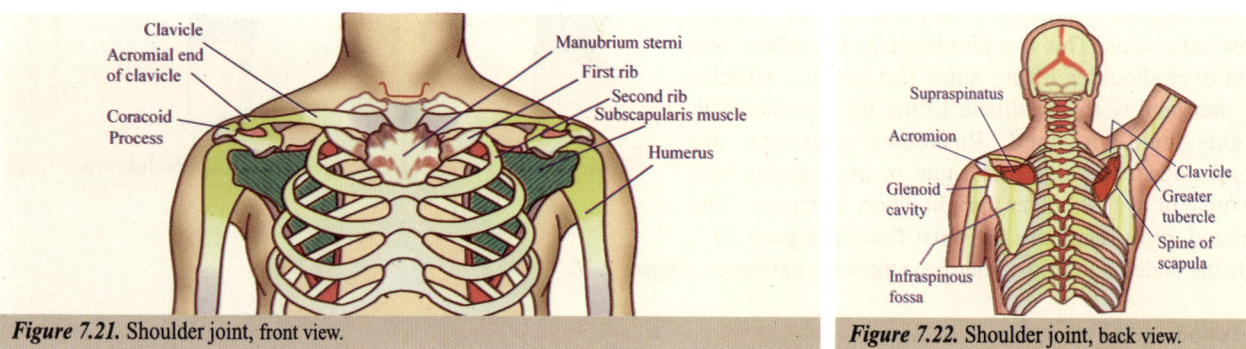

Figure 7.21. Shoulder joint, front view.   *Figure 7.22.* Shoulder joint, back view.

7.4.1. APPLIED ANATOMY
o   The shoulders are intermediate joints between the spinal axis and the upper limbs, *Figures 7.21* and *7.22*.
o   Unlike the hips, which are directly articulating with the spinal axis, there is no direct bony connection between the shoulders and the spinal axis. The arm forces transmit to the spinal axis via the clavicles and scapulas. The **clavicles** are similar to the pubic bone of the pelvis. They form bridges over the vessels and nerves in the front of the arms. The **scapulas**, or shoulder plates, are similar to the Ischium and Ilium of the pelvis. They transmit forces from the shoulders to the spinal axis in the back of the arms.
o   The clavicles and scapulas are suspended to the spinal axis by muscles and tendons that permit greater degree of mobility of the shoulders during transmission of forces, *Figure 7.22*.
o   The intermediate position of the shoulders, between the arms and the spinal axis, makes it possible to exercise the shoulders by either resisting forces applied to the arms (such as lifting weights, pulling loaded cables, or moving the arms themselves) or resisting one's own bodyweight while the arms are kept fixed to external objects (such as Pushups and Chin-ups). The direction of resistance determines which side of the shoulders is exercised.
o   The shoulder proper is a ball and socket joint between the upper arm and the shoulder plate. The ball is the head of the humerus and the socket is the glenoid cavity that is engraved into the lateral upper projection of the shoulder plate. The shoulder proper can only rotate within the limiting range of the gliding spherical surface of the ball on the inner surface of the glenoid cavity.
o   Further rotation requires the shoulder plates to slide on the chest cage with their muscular suspensions in order to rotate the entire shoulder joint, en bloc. The rotation of the scapulas allows raising the arms overheads.
o   By way of the soft tissue suspension of the shoulders to the spinal axis and the semi-spherical gliding of the ball and socket joints, the shoulders can be elevated, rotated, flexed, extended, adducted, and abducted. The hips cannot be elevated or lowered but can perform the other five actions.
o   In order to exercise the shoulder muscles, the following peripheral and axial muscles participate in muscular balance during resistance training:
o   **Peripheral muscles** are the arms muscles that convey the arm forces to the scapula. These muscles are the Biceps, the Triceps, and the Coracobrachialis. The scapular muscles convey the forces from the three surfaces of the shoulder joints to the scapulas. These muscles are the Infraspinatus, the Supraspinatus, the Subscapularis, and the Teres.

o **Axial muscles** are the Trapezius, the Levator scapulae, the Rhomboids, and the Latissimus dorsi. These transmit the scapular forces to the back of the spinal axis. The front components of the scapular forces are transmitted to the spinal axis by the Serratus anterior and the Pectoral muscles through the chest cage. The Scalene and Sternomastoid muscles pull the chest cage upwards towards the spinal axis.
o **Muscular balance:** The balance between the front and back transmission of scapular forces to the spinal axis determines the curvature and relative position of the clavicles and chest cage with respect to the spinal axis. The balance between the forces acting on the shoulder proper, between upper arm and scapula, determines the range of mobility of the shoulder in the three directions.

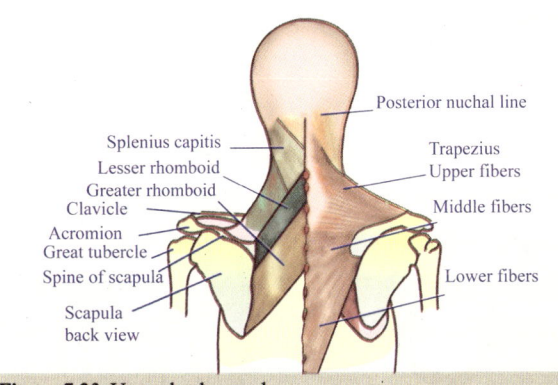

Figure 7.23. Upper back muscles.

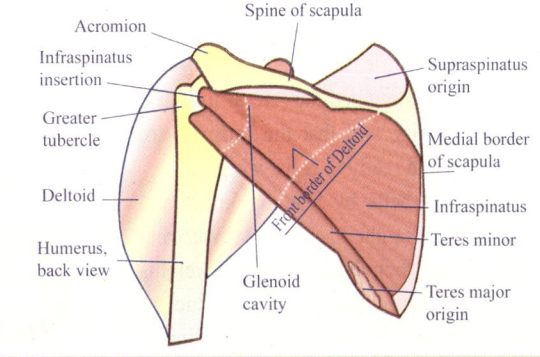

Figure 7.24. Infraspinatus and Deltoid.

7.4.2. SHOULDER ELEVATION

Shoulder elevation, or shoulder shrugging, is carried out by sliding the scapulas upwards along the spinal axis with minimal motion within the shoulder joints. The force of elevation arises from the muscles that attach to the upper spines and the back of the skull and the upper borders of the scapulas.

The main shoulder elevators are the upper fibers of the Trapezius muscle. These pull upwards the scapular spine, the acromion process, and the lateral tip of the clavicles, *Figure 7.23*. The medial upper tip of the scapula is elevated by the Levator muscle of scapula and Rhomboid muscles. The Deltoid and Infraspinatus maintain external rotation of the shoulder thus prevent caving in, *Figure 7.24*. Shoulder elevation is very crucial to lifting since the active muscle lifters are large, with diverse directions, and attach directly to the spinal axis. The Trapezius shrugs the shoulders aggressively during lifting from the lower border of the chest to the shoulder level. During early phases of lifting objects from the floor, the Trapezius stretches and contracts by isometric contraction until substantial shoulder elevation is needed. Here, the pre-stretched Trapezius amplifies the stretch reflex signals and generates vigorous contractile force that moves the heavy weight to the shoulder level and above. The Trapezius not only elevates the shoulders with weights held by the hands, but also resists the vigorous accelerating drive generated by the legs and spinal erectors that create great body momentum. Weak and untrained shoulder elevators cause hunching of the upper spines in the young, old, women, and people with soft bones (osteomalacia and osteoporosis). Beginners and unconditioned people experience discomforting soreness at the back of the neck, when they start practicing Weightlifting due to the contraction of the Trapezius on the back of the neck and the skull.

7.4.2.1. Shoulder Shrugging
Purpose
Shoulder shrugging by dumbbells, *Figure 7.25*, or barbells, works out the upper fibers of the Trapezius, selectively. The dumbbells offer better control of individual muscles. These exercises should be only practiced by beginners or during rehabilitation for the sake of increasing muscle tone and size. There are other superior exercises, which shrug the shoulders better and stronger such as the pulls of Clean, Snatch, and Deadlift.

Execution
The exercise is performed while standing upright with straight and hardened spinal erectors and abdominal muscles, retracted scapulas, and thrust chest. In order to judge whether the scapulas are well retracted or not, you should feel the muscles under the armpits hardened and both arms pushed out to the sides, away from the body as in *Figure 7.25*. In this upright posture, the shoulders are elevated and lowered while the elbows remain straight.

7.4.2.2. One-Hand Dumbbell Side Bends
Purpose
Holding weight in one-hand and bending the body to the opposite side works out the Trapezius, the vertebral muscles between the transverse processes, and the abdominal oblique muscles, *Figure 7.26*. The Trapezius fibers, on the side of the

loaded arm, can be contracted either by shortening by elevating the shoulder, or isometrically by maintaining relative fixed positions of the shoulder bones. The opposite side of the body is tilted by the combined contraction of the muscles in between the transverse processes of the spinal axis, the abdominal oblique muscles between the chest cage and the pelvis, and the Quadratus lumborum muscles between pelvis and lower rib and transverse processes of the lumber vertebra. This lateral flexion exercise is important in conditioning the balance of the lateral sides of the spinal axis that are seldom trained in all weight training exercises.

Execution
o Lateral bending with weights is a serious physical activity and has to be approached with thorough warm-up of the torso. Before you lift the dumbbells, make sure that you have stretched the lateral muscles, without weights, and that the muscles are warmed up and ready to resist weights.
o Lift the dumbbells by bending knees and maintaining straight back. Remember that people injure their back with lightweights more than with heavy weight due to underestimating the seriousness of lifting.
o After assuming straight upright posture with lordotic back and thrust chest, bend slowly to the opposite side of the dumbbell held arm. You will increase the angle of bending with training. Yet, as a beginner, you should not exaggerate bending in order to avoid tearing the fibers of these unused muscles or herniating spinal discs.

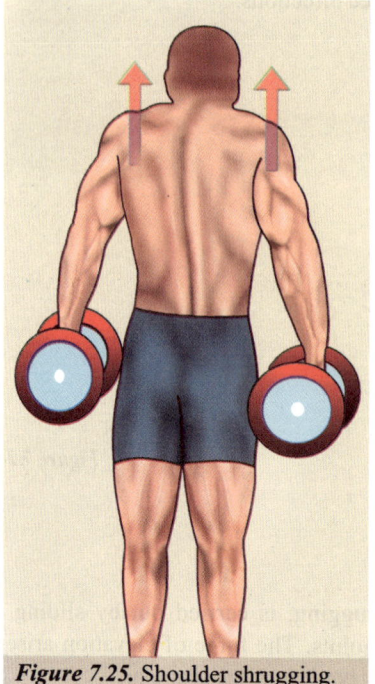

Figure 7.25. Shoulder shrugging.

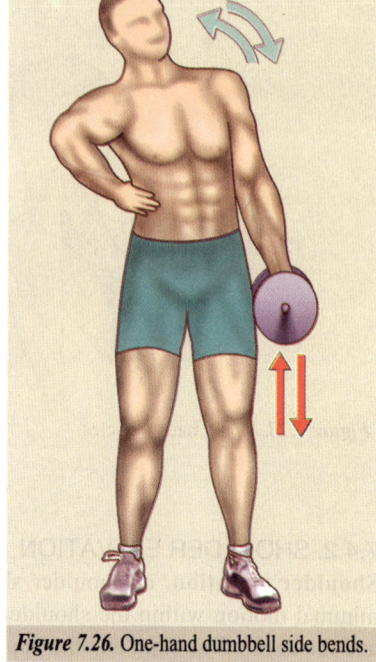

Figure 7.26. One-hand dumbbell side bends.

7.4.3. SHOULDER EXTERNAL ROTATION
o **Shoulder rotation is carried out by rotating the ball of the head of the humerus on the socket of glenoid cavity.** Lateral or external rotation comprises of the front surface of the arms turning to the outside. Inside turning comprises medial or internal rotation.
o **External rotation** is carried out by the combined actions of the Deltoid posterior fibers that are inserted at the lateral border of the middle of the humerus, and the Infraspinatus that is inserted at the greater tubercle of the humerus, *Figure 7.24.* The external rotators are thus located behind the humerus.
o The Infraspinatus is one of the four rotator cuff muscles and helps anchor the ball of the humerus into its socket, when the Deltoid performs rotation. Injury or weakness of the Infraspinatus can be suspected in motions that throw the elbow behind the shoulders. This happens in Bench Press or deep Push-ups that force the ball posteriorly against weak or damaged Infraspinatus.
o Strengthening the posterior Deltoid, by external rotation and rowing compensate for the weak Infraspinatus. External rotation is encountered in combination with other muscular actions such as in the Snatch lift, where the arms rotate externally above shoulder levels. There are many exercises that strengthen the two external rotators. The following are common shoulder exercises that enhance external rotation:
  1. One-hand dumbbell rows.
  2. Bent-over lateral arm raises.
  3. Bent-over rows.
  4. T-bar bent-over row.
  5. Seated cable rows.

7.4.3.1. One-Hand Dumbbell Rows
Purpose
Dumbbell rowing, *Figure 7.27,* works out each side in isolation and can be used to create impressive size, definition, and strength of the back Deltoid.

Execution
o It is performed while leaning forwards, bending on a bench, or without the support of a bench. The lower back is the weakest link in this posture. Thus it must be arched in and maintained hardened.

o   The dumbbell is pulled slowly from the floor upwards until the elbow reaches maximal elevation. It is then lowered slowly to the floor. Touching the floor with each lift increases the range of motion. The body should maintain still, bent posture. If the body bounces upwards and downwards then other muscles are aiding the shoulder extensors.
o   The elbows can point into three different directions. The elbow may point away from the body. This is called "transverse abduction" because the upper arms are abducted in plane that is transverse to the body axis[3].
o   If the elbow points backwards during pulling, then other back muscles assist the posterior Deltoid and Infraspinatus such as the Latissimus dorsi. The backward elbow pulling extends the shoulder.
o   Leaning such that the back is kept horizontal guarantees posterior Deltoid workout without the assistance of the lateral Deltoid. This kick in during shoulder abduction, while the body is in oblique or upright posture.

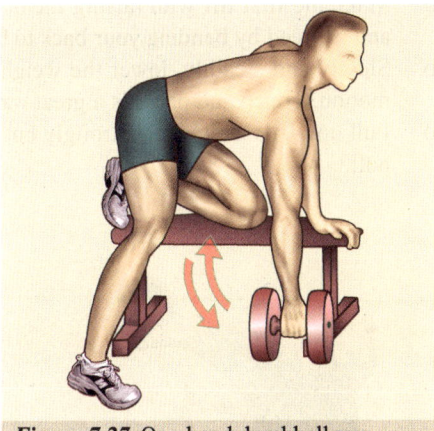

Figure 7.27. One-hand dumbbell row.

7.4.3.2. Bent-Over Lateral Arm Raises
Purpose

Arm raises with dumbbells, *Figure 7.28*, or cables, *Figure 7.29*, are sometimes practiced for the sake of change and symmetry, particularly when other exercises seem to create imbalance. One-hand held dumbbells or cable handles can pin point the weak and sluggish muscles and emphasize the side that need more exercise in order to catch up with the whole body.

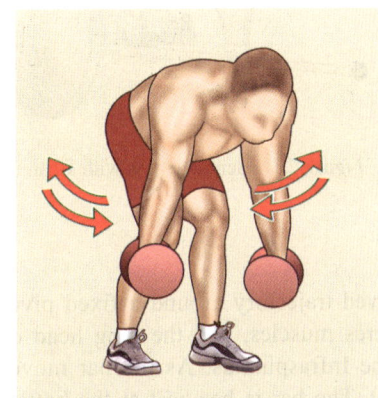 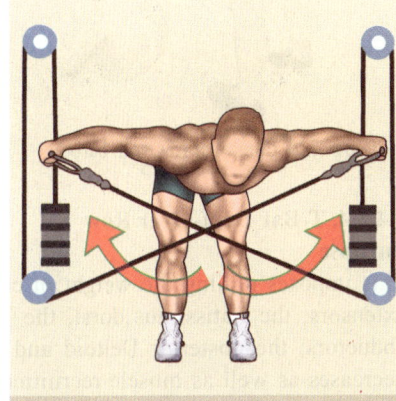

Figure 7.28. Bent-over lateral arm dumbbell-raises.   *Figure 7.29.* Bent-over lateral arm cable-raises.

Execution
o   The dumbbells or the cables have to be pulled with the body kept still while the arms are abducted transversely.
o   The torso has to assume the horizontal position if transverse abduction is to be achieved. If the torso rises and falls during pulling or raising, then neither the Infraspinatus nor the posterior Deltoid would be worked out through full range of motion, though they might benefit from the jerky motion of the body.
o   Slow and steady motion is the essence of arm raises since these aim at enhancing muscular control, size, and strength.

7.4.3.3. Bent-Over Rows
Purpose
o   There are many modifications to this exercise that alter its target muscle. Leaning forwards until the back assumes horizontal level and pulling the barbell from the floor, works out the posterior Deltoid and Infraspinatus.
o   The close or Clean handgrip increases the range of motion.
o   The wide or Snatch handgrip increases isometric contraction, but limits the range of motion.
o   Leaning forwards obliquely works out the lateral Deltoid head.
o   Pulling with elbows pointed backwards and kept close to the sides, involves the Latissimus dorsi.
o   Retracting and spreading the scapulas during pulling and lowering the weight works out the Trapezius middle fibers by concentric contraction, instead of the isometric contraction have the scapulas been kept fixed.
o   Lowering and raising the torso, while pulling and lowering the weight, works out the spinal erectors, Hamstrings, and Glutei with concentric contraction.

Execution
o   These are performed by pulling a barbell from the floor upwards while bending over the barbell, *Figure 7.30.* Since lifting is performed with the back bent horizontally, therefore thorough warm-up and light start are mandatory in order to avoid serious injury.
o   Start the first lift by full Squatting to the barbell. This way you can probe the flexibility and readiness of your Hamstrings and lower back.

---

[3] Transverse plane is a plane that divides the body into upper and lower portions.

- o Make the first lift with raising the back upright before assuming the bent-over posture. Then bend your knees slightly and proceed by bending your back to horizontal level.
- o Slowly and steadily, lower the weight. You can touch the floor each lift if you enjoy perfectionism and full range of motion. Touch and pause is a great way of enhancing muscular control.
- o Pull upwards slowly and strongly but remember to tighten your lower back and thrust your chest before and during the pull.

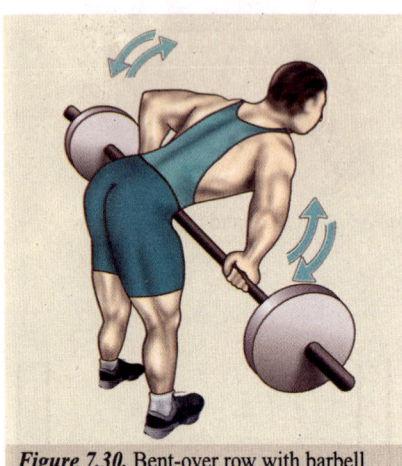
Figure 7.30. Bent-over row with barbell.

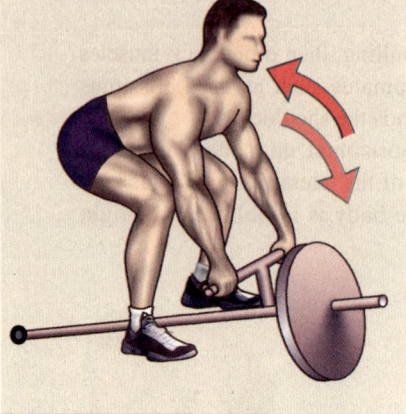
Figure 7.31. Bent-over row with T-bar.

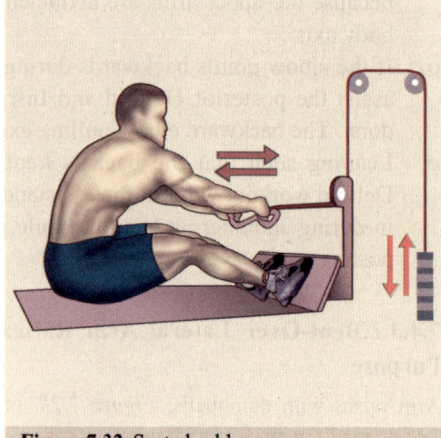
Figure 7.32. Seated cable row.

7.4.3.4. T-Bar Bent-Over Row
Purpose
This imposes pulling the weight in curved trajectory around a fixed pivot, *Figure 7.31*. The T-bar works the shoulder extensors; the Latissimus dorsi, the Teres muscles, and the long head of Triceps; along with the transverse shoulder abductors; the posterior Deltoid and the Infraspinatus. As the bar moves upwards, the horizontal lever arm of force decreases as well as muscle recruitment. The bar is heaviest at the bottom. Such variation in resistance lends different adaptation of the neuromuscular control.

Execution
- o Like bent-over row, warm up and start light to avoid injury. Since you are pulling upwards and backwards, your back is exposed to both shear stress and compression. This requires very attentive back hardening in lordotic posture.
- o Rowing can also proceed in three elbow directions. Elbows moving close to the sides of the body enforce shoulder extensors. Elbows pointing away from the body emphasize shoulder transverse abduction. Elbows directed in the middle between the sides of the body and the transverse plane, at the chest, balance extensors and abductors.
- o Elevating the hips and lowering the chest levels engages the middle scapular muscles than the upper muscles. This is more desirable since the middle scapular muscles are seldom trained sufficiently.

7.4.3.5. Seated Cable Rows
Purpose
- o Seated cable rowing is very common and useful exercise, *Figure 7.32*. The major advantage of this exercise is the ability to work out the desired muscles, for long time and at desired progressive pace, without draining your energy resources in postural balance.
- o The close hand griping on the cable handle increases the range of shoulder transverse abduction. Also, as is the case with bent-over rows, this exercise can be modified to work out the transverse shoulder abductors (posterior Deltoid and the Infraspinatus), the shoulder extensors (Latissimus dorsi, Teres muscles, and long head of Triceps), the spinal erectors, and the scapular retractors (middle Trapezius fibers and Rhomboids).
- o Its disadvantage lies in the lack of adequate tone on the spinal erectors unless the person remembers to assume erect upright back. Pulling with the rounded back is dangerous.
- o Slow pulling and slow return of the cable enhance isometric contraction and causes fast growth of the muscle size.
- o Jumping to seated cable rows, prior to warm-up and with heavy weight, invite troubles because the cable pulls perpendicular to the spinal axis and can easily cause severe disc herniation.

Execution
- o Seated cable rowing can be performed with both or one-handed. The latter is asymmetric and requires great attention to spinal integrity.
- o Although the seated position eases the exercise, yet the full range of motion should not be compromised. Rowing should proceed with upright torso posture or slightly leaning forwards. The elbow should extend from full extension to

full flexion. The torso might move after the end of elbow action or during it. Still torso emphasizes shoulder extension while bouncing the torso adds more toning to the spinal muscles.

7.4.4. SHOULDER INTERNAL ROTATION

Internal rotation of the shoulder is carried out by the combined action of the **Pectoralis major, Subscapularis** (both are shoulder transverse adductors), **Latissimus dorsi, Teres** (both are shoulder extensors), and **anterior fibers of Deltoid** (shoulder flexor), *Figures 7.21, 7.22* and *7.24*. All internal rotators are inserted to the front of the humerus. Two of them (Deltoid and Pectoralis major) originates from the front of the chest and shoulders. The other four (Teres, Subscapularis, and Latissimus dorsi) originate from behind the chest. Thus, internal shoulder rotation encompasses the use of the shoulder proper, chest, and back muscles. The following are common exercises for enhancing shoulder internal rotation:

Anterior Deltoid exercises	Subscapularis exercises	Pectoralis major exercises
o Barbell Shoulder Press.	o Dumbbell flyes.	o Bench Press.
o Seated Shoulder Press.	o Incline dumbbell flyes.	o Inclined Bench Press.
o One-hand Shoulder dumbbell Press.	o Inclined dumbbell Press.	o Pushups.
o Dumbbell front raises.	o Cable flyes.	o Parallel bar dips.
o Cable front raises.	o Deck flyes.	
	o Pullover.	

These exercises share one common feature, that is, they involve **"pushing or Pressing"** the weight by both arms. These are the most famous weight training exercises and rightfully so. The following five exercises emphasize strengthening of the **anterior Deltoid**.

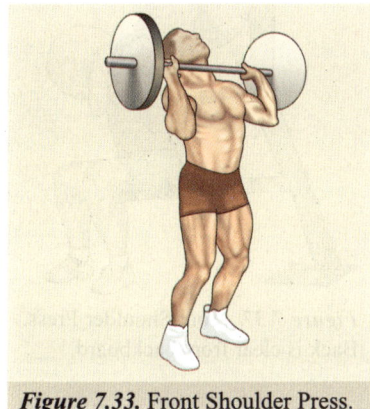 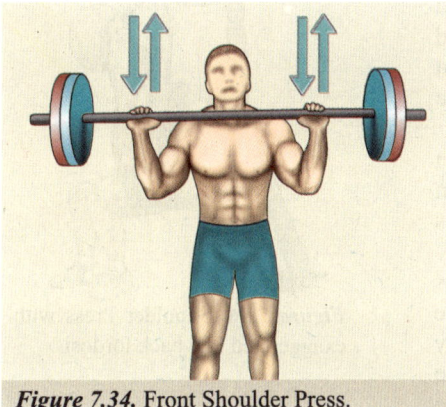 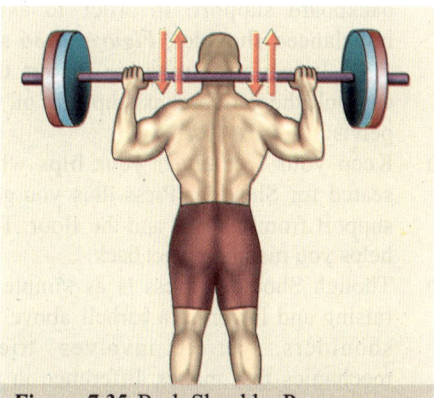

Figure 7.33. Front Shoulder Press.   *Figure 7.34.* Front Shoulder Press.   *Figure 7.35.* Back Shoulder Press.

7.4.4.1. Barbell Shoulder Press
Purpose
Shoulder Press with barbell works out the front fibers of the Deltoid, *Figures 7.33* and *7.34*.
o **From the early years of training, Weightlifters practice shelving the bar on the shoulders and over the** sternomandibular joint, at the root of the neck.
o Lifting the bar from this location with the elbows lowered below the shoulders works out the **Supraspinatus** muscles intensely. These muscles, one on each side, arise from the back of the scapulas, from above the scapular spine, and run over the shoulder joint where they insert into the greater tubercle of the humerus, *Figure 7.22*. Adults who started training after the age of eighteen, those who do not have regular daily training routine, or beginners have to be very careful in lifting heavy weight with the elbows below the shoulders. In this posture, a weak Supraspinatus can snap torn causing life long shoulder problem of torn rotator cuff. Gradual and progressive regular training is required to strengthen the Supraspinatus.
o The fame of Front Shoulder Press stems from its **multiple target of major muscles**. The Supraspinatus starts anchoring the shoulder ball, the front Deltoids flex the shoulders by moving the upper arms forwards and upwards. The upper Trapezius kicks in and rotates the scapulas to the sides by pulling their upper and outer tips. The Triceps extends the elbow. The spinal erectors contract isometrically to erect the spinal axis.
o **Standing Shoulder Press** is very taxing on the cardiovascular system but is a fundamental exercise for Weightlifters. With training, standing Shoulder Press conditions the sympathetic nervous system to adapt to such strenuous activity. All postural muscles work harder during standing Shoulder Press. Weightlifters practice shoulder Press after the Clean lift from the floor and thus have to perform high shoulder flexion (elbows are raised to the Shoulder level under the bar), followed by lowering the elbows to initiate the Shoulder Press.

WEIGHT TRAINING

o Shoulder Press from **behind the shoulders** still works out the front Deltoid but puts the posterior Deltoid, Infraspinatus, and middle Trapezius under constant isometric tension in order to retract the scapulas backwards, *Figure 7.35*. The Supraspinatus are less stretched with back Shoulder Press since the elbows are slightly elevated more than in the front shoulder position. The retracted scapulas, in back Shoulder Press, are desired for increasing tone of the scapular retractors.

Execution
o Barbell Shoulder Press should not be performed without prior lifting from the floor, in the same session. Lifting from a rack, without prior warm-up by lifting from the floor, exposes the lower back into acute and intense shear stresses.
o Lifting from a rack can follow lifting from the floor, for the sake of reducing the load volume.
o With the barbell loaded on the front of the back of the shoulders, harden the lower back and thrust the chest prior to initiating the Shoulder Press.
o The very early few millimeters of the Press pre-stretch the Deltoids and enhance subsequent lifting. Push upwards slowly with the shoulder, and not the legs or the torso. These work in the Jerk lift.
o As soon as the bar passes the level of the eyebrow, the pushing should be directed backwards, in the case of front shoulder Press, and forwards, in the case of back Shoulder Press.
o Fully extend the elbow overheads, in order to avoid shortening of the shoulder ligaments and tendons. You can pause at the top to gain more shoulder stability.
o Lower the bar slowly in reverse sequence. Preferably, the bar should be lowered to the shoulders. Repeat the Press from three to eight times.
o Reduce the number of repetitions as the weight increases.

7.4.4.2. Seated Shoulder Press
Execution
o **This should be done with little or no** backboard support, in order to avoid imbalanced shoulder, *Figures 7.36* and *7.37*. It requires strong hip flexors that can pull the vertebral axis upright on the pelvis.
o Keep your feet under your hips when seated for Shoulder Press thus you gain support from the seat and the floor. This helps you maintain erect back.
o Though Shoulder Press is as simple as raising and lowering a barbell above the shoulders, yet it involves tricky mechanics that makes difference in the final outcome. The beginning of the

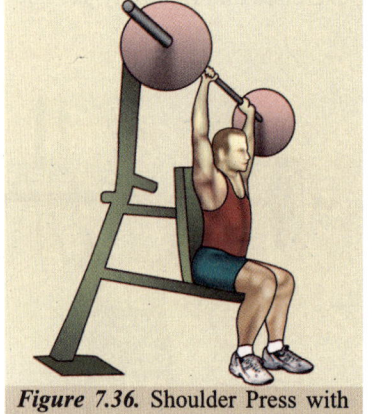
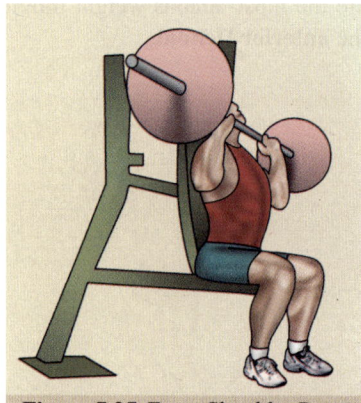

Figure 7.36. Shoulder Press with exaggerated low back lordosis.

Figure 7.37. Front Shoulder Press. Back is clear from backboard.

Press should start with well-erected back, whether standing or seating and well thrust chest. These two actions facilitate blood flow to and from the arms, head, and chest.
o The thrust chest supports the Deltoids and the Supraspinatus when they initiate the Press from the shoulders, upwards, to the chin level.
o In the front position, the head should be kept flexible, moves backwards when the bar passes the neck. This prevents hitting the chin, nose, or forehead. The bar then moves forwards when it passes the level of the eyebrows in order to maintain the bar center of mass over the body axis. Keeping rigidly stuck head, during raising and lowering the weight, causes muscular deformity of the shoulder and upper back.
o Slow lifting and lowering enhances isometric contraction and induces fast muscular growth in addition to enhancing adaptation to stretching of ligaments and tendons.

7.4.4.3. One-Hand Shoulder Dumbbell Press
Purpose
o Shoulder dumbbell Press is the golden standard in shoulder Strengthening, *Figure 7.38*. One can balance weak shoulders by increasing the number of sets on the weaker side.
o One can also increase flexibility by lowering the dumbbell very close to the clavicle and rotate the arms while raising and lowering the weight. This exercise forces the Supraspinatus to work hardest since there is no limiting bar that ties the two arms transversely. Thus, light and high repetition shoulder Press, with dumbbells can greatly strengthen this important rotator cuff muscles.
o Pressing by one-hand increases the isometric tone of the fixed shoulder. Simultaneous arms raising and lowering, alternatively, enhances the motor control of the Trapezius, Deltoid, and Supraspinatus. With one-hand Shoulder Press, you can develop greater edge in competitive sports that require strong shoulders.

Execution

o Shoulder Press with dumbbells can be performed while standing or seating. It can be performed with the hand fists directed forwards or medially. It can also be performed with elbows directed forwards or laterally, to the outside.

o The posture of the hand fists determines the tension on the rotator cuff muscles. Front elbows posture stretches the Supraspinatus muscle. Lateral elbows posture stretches the Subscapularis muscles.

o Regular stretching of the rotator cuff muscles is paramount to shoulder mobility and integrity. This cannot be achieved without gradual, progressive, and regular training.

7.4.4.4. Dumbbell Front Raises
Purpose

This front Deltoid strengthening exercise is practiced by some weight trainees using one dumbbell, in one or both hands, and raising and lowering the dumbbell, with extended elbows, from the waist level to the shoulder level, *Figure 7.39*. Though this exercise works out the front Deltoid, yet it exaggerates upper body hunching. It enhances the definition of the front fibers of the Deltoid and fosters neuromuscular control of the shoulder joint. It almost eliminates the assisting action of the lateral Deltoids, by way of imposing two hands gripping of the dumbbell.

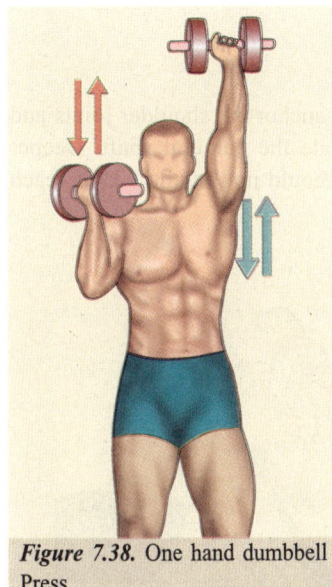

Figure 7.38. One hand dumbbell Press.

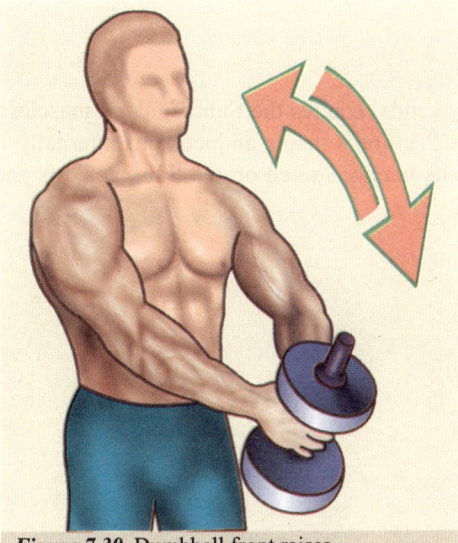

Figure 7.39. Dumbbell front raises.

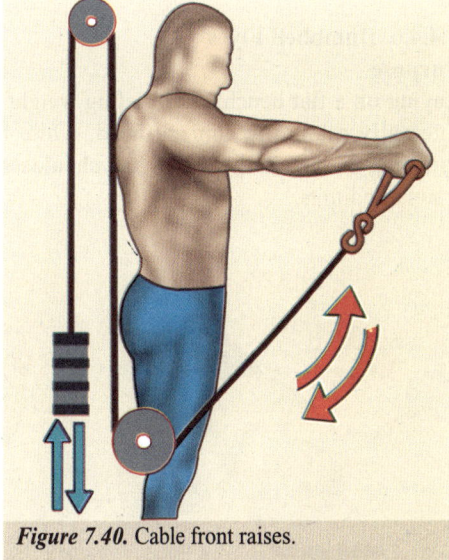

Figure 7.40. Cable front raises.

Execution

o Holding a weight in front of the body and lifting it upwards and then reversing the motion is called **"front raises"** if the elbows are kept extended during the raising. Thus, only shoulders are bent, or flexed, during lifting the weight.

o If lower back or upper back are forgotten and thrown into kyphotic posture, then the exercise would do more harm than good. The chest should also be kept in extreme upward thrust to compensate for the momentum of front raising.

o Light weight with slow and proper technique will accomplish the goal of this exercise, which is the exaggeration of the definition of the front Deltoid and the stimulation of sluggish muscle bundles.

7.4.4.5. Cable Front Raises
Purpose

These convenient exercises require minimal preparation to work out the front Deltoid muscle, *Figure 7.40*. It dedicates the whole body energy for the workout of few muscles, to the most. The Trapezius stabilizes the scapulas isometrically while the front Deltoid raises the arm. The elbow is kept extended during raising and lowering the arm. Like all one hand exercises, cable front raises enhance motor control and allow impressive development of the working muscles.

Execution

Cable front raises differ from dumbbell front raises in the direction of pull and the asymmetry of action. Since the cable is directed obliquely, the shoulder has to engage both the front Deltoid and the scapular retractors to account for the oblique trajectory of forces.

Slow and steady raising, with the shoulder acting as the only effector muscle, would dramatically enhance the front Deltoid and foster greater neuromuscular control. With one cable, you cannot conceal asymmetric balance with the other arm and thus you have to deal with realistic arm condition.

7 WEIGHT TRAINING

The next six exercises emphasize strengthening of the **Subscapularis** muscle. The Subscapularis is one of the four rotator cuff muscles and acts as internal rotator and stabilizer of the shoulder. It passes from the front of the scapula to the front surface of the shoulder joint, under the tendon of the short head of Biceps to reach the lesser tubercle of the humerus, *Figure 7.41*. Although the Subscapularis and the Pectoralis major act as internal rotators, the former acts closer to the joint on the lesser tubercle. The Subscapularis passes backwards under the coracoid process, whereas the Pectoralis acts farther away from the joint on the crest of the greater tubercle and passes forwards above the tendons of the Biceps. Thus, the two muscles work in synergy to rotate and adduct the humerus. One pulls the humerus backwards and inwards from the top of the humerus, while the other pulls forwards and inwards from a lower point down the humerus.

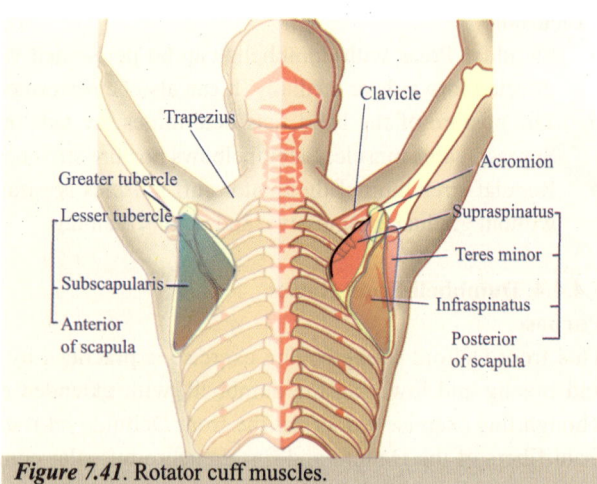

Figure 7.41. Rotator cuff muscles.

7.4.4.6. Dumbbell Flyes
Purpose

Laying on a flat bench and resisting weight by hands requires the Subscapularis muscles to anchor the shoulder joints and internally rotate the humeral head, while the Pectoralis major adducts and internally rotate the humeral shaft. Deeper lowering of the elbows below the shoulders puts intense stretch on the Subscapularis and should not be allowed to reach traumatic limits.

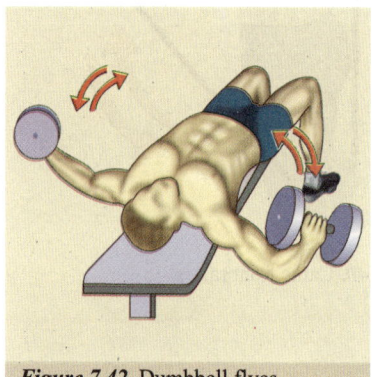
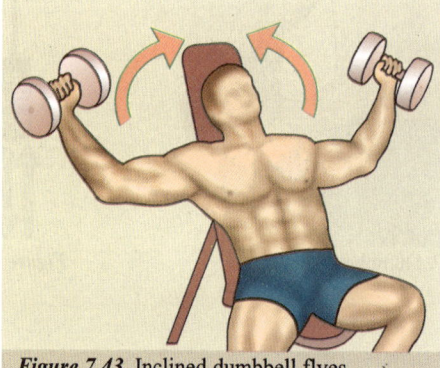
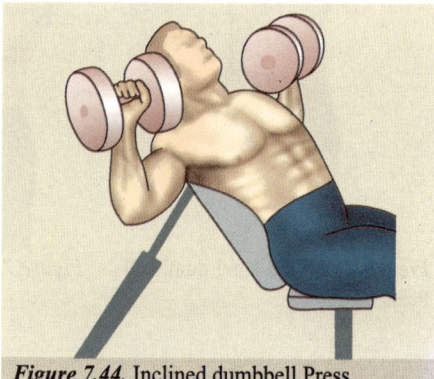

Figure 7.42. Dumbbell flyes.   *Figure 7.43.* Inclined dumbbell flyes.   *Figure 7.44.* Inclined dumbbell Press.

Execution
o   These are performed by holding two dumbbells, one in each hand, while lying on a bench, *Figure 7.42*.
o   Spread the arms to the sides, transversely on the body axis. The hand fists may be directed to the inside- medially or downwards with respect to spinal axis. Thus, the dumbbell axis is either longitudinal or transverse with respect to the body axis. Spreading the arms can proceed laterally as far as the shoulder joint can tolerate but not beyond or below chest horizontal level.
o   You can pause briefly at the bottom in order to stretch the Subscapularis and Pectoralis major, or you can proceed reversing the motion and elevating the arms.
o   Raising the dumbbells upwards can be accompanied by some degree of bending of the elbows.
o   The dumbbells should be let loose without hesitation if any tense feeling or pain is experienced at the shoulder. Distraction should be minimized during performing of this high-risk exercise in order to maintain focus on contracting active muscles.

7.4.4.7. Incline Dumbbell Flyes
Purpose

These shift the resistance to the clavicular fibers of the Pectorals major and anterior Deltoid in addition to working out the Subscapularis, *Figure 7.43*. Its rationale is based on enhancing the bridging of the clavicle over the vital vessels and nerves to the arms and head thus enhances upper body strength. The flyes differ from Shoulder Press in their transverse motion across the body axis. This posture requires isometric contraction of the Biceps and Triceps to maintain fixed elbows.

Execution

o   With inclined bench flyes, you have the opportunity to enhance upper chest bulging, or thrusting, by strengthening the clavicular fibers of Pectoralis major and Pectoralis minor. Thus maintaining lordotic lower back will allow full stretching of the Subscapularis muscles and enhances chest upward bulging.

o   With hand fists facing medially, to the inside, the Biceps brachii are less tense and most of the weight falls on the chest adductors to bring the arms upwards and forwards. These are the Subscapularis and Pectoralis major.

o   With hand fists facing forwards, the Biceps are stretched and the arms are more secure in spreading to the sides under the tone of the Biceps.

o   Flyes are slow motion exercises that focus on enhancing wide range of motion of privileged muscles such as the Subscapularis. There is no need to increase speed or perform abrupt moves.

7.4.4.8. Inclined Dumbbell Press
Purpose

This is another great exercise of the Subscapularis, anterior Deltoid, clavicular head of Pectoral muscles, and the Triceps, *Figure 7.44*. The inclined position shifts the resistance away from the Supraspinatus to the Subscapularis. It is intended to enlarge and strengthen the upper chest muscles in order to enhance arm and head perfusion.

Execution

o   The dumbbells are Pressed upwards and lowered with steady and preferably slow motion. As with upright shoulder Press, this exercise can be used to develop very strong and massive shoulder and upper chest.

o   The Press motion differs from the flyes motion in that; Pressing is directed upwards, while flyes are spreading laterally, in curved trajectory.

o   Performing this exercise two or three times per week, with minimum of three sets at over 60% 1RM, can greatly enhance shoulder function in just few weeks.

7.4.4.9. Cable Flyes
Purpose

This exercise facilitates the working out of shoulder rotators by its easy access and uniform resistance, **Figure 7.45**. The standing position shifts the resistance from the upper Pectoral fibers to the lower ones. Cable flyes with acute forward leaning, to horizontal back position, can shift the resistance towards the middle Pectoral fibers.

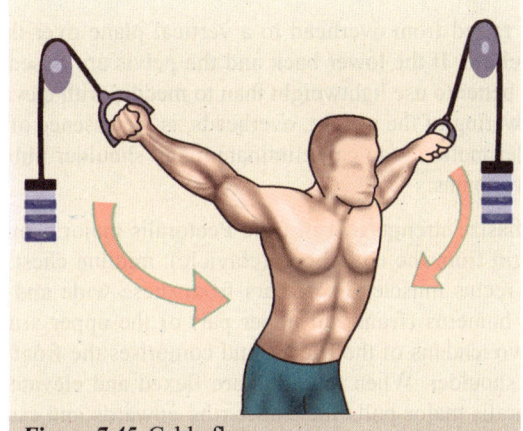
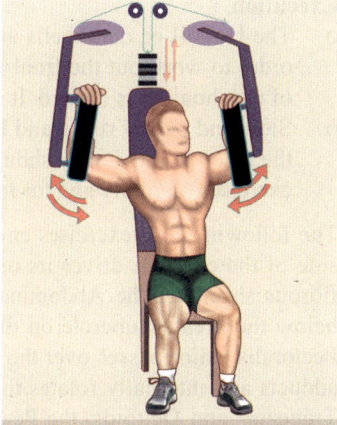

Figure 7.45. Cable flyes.   *Figure 7.46.* Pectoral deck flyes.

Execution

o   The level of the cable pulleys determines which section of the chest that performs the resistance.

o   The cables are pulled, slowly and steadily, from the sides towards the middle with extended elbows. The elbows might be kept slightly bent, but should remain in their initial angle, during the course of pulling and returning of the cables.

o   Maintain retracted scapulas and thrust chest in order to avoid habitual kyphosis.

o   Full range of motion comprises of pulling medially until the two hands come very close together and then return the cable until both arms are stretched to the sides, but not far, behind the chest.

7.4.4.10. Deck Flyes
Purpose

These are unique in applying the force to the medial side of the forearms with both arms externally rotated by the limiting deck handles, *Figure 7.46*. This is of greatest importance to people with hand or wrist injuries or inherited deformities. Most of the adduction of the shoulder is shifted to the Subscapularis and Pectoralis major since the externally rotated and transverse arms inactivate the Deltoids by moving their points of insertion far to the back of and above the upper arms.

Execution

o   The backboard support and arm decks make this exercise one of the safest weight training exercises. Another trick to make it safer is to initiate the loading with both elbows in order to avoid twisting the lower back, had only one elbow being used.

o   Also, if you maintain normal range of motion, you would not overstretch the Subscapularis. Normal range means maintaining the elbows in the range from the sides of the body to the front, and not behind the body. You can increase

WEIGHT TRAINING

that range if you advance in training and gain more experience in recognizing your limits of flexibility and strength.
o   Another great tip in performing this exercise is the pushing of the decks with palms of both hands, instead of the elbows. In this case, the Biceps brachii is short and strong and the chest is in exaggerated bulging posture. That means that the Pectoralis major muscles are fully stretched during resistance. This way you gain both shoulder flexibility and strength.

7.4.4.11. Pullover
Purpose
This exercise is a rare tool in the repertoire of peripheral weight training. It permits overhead lifting in supine position. It assists in reversing shoulder imbalance due to shortened shoulder adductors and extensors (Pectoralis major, Latissimus dorsi, Subscapularis, Teres, and long head of Biceps muscles), *Figures 7.47* and *7.48*. The extreme elongation of the shoulder adductors may reverse the shortening of these muscles and facilitate proper posture. The abdominal muscles and the long head of the Triceps work out during the rising of the weight from overhead to a vertical plane.

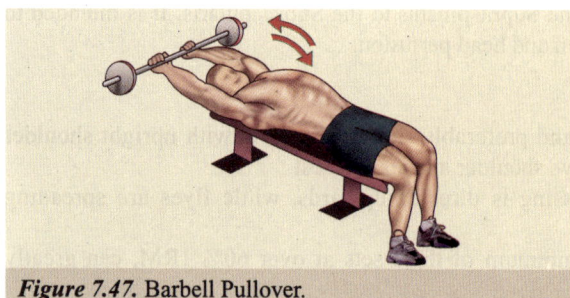
Figure 7.47. Barbell Pullover.

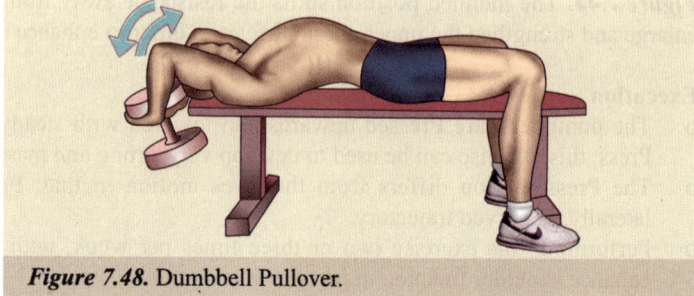
Figure 7.48. Dumbbell Pullover.

Execution
o   The barbell or dumbbells are raised from overhead to a vertical plane over the shoulders or even to the abdomen in order to work out the front Deltoid. If the lower back and the pelvis are raised off the bench then the range of motion of the shoulder is limited. It is better to use lightweight than to meddle with elevating the pelvis off the bench.
o   Slow and steady rising and lowering of the weight, overheads, is the essence of this stretching exercise. If you focus on the smooth and steady shoulder motion, you can eliminate many shoulder imbalance problems, with performing these exercises regularly and for few months.

The following four exercises emphasize strengthening of the Pectoralis major. This muscle covers the entire front of each side of the chest. It drives its origin from the collarbone (clavicle), midline chest bone (sternum), upper six ribs, and the fibrous sheath of the Abdominal rectus muscle. The fibers from these wide and multiple origins converge on the crest below the greater tubercle on the humerus (front and upper part of the upper arm bone), *Figure 7.2*. The tendon of the Pectoralis major passes over the two tendons of the Biceps and comprises the front flap of the armpit. The Pectoralis major adducts and internally rotates the shoulder. When the arms are flexed and elevated by the strong combined action of the Trapezius and Deltoids, the Pectoralis major pulls the upper ribs upwards and outwards, towards the shoulders, with the help of the Pectoralis minor. The latter pulls the ribs towards the coracoid process of the scapula.

7.4.4.12. Bench Press
Purpose
This is a universally known exercise that works out the Pectoralis major, Subscapularis, Triceps, and anterior Deltoid, in addition to the Serratus anterior.

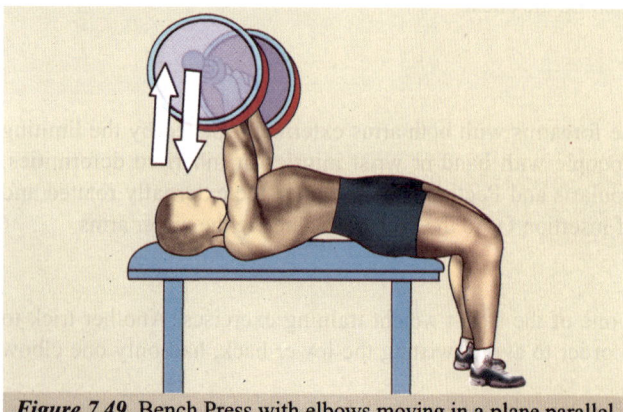
Figure 7.49. Bench Press with elbows moving in a plane parallel to the body axis.

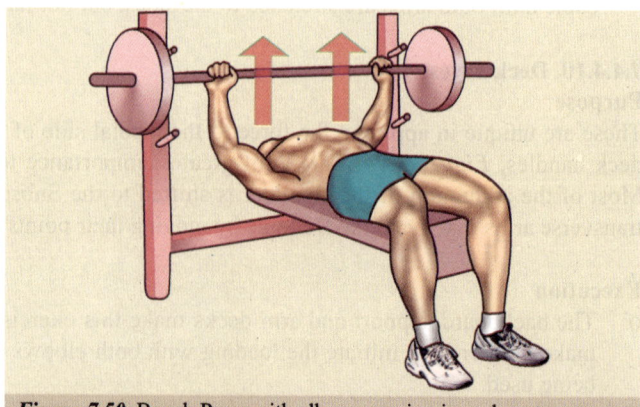
Figure 7.50. Bench Press with elbows moving in a plane transverse to the body axis.

Execution
o The Bench Press is performed on a flat horizontal bench, *Figures 7.49* and *7.50.* During Pressing, the body abuts the bench at the shoulder plates. The buttocks and the feet may take support from the floor.
o Arching the lower back upwards in this supine position guarantees proper spinal support during forceful lifting by the chest. Recall that contracting the chest muscles increases upper body venous pressure and hence increases intracerebral fluid pressure, which in turn affects spinal perfusion. This is aggravated by kinked spinal cord, in the case of rounding the back posteriorly. The erect and concave lower back assists in elevating the ribs and thrusting the chest thus facilitating the generation of force by increasing the size of the chest cavity.
o Close hand gripping of the bar in Bench Press increases the Triceps range of concentric contraction while wide hand gripping increases the isometric contraction on the Pectoral and Subscapularis muscles. The wide handgrip forces the shoulder balls to rotate in their sockets such that the Subscapularis muscles are overstretched.
o Also, pointing the elbows away from the body, in a plane transverse to the body axis, places the shoulder balls directly and evenly under the Subscapularis and thus facilitates the adduction of the shoulders by the Pectoral fibers with minimal Deltoid assistance, *Figure 7.50.* Pointing the elbows downwards, parallel to the body axis, shifts the pressure to the front Deltoid and Trapezius with little Pectoral contribution.
o Pressing the weight upwards, with both arms, is done by the adduction of the upper arms from the sides. It requires strong stabilization of the scapulas. Remember that the scapulas are not in direct contact with spinal axis. The muscle that anchors the scapulas to the chest wall is the Serratus anterior. Thus, when the shoulders lift weights, the scapulas are anchored in places as follows.
  i. The upper Trapezius pulls the upper and lateral corner of the scapulas in upward and medial direction.
  ii. The Latissimus dorsi pushes the lower and lateral border of the scapulas in medial and forward direction.
  iii. The Serratus anterior pull the medial edge of the scapulas to the front ribs.
  iv. The middle Trapezius pushes the scapulas forwards.

Muscular imbalance issues:
o Since the travel distance in Bench Press is short and does not require complex lifting technique, strength seems to be the major determining factor in maximizing the Bench Press. Such strong and massive upper arms and chest muscles can undermine other lifting technique such as the Clean and the Snatch.
o A stiff and short Subscapularis interferes with shoulder flexion during the Clean and prevents the bar from reaching the top of the Deltoids. The strong and short Subscapularis can bring the bar falling downwards before finishing the overhead Snatch, unless strong posterior Deltoid and Infraspinatus counteract the action of the Subscapularis.
o To test the stiffness and shortening of the **Subscapularis** and the **Pectoralis major**, one has to perform the front Squat and overhead Squat and assess the ability to flex the shoulders, when descending deep in the front Squat, and the stability of the arms above the shoulders, during deep overhead Squat. If the two muscles outpace the **Infraspinatus and posterior Deltoid** in strength and tone, it would be very difficult to assume fully flexed or upright extended shoulders in those two exercises.
o **One-hand dumbbell Press,** from flexed shoulders to fully extended overhead shoulders, strengthens and stretches the Subscapularis. When the shoulder is fully flexed, with bent elbow elevated to horizontal while standing or seating and the dumbbell sits on the top of the shoulder, the front Deltoid pulls the humerus upwards against the Subscapularis' pull and thus reduces the tone in the latter muscle and eases shoulder flexion, *Figure 7.38.*
o The shoulder Press can be strengthened beyond average training norms by concentrated strengthening of the individual muscles: the Triceps, the Pectoralis major, and the Subscapularis, by one-hand dumbbell Presses, *Figure 7.38,* elbow extension, *Figure 7.15* thru *7.18,* and flyes, *Figure 7.42.* One-hand resistance exercises utilize the whole cardiac output and oxygen consumption in strengthening individual muscles thus build up the ingredient components of strong Bench Press.

7.4.4.13. Inclined Bench Press
Purpose
Inclined Bench Press targets the upper fibers of the Pectoralis major (clavicular head), the front Deltoid, and the Subscapularis in addition to the Serratus anterior and the Triceps, *Figure 7.51*. The barbell inclined Press differs from one-hand dumbbell Press in that the limiting bar restricts shoulder adductors, while dumbbells allow strengthening free and balanced adductors in addition to enhancing motor control. However, dumbbells do not have racks to support them as with barbells (racks for dumbbells are not invented yet).

Execution
o On the inclined bench, the shoulder plates and the buttocks abut the bench, while the lower back forms a bridge over the upper and lower contacts with the bench.

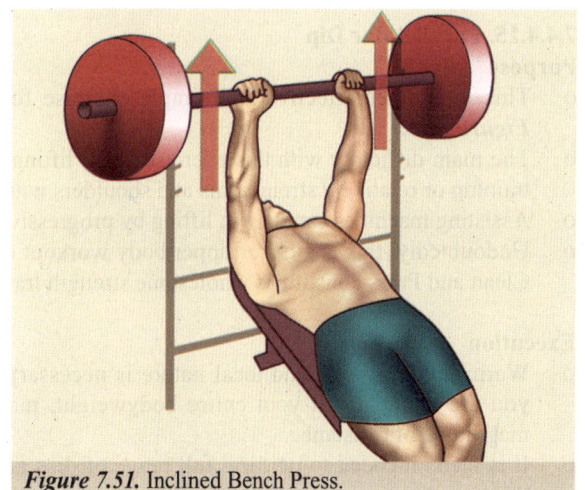

Figure 7.51. Inclined Bench Press.

o Load the barbell off the rack and pause to adjust your bounds prior to starting. The bar should be evenly gripped by both hands. It should be placed vertically over the shoulders.
o Slowly and steadily, lower the barbell until it touches the chest. It is advised to use lightweight and descend to the chest rather than performing partial descent.
o Wide handgrip with elbows moving in a plane transverse to the body axis brings the clavicular head of the Pectoralis in line with vertical Press.
o Close handgrips with elbows, pointed along the body axis, shift the resistance towards the front Deltoid.

7.4.4.14. Pushups
Purpose

This is the most basic and effective exercise for strengthening the Triceps, the Pectoralis major, the Subscapularis, the Serratus, and the abdominal muscles, *Figure 7.52*. The Pushups can be performed anywhere, with great results on the strength and size of the upper body.

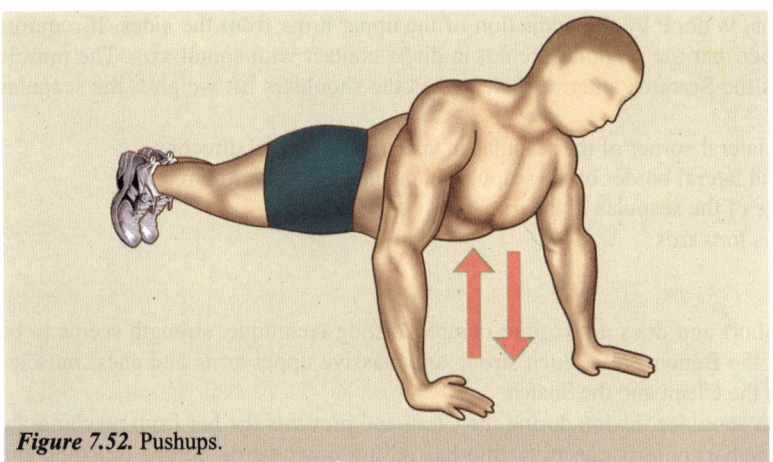
Figure 7.52. Pushups.

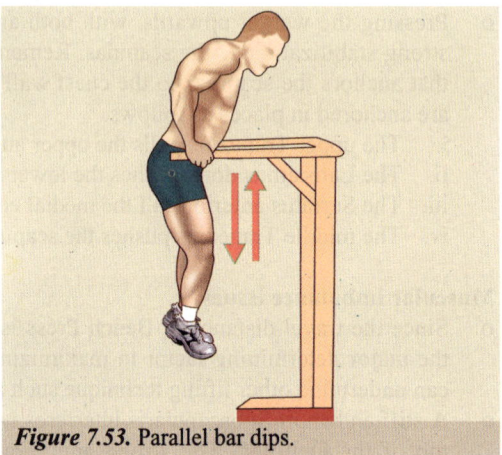
Figure 7.53. Parallel bar dips.

Execution
o The hand stance can vary from close to wide, and the feet level can vary from the horizontal level of the hands to as high as upside down Pushups, with the legs falling vertically above the hands.
o Elevated feet emphasize the strengthening of the upper chest than the lower chest.
o Elbows pointing to the outside eliminate the action of the anterior Deltoid and emphasize the Pectoral muscles.
o Elbows kept to the sides of the body emphasize strengthening of the anterior Deltoid.
o Very wide hand stance fosters stretching of the Pectoral muscles.
o Very narrow hand stance enhances Triceps strength and anterior Deltoid.
o Pushups with both hands supported by elevated objects, while the chest dips below the hands levels, are also practiced for stretching the Subscapularis and Pectoralis major. Close hand stance with elbow pointed backwards, shifts the resistance towards the front Deltoids.
o You do not have to perform perfect, full range of motion, pushups in order to get strong. High repetition of very low Pushups is of great effect in strengthening, despite the limited range of motion of ascent. Deep pushups overstretch the Subscapularis, Pectoralis, and Triceps.

7.4.4.15. Parallel Bar Dip
Purpose
o This is another effective and simple exercise for the Triceps, front Deltoid, Subscapularis, and Pectoralis major, *Figure 7.53*.
o The main difficulty with this exercise is the lifting of the whole bodyweight that requires good warm-up and advanced training or relatively strong arms and shoulders with respect to the bodyweight.
o Assisting machines can help in lifting by progressive increase in resistance.
o Undoubtedly, this is a major upper body workout of moderate intensity. Combining the parallel bar dip with Squat and Clean and Press constitutes wholesome strength training routine of the major body muscles and joints.

Execution
o Warm-up of general and local nature is necessary before embarking on this whole body, demanding exercise. Since you are about to lift your entire bodyweight, make sure that you have advanced to this level and can handle this magnitude of resistance.
o It is recommended to perform full range of dips as often as possible. However, sometimes you might have to increase the repetition at the expense of limiting the range of motion.

o The wide parallel bars shift the resistance towards the Subscapularis and the Pectoralis major, the main shoulder adductors.
o The close parallel bars require more front Deltoid (shoulder flexor) and Trapezius (elbow extensor).
o Slow lowering of the body enhances eccentric contraction and speeds muscle growth and strength.
o Dipping deep and pausing briefly enhances stretching of the Pectoralis, Subscapularis, and anterior Deltoid.

7.4.5. SHOULDER ADDUCTION AND EXTENSION

Shoulder adduction is the attraction of the arms from the sides towards the body. This comprises of the rotation of the ball head of the humerus on the socket cavity of the scapula, at the shoulder joint. Shoulder adduction is carried out by the combined actions of the following muscles.
o The back adductors of the shoulders: the Latissimus dorsi, the Subscapularis, and the Teres major, *Figures 7.13, 7.14* and *7.21*.
o The chest adductor of the shoulder: the Pectoralis major, *Figure 7.54*.
o The arm adductors of the shoulder: the Coracobrachialis muscle, Biceps brachii, and long head of Triceps, *Figures 7.13* and *7.54*.

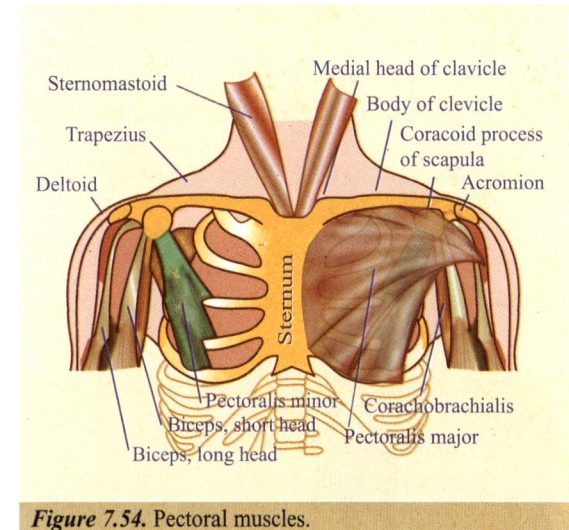

Figure 7.54. Pectoral muscles.

Since most exercises are performed with elbow flexion, the Biceps is often strengthened during arms adduction. The main reason for having all these muscles, performs apparently similar actions, is that the shoulder joint is adducted in multiple planes as follows.
o **Transverse adduction** is carried out in a plane perpendicular to the body axis. This is the case of bringing the spread arms from the outside to the middle as in Dumbbell Flyes, Bench Press, and Pushups.
o **Longitudinal adduction** is carried out along the body axis, in either an anterior-posterior plane[4] along the spinal axis or a right-left plane along the spinal axis. The adduction of the arms from anterior to posterior is called "shoulder extension". The redundancy in nomenclature in describing shoulder motion is attributed to the redundancy in actions of the shoulder muscles.
o Some adductors work most in certain planes but less in the others. The multiplicity of adductors guarantees smooth shoulder mobility in different planes of motion.

In addition to the previously described exercises of shoulder adduction, the following two exercises combine shoulder adduction and extension.

7.4.5.1. Chin-Ups
Purpose
o Pulling the bodyweight upwards by gripping on a fixed object requires fixation of the scapulas to the chest cage, adduction of the shoulders on the scapulas, and flexion of the elbows.
o The Trapezius lower fibers pull the scapulas downwards in order to fix the scapulas during ascending. Weaker lower Trapezius prevents fixation of the scapulas.
o The Latissimus dorsi, Teres major, long head of Triceps, and Subscapularis pull the humerus towards the scapula and the pelvis.
o The Pectoralis major pulls the humerus towards the chest.
o The Biceps flexes the elbows. The weakest links in chin-ups is the Biceps in athletes, and the major adductors in non-athletes.

Execution
o Close grip Chin-ups, with elbows pointing forwards, eliminate most of the action of the Pectoralis major by making the direction of its fibers perpendicular to the plane of rotation of the humerus and thus shifts the resistance to the other back muscles, *Figure 7.55*.
o Wide grips increase the chest participation in upward pulling by forcing the elbows to point to the sides and thus aligning the Pectoral pull along the plane of rotation of the humerus, *Figure 7.56*.
o Overhand gripping reduces the Biceps flexing power and increases its supination power, in addition to forcing the elbows to point to the sides thus increases the participation of chest adductors.
o Underhand gripping enhances the Biceps flexing power and facilitates upward pulling. In addition to enhancing the back adductors of the shoulders and the Triceps adduction, underhand gripping reduces the action of the chest adductors of the shoulders.

---
[4] Vertical plane that passes from anterior to posterior is called "sagittal plane". It divides the body to night and lift portions.

7.4.5.2. Cable Pulldown
Purpose

This is another versatile exercise that is useful in progressive enhancing of training intensity, *Figure 7.57*. Instead of lifting your entire bodyweight, you can play with whatever weight you can pull. You can perform few sets and many repetitions until you accomplish the desired strength and size of the shoulder adductors. It is therefore a substitute of the Chin-ups. The following muscles can all be strengthened and enlarged in size, over few months, by high volume and intensity of Cable Pulldown.
o   The back adductors of the shoulders: Latissimus dorsi, Subscapularis, Teres major, and lower Trapezius.
o   The chest adductors of the shoulders: Pectoralis major.
o   The arm adductors of the shoulder: The long head of Triceps.

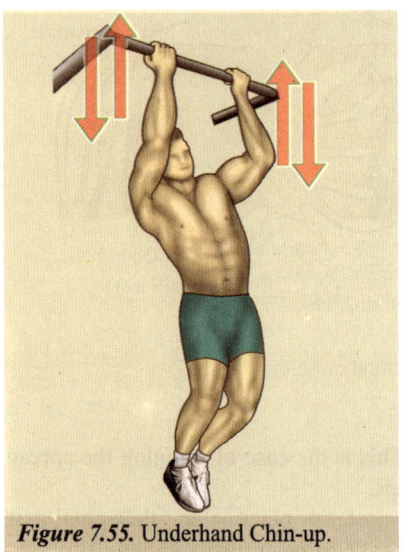
Figure 7.55. Underhand Chin-up.

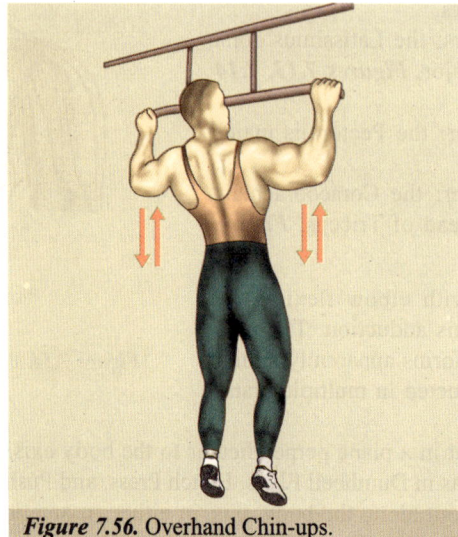
Figure 7.56. Overhand Chin-ups.

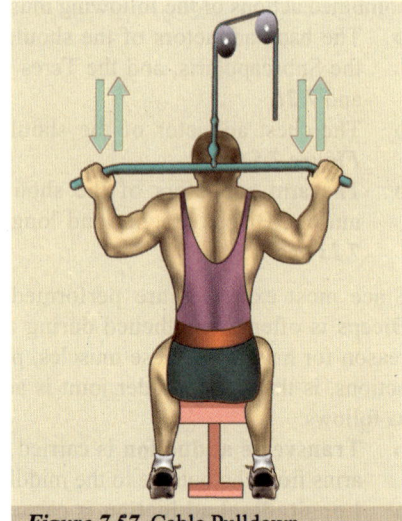
Figure 7.57. Cable Pulldown.

Execution
o   The wide grip Pulldowns work out both chest and back adductors while the close grip, with elbows pointing forwards, diminishes the participation of the chest adductors.
o   Pulling downwards, behind the shoulders, increases the role of chest adduction of the shoulders, by the way of the transverse plane of elbow motion. The bad reputation of behind-shoulder Pulldown is attributed to the fact that many people engage in weight training late in life after the shoulders have long been stiffened by short ligaments and tendons. These acquired deformities might benefit from gradual and progressive resistance training rather than avoiding exercises that do not seem fitting the individual.
o   The Pulldown can be executed in many ways as regard to the trajectory and the acceleration of the pull. Steady and slow pulling, and returning of the loaded cable, can significantly hasten muscular development by combined isometric, concentric, and eccentric contraction.
o   The common mistakes that many people make in the Cable Pulldown is the hunching of the upper back, the yanking of the cable, the bouncing of the torso, and the stiffening of the head during pulling.
o   You can avoid back hunching by remembering that even seated exercises require attentive thrusting of the chest.
o   Yanking the cable might cause it to snap torn and will eliminate the pre-stretch isometric contraction that occurs in slow pulling. Pre-stretching enhances neural control of muscular recruitment.
o   You should minimize bouncing the torso especially during the most of load volume. You can bounce if you are trying new and heavy weight. You should bounce the head such that the bar trajectory stays close to vertical. Thus, when the cable handle reaches the level of the eyebrows the head can advance forwards between the arms, during the ascent phase. The motion is reversed during the descent phase.
o   With Pulldowns, you have great opportunity to enhance you arms and back beyond common norms. With easy seating, manageable weight addition, and simple technique you can remedy many musculoskeletal deformities with long and patient training.

7.4.6. SHOULDER ABDUCTION
Shoulder abduction, the reverse of adduction, involves lateral movement of the arms, away from the midline of the body, and is carried out by the combined action of the lateral and anterior fibers of the **Deltoid, Supraspinatus, Serratus anterior, Levator scapulae, and upper Trapezius**. The Deltoid and Supraspinatus abduct the shoulder joint proper. That involves the rotation of the humeral ball on the glenoid socket. The Serratus anterior drags the medial border of the scapula outwards to the sides while the upper Trapezius and Levator scapulae rotate the upper border of the scapula in order to direct the glenoid socket laterally and upwards.

Shoulder abduction is encountered very often in lifting weights from the waist level to shoulder level. The Snatch lift utilizes shoulder abduction most. The following three exercises are common examples of weight training for shoulder abduction:
o   Lateral dumbbell raises.
o   Lateral deck raises.
o   Upright barbell row.

7.4.6.1. Lateral Arm Raises
Purpose
It is evident from the unusual position of the arm during abduction that this exercise is unique in working out muscles that seldom participate in every day physical work. The only time you may use the lateral Deltoid in daily activity is when you try to push something to the side, by the side of elbow.   Enlarged lateral Deltoids lend the upper body athletic appearance of masculinity.

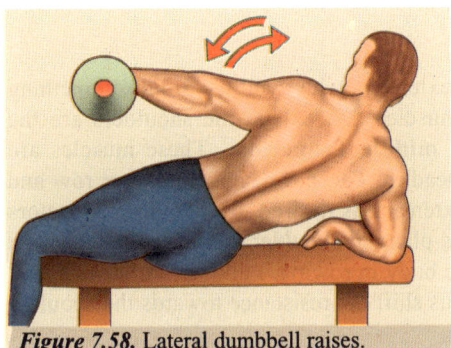
Figure 7.58. Lateral dumbbell raises.

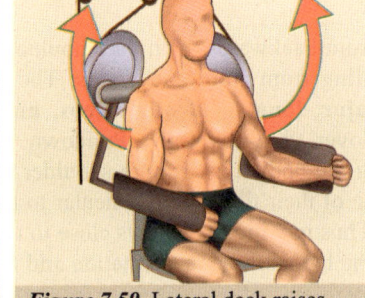
Figure 7.59. Lateral deck raises.

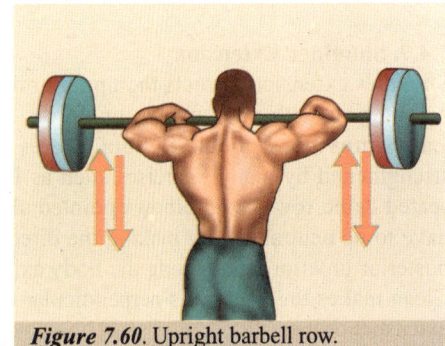
Figure 7.60. Upright barbell row.

Execution
o   Lateral raises can be performed by applying resistance to the lateral motion of the upper arms, *Figures 7.58 and 7.59*. Dumbbells or cables held in hands, or loaded decks of specially designed machines pushing against the lateral sides of the upper arms, can strengthen the five muscles that abduct the shoulders.
o   During all postures of shoulder abduction, the chest should bulge in upward thrust posture in order to prevent shoulder deformities, during the contraction of the Deltoids. Even when you lay on your side to perform arm abduction, you should thrust your chest to the front.
o   Use lightweight to be able to initiate muscular contraction without acute stressing. Increase the weight gradually, as long as the technique is intact and the motion is smooth.
o   During laying down lateral raises, you should not reach vertical arms. All what you need is an acute angle between the horizontal and the vertical.
o   Slow and steady motion is the essence of this stretching exercise.

7.4.6.2. Lateral Deck Raises
Purpose
This differs from one-hand dumbbell raises in its symmetric posture and easy arrangement of the machine. You can accomplish a lot in little time, *Figure 7.59*. You can also perfect the chest thrust with the aid of the backboard. Its greatest benefit is for those with hand, wrist, or forearm injuries that require local resting of these parts.

Execution
o   While seating, thrust your chest upwards and throw your shoulder backwards.
o   Adjust the deck arm pads to abut against the forearms, with bent elbows. The forearms will be kept horizontal to the vertical upper arms.
o   While slowly and steadily abducting your shoulder, maintain the initial chest, shoulder, and head positions. The shoulder proper should be the only joint that moves, until the upper arms approach the horizontal level of the shoulders. Recall that abduction is purely a lateral motion. Thus, your elbow should start from the very side of your chest and remain in that vertical plane (coronal or right to left and vertical plane), without advancing forwards.
o   Your elbows can reach as high as the shoulder level or exceed that if you have the strength and flexibility to maintain extreme elevation.
o   You can even limit your range of abduction into the angles that you feel require special strengthening.

7.4.6.3. Upright Barbell Arm Rows
Purpose
Holding a barbell in both hands while standing and moving the barbell upwards and downwards, in front of the body, works out the lateral and anterior heads of the Deltoid, *Figure 7.60*. Upright arm rows produce impressive results in toning

and strengthening the lateral Deltoid, which wastes away very fast with inactivity and causes the common appearance of narrow shoulder width. Of course, large and strong lateral Deltoids have to be acquired along large and strong Trapezius and upper arm, which all add to the athletic look of the shoulders. Weightlifting exercises that are equivalent to upright arm row are the military, power, and classic; Clean and Snatch lifts, with handgrips that vary from very close grip-span to very wide grip-span. In addition to the strengthening the shoulder abductors, the Weightlifting exercises work out the legs and back along with the shoulders thus reduce the redundancy in exercise planning.

Execution
o   Hold a barbell with narrow handgrip at the middle of the bar. You can also do that with a plate or a dumbbell.
o   Maintain lordotic lower back and thrust chest before commencing the rowing.
o   Pull upwards by bringing the barbell close to your body. Slow and steady motion enhances growth of strength and mass. Ballistic motion is dangerous in this short range of motion.
o   Lowering the barbell slowly is more beneficial in enhancing the eccentric contraction and permitting greater control on overcoming resistance.
o   If the bar is kept at a distance from the body then the front Deltoid exerts most of the resistance.

7.4.7. Shoulder Extension
Shoulder extension attracts the upper arms from backwards. You use shoulder extension when you try to kick something behind you with your elbow, or during pulling from front backwards. The muscles that extend the shoulders are the **Latissimus dorsi, back Deltoid, Teres major, long head of Triceps, and middle Trapezius.** These muscles are strengthened by many exercises such as Pullover, chin-ups, Cable Pulldown, Deadlift, Clean, Snatch, Bent-over row and seated cable rows, with elbows pointed along the body axis. If pure shoulder extension is desired, the shoulder adductors have to be neutralized by making the direction of their fibers perpendicular to the plane of shoulder rotation. The latter is a posterior-anterior plane along the body axis. Thus moving the elbows close to the body in rowing, Pullover, Pulldowns, and Clean makes the Pectoralis perpendicular to the humeral plane of rotation and thus shift the resistance towards the shoulder extensors proper.

7.4.8. SHOULDER FLEXION
Shoulder flexion brings the arms upwards and forwards from the sides of the body. As in the case of extension, pure shoulder flexion requires elimination of the chest adductors by moving the arms in an anterior-posterior plane along the body axis. The muscles that flex the shoulders are the **Deltoid** (anterior and lateral heads), **Biceps brachii**, and **Coracobrachialis**. It is very important to remember these three muscles when trying to remedy problems associated with inability to flex the shoulders, as in the case of front Squat. Strong shoulder adductors (Pectoralis, Subscapularis, Latissimus dorsi, Teres, and long head of Triceps) can impede the full flexion of shoulders during front Squat. Long and hard strengthening of the Biceps, Deltoid, and Coracobrachialis muscle is required to balance the strong actions of the adductors.

7.5. STRENGTHENING THE HIPS

The hips differ from the shoulders in their direct bony articulation with the spinal axis through the junction between ilium and sacrum bones, *Figure 7.61*. This bony configuration precludes the hips from elevation along the spinal axis and thus makes the hips more stable during mobility. As all socket and ball joints, the hips adduct, abduct, flex, extend, and rotate.

In order to work out the hips, the following peripheral and axial muscles participate in muscular balance.

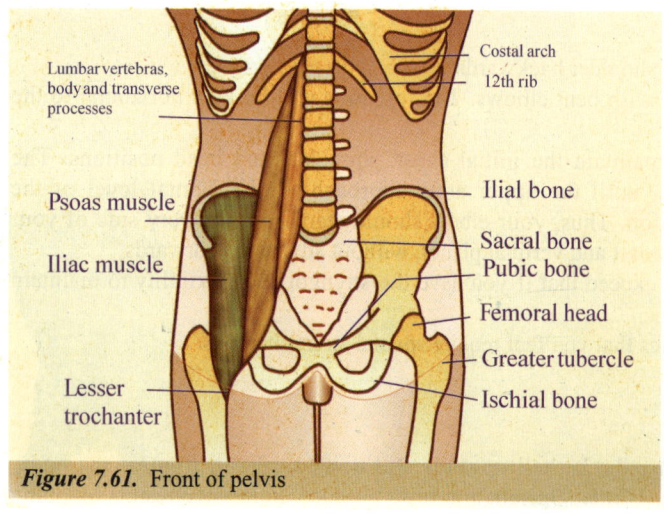
Figure 7.61. Front of pelvis

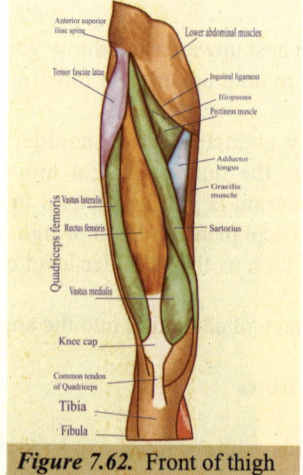
Figure 7.62. Front of thigh

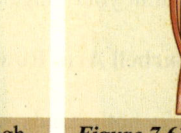
Figure 7.63. Back of thigh

o **Peripheral muscles:** the Quadriceps and Hamstrings transmit the forces from the feet to the pelvis through the knee joints, *Figures 7.62* and *7.63*. In front Squat and overhead Squat, the shoulder muscles also transmit the forces from the hands to the spinal axis.
o **Axial muscles:** The spinal erectors, hip flexors, and gluteal muscles support the spinal axis and pelvis during hip exercises, *Figures 7.61* thru *7.63*.
o **Muscular balance:** All forces acting on the front of the hip joint are transmitted to the spinal axis through the Iliopsoas muscles, adductor muscles of the thigh, and the Rectus femoris and Sartorius muscles. On the back of the hip, forces are transmitted to the spinal axis via the gluteal muscles and the hip abductors. The spinal erectors react to the balance between the front and back hip muscles.

The Iliopsoas muscles originate from the lumbar vertebras and their transverse processes and from the iliac bone. They insert into the femur lesser trochanter. The adductor muscles of the thigh originate from the pubis and insert into the femur, except the Gracilis muscles that inserts into the tibia.

7.5.1. HIP EXTENSION
Hip extension maintains upright posture by pulling the top of the pelvis backwards on the thighs. The prime hip extensors are:
o Gluteus maximus muscle.
o Hamstrings: Semitendinosus, Semimembranosus, and long head of Biceps femoris.
o Adductor magnus, ischial fibers.

During hip extension, the femoral heads are anchored in their sockets by the actions of the following hip abductors: **the Gluteus medius, the Gluteus minimus, the Piriformis, the Obturator externus, the two Gemellus muscles**. These abductors draw the femoral shaft medially and forwards and thus anchor the femoral head in the Acetabular fossa. This is a socket in the pelvic bones, formed by the union of the three bones: Pubis, Ilium, and Ischium.

Hip extension can be strengthened by the following common exercises:
1. One-legged hip extension.
2. Goodmorning back extension.
3. Horizontal back extension.
4. Dumbbell Squat.
5. Inclined Leg Press.
6. Deadlift.
7. Back Squat.
8. Front Squat.

7.5.1.1. One-Legged Hip Extension
Purpose
This can be done either by horizontal floor hip extension, where the weight of one leg is used as a resisting force, or by cable hip extension, *Figures 7.64* and *7.65*. The floor exercise allows long and hard training of the hip extensors since most of the postural energy is saved. The upright cable hip extension enhances postural control but requires an extra machine, which diminishes its popularity. It is suitable for overweight people since it also works out the other hip abductors, in addition to eliminating the need for crawling to the floor.

Execution
o Hip extension with one leg is performed with straight knee during the backwards and upwards raising of the whole leg.
o Before initiating any leg elevation, you should tighten your belly and lower back. Since this is an asymmetric exercise, it requires some warm-up prior to its execution.
o The extent of backward extension depends greatly on the conditions of your spinal discs and the flexibility of the spinal ligaments. You should never attempt to perform this exercise with any spinal discomfort or recent injury. This might worsen herniation of injured discs.

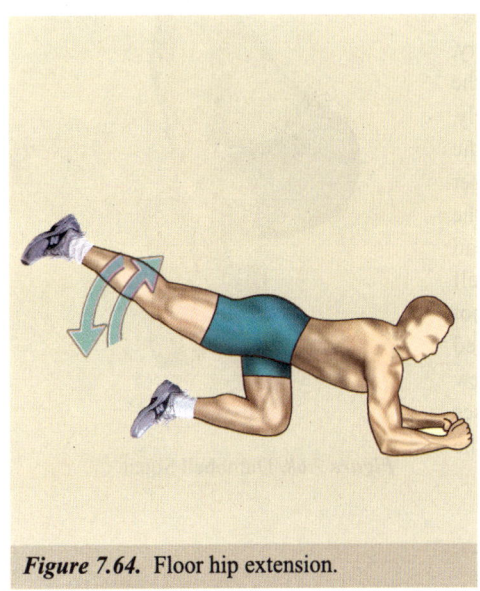
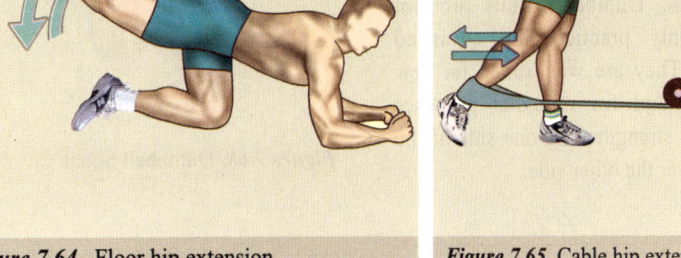

Figure 7.64. Floor hip extension.   *Figure 7.65.* Cable hip extension.

o Isometric and eccentric contractions can be greatly enhanced by pausing and slowing the return of the leg. Both contractions are required in enhancing spinal strength.

7.5.1.2. Goodmorning Back Extension Purpose

This exercise must be performed as long as you walk on this planet. The cumulative strengthening effect on the spinal erectors and hip extensors will guarantee that you maintain the human upright posture, with less visits to orthopedic doctors. Above all, daily training even for few minutes will enhance your understanding of the behavior of these postural muscles. The few basic facts that may ease your understanding of the back erectors are:

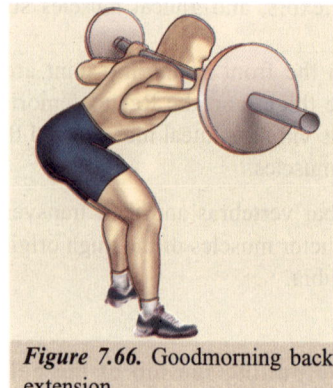
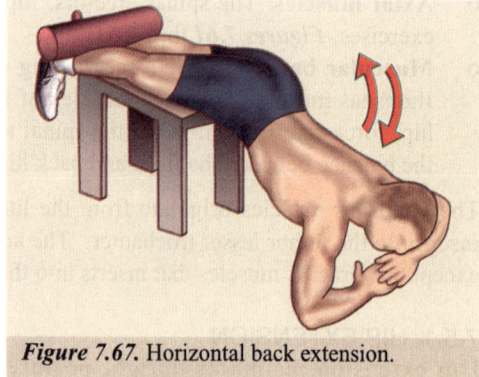

Figure 7.66. Goodmorning back extension.

Figure 7.67. Horizontal back extension.

o The back muscles do not fare well without mobility.
o The back muscles do not tolerate abrupt forces without progressive training.
o The back muscles are not always severely injured when they cause acute and annoying pain.
o The long dismissal of strengthening of the back muscles can cause life long crippling injuries.

Execution

o Goodmorning extension is performed without weight or by putting weight on the back of the shoulders and bending forwards, with slightly bent knees and concaved back, *Figure 7.66*.
o You can bend as far as you want as long as you keep concave back and as long as you maintain progressive and regular training.
o Stiffed and straight legs work out the Hamstrings intensely since they elongate the Hamstrings at the knee joints. In this position of straight knee, care must be taken when bending to avoid rupturing the overstretched Hamstrings.
o Slow and cautious leaning should be practiced. Yet, very slow motion can lead to hesitation and distraction.

7.5.1.3. Horizontal Back Extension

This is performed by lying prone, face done, on a special bench that has support for lower legs[5] at the ankles. The upper body hangs freely outside the bench, *Figure 7.67*. This exercise eases knee pressure and eliminate postural tension by using the lower limbs for stretch instead of compression, as in the case with the Goodmorning exercise. Here the upper body is used to generate resistance force on the back and hip extensors. Its convenience allows long and hard back stretching, with less energy expenditure. Thus, it reduces overtraining due to excessive load volume. The exercise can be made intense by increasing speed of motion or holding weight in hands, or behind the shoulders.

7.5.1.4. Dumbbell Squat

This is one of the oldest know strength training exercise, *Figure 7.68*. It used to be performed as one-hand Clean and Press or Snatch in the Olympic games until 1920. For the sake of symmetry, you can lift the two dumbbells from the floor to full leg extension. Alternatively, you can proceed with full lift to the shoulder level to work out both the upper body and legs. You can even Snatch the dumbbells from the floor to overhead level, depending on the dumbbell weights. Dumbbell Pulls are not commonly practiced by advanced lifters. They are well suited for new comers and for remedial purposes such as strengthening one side of the body over the other side.

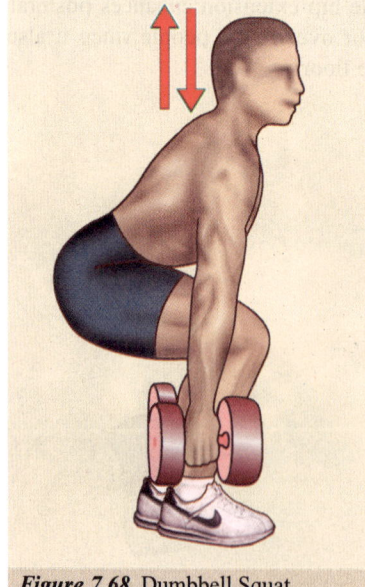
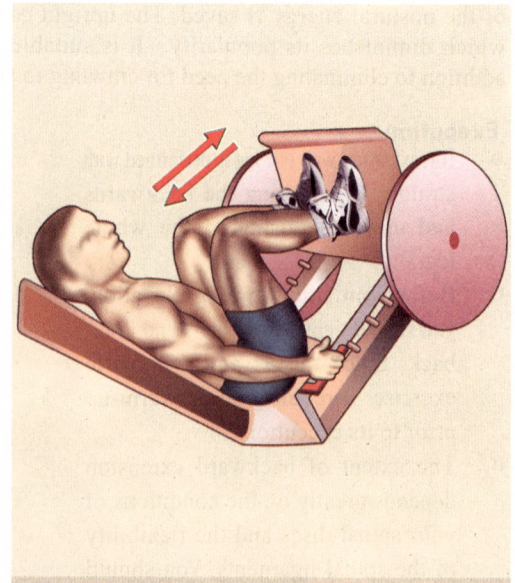

Figure 7.68. Dumbbell Squat.

Figure 7.69. Inclined Leg Press.

---

[5] Lower leg refers to the region between knee and ankle. Lower limb refers to the whole leg.

7.5.1.5. Inclined Leg Press
Purpose
This works out the hip extensors by concentric contraction, while the spinal erector contracting isometrically to fix the torso, *Figure 7.69*. The inclined upward Leg Press, with the heart positioned below the point of force application, facilitates venous return and makes this exercise well tolerated by many people. Leg Press can be used to enhance greater range of motion of the knees by lowering the platform until the calves touch the thighs.

Execution
o   The exercise is performed by pushing the loaded carriage by both feet, while the torso abutting the inclined back support.
o   Slow motion in pushing and lowering the platform enhances eccentric as well as concentric contraction.
o   Close feet-stance and close knees emphasize front thigh muscles.
o   Widely separated knees, regardless of the feet-stance, enhance hip adductors.
o   Full descent with carriage enhances knee and hip flexibility and can be used to rectify long acquired shortening of their ligaments and tendons.

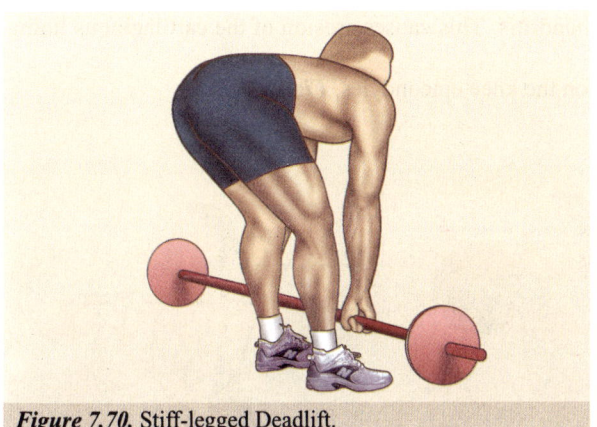

Figure 7.70. Stiff-legged Deadlift.

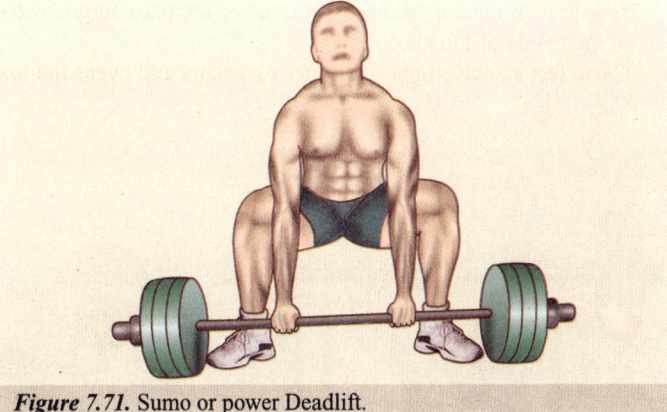

Figure 7.71. Sumo or power Deadlift.

7.5.1.6. Deadlift
Deadlift was also described in details in Chapter Five.

Purpose
This works out hip and back extensors through application of force on the arms and shoulders. The shoulder elevators transmit the forces from the arms to the axis by isometric contraction.
The reason for the popularity of the Sumo Deadlift is the intense stretching effect on the hip adductors and the upper Trapezius that induces a feeling of tight upper and lower body after the exercise.

Execution
o   Stiff-legged Deadlift emphasizes the Hamstrings stretch more than bent-legged Deadlift, *Figure 7.70*.
o   The Sumo Deadlift on the other hand, emphasizes the hip adductors and gluteal maximus by spreading the upper legs[6] to the sides, *Figure 7.71*. It puts intense stretch on the upper Trapezius, particularly when the lifter retracts the scapulas by the middle fibers of the Trapezius and pulls the Deadlift with upper fibers of the Trapezius.
o   The close handgrips of the Sumo Deadlift lowers the clavicles below their normal position and overstretches the Trapezius upper fibers.
o   The Deadlift is executed by hyperextended back, thrust chest, and retracted scapulas.
o   The early upward drive of the barbell must proceed slowly by the Quadriceps and Hamstrings contraction. The upper body remains in isometric contraction, for the sake of transmitting the forces of leg drive to the spinal axis and the arms that are suspending the barbell.

7.5.1.7. Back Squat
Squat was also described in Chapters Five and Six.

Purpose
This is the mainstay for exercising the knee, hip, and back extensors. Squatting every workout, even for as little as three or four sets, is the wisest plan you can embark on in maintaining robust body extensors. The back Squat loads the barbell right on the scapular spines thus eliminate the need for shoulder extension or adduction, as is the case with the Deadlift.

---

[6] Upper leg refers to the region between the hip and knee. Lower leg refers to the region below the knee. Lower limb refers to the legs in general.

7 WEIGHT TRAINING

Execution
o Since squatting requires back, hip, and knee extension, thorough warm-up of these regions guarantees better Squat technique without injury. The thrust chest and retracted scapulas guarantee that the weight of the barbell falls on the line of action of the spinal erectors.
o Caved in chest or lax scapulas are judged by dropped shoulders and lax arm support of the barbell. These cause the weight of the barbell to compress the spinal discs, misalign the spinal joints, and could cause sprain or strain and future back stiffness.
o The lumbar spines are best kept concave since they form the critical link between the upper body and the pelvis. After practicing the Squat for few days, your body extensors might relax their tone and you will not experience the stubborn stiffness of the first time you have Squatted with weights. Even top lifters experience hypertonic muscular contraction when performing unaccustomed activities. That is because the high sympathetic activation of muscles that is new to unaccustomed recruitment of muscle fibers.
o Weightlifters squat to buttocks-on-heels depth and bounce at the bottom to overstretch the Quadriceps tendons. Novice lifters have to work around flexibility progressively, with lightweight, until the ankles, knee, hips, and back regain full range of motion under resistance.
o Wide feet stance during Squatting shifts some resistance to the hip adductors, the inner muscles of the thigh, *Figure 7.72*. It loads the lateral condyles of the femur more than the medial condyle, thus facilitates squatting to people with medial meniscus injuries or medial condyle osteochondritis. This causes erosion of the cartilaginous lining of the inside of the knee.
o Close feet stance emphasizes knee extensors and evens the load on the knee epicondyles, *Figure 7.73*.

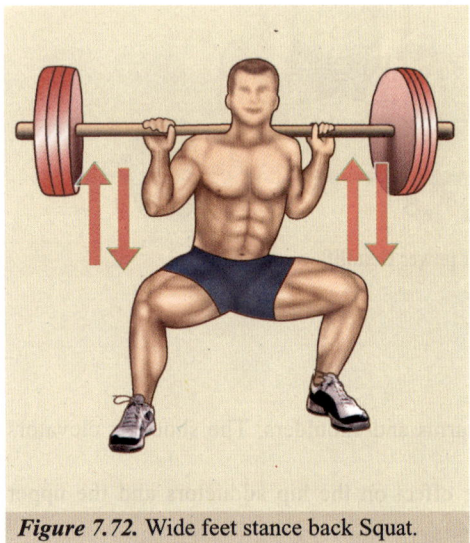
Figure 7.72. Wide feet stance back Squat.

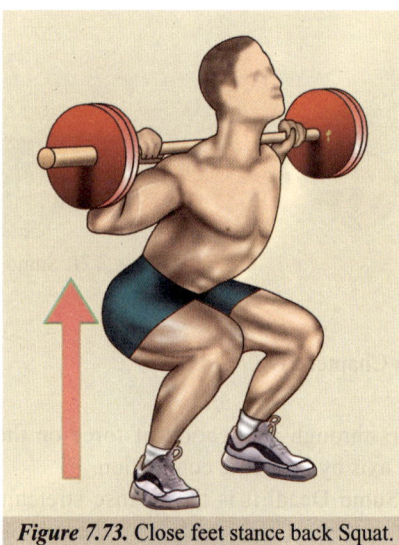
Figure 7.73. Close feet stance back Squat.

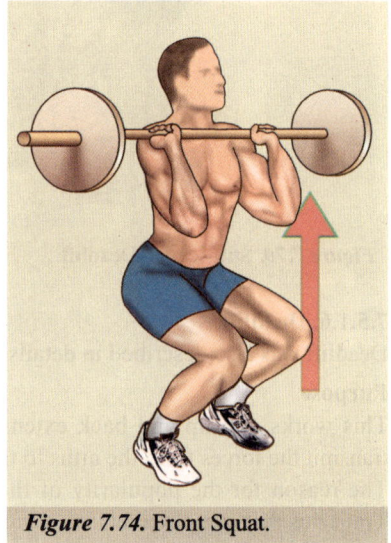
Figure 7.74. Front Squat.

7.5.1.8. Front Squat
Purpose
The front Squat should not be confused for front exercising of the thighs. The only advantage of front Squat over back Squat is the emphasis on the shoulder flexion during squatting in addition to loading the weight in front of the spinal axis. The front Squat is formidable to people that started lifting at adult age. It requires very strong shoulder flexor (anterior Deltoid) in comparison to the shoulder adductors. The Subscapularis is the key muscle in pulling the upper arms downwards and thus prevents the arms from supporting the weights on the front of the shoulders, *Figure 7.74*. Since the weight is loaded on the clavicles and the outer tips of the scapulas, both scapulae elevator and chest elevators have to balance the upper body during the transfer of forces from the shoulders to the spinal axis. No other exercise would need your full awareness of shoulder balance like the front Squat. When it becomes apparent that you have a problem raising the elbows, while squatting, then you have uncovered the hidden secret of weak and unbalanced shoulder flexors, in opposition to strong and short chest adductors. The latter pulls the upper arms medially and to the center of the chest, while the former pulls them upwards and to the upper tip of the shoulder. While working around strengthening the shoulder flexors (Deltoid), you should contemplate strongly spreading the scapulas to the sides and concaving the lower back. This posture elevates the entire shoulder and thus weakens the Subscapularis, by narrowing the range of adduction, when the scapulas are spread laterally.

7.5.2. HIP FLEXION
o Hip flexors bend the thighs upwards on the front of the pelvis. When the thighs are fixed, as in standing, sitting, or walking, the hip flexors pull the front of the pelvis downwards to the thighs, thus enhance lumbar concavity.

o The hip is flexed by the combined actions of **Iliopsoas, Tensor muscles of fascia lata, Rectus femoris, Sartorius, Adductor longus, Adductor brevis, and Pectineus**. The hip flexors fan around the pelvis to grab its front, side, and back. It is very clear from the fanning of the hip flexors that they are fundamental muscles of stabilizing the pelvic platform on which the spinal axis stems upwards.
o The Iliopsoas pull the lumbar vertebra at the back of the pelvis towards the upper thigh, *Figure 7.61.*
o The muscles of Tensor fascia lata, Rectus femoris, and Sartorius pull the side of the pelvis towards the thigh, *Figures 7.62* and *63*.
o The remaining three adductors pull the front of the pelvis towards the thigh.

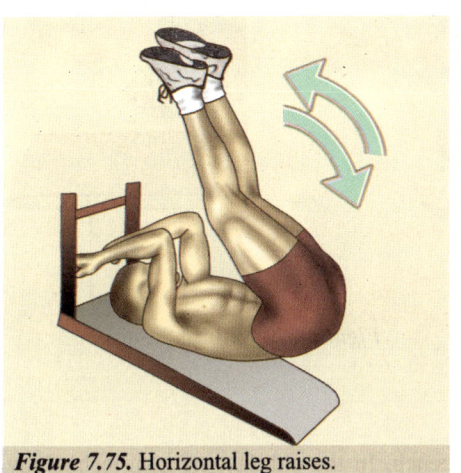
Figure 7.75. Horizontal leg raises.

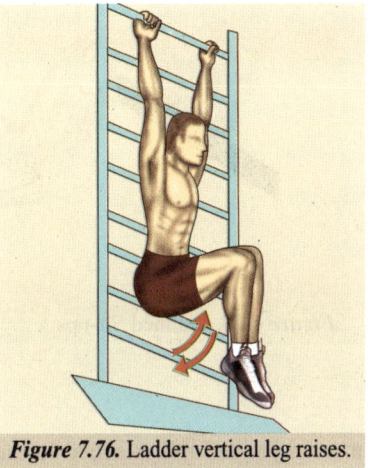
Figure 7.76. Ladder vertical leg raises.

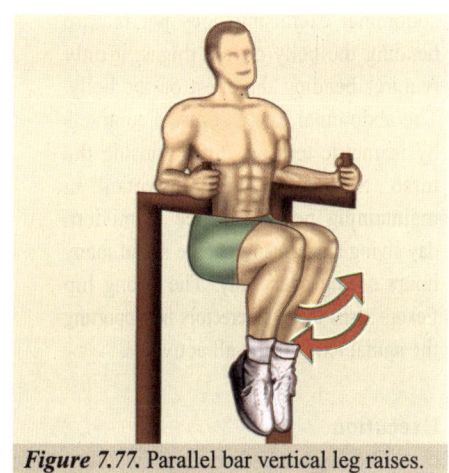
Figure 7.77. Parallel bar vertical leg raises.

Hip flexion is exercised by the following common exercises:

1. Horizontal leg raises.
2. Ladder vertical leg raises.
3. Parallel bar vertical leg raises.
4. Inclined Sit-ups.
5. Vertical Sit-ups.

7.5.2.1. Horizontal Leg Raises
Purpose
Lying on the back and fixing the upper body, by gripping a supporting object, allows the person to raise the legs and bend the thighs on the belly. This strengthens hip flexors. Farther elevation of the buttocks from the ground or bench works out the **abdominal Rectus muscles**, *Figure 7.75.*

Execution
o Horizontal leg raises can be performed with straight or bent knees, horizontal or inclined surface, with legs kept together or spread apart.
o The ability to lift the entire lower body on the thoracic spines tests the strength of the shoulders and elbow flexors, abdominal rectus, and hip flexors. This is achieved by elevating the buttocks and lower back off the floor or bench, while the hands are clenching onto a fixed overhead bar.
o Raising one leg at a time enhances neural control of the hip flexors.
o Raising the legs upwards and then performing a twisting motion with the legs, around the longitudinal axis, strengthens the abdominal oblique muscles. This is done by placing one leg on the top of the other, instead of lifting them side-by-side. The twisting motion is very effective in tightening the sides of the belly.

7.5.2.2. Ladder Vertical Leg Raises
Vertical leg raises are performed by supporting the body by hand gripping on a ladder, *Figure 7.76*. The ladder-raises stretch the shoulder adductors and extensors. The stretched upper body makes it hard to work out the hip flexors unless the upper body is relatively strong. The vertical position of the chest makes breathing more taxing. In addition, the weight of the lower body is entirely being lifted by the Iliopsoas. Here, the spinal joints are not supported by a bench, as is the case horizontal leg raises. Thus, the spinal erectors are activated in order to support stretching and straightening the spines.

7.5.2.3. Parallel Bar Vertical Leg Raises
The parallel bar raises contract the shoulder extensors, and decrease the efficiency of hip flexion. These differ from ladder leg raises in reducing the upper body stretch, and from the horizontal raises in imposing spinal stretch and heavy resistance to the Iliopsoas. For people with strong upper body, this sort of leg raises can be utilized in trimming the abdominal oblique

muscles. This is achieved by raising one leg on the top of the other and twisting the pelvis, during leg raises, *Figure 7.77*.

7.5.2.4. Inclined Sit-ups
Purpose
These differ from leg raises in using the upper bodyweight to induce resistance. The main purpose of this exercise is strengthening the hip flexors, not the abdominal rectus, *Figure 7.78*. Pure abdominal exercising does not require bending the belly on the thighs, it only requires bending the chest on the belly. The abdominal Rectus muscle contracts by isometric tension, during raising the torso. Sit-ups are very important in maintaining pelvic balance in modern day living since many people spend many hours sitting every day. The strong hip flexors assist the back erectors in supporting the spinal axis during all activities.

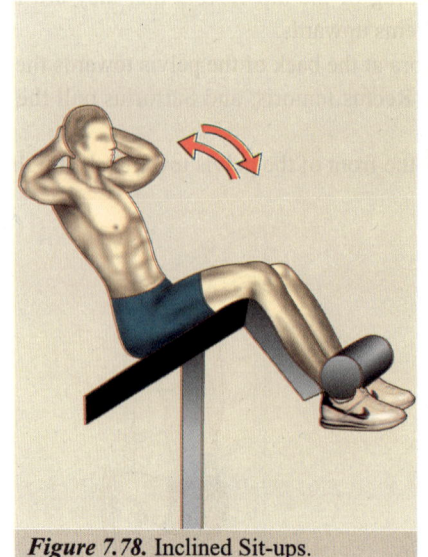
Figure 7.78. Inclined Sit-ups.

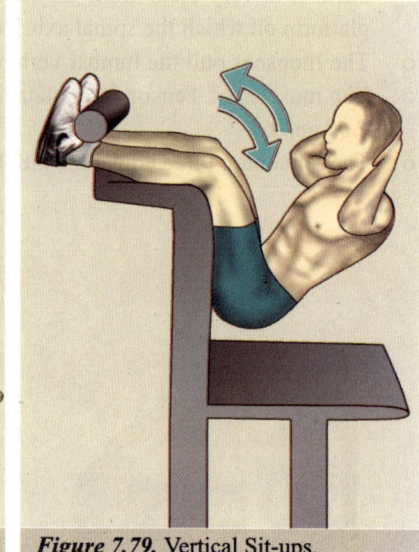
Figure 7.79. Vertical Sit-ups.

Execution
- The legs are fixed by the feet, under a cross padded roll attached to the bench. In the old days of gym technology, wooden benches were used. Full range Sit-ups on hard surface cause ulcers at the tip of the sacrum, due to raising and lowering the upper body on fixed pelvis, on hard surface.
- Sit-ups are performed on flat, inclined, or vertical surfaces provided that there is some sort of support gripping of the feet. Flat bench or floor Sit-ups are easy and should be performed in days of high load-volume days.
- You do not have to labor hard in order to work out the whole range of motion. Strengthening a particular angle, of the whole range in a particular set of exercise, minimizes exhaustion.
- Remember that the abdominal Rectus is contracting mostly isometrically during Sit-ups. Yet, you can activate the abdominal oblique muscles by advancing one shoulder ahead of the other while sitting-up.

7.5.2.5. Vertical Sit-ups
Purpose
These differ from oblique Sit-ups in increasing the effect of the upper body weight on the hip flexors, *Figure 7.79*. The lower position of the upper body enhances venous return and stretches the cardiac ventricles. It also mobilizes the guts upwards thus relieves the lower abdominal muscles from constant pressure. The abdominal muscles work harder in vertical Sit-ups than in any other exercise.

Execution
- You should never attempt to perform these Sit-up exercises without thorough warm-up. Although you are not lifting from the floor, the Iliopsoas muscles counteract the spinal erectors, *Figure 7.80*. Intense contraction of the Iliopsoas without warming up the spinal erectors can cause serious back injury.
- Perform at least three sets of unweighted Goodmorning, of at least ten repetitions per set, prior to embarking on any Sit-up exercise.
- The legs are fixed by the feet under a cross padded roll attached to the bench.
- The upper body can hang vertically downwards or lay on a flat bench.
- Elevating the upper body with twisting motion can enhance the oblique abdominal muscles intensely.

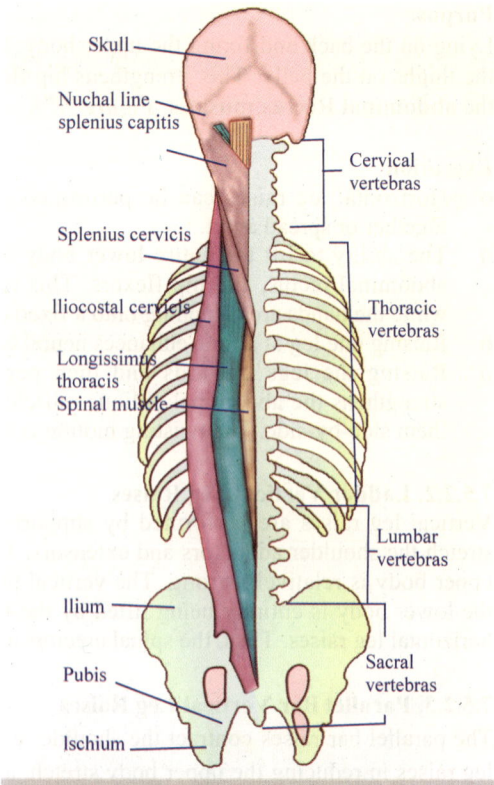
Figure 7.80. Spinal erector muscles.

7.5.3. HIP ADDUCTION
o   Hip adductors are the inner muscles of the upper thighs that pull the femur, the bone of the upper legs, medially, *Figure 7.62*. These muscles are **the Adductor magnus, the Adductor longus, the Adductor brevis, the Pectineus, the Gracilis, and lower fibers of Gluteus maximus.**
o   The Adductor magnus originates from the ramus and tuberosity of Ischium, the two bone projections we sit on.
o   The subsequent four adductors originate from the pubic bone.
o   The Gluteus maximus originates from the Ilium, Sacrum, and Coccyx.
o   Thus, each of the five bones of the pelvis (Ischium, Pubis, Ilium, Sacrum, and Coccyx) contributes to hip adduction. All the adductors insert on the back of the femur, except the Gracilis that inserts medial and upper to the tibia.

The hip adductors work out during wide feet-stance of the Squat and power Deadlift, but special exercises are sometimes performed to strengthen the hip adductors.

7.5.3.1. Cable And Machine Hip Adduction
These are performed using cable or machine decks to apply force to the inner side of the legs, while pulling the legs medially. The cable adduction is executed in standing position, *Figure 7.81*. The loaded cable pulls the ankle laterally, while the adductors resist, by dragging the leg medially. The seated machine hip adduction applies forces by loaded decks on the inner sides of the thighs. The hip adductors draw the thighs inwards. These are special exercises that are intended for general conditioning of beginners, late starters, rehabilitation, and when deformities or imbalance are targeted for correction.

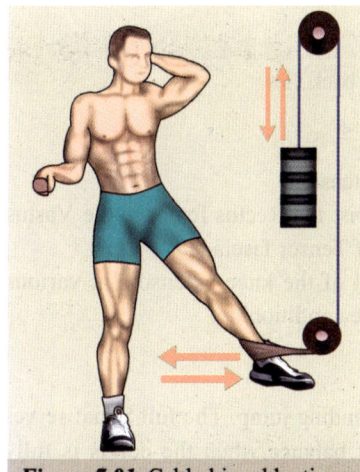
Figure 7.81. Cable hip adduction.

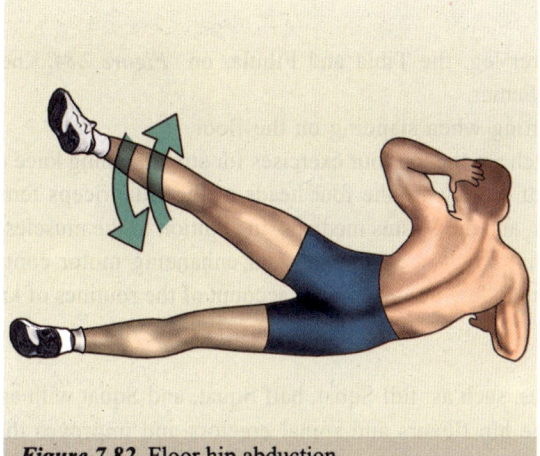
Figure 7.82. Floor hip abduction.

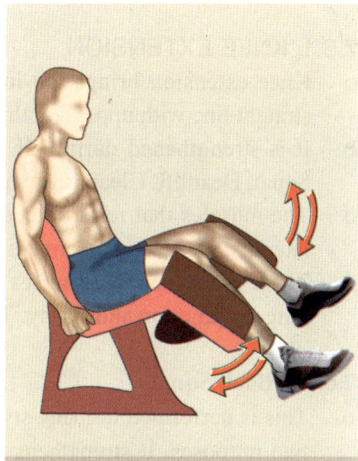
Figure 7.83. Machine hip abduction.

7.5.4. HIP ABDUCTION
o   Hip abductors pull the femur laterally and anchor the femur head into its socket. The major task of hip abductors is evident during running. The hip abductors anchor the femur head of the supporting leg. In the same time, they abduct the advancing leg in order to prevent the pelvis from dropping, during running.
o   Running works out the abductors of the leg that is supporting the bodyweight, by pulling the pelvis towards its side in order to maintain the spinal axis upright. The alternate shifting of the abduction from side to side during running is a determining factor in long distance endurance running, where the hip abductors adapt by developing highly efficient aerobic cellular respiration and slow twitch muscle fibers.
o   The combined actions of the following muscles abduct the femur shaft and compress the femur head: **Gluteus maximus, Gluteus medius, Gluteus minimus, muscles of Tensor fascia lata, Sartorius, Gemellus superior, Gemellus inferior, Obturator internus, Obturator externus, and Piriformis.**
o   These muscles originate from the Sacrum, Ilium, and Ischium. They are inserted on the upper back of the femur.
o   Hip abductors work out during squatting and deadlifting with close feet-stance by anchoring the hip balls into their sockets.

7.5.4.1. Floor And Machine Hip Abduction
o   Floor hip abduction is convenient and allows long and hard aerobic workout, for fat burning and hip trimming, *Figure 7.82*. The floor abduction utilizes the weight of the entire leg, as resisting force, to strengthen the abductors.
o   Machine hip abductors enhance the anaerobic strengthening of the muscles and increase their size and strength, *Figure 7.83*. The abductors are trained by applying forces at the outer sides of the legs, while resisting by pushing laterally.

7.6. STRENGTHENING THE KNEES

o   The knees are hinge joints that can only move in one plane of flexion and extension with very limited ability to rotate, *Figure 7.84*.
o   The knees cannot abduct, adduct, or elevate. The lateral and medial attachments of ligaments and muscles prevent the knees from abduction and adduction that is prohibited by the very design of its bony articulation.
o   The internal cruciate ligaments prevent the lower knee bone, the Tibia, from translation on the upper knee bone, the Femur. Thus, the knees are very insecure joints that can be easily injured by adduction, abduction, translation or rotation.
o   If exercise can do any good to the health of the knees, it can improve their strength and response to voluntary control, but exercise cannot prevent injuries due to reckless use of the knees or freak accidents that violate the anatomy of the knees.
o   Exercise can develop very strong extensors and flexors around the knees in proportion to the bodyweight. Yet, heavier bodyweight will undoubtedly put the knees at higher risk of twisting or wearing out.

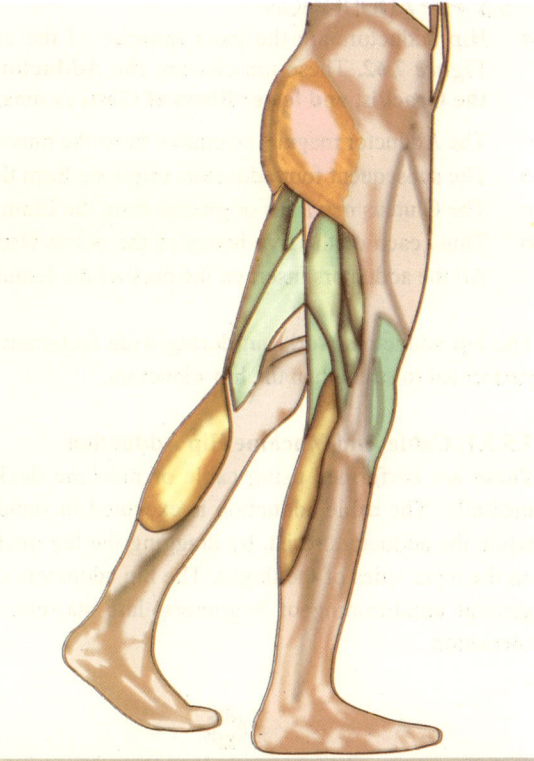

Figure 7.84. Knee, back view.

7.6.1. KNEE EXTENSION
o   Knee extension brings the lower leg, the Tibia and Fibula, on straight line with upper leg, the Femur.
o   It is strengthened during all lifting when standing on the floor Squat, Deadlift, Clean, and Snatch are the top four exercises for strengthening knee extension.
o   The muscles that resist forces of gravity are the four heads of the Quadriceps femoris: the Rectus femoris, the Vastus lateralis, the Vastus Intermedius, and the Vastus medialis, in addition to the muscles of Tensor fascia lata.
o   There are so many exercises that target strengthening and enhancing motor control of the knee extensors at various ranges of motion and agility. The following is a concise account of the routines of knee conditioning.

7.6.1.1. Back Squat
o   This is performed in many styles, such as: full Squat, half Squat, and Squat with ascending jump. The full Squat serves two purposes. It strengthens the hip flexors and spinal erectors and improves their balance when the pelvis is fully lowered below the knee levels. Secondly, it stretches the Quadriceps tendon to extreme. It thus induces the tendon ganglions to adapt by higher threshold of firing the termination signals of shutting the resisting muscles off.
o   The half Squat enhances the eccentric muscular contraction by setting brakes amidst the range of extension. Heavy half Squat is traumatizing to the knee structures and can cause a career ending knee injury.
o   The jump Squat is superb in enhancing neural recruitment of the Quadriceps.

7.6.1.2. Front Squat
Front Squat requires dual recruitment of the shoulders and knees. The mid-body carries extra burden of concerting such dual recruitment. It is mainly a neuromuscular conditioning exercise. It requires continuous problem-solving efforts, to remedy inflexibility and imbalance despite apparent strength. Front Squat can be performed with Clean from the hang in order to minimize instability due to inactive shoulder extensors and flexors.

7.6.1.3. One-Leg Stepping On A Block With Weights
This is an excellent asymmetric exercise that works out the hip abductors and the knee extensors, simultaneously. Its unique advantage is the specificity of neural control of individual heads of the Quadriceps. Stepping on a raised block, with a barbell loaded on the back of the shoulders, requires maximal recruitment of the Quadriceps, from fully relaxed status of standing upright. It differs from Squat in that the latter increases recruitment progressively and monotonously.

7.6.1.4. Deadlift
Deadlift engages the scapulas in transmitting the weights to the knees. Well-trained lifters use the Deadlift to exercise the knee extensors by lifting with upright torso and concave lumbar region. Lifting with inclined torso raises the hips too high above the knee level and enhances Hamstrings resistance over Quadriceps resistance.

7.6.1.5. The Clean and Snatch
These are one step better than the Deadlift in that they strengthen the upper body and generate virtual forces due to whole body acceleration over the bent knees. For the Clean and Snatch to benefit knee function, full squatting has to be practicing in the starting position as well as in the final phase of squatting under the bar.

7.6.1.6. Seated Knee Extension
This is unique in eliminating the Hamstrings action on supporting to the knees from behind. Thus the Quadriceps extends the knees while the anterior cruciate ligament prevent anterior translation of the tibia on the femur. It is a great rehabilitation exercise for inner knee structures. Knee extension is carried out on a bench with weight loaded on the front of the lower leg. The knee is extended against resistance while the entire body kept still with the hands gripping the side support of the machine, *Figure 7.85*.

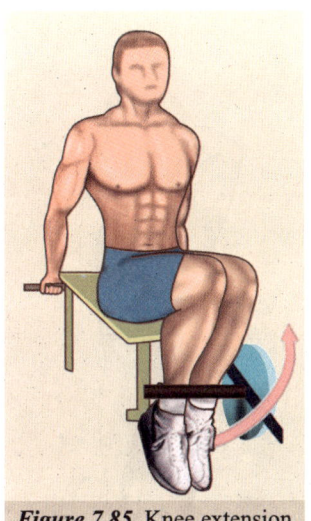
Figure 7.85. Knee extension.

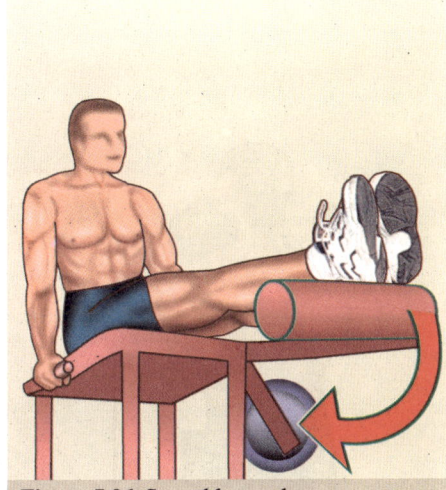
Figure 7.86. Seated leg curls.

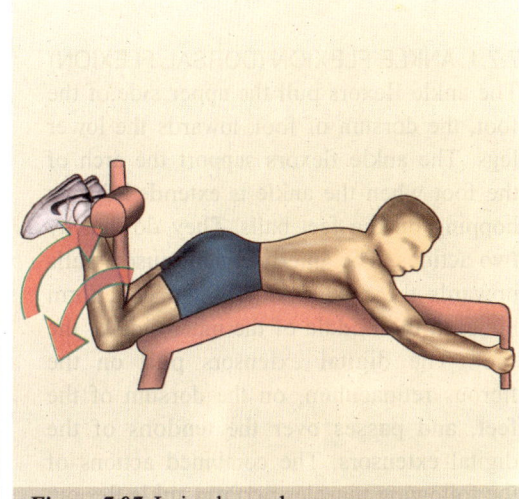
Figure 7.87. Lying leg curls.

7.6.2. KNEE FLEXION
o   Knee flexion comprises of bending the lower leg backwards on the upper leg. The knee flexors balance the extensors in supporting the hinge configuration of the knee joint.
o   Thus when you lean forwards or run, the knee flexors prevent your upper body from falling forwards by pulling the back of the thighs to the lower legs.
o   During running, knee flexors facilitate lifting the body to higher elevation, instead of being dragged on the surface of the ground.
o   The following five muscles participate in knee flexion: Hamstrings, Gracilis, Sartorius, Popliteus, and Gastrocnemius. Each muscle has a specific role to play.
o   The Hamstrings coordinate knee flexion and hip extension. The Gracilis transmits the adduction forces of the hip to the knee thus assist in maintaining the tibia and femur alignment. The Sartorius is an external rotator of the leg. The Popliteus is a medial rotator of the tibia and is used to unlock an extended knee. The Gastrocnemius coordinates knee flexion with ankle extension.

7.6.2.1. Leg Curl
Leg flexion machines apply forces to the back of the lower legs, while the lower legs are curled on the back of the thighs. Knee flexion curls are important in alleviating shortening and stiffness of the knee flexors that impede knee extension. Seated knee flexion, *Figure 7.86,* stretches the Hamstrings more than lying knee flexion because the ischial bones are displaced farther away from the knees when the person is seated. Since the knee extensors are mostly inactive during seated flexion, the internal posterior cruciate ligament is the main opponent to posterior knee translation by the pull of the Hamstrings and Gastrocnemius on the tibia. Lying prone during performing leg curls, *Figure 7.87,* works out the Hamstrings very hard, since they are shortened by hip extension and lack sufficient stretch reflex. Lying leg curls work similar to concentrated Biceps brachii[7] curls by imposing more strain on the Gastrocnemius, short head of Biceps femoris, and Semimembranous muscles.

---

[7] Biceps brachii is the front muscle of the upper arm. Biceps femoris is one of the three muscles of the back of the thigh.

7. WEIGHT TRAINING

7.7. STRENGTHENING THE ANKLE

o   Like the knees, the ankles are hinge joints that mostly perform flexion and extension.
o   Unlike the knees, the ankle joint is supported on each side with bony projection. These are the medial downward projection from the tibia and lateral downward projection from the fibula. The two bony projections, one on each side of the ankle joint, serve multiple functions.

   i.   They support the hinge joint articulation.
   ii. They also work as pulleys for the tendons of the muscles of the lower leg.
   iii. The bony projections create tunnels for passage of major vessels and nerves from the lower legs to the feet.

o   The narrow space of the ankle joint hosts the major tendons that control body balance on the ground during motion and standing. Due to the great weight that the ankles carry, it is easy to strengthen the ankles than any other joint in the body. Running and hopping on the feet- balls strengthen the ankle extensors.

7.7.1. ANKLE FLEXION (DORSAL FLEXION)

The ankle flexors pull the upper side of the foot, the dorsum of foot, towards the lower legs. The ankle flexors support the arch of the foot when the ankle is extended during hopping on the feet balls. They do that by two actions. The anterior tibial muscle pulls upwards the medial side of the cuneiform bone, in the middle of the inner side of the foot. The digital extensors pull on the fibrous retinaculum, on the dorsum of the feet, and passes over the tendons of the digital extensors. The combined actions of the following muscles perform ankle flexion: **Tibialis anterior, Extension digitorum longus, Extensor hallucis longus, and Peroneus tertius.**

Dorsiflexion supports hooking the feet under a support bar during inclined Sit-ups and works most during kicking a football with the dorsum of foot. Ankle flexion is worked out by isometric contraction during calf raises, *Figures 7.88* and *7.89*. There are not gym exercises that work out the ankle flexors by concentric contraction since this requires putting weights on the dorsum of the feet and lifting them, by raising the toes upwards.

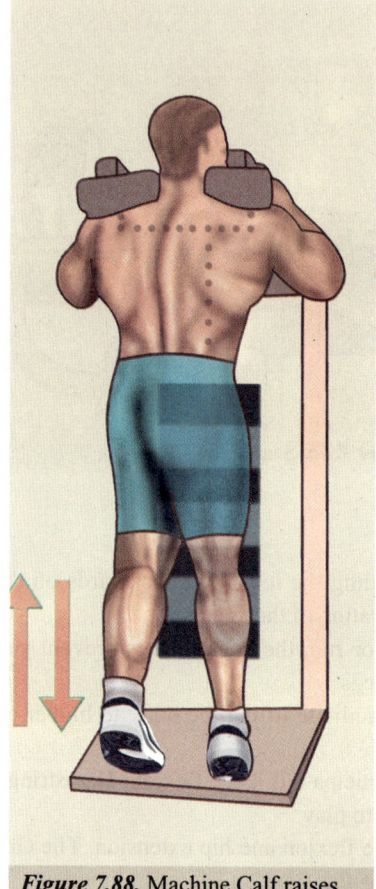

Figure 7.88. Machine Calf raises.

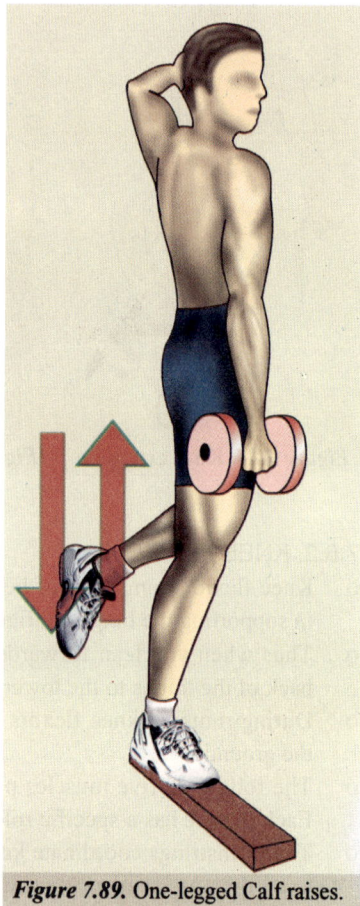

Figure 7.89. One-legged Calf raises.

7.7.2. ANKLE EXTENSION (PLANTAR FLEXION)

o   The ankle extensors raise the whole body on the feet balls by raising the under surface of the feet, the plantar surface or sole of foot, away from ground.
o   The ankle extensors are vital to mobility, agility, and coordination.
o   The combined actions of the following muscles produce ankle extension: **Gastrocnemius, Soleus, Plantaris, Tibialis posterior, Flexor hallucis posterior, and Flexor digitorum longus.**
o   The Gastrocnemius coordinates knee flexion with ankle extension and works out most during ballistic contraction such as jumping.
o   The Soleus is an ankle extensor proper and performs most of the extension during slow contraction in addition to turning the foot outside (eversion).
o   The Tibialis posterior assists in extension in addition to turning the foot inside (inversion) and maintaining the arch of the foot from collapsing on the blood and nerve supply to the sole.
o   The flexors of the toes also support the foot arch with farther extension under the sole.

Calf raises, *Figures 7.88* and *7.89*, are performed occasionally to enhance definition and mass of the muscles of the lower legs. These exercises have to be performed for long time in order to show any substantial results in people with thin lower legs.

7.8. STRENGTHENING THE ABDOMINAL MUSCLES

o   The abdominal muscles are located in the front sheath of the visceral contents of the abdominal cavity. They play vital role in regulating the homogeneous flow of gases, fluids, and solids within body cavities.
o   The abdominal muscles act as elastic membranes that dampen vibration and enhance wave propagation such that the inner milieu of the body maintains stability. Strong abdominal muscles prevent herniation (bulging to the outside) of the abdominal contents, when sudden excessive expiration takes place, as in coughing or sneezing.
o   They mobilize the guts by applying constant high tone that forces intestinal gases to move downwards or upwards the intestine thus facilitating the passages of digested food within the intestine.
o   The most vital functions of abdominal muscles though are enhancing circulation and breathing. The ability to control the intraabdominal pressure by strong and toned abdominal muscles assist in creating the negative pressure on the chest cage during inspiration and the positive pressure during expiration.
o   It also assist venous return from the limbs to the heart thus relieves congestion of the pelvic organs and the spinal cord.

The abdominal muscles consist of the front **Rectus abdominis** and the side Oblique and transverse muscles, **the External oblique, the Internal oblique, and the transversus abdominis.**
o   The Rectus abdominis originates from pubic crest of the pelvis and inserts into lower front ribs and the xiphoid process of the chest. It runs in the front of the belly and flexes the spinal axis by pulling the chest cage to the pelvis.
o   The two oblique muscles (External oblique and Internal oblique) originate from the lower front and back ribs, lumbar fascia, ilium, and Inguinal ligament and insert into the fascia of Rectus abdominis, ilium, inguinal ligaments, pubic crest, conjoint, and ribs, and linea alba. They run perpendicular to each other across the sides of the belly. They pull the chest cage to the side towards the pelvis by flexion and rotation by way of their perpendicular direction.

7.8.1. FLOOR ABDOMINAL CRUNCHES
o   Abdominal crunches are performed while lying supine and raising the head and chest on fixed lower back, *Figure 7.90*.
o   If the entire torso departs the floor then the hip flexors have to work hard. This fatigues the body and undermines your ability to exercises the rectus abdominis muscles. It is thus very simple and easy to work the front abdominal muscles, long and hard, if you curtail your appetite of lifting your entire torso and content yourself with mere abdominal workout, for the time being.
o   The lower back and lower thoracic vertebras have to stick to the ground during the entire abdominal crunches.

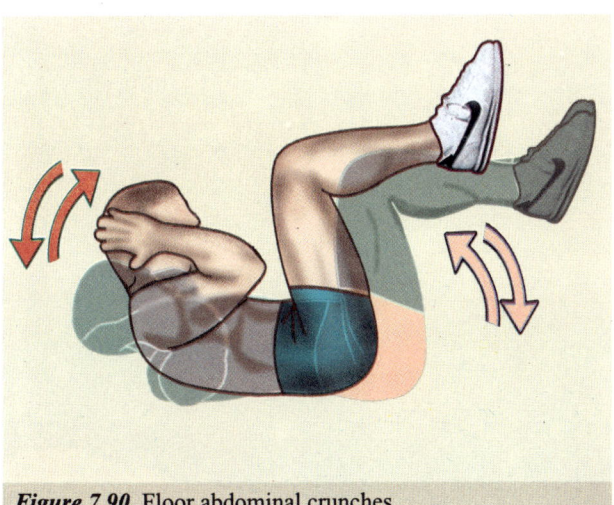
Figure 7.90. Floor abdominal crunches.

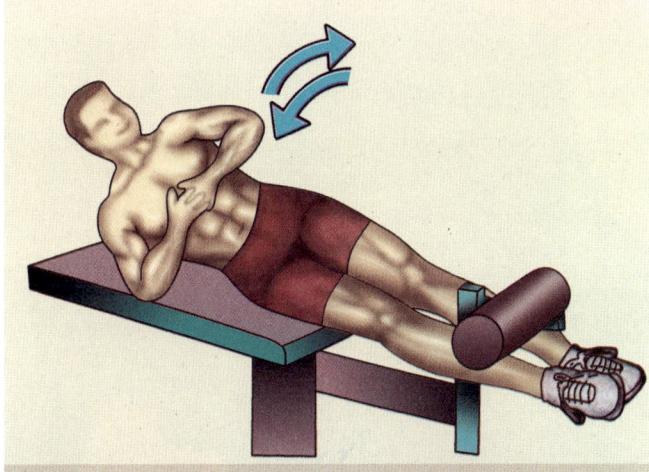
Figure 7.91. Oblique bends.

7.8.1.1. Oblique Bends

Oblique side bends are performed on a bench that has leg support, *Figure 7.91*. They can also be performed during floor crunches lying on the side of the body. This lateral lying position brings the oblique abdominal muscles into line with pulling the upper body weight. Of course, both sides have to be exercised separately since these are side muscles, while the rectus muscle can work solely with front crunches.

7.8.1.2. Trunk Rotation

This exercises the oblique abdominal muscles by twisting the chest on the pelvis along the spinal axis, *Figure 7.92*. The upper body may be kept fixed to the machine support or by using the upper body momentum to counteract the lower body motion. This exercise is equally useful to massaging the spinal joints and muscles and ligaments in between the transverse processes of the spines.

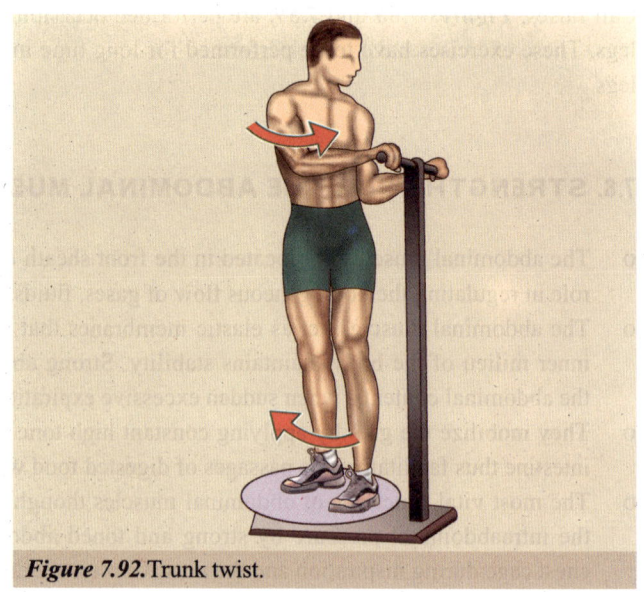

Figure 7.92. Trunk twist.

Chapter 8
The Snatch Lift

8.1. STANDARD SNATCH TECHNIQUE

The snatch lift comprises of lifting a barbell from the floor overhead with monotonous motion, without pauses or apparent shoulder pressing, in the interim. The variation in the style of lifting lies in the descent process of Squat versus leg spring.

8.1.1. PREPARATION
o   Stand over the barbell with the feet balls positioned under the bar, shoulder-width apart, or slightly wider, **Figure 8.1**. Close feet stance causes imbalance during performance. Wide feet stance impedes deep descent under the bar.
o   Before descending to grip the bar, try to relax every muscle in the body, particularly the thighs, lower back, and shoulders, **Figure 8.2**.
o   Squat down and grip the bar with wide overhand grip, **Figure 8.3**.
o   Position the shoulders over the bar with the back arched tightly inwards, in lordotic posture. Keep arms straight at the elbows, with elbows pointed laterally, **Figure 8.4**.

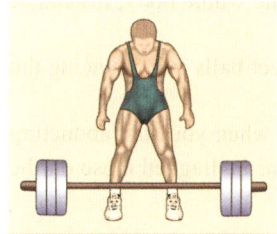
Figure 8.1. Standing over the bar.

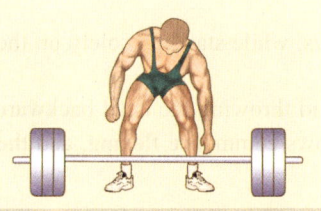
Figure 8.2. Descending to grip the bar.

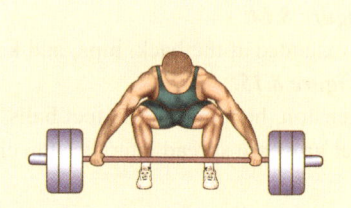
Figure 8.3. Adjusting handgrips.

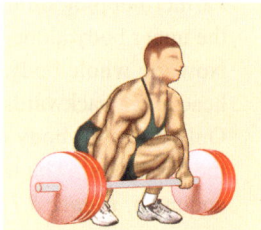
Figure 8.4. Adjusting posture of start position.

8.1.2. INDUCTION OF ACCELERATION
o   Before attempting to lift, exaggerate lordotic back, thrust the chest forwards and upwards, throw the shoulders backwards, and straighten the elbows, **Figure 8.5**.
o   Pull the bar upwards, off the floor by extending the hips and knees while maintaining very tight upper body, **Figure 8.6**.
o   Farther ascent is induced by leg drive, with very still upper body. The back stays inclined and concave. No elbow bending, no shoulders caving in, and no lower back laxity are allowed, **Figure 8.7**.
o   As the bar reaches the knees, the back assumes active arching inwards. The inclination angle of the back, with vertical, slightly narrows. The chest farther advances in thrusting as the scapular muscles over-tighten, **Figures 8.7** and **8.8**.

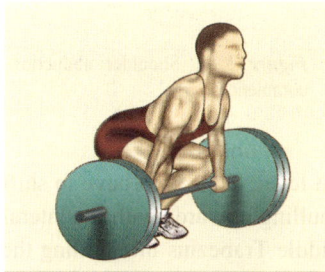
Figure 8.5. Final start position.

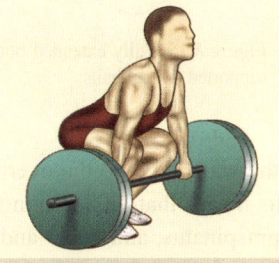
Figure 8.6. Tightening for lift.

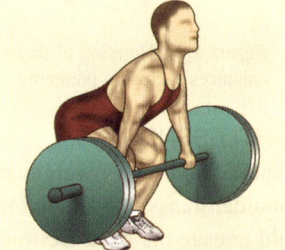
Figure 8.7. Deadlifting under the kneecaps.

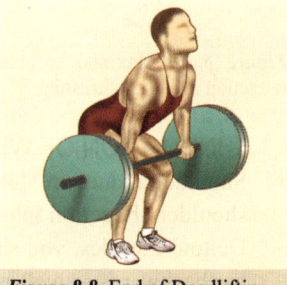
Figure 8.8. End of Deadlifting.

8.1.3. INDUCTION OF SPEED
o   As the bar passes the over the kneecaps, vigorously raise the shoulder plates, while dragging the bar as close to the legs as possible, **Figure 8.9**.
o   When the bar passes over the upper thighs, employ the forward kick by the hips and the backward shrug by the shoulders, **Figure 8.10**. The timing and magnitude of combined **"hip-kick and shoulder shrug"** are crucial to lifting.

o   As the bar reaches the groin region, the knees are still slightly bent, while the upper body almost reaches upright posture, *Figure 8.11*.
o   Further elevation of the bar is achieved by vigorous shoulder shrugging, *Figure 8.12*.

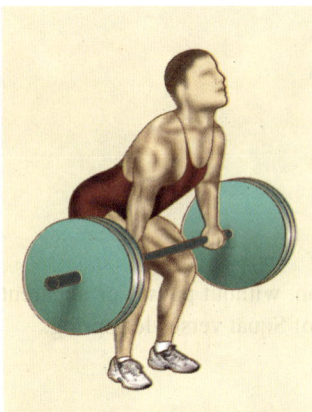 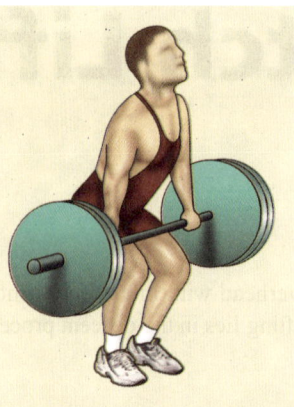 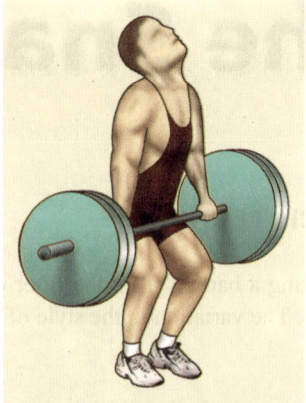 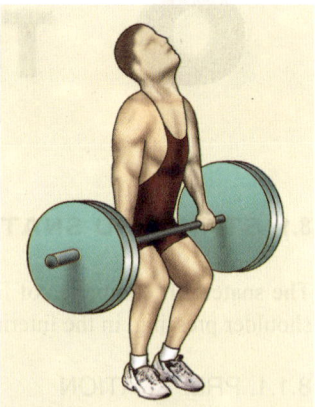

Figure 8.9. Maximal scapular tightening.   *Figure 8.10.* Forward Hip kick and backward shoulder shrug.   *Figure 8.11.* Upright straightening of the upper body.   *Figure 8.12.* Maximum shoulder shrugging.

8.1.4. INDUCTION OF MOMENTUM

o   In order to generate farther momentum, vigorously retract the shoulder plates, thrust the chest upwards and bounce the upper body backwards, *Figure 8.13*. Recall that the arms are still solidly tight and straight, at the elbows, and the shoulders are maximally shrugged.
o   Farther hopping on the feet balls, with straight arms, would enhance backward bouncing of the whole body, instead of the upper body alone, *Figure 8.14*.
o   Now the whole body is extended at the back, hips, and knees, while standing solely on the feet balls and bouncing the head away backwards, *Figure 8.15*.
o   Only after full body extension, hopping on the feet balls, and throwing the head backwards, when you start abducting the shoulders[1]. The upper arms are spread laterally, the elbows commence flexing, and the bar is dragged close on the abdomen, *Figure 8.16*.

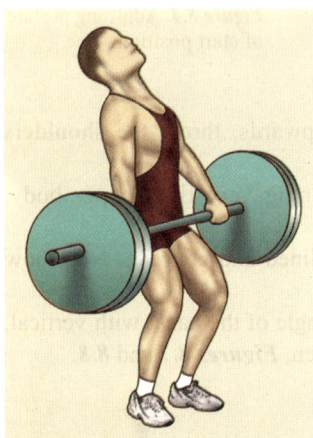 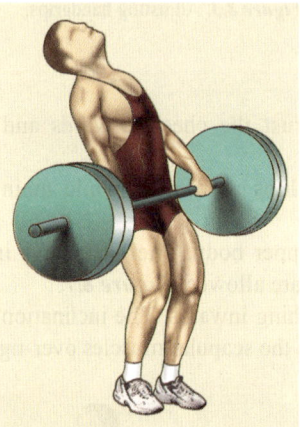 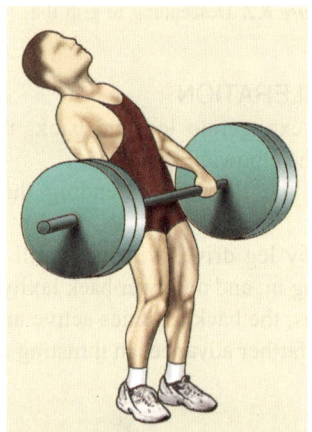 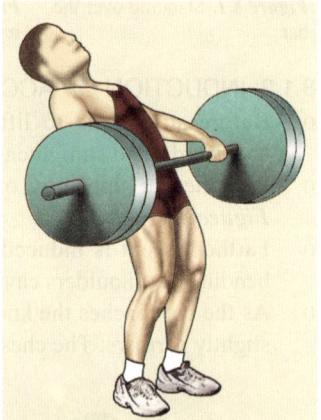

Figure 8.13. Maximal scapular retraction and chest thrusting.   *Figure 8.14.* Hopping of feet ball enhances backward bouncing.   *Figure 8.15.* Fully extended body supported on feet balls.   *Figure 8.16.* Shoulder abduction commences.

8.1.5. INDUCTION OF WEIGHTLESSNESS

o   Shoulder abduction alone cannot pull heavy weight from the waist level to the overhead level. Thus, you have to shift shoulder abduction into shoulder transverse adduction. This means that, in addition to pulling upwards with the lateral Deltoid muscles, you should engage the back Deltoid, Supraspinatus, and upper and middle Trapezius into pulling the bar backwards as well as upwards, *Figure 8.17*.
o   Now, the bar is approaching the shoulder level and the hips are advanced under the bar. No farther vigorous upwards lift is possible at this position. Thus, the knees are prepared to flex into squatting while the elbows have reached the shoulder level, *Figure 8.18*.
o   While the arms guide the bar backwards and upwards, the hips return backwards, but descend as the knees flex. Here, the heels should have landed onto the floor to prepare for full squatting, *Figure 8.19*.

---

[1] Shoulder abduction means moving the upper arm to the outsides, laterally. This can bring the elbows as high as the shoulder level, to the side.

o   While the hip sink downwards between the lower legs, the upper arms are throwing the bar over and behind the head. The upper body has to advance forwards, in the meantime, in order to enhance shoulder elevation, *Figure 8.20*.

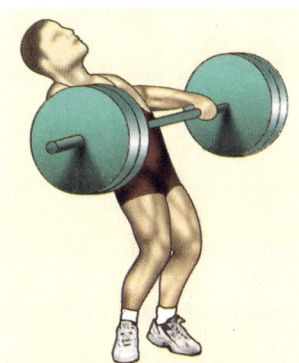
Figure 8.17. Transverse shoulder adduction draws the bar closer to the body.

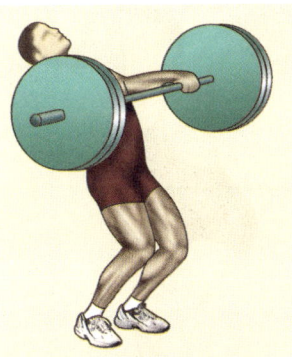
Figure 8.18. Beginning of descent by knees flexion.

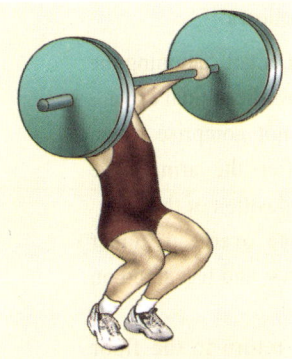
Figure 8.19. Sinking of the hips.

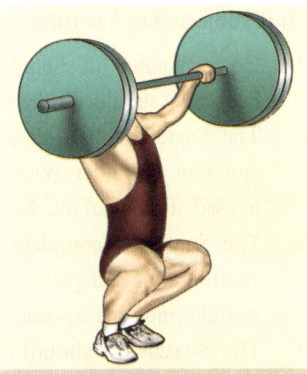
Figure 8.20. Advancing the upper body while squatting.

8.1.6. OVERHEAD SQUATTING

o   As the bar moves upwards and backwards, the upper body advances downwards and forwards. The arms catch the bar at arms length over shoulders, while moving into the Squat position, *Figure 8.21*.
o   Bar catching is stabilized by adjusting muscular contraction in order to balance the centers of mass on a vertical plane through the feet balls. Here, the Trapezius, Deltoids, Triceps lock the bar over the spinal axis. The balance between the Subscapularis and Supraspinatus determines the ease of tolerating this posture. In addition, the balance between the Iliopsoas and the back erectors determines the lower body stability during overhead Squat, *Figure 8.22*.

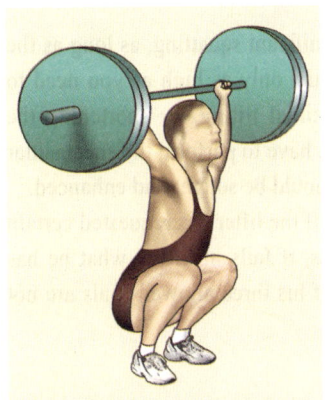
Figure 8.21. Bar catching in overhead Squat.

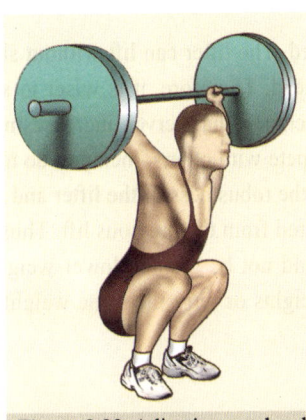
Figure 8.22. Adjusting overhead Squat.

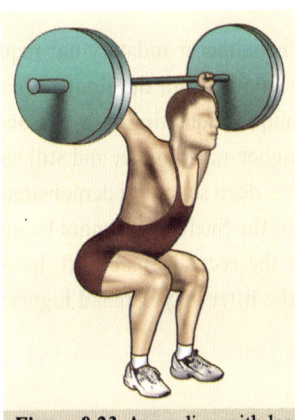
Figure 8.23. Ascending with leg drive.

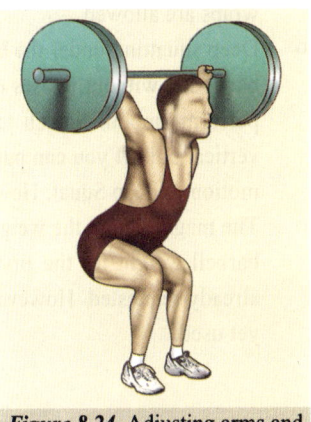
Figure 8.24. Adjusting arms and body posture.

8.1.7. FINAL ASCENT

o   As soon as the bar is caught and stabilized in overhead squat, on the locked out arms, ascent commences with tightening the upper Trapezius, Deltoids, and Triceps while the Quadriceps and Glutei initiate the upward ascent with the bar. Here, the torso will incline on the vertical line in order to compensate for the hip elevation, *Figure 8.23*.
o   As the knees extend over horizontal thigh level, locked upper body maintains the center of masses vertical on the feet balls. Manipulation of the chest thrusting, back-lordosis, and shoulder rotation, balances the final phases of ascent, *Figure 8.24*.
o   Final lower body extension is only possible if the shoulder proper could still sustain the final work of upward descent. Now the bar is high overhead and the heart has to pump blood to higher level of tightly contracted muscles, *Figure 8.25*.
o   Snatch is completed by full-extended body and arms with the bar placed an arm-stretch overhead, *Figure 8.26*.

8.1.8. BARBELL RETURN TO THE FLOOR

Bend knees slightly. Lower the barbell, very close to your body, to mid-thigh position. Slowly lower the bar to the floor with taut lower back and trunk. Advanced athlete may drop the bar from the final Snatch position. Bar throwing may be practiced to reduce the stress or fatigue involved in lowering the bar, as prescribed. Use rubber Weightlifting plates on a Weightlifting platform if this unloading method is used.

8. THE SNATCH LIFT

8.2. CONTEST RULES OF THE SNATCH LIFT

In order to standardize competition, a correct Snatch lift is subjected to few rules, as follows.

- Correct Snatch lift should not entail stationing the bar on the shoulder, prior to overhead final drive.
- The Snatch motion should not comprise of an apparent shoulder push, after the arms have paused at the final overhead position of the bar.
- The Snatch is complete once overhead, under control, arms straight at elbows, and feet stand on straight line, side-by-side.
- The Snatch lift should not return to the floor after initial upward advancing of the lifting has commenced. Thus, once lifting proceeds, the bar should proceed upwards is smooth motion, without midway stations or pauses other than the final overhead stop.

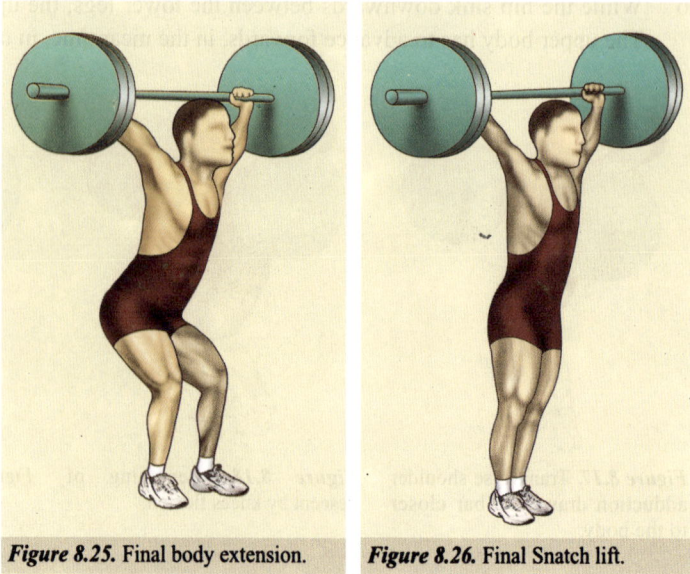

Figure 8.25. Final body extension.   *Figure 8.26.* Final Snatch lift.

- The upward Snatch motion can involve lifting overhead, and descending in Squat, but should not involve elbow bending, once the bar reaches overhead. Thus, the whole body can descend with the bar caught in both hands, with straight and locked arms. Yet, the bar should not descend with bending elbows, before final signaling from the judges.
- Correct contest Snatch lift is a single lift. If the lifter repeats the lift after returning the bar to the floor, the second lift is not counted and the first lift might be defaulted for breaking contest rules.
- Snatch lift cannot be performed with wrist straps. The lifter may wear standard knees, wrists, or elbow wraps, but no hand wraps are allowed.
- Deep squatting under the bar is neither mandatory nor required. The lifter can lift without significant squatting, as long as the bar is lift without pauses or stations, from the floor to overhead. Therefore, it is wiser to squat only as high as you need to perform smooth Snatch technique. Squatting is a personal choice that serves increase maximal lifting, by shortening the vertical pull. If you can pull higher and stronger and still compete with others, then you do not have to perform the spectacular motion of deep Squat. However, deep squatting demonstrates the robustness of the lifter and should be sought and enhanced.
- The magnitude of the weight of the Snatch lift cannot be lowered from the previous lift. Thus, if the lifter has requested certain barbell weight for the first or the second Snatch lift, he would not be granted lower weights, if fails in lifting what he has already requested. However, the lifter may demand higher weights or retry the same weight if his three allowed trials are not yet used.

8.3. TRAINING PRACTICE ON THE SNATCH LIFT

Weightlifters do not practice the standard Snatch each training session. They have to work on enhancing the different phases of the lift, in addition to the general requirements of strength, flexibility, coordination, and recuperation. Therefore, weightlifters may resort to spice their training plan with variations of style of execution and level of intensity that serve the purpose of enhancing the neuromuscular performance of the Snatch, as follows.

- During training, you are absolved of the stringent rules of contest. You have the options to refining the Snatch lift with various methods of execution.
- You can perform the Snatch with a Barbell, Dumbbell, plate, or any manageable object.
- You can break down the different phases of the Snatch to Deadlift, Hang Snatch, or Shoulder Press and Overhead Squat.
- You can perform Snatch in military, power, or standard style.
- You can vary the handgrip from close, shoulder-width, to standard handgrip width.
- You can perform more than one lift in a set, usually three repetitions per set.
- The norm of training practice is relying mainly on the standard Snatch style and supplementing that with enhancing variations of the technique. The standard style of the Snatch is performed, on average, four to six sets per session, with weight in the range 60% to 90% 1RM. The accessory exercises are performed in groups of three to four sets, once or twice weekly.

THE SNATCH LIFT

8.4. SPECIFIC FEATURES OF THE MECHANISM OF EXECUTION OF THE SNATCH

8.4.1. ARM USAGE IN TRANSFER OF FORCES

o   For so long, Weightlifters have realized that the arms are best used as *transfer rods*. The arms are the weakest parts of Weightlifters and are best put to use only as straight, stiffed limbs, during most of the lifting processes, *Figure 8.27*.

o   Straight limbs can stand tension by virtue of the strength of their ligaments, tendons, and supporting fibrous tissues. Since the arm muscles are long and contain few pinnas, they are not specialized in strong muscular contraction, as is the case with the lower limbs. Thus, the upper limbs are utilized for their **ligaments**, whereas the lower limbs for their muscles.

o   Thus significantly heavy weights are driven up by **axial and paraxial muscles**. The strength of these big muscles is transferred to the bar via the arms. This contradicts the common usage of the arms by lay people, in pulling.

o   Performing this trick, of straight arms during lifting, is easy said than done. Lifters tend to resort to the **basic instinct** of bending the arms prematurely to approximate the bar to its final destination. Since the arm will definitely fail to lift the extraordinarily heavy weight, the lifter may drop the weight in submission to the failed arms.

o   With lengthy and regular training, the Biceps and the Triceps muscles will develop enough strength to keep the arms as straight as possible. Weaker arm muscles trigger early firing of the tendon organs to terminate the lift.

o   Another explanation of the failure of bent arms, during lifting, is **vascular** in origin. Bent arms require the clavicles to fall downwards and restrict the major veins to the arms. Venous congestion of the arms during lifting is numbing to the peripheral nerves and leads to failure of lift.

o   The **central motor control** of the extrapyramidal[2] system is overwhelmed by the complex involvement of the so many joints, when the arms are bent. The communication between the central system and the peripheral motor effectors conveys information about the speed of motion, the acceleration of motion, the magnitude of strength, the relative position of each joint, and specific muscles that need get involved. The central system processes this information to determine the proper recruitment order and speed. Bending the arms complicates this information and overloads the brain to failure. Advanced lifters learn to engage only few groups of muscles in each phase of the lifting. Thus learning how to dissect the lift into its basic phases is of profound help to advance training, *Figures 8.27* thru *8.29*.

o   Inexperienced beginners always bend the arms lifting, unaware of the fact that lifting entails two processes. First is to equalize the weight of the bar without

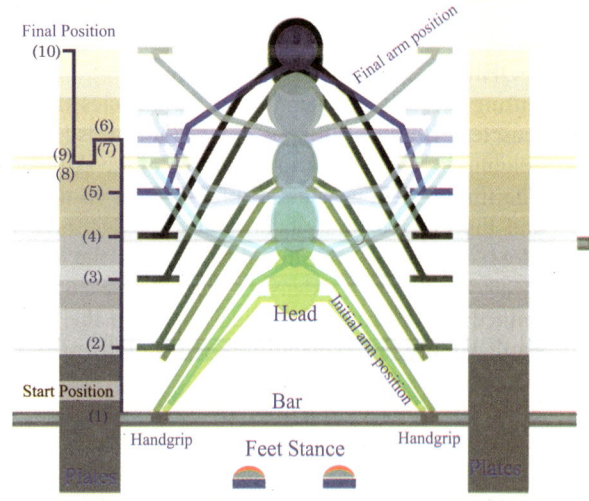

Figure 8.27. The arm pull during Snatch (front view): 1- Start position, 2- Deadlift and acceleration, 3- Beginning of speeding, 4- Maximal speed, 5- Shoulder abduction (weightless bar), 6- Maximal height of weightless bar, 7- Lifter descends under a suspended bar, 8- Dipping of the bar and the lifter, 9- Retrieval and ascent, 10- Final height of lift.

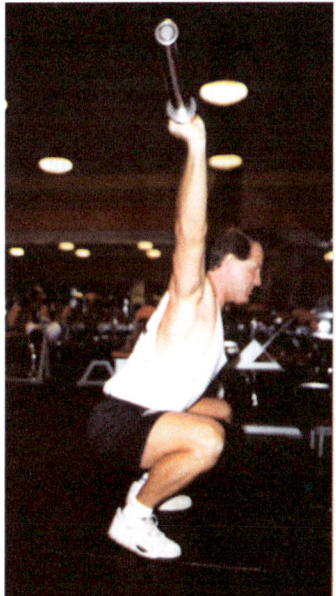

Figure 8.28. Learning to balance a bar vertically above the lower back, mid feet, and hip joint, during Overhead squatting requires regular training.

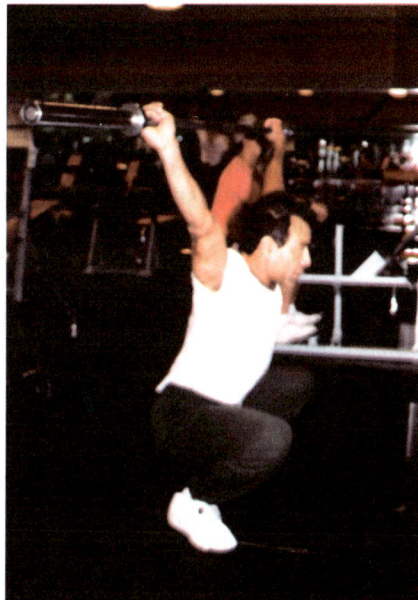

Figure 8.29. Thrusting the chest and erecting the lower back facilitate shoulder elevation and scapular retraction.

---

[2] The pyramidal neural tract coveys motor signals from the brain motor neurons to the spinal neurons. The "pyramidal" feature originates from the shape of cross section of the tract in the dissected brain. The extra-pyramidal neural tract originates from many areas in the brain. It modifies the pyramidal action through the spinal gamma neurons. The extra-pyramidal tract displays the effects, of rest, sleep, anxiety, stress, brain imbalance, and other vital functions, on neuromuscular control. When you struggle to perform, flex, or bend, it ts due to extra-pyramidal upset. A warm bath and adequate stretching will undoubtedly restore your ability to master your muscles and suppress the overriding activation of a stressed brain.

any movement. Second is to put the bar into ascending motion. If arms are bent during the first phase of equalization, very little strength will remain in the arms to proceed with the second phase of ascent. Experienced trainees learned to keep the elbows straight as long as the bar is still moving up. Even in their worst days, experienced lifters can lift better than inexperienced trainees, thanks to this arm trick.

8.4.2. ORIGIN OF LIFTING FORCES

o Lifting forces are generated by the muscles that take their origin from the **vertebral column**, the axial or primary muscles. Because lifting is directed upwards (cephalad), the force has to originate from a point higher on the vertebral columns. This is the occipital portion of the skull and upper back of neck, the Nuchal line.

o The line of action of these forces passes to the arms through the scapula and the clavicle thus incorporates the Deltoids in its way to the arms. Most probably, the initial sensor of the magnitude of the weight is located in the neck extensors. This can be easily explained in terms of the immediate location of the neck between the arms and the axial column. Farther more, all Weightlifters are well characterized by the heavily built neck muscles.

o Since the point of origin of the lifting force lies behind the skull, lifters realize that the skull can be used in leverage action to generate momentum. That aids the person in lifting weights far exceeding his own body weight, *Figure 8.30*. The backward head bouncing during lifting starts when the bar clears the knees and when the speeding process is advanced. Now with head thrown back and the arms kept straight and hardened at the elbow, the bar is falling very close to the body. This posture maintains shorter arm of resistance, while the longer arm of force is getting longer. The *arm of resistance* is measured as the horizontal distance between the vertical that passes through the middle point of the bar and the vertical that pass through the base of the big toes. The *arm of force* is the horizontal distance between the latter vertical and the vertical that passes through the base of the skull. As the skull is through backwards, the force-arm is growing, as well as the force of pulling.

o Bouncing the head backwards without falling is a skill that develops over time. This is gained by conditioning the nervous system coordination and the muscular strength to synchronize each element of the combination of pull-head bouncing-squatting.

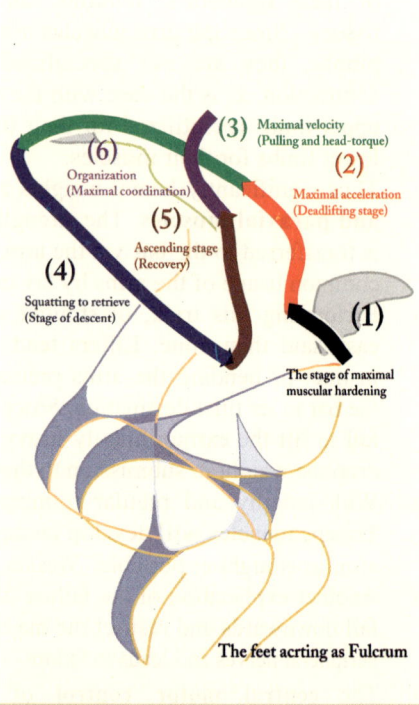

Figure 8.30. The head motion during lifting,

8.4.3. MOMENTUM OF HEAD BOUNCING

The Glutei, Hamstrings, and Spinal erector muscles generate backward bouncing of the head around the knee and upward elevation on the knees. The Quadriceps generates forward bouncing and upward elevation around the knees. These two actions around the knees, during leg drive, produce a combination of an upward force of lifting and a couple of two opposing but equal forces. The "couple" is another name for the "torque" and represents the tendency of force to rotate the body when acting remotely around a point. The direct force generated by the Quadriceps at the knees acts directly on the knees by extending them. The remote force generated by the action of the other three extensors on skull bouncing acts remotely at the knees, trying to flex them. The generated moment equals the muscular force, multiplied by the horizontal distance between the head and the knee. That moment is a property of the couple or torque.

8.5. LEARNING THE SNATCH LIFT

8.5.1. DISCOVER YOUR ABILITY TO PERFORM FORMIDABLE MOVEMENTS

The effort taken in learning the Snatch lift results in a gratifying feeling of accomplishment. That is because the Snatch lift challenges the ability of the upper and the lower body girdles to perform in harmony. Any imbalanced joint manifests clearly in this lift. What else is more gratifying than seeing the results of your planning become reality? After few weeks practicing, the lifter discovers the immense ability of the body to perform quick, symmetrical, harmonious, and powerful lift.

8.5.2. INDIVIDUAL VARIATION IN LEARNING AND OBJECTIVITY

o The main problem confronting self-learners is the lack of objectivity due to the lack of immediate input from an outside observer, a coach. There are many cases when the learner possesses exquisitely keen ability to execute perfect technique by a mere glance of observation. Yet, the majority of people would not grasp even few of the many features of proper lifting, on short observation. The previous habits in the person's life override his or her ability to quickly grasp the new modification in performance.

o Coaches can easily pinpoint the dominant traits, in new learners, of total unacquaintance of the mechanics of lifting. After explaining to beginners how to stand close to the bar, overextend the back, drop the hips to the knee-level,

straighten arms, thrust chest, and proceed slowly with hardened muscles, not even a single rule would be followed, in the first few trials after explanations. It would take constant reminding and reasoning, with new learners, to instill the new habits into their higher center of automatic control of motor execution. Sometimes, few days or weeks might go by before the new learner begins to initiate newly learned habits with little or no reminding.
- New learners have their prejudice toward practical execution of motor skill. Many have been taught to believe that lifting is as easy as any naturally acquired skill, such as walking and eating. What enforces these prejudices is the attitude of many fitness trainers that confuse body form for performance. The new learner makes his utmost goal in lifting the weight to his chest; with total disregard to all told rules. With persistent reminding, he starts to incorporate one or few rules at a time, depending on his ability to relax his mind and suppress his driving emotion.
- Some learners feel satisfaction in just becoming able to execute the least rules possible and hope to complete the rest in latter sessions. Many would renege on certain rules, repeatedly and for many months or even years. This could be attributed to many factors in the personal life that reduce the strength of some groups of muscles and force the lifter to skimp the rules of proper lifting. An example of the latter case, a school student who spends many hours sitting would suffer from major upper body weakness, compared to a warehouse worker who lifts most of his time on the job in addition to training. Another example is that of a frequent reader of Bodybuilding publications who trains different parts of his body, on consecutive days, and finds himself struggling with the gruesome effort of whole body exercise, in a single workout.
- Thus, learning has to account for all factors that shape the person's life and affect his mind and body to deal with the mechanics of lifting. A gradual insertion of one rule at a time is the best approach to conquer the grounds in the learning process. It is very beneficial to deepen your insight into your own makeup. Ask yourself, what is lacking in you that makes you different from your role model? Remember that long term planning can get many people, including yourself, to any advanced level they aspire to.
- When you fail to execute some rules, remember that you are still learning. I hate to tell you that learning is a life long process. The elitist of all athletes submits to that very fact about learning, until the end of life. By the time, you learn all the rules of proper lifting; you confront new issues of striving to get stronger and stronger with time. If you strike the right balance of proper knowledge and behavior, you distinguish yourself from others by your very individual ingenuity.

8.5.3. LEARNING WITH DUMMY OBJECTS
- Learning a new lift has to start with ridiculously light objects. A rope or a light wooden rod may help simulate the bar and coordinate visual sensation with motor activity.
- The ultimate goal of light weight execution is to master the timing of five distinctive phases of the Snatch motion. The five phases are alternating combination of stability, of one half of the body, accompanied by mobility, of the other half, in successive alterations cadence, as follows.
    i. The first phase is the equalization of the inertia of the external weight by tightening major muscles prior to initiating motion. This is the phase of **"start position"**.
    ii. The second phase is the isometric tension of the upper body, when the lower body is extending. This is the phase of **"acceleration"**.
    iii. The third phase is the upper body extension, when the lower body reaches maximal stability. This is the phase of **"speed"**.
    iv. The fourth phase is lower body flexion, while the upper peripherals are extending. This is the phase of **"descent"**.
    v. The fifth phase is the extension of the lower body, while the upper body reaches maximal stability. This is the phase of **"ascent"**.
- As the weight gradually increases, the nervous sensors of muscles and tendons will reset their firing potential to new levels. Acquisition and adaptation to such compound motion resides in modifying motion reflexes, not just cognition.
- The longer is the period of practice with light weight, and the gradual is the increase of the external weight, the more predicable is the response of the balance sensors. This is particularly true in the Snatch lift, which differs from all other locomotive activities.
- The Snatch requires robust contraction of the shoulder and the leg muscles, a wide range of motion with strong flexible joints, and a tip-top axial musculoskeletal fitness.
- Even after many years of training on the Snatch lift, the lifter has to refresh the memories of his muscles, joints, and tendons, by executing the Snatch mechanism with very light weight.

8.6. START POSITION OF THE SNATCH

8.6.1. ANALYSIS OF THE START POSITION OF THE SNATCH
- In order to transmit muscular forces to the bar, the body has to assume distinctive posture that optimizes the leverage action of the muscles on joints. With completely tightened and still upper body, your lower body initiates the upward drive, by strong extension motion. Low body extension entails overextended back and concentrically contracting Glutei and Quadriceps, in order to equalize the weight of the bar.

8 THE SNATCH LIFT

- In order to master this crucial technique of initiating lifting, your back will have to simulate an inclined flat and solid board, *Figure 8.31-A*. The flat board comprises of the Trapezius on the top of the back, the Deltoids on the sides of the shoulders, the Latissimus dorsi on the sides of the back, and the shoulder plates in the center of the flat surface.
- The Trapezius will bulge on the sides of the neck, *Figure 8.31-B*.
- The Latissimus dorsi will fill the gap between the arms and the chest and push the arms away from the body, to the outside, *Figures 8.31 and 31-D*.
- The Deltoid will fill the side view of the shoulders.
- The flatness of the back is viewed from the side as a straight line, inclined with the vertical, between 30 to 45 degrees, *Figures 8.31-A* and *-C*.
- The thighs can initiate the upward derive from slightly above the knee level. Yet, squatting below the knee levels is a common habit in stretching the knees, *Figures 8.31-E* thru *-G*.
- Any temptation to compromise the flatness of the back or the tightness of its muscles will lead to losses in transferring the forces from the legs to the rams, passing by the spinal axis.

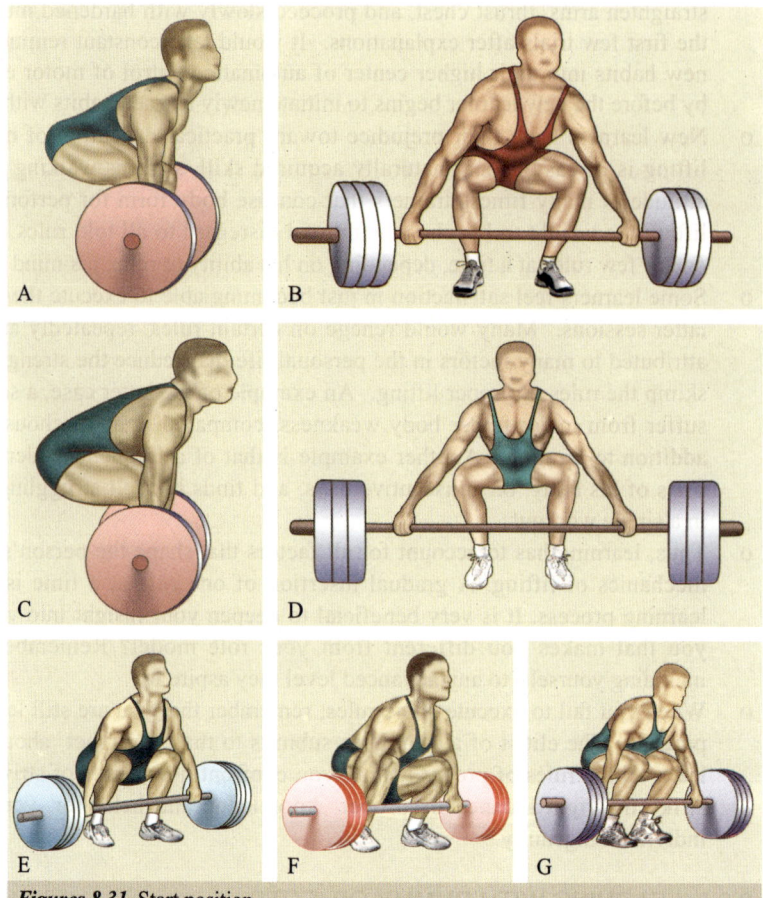

Figures 8.31. Start position.

8.6.2. STRENGTHENING THE START POSITION OF THE SNATCH
The start position of the Snatch can be enhanced with various methods of training, as follows:
- Regular execution of the standard Snatch, at least three sessions weekly.
- Deadlift and pulls with Snatch posture and hand griping.
- Squat with variation in depth, intensity, and style. This exercise enhances major axial muscles.
- Goodmorning exercise for strengthening back erectors.
- Sit-ups with weights for strengthening the Iliopsoas. This helps stabilizing the pelvis by pulling the lumbar vertebras forwards, towards the thighs.
- Biceps and Triceps strengthening for the sake of strengthening the elbow stability, during stretching prior to lifting.

8.7. PHASE OF ACCELERATION OF THE SNATCH

8.7.1. ANALYSIS OF THE PHASE OF ACCELERATION OF THE SNATCH
- As soon as the weight of the bar is equalized, by whole body tightening, the Trapezius initiates the first vigorous contraction in breaking the deadlock, of a heavy bar weight abutting the floor. During Trapezius shrugging, the entire scapular muscles work hard to stabilize the scapulas and thrust the chest forwards and backwards, *Figures 8.32*.
- The lower back assumes lordotic and tight posture, *Figure 8.32-A*. Some lifter has the ability to compromise the low back concavity and lift with straight lower back, with few or no problems, *Figure 8.32-C*.
- The arms are tightly extended at the elbows and strongly adducted to the spinal axis by the Latissimus dorsi.
- The hips are elevated faster than the chest and head. Thus, the back inclination approaches the horizontal, from that of the start position. The early elevation of the hips throws the chest forwards and increases the stretch on the Hamstrings, *Figure 8.32-C*.
- The bar must move very close to the shins, even though the chest has assumed more forward position, from that of previous position.
- The thrust chest and retracted scapulas are judged by the advance of the chest, ahead of the shoulders, and the flattening of the two scapulas, *Figures 8.32-E* thru *-G*.
- Pictures alone cannot demonstrate the speed of lifting. In this phase, speed starts from null at the floor and gradually increases, but remains minimal, up to the kneecaps. Your goal in this phase is not to move fast, but to maintain changing speed.
- All muscles above the waist level contract by mere isometric contractions. If there is any relative slow motion in the upper body, it will be in the exaggeration of the lordosis curvature of the lower back and the farther retraction of the

scapulas. Advanced lifters master these two, slow and strong, relative motions. Lordosing the lower back and thrusting the chest bring the arms closer to the spinal axis and thus eliminate horizontal shear stresses.
o The hands clench the bar tightly in neutral posture, allowing the bar to hang vertically of the arms.
o The elbows are tightened by the opposing actions of the Biceps brachii and the Triceps.
o The shoulders are widely spread laterally, in order to maintain elevated clavicles and permit vital passages through the neck outlet, to and from the chest and arms, *Figure 8.32-D*.
o The heels are stuck solid on the ground, yet the mid-feet are strongly arched, bridging the space between the heels and the feet balls. This feet posture is learned from the alert state of performing vigorous dynamic work. This is not the case in stationary exercises such as the Deadlift.

8.7.2. STRENGTHENING THE PHASE OF ACCELERATION OF THE SNATCH

Breaking the deadlock, by setting the barbell into motion, requires very strong axial muscles as well as strong-arm muscles.
o The Deadlift exercise is crucial in strengthening the muscles that induce acceleration.
o The Squat in crucial in enhancing leg drive.
o The Goodmorning fosters greater stretchability of the spinal ligaments and muscles.
o The Bench Press strengthens scapular retraction.
o The forearm reverse and Biceps curls are paramount to strengthening elbow flexion and wrist extension.
o The Leg Press can strengthen flexibility of fully flexed knees and hips.

8.8. PHASE OF INITIATING MOMENTUM OF THE SNATCH

8.8.1. ANALYSIS OF THE MOMENTUM INITIATION OF THE SNATCH

Your next task commences as the bar (rope or rod) approaches the kneecaps. You then have to get ready to mere torso extension. This is accomplished by vigorously contracting the Hamstrings, the Glutei, and the back erectors in order to bounce your entire upper body backwards. The main reason for commencing this phase after the bar clears the knees is that the travel from here to the shoulders is obstacle-free. Below the knees, one cannot move fast since the knees protrude in the way of pulling the bar.
o As the bar clears the knees, the Glutei and the back erectors vigorously contract. The bar will be driven upwards solely by means

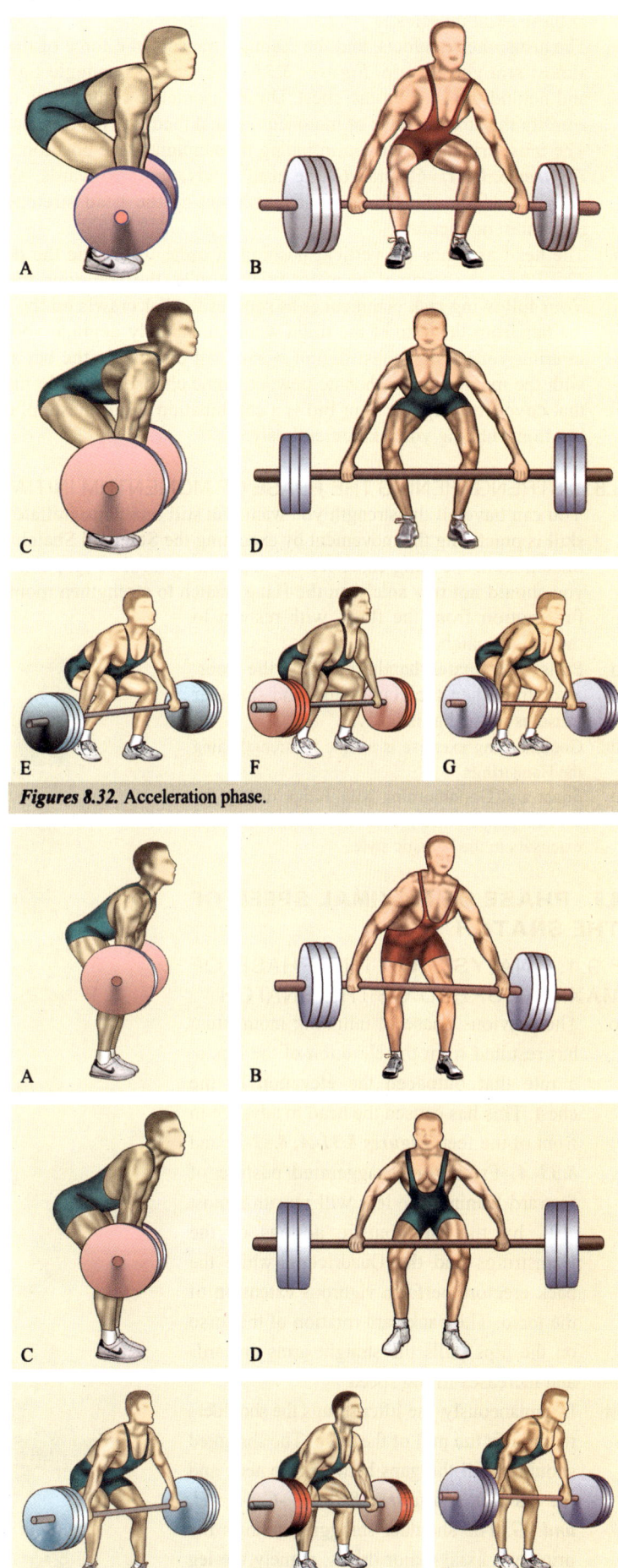

Figures 8.32. Acceleration phase.

Figures 8.33. Initiating momentum.

THE SNATCH LIFT

of these axial muscles.
- The arms, the shoulders, and the scapulas transmit the force of the axial muscles to the bar. The arms have to maintain almost straight posture, *Figures 8.33*. The scapulas snuggle tightly to the chest cage. The shoulders spread laterally and behind the front of the chest. During isometric contraction, the upper body experiences extreme stretch. This will amplify the stretch reflex of motoneurons and facilitate neuromuscular control of maximal strength.
- The most critical posture in initiating momentum is the position of the head with respect to the feet balls. Note that in *Figures 8.33-A, -C,* and *–G*, the head is advancing forwards, ahead of the feet. In the same time, the lower back is deeply lordotic. The forward advancement of the head stretches the Hamstrings maximally and helps initiate the maximum momentum.
- The head assumes the vertical position in order to elevate the posterior Nuchal line of the skull to the highest level. This line is the origin of the major axial muscles, the Trapezius and Capitis longus.
- Your following task commences as soon as the bar crawls on the thigh, *Figures 8.33-D*. Any slightest displacement of the bar from the skin of the thigh would drastically degrade your lifting ability. You have to strike a balance of not injuring your skin, in that region, versus not distancing the bar away from your body. Some lifters paint their thighs with the magnesium carbonate powder, some choose smoothly machined bar, other train wearing long training trousers that cover the thighs. Your bid is a combination of all these, plus extra conditioning of the upper body to prevent the bar from rubbing your skin relentlessly.

8.8.2. STRENGTHENING THE PHASE OF MOMENTUM INITIATION
- You can have all the strength you want, yet still unable to initiate sufficient momentum. The best way of mastering this skill is practicing the movement by executing the Standard Snatch style, on regular basis.
- Snatch from the hang enhances the muscular control of scapular muscles during the forward leaning of the torso. Yet, you should not rely solely on the Hang Snatch to strengthen momentum initiation. You must increase the proportion of full motion from the floor, with respect to the Hang Snatch.
- Pulls with Snatch handgrips, from the floor, also strengthen the Hamstrings and scapular muscles in the ballistic style.
- Goodmorning exercise is unique in strengthening the Hamstrings.
- Squat and Goodmorning with Jump, during the ascent phase, strengthen the back and hip extensors in the ballistic style.

8.9. PHASE OF MAXIMAL SPEED OF THE SNATCH

8.9.1. ANALYSIS OF THE PHASE OF MAXIMAL SPEED OF THE SNATCH
- The previous phase of initiating momentum has resulted from the elevation of the hip, at a rate that outpaced the elevation of the chest. This has caused the head to advance in front of the feet, *Figures 8.31-A, 8.32-A,* and *8.33-A*. From this exaggerated posture of forward leaning, the legs will remain almost still, by the antagonistic actions of the Hamstrings and the Quadriceps, while the back erectors perform vigorous extension of the torso. The backward rotation of the torso on the hips pulls the straight arms upwards and increases lifting speed.
- Instantaneously, the lifter shrugs the shoulders to amplify the pull of the torso. The shrugged shoulders fill the gaps between the neck and the shoulders, *Figures 8.34-A, -C, -F, -H, and -G*. The shoulder shrugging follows the prior two axial major drives, namely the leg drive and the back erection drive. The drive of shoulder shrugging originates from the Trapezius.

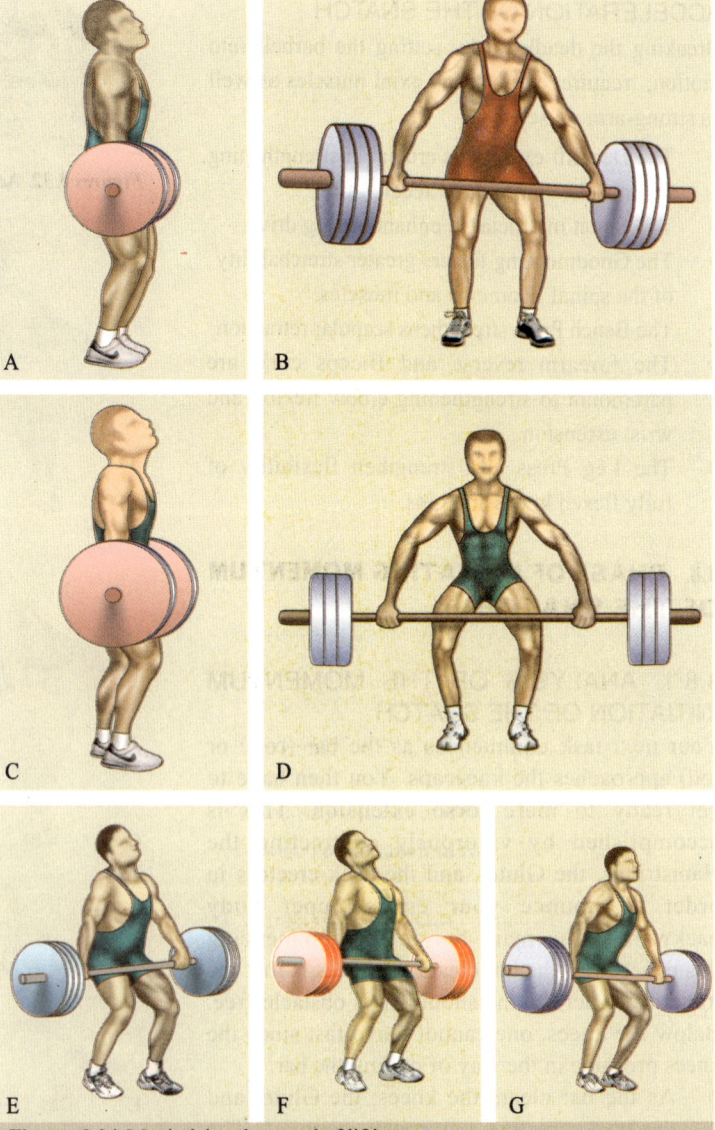

Figures 8.34. Maximizing the speed of lifting.

That of the legs originates from the Quadriceps and Glutei. The back erector drive originates from the Hamstrings and spinal erectors, *Figures 8.35*.
o   As the bar approaches the upper thighs, the legs, the torso, and the head, all fall on a vertical plane on the feet balls, *Figures 8.34-A* and *-C*. The bar is dragged very closely on the thighs. This phase is very brief, since the barbell is speeding upwards with the multiple actions of leg, torso, and shoulder drives.
o   As we see from *Figures 8.34-E* thru *-G,* the shoulders are spread laterally behind the chest, which is thrust upwards and forwards. This posture is critical to elevating the clavicles over the vital vessels and nerves that traverse the upper chest to reach the arms and brain.
o   The elbows are also still extended and tightened for two reasons. First, straight elbows efficiently transfer the axial forces to the barbell. Second, tight elbows can initiate the subsequent flexion by the Biceps brachii, Brachialis, and Brachioradialis.
o   The feet are supported on the heels and feet balls as long as the head is along or in front of the vertical plane on the feet balls. If the head bounces backwards behind that plane then the heels have to be elevated in order to torque the hips forwards, opposite to the head direction.

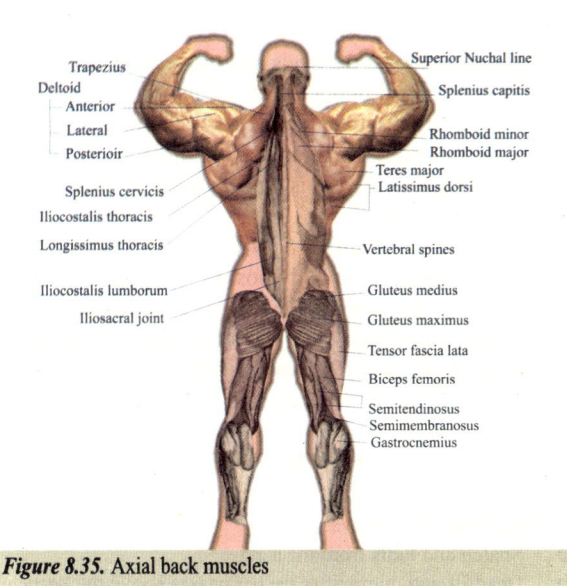

Figure 8.35. Axial back muscles

8.9.2. STRENGTHENING THE PHASE OF MAXIMAL SPEED

Maximizing the lifting speed, from the low thigh to high thigh levels, requires strong torso extension, strong shoulder shrugging, strong scapular retraction, and strong elbow flexion and extension. Theses can be strengthened by the following exercises.
o   Standard Snatch, Power Snatch, and Snatch from the hang.
o   Pulls with Snatch grips.
o   One-hand dumbbell Shoulder Press.
o   Goodmorning with jump.

8.10. PHASE OF MAXIMAL MOMENTUM OF THE SNATCH

8.10.1. ANALYSIS OF THE PHASE OF MAXIMAL MOMENTUM OF THE SNATCH

o   The set of actions that occurred above the knees resulted in using the inertia of the upper body in order to create ballistic lifting motion. The peak of this motion occurs when the entire body assumes an exaggerated full extension while hopping on the feet balls and inclining backwards. The backward inclination balances the weight of the barbell plus the virtual forces due to increased amount of motion, that is momentum, *Figures 8.36*.
o   The fully extended upper body brings the bar onto the anterior superior iliac spines. These are two bony projections, one on each side, on the front of the pelvis and at the belt line of the waist. At this location, the bar divides the body into two equal halves. The hips fall slightly under the bar level and the shoulders fall above it. The bar is, therefore, used as a rotation axis. The upper body rotates backwards, with respect to the bar, by the strong Trapezius shrugging. The

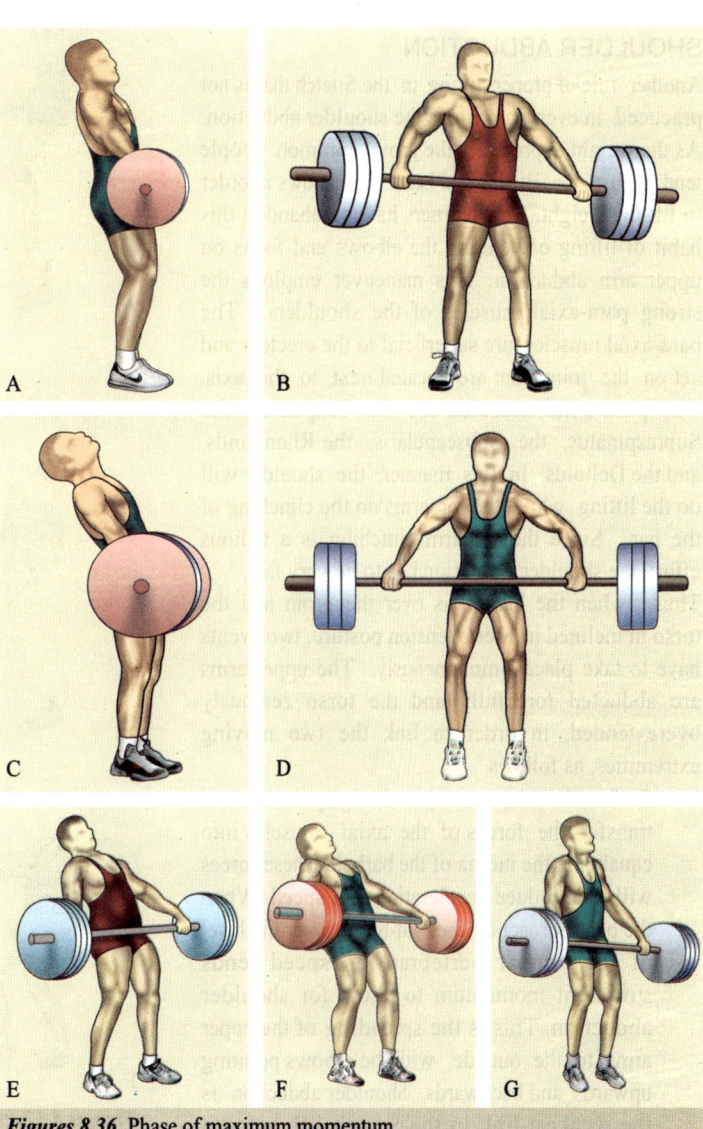

Figures 8.36. Phase of maximum momentum.

8 THE SNATCH LIFT

lower body thrusts forwards, under the bar, with the strong contraction of the Glutei and Gastrocnemius. The latter muscles elevate the heels and move the knees forwards.

o The backward bouncing of the upper body and the forward thrusting of the buttocks can only be beneficial if the arms are still tightly extended. This is the most critical trick in the Snatch technique. For lay people, this brief and dynamic body posture is very difficult to imagine, since it defies the norms of static balance of forces encountered in everyday life. Dynamically, it is well thought of way of utilizing the body inertia to generate forces greater than the magnitude of bodyweight..

o The lifters in *Figures 8.36-C* and *-D* do no hop on their feet balls, since their heels are still anchored to the floor during the fully extended body posture. This can be explained by the fact that individual variation does exist in performance. Some lifters jump on the whole feet soles, instead of elevating the heels only.

o Light lifters have the great advantage of flat belly that allow the bar to move very close to the vertebral axis, *Figures 8.36-A, -C,* and *-D*. Heavy lifters with large waist size have to exaggerate backward bouncing in order to bring the bar closer to the vertebral axis on the bulging abdomen, *Figures 8.36-E* and *-F*.

8.10.2. STRENGTHENING THE PHASE OF MAXIMAL MOMENTUM

Maximum momentum requires very strong Trapezius, Spinal erectors, Buttocks, and Gastrocnemius. These are strengthened as follows.
o Snatch and Pulls from the hang.
o Deadlift with jump after the bar passes above the kneecaps.
o Goodmorning with jumps during the upward stroke of torso extension.
o Calf raises with jump in place or with advancing forwards.

8.11. PHASE OF SHOULDER ABDUCTION OF THE SNATCH

8.11.1. ANALYSIS OF THE PHASE OF SHOULDER ABDUCTION

Another rule of proper lifting in the Snatch that is not practiced in everyday life is the shoulder abduction. As the weight approaches the groin, common people tend to use the Biceps and bend the elbows in order to lift the weight. New learners have to abandon this habit of lifting of bending the elbows and focus on upper arm abduction. This maneuver employs the strong para-axial muscles of the shoulders. The para-axial muscles are superficial to the erectors and act on the joints that are located next to the axis. The para-axial muscles are the Trapezius, the Supraspinatus, the Subscapularis, the Rhomboids, and the Deltoids. In this manner, the shoulder will do the lifting while the forearms do the clinching of the bar. Since the forearm clinching is a tedious effort, the shoulder abduction has to be very fast.

Thus, when the barbell is over the groin and the torso in inclined in overextension posture, two events have to take place simultaneously. The upper arms are abducted forcefully and the torso zealously overextended, in order to link the two moving extremities, as follows.

o So far, the arms were used to grip the bar and transfer the forces of the axial muscles into equalizing the inertia of the barbell. These forces will then induce acceleration and speed. When the bar approaches the mid-body, over the level of the lumbar vertebras, its speed lends sufficient momentum to allow for shoulder abduction. This is the spreading of the upper arms to the outside, with the elbows pointing upwards and backwards. Shoulder abduction is the weakest link in the Snatch lift, since it

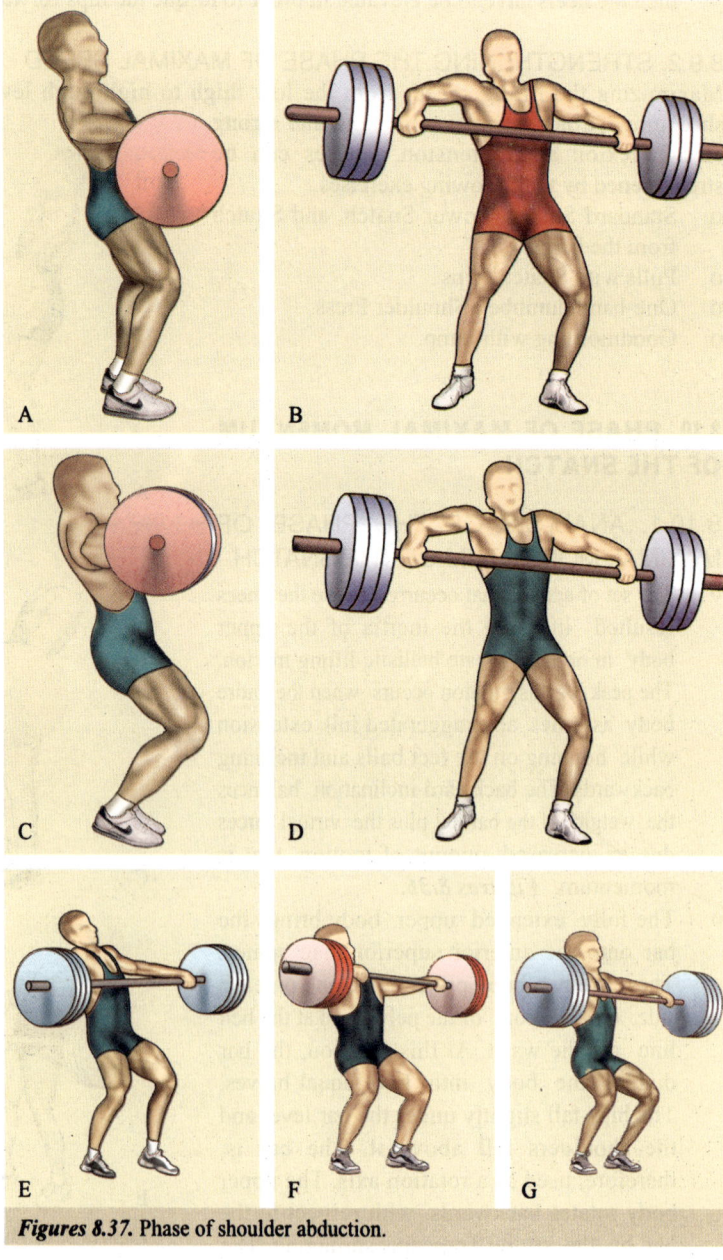

Figures 8.37. Phase of shoulder abduction.

entails the smallest and the more distal paraxial muscles, the Deltoids and Supraspinatus.
- o   While the upper Trapezius shrug the scapulas upwards, and the middle Trapezius retracts them medially, the lateral Deltoid pulls the upper arms upwards, *Figures 8.37*.
- o   The back Deltoids pull the bar close to the body thus facilitates the action of the wrists. Up to this point, the wrist should remain neutral, no extension or flexion. The wrists cannot perform extension with such very heavy weight. They have to wait until the Deltoid finishes the job of shoulder abduction and the whole body dips under the barbell. In other words, the wrists have to wait until the barbell feels weightless. This state is created by the balance between upwards acceleration generated by muscular forces and downward acceleration generated by gravity.
- o   Shoulder abduction is hindered by the bounds of human anatomy. The shoulder sockets, - the glenoid cavities-, are less than half spheres in curvature. Thus, the range of shoulder abduction is comprised of the combined elevation of the upper arms and the lateral motion of the scapulas. This will bring the bar no higher than the upper chest level.
- o   Bending the knees can aid in farther ascent of the barbell with respect to the body, by lowering the body downwards while the bar is being suspended in the hands. This is performed while the feet are still standing on their balls, *Figures 7.37-C* and *-E*.
- o   Advanced lifters train heavily on bringing the bar very close to the chest cage during this phase. That is because the Deltoids cannot stand extreme torque by the front displacement of the bar. From the close location at the chest, the bar will be snatched easily upwards and overheads. The back Deltoids and the middle Trapezius muscles perform the approximation of the barbell to the chest cage.
- o   Maximum lifting can only be achieved by keeping the head the farthest, backwards, *Figure 7.37*. This guarantees that the center of body mass falls behind the feet balls when the center of barbell mass falls in front the feet balls.
- o   Objectively, the lifter has to find simple ways to perform the ideal technique of optimum bar trajectory. For example, the lifter might focus on bringing the bar to the center of the lower chest while the head is thrown backwards and prior to descent. Advanced lifters aim at guiding the bar backwards, rather than upwards. Since the bar is already speeding upwards, while the body is bouncing from front backwards, therefore backward pulling, as felt by the lifter, will translate into farther ascent of the bar.

8.11.2. STRENGTHENING THE PHASE OF SHOULDER ABDUCTION

Shoulder abduction is accomplished with the combined actions of the upper Trapezius, the Supraspinatus, the lateral Deltoids, the Biceps, the Triceps, and the forearm muscles. Theses muscles are strengthened by the following assisting exercises.
- o   Snatch and Pulls from the hang, with emphasis on both components of eccentric and concentric contraction.
- o   Biceps and Triceps strengthening exercises.
- o   One-hand Shoulder Press.
- o   Lateral dumbbell arm raises.
- o   Bent-over rows.

8.12. PHASE OF DESCENT OF THE SNATCH

8.12.1. ANALYSIS OF THE PHASE OF DESCENT OF THE SNATCH

Descending under the upward speeding barbell is achieved by squatting with both legs. This technique is less than 50 years old. Before that, leg spring was the dominant technique of descent under the bar. That comprised of lunging by one leg under the bar and backwards behind the lifter. This task of simultaneous arm abduction and leg flexion is the major challenge in the Snatch lift. It becomes the most formidable task as the lifter exceeds the second decade of life, without previous whole body training. Jumping under a moving object, in a frog-squatting position, defies all ordinary laws of everyday life. Yet, in the world of fitness, the boundaries of performance are stretched beyond familiar limits. The awesome features of the axial muscles of multi-pinnate groups of fibers, diverse attachments of their pinnas tendons and bones, are utilized to the maximum in performing extraordinary combinations of squatting, back overextension, and arms abduction. The

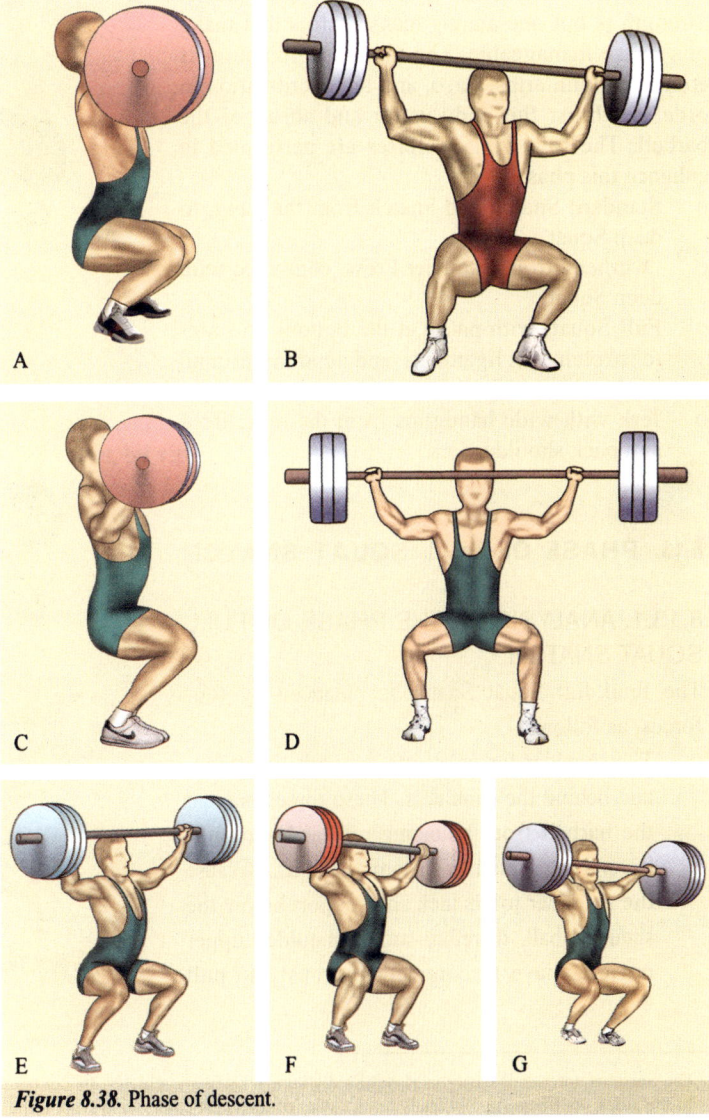

Figure 8.38. Phase of descent.

muscles with lesser pinnate features, such as the arm and lower leg muscles, are used as tensile strings or supporting levers but not as driving force. The following are the features of this phase.
- o This is an optional phase of performance. Its purpose is to augment barbell ascent and whole body descent such that the bar can be supported by straight arms, overhead. The legs have the power that can elevate the bodyweight and the weight of the barbell by concentric contraction. The arms can only support lifting the barbell weight with isometric contraction.
- o In order to descend under the bar while sustaining lifting, the bar has to clear the face area, in its way backwards and upwards. The head was already receding backwards behind the thrust chest.
- o The lifter performs two instantaneous movements. Drop the hips, downwards and backwards, and throw the barbell backwards and upwards, *Figures 8.38-A, -C, -E-G*. These combined motions of *"dip and throw"* causes the barbell to descend slightly before the arms catch it overhead
- o The knees are bent and the heels land on the ground in order to establish wider base for standing.
- o The Iliopsoas pull the lumbar spines forwards while the spinal erectors maintain lordotic lower back. This lower back lordosis advances the torso ahead under the bar.
- o The back Deltoids, the Triceps, and the Trapezius support the arm motion during guiding the barbell form front of the chest to above the eyebrows.
- o The most formidable motion in this phase is the balance of the Subscapularis and the front Deltoid. If the Subscapularis muscles were short and spastic, they would draw the arms forwards and prevent overhead stability, during this phase of backward throwing of the barbell. Strong front Deltoids help stabilize the arms overheads.
- o Another balance that plays actively during this phase is that between the Serratus anterior and the upper Trapezius. The Serratus anchors the scapulas to the chest cage,[3] whereas the upper Trapezius pulls the upper borders of the scapulas medially and upwards.

8.12.2. STRENGTHENING THE PHASE OF DESCENT OF THE SNATCH

Descending under a moving weight requires well-coordinated shoulders, spinal axis, and pelvis. Strength is but one among many factors that make this phase manageable. The visual coordination is combined with arms, torso, and leg coordination in order to thrust the body under and ahead of the barbell. The following exercises are performed to enhance this phase.
- o Standard Snatch and Snatch from the hang, to deep Squat.
- o Overhead front Shoulder Press, combined with deep Squat.
- o Full Squat, with pause at the bottom, in order to stretch the ligaments and tendons around the knees and hips.
- o Jerk with wide handgrips from the rack, front and back shoulder Jerk.

8.13. PHASE OF FULL SQUAT SNATCH

8.13.1. ANALYSIS OF THE PHASE OF FULL SQUAT SNATCH

The final full Squat Snatch is balanced by four forces, as follows.
- o The shoulder forces elevate the barbell upwards and behind the shoulders. These forces prevent the barbell from bouncing too far backwards, beyond the shoulders anatomical limits. Because the shoulder joints lack any support below the shoulder ball, therefore strong shoulder upper muscles have to contract vigorously to pull

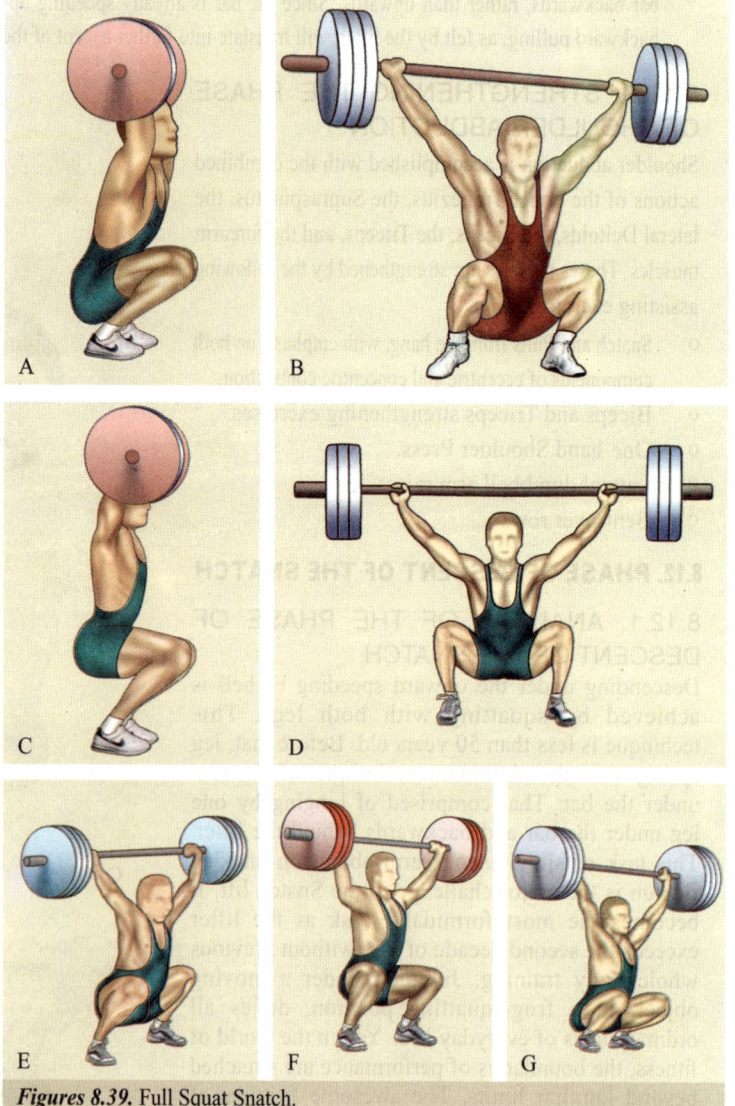

Figures 8.39. Full Squat Snatch.

---

[3] The Serratus anterior is easily used, yet hardly known by many athletes. Its contraction brings the scapulas to fill under the armpits. It thus pushes the arms to the sides. Its fibers run obliquely on the sides of the chest cage, wind around the chest, and pull the scapular medial border to the sides. You activate the Serratus anterior when you want to show a wide upper back and chest size.

the shoulder balls into their sockets and prevent downward dislocation, *Figures 8.39-B and -D*. These muscles are the Deltoids and Supraspinatus.
- o   The back extension forces support the scapulas and thrust the chest forwards. These forces align the overhead-extended arms, over the scapulas, with the spinal axis, *Figures 8.40-A* and *-C*. Thus, the center of mass of the external weight falls vertically on the mid-chest spines, mid-thigh point, and mid-feet. Any laxity in the back extension can result in toppling the balance of weights and cause fall, *Figures 8.39-C* and *-F*.
- o   The hip flexion forces pull the pelvis and the spinal axis forwards and downwards. The Iliopsoas draws the abdomen tightly to the thighs and arch the lumber spines inwards, *Figures 8.39-A, -C, -E,* and *-G*. Weak Iliopsoas cause the pelvis to dip backwards and downwards and throw the entire body and weight backwards, during fall.
- o   The leg forces support the combined weight of the bar and the bodyweight. The Quadriceps draw the femur to the lower legs while the hip adductors draw the femur to the pelvis. The Hamstrings and Tensor fascia lata draw the pelvis to the lower legs. The Glutei support the lateral and posterior aspects of the hip balls. The combined forces of these muscles support the ankles, knees, and hips during full Squat, as well as during ascent.

Strong muscles do not guarantee successful performance.[4] Neuromuscular control is paramount to performance during this brief and intense phase. Weightlifters learn to master this phase with trial and error, in constant effort to tweak the balance of the four forces, described above. The following tips are helpful in mastering this phase.

- A.   The most important tip in executing full Squat Snatch is the **forward chest thrust**, as soon as the bar passes overhead. This is an objective move on the part of the lifter that aims at positioning the bar and the arms behind and above the chest
- B.   The second tip is to **quickly lock the shoulders**, elbows, and wrists, in overhead-extended arm posture, as soon as the bar is felt to reach its highest level. Such arm locking prevents any perturbation of the overhead weight. Due to the relative weakness of the upper body and the great torque of any overhead perturbation, the quickly locked arms constitute a solid transfer lever between the barbell and the spines.
- C.   The third tip is **pay greatest attention to the control of the knees and hips**. Maintaining these joints under highest mental concentration will enable the lifter to maneuver squatting, dipping, and ascending. You can increase the level of attention by squatting higher than full Squat, then take over the tone of the muscles of the thighs and buttocks, by adjusting the depth of squatting.

8.13.2. STRENGTHENING THE PHASE OF FULL SQUAT SNATCH
Full squatting during the execution of the Snatch requires regular practice for flexibility, balance and strength. The following are recommended exercises for enhancing this phase.
- o   Full Squat Snatch, from the floor or from the hang.
- o   Shoulder Press, with Snatch handgrip, while squatting fully.
- o   Overhead Squat and advancing with the feet in "Penguin walking". This entails elevating the arms overhead during full Squat and advancing forward with alternating feet.
- o   One-hand Shoulder dumbbell Press.

8.14. PHASE OF FULL ASCENT OF SNATCH

8.14.1. ANALYSIS OF THE PHASE OF ASCENT OF THE SNATCH
- o   The final phase of the Snatch of ascent commences when the bar reaches its final destination overhead and the body has been stabilized. Ascent is initiated by farther tightening of the shoulders and locking of the arms, farther thrusting of the chest, and farther arching of the lower back.
- o   The most difficult part of ascent is getting the middle portion of the Trapezius to retract the scapulas, at its upward border, the Serratus anterior to fix the inner portion of the scapulas, and the Latissimus dorsi to support its lower tips. If these three groups of muscles were trained to deal with such fully extended torso and fully flexed legs, then the ascent is driven by the back erectors, Glutei, and Quadriceps. If the scapular muscles are not well conditioned then any effort to ascend from full Squat will end in leaning forwards and toppling the barbell to the floor. The barbell may fall in front of the body or from behind it.
- o   Most probably, if the initial effort to ascend with weight constitutes concerted balance of the legs, back, and shoulders, then subsequent efforts will rely solely on strength, rather than on muscular balance. The head and hip masses will be utilized during ascent to balance the arms with the barbell placed over the mid-chest spines.

---

[4] Muscles exert physical strength by the combined neural control of voluntary and involuntary nervous system. Flexion and extension reflexes operate between segments of the spinal neurons and adapt to long training. Higher voluntary neural control is crucial in preventing overtone and permitting the individual to achieve voluntary control on his joints and limbs. Parkinsonism syndrome vividly demonstrates the overwhelming interference of overtone during rest. Parkinsonism patients can perform voluntary muscular actions almost like normal people, but cannot sit restfully without tremors.

- o The arms and shoulders will remain locked, from bottom to top. The legs will drive the bodyweight and barbell weight upwards, while the upper body sustains isometric contraction, supporting the barbell during ascending.
- o The Snatch is complete when the knees extend fully; the arms and shoulders are locked in overhead extension, and both feet on the ground, heels to toes.
- o In contests, the weight can be dropped to the floor only after the Judge gives the sign to terminate the lift. Dropping the weight should not be for the purpose of slamming the weight to the floor, but rather for relieving the body from the stress. Violent slamming of the weight to the floor might bring unwanted consequences, legal as well as injury.

8.14.2. STRENGTHENING THE PHASE OF ASCENT OF SNATCH

Ascending from full Squat, with overhead held weight requires regular training of the shoulders, back, and legs. After few weeks of training, the new lifter would have master a new skill of using the axial and paraxial muscles, as first and second choices, respectively, prior to ever resorting to peripheral joints. He or she also will become convinced that the lower body is best equipped to equalize motionless objects in order to initiate external motion, while the upper body is fit for guiding moving objects to proper course of motion. In everyday living, such learned lesson is invaluable. When force is imparted on objects, the lower body has to be hardened -in slight flexion at all joints- prior to any upper body resistance. The following exercises are recommended for enhancing ascent phase of the Snatch.
- o Regular Snatch with full squatting.
- o Overhead Squat with "Penguin walking".
- o Shoulder Press with barbell combined with overhead squatting.
- o One-hand Shoulder Press.
- o Front shoulder Jerk.
- o Squat and Deadlift.

8.15. TEACHING THE SNATCH LIFT

8.15.1. FRAMEWORK OF TRAINING FOR THE SNATCH

Teaching adds objectivity to the defiant behavior of the strong and youthful trainees. The coach has to lay down the framework of the entire process of training, in simple and clear words. This can be summarized as follows.
- o The first component of Weightlifting training is practicing the proper technique of lifting, with no weight or just the bar without plates. This might re quire few sets in the beginning, yet it is a constant component of all subsequent training sessions. All training sessions will start with light warm-up but with less number of sets, as the lifter advances.
- o The barbell weight increases only when the technique is deemed appropriate for advancing in lifting. It does not make any sense to try to challenge yourself with lifting heavier weights if the technique of previous lifts was flawed.
- o As the technique is being mastered, individual deficits become more evident. These should be assessed and managed with future assisting exercises.
- o Other than the quality of execution of the technique of lifting, the load volume has to be considered in deciding to increase the barbell weight. The lifter should not try to lift heavy on every occasion, or lift light for long time. Progressive increments in weight increase resistance and strength.
- o The load volume is the accumulated net of whole lifts of all sets and sessions, of certain interval of training. Thus, there is weekly load volume, monthly load volume, annual load volume, and cycle load volume. Maximal lifting weights occur on monthly basis. Minimal lifting weights, below 70% 1RM, occur more often, on weekly basis. New trials of lifting are super-maximal that occurs around contests or every few months.
- o Training sessions are described according to their intended goals. A training session can be described as "strengthening session" when the load volume for that session is high. A training session can be described as "restful session" when both intensity and volume are low, with emphasis on practice of better technique. A training session can be described as "intense session" when many sets of few repetitions are performed at high intensity, over 80% 1RM. Finally, a training session can be described as "assisting sessions" when remedial exercises are practiced to deal with individual muscle deficits.
- o Progress occurs on many levels. The lifter can advance in performing balanced technique in few months of training. After a year or so, the technique becomes more automated, with few accidental mistakes. Advance in developing strength fluctuates over the years. Strength reaches plateaus in various stages of life depending on age, nutrition, rest, intensity of training, and balance of training. Advance in tolerating vigorous activity is very dependent on continuity of training. At certain age, interruption of training might lead to irreversible decline in tolerance to vigorous training.
- o The young trainees have to be informed about the essential need for long training, over many months, in order to reach certain goals, without injuries. Champions are not made in six months or even a year. Many months will be spent in mastering the technique, building strength, dealing with individual deficiencies, and instilling habitual solid mannerism essential for proper lifting. Beginner trainees incline to lifting heavier and sooner, each time they workout. Part of the reason is to please the trainer and convey their sense of appreciation to his effort. Another part is attributed to the lack of understanding of the recovery process of the body and how strength is being acquired.

8.15.2. HEAVY LIFTING VERSUS FINE MOVEMENTS
The second task of the coach is to explain to beginner trainees the basic rules of applied anatomy of lifting. That entails the groups of muscle that are best suited for heavy lifting, which are different from those that deals with fine movements.
- o   In developed societies, muscles suited for heavy lifting are wasted in common people. With many decades of prosperous industrialization, many people have lost touch with essential daily physical activity.
- o   The arms and shoulders are the weakest lifting muscles, yet the best in performing fine movement such are using a screwdriver, or turning an object in an awkward location. Though arms and Shoulders are strengthened by Weightlifting, every effort is made to minimize their injury. Such effort will allow the person to train regularly and focus on the strengthening of major muscles, without being annoyed with painful wrists or frozen shoulders.
- o   The best lifting muscles are the deep muscles, located very close to the vertebral spines and support back erection during overextension. Strengthening the muscles of heavy lifting differs from Bodybuilding in that the latter deals with superficial muscles, more than deeper groups. Even very advanced Bodybuilders err in developing huge peripheral muscles in relation to axial muscles.
- o   When peripheral muscles exceed axial muscles in strength, the lifter relies more on the peripheral muscles. This would definitely result in injuries to the spinal structures. Peripheral muscles generate enormous virtual forces on the spinal axis, by virtue of the long-arm of force, between the periphery and the spinal axis. To make use of this understanding of the muscles of lifting, the trainee is to be taught to use each group of the lifting muscles in a proper timing manner.

8.15.3. DRIVING FORCES IN MULTI-JOINTED MACHINES
- o   In any multi-jointed moving machine there should be only few, or better be one, driving force, acting at a single driving joint. The rest of the joints should maintain stabilizing posture.
- o   That is because, if more than one driving force work simultaneously, their net resultant may vanish. This can be simulated by two or more persons trying to push an object in different directions. This may result in opposing forces, with minimal net resultant.
- o   Another reason for relying on one single joint for induction of efficient motion is that, the human brain operates mostly at a single focus of attention. The single working joint operates at optimal neural attention and thus achieves the desired task. Distraction causes the neural system to engage many joints, which results in haphazard motion.
- o   Let only one force drive the whole "show". This puts the mind at ease in figuring out the rest of the joints. The "one task at a time" approach applies to other aspects of the training.
- o   The trainee is instructed to approach the bar relaxed, refrain from frowning,and focus on the memories of prior lessons of lifting. Such rituals of mental concentration help recruit the proper muscular sequence during vigorous training.

8.15.4. COMMON MISTAKES IN THE EXECUTION OF THE SNATCH
- o   During the execution of the different phases of lifting, the trainee should be informed of the level of his compliance with technical rules of lifting. The deviation from proper lifting should be rectified according to prioritized list of options. The default of highest priority should be tackled first, in isolation of the other defaults. Trying to rectify multiple mistakes, simultaneously, results in protracting the effort of learning.
- o   As soon as the lifter shows improved compliance with the default under consideration, he should be complemented for paying attention. This enforces the increased level of attention to that specific error in execution. Then, the default next in the priority list can be tackled. Sometimes, the lifter experiences significant difficulty in executing specific motion, even after many trials. Here, one should opt to proceed to the next default and hope that, as times passes, the lifter might overcome his difficulty. Alternatively, the coach might figure out a different approach to rectify such incompliant performance. Such new discovery, of alternative solution to protracted defaults, may lie in uncovering individual deficits in strength, flexibility, or perception, on the part of the lifter.
- o   The commonest default in the Snatch lift is **the displacing of the bar away from the body**. Many beginners reach the age of training for Weightlifting with no background on the subject of mechanical balance of forces. The slightest displacement of the bar from optimum trajectory results in shear stress and torques that topple the body and the barbell to the ground, as follows.
    - i.   Shear stresses at the wrist can incapacitate the lifter for weeks and prevent him from lifting any object, due to painful and inflamed wrist.
    - ii. Shear stresses at the lumbar spines may cause longer disability or even permanent injury.
    - iii. Shear stresses at the shoulder plates can be annoying for few days.
    - iv. Shear stresses at the shoulders may disrupt the rotator cuff muscles or traumatize the ligamentous structures of the shoulders.
- o   The second common error in lifting is the **limited sagittal (front to back) displacement of the hip, chest, and head.** This is the style of lifting of stiff, elderly, or unconditioned people. The horizontal displacement of the hip, behind the vertical line of centers of masses, and the horizontal displacement of the head and chest in the opposite direction, are

THE SNATCH LIFT

good measures of the ability of the lifter to generate torque. A lifter who was not told of simplifying the driving force would often try to drive the barbell with both arms and legs. This results in inefficient utilization of the axial muscles. The axial muscles operate effectively when the head-and-hip vector rotates around the vertical axis, with the spinal axis working as a lever. The rotation of the weights of the head and pelvis, around a center, creates angular momentum, in addition to the translation momentum induced by the upward pulling. Lifters, who tend to lift with stiffed upright posture without horizontal displacements of the hip, head, and chest, have to rely on their arms and shoulders, with definite failure in lifting sub-maximal weights.

o The third common mistake in the Snatch lift is the **cushioning action of descent under the bar**, after the arm-abduction has reached its peak effort. Many beginners are apprehensive of performing leg flexion during overhead lifting. That is because, neither the shoulders are used to elevation as the legs bend, nor the legs are used to resist weights as the arms are placed overhead.

8.15.5. LANDMARKS OF PROGRESS IN THE SNATCH

o The main landmark that signals the efficiency of the teaching process is the new acquisition of **skillful head movements**, *Figure 8.40.* Beginners lift the bar above the shoulder level with the head kept behind the vertical plane of the bar and the feet. As the trainee gains confidence, he or she starts pushing his or her head under the bar, as soon as it clears the head. Advanced lifters master perfect timing of inserting the head under the bar, or even in front of its vertical plane. The head motion signifies the confidence of the lifter in his ability to put his shoulders in extreme extension under overhead heavy weight. It also signifies the developing of nervous coordination of the big muscles, joints, equilibrium, and visual sensation. Ordinary people have hard time developing good head control, while lifting above the shoulders. That is because most people, including Bodybuilders and Powerlifters, do not practice over-head lifting in standing of free-squatting position.

o Lifting while seating or standing still differs from lifting during whole-body motion. In the latter, the relative locations of the joints are changing and the brain is overloaded with influx of signals regarding these affairs. With training, such whole-body motion aids in recruiting proper muscles for proper balance. Thus, lifting above the shoulder while in motion, as in the Snatch lift, requires not only well-conditioned and **balanced shoulders,** but also shoulders that can perform effectively when the whole body is moving.

o In the first few years of training, a lifter might strike the bar against his chin, nose, or forehead. An unpleasant cut above the nose could result from hasty and fast lifting of light weight. As the lifter develops **strong back erectors**, the lower back possesses distinguished over-extension posture, which helps thrust the chest upwards. This prevents many collision accidents between the bar and the prominent parts of the face.

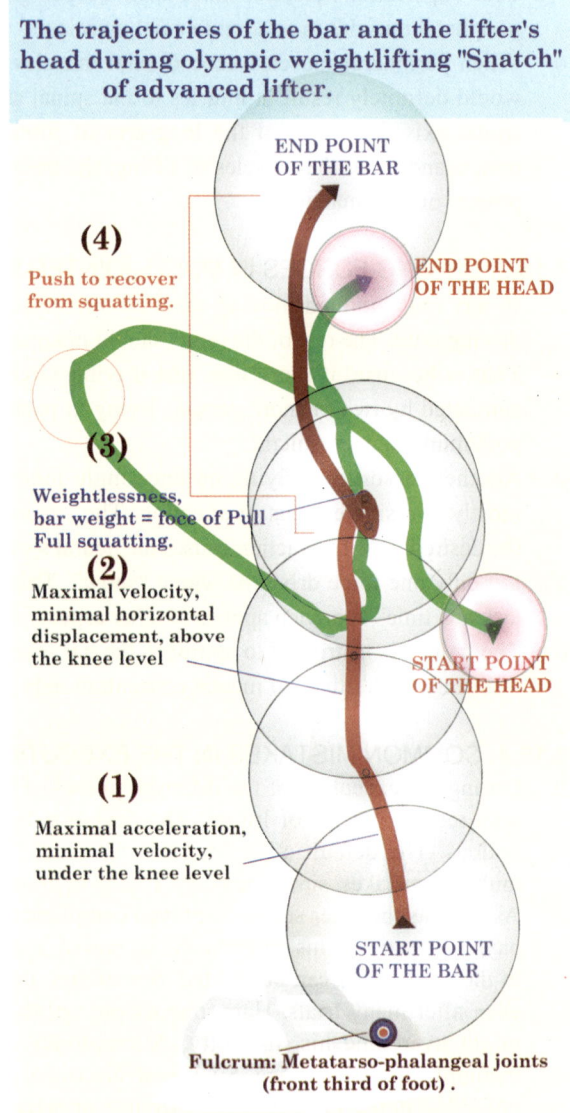

Figure 8.40. Bar trajectory of the Snatch lift.

o Training on the Snatch for long time, months or years, results in distinctive gains in the posture. The upper scapular muscles become significantly developed and help the person pick up objects from the floor with noticeable ease.

o The long duration of isometric contraction of the elbows, during the Snatch, enhances exquisite balance between the elbow flexors and extensors. This gives the lifter greater ability in controlling the elbow actions.

8.15.6. TWEAKING THE SNATCH LIFT

After few years of training, the lifter develops concrete understanding of the essence of the Snatch lift. Later, he will resort to such solid conviction, every time he confronts troubles in executing the lift. He would have learned that the Snatch, though seems formidable to untrained spectators, could be easily executed when few rules are rigorously adhered to.

- o The *first rule* is that the Snatch is driven upwards by the lower body. That **upward drive** cannot be effective unless the upper body conveys it to the arms that hold the bar without losses. Any upper body laxity, during the upward drive, would increase losses. In addition, the angles between the thighs and torso, the torso and arms, the scapulas and the chest cage are particularly crucial to effective transfer of forces, between the pelvic girdle and the shoulder girdles.
- o The *second rule* is that the back muscles between and above the two scapulas complete the drive force above the mid-thigh level. The **scapular muscles** that mediate arm-spine transfer of forces are the Supraspinatus, the Trapezius, the Rhomboids, the Levator scapulae, the Infraspinatus, the Subscapularis, and the Serratus anterior. These muscles are the greatest assets to the lifter during the Snatch. They not only transfer the spinal forces to the arms, but also support bridging the collarbones over the chest cage and the scapulas, in order to allow for passage of blood to the brain and the arms. Weak scapular muscles hinder the Snatch. These muscles are the focus of the strengthening exercises for the Snatch.
- o The *third rule* is that not only upward drive force is needed to snatch, but also a torque of the torso on the hips is crucial to lifting. The torque is produced by the Glutei thrusting the hips forwards, and the back erectors thrusting the head and chest backwards. Without the **angular momentum** generated by that torque, Weightlifter would not be able to lift weight heavier than the average population. The torque around the major joint is the essence of the sport of Weightlifting. It is greatly affected by aging, stiffness, neuromuscular condition, and hesitation to perform.
- o The *fourth rule* is that any departure from **vertical ascent** of the bar compromise effective lifting. Thus, the lifter has to master the generation of great angular momentum of the body while, in the same time, prevents the barbell from producing any counteracting angular momentum. In *Figure 8.38,* the head trajectory bounces from front backwards, then to the front again, while the bar trajectory follows vertical descent, as much as possible. There is no mean to avoid the small displacement of the bar trajectory around the shoulders. Yet, every effort has to be made to maintain vertical bar trajectory.

8.15.7. ASSISTING THE SNATCH LIFT
Each phase in the execution of the Snatch lift presents specific signs of strength or weakness of muscular coordination
- o Inefficient upward drive requires strengthening the lower body, when the upper body performs similar actions to the Snatch. The Deadlifts, the Pulls, and leg exercises become the center of attention in the planning of assisting exercises.
- o When the upper finalizing drive is deficient, the upper back and shoulder require more attention. The Snatch from the 0hang, the Shoulder Press with overhead squatting, and the exercises that strengthen the shoulder girdle and arms, all enhance the upper body drive of the Snatch, from the waist to overhead.
- o When the ability to generate torque is lacking, the practice of the whole technique would be recommended to stimulate coordinated agility. Torque during the Snatch lift cannot be generated effectively with hyper-spastic legs, back, or shoulder muscles. These muscles must be well rested, massaged, and stretched properly in order to be able to coordinate the powerful torque, of the torso on the hips.
- o The departure of the bar from the vertical plane of centers of masses signifies imbalance of a linking group of muscles that generate horizontal forces. The Glutei, Quadriceps, Hamstrings, back erectors, and back scapular muscles are the main keepers of the vertical trajectory of the bar

8.15.8. PROPER SEQUENCE OF THE SNATCH IN TRAINING SESSIONS
The order in which the Snatch lift is executed is subjected to some considerations, in regard to the required muscular strength, the balance of the various joints, and the goal of executing certain versions of the Snatch.
- o Heavy standard Snatch has to follow thorough warm-up in order to ensure that all muscles and joints are equally ready for aggressive vigorous work.
- o It cannot be executed after partial exercises, such as Squat, Bench Press, or isolated muscle exercises.
- o If the Snatch were light, steady, or modified to serve strengthening, it would be possible to execute it out of that order. The problem of executing the Snatch after partial exercises is the ensuing of overtone in the exercised muscles. The increased tone degrades the balance of the Snatch lift.
- o Serious shoulder injuries might result, if standard Snatch with deep Squat follows Bench Pressing or Biceps exercises. That is because the Snatch requires full stretch of the pectoral and Biceps tendons and muscles during overhead extension.

8.16. HIGHLIGHTS OF CHAPTER EIGHT

1. In any multi-jointed moving machine there should be only few, better be one, **driving force** at a single joint, while the rest of the joints are only subjected to tensile stabilizing force. That is because if more than one driving force work simultaneously, their net resultant may vanish.

THE SNATCH LIFT

2. The *first rule* is that the Snatch is driven upwards by the lower body. That **upward drive** cannot be effective unless the upper body conveys it to the arms that hold the bar without losses. Any upper body laxity, during the upward drive, would increase losses. In addition, the angles between the thighs and torso, the torso and arms, the scapulas and the chest cage are particularly crucial to effective transfer of forces, between the pelvic girdle and the shoulder girdles.

3. The *second rule* is that the back muscles between and above the two scapulas complete the drive force above the mid-thigh level. The **scapular muscles** that mediate arm-spine transfer of forces are the Supraspinatus, the Trapezius, the Rhomboids, the Levator scapulae, the Infraspinatus, the Subscapularis, and the Serratus anterior. These muscles are the greatest assets to the lifter during the Snatch. They not only transfer the spinal forces to the arms, but also support bridging the collarbones over the chest cage and the scapulas, in order to allow for passage of blood to the brain and the arms. Weak scapular muscles hinder the Snatch. These muscles are the focus of the strengthening exercises for the Snatch.

4. The *third rule* is that not only upward drive force is needed to snatch, but also a torque of the torso on the hips is crucial to lifting. The torque is produced by the Glutei thrusting the hips forwards, and the back erectors thrusting the head and chest backwards. Without the **angular momentum** generated by that torque, Weightlifter would not be able to lift weight heavier than the average population. The torque around the major joint is the essence of the sport of Weightlifting. It is greatly affected by aging, stiffness, neuromuscular condition, and hesitation to perform.

5. The *fourth rule* is that any departure from **vertical ascent** of the bar compromise effective lifting. Thus, the lifter has to master the generation of great angular momentum of the body while, in the same time, prevents the barbell from producing any counteracting angular momentum. In *Figure 8.38,* the head trajectory bounces from front backwards, then to the front again, while the bar trajectory follows vertical descent, as much as possible. There is no mean to avoid the small displacement of the bar trajectory around the shoulders. Yet, every effort has to be made to maintain vertical bar trajectory.

Chapter 9

The Clean & Jerk

9.1. STANDARD TECHNIQUE OF THE CLEAN

The Clean is a freestyle lift of a barbell from the floor to the shoulders. It is performed without wrist raps, racks, or assisting devices, other than the barbell. The lift proceeds from the floor to the shoulders in various styles of lifting. If the lifter remains standing after the full upward pull, with slight dipping by the knees and hips, then the barbell has to travel upwards with strong arm and shoulder pull. This high pull Clean is termed **"Power Clean"**. The Power Clean is a basic upper back strengthening exercise. If the lifter refrains from dipping after the full upward pull, continues on pulling the barbell to the shoulders, without lowering the torso, then the Clean is termed **"Military Clean"**. The Military Clean is a basic strengthening exercise for the arms and shoulders. Competitive Clean lifting requires significant dipping of the torso under the barbell after the full upward pull, in order to compensate for the relative weakness of the upper body. The deep squatting under the bar after aggressive pulling is called **"Full Squat Clean"**. The Full Squat Clean is a basic exercise for strengthening full body extension and flexion.

9.1.1. PREPARATION
o   Stand over the barbell with the feet balls positioned under the bar, shoulder-width apart, or slightly wider, *Figure 9.1*. Since the Clean lift is conducted with narrower handgrips, compared to the Snatch, therefore the feet stance should be as wide as the arms could allow the knees to remain to the inside of the elbows, during the low phases of lifting.
o   As with the case of the Snatch, before descending to grip the bar, try to relax every muscle in the body, particularly the thighs, lower back, and shoulders, *Figure 9.2*.
o   Squat down and grip the bar with slightly wider than shoulder-width overhand grips, *Figure 9.3*. If you can flex the shoulders and extend the wrists with wider handgrips, when the bar is placed on the front of the shoulders, then you can shorten the vertical travel. Close handgrips increase the travel distance whereas wide handgrips make shoulder and elbow flexion difficult to execute.
o   Position the shoulders over the bar with the back arched tightly inwards in lordotic posture. Keep arms straight at the elbows, with elbows pointed laterally, *Figure 9.4*.

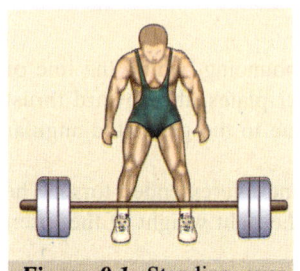

Figure 9.1. Standing over the bar.

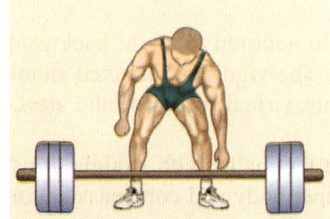

Figure 9.2. Descending to grip the bar.

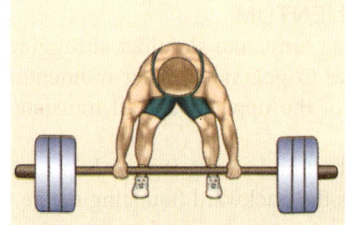

Figure 9.3. Adjusting handgrips.

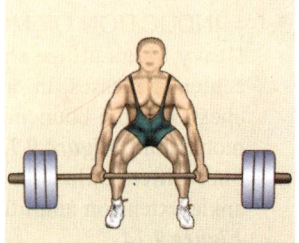

Figure 9.4. Adjusting posture of start position.

9.1.2. INDUCTION OF ACCELERATION
o   Before attempting to lift, exaggerate lordotic back; thrust the chest forwards and upwards. In the front view, this posture results in closing the gap between the abdomen and thighs and bulging of the upper chest. Throw the shoulders backwards, and straighten the elbows, *Figure 9.5*. These will appear separated from the chest, due to the bulging of the Latissimus dorsi between the sides of the chest and the arms.
o   Pull the bar upwards off the floor, by extending the hips and knees while maintaining very tight upper body, *Figure 9.6*. Many advanced lifters deepen their Squat on the bar, prior to the final tightening of the body, in order to induce maximal stretch of the thighs and back, *Figure 9.7*.
o   Farther ascent is induced by leg drive, with very still upper body. The back stays inclined and straight. No elbow bending, no shoulders caving, and no lower back laxity are allowed, *Figure 9.8*. The Clean grip causes the Trapezius to spread widely over the shoulders and support the scapulas during this early phase of equalization of the heavyweight, *Figure 9.8*.

THE CLEAN & JERK

o During the very early motion of the bar, below the kneecaps, the isometric contraction is the dominant source of induction of acceleration, with minimal lower body concentric contraction.

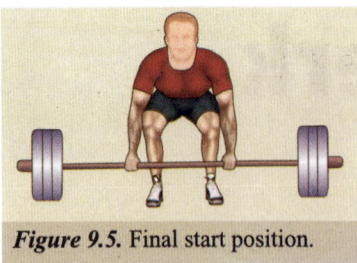
Figure 9.5. Final start position.

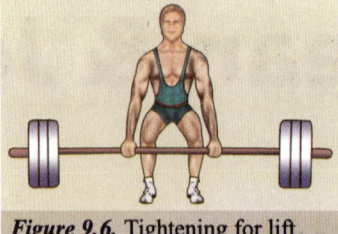
Figure 9.6. Tightening for lift

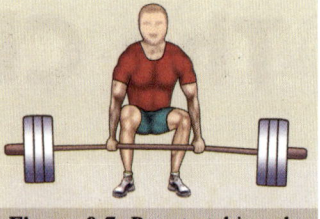
Figure 9.7. Pre-stretching the lower body.

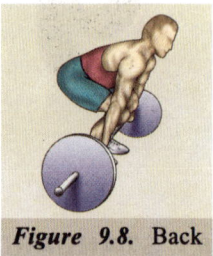
Figure 9.8. Back posture.

9.1.3. INDUCTION OF SPEED
o As the barbell clears the kneecaps, vigorously raise the shoulder plates, while dragging the bar on the thighs.
o Lifters with heavy bodyweight utilized their inertial energy as soon as the bar clears the kneecaps, *Figure 9.9*. This posture differs from that of *Figure 9.10*, in that the heavy lifter can afford forward leaning with extremely heavy weight. It also differs from that of *Figure 9.11*, in that, the heavy lifter can sustain widely spread shoulders. The backward leaning and the shoulder elevation will help in generating great inertia that induces speed, *Figures 9.10* and *9.11*.
o Lifters with short and strong legs rely mostly on the leg drive to induce maximal speed, *Figure 9.10*.
o Lifters with tall legs and torso have to utilize the strong upper back muscles in order to compensate for the farther travel of the bar, *Figure 9.11*.
o The early elevation of the hips, compared to the chest and shoulders, tightens the Hamstrings and prepares them for generating backward torque around the hips, *Figure 9.12*.

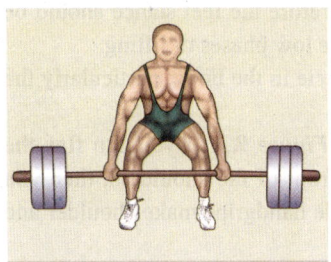
Figure 9.9. Inertial utilization in a heavy lifter.

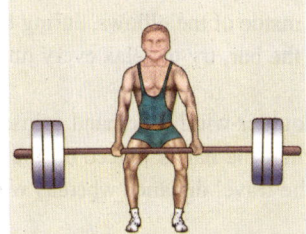
Figure 9.10. Leg drive in a short lifter.

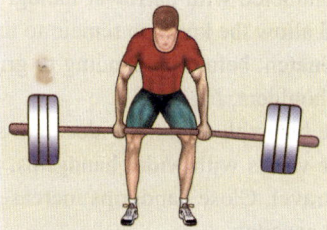
Figure 9.11. Upper body drive, in a tall lifter.

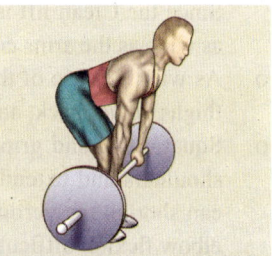
Figure 9.12. Hamstring tightening by forward leaning.

9.1.4. INDUCTION OF MOMENTUM
o Heavy lifters utilize strong arms and shoulder shrugging, in addition to slight backward bouncing behind the line of center of masses, in order to generate farther momentum. The vigorous retracted shoulder plates, the upward thrust chest, and the bouncing of the upper body, all translate into virtual forces on the arms due to the generated angular momentum, *Figure 9.13*.
o Short lifters utilize the short and strong legs to hop on the feet balls, with straight arms and overextended torso. The ankle extension amplifies the backward bouncing of the upper body and compensates for the light weight of the lifter, *Figure 9.14.*
o Tall and light lifters rely heavily on the scapular muscles as well as on hopping on the feet balls, in order to generate angular momentum, *Figure 9.15*.

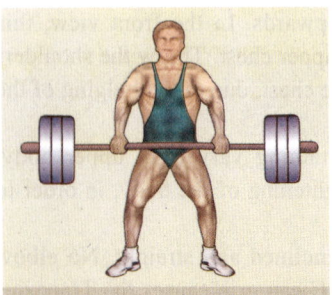
Figure 9.13. Maximal Trapezius shrugging.

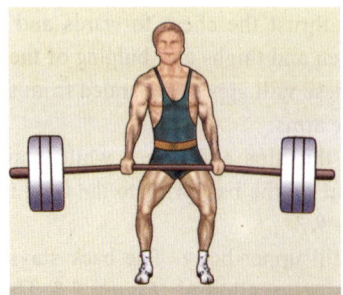
Figure 9.14. Hopping of feet balls and backward bouncing.

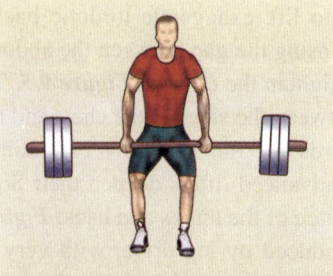
Figure 9.15. Relying heavily on upper body strength.

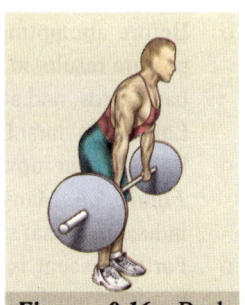
Figure 9.16. Back lordosis.

- o   The straight elbows and lordotic lower back are essential in translating the angular momentum into virtual forces at the gripping hands, *Figure 9.16*.

9.1.5. INDUCTION OF WEIGHTLESSNESS
- o   The external weight of the barbell has to come to a state of relative weightlessness in order to enable the shoulders and the legs to perform simultaneous flexion. Flexion brings the whole body under the bar in squatting position.
- o   The state of weightlessness is initiated by the previous legs and back drives. Now, the shoulders commence three consecutive actions in order to finalize the state of weightlessness, as follows.
- o   The shoulders move from the shrugging state of *Figures 9.13* thru *9.16* to a progressive cadence of abduction, transverse adduction, and flexion. In layman words, shoulder shrugging proceeds to spreading the elbows sideways, pulling backwards, then flipping the elbows under the bar to elevate the weight.
- o   Shoulder abduction alone cannot pull heavy weight from the waist level to the shoulder level. Thus, you have to shift shoulder abduction into shoulder transverse adduction. This means that, in addition to pulling upwards with lateral Deltoid muscles, you should engage the back Deltoid, Supraspinatus, and upper Trapezius into pulling the bar backwards as well as upwards, *Figures 9.17* thru *9.20*. Transverse shoulder adduction is accomplished by the retraction of the scapulas and the adduction of the upper arms, upwards and backwards. The elbows will flip under the bar with strong and vigorous shoulder flexion. The advantage of transverse shoulder adduction is the higher elevation of the barbell and the lesser need for deep squatting.

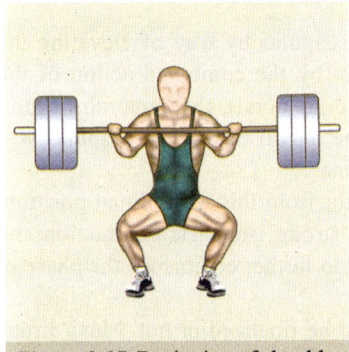
Figure 9.17. Beginning of shoulder flexion and descent.

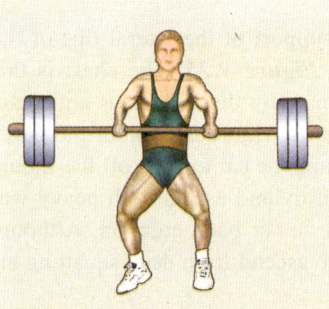
Figure 9.18. Beginning of transverse shoulder adduction and descent.

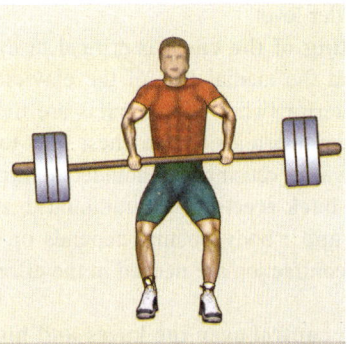
Figure 9.19. Beginning of shoulder elevation and abduction and descent.

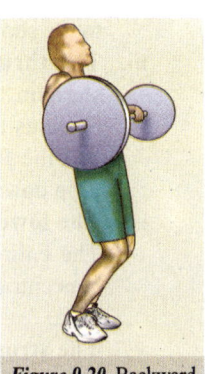
Figure 9.20. Backward bouncing.

- o   Light weight lifters might not have such horizontal muscular strength of the scapulas. They utilize shoulder extension and back bouncing to finalize the weightlessness state. Shoulder extension is accomplished mostly by the Latissimus dorsi and the Triceps, *Figure 9.18*. The disadvantage of mere shoulder extension is the low elevation of the bar and the need for deep squatting and strong shoulders.
- o   Tall lifters might not have the luxury of strong transverse shoulder adduction or efficient shoulder extension. They rely mostly on shoulder abduction prior to flipping the elbows under the bar, *Figure 9.19*. Shoulder abduction requires strong Deltoids, Supraspinatus, and upper Trapezius, in addition to greater arm strength.
- o   While the shoulders finalize the weightlessness state, the back erectors pull the torso backwards, with the weight held in both hands. The knees begin to flex as soon as the weight of the barbell is equalized enough to permit safe descent under the weight, *Figure 9.20*.

9.1.6. DESCENT UNDER THE BAR
- o   Descending under the barbell, after strong and vigorous upward pulling, is the most ingenious modification made in the technique of the Clean lift in the last half century. This modification necessitated developing strong and massive thigh muscles in order to endure the enormous downward forces of squatting and upward forces of ascending with the barbell. Descending under the bar is an optional choice in contest. You can lift the bar as high as you want without squatting, as long as you follow the technical rules of the Clean lift. Descending only serves enhancing the lifting power through generation of momentum, torque, and vertical translation, of the barbell to the lowered shoulders.
- o   As the bar moves upwards and backwards and the upper body advances downwards and forwards, the arms flip under the bar to catch it at the lowered shoulders, while moving into the Squat position. Heavy lifters can execute very high pull with squatting to parallel, *Figure 9.21*. Short lifters can descend deeply under the bar due to their short legs and arms, *Figure 9.22*. Most lifters cannot pull at this phase with even strength on both sides, *Figure 9.23*. The latter figure illustrates the effort of a tall lifter trying to pull the bar high in order to avoid deep squatting.
- o   In training, Weightlifters perform "high power pulling" for the sake of strengthening the upper scapular muscles, *Figure 9.24*. High pulling is not recommended for extended period of time since it causes stiffening of the shoulder and knee joints.

9 THE CLEAN & JERK

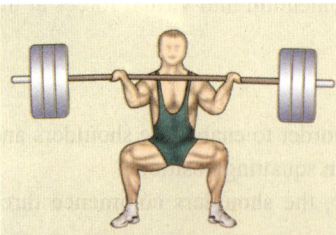
Figure 9.21. Completing shoulder flexion.

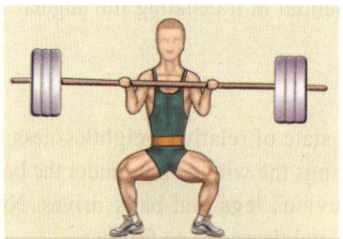
Figure 9.22. Pulling and descending.

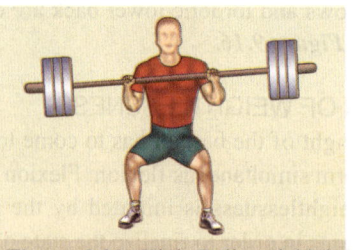
Figure 9.23. High Pull and high Squat.

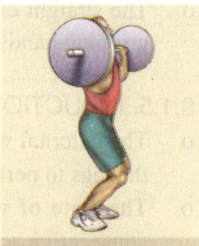
Figure 9.24. Power Pull.

9.1.7. FULL SQUAT CLEAN
o   The most critical tasks in this phase are the following five actions.
   i.   **The close dragging of the bar on the upper chest** is achieved by strong elbow flexion and shoulder extension. The elbow flexion is achieved by the Biceps brachii, the Brachioradialis, and the wrist extensors. The shoulder extension is achieved by the Latissimus dorsi, long head of Triceps, Infraspinatus, and Teres muscles. The combined actions of these muscles pull the bar close to the upper chest, *Figures 9.21* thru *9.24*.
   ii. **The strong and fast flipping of the elbows** under the bar is achieved by the vigorous contraction of the Deltoid, Biceps brachii, and Coracobrachialis. The combined actions of these muscles elevate the bar from low chest level to the shoulder level.
   iii. **The thrusting of the chest** is critical to the support of the lateral tips of the scapulas by way of elevating the sternum and the medial tips of the clavicles, *Figure 9.25*. The chest is thrust by the combined action of the Serratus anterior (when the scapulas are tightened by the Trapezius and Latissimus dorsi), the Pectoralis minor, and the Sternomastoids. If the chest fails to thrust vigorously under the bar, the lateral tips of the scapulas will drop downwards, causing the shoulders to drop and the bar to slide off the shoulders.
   iv. **The lower back erection** is paramount to stability and ascent with heavy weight from this front Squat position. The entire upper body posture depends on the lower back erection. Although strong isometric contraction and concentric contraction are needed in the effort to ascend from deep squatting and to farther commence the phase of Jerk.
   v.   **The strong control over the knees and hips** determines whether the lift would be finalized or not. Many lifters plan to squat under control, instead of dipping deep and fast, *Figure 9.26*. Although strong legs are great assets to the recovery from deep and fast squatting, yet upper body strength is also needed to facilitate respiration, heart beating, and arm elevation. Controlled squatting offers the advantage of increased ability to continue the lift, all the way to overhead Jerk, *Figure 9.27*. These five tasks have to be undertaken simultaneously and swiftly in order to prevent the barbell from generating greater downward momentum.

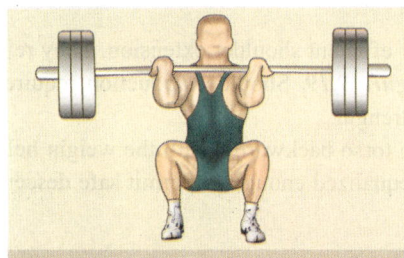
Figure 9.25. Ideal Squat Clean.

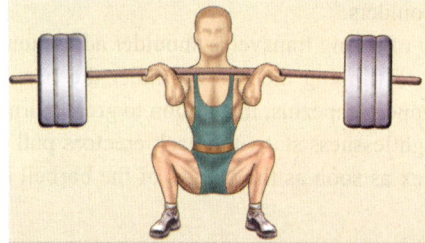
Figure 9.26. Full Squat Clean with deep and fast descent under the bar.

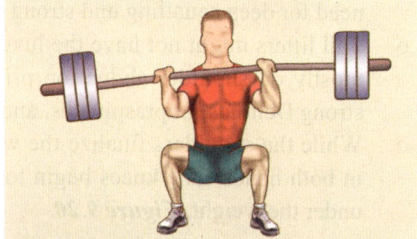
Figure 9.27. Parallel Squat Clean with controlled descent under the bar.

9.1.8. ASCENT FROM THE CLEAN SQUAT
o   The recovery from the Clean Squat is a tedious work of balance between the shoulder girdle, the lower back, and the pelvic girdle. The five tasks, described in *Section 9.1.7*, will concert the unfolding of the body from the full flexion position of deep Squat. The experience of the lifter plays into picking one task before the other. As shown in *Figures 9.26* and *9.27*, advanced lifters struggle with the decision of initiating the five tasks of ascending form full flexion. The body flaws become transparent in this phase of strength, balance, and flexibility, as seen from the departure of the bar from horizontal level, in the last two figures.
o   Fast and deep squatting protracts ascent with heavy weight and might cause serious stresses, *Figures 9.26, 9.28* and *9.29*. On the other hand, controlled high squatting makes ascending more manageable, *Figure 9.30*. In *Figure 9.29*, you can notice the sinking of the Trapezius behind the bar, whereas the Deltoids and the Biceps brachii bulge under the bar to prevent its fall. This posture is costly, particularly during the initiation of the Jerk lift. That is because the elbows have to drop and the scapulas to descend, in order to align shoulders and arms under the bar for upward jerking. In *Figure 9.30*, the Trapezius is protruding over the shoulders and the bar, while the elbows are lower than the

previous figure. Thus, the controlled squatting, in the Clean of *Figures 9.25* and *9.27,* results in more manageable upper jerking of the barbell.

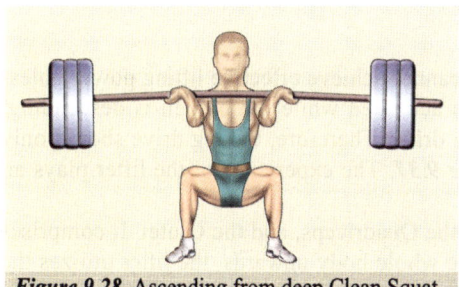
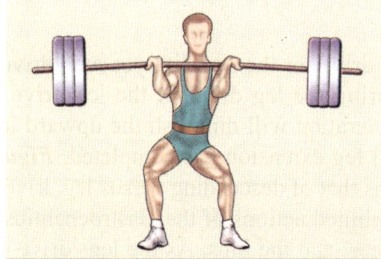
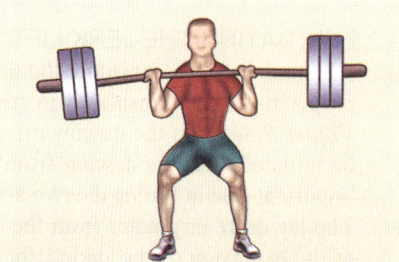

Figure 9.28. Ascending from deep Clean Squat.

Figure 9.29. The consequence of squatting deep and fast.

Figure 9.30. Strong and control ascent.

9.1.9. FINALIZING THE CLEAN
o   The Clean lift is final when the body extends fully under the bar. In contest, the Weightlifter has to bring the knees to full extension, with the bar supported on the shoulders and both feet are flat on the ground, *Figures 9.31.*
o   The subsequent phase of the Jerk cannot commence before arranging the arms, scapulas, chest, and shoulders under the bar, *Figure 9.32*. Although the elbows have to be lowered, yet the shoulders must remain elevated under the bar to prevent it from sliding on the chest.
o   Some lifters perform simultaneous lowering of the elbows and extending of the legs, *Figure 9.33*. This way the lifter simplifies the arranging process in preparation for the Jerk. The initial elevation of the bar from the chest, after full knee extension, shown in *Figure 9.34,* can only be tolerated in contest if it was a continuation of the ascent from the Clean. However, elevating the bar in attempting the Jerk results in defaulting the lift, if the attempt is not completed in the first trial of elevation.

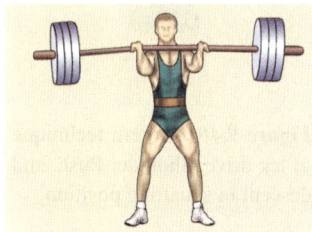
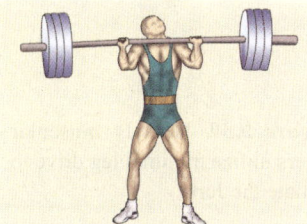
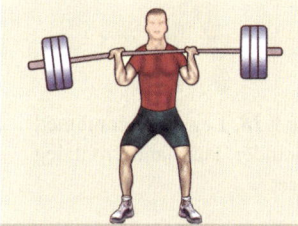
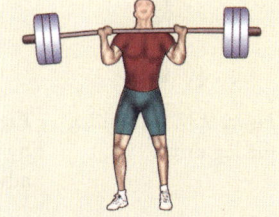

Figure 9.31. Full leg extension with tightly flexed shoulders and elevated elbows.

Figure 9.32. Lowering the elbows and retracting the scapulas with aggressive chest thrusting.

Figure 9.33. Controlled leg extension simultaneously performed with elbow dropping.

Figure 9.34. Aligning the shoulders and elbows under the bar.

9.2. STANDARD TECHNIQUE OF THE JERK

In formal Weightlifting contests, the Jerk lift is the second part of the Clean and Jerk lift. There is no only-Clean lift in contests. This is not the case in training for Weightlifting. In training sessions, the lifter has the freedom to plan his workout anyway he wishes. However, many prefer to perform the two parts of the lift, even in training, in order to maintain muscular balance. The Jerk lift drives its name from the strong leg drive utilized in mobilizing the weight of the barbell from the shoulders. The Jerk differs from the Shoulder Press in that the Press is initiated by shoulder drive, utilizing the front and lateral Deltoids and the Triceps. In the old days, the Shoulder Press was performed with significant bouncing of the torso in initiating the Press.

9.2.1. PREPARATION FOR THE JERK LIFT
o   After full recovery from the Clean ascent, the preparation for the Jerk takes the form of slightly lowering the elbows, thrusting the chest, lordosing the lower back, and unlocking the knees, *Figure 9.35*.
o   With the bar firmly seated on the shoulders, the entire body of the clavicles, and the palms of the hands, the lifter performs four active tasks.
  i.   Arch the lower back farther inwards, while tightening the back erectors and the abdominal muscles.

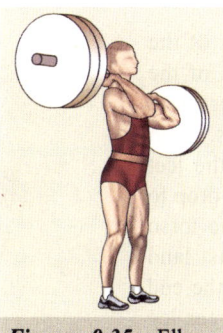
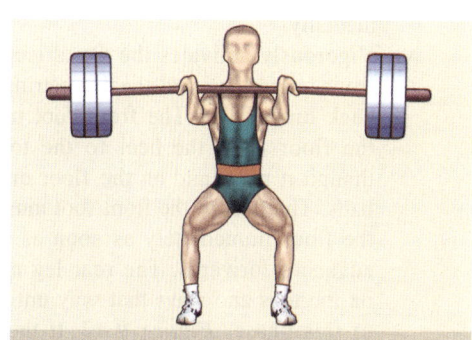

Figure 9.35. Elbow position for the Jerk.

Figure 9.36. Descending to initiating the leg drive for the Jerk.

ii. Thrust the chest cage farther upwards and forwards, in order to ease the burden on the shoulder structures.
iii. Dip with the legs by bending the knees and throwing most of the weight on the feet balls.
iv. Farther hardening of the cervical spines and elevating the head slightly backwards and upwards.

9.2.2. INITIATING THE JERK LIFT

o   Although the legs constitute the main drive for the Jerk lift, yet such drive cannot achieve effective lifting power unless proper timing is considered in triggering the leg drive. If the leg drive is activated while the barbell is descending, *Figure 9.36*, then the downward acceleration will diminish the upward leg drive. Therefore, the leg drive should only be initiated after the descent from full leg extension has completed, *Figure 9.37*. The experience of the lifter plays an important role in timing the two actions that of descending versus leg drive.

o   The leg drive originates from the combined actions of the Gastrocnemius, the Quadriceps, and the Glutei. It comprises of the extension of the ankles, the knees, and the hips. As the legs drive the whole body upwards, the lifter utilizes the combined momentum of his bodyweight and the barbell weight to lift the barbell from the chest. The lifter has to aim his push upwards and backwards while, in the same time, sneaks one of his legs forwards, *Figures 9.37* and *9.38*.

o   Heavyweight lifters can generate effective shoulder push without the need for significant descent for leg drive, *Figure 9.39*. In this case, the massive scapular and shoulder muscles allow for plenty of room for the scapulas to descend and overstretch the Deltoids and the Trapezius. The stretch reflex, in these major muscles, suffices the lifting of the heavy weight from the shoulders.

o   The modern technique of overhead Jerk and Squat descent is exquisitely difficult, *Figure 9.40*. In this new Jerk style, the lifter utilizes both leg and shoulder drive then dips under the bar by bending knees, hips, and ankles, instead of lunging one leg in front of the body and the other to the back.

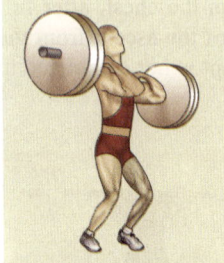
Figure 9.37. Maximizing the leg drive.

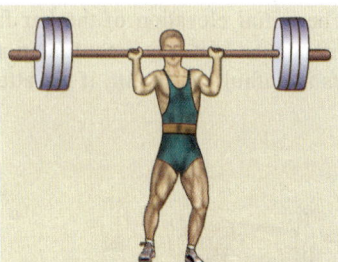
Figure 9.38. Leg drive combined by Shoulder Push and front leg advance.

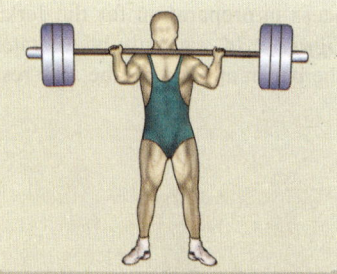
Figure 9.39. Heavily muscular lifters utilize minimal leg drive to initiate the Jerk.

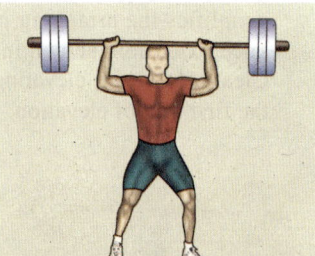
Figure 9.40. Modern technique of leg drive, Shoulder Push, and descent in squatting position.

9.2.3. SHOULDER DRIVE AND LEG LUNGING

o   The shoulder drive can only be effective if the head clears the way for the bar to ascend, the torso attacks forwards and under the barbell to prevent its fall, and the shoulders push the bar backwards and upwards. If the lifter tries to push the barbell only upwards, he would then translate the barbell horizontally. That is because the barbell, as well as the whole body will be moving forwards. Subjectively, the lifter has to push the weight close to his face, *Figure 9.41*.

o   As soon as the bar clears the face area, the lifter performs four active tasks.
i.   Vigorously extends the elbows and locks both the shoulders and the elbow under the bar
ii. Advances his torso under the bar, with tightly arched lower back and thrust chest.
iii. Swiftly advances the head forwards in order to allow the upper Trapezius pull the shoulder plates tightly, upwards and medially.
iv. Vigorously activates the Quadriceps of the front lunged leg and the Hamstrings of the back lunged leg. The front foot must abut the floor from the heel to the toes, even though it may land on the floor on the feet balls. The heel of the front foot must drop to the floor immediately as soon as the torso advances forwards. The rear leg must land on the toes and stays that way until the end of this phase, *Figure 9.42*. If the rear leg lands on the heel, it will then lock the entire leg at the hip and knee joint and therefore,

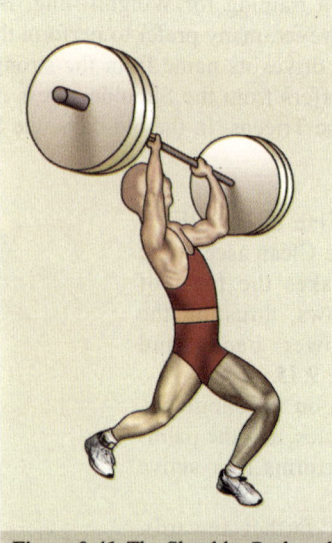
Figure 9.41. The Shoulder Push and leg lunge.

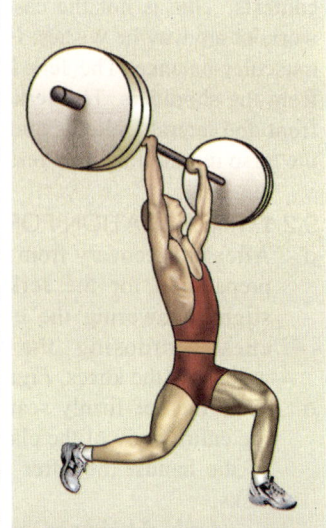
Figure 9.42. Elbow extension and torso advance.

impede any ability to maneuver during this transient motion. Thus, the front foot is used for support whereas the rear foot is used for balance.
- o Leg lunging is a technical choice, rather than a requirement in formal Weightlifting competition. The legal requirement for validation of the Jerk lift is the monotonous and smooth lifting of the barbell without elbow pressing, stationing, or advance and retreat motions. Therefore, the lifter can execute the Jerk lift either by leg lunging or squatting. Lunging the legs involves springing, which displaces the center of masses, whereas squatting maintains minimal displacement of the center of masses, since the feet remain anchored to the ground.

9.2.4. STABILIZING THE JERK MOTION
- o The upward mobilization of the barbell, from the shoulder level to overhead, occurs in a ballistic fashion, whether the leg lunging or the Squat dipping is used to advance the body under the bar. The Jerk is defaulted if initiated by mere Shoulder Press. In order to stabilize the heavy moving barbell, the ballistic motion of the barbell has to be dampened by multi-joint cushioning action. The experienced lifter masters the cushioning action that prevents acute trauma to the elbow, shoulders, and spines, as follows.
- o The upward Shoulder Push and elbow extension have to be synchronized with the body advance and descent under the bar, *Figure 9.43*. Premature locking of the elbows or shoulders before adequate body descent can cause serious shoulder injury. Many lifters even delay arm locking until full body descent and arm extension are achieved. That might result in slight drop of the bar trajectory prior to arm locking.

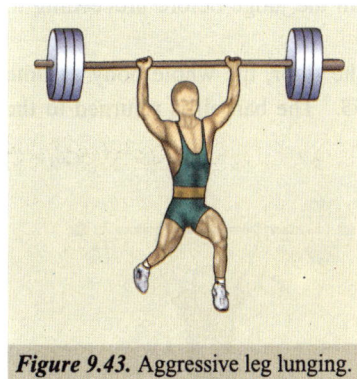
Figure 9.43. Aggressive leg lunging.

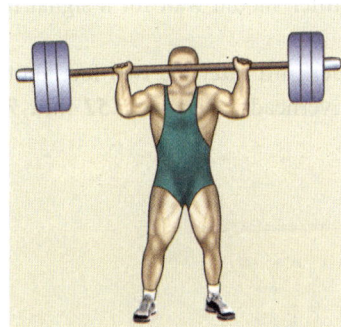
Figure 9.44. Aggressive Shoulder Push.

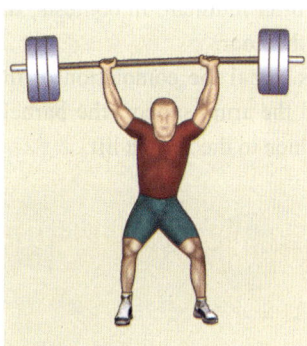
Figure 9.45. Squatting for the Jerk.

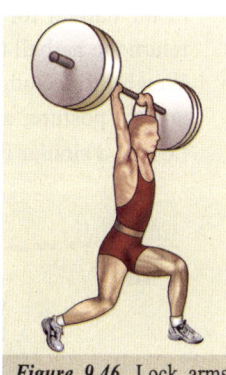
Figure 9.46. Lock arms and torso advance.

- o In order for the stabilization of the Jerk motion to be successful, the bar trajectory has to bring the center of mass of the bar close to the vertical plane of the center of mass of the moving body of the lifter. In *Figure 9.44,* the lifter emphasizes pushing the bar very close to his face in order to ensure its vertical ascent. The slightest deviation of the two centers of mass may generate torque that far exceeds the torque ability of the shoulders.
- o As the bar clears the face area, the lifter utilizes the shoulder and pelvic girdles to move the center of mass of the bar behind the head and dip with hip and knee flexion, with lower back lordosis, *Figure 9.45*. The thigh and buttock muscles can perform effective dampening action to the motion by controlled leg flexion. The shoulders participate in the dampening action by sliding the scapulas on the chest cage with the action of the Trapezius muscles.
- o The old days technique, of slamming the lunged front foot on the floor, is obsolete. Modern Weightlifters can execute leg lunging quietly, yet fast and vigorously, *Figure 9.46.* The stabilization of the Jerk motion is finalized when the front foot is tightly anchored to the ground, the rear foot is balanced on the bases of the toes (feet balls), the arms are locked on the overhead barbell, and the entire body is free from gross shakes or tremors. This stable state is only subjective and instantaneous. In the overhead Jerk and Squat, both feet will be anchored on the ground, whereas the pelvis performs the balancing feedback with the head motion.

9.2.5. RECOVERING FROM THE JERK MOTION
- o This comprises of straightening the whole body under the barbell in full extension, with the weight held in hands overheads. In the leg lunging position, recovery proceeds in three-foot motions. First, the front leg extends at the knees. It is then dragged backwards, just few inches, *Figure 9.47*. In this move, the front foot is used as stable and strong support platform while the rear foot maneuvers for balance. Second, the rear foot is dragged forwards, almost to all the way under the body, *Figure 9.48.* In these two moves, the upper body is locking the weight of the barbell with strong isometric contraction. Third, the whole body shifts its weight once again on the front foot while the rear leg is dragged forwards. Now, the two feet should be together under the body.
- o Powerful lifters can recover in two-foot moves, instead on three, due to their massive musculature and limited leg spring, *Figure 9.49.*
- o Recovering from overhead-Jerk Squat requires exquisite strength and balance of the shoulders, back, and legs. The lifter locks the shoulders on the barbell by vigorous contraction of the Trapezius, the Deltoids, and the Triceps. Then he thrusts the chest and arches the lower back inwards in order to utilize upward leg drive, *Figure 9.50.*

THE CLEAN & JERK

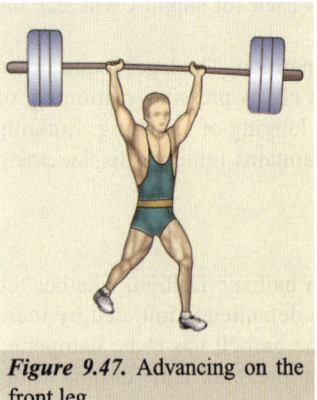

Figure 9.47. Advancing on the front leg.

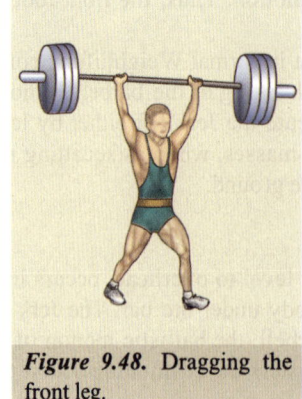

Figure 9.48. Dragging the front leg.

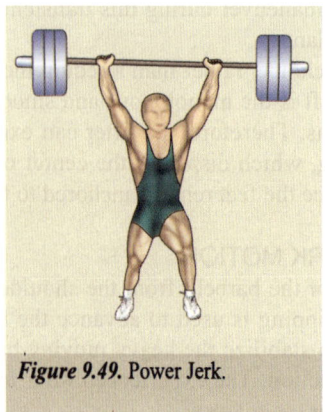

Figure 9.49. Power Jerk.

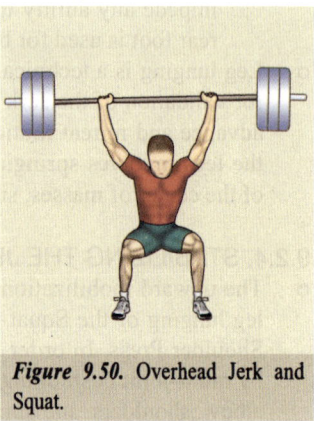

Figure 9.50. Overhead Jerk and Squat.

9.2.6. FINAL JERK LIFT

o The Jerk lift is complete when the bar is overhead with whole body extension in stable posture. The two feet should be abutting the floor. The knees, hips, back, shoulders, and elbows should be extended. The body should appear in control of the barbell for a brief moment. In contests, the lifter should wait for a signal from the judge before proceeding to return the barbell to the floor.

o Weightlifting judges signal the completion of the Jerk lift after the two feet abut the floor, the whole body assume upright posture, and the arms support the barbell overheads, *Figures 9.51* thru *9.53*. The barbell is returned to the floor in a similar fashion to the Snatch lift.

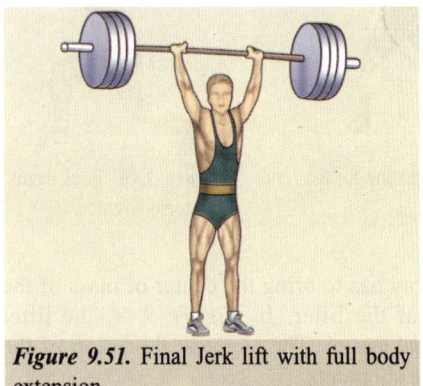

Figure 9.51. Final Jerk lift with full body extension.

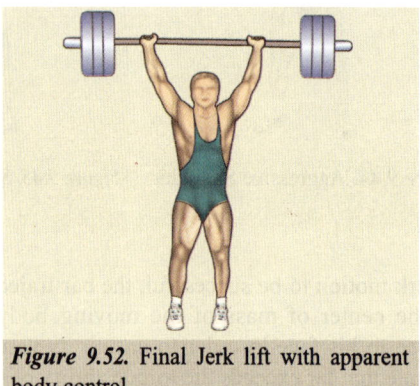

Figure 9.52. Final Jerk lift with apparent body control.

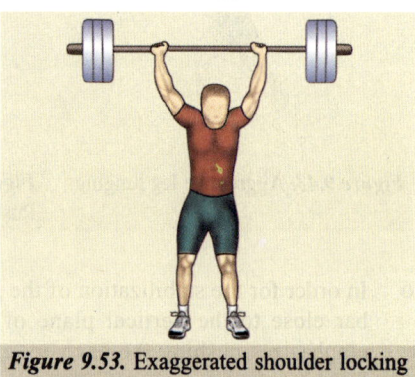

Figure 9.53. Exaggerated shoulder locking in the final Jerk lift.

9.3. CONTEST RULES OF THE CLEAN AND JERK LIFT

In order to standardize competition, the Clean and Jerk lifts are subjected to few rules to qualify for correct lifts.

o The Clean and Jerk is a two-stage lift. In the Clean, the barbell is lifted from the floor to the shoulders. After a brief pause, the barbell is driven from the shoulders to an arm length, overheads. The lift is complete when the feet are in line, side by side, and the bar is under control. The Jerk should not be initiated during the ascending in the Clean from the floor, but rather after pausing at the completion of the Clean.

o Correct Clean lift should proceed upwards once the initial pull is initiated. Retreat or retrial defaults the Clean. The initial pull is judged by the intention of the lifter to commence the Clean, in the allotted time permitted by the contest rules.

o The Bar should proceed upwards without pausing, in the distance between the point of beginning and the shoulders. Pausing at the thighs, and then proceeding with thigh push and shoulder shrug, defaults the Clean lift.

o The elbows are not allowed to touch the knees or thighs, during full Squat descent after the barbell is lifted from the floor. This does not apply to abutting the arms on the sides of the knees during the start position.

o The ascent from full Squat to upright in the Clean is not stringently regulated. The lifter can bounce up and down to initiate ascent, if fails to ascend under tight control immediately after the Squat is completed.

o The Jerk commences only after the two feet are together, in line, and the barbell is supported on the shoulders, in upright posture.

o Once the jerk is initiated, it should not retreat or retried. Shoulder Press is slow and can be easily spotted and defaulted. The Clean and Jerk is complete with the barbell overhead, under the controlled support of the lifter, with fully extended body.

9.4. TRAINING PRACTICE ON THE CLEAN AND JERK LIFT

9.4.1. DISSECTING THE MOTION OF THE CLEAN AND JERK

As with the case of the Snatch lift, Weightlifters do not practice the standard Clean and Jerk each training session. They also have to work on enhancing the different phases of the lift, in addition to the general requirements of strength, flexibility, coordination, and recuperation. The common phase of pulling from the floor applies to both the Clean and the Snatch strengthening. The Pull is executed with variable handgrip width, variation in the travel height, and variation in the mode of muscular contraction, as follows.

o The initiation of the Pull has to be mastered religiously, by lowering the hips, thrusting the chest, lordosing the lower back, and tightly extending the elbows, *Figures 9.54* and *9.58*.
o The upper body must remain in tight isometric posture, while the leg drive is being executed, *Figures 9.55* and *9.59*.
o The shoulder drive commences with combined lateral abduction and transverse shoulder adduction. This is performed by pulling the upper arms, backwards and upwards, combined by shoulder shrugging or elevation, *Figures 9.56* and *9.60*.
o Farther shoulder drive is induced by shoulder abduction, combined by shoulder shrugging or elevation, *Figure 9.57*.
o Shoulder extension is executed by pulling, while the elbows are maintained close to the sides, *Figure 9.61*. This final posture precedes flipping of the elbows under the bar, prior to squatting to retrieve the bar.

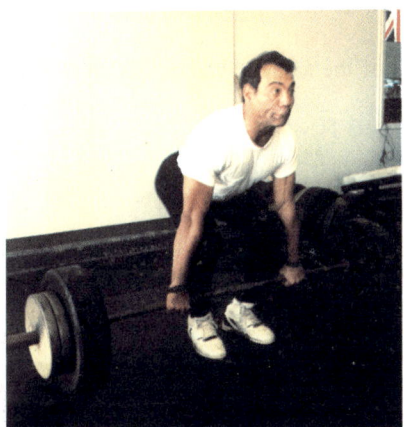

Figure 9.54. Start position for the Deadlift Clean.

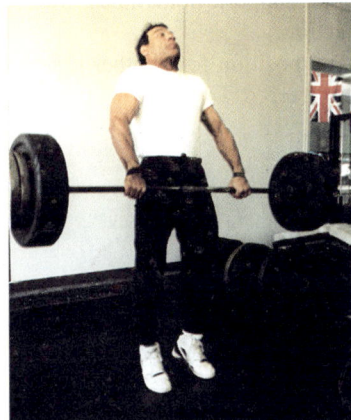

Figure 9.55. Clean Pull after lower body drive.

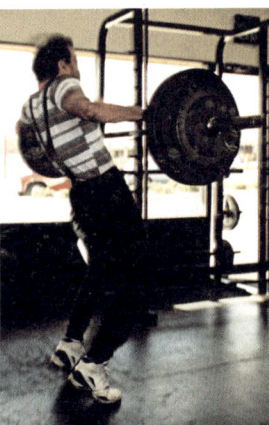

Figure 9.56. Shoulder drive with arm abduction and transverse adduction.

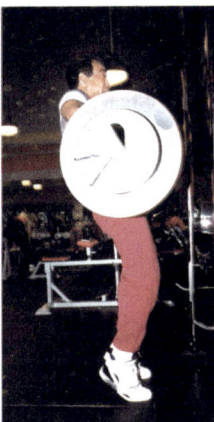

Figure 9.57. Shoulder drive with arm abduction.

The full Clean and Jerk motion is dissected in training practice, as follows.
o During training, you are absolved from the stringent rules of Weightlifting contest. You have the options to refining the Clean and Jerk lifts with various methods of execution.
o You can execute the Clean and Jerk lifts with a barbell, dumbbell, plate, or any manageable object.
o You can break down the different phases of the Clean lift into Deadlift, Hang Clean, Bent-over row, or Military Clean.
o You can break down the Jerk lift into shoulder pushing with heavy weight, front Jerk, back Jerk, or Jerk while squatting.
o You can work on enhancing the isometric contraction, from the kneecaps to the lower chest, in the Hang Clean. Alternatively, you can enhance the eccentric contraction during lowering the bar in the Hang Clean.
o You can vary the handgrip from close, shoulder-width, to standard handgrip width in order to emphasize different areas of the scapular muscles.
o You can perform more than one lift in a set, usually three repetitions per set.
o The norm of Weightlifting training is practicing the standard Clean and Jerk lifts and supplementing these with enhancing exercises of variations of the technique. The standard style of the Clean and Jerk is performed, on average, six to eight sets per session, with weight over 60% 1RM. The accessory exercises are performed in groups of three to four sets, once or twice weekly.

9.4.2. HANG CLEAN
o The Hang Clean is not a standard exercise that serves complete strength training. Since, in the Hang Clean, the lower phases of the Clean lift are skipped, therefore the sole training on the Hang Clean can result in serious stiffness and shortening of the ligaments and tendons of the knees, hips, back, and shoulders.
o This exercise can be performed after the Classical Clean as a way to strengthen the elbow and shoulder flexors. These are the Biceps brachii, Brachialis, Coracobrachialis, Deltoids, and Supraspinatus.

9 THE CLEAN & JERK

- o The Hang Clean can be executed with full Squat after the pull, with military Pull, or with protracted isometric contraction of the Biceps, prior to final ballistic pulling.
- o The Hang Clean is performed with overhand grip, slightly wider than shoulder width. The barbell can be lifted from the floor to the hang position, or from racks or blocks. The floor lifting is advantageous in stretching the back progressively prior to the Clean. The hoisted position can cause acute back injury if the Hang Clean were not preceded by standard Clean. That is because lifting from the Hang was not preceded by progressive preparation and warm-up.
- o The Hang Clean cannot be performed without bending the knees and hips in order to lower barbell to the low-thigh level. This is accompanied by great leaning forward with the torso, in order to generate momentum by the Hamstrings and back erectors. If the knees and hips were not bent, then the lifter would be performing mere shoulder shrugging in order to initiate the Clean. This defeats the purpose of the Hang Clean, which is set to strengthen muscles by impulsive stretching, rather than by controlled tension contraction.
- o The pull of the Hang Clean is initiated with thrust chest, shoulders vertically over the bar, and the back arched tightly. Arms are tightly straightened at the elbows, until full momentum is generated by the bouncing of the torso.
- o Shoulder shrugging increases as momentum increases. Arm pulling commences when the shoulders are maximally shrugged and the whole body is supported on the feet balls and thrown backwards *Figure 9.55.*
- o Arms pulling comprises of aggressive elevation of the upper arms and abducting them. This forces the elbows to move out, to the sides, keeping the bar close to the body, *Figures 9.56, 9.57,* and *9.61*. As the bar is drawn upwards and backwards, the torso must dip forwards and downwards under the bar, while rotating the elbows around the bar.
- o The bar is caught on the shoulders while moving into squat or slight dipping position. Usually, lifters ascend with the barbell as soon as they feel the bar is under good support. Sometimes, lifters protract the Squat or dipping posture in order to exercise stretching and isometric contraction.
- o After ascent, the bar can be lowered to the hang position for another repetition of the same exercise, for up to three times.

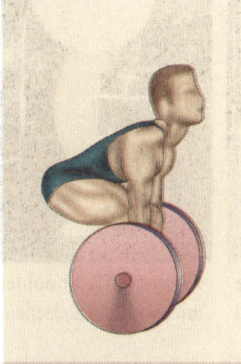

Figure 9.58. Adjusting the start position, side view.

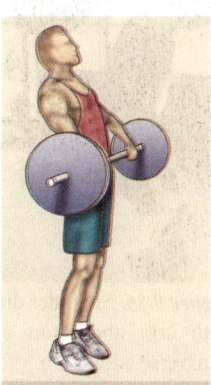

Figure 9.59. Clean Pull after lower body drive, side view.

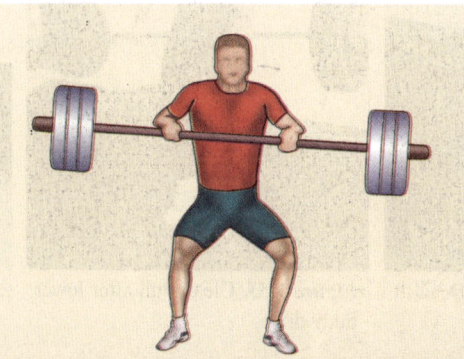

Figure 9.60. Shoulder drive with arm abduction and transverse adduction, during commencing squatting under the bar.

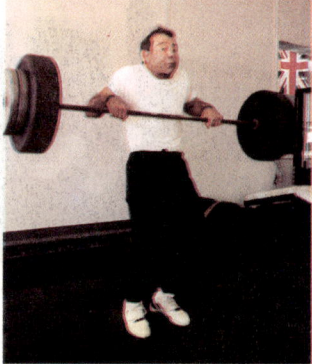

Figure 9.61. Shoulder drive with arm extension in preparation for vigorous shoulder flexion and elbow flipping under the bar.

9.4.3. HANG PULL
- o This is another partial assisting exercise for strengthening the Supraspinatus and Deltoid muscles. The advantage of executing the pull from the Hang is the concentrated stressing of the lateral and posterior fibers of the Deltoids and the Supraspinatus, in addition to the minimum load volume required for short ascent.
- o The barbell is pulled either after initial Deadlift or from hoisted position, over racks or blocks. The bar is held in overhand grip, as in the standard Clean. The knees and hips are slightly bent at the beginning of the pull. The rest of the pull proceeds as in the Hang Clean but the motion ends before rotating the elbows, *Figures 9.56, 9.57,* and *9.61.*
- o The Hang Pull can be performed with protracted isometric contraction pause at the top of the motion, or eccentric contraction deceleration during lowering the barbell. These two modifications result in greater arm and shoulder strength, massive gain of muscle size, and strong ballistic pull of the Clean and Snatch lifts.
- o The Hang Pull has to assist the standard full motion Clean in order to balance the shoulder muscles and to prevent the stiffness of the lower body. Thus, the Hang Pull can be alternated with the Hang Clean between sessions, whereas the standard Clean constantly precedes each of them.

9.4.4. HIGH PULL
- o The High Pull is performed from the floor, with the handgrips, feet stance, and start position of the Clean, *Figures 9.54* thru *9.57.* This is very essential piece of teaching the Clean lift. All beginners can quickly learn how to master the Clean lift if they practice on few sets of High Pull. This eliminates the apprehension of the complexity of the elbow, chest, back, and head motions of the Clean. The straight upward direction of the Pull puts the mind of the beginner at

ease, by realizing the simplicity of straight-line motion. The subsequent back bouncing, shoulder flexing, and torso dipping, are completely eliminated with the Pull. These three motions will be inserted later, systemically, in order to enhance the automatism of the technique.
o   The High Pull is an advanced phase with respect to the Deadlift, yet a muted phase with respect to the full Clean. In this sense, the High Pull can be performed with weight greater than that of the Clean and at speeds greater than that of the Deadlift. Its main purpose is the enhancement of the axial muscles, from the knees to the back of the skull.
o   The High Pull must be practiced at least twice a week, in order to excel in lifting from the floor. The High Pulls not only condition the axial extensors for vigorous body erection, but also strengthen the skeletal axis to stand excessive virtual forces.

9.4.5. PUSH PRESS
o   Lifting the barbell from the shoulder overheads, with leg drive, is called **"Push Press"**. It differs from the Shoulder Press in that the latter does not utilize leg drive. The leg drive prevents the rotator cuff muscles from snapping torn when the shoulder joints try to rotate the upper arms, from below the shoulder level, upwards. Instead, the Deltoids will engage vigorously as soon as the barbell is pushed upwards, from the shoulders, by the leg drive. Thus, the Supraspinatus are spared the acute stress of lifting the barbell, as in the Shoulder Press, and can now participate in the Push Press with shorter and stronger fibers.
o   The Push Press aims at strengthening the Serratus Anterior, Deltoid, and Triceps, in addition to the dynamic stretching of the shoulder ligaments and tendons that exceeds that of the Shoulder Press.
o   Although the Shoulder Press is conducted by the shoulder girdle, it requires utmost support of the legs, back, and chest. The knees should start with initial bend in order to allow for adjusting balance of the upper joints and posture. The lower back must arch in, tightly, while the chest thrusts upwards and forwards. This guarantees the retraction of the scapulas at the back of the chest and, consequently, the firmness of the shoulders under the bar.
o   In order for the Push Press to be effective, the chest has to remain thrust while dipping by the whole body by bending the knees and hips. In addition, the shoulders should dip downwards but not forwards. Forward dipping of the shoulders wastes the leg drive by creating two opposing forces at the barbell.
o   In beginners and Bodybuilders, the shoulders may relax its flexion under the bar during the dipping action. This laxity may result in very ineffective leg drive. Advanced lifters increase shoulder flexion by maintaining elevated elbows while dipping for leg drive.
o   For optimum timing of the Push Press, the upward leg drive must wait until the downward dipping is ceased, before kicking in. Experienced lifters master the vigorous tightening of the upper body prior to the induction of leg drive. Thus, when the leg drive is set into action, it imparts its effect on tightly supported barbell on the lifter's shoulders.
o   The effective leg drive is immediately followed by upward Shoulder Press. The front Deltoid, Biceps brachii, and Triceps contract vigorously, without changing length, until the leg drive has moved the entire body and the barbell to peak height. This occurs as the hips, knees, and ankles all extend fully on the top of the feet balls. Thereafter, the shoulder and arm muscles contract concentrically and move the bar upwards and backwards, *Figures 9.40* and *9.44*. When the bar clears the face area then the lifter has few choices to make in finalizing the Press.
o   The lifter can lock the lower body in rigid extension and continues the Shoulder Press by farther contracting the Deltoids and Triceps. In the meantime, the bar is pushed to the back; an arm stretch over the nape of the neck while the head advances forwards. This is called **"Shoulder Push Press"**. This is only a strengthening exercise for the Triceps and Deltoid. It is not permitted in Weightlifting contests.
o   Another choice is to dip with the torso by bending the knees and hips while pressing the bar upwards and backwards and advancing the head forwards. The dipped body soon extends into upright posture, as soon as the arms lock on the barbell in full overhead extension. This is called **"Power Jerk"**.
o   A third choice is to dip with torso by springing with one leg forwards and the other backwards, while the bar is driven upwards and backwards. The legs will soon return together to line, *Figures 9.43, 9.47, 9.48,* and *9.51*. This is called **"Split Jerk"**.
o   The fourth choice is to dip with the torso into deep Squat while the bar is driven upwards, *Figures 9.45* and *9.50*. This is can be called **"Overhead Squat Jerk"**.

9.4.6. SPLIT JERK
o   This is the most widely practiced style of jerking the barbell from the shoulders overheads. It must be emphasized that the leg split or lunge is an optional choice and is not a contest requirement for valid, complete Jerk lift. The leg split serves the purpose of minimizing the stress on the shoulders, during the Shoulder Press, by imparting impulsive force on the barbell, then dipping with the body and extending the elbows.
o   The main reason that Weightlifters practice Split Jerk in training is the need for conditioning the shoulders, head, and chest for ballistic impulsive motion. This differs from steady Shoulder Press in that the Jerk motion generates greater momentum, utilizing the greater strength of the lower body over the upper body.
o   The Jerk might become formidable if the shoulder joints cannot rotate the upper arms upwards, in addition to assuming fully shrugged position. The upper arms have to be stabilized in a position very close to the ears, *Figures 9.51*

9 THE CLEAN & JERK

thru *9.53*. The Press is accomplished by the combined vigorous contraction of the upper Trapezius, the Supraspinatus, the back Deltoids, the Triceps, the Serratus anterior, and the Latissimus dorsi. These muscles cannot be activated with such vigor during steady Shoulder Press. This mainly relies on the sustained contraction of the anterior Deltoid.

o The Split Jerk is always performed, in training practice, after the Clean from the floor. It can be executed from the rack, in the form of front-shoulder, or back-shoulder, Split Jerk. The front-shoulder Jerk is of particular importance since it strengthens the muscles that stabilize the scapulas when the shoulders are elevated and semi-flexed. The back-shoulder Jerk is easier than the front one but utilizes the lateral Deltoids more the anterior Deltoids and does not emphasize strengthening the muscles of chest thrusting, during shoulder pushing.

9.5. PROPER LIFTING TECHNIQUE FOR THE CLEAN AND JERK

9.5.1. PROPER TECHNIQUE FOR THE CLEAN

o Weightlifters tackle the task of heavy ballistic lifting with vivid imagination of the **systemic breakdown** of the lift. This approach to lifting reduces the overwhelming apprehension of performing complex and tedious physical work. The complexity of heavy, full range lifting stems from the diverse nature of motion of the joints. The wrists, for example, cannot perform flexion or extension with very heavy weight. In addition, the knees cannot perform any abduction or adduction and, therefore, the limitations of the knees are critical in planning the sequence of motion of lifting. The shoulders are very mobile, yet weaker than the hips. Therefore, executing a specific technique in the different phases lifting ensures powerful lifting and less traumatic outcome.

o The first step in the breakdown of the Clean is the **Deadlift phase**. This is executed with overhand grips, about shoulder width apart, and with elbows aimed midway, between laterally and backwards. The thrust chest and retracted scapulas place the Deltoids vertically over the bar, *Figure 9.4*. The initiation of the Deadlift motion in the Clean lift does not differ from that of mere Deadlift exercise. Yet, after one or two inches of ascent, the Clean motion deviates from the Deadlift exercise.

o The drive for the Deadlift of the Clean is initiated with the hips slightly elevated over the horizontal level of the knees. Farther elevation of the hips exceeds the rate of elevation of the torso. By the time the barbell reaches the kneecaps, the knees should have been extended more than the hips, *Figures 9.5* thru *9.7*. Thus, fast rising of the hips, compared to the torso, positions the torso in a "lean-over" position, with the **head advanced**, way in front of the front of the feet.

o The second step in the breakdown of the Clean is the **Pull**. This is initiated by the vigorous **contraction of the Hamstrings**, while the entire back maintains rigid leverage between the arms and the hips. As the Hamstrings pull the entire torso backwards, the arms remain tightly extended and the knees and ankles farther increase their extension. When the torso has reached upright posture, the whole body should be fully extended. As the head crosses the vertical plane of the feet balls, the heels are raised and the Glutei are vigorously contracted, *Figure 9.14*.

o Now, the two major muscle groups, the Glutei at the hips and the Trapezius muscles at the shoulders, generate the **pulling torque**. The Glutei thrust the hips forwards, while the Trapezius thrust the shoulders backwards. In the meantime, the ankle is amplifying the torque by elevating the heels and rotating the entire body backwards on the feet balls, *Figures 9.18* and *9.19*.

o The second portion of the Pull is executed by shoulder shrugging, shoulder abduction, and shoulder extension. This is the **weakest link** in the Clean, since the arms and shoulders are much weaker than the legs and hips. Therefore, the arm and shoulder pulling have to be augmented with **quick descent** of the torso by squatting. The descent of the torso is supported by the vigorous isometric contraction of the lower legs, in full flexion position, and the robust rotation of the elbows under the bar with subsequent isometric contraction, in full flexion.

o The **squatting and elbow flipping** under the bar is only possible if the chest is thrown in vigorous thrust, and the lower back in vigorous lordosis. These two actions ensure the upright support of the loaded torso on the squatting pelvis. The two actions also enable the squatting lifter to ascend with the weight and, furthermore, continue with the Jerk lift.

o The **unfolding of the body** from full front Squat requires aggressive concentric contraction of the Quadriceps, Glutei, Erector spinae, and Deltoid.

9.5.2. PROPER TECHNIQUE FOR THE JERK

The Jerk differs from Shoulder Press in the initiation of upward drive. The drive for the Jerk originates from the muscles of the lower body, namely, the Quadriceps and the Glutei, *Figure 9.62*. The Olympic Shoulder Press was initiated by the Glutei and the Deltoids, *Figure 9.63*. The Jerk is executed as the Clean ends, as follows.

o Place a barbell on your shoulders by tightening the front Deltoids and semi-flexing the upper arms. This brings the elbows to the front of the body, *Figure 9.35*. The bar must sit on the sternoclavicular joints, at the base of the neck, and push the anterior structures of the neck backwards. This sounds like a strangulation technique! However, with training the musculature and bones of the root of the neck, will develop and tolerate such action. In addition, the throat and front neck will desensitize to the pressure of the bar. Any untoward effect results in shutting off the shoulder muscles and, consequently, lowering the bar with the elbows away from the neck, *Figures 9.25, 9.31, 9.32,* and *9.36*.

- o The front-shoulder positioning of the bar is very taxing, due the great effort made by the scapular muscles to **maintain the clavicles in high bridging position** over the vital vessels, air passages, and nerves, at the root of the neck and chest outlet. The lifter will find that strengthening shoulder and scapular muscles is very vital to enhancing the front shoulder positioning in the initiation of the Jerk.
- o The bar is gripped with **overhand grip** at a comfortable width. Close handgrips overstretch the Supraspinatus muscles, at the upper back of the shoulder joints. Wide handgrips overstretch the Subscapularis muscles, at the upper front of the shoulder joints.
- o Since the Jerk is mainly driven by the leg and shoulders, therefore there is no need to exert the arms or hands in the initiation of the Jerk. As the bar is entirely supported by the shoulders and the front upper chest, therefore the arms and hands should be minimally activated. These will be dearly needed in the upper phases of the Jerk. Advanced Weightlifters master the great **silencing of the arms and hands** contraction, during the start position of the Jerk. They greatly appreciate the tremendous efforts of the arms and hands in the Jerk lift when the barbell is impulsively pushed above the head, *Figure 9.41* and *9.42*.

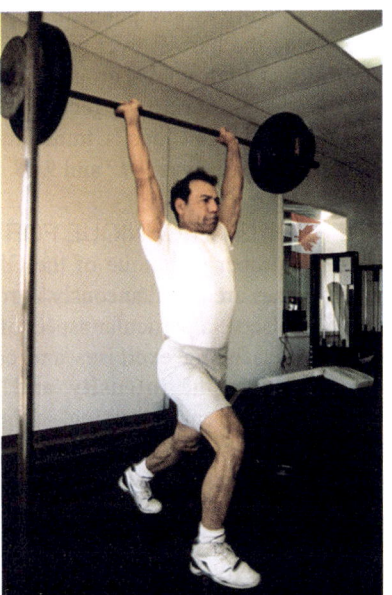
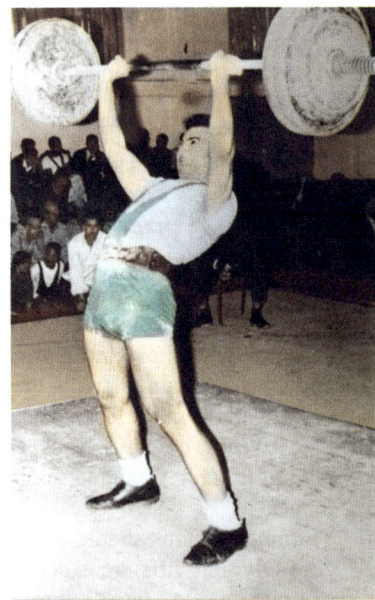

Figure 9.62. Split Jerk. The front foot is flatly anchored to the floor, while the rear foot balances the body over the metatarsal heads.

Figure 9.63. Olympic Press was eliminated from Olympic games after 1972. The pelvic thrust was widely used to enhance the Press.

- o In order to avoid aborting the Jerk lift prematurely, before full arm extension overheads, the execution of the leg drive has to be practiced very frequently. This serves the purpose of acquiring the sense of **timing of the descent and the upward drive** and the feeling of the relative positioning of body parts. The hips and shoulders have to fall vertically over the heels. This can be achieved by slow and powerful descent while paying utmost attention to descending downwards, without forward or backward displacements of the hips or shoulders.
- o Although the heels carry the entire weight, of the body and barbell, yet the feet arches will be vigorously tightened and contracted when the real impulsive motion commences. For now, the feet are anchored tightly to the floor until the bar is pushed off the shoulders.
- o The **leg drive** is executed by lowering the body by bending the knees and hips. Simultaneously, with the descending of the body, the head is rotated slowly and gradually backwards, whereas the chest increases thrust, and the lower back increases lordosis. When the descent ceases and the upward drive begins, the head should be out of the way of the upward trajectory of the bar. In the beginning, you might err by sticking your head in the way and incur a hit at the chin or nose. Alternatively, you might try to move the bar forwards to avoid hitting your chin, thus, resulting in ineffective leg drive.
- o The trickiest phase of the Jerk Push is the **synchrony of the leg and shoulder drives**. You should not attempt to push with your shoulders while performing the descent. You also should not attempt to push with shoulders while the leg drive is gaining momentum. Again, you should not initiate the leg drive while descending. What you should do is to focus greatly on the thighs, lower back, and shoulders. As soon as the thighs finish their impulsive upwards drive, the back engages by straightening from lordosis, followed by shoulder pushing. The three actions of the thighs, back, and shoulders should proceed in cadence, without pauses. This is the intimate transfer of muscular forces into the external weight of the barbell.
- o As the barbell moves ballistically upwards, the head should be entirely off the way. This impulse generates weightlessness state and permits the lifter to lunge the front leg, with bent knee, while the other leg is lunged, with straight knee, backwards. The front foot has to advance while the rear foot retreats, in order to **advance the torso** under and in front of the barbell. Because the state of weightlessness is very brief, the lifter has to assume a supporting posture to the acute compression by the external weight, while standing on sprung legs. Therefore, the arms assume rigid and strong overhead extension, the back of the shoulders is shrugged and elevated vigorously, the lower back is excessively tightened, and the front leg Quadriceps is combined with the rear leg Hamstrings in vigorous isometric contraction. This posture prevents the barbell from shaking or losing balance, *Figures 9.43* and *9.49*.
- o As soon as bar is balanced over the shoulders and hips, push to extend your front leg and take a step or two

backwards. When your front foot is about halfway straightened, step forwards with your rear foot to bring both feet in line together. Maintain upward pressure on the barbell over your hips and shoulders. The common mistakes occur in **retuning the legs** either by lifting the feet high above ground or relaxing upper body support to the weight. You should drag your feet very close to the ground during the recovery from the split-leg position. In the meantime, pay utmost attention to the arms, shoulders, back, and hips. Utmost attention can put your entire muscles in a state of "fight" and create "steel-locking" of the joints, *Figures 9.47* and *9.48*.

9.5.3. TRAINING PRACTICE ON THE PROPER TECHNIQUE FOR THE CLEAN AND JERK

o Beginner Weightlifters start practice the proper technique of the Olympic lifting as a **core segment** of the training session. The basic strength building exercises are simultaneously introduced as **assisting exercises** to the core segment. The assisting exercises have to be picked to serve a particular aspect of the Olympic lifts.

o The process of picking and eliminating, assisting exercises and core Olympic exercises, evolves as the beginner becomes acquainted with the relationship of the **intensity and volume** of training load. The most significant modification, in the beginner's perception of strength training, is the realization that physical strength develops over many weeks, not days. Thus, each single training session must fit into the big picture of a weekly, monthly, and annul plan of training. Training sessions should last approximately 90 minutes and should end there, even if the lifter can last longer.

o Training sessions should include a **balanced variety of exercises** in each segment, core or assisting segments. The core Olympic lifts are executed in groups of five to eight sets each, of one to three repetitions per set. The assisting exercises are executed in groups of four to six sets, of three to eight repetitions per set. The combination of freestyle lifting and assisting exercises will accompany all training sessions, for the entire life of practice of the lifter, except the few weeks prior to contest. Prior to contest, lifters practice freestyle lifting only, in order to allow for fast recuperation and heighten the neuromuscular coordination.

o Beginners should be taught the concept of **progressive incremental resistance** as a mean to enhance muscular strength. That is acquired by explaining the rationale of increasing the barbell weight within each exercise group. The weight should only increase when the previously executed set indicates that the lifter is comfortable with the technique and speed of lifting. If the weight of the barbell has to increase, it should do that every other set or two. Otherwise, the lifter should content himself or herself with light and smooth performance, rather than straining his joints or compromising the technique. In addition, the increase in weight should range from five kilograms, for light weightlifters, to twenty kilograms, for heavy Weightlifters. If, after increasing the weight, the technique deteriorates, then it is advised to terminate that group of exercise and proceed with the next group. It should be clear that barbell weight is changed between sets, of a particular group of exercises.

9.6. PROS AND CONS OF EXPLOSIVE WEIGHT TRAINING

9.6.1. RISK FACTORS

o Explosive weight training comprises of **generating momentum** by fast body motion in order to produce greater lifting forces. Examples of explosive exercises are the Snatch, the Clean and Jerk, the Power Clean, the Jump Squat, and the Push Press. The apparent danger of fast motion, during lifting, is greatly reduced by lengthy, progressive, and incremental preparation. That danger becomes reality when the lifter ignores regular and relevant training. Any interruption in training should be factored in the safety of explosive training.

o Explosive weight training requires long training and conditioning in order to develop the neuromuscular coordination, musculoskeletal strength, and connective tissue tolerance to impulsive forces. This sort of training prepares the body for the exorbitant, potentially traumatic forces by way of enhancing fast twitching muscles and responses. On the other hand, controlled high-tension resistance exercises enhance slow twitching muscles, yet compromise **balance and fast response**. Neuromuscular reflexes adapt to compound, fast and complex motions differently from simple motions.

o Proper training prevents incurring trauma, both acutely and cumulatively, to muscle tissue, fascia, connective tissue, and bony structures. **Progressive incremental training**, on extremes of acceleration and deceleration forces placed on involved structures, leads to strengthening those structures in accordance to the magnitude of resistance. In addition, the relatively long breaks and rest intervals, between exercise sets and training sessions, allow for greater recuperation. This is not the case in controlled high-tension exercises that are performed for high number of repetitions and that emphasize highly toned muscles. High repetitions reduce the recuperation interval. In addition, highly toned muscles impede circulation and neuromuscular control.

o The apparent forced hypertension of the lumbar spine, in explosive training, might be extremely over and beyond the norms of the population at large. Yet, Weightlifters have devised many effective ways of **strengthening the spinal joints** beyond the imagination of lay people. The prevalence of spinal injuries -such as lumbar sprain, strain, disc injury or spondylolysis- among Weightlifters, is extremely lower than that in the population at large. This is based on the author's personal observation, since the population of Weightlifters is not that vast. In addition, the many years spent in freestyle lifting offer the lifter great educational experience on the nature of the spinal function. The neurological studies on spinal stresses, torques, and electromyographic activity, during explosive training, might yield

- some scary data, yet do not account for the realistic outcome of many years of proper training of young lifters. Many Weightlifters lead very gratifying life after many years of training and competing, *Figures 4.13* thru *4.15,* and *4.17*.
- o It might be true that performing Olympic lifts provides little benefit to athletes in their training programs for any sport other than Olympic lifting, since **motor skills** are, generally, not transferable across sports. Yet, accomplishing high strength in Olympic lifting alone greatly impacts the musculoskeletal posture and mobility for many years to come.
- o The main gain of regular training is the concrete appreciation of the progress made in physical strength. The lifter will go through specific landmarks of developing and evolving, during practicing freestyle lifting. With recuperation and many trials and errors, Weightlifters can ascertain accurately the **tensile strength** of their ligaments, tendons, and muscles. I should emphasize that lifting weight is stringently regulated by feedback safety mechanism, by the brain and the peripheral nervous system. Lifters practice by dissecting the motion of lifting, systemically, and master the progression, or the bail out, of each step of the motion. Thus, the fear of exceeding the limits of structures apply mostly to untrained folks, not to Weightlifters.
- o Injuries due to explosive training occur more frequently during **off-training** periods than during training. The main reason is the great need for rest, nutrition, and massage, in a cyclic fashion, according to the periodization of load intensity and volume. Another factor in incurring off-training injuries is the lack of warming up or preparation of highly fatigued muscles, prior to performing other physical activities. The recuperating muscles, in between training sessions, can be inadvertently injured if not allowed to adequately rest and regenerate.
- o The obsession with fear of cumulative injuries, due to explosive lifting, is negated on grounds that injuries occur only when **anatomic or physiologic limits are breached**. Thus, as long as explosive training differs from controlled training only in intensity, due to induced momentum and not in anatomic or physiologic breach, therefore both methods of training are equally risky, as far as predisposition to injury is concerned.
- o Explosive ballistic exercises not only increase the tensile strength of soft tissues and density of bone, but also foster **distribution of strength and bone density,** in locations and directions that are pertinent to functional motion. While controlled-velocity exercises also enhance strength and bone density, these are merely executed in the directions that the lifter perceives as preferred. For example, performing Shoulder Press with controlled velocity emphasizes the Deltoids and Trapezius muscles, with low tension on the surrounding ligaments, tendons, and bone. Here, the muscles of the lower back and legs are tightened isometrically and are thus, prevented from dynamic neuromuscular recruitment. On the other hand, the Shoulder Push exposes the entire body into impulsive stretching forces that simulate real living activities. The leg and shoulder drives of the Shoulder Push induce greater recruitment activities of various muscles and thus, prevent locking of joints and occurrence of spastic acute injury. Spastic injuries of controlled velocity exercises are attributed to the great isometric contraction of supporting muscles for longer times, than in explosive exercises.

9.6.2. NECESSITY OF BALLISTIC WEIGHT TRAINING
- o Ballistic lifting movements are necessary in enhancing athletic performance by **simulating movement** patterns of velocity and acceleration. The synchrony and briefness of ballistic motion require the high engagement of the neuromuscular system. Training enhances voluntary control of motor skill. Of course, controlled velocity exercises must be used as assisting exercises in enhancing the weak links of the ballistic lifts. Squat, Deadlift, and Goodmorning exercises are examples of controlled velocity exercises that assist the Clean and Jerk and the Snatch.
- o Heavy ballistic lifting induces greater recruitment of **fast twitching muscle fibers** and requires great silence in the muscles, prior to the stormy contraction. Thus, muscular hypertrophy and spasm impede ballistic lifting. This differ significantly from controlled speed exercises that induce slow twitching muscle fibers and cause higher muscular spasm and swelling. Swollen and spastic muscles are less responsive to real living motor demands. Yet, the two modes of exercises are needed alternatively. The latter mode of exercise strengthens muscles lagging in strength behind the rest of the body. Enhancing the slow twitching muscle fibers expands the population of smaller neural axons and cell bodies in the spinal cord, due to the hypertrophy of this fiber type by controlled light lifting. The slow muscle fibers are the first to kick into action, due to their low threshold of stimulation, and thus, spare the powerful fast fibers for greater intensity lifting.
- o **Heavy lifting** stimulates fast twitching muscle fibers. It has to be performed in few repetitions, since these fibers are deficient in mitochondria, and therefore low on endurance. **Light lifting** stimulates slow twitching muscle fibers. It can be performed at high repetitions, since these fibers possess greater density of mitochondria, and therefore high on endurance. Combination of heavy and light lifting enhances both muscle fibers and elevates the plateau of net force, ballistic plus isometric contraction.
- o The simultaneous induction of **multiple joint** movements, in Olympic lifting, enhances the lifter's ability to impose control on major muscles, in concerting fashion. This differs from controlled speed exercises where the lifter pays attention to one or two joint movements, in comparison to four or more joints that set in motion in Olympic lifting. Even if the specificity of movement is not transferable from Weightlifting to other sports, yet the enhanced simultaneous muscular control is a substantial gain of freestyle lifting.
- o Ballistic Weightlifting is not an optional choice in heavy lifting. It is a necessity. Since Olympic lifts travel full range, from the floor, overheads, they cannot be executed by controlled-speed high-tension contraction. The formidable link in full range lifting lies in the arm and shoulder elevation of weights, from below shoulder level, overheads. Ballistic

motion merely circumvents this weakness by **imparting the momentum** generated by major axial muscles on the bar during this formidable phase of lifting. Weightlifters do not perform ballistic motion for spectacular show up, but rather for mechanical necessity.
o   It is very evident that momentum generation by the Quadriceps, the Hamstrings, the Glutei, the Erector spinae, and the Trapezius is accomplished by the massive recruitment of **slow twitching muscle fibers**. These are strengthened by controlled-speed high-tension exercises. Since these muscle fibers are easily activated and can endure longer aerobic energy production, they are capable of producing adequate momentum prior to the initiation of ballistic motion. The imparted momentum, of the leg-back-shoulder torque, enables the fast twitching muscle fibers to perform the vigorous and brief contraction that circumvent the weakness of the arms and shoulders. Therefore, all ballistic motions occur either when the barbell is closely below or above the shoulders level. These are the phases of elbow flipping under the bar in the Clean, overhead elbow extension under the bar in the Jerk, and overhead arms elevation in the Snatch.

9.7. ERRORS IN THE CLEAN AND JERK

9.7.1. THE CLEAN FAULTS, CAUSES AND CORRECTIONS

Performance faults are not amenable to immediate correction. Planning for long and regular effort to rectify the anatomical and functional causes should entail alerting the lifter to the deviation from proper technique and incorporating assisting exercises to remedy the deficit, as follows.

9.7.1.1. Premature Elevation Of Hips Before Raising Bar
This may be caused by insufficient thigh and hip strength, lack of knee and hip flexibility, weak back erectors, or weak shoulder shrugging muscles, as follows.
o   The long-term correction of premature hip elevation should encompass regular axial strength exercises. Examples of these exercises are the Power Clean and Military Clean, with deeply lowered hips at the start position.
o   Flexibility-enhancing exercises promote the range of motion of the knees, hips, and back. Examples of these exercises are lifting weight from the floor with feet standing on blocks, deep squatting, Jump Squat, and Jump Goodmorning.
o   Spastic leg and back muscles must be relieved by stretch, massage, rest, or hot sauna. Many Yoga exercises are very effective in rendering spastic muscles relaxed and enhance restful sleep. This hastens buildup of strength.

9.7.1.2. Forward Displacement Of Bar Trajectory
Displacement of bar trajectory, in front to the center of mass of the lifter, generates torque that tends to rotate the body forwards. This is caused by either insufficient scapular pull during ascent, premature elbows or arm bending, or insufficient backward toque of the torso on the hips. These result in early movement onto toes, as the bar ascends below the knee.
o   The insufficient scapular balance during ascent diminishes the transfer of leg-back drive to the arms and results in forward leaning of the body. This deficit is rectified by assisting exercises such as High Pull, Hang Clean, and Bent-Over Row.
o   Premature arm bending loosens the transfer leverage, between the shoulders and the bar, and results is allowing the bar displace forwards. This can be prevented by strengthening isometric contraction of the arms in Hang Clean, Hang Pull, Chin-ups, and Deadlift.
o   Insufficient torque of the torso prevents the hips from advancing forwards, and the head from retreating backwards enough to pull the bar close to the body. This is assisted by Hang Clean with full Squat, Jump Goodmorning, and High Pull.

9.7.1.3. Backward Displacement Of Bar Trajectory
Backward displacement of the bar forces the whole body to move backwards. This is caused by aggressive back and shoulder pull in excess to leg support. This happens when the lifter attempts to lift new weight record, after returning from long interruption of training, or when the training plan is inadequately compressed in time interval. Corrective measures include standard axial training and adequate accumulation of load volume, in order to allow for developmental progress of major muscle strength and coordination.

9.7.1.4. Insufficient Torso Torque
The torso torque pulls the barbell upwards and inwards, towards the body. The forces that generate the torso torque originate from the Gastrocnemius, the Hamstrings, the Quadriceps, the Glutei, the back Erectors, and the Trapezius. Thus, any delay or rush in the actions of the ankles, knees, hips, or spines could result in inadequate torque. Thus, corrective measures must emphasize these joints by simulating exercises. Regular practice on the standard Clean and Jerk, Power Clean, Hang Clean, High Pulls, and Goodmorning are the mainstay in enhancing the skill and strength of generating torque by the torso.

9.7.1.5. Insufficient Full Body Extension
Full body extension represents standing on the feet balls with extended ankles, straight knees and hips, hyperextended back, straight arms, and shrugged shoulders. The center of mass of the lifter is thrown behind the feet balls, whereas the center of mass of the barbell remains over the feet balls. The reason that the body does not fall backwards, despite its exaggerated back bouncing, is that the barbell pulls the body downwards and forwards, by means of its prior state of motion. The body can easily fall backwards if the lifter is not well trained on such coordinative technique.

Insufficient full extension can result from weak body extensors, improper technique, or excessively heavy weight. Axial exercises for strength and flexibility on similar activities build up this overall strength.

9.7.1.6. Insufficient Shoulder Flexion
Pulling the bar from mid-abdomen level to the shoulders requires strong-arm flexors and shoulder flexors. The arm flexors are the Biceps brachii, Coracobrachialis, Brachialis, and Brachioradialis muscles. The shoulder flexors are the front Deltoids and Supraspinatus. These muscles rack and secure the bar on the shoulders provided that; the chest thrust and back lordosis are maintained actively and strongly.
- o Inadequate upward pull, by the leg-back-shoulder drives, hinders the efforts of the shoulder and arm flexors to rack and secure the bar on the shoulders. This causes the bar to fall short of the shoulders and slides downwards on the arms, downwards. Assisting exercises of the upper scapular muscles, shoulders, and arms foster the pull strength.
- o Collapsed chest results from imbalanced scapular muscles or lax lower back. This causes the shoulders to drop, with the bar racked on them, with acute kyphosis on the thoracic spines. One-hand dumbbell exercises are of great value in enhancing shoulder thrust by strengthening the Serratus anterior, Pectoralis major and minor, and shoulder rotator cuff muscles.
- o Inflexible ankles, knees, hips, or lower back hinders adequate descent of the torso under the bar. Such delay in vertical drop of the body wastes the upward pull and shifts the burden on the arms and shoulder flexors. Stretching exercises of the legs and back in full flexion are helpful in enhancing deep descent during the Front Squat of the Clean.
- o In the full Squat Clean, the back is thrown into tight lordotic stand while the elbows shoot, and the body drops under the bar. If the back slacks, the lifter will lurch forwards, the elbows may drop on the knees, or the bar will dump ahead.

9.7.1.7. Inadequate Support Of Full Body Flexion
Full body flexion occurs in full squatting and elbow elevation under the bar. Inadequate support in that position results in the elbows touching the knees. This is defaulted in formal Weightlifting contests. It results from many causes, as follows.
- o Fast, uncontrolled descent does not allow the back, chest, and shoulders to activate fast enough to prevent collapse of the elbows on the knees.
- o Insufficient pull, back lordosis, chest thrust, or shoulder flexion prevent upright erection of the torso on the pelvis. Strengthening axial erection of the spines requires many months, or even years, of serious training in order to develop spinal strength and flexibility. The cumulative effects of performing the Clean, the Pull, the Deadlift, the Goodmorning, and the Squat result in greater enhancement of the spinal erection.
- o Weak arm flexors prevent the racking and securing of the bar on the shoulders. Strengthening the arm flexors assist in transferring the axial pull from the torso to the bar and pulling the bar, upwards and inwards on the top of the shoulders.

9.7.2. THE JERK FAULTS, CAUSES AND CORRECTIONS
9.7.2.1. Insufficient Leg Drive
Failure to maximized leg drive results from:
- o Unstable leg stance, such as raising the heels or toes during dipping, diminishes the upward extension of the thigh and hip muscles and generates horizontal shear stresses. This requires paying great attention to feet stance prior to descending for initiating the leg drive.
- o Shallow descent does not allow for adequate Quadriceps and Gluteal power output. Optimum descent is learned by experience since deep descent might also greatly weaken concentric muscular contraction. Since descent is executed by knee and hip flexion plus lower back lordosis, it can be strengthened by regular practice on the Front Jerk and Front Squat. These two exercises engage chest thrusting in the process of descent for leg drive. That is not the case in back Shoulder Jerk or Back Squat.
- o Deviation from vertical descent can result from chest collapse, lower back laxity, inadequate shoulder flexion, or unstable feet stance, during descending for leg drive. Corrective measures include slow controlled descent in order to preserve the coordination of the shoulders, back, and legs on the feet. Also, strengthening the relevant joints by simulating movements is paramount to achieving functional strength.
- o Generation of opposing forces by mistiming body descent and shoulder push. Descent intends to pre-stretch leg, hip, and back muscles and to allow space for aggressive concentric muscular contraction. This should not coincide with activities at the chest, shoulders, or arms, other than tight support of the bar. The shoulders should not attempt to push prior to the initiation and completion of the leg drive.

THE CLEAN & JERK

9.7.2.2. Forward Displacement During Shoulder Push
The anatomic design of the upper limb joints allows them to rotate in order to translate handheld objects into vertical trajectory. The rotation of the upper arms on the shoulder joints forces the bar trajectory to move forwards, rather than upwards. The consequences of this anatomical restraint are as follows.
- o   In order to direct the bar upwards, with respect to the body, the body has to advance forwards and downwards under the bar.
- o   This is helped by the lifter aiming the Shoulder Push backwards and upwards, by the actions of the Deltoids. Logically, beginner Weightlifters perceive shoulder pushing as an upward pushing. Yet, body anatomy does not support vertical-piston lifting, but rather support rotational leverage lifting.
- o   Forward displacement worsens by collapsing chest, dropping elbows, or softening of the lower back. Strengthening training is not a substitute to attentive performance during brief transient motion.

9.7.2.3. Flawed Leg Split
Leg lunges serve lower and advance the body under the bar. Too much drop in the leg split could shift the centers of masses significantly, weaken the leg recovery and support, and extend the distance between the sprung feet. Also, limited drop in the leg split puts more burden on the arms and shoulders on elevating the weight. Corrective measures include strengthening and technique enhancement of the motion. Strengthening of the leg split includes strengthening the shoulder push by heavy half squatting and front Shoulder Jerk heaves. Both exercises combine shoulder, back, and leg strengthening and speed. Also, keep in mind that overtraining and stressed joints lead to flawed leg lunging. This requires rest, volume reduction, stretching exercises, and restoration of normal tone and comfort during joint usage.

9.7.2.4. Backward Displacement Of Bar During Overhead Arm Extension
The balance between Shoulder Pushing, leg lunging, and torso dropping determines the final position of the bar overheads. The synchrony of the three actions is gained by regular and long training. Yet, excessive weight or poor performance contributes to exaggerated backward displacement of the bar, at the end of the arm extension. In that imbalanced and dangerous position, the lifter has to bail out by releasing the weight and escaping, by darting forwards.

9.7.3. GENERAL TIPS ON TECHNIQUE
- o   Maintain solid **foot contact** with the platform during the slow and strong phases of initiating the ballistic motion, as well as during the phases of catching at the end of ballistic motion. Solid feet stance eliminates shaking of joints and suppresses the firing of proprioreceptors during imbalanced states. This permits the major muscles to maximally contract without interruption termination signals from the nervous system
- o   Keep feet slightly wider than hip width. This accommodates the oblique articulation of the femur with the pelvis. In Full Squat, narrow feet stance requires greater unlocking effort on the knees, hips, and lower back. One or two inches increase in the **feet stance**, over hip width, dramatically enhances the control on ascent.
- o   The most determining motion in the Clean is maintaining the bar very **close to the body**. Only when the bar is below the kneecaps, when it has to stay apart from the shins. Over the thighs, the bar almost scrubs the skin as the torso generates momentum. At the groin, instead of moving the bar into the groove between the thighs and the low abdomen, the lifters thrusts his buttocks forwards, thus maintains vertical ascent of the bar. Over the mid-abdomen, the bar once again scrubs the lifter's cloth. At the upper abdomen, the lifter would have elevated the shoulders and arms and, thus, move the chest cage upwards and backwards. Here, the bar moves over the lower costal ribs of the chest. The sliding of the scapulas over the back of the chest cage allows the elbows to move backwards and to maintain the bar close to the body.
- o   The **arms** hang loosely before lifting starts, in order to eliminate any spasticity and to allow for maximum blood perfusion. When lifting starts and until the bar reaches the groin region, the arms assume solid isometric contraction. This does not only serve as good transfer lever, but also prepares the arms for the incoming vigorous flexion. The isometric contraction stimulates the pre-stretch reflex of the arm muscles and amplifies recruitment. The Deltoids will abduct the arms when the bar is pulled from the groin to mid-abdomen. The long head of Triceps, aided by the Latissimus dorsi and other back adductors and extensors, will pull the upper arms when the bar moves from mid-abdomen to mid-chest region. The Biceps brachii, Brachialis, Coracobrachialis, and Brachioradialis pull the forearms when the bar reaches high chest level. Thus, the elbows draw spiral curve, from lateral pointing, backward pointing, to backward-forward flipping, in a quarter or circle curve. This elbow motion is referred to as "screwing the elbows under the bar".
- o   The **overall explosive** lift does not begin and end with explosive contraction. It rather begins with strong contraction of massive amounts of slow twitching muscle fibers of the Quadriceps, Glutei, back Erectors, and Trapezius. This slow and strong phase initiates the most difficult motion of accelerating the barbell and the body. The explosive motion ends by capitalizing on the previous phase and utilizes the speed at the end of the accelerated phase. This ballistic phase of the motion relies mainly on the fast twitching muscle fibers of the major axial muscles. This phase overcomes the weakest link of arm pulling and flexion.

9.8. MANAGING TRAINING LOAD INTENSITY AND VOLUME

o   In order to quantify the intensity of resistance, lifters use either the **percentage** of the maximum weight they can lift or **absolute** poundage, in relation to the maximum poundage they can lift. For example, the expressions 50% 1RM, or 85% 1RM refer to the intensity of resistance, in percentage of the one repetition of maximum lift of that particular exercise. Also, the expressions –50 kg, -20 kg, or –10 kg refer to the absolute weight of the lift, in magnitudes less than the maximum. Thus, if the maximum lift is 100 kg then the previous expressions refer to lifts of 50 kg, 80 kg, and 90 kg, respectively. Training with intensity in the range from 70% to 90% serves the purpose of enhancing strength provided that, longer intervals of recuperation are allowed. Training intensity in the range 50% to 60% enhances muscular mass, provided that; greater number of repetitions is performed.

o   The cumulative effects of training with submaximal lifts represent the **load volume**. The load volume correlates linearly with overall strength and is used as an index for progress in training. The number of exercise groups, sets per group, and repetitions per set, determine the load volume of a particular training session. The load volume of the weekly number of sessions is added to yield weekly load volume. These are added to give monthly load volume, and so on.

o   Weightlifting training proceeds in **cycles** of variation of load volume. Thus, you do not have to lift heavyweights throughout the entire cycle. The cumulative effects of these submaximal lifts, between 70% and 90%, will build strength of tendon, ligament, and muscles, using two to five repetitions per set.

o   **Maximal lifts** are performed periodically, in one out of ten lifts, not every session or week but rather every cycle. The cycle consists of six to twelve weeks, with progressively increasing weekly load volume. The weekly load volume begins at intensity of 70% for eight sets, of three repetitions per set. Incremental weekly, or biweekly, addition of 5% will bring intensity to 90%, by the end of the cycle, where the number of repetitions decreases down to single lifts. The short 6-week cycle are intended for advanced training for preparation to contest and not used throughout the year.

o   The training cycle is repeated with weekly **higher percentage,** on the assumption that the maximum lifts are getting higher too. The cycle load volume increases as the lifter gains strength, cycle after cycle. This concept of defining the load volume as a numerical index in progressing in developing strength is very helpful in documentation, comparison of performance, and assessment of training plan. It also predicts and explains the development of overtraining.

o   The Clean and Jerk lifts are **major strengthening** exercises for the legs, back, and shoulders since these can be executed with heavier weights than the Snatch. The progressive folding and unfolding of the body from Start position, full extension pulling, full squatting Clean, ascending, dipping, to shoulder pushing, all constitute global strengthening of axial and peripheral muscles, tendons, ligaments, and bones.

9.9. HIGHLIGHTS OF CHAPTER NINE

1. If the lifter remains standing, during the Clean lift, with slight dipping by the knees and hips, then the barbell has to travel upwards with strong arm and shoulder pull. This high pull Clean is termed **"Power Clean"**. The Power Clean is a basic upper back strengthening exercise. If the lifter refrains from dipping, continues pulling the barbell to the shoulders without lowering the torso, then the Clean is termed **"Military Clean"**. The Military Clean is a basic strengthening exercise for the arms and shoulders. Deep squatting under the bar after aggressive pulling is called **"Full Squat Clean"**. The Full Squat Clean is a basic exercise for strengthening full body extension and flexion.

2. Before attempting to lift, **exaggerate lordotic back; thrust the chest forwards and upwards**. In the front view, this posture results in closing the gap between the abdomen and thighs and bulging of the upper chest. Throw the shoulders backwards, and straighten the elbows. The elbows will appear separated from the chest with the bulging of the Latissimus dorsi between the sides of the chest and the arms.

3. During the very early motion of the bar, below the kneecaps, the **isometric contraction** is the dominant source of induction of acceleration, with minimal lower body concentric contraction.

4. During lifting from the floor, shoulder abduction alone cannot pull heavy weight from the waist level to the shoulder level. Thus, you have to shift shoulder abduction into shoulder transverse adduction. This means that, in addition to pulling upwards with lateral Deltoid muscles, you should engage the back **Deltoid, Supraspinatus, and upper Trapezius** into pulling the bar backwards, as well as upward.

5. Descending under the barbell, after strong and vigorous upward pulling, is the most **ingenious modification** made in the technique of the Clean lift in the last half century. This modification necessitated developing strong and massive thigh muscles, in order to endure the enormous downward forces of squatting and upward forces of ascending with the barbell. Descending under the bar is an optional choice in contests

6. You can lift the bar as high as you want without squatting, as long as you follow the technical rules of the Clean lift. Descending only serves **enhancing the lifting power** in addition to the momentum generation, the torque generation, and the vertical translation.

7. **The thrusting of the chest** is critical to the support of the lateral tips of the scapulas, by way of elevating the sternum and the medial tips of the Clavicles. The chest is thrust by the combined action of the Serratus anterior (when the scapulas are tightened by the Trapezius and Latissimus dorsi), the Pectoralis minor, and the Sternomastoids. If the chest fails to thrust vigorously under the bar, the lateral tips of the scapulas will drop downwards causing the shoulders to drop and the bar to slide off the shoulders.

8. **The lower back erection** is paramount to stability and ascent with heavy weight from front Squat position. The entire upper body posture depends on the lower back erection. Both strong isometric contraction and concentric contraction are needed in the effort to ascend from deep squatting and farther commence the phase of Jerk.

9. **The strong control over the knees and hips** determines whether the lift would be finalized or not. Many lifters plan to squat under control, instead of dipping deep and fast. Although strong legs are great assets to the recovery from deep and fast squatting, yet upper body strength is also needed to facilitate respiration, heart beating, and arm elevation. Controlled squatting offers the advantage of increased ability to continue the lift, all the way to overhead Jerk.

10. **Fast and deep squatting** protracts ascent with heavy weight and might cause serious stresses, *Figures 9.26, 9.28* and *9.29*. On the other hand, controlled high squatting makes ascending more manageable, *Figure 9.30*. In *Figure 9.29*, you can notice the sinking of the Trapezius behind the bar, whereas the Deltoids and the Biceps brachii bulge under the bar to prevent its fall

11. Although the legs constitute the main drive for the Jerk lift, yet such drive cannot achieve effective lifting power unless **proper timing** is considered in managing the leg drive. If the leg drive is activated while the barbell is descending, *Figure 9.36*, then the downward acceleration will diminish the upward leg drive. Therefore, the leg drive should only be initiated after the descent from full leg extension has completed, *Figure 9.37*. The experience of the lifter plays important role in timing the two actions that of descending versus leg drive.

12. The **shoulder drive** can only be effective if the head clears the way for the bar to ascend, the torso attacks forwards and under the barbell to prevent its fall, and the shoulders push the bar backwards and upwards. If the lifter tries to push the barbell only upwards, he would then create a curved trajectory for the bar. That is because the whole body will be moving forwards to land on the front lunging leg. The lifter has to push the weight close to his face, *Figure 9.41*.

13. **Leg lunging** is a technical choice, rather than a requirement in formal Weightlifting competition. The legal requirement for validation of the Jerk lift is the monotonous and smooth lifting of the barbell without elbow pressing, stationing, or advance and retreat motions. Therefore, the lifter can execute the Jerk lift either by leg lunging or squatting. Lunging the legs involves springing, which displaces the center of masses, whereas squatting while jerking maintains minimal displacement of the center of masses since the feet remain anchored to the ground.

Chapter 10 Endurance versus Strength

10.1. PHYSICAL ENDURANCE & STRENGTH

10.1.1. INHERENCE AND NURTURE

The ability of the biological system of organs to persevere, for minutes and hours, **expending energy** and generating forces, depends on inherent capacity of managing energy resources, as well as on the acquired skills and adaptation to nurturing activities. Inherent traits are expressions of genes that control chemical processes, which, in the end, lead to structural changes and dynamic physical work. Acquired skills modify genetic expression and tweak inherent traits in a manner that allows better adaptation to changing environment.

The **biological system** comprises the structural framework of genetic activities that aim at the unique goal of energy utilization. It provides adequate exchange of gases with the atmosphere, adequate flow of fluids within the body, adequate shuffling of chemical ingredients, from one specific process to the other, and finally orchestrates the global operation of performing external work. The biological system thus requires a **mass of organs** to perform its **metabolic processes,** and a **delivery system** to sustain such processes, in conjunction with a **ventilation system**. The interaction of these four entities (mass, metabolism, delivery, and ventilation) determines the level of endurance and strength of the biological system, *Figure 10.1*.

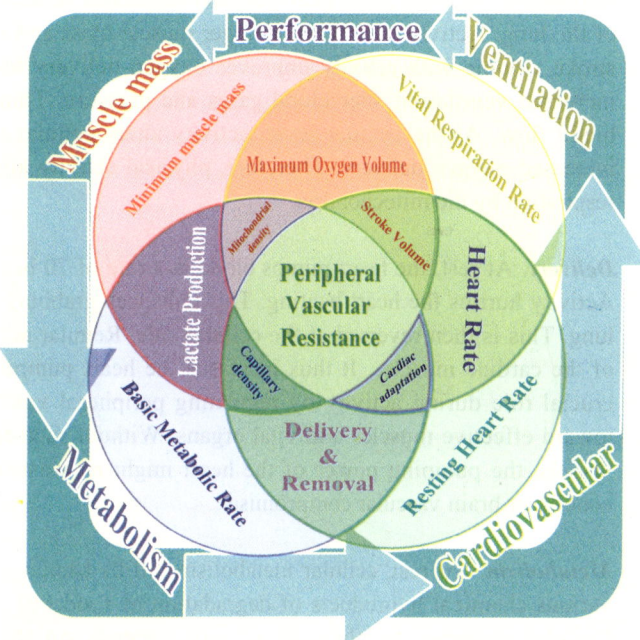

Figure 10.1. Overlapping of biological functions during energy expenditure.

In physical fitness, **endurance** refers to the tempo of the process of energy expenditure. High endurance amounts to slow rate of energy production that lasts for longer duration, until energy resources are depleted. **Strength**, on the other hand, refers to intensity of energy expenditure that proceeds at fast rate, for brief duration. The regulation of energy expenditure is achieved by neural and hormonal control of the biological machinery of power production. Despite the complexity of the interplay of great number of variables involved in energy regulation, few fundamental variables greatly impact the effect of endurance and strength training on our biological system. At least four variables, each relates to one of the four basic entities the biological system, can be clearly studied for enhancement and evaluation of physical performance. The four variables are:

o **Maximum oxygen consumption** accounts for the effect of ventilation on physical performance.
o **Maximum cardiac output** accounts for the role of the delivery system on energy production.
o **Maximum lactate accumulation** represents the role of metabolism in physical work.
o **Mechanical efficiency** accounts for the transfer of chemical energy into mechanical energy, by the muscle mass.

10.1.2. OPTIMIZATION OF ENERGY EXPENDITURE

Optimization of the four basic entities of the biological system amounts to maximizing utilization of energy, which is the ultimate goal of all living organisms. Strength and endurance training modifies the power production capability of the system through **energy regulation**. It modifies genetic expression of **protein synthesis**. Thus, new muscle fibers are generated and new enzymes with higher activities are produced. The growth in the smooth muscle fibers is expressed in thicker heart muscles, new blood capillaries, and more compliant and flexible vascular arterial network. The growth in skeletal muscle mass is expressed in bigger and stronger muscles, heavier bones, and improved recruitment. The growth in the enzymatic capacity is demonstrated by microscopic changes in cellular elements with higher densities of mitochondria and contractile muscle protein.

However, maximum endurance and maximum strength are mutually exclusive, since each tackles the **rate of expending** of one, and only one thing, that is energy. We have to choose our desired combination of strength and endurance. Running for longest distances, for example, precludes us from lifting heaviest weights. Yet, all physical activities have various proportions of endurance and strength. **Low endurance** lowers the threshold for physical and mental fatigue during activity and prolongs recuperation from stressful activities. **Low strength** destabilizes the coherence of the framework of the system and undermines the pumping power of the heart and the respiratory effort of the chest and diaphragm are vary during rest and activity, as follows:

The four basic entities that characterize physical performance are:

o *Ventilation.* At rest, respiratory ventilation proceeds at a tidal rate sufficient to fulfill basic metabolic needs of cellular respiration. Activity alters heart rate and stimulates ventilation in order to catch up with the increasing blood perfusion of the lung. Activity also recruits larger muscle mass and requires higher oxygen consumption. The increased cardiac stroke volume with activity improves oxygen delivery to growing muscular recruitments. In addition, activity and increased ventilation alter blood gases and pressure. Thus, activity affects peripheral vascular resistance to greater blood flow. At the cellular level, activity alters cellular mitochondrial density, which in turn affects utilization of increased oxygen delivery. Therefore, physical activity affects both, mechanical ventilation by the lungs and cellular respiration by the mitochondria.

o *Delivery.* At rest, the heart pumps blood at a rate of 70 beats/min. Each heartbeat delivers 70 ml of blood to the body. Activity hurries the heart beating. This enhances grabbing more oxygen and removing more carbon dioxide from the lung. This is then reversed at the cellular side. Regular activity affects cardiac muscle thickness and capillary density of the cardiac muscle. It thus increases the heart pumping power and stroke volume. Neural central control plays crucial role during activity by regulating peripheral vascular resistance. This neural regulation directs blood flow toward effective muscles and vital organs. Without such regulation, in the form of dilation and constriction of blood vessels, the pumping power of the heart might be wasted in fruitless work that causes heart failure, loss of motor control, or brain vascular compromise.

o *Metabolism.* At rest, cellular metabolism fulfills basic metabolic needs such as heat production and the provision of various chemical byproducts of degradation of foodstuff. Activity increases cellular metabolism and its byproducts. Cellular response to physical activity depends on the mitochondrial population that determines the rate of accumulation of byproducts, and the capillary density that affects the rate of removal and delivery of metabolic needs. The net result of this balance is the fate of lactate accumulation during activity. Lactate affects muscle performance and peripheral vascular resistance, through altering the concentration of protons (hydrogen ions) and acidity in the immediate fluid medium. The interaction between cellular metabolism and cardiovascular system determines the ability of cellular and systemic functions to proceed optimally, for desired levels of endurance and muscular mass. Thus, cellular functions affect the performance of organs, as well as systemic chemical and mechanical functions of the body as a whole.

o *Muscle mass.* At rest, a minimal portion of the muscle mass is recruited to maintain posture, to frequently turn the body in place to avoid ischemia (reduced blood flow), to generate basic heat requirement, and to aid in scaffolding passages of major blood vessels and nerves. Activity increases oxygen consumption and lactate production by muscles. The increased cardiac stroke volume, and capillary and mitochondrial densities, by regular activities, enhance the interrelationship between muscular metabolism, oxygen supply, and byproducts removal. These three adaptive variables regulate the generation of the kinetic energy by means of musculoskeletal arrangement of levers, joints, active elements, and supporting elements. The acquired skill of the individual, in addition to inherent motor and sensory abilities, influence the transformation of energy and the production of intricate physical performance. Skillful performance modifies the neural central control of the peripheral vascular resistance, which allows muscles to exert their most power at lowest cost of energy utilization. Well-train athletes can execute complex motions with great grace and minimum effort, by synchronizing muscular recruitment and circulatory needs, simultaneously and instantaneously. Skill and efficiency are vividly appreciated in some sports, more than in others. In swimming, for example, performance may make the difference between living and drowning. Various strength and endurance activities determine the optimum muscle mass for maximum oxygen consumption.

10.1.3. OPTIMIZATION OF ENERGY EXPENDITURE IN OLYMPIC WEIGHTLIFTERS

To demonstrate the significance of optimum muscle mass for maximum strength, the author presents the data from the Olympic games of Atlanta, 1996, as follows.

o **Relative strength** is defined as the ratio of the maximum lift to the bodyweight of the lifter. Relative strength is inversely and linearly proportional to bodyweight. *Figure 10.2* presents the data of 217 Olympic Weightlifters. The figures shows steady decline in relative strength as bodyweight increases. Optimum bodyweight for male Weightlifters falls within the range of 65 to 75 kg. Up to bodyweight of 80 kg, top Weightlifters can lift 2.8 times their bodyweight, in the Clean and Jerk lift, and 1.8 times their bodyweight, in the Snatch lift. Over 110 kg bodyweight, drastic decline in relative strength is the rule.

o **Absolute strength** can be quantified by the maximal lift in Olympic games. The increase in absolute strength plateaus over bodyweight of 120 kg and is linearly proportional to bodyweight in the region under 75 kg. *Figure 10.3* shows the absolute increase in strength with bodyweight, up to 80 kg bodyweight. Over 120 kg bodyweight, absolute strength plateaus. Maximum lifts are 260 kg in the Clean and Jerk and 215 in the Snatch.

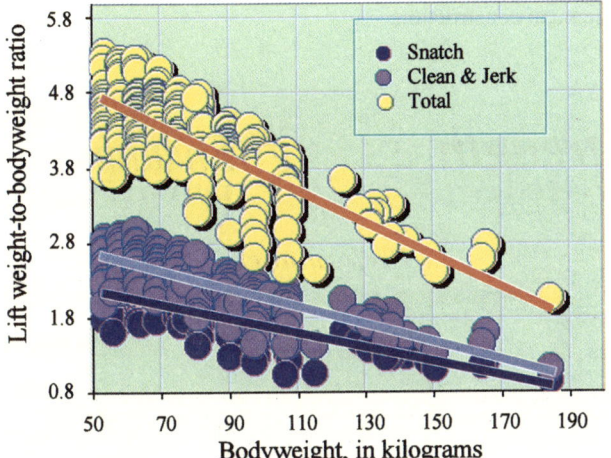

Figure 10.2. Relative strength in Atlanta 1996 Olympic games. Variation of lift-weight to bodyweight ratio with lifter's bodyweight, for 217 Weightlifters.

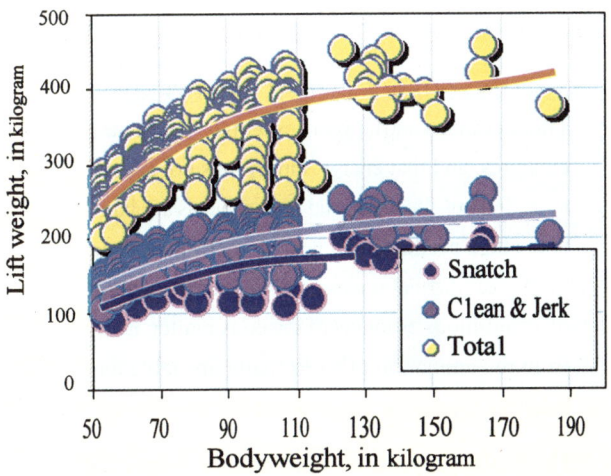

Figure 10.3. Absolute strength in Atlanta 1996 Olympic games. Variation absolute lift-weighs with lifter's bodyweight, for 217 Weightlifters.

o The **specificity** of movement can be deduced from the comparison of the absolute strength in the Clean and Jerk to the Snatch lifts. The difference between the two lifts lies in the function of the shoulders and the cardiovascular work done, during the lifting process. *Figure 10.4* shows that there is a constant ratio of 1.2 between the maximum lifts of the Clean Jerk and that of the Snatch lift, regardless of the bodyweight. Since the Snatch expresses upper body strength while the Clean Jerk represents lower body strength, it seems than Olympic Weightlifters can achieve high body proportion, even when their bodyweight exceeds the norms. This is an apparent accomplishment of strength training.

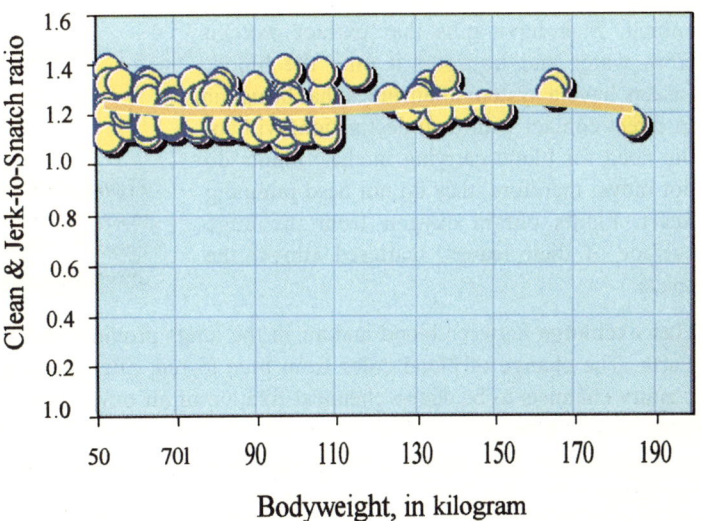

Figure 10.4. Atlanta 1996 Olympic games: Clean & Jerk-to-Snatch ratio for 217 Weightlifters.

o **Aiming for higher optimum**. The ability to raise the optimum level of energy expenditure, such that both endurance and strength exceed the average norms of the general population, is the main impetus for athletic sports. The persistence of athletes to break previous records of strength, speed, distance, height, and coordination, attained by predecessors, attests their faith in better combination of strength and endurance. Many modern Olympic Weightlifters resort to simplicity in training, training longer in interrupted sessions, and pushing the boundaries of flexibility, speed,

10 ENDURANCE VERSUS STRENGTH

endurance, and strength. This determined endeavor can only lead to success when supported by sound scientific basis. Training, rest, and nutrition are the pillars of this endeavor. In addition to professional training planning, Weightlifters emphasize nutritional habits of least amount of food consumption and highest protein building quality. This persistence in advancing human health has proven fruitful in discovering the basic principles for planning sound and effective strength training programs.

10.2. VENTILATION, PERFUSION, AND CIRCULATION

The process of delivering atmospheric oxygen to the cells, for the purpose of energy production, entails many physical and chemical processes. The body provides the structural frame and the regulating system to allow for the physical availability of air into the alveoli of the lungs. From there, the body possesses many chemical means to extract the oxygen from the air and deliver it to the cells. The cells then perform cellular respiration, utilizing intricate physical and chemical processes. The cells utilize physical barriers to compartmentalize various biochemical substrates and reactions. The overall outcome is the production of energy and water. Portion of that energy is converted into kinetic energy for the mobility of the animal. Another portion is utilized for regulating the thermal environment of the animal. A third portion of the energy produced will be stored on chemical compounds for the tasks of basic biochemical construction.

10.2.1. GAS EXCHANGE IN REST AND EXERCISE

o The fact that ventilation is essential for moving creatures, and that energy supply was not created in the form of fluid and solid food alone, is attributed to the **high production** of heat by moving animals. Such great thermal production requires the removal of voluminous amounts of gaseous matter, away from the animal, in order to maintain stable and balanced immediate environment for active living.

o The main purpose of ventilation is capturing **gaseous oxygen** from the air and fixing it onto blood elements that carry it away to remote cells. All animals possess a ventilation system that is regulated by central nervous system, in accordance with the level of activity of the animal. Fish have gills that extract oxygen from water and transport it onto the blood. Insects have a system of air tubes that bring air in direct contact with final destination, without the need for blood carrying media. Plants do not move, therefore, they do not need pumping heart. Plants obtain oxygen from the huge surface of their leaves, scattered allover the space.

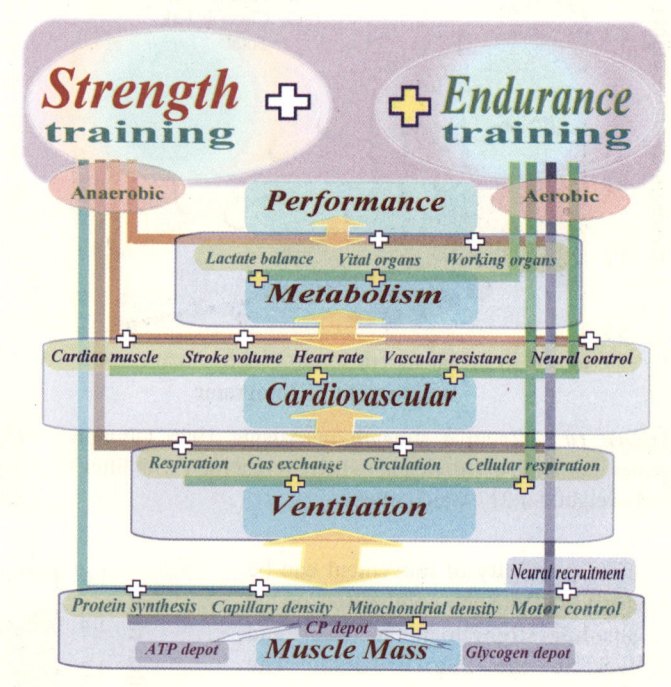

Figure 10.5. Effects of endurance and strength training on muscle mass, metabolism, cardiovascular system, and ventilation.
Pluses "+" signify enhancement, increase, or stimulation. White "+" are effects of strength and yellow "+" for endurance.

o **Gas exchange** between blood and air in the lungs provides the body with vital chemical energy that sustains life on Earth. The change of blood color from blue to red, after passing through the lungs, was proven by the eighteenth-century chemists to be due to chemical fixation of air oxygen by pigments in the red blood cells. These pigments were later called "hemoglobin". The hemoglobin links the oxygen carrying capacity of the blood to the maximal energy expenditure by living human cells. Oxygen saturation of hemoglobin depends on the rate of oxygen and carbon dioxide exchange in the lungs, during ventilation, and rate of blood flow through the lungs, during perfusion.

o Restful lungs receive about 71.4 ml of blood, with each heartbeat of 0.86 seconds duration. This amount of blood perfuses a network of narrow capillaries that line the walls of 300 million alveoli. The blood capillaries have average diameter of 0.3 mm, totaling about 100 square meters of surface area, of air-fluid surface of gas exchange. During exercise, heart rate increases from 70/min to a maximum of 190/min. This fast beating shortens the transit time of blood, in the lungs, from 0.86 sec to as low as 0.31 sec. However, the diminished gas exchange, due shortening of the pulmonary transit, is compensated by the opening of new capillary bed, by means of **sympathetic stimulation**.

o **Cardiac output** increases with activity from 5 liters per minute, during rest, to maximal output of up to 30 liters/min, during vigorous activities. Such increase is attributed to the increase of stroke volume from 70 ml/beat to 158 ml/beat, in addition to the increase in heart rate.

- o **Respiration rate** also increases with exercise, from 12/min up to 60/min. This results in increasing air ventilation from eight liters/min up to 100 liters/min. The combined increase in ventilation and cardiac output increases oxygen uptake in the lungs from 0.31 liters/min up to 5 liters/min. The net increase of oxygen delivery to muscle cell can amount to 500 times that at rest. This is accounted for by increase in blood flow, by six folds and oxygen uptake by fifteen folds. In addition, activity also increases both oxygen extraction by active muscle cells and blood pooling by sympathetic regulation.

10.2.2. MAXIMAL OXYGEN CONSUMPTION OR $VO_{2\,MAX}$

- o Maximum oxygen consumption sets the upper limit for any physical work that can be done by a biological system. That is because physical work utilizes the **combustion energy** of oxygen and hydrogen interaction. Hydrogen originates from the food intake, whereas oxygen is delivered from the atmosphere to the cells.
- o $VO_{2\,max}$ is limited by pulmonary and cardiovascular functions, which orchestrate **delivery** of oxygen from lungs to cells, *Figure 10.5*.
- o Maximum oxygen consumption is directly related to maximum power production by muscles. Adaptations in the trained muscles play significant role in the rate of **oxygen utilization**, during maximal ventilation, yet muscles can consume any amount of oxygen delivered by the cardiovascular system.

10.2.3. MECHANICS OF VENTILATION

Lung ventilation is dependent on the nervous system, musculoskeletal system, and blood chemistry and pressure, as follows.

- o The central nervous system controls the **involuntary** rhythm of the diaphragm, through the phrenic nerve. This originates from the central respiratory center, in the brain stem.
- o The central nervous system also controls the **voluntary** skeletal muscles of the chest cage, through the pyramidal tract. These are the accessory muscles of respiration.
- o Pressure and chemical **sensors** are located in the walls of major blood vessels. These sensors convey signals from the vascular system to the central regulating nervous system, through the vagus nerve. The conditions of pressure sensors and chemical sensors determine the speed and efficiency of firing. This mainly depends on the age of the individual and the conditions of the vascular walls. Cholesterol plaques deposit at the vascular walls in pathological conditions such as atherosclerosis, obesity, and hypercholesterolemia. These deposits deform the pressure and chemical sensors and negatively impact the response of the ventilation, cardiac, and vascular responses to activity, or even during rest.
- o The **nervous regulation** imparts its effect on the motion of the diaphragm, ribs of the chest cage, the blood vessels of the interstitial tissue of the lungs, and the heart. The nervous system regulates the muscular forces that move the diaphragm, upwards and downwards. In the meantime, the nervous system also regulates the forces that support the chest against the piston action of the diaphragm, of suction and compression. During automated restful breathing as well as during violent ventilation, there are different levels of muscular engagement that take place under those different breathing activities. The diaphragm, intercostals muscles (between ribs), abdominal muscles, and chest and shoulder muscles, all play specific roles in assisting ventilation, in rest and activity. In addition to the spontaneous ventilation activity, animals can override the central respiratory command and commandeer respiration, from cessation to hyperventilation, and from shallow to deep and vigorous breathing.
- o **Ventilation during activity.** Resting humans breathe about ten to fourteen times per minute, each breath nets about 500 ml of air. This volume of breathing air is referred to as "tidal volume". Resting ventilatory volume per minute averages six to eight liters of air. Vigorous respiration can increase breathing volume to 2500 ml/breath, and breathing rate to more than 25/min. Thus, vigorous exercise may increase ventilatory volume per minute over 20 times that during rest. The respiratory nervous system controls ventilation by increasing the tidal volume at moderate level of activity, while increasing breathing frequency at vigorous activity. Higher brain functions of volition enable animals to control ventilation regulation to great extent. The balance between the depth and the frequency of ventilation is affected by muscle mass, metabolism, cardiovascular performance, and efficiency of physical work.
- o **Aging and ventilation**. This mainly increases residual lung volume due to loss of elasticity of the supporting and active elements of ventilation. Lungs become less dynamic during activity. No changes occur in gas exchange function, total lung capacity, or tidal volume.

10.2.4. CIRCULATION

- o **Delivery**. Higher animals utilize blood medium to transport oxygen, nutrients, metabolic byproducts, hormones, buffering ions, and heat between the muscles and other cells of different organs. The blood contains 50% to 60% fluid medium, per volume, that carries various kinds of particles and dissolved chemicals, and formed cells.
- o The **formed cells** regulate selective transport of gases, ions, and other byproducts, during their passage through the body filters of lungs, kidneys, liver, and capillary membranes. The cellular walls of the red and white blood cells

provide the biological system an effective mean of selectively transporting ions, whenever and wherever the system deems appropriate.

- **Hemoglobin**. This is a complex organic compound of iron ions and globin protein. Hemoglobin is contained within the red blood cells, at a concentration of 12 to 16 gram hemoglobin per 100 ml of blood. Hemoglobin concentration is lower in women than in men. Hemoglobin is the main blood pigment that carries oxygen molecules on its iron atomic bonds. It strongly binds to oxygen at the lungs and releases oxygen at locations of reduced oxygen saturation, at terminal cells. One-gram of hemoglobin binds to 1.34 ml volume of oxygen, at sea level pressure.[1] The difference in hemoglobin concentration among athletes amounts to difference in oxygen carrying capacity and in utilization of the $VO_{2\,max}$.

- Muscles and other tissues are affected by the rate of delivered nutrients and fuel, and removal of byproducts. Thus, overall performance is heavily affected by the concentration of oxygenated hemoglobin in blood. Diseases that affect the ability of hemoglobin to carry and release oxygen hinder physical performance. These diseases are caused by defects in the wall of the red blood cells, defects in the synthesis of hemoglobin, inadequate synthesis of hemoglobin, or toxic activities. Cigarette smoking and monoxide poisoning are examples of toxic effects of inhaled substances. Both diminish the ability of hemoglobin to carry adequate oxygen to the cells. Iron deficiency anemia is an example of nutritional deficiencies that cause reduced synthesis of hemoglobin. Pernicious anemia that is caused by nutritional deficiency occurs in strict vegetarians, due to the defective synthesis of red blood cells caused by deficient vitamin B_{12}. Preventing anemias caused by poor nutrition is an area where improvement can be made in strength and endurance training.

- **Partial arterial saturation**. Vigorous exercise reduces the transit time of gas exchange in the lungs. This affects oxygen diffusion more than carbon dioxide diffusion, which is more readily capable of diffusing than oxygen. Decline in the percentage of oxygen loaded on hemoglobin results from that short transit time and poor opening of dormant circuits of pulmonary capillaries, despite higher cardiac output and $VO_{2\,max}$. The role of sympathetic activity, in regulating increases in pulmonary capillary bed, explains the paramount importance of rest, training, and nutrition.

- Adequate **rest** enables the nervous system to suppress hyperactivity that dominates fatigued and restless individuals. In addition, **nutrition** provides the nervous system the essential nutrients for the ongoing complex activities of the nervous system. **Training** enhances the muscular, nervous, and skeletal elements of the biological system, by means of enhancing cellular cycling of substrates for energy production. Such cellular cycling provides the metabolic pool with sufficient amounts and varieties of byproducts for synthesis and regeneration of cellular components.

10.2.5. METABOLISM

- **Fueling.** As muscles perform physical work, they burn fuel and produce byproducts. The fuel utilization process operates on two levels, anaerobic and aerobic. Anaerobic fuel burning occurs in the cytoplasm of cells. This is a fast, yet inefficient mean of energy production. Anaerobic burning produces lactates, which are end products of glucose breakdown. Lactates are of no farther use to the muscles and must exit to the circulation, for processing in other locations. Aerobic fuel burning occurs in the mitochondrial apparatus of the cells. This is slow, but efficient mean of energy production. It produces plenty of useful byproducts for synthesis of many sorts of biological compounds.

- After long periods of training of months or years, the body adapt to the production of byproducts by building up new cellular oxidation factories. These are mitochondrial granules in the cytoplasm of cells. Mitochondria oxygenate the metabolic byproducts of carbohydrates, fats, and protein, in order to produce energy. The trained person can tolerate much greater production of lactates than the untrained. Training increases the expression of Nitric Oxide Synthase (NOSase) enzyme, which fosters release of the gas that dilates blood capillaries. A high lactate threshold is due to adaptive improvement of the muscle's ability to generate energy by anaerobic oxidation, yet maintain adequate aerobic process.

- Untrained folks do not have adequate mitochondrial density, stored muscle glycogen, or adequate NOSase and, therefore, have limited anaerobic generation of energy. They tire quickly and cannot generate greater muscular power. As physical work persists, the trained person develops greater ability to mobilize fat depot and pumps fatty acids to working muscles. These are utilized in aerobic endurance physical work. The glycerol portion of the mobilized fat is converted by the liver, kidney, and intestine into glucose that is consumed in energy production.

- **Efficiency of burning.** The chemical energy utilized by biological systems originates from food and air intake. The biological factory of hormones, enzymes, and catalysts conducts all chemical reaction that transforms chemical energy into kinetic energy. This requires expansion in the volume of matter, in order to create **displacement in space**. Thus, heat energy must be produced in order to generate muscular contraction, and hence kinetic energy. Like most efficient engines, biological systems run at an efficiency of about 40%. Thus, 40% of the ATP energy can be transformed into kinetic energy. The remaining 60% of chemical energy goes for heat production.

- **Inherent efficiency in fiber type.** Muscle fibers fall into two distinct types, in regard to their rate of expending

---

[1] "Review of physiological chemistry" 15th edition, by Harold A. Harper, Lange Medical Publications, Los Altos, Ca (1975) page 221.

energy, size of motor unit, and threshold of firing. Smaller motor units are recruited first, with successively larger units firing at increasing muscle tension levels. Slow twitch units are called "Type-I" fibers. These tend to be smaller and produce less overall force than the intermediate and fast twitch units. These are called "Type-IIA" and "Type-IIB", respectively. The difference in the speed of contraction between Type-I units and Type-II units may be attributed to different degrees of enzymatic activity of myosin ATPase. This enzyme regulates muscular contraction by the Actin-Myosin complex. In addition, the slow twitch fibers have a very poorly developed sarcoplasmic reticulum, when compared to fast twitch fibers, and can, if stimulated, quickly release calcium to trigger contraction. The fast twitch fibers also possess Troponin with higher affinity for calcium and, therefore, can contract more vigorously. The two muscle fiber types also differ in their capillary, mitochondrial, and glycogen densities. Thus, their ability to extract oxygen, and get rid of byproducts is also different.

10.2.6. PERFORMANCE

o **Physical work**. Performing effective physical work requires learned skills. These are gained by training on utilizing the biological system in producing power at optimum ventilation and cardiac output, while maintaining below threshold level of blood lactate. Producing powerful muscular forces, with proper technique of execution, minimizes wasted energy. Unskilled technique dissipates energy in the form of heat strain of musculoskeletal system and over stressing of pulmonary and cardiovascular systems. The role of training skill is apparent in the neuromuscular coordination and the autonomic regulation of cardiovascular system.

o **Physical adaptation**. Regular training for many years will undoubtedly alter anatomical structure of an individual, as long as training is maintained. Bones, muscles, ligaments, and tendons adapt to specialized training in a pattern that affects the outlook of the athlete and imposes distinctive feature on his or her appearance. Physiological adaptation to training is prominent as well. Trained athletes attain higher technical perfection that enables them to break down technical execution of motion into simple distinctive tasks, without burdening the brain with distracting details. In addition, advanced training increases the body's ability to utilize maximal ventilation better than untrained persons do. The latter usually fails to attain maximal oxygen consumption when performing hard work. A reliable index of endurance is the product (VO2 max x lactate threshold) that can be attained during peak endurance performance.

o **Biological limitation on performance**. Aside from the development of muscle cells, in response to strength and endurance training, there is upper ceiling to peak performance, imposed by biological limitation. The muscles of the heart and the diaphragm expend more energy at peak performance. If muscular development exceeds that of the heart and the respiratory muscles, then the former will steal most energy expenditure from the latter, resulting in cardiopulmonary incompliance. Though the diaphragm has a high density of Type-I fibers, a high capillary density, and high concentration of oxidative enzymes, compared to skeletal muscles, its adaptation to training cannot result in massive hypertrophy. Such hypothetical state could impede endurance work by the relative diminishing of mitochondria density, with respect to the density of contractile fibers, of hypothetically hypertrophied diaphragm.

o Engaging **accessory respiratory muscles** during high intensity training is limited with the ability of skeletal muscles to endure protracted powerful work. Thus, breathing becomes more demanding at high ventilation rates and training intensities, due to fatigue of respiratory and cardiac muscles. Strengthening accessory muscles of respiration and enhancing their endurance is an area where training can make difference in enhancing performance. Learning to pace your breathing rhythm with technical movement, during training, minimizes steal of energy expenditure from cardiac and respiratory muscles. Long training leads to adaptation of the neural centers of regulation of respiration, circulation, arousal, and motor control, and facilitates the automation of the performance process.

10.3. RUNNING FOR ENDURANCE AND STRENGTH

10.3.1. BURNING FUEL DURING ACTIVITY

o **Whole body performance**. Running constitutes the basic sort of aerobic activity that lubricates the engine of life. The simplicity, accessibility, and effectiveness of running, on controlling energy expenditure, make running a common remedy for many maladies. This is attributed to the process of moving large muscle mass, consuming large volumes of oxygen, and imposing heavy demands on the heart capacity. The whole body performance, during running, makes the analysis of running style very informative about the cumulative effects of living activities on the physiology and anatomy of the runner.

o **Energy flow**. Running requires constant energy expenditure by the entire body. It draws its hydrogen energy from the stored body depots and its oxygen from breathing. The efficiency of burning is under the mercy of cellular ingenuity to prepare proper ingredients of burning and introduce them into harmonious and meticulous chemical reactions. The early eighteenth century belief that lungs are the only oxidation sites in the body was discarded by observing that plants and microorganisms perform biological oxidation without lungs.

o All conventional burning involves oxygen and hydrogen. Additionally, all produce carbon dioxide and water plus thermal energy. In its primitive nature, thermal energy amounts for change in volume of mater and, therefore, a significant portion of thermal energy is converted into kinetic energy. That is **motion**. The change of volume of hot water in steam trains drives its wheels. The change in volume of burning gasoline in automobile engines drives its wheels. The change in volume in muscle proteins by energy expenditure causes its fibrous protein to slide and generate muscular force. Thus, heat is the essence of motion of macroscopic objects. Since heat results from the motion of electrons, therefore, one can conclude that there is no macroscopic motion without heat and there is no heat without microscopic motion.

- **Force flow.** Energy knows no direction, but a quantity that increases or decreases in amount, depending on expending or depositing processes, such as activity and food intake, respectively. Unlike energy, forces act in specific directions, though it is generated by energy. The direction of force is produced by the material object that expends energy. Muscles convert chemical energy to kinetic energy and determine the magnitude and direction of forces. Musculoskeletal leverage provides such directions to muscular forces. Muscles act on bones through tendons. Ligaments bind joints to maintain cohesion of body parts under the actions of forces. In addition, cartilages dissipate friction losses to prevent excessive local heat destruction by moving parts. Running reveals the harmonious nature of such flow of forces and shed light on performance of many structures in the body.

10.3.2. DYNAMIC FORCES IN RUNNING
Running involves three main dynamic forces, as follows.
- **Pelvic torque.** This is generated mainly by the Iliopsoas contraction of the advancing leg and the Glutei contraction of the retreating rear leg. The contraction of the hip flexor and the hip extensor, of alternative legs, generates a torque of two, off-line, equal, but opposite forces. That couple twists the pelvis in the horizontal plane, lunges the two legs in opposite directions, and displaces the center of gravity. The effort to compensate for the vertical drop of the body, while producing pelvic torque, equals the potential energy stored in bodyweight that is displaced vertically. That is source of energy expenditure during running, since a person with lighter weight carries lower potential energy than those with heavier weight.
- **Shoulder torque.** This maintains body balance by turning the shoulders in a direction opposite to the forward thrust couple of the pelvis. The back erectors, abdominal muscles, and scapular muscles generate this second dynamic force of running. This is produced by twisting the vertebral column, retracting one scapula, and detracting the other scapula. The shoulder, on the side opposite to the advancing leg, advances forwards, while the other shoulder moves backwards. If the torso is strong, the two couples (torques) work on the spinal ligaments by stretching and relaxing them. If the torso is weak, the two couples induce a lot of disturbance in the disc capsules, along the vertebral column, and might weaken their support.
- **Pelvic stabilization.** As the legs spread during the forward thrust, the body center displaces vertically. The runner compensates for the vertical displacement by changing the angles of the hip, knee, and ankle to maintain minimal vertical displacement, in order to avoid bumpy running. Stabilizing the pelvis on the hips is achieved by the abductors, rotators, and extensors of the hip joints. That elevates the pelvis on the supported leg, while the other leg departs the ground.
- Analyzing the three dynamic elements among runners reveals a lot of information about the requirements of modifying his or her strength training plan in order to remedy accumulated body flaws. The groups of muscles that generate various dynamic forces of running produce endless postural curves, and lines of inclination, that all points out to lax ligaments, deformed bones, and imbalanced muscles. The following are examples of individual variation in running and their deduced causative maladies.

10.3.3. MUSCLE MASS AND DISPROPORTION IN RUNNERS
- **Heavily built runner**. In *Figure 10.6*, a well-built and heavy runner concentrates mostly on stabilizing his pelvis by reducing torso inclination and twisting, plus reducing arm swinging. The heavily built runner can hardly flex or extend his hips, yet can flex his unsupported knees, while the entire body performs minimal mobility. This cautious act prevents the strong forces of momentum and contraction of bulky musculature from injuring his back, while running. Optimum body proportions enable this runner to maintain near upright posture with erect lower back. His confidence in the strength of various joints permits him to flex his knees beyond 90 degrees and land vigorously on the other leg with maintained upright posture. This runner could benefit greatly from weight reduction and full range of motion stretching of major joints.
- **Slim and tall runner.** In *Figure 10.7*, a slim and tall runner has no difficulty swinging arms and legs. His balanced body proportions enable him to maintain perfect body posture without hunching upper back or leaning forwards. The weaker lower body of this tall runner, despite optimum bodyweight, makes him avoids exaggerated bending of his knees. He takes advantage of his strong upper body to maintain perfect torso posture. The limited bending of his knees may enable him to endure longer running, but would stiffen his ligaments in that narrow range of motion. This runner could benefit greatly from regular and long strengthening of the lower body and back erectors. Progressive incremental resistance training, for these chronic cases of muscular disproportion, has to proceed at slow rate, of many months or years. The slow rate of training enables the bony development to catch up with soft tissue hypertrophy.

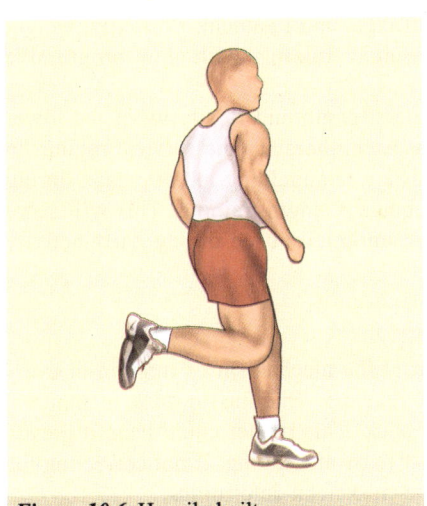
Figure 10.6. Heavily built runner.

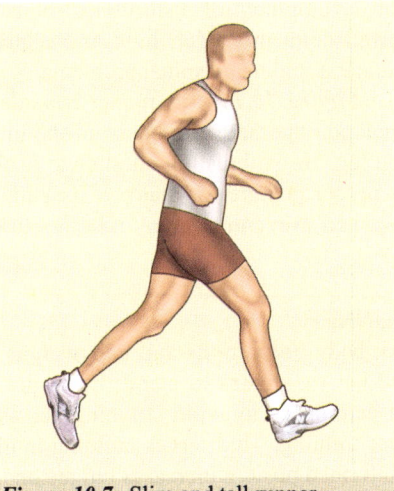
Figure 10.7. Slim and tall runner.

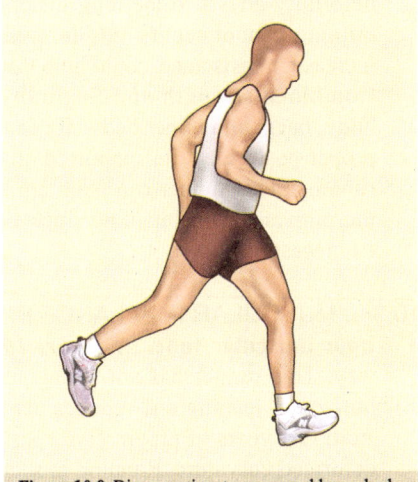
Figure 10.8. Disproportionate upper and lower body.

o **Disproportionate upper and lower body.** In *Figure 10.8*, a runner with weak upper body and heavy lower body leans forwards to displace his center of gravity further ahead, in order to drag his heavy lower body. His weight interferes with his flexibility to freely bend his knees. This runner could benefit greatly from persistent upper body training at slow rate. Developing upper body strength is much easier than developing strong legs and back. That is because the lower body requires much heavier weight to develop muscular mass and bone strength.

10.3.4. MUSCLE MASS AND FLEXIBILITY ISSUES IN RUNNERS

o **Extensive weight training and heavy bodyweight.** In *Figure 10.9*, a runner with noticeable extensive weight training has difficulty reaching normal range of motion at the shoulders, vertebras, and pelvis. His weight training gives him the advantage of maintaining perfect alignment of axial joints, yet deprives him from adequate range of motion. Improving range of motion of strong physiques requires special weight training since stretching without weight will not overcome the strength of strong and short ligaments, unless stretching is very well planned by experienced coach.

o **Extensive weight training and proper bodyweight.** In *Figure 10.10*, a weight-trained runner achieves better range of motion than previous runner and is able to swing limbs and torso more easily. The combination of proper weight training and light bodyweight enables the person to run with less fear of straining joints or spines.

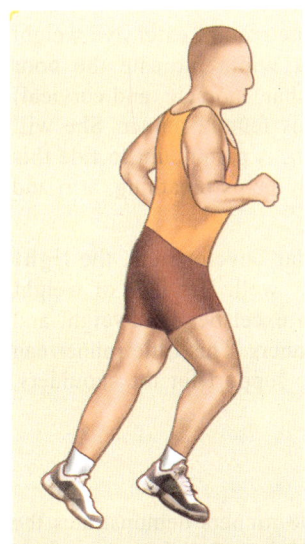
Figure 10.9. Extensive weight training and heavy bodyweight.

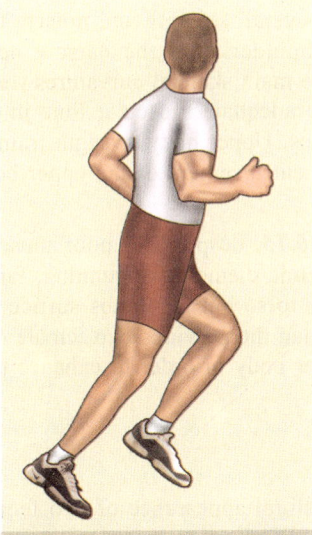
Figure 10.10. Extensive weight training and optimum bodyweight.

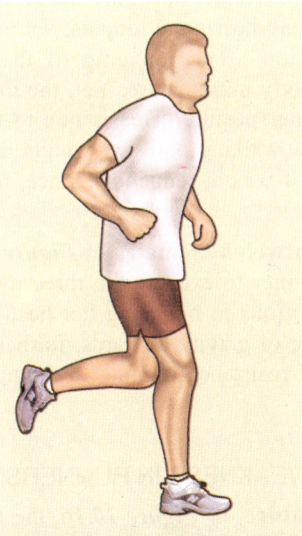
Figure 10.11. Lower back deformity.

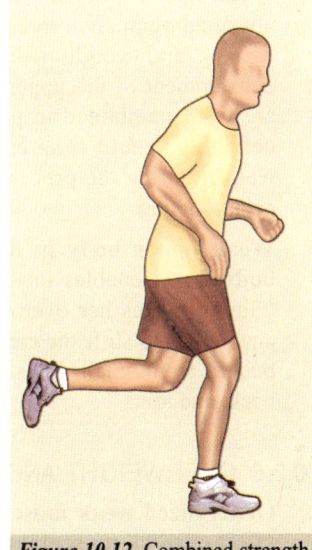
Figure 10.12. Combined strength and flexibility.

o **Lower back deformity.** In *Figure 10.11*, a runner with lower back deformity is maintaining his back in rigid convex posture, evident from the retreat of the abdomen and the backward curvature of the back. Weight training of the lower back and pelvis, from early years of life, would have prevented the **convexity of the lower back** during running. The imbalance between hip flexors (Iliopsoas) and back erectors (spinal erectors, Hamstrings, Glutei) caused this runner to freeze his pelvis and rely on knees and shoulder to balance his gait. The demonstration of such advanced lower back

10 ENDURANCE VERSUS STRENGTH

deformity attests to the long history of development of distortion of bone, cartilage, and ligament. Presently, weight training cannot rectify this long-incurred deformity. Yet, light and regular weight training, with slow progressive increase in resistance, could help this runner avoid many spinal problems.

o **Combined strength and flexibility.** In *Figure 10.12,* this runner has adequate strength and flexibility in the lower body, back, and upper body. He can maintain the three curvatures of the lumbar back, thoracic, and cervical regions in proper posture, while supported on one leg. He is thrusting chest cage forwards and maintaining lordotic back during running. This runner can maintain his proper posture for many years with adequate strength training. This will serve the purpose of maintaining thick bones and preventing many muscles that are minimally used during daily activity from wasting away.

10.3.5. MUSCULAR IMBALANCE IN RUNNER

o **Poor muscular tone.** In *Figure 10.13*, body proportions and bodyweight impact the mechanism of running in every way. This runner has not strengthened her **extensors** to stand the slightest bouncing. She has to stick to minimal horizontal leaning and reduces her forward thrust to avoid straining her weak back. This runner could benefit greatly from few years of progressive resistance training. That serves building muscular mass and toning, if not correcting the deformed curvature. Running in such deformed posture increases fatigue and worsen skeletal deformities.

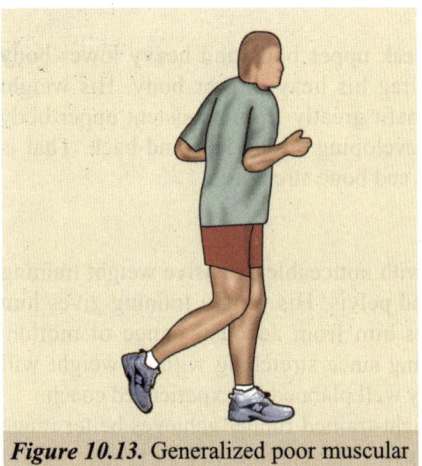
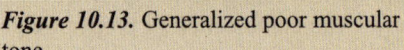
Figure 10.13. Generalized poor muscular tone.

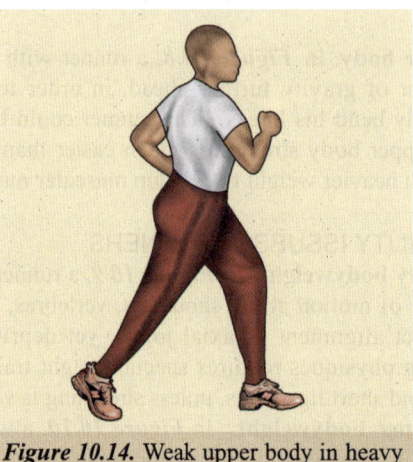
Figure 10.14. Weak upper body in heavy female.

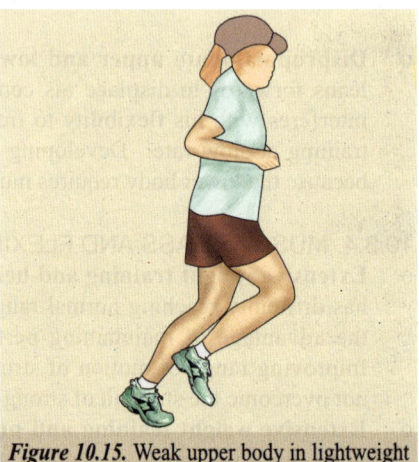
Figure 10.15. Weak upper body in lightweight female.

o **Weak upper body in heavy female.** In *Figure 10.14*, an untrained female has much stronger lower body. She does not mind aggressive thrust and horizontal torques, yet her overall strength and **muscle tone** require extensive weight training and weight reduction. The rounding of the shoulders and the narrow neck width indicate the poor development of the upper body musculature. Yet, the three main skeletal curvatures (lumbar, thoracic, and cervical) are well maintained in proper posture. This is due to the adequate muscular tone in this female runner. She will definitely benefit from brisk walking until her weight drops. Upper body strength training is paramount to tide this woman during the process of weight reduction. Since, the enhancement of the upper body helps breathing, arm and neck function.

o **Weak upper body in lightweight female.** In *Figure 10.15*, despite her poor muscular development, the **light bodyweight** enables this runner to execute the three dynamic elements of running, fairly well. Her lack of weight training makes her over cautious in bouncing her head or torso but her limbs suffice to excel her lightweight and enable her to shift the center of gravity forwards, further than the previous two female runners. This little runner can benefit from small doses of resistance training to the upper body in order to enhance the support for the shoulders, neck, and arms.

10.3.6. OVERWEIGHT AND WEAKNESS IN RUNNERS

o **Generalized weak musculature.** In *Figure 10.16,* the postural appearance of two female runners demonstrates the effect of **weak musculature** on the mechanism of running. Weak spinal muscles prevented these female runners from aggressive thrusting using pelvic muscles. They have to avoid aggressive thrust to reduce hyperextending their weak back. They also have to avoid shoulder twisting since the scapular muscles are not well strengthened for such twisting. Finally, they have to drag their legs closer to the ground to reduce vertical displacement that requires overall torque of major joints in the body. Strength training would have remedied many of their limitations in addition to helping in weight reduction. Axial training in particular would enhance spinal strengthening, within few weeks, and starts a chain reaction of progressive development in tone, cardiovascular, and pulmonary functions.

o **Pelvic stabilization in heavyweight and lightweight females.** *Figure 10.17* demonstrates **pelvic stabilization** in overweight and normal weight runners. The overweight runner has difficulty preventing the pelvic drop on the supported leg. The rear leg is dragged and laterally rotating (deviated foot) due to the lax adductors of the hips. The other lightweight female performs perfect pelvis stabilization with very graceful leg motion. Strength training would enhance the musculature around the major joints and prevent such laxity during running. The heavy female, in this figure, may incur serious injuries to the ankles, knees, and hips due to the low tone and weakness of the supporting muscles.

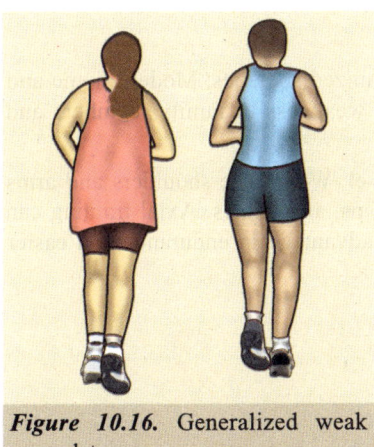
Figure 10.16. Generalized weak musculature.

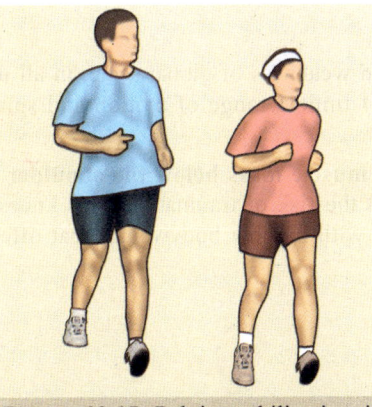
Figure 10.17. Pelvic stabilization in heavyweight and lightweight females.

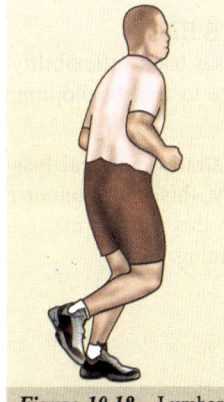
Figure 10.18. Lumbar weakness in overweight male.

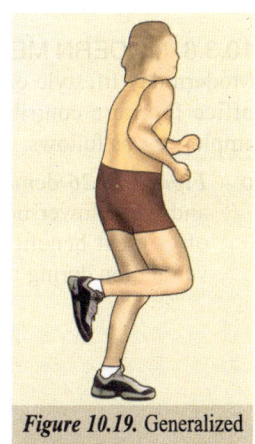
Figure 10.19. Generalized skeletal deformities.

o **Lumbar weakness in overweight male.** *Figure 10.18* demonstrates the effect of **overweight, weakness, and imbalance** due to lack of strength training. This heavy runner does not have the strength to spring legs, swing shoulders, or assume proper running curvatures. This runner can benefit greatly from axial training in order to enhance the lumbar lordosis. His heavyweight and height could cause serious trauma to the knees and lumbar spines. Only regular and long training can benefit these cases of long neglect and overweight.

o **Generalized skeletal deformities**. *Figure 10.19* demonstrates the effect of **weakness and imbalance** due to skeletal deformities and lack of strength training. This runner demonstrates apparent lumbar, thoracic, and cervical loss or proper curvatures. Her running posture is completely counterproductive. This runner may benefit from long and regular planning of strength training in order to halt the progression of farther caving of the chest, lower back, and neck spines.

10.3.7. LUMBAR DEFORMITIES IN RUNNERS

The very common problem of neglecting strengthening the back extensors is very florid in the following six runners, in the form of weak back muscles.

o In *Figures 10.20* and *10.21*, the long-term neglect of strength training caused these runners to **waste scapular muscles**, shoulders, and arms. Their strong lower body is laboring to thrust a crumbled upper body and a weak vertebral axis. Note the close age range, similar muscular pattern, and opposite sex.

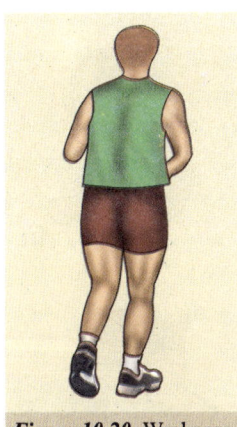
Figure 10.20. Weakness of lumbar and scapular muscles in female.

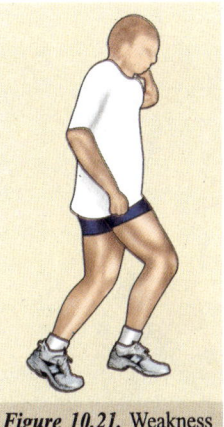
Figure 10.21. Weakness of lumbar and scapular muscles in male.

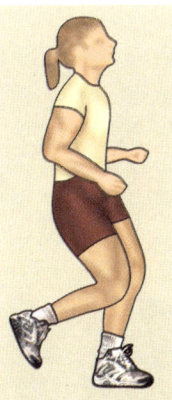
Figure 10.22. Advanced lower back deformity in female.

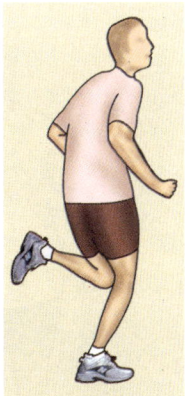
Figure 10.23. Advanced lower back deformity in male.

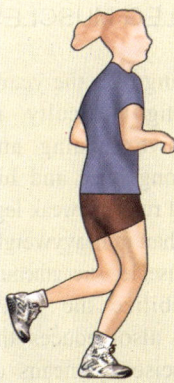
Figure 10.24. Limited range of motion and inflexibility in female.

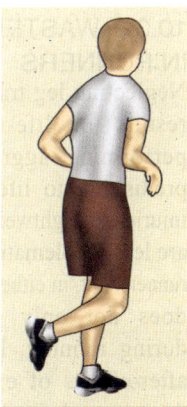
Figure 10.25. Limited range of motion and inflexibility in male.

o *Figures 10.22* and *10.23* demonstrate two runners with **advanced lower back deformity** and upper body weakness. Running exacerbates lower back instability. They should have planned lengthy and extensive training exercises in

order to be able to maintain proper lower back erection while running. Note also the close age range, similar muscular pattern, and opposite sex.
- o *Figures 10.24* and *10.25* show two runners with noticeable **limited range of motion and inflexibility** despite proper body proportion. Strength training helps vitalize muscles and prevents ligaments from freezing at short and limited range of motion. Note also the close age range, similar muscular pattern, and opposite sex.

10.3.8. MODERN MEN'S BACK

Modern day lifestyle causes back inflexibility and weakness of global scale, in all urbanized societies. Modern home and office furniture contribute to the development of limited range of motion and spinal weakness in family members and employees, as follows.

- o *Figure 10.26* demonstrates classical **loss of muscle mass below the shoulder level**. With large shoulders and arms and weak lower body, this male runner runs the risk of traumatizing his knees, hips, and ankles. Axial training can offer great benefit to this runner, especially with his low bodyweight that offers advantage in endurance and easier ventilation during training.

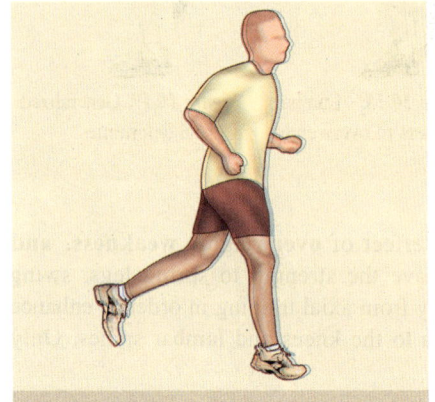
Figure 10.26. Poor muscular development of the lower body.

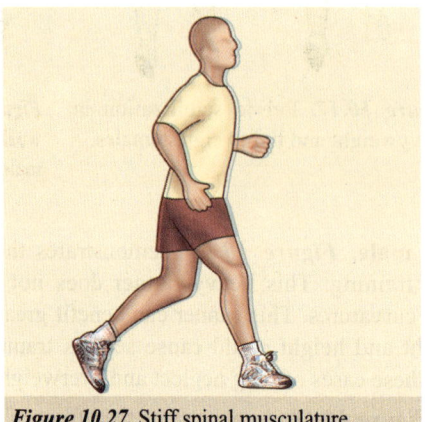
Figure 10.27. Stiff spinal musculature.

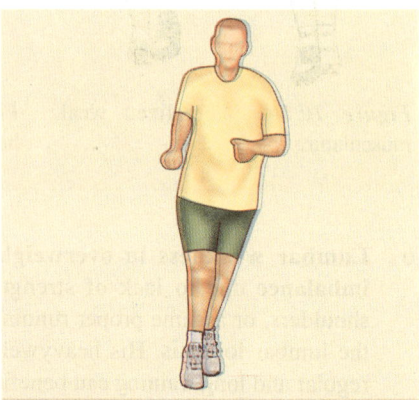
Figure 10.28. Imbalanced scapular musculature.

- o *Figure 10.27*, a runner exhibits a stiff vertebral column preventing leaning forwards. Although maintaining an upright erect back is a desired trend in running, keeping **stiffened back** is not. Proper ventilation requires elastic chest cage and torso, in order to reach maximum oxygen consumption. This runner benefit greatly from stretching strength training to enhance the range of motion of scapular, spinal, and pelvic joints.
- o In *Figure 10.28*, in contrast to the previous two runners (note their dropped shoulders in relation to the lower ear lobes), this runner overcomes his weak upper body by shrugging his shoulders, in order to be able to twist the torso, to counteract the twist at the pelvis, and keep the head properly leading his front foot. **Shoulder shrugging** stems from imbalanced scapular muscles. Axial strength training can offer these three runners the greatest benefits that far exceed those from peripheral exercises. Few sets of Clean, Snatch, Pulls, Deadlift, and Squat, scattered over the week, can show good results in few months.

10.3.9. WASTED LEG MUSCLES IN RUNNERS

Neglecting leg training over the years, results in life long difficulty in performing aggressive running and predispose to life long knee and hip injuries. In lightweight runners, weak legs are less problematic than in heavyweight runners. Yet, in either case, leg strengthening does not only stabilize the joints during running, but also reduces the after-effects of exercise by means of the enhanced circulation around the knees and hips. After running, well-trained and strengthened legs, allow the person to resume normal life activities and sleep comfortably with little annoying ischemic pain, unless organic injury exits The following examples support this argument.

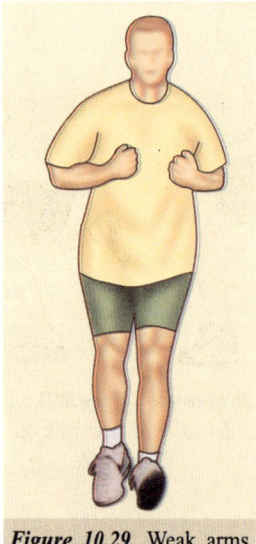
Figure 10.29. Weak arms and legs.

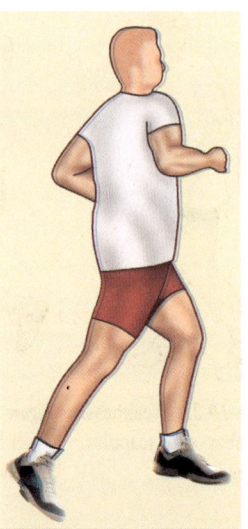
Figure 10.30. Stiff and disproportionate body.

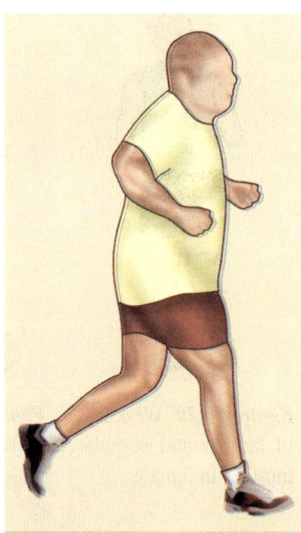
Figure 10.31. Truncal obesity and leg wasting.

o *Figure 10.29.* shows a tall and heavy lifter running on skinny legs, as compared to the waist size. The weak arms and legs force him to bend his elbows in excess, and maintain narrow span between his feet. Though running enhances the cardiovascular performance of this runner, he can be helped by axial training with progressive increase in resistance.

o *Figure 10.30.* shows a heavy runner with well-built arms and shoulders, yet his entire **body is too stiff** to run properly. His legs are too stiff to bend and his lower back is too stiff to assume extension. The apparent wasting of this runner's gluteal muscles makes him throw his bodyweight on the supported leg and drop his rear foot to the ground. The runner advances forwards with great lateral bouncing, from side to side, due to the weak pelvic support. This runner could benefit greatly from planning a lengthy weight-training program that targets the pelvic muscles. The Goodmorning, Deadlift, Pulls, and Sit-ups are examples of exercises that can help stabilize the pelvic girdle.

o *Figure 10.31* shows a runner with weak legs and arms plus **heavy weight around the waist**. Neither are his legs bending properly, nor is his back capable of extending. This runner is subjected to high risk of back and knee injuries more than any other runner, shown above, is. The heavy weight causes the knee surfaces to rub haphazardly against each other, causing meniscus and cartilage injuries. The big waist size predispose to spinal injuries. Running is more traumatic to this individual than mere walking or weight training. His best bid is regular aerobic training and toning weight training until his waist size is reduced. This must proceed along with dietary discipline to reduce weight. The three runners would benefit from lower body training, over many months to years, in order to revitalize the wasted musculature.

10.3.10. MUSCULOSKELETAL STIFFNESS
Maintaining proper bodyweight by regular aerobic exercises, such as running, is not a substitute for strength training. Strength training enhances individual muscles and muscle groups thus prevents sneaky and hidden flaws from insidiously growing out of proportion. The following six figures demonstrate the progression of musculoskeletal stiffness in runners with optimal bodyweights

o *Figures 10.32* and *10.33* show light bodyweight runners with **stiffened back extensors** and shoulders that interfere with the ability of torso to generate upper body torque. Both runners compensate by exaggerating leaning to the side or the front. The slightest of strength training offers these runners much better control on the pelvis, spines, and shoulders.

o *Figure 10.34* presents a light weight runner with **stiffened pelvis and lower back** that forces him rely more on his knees and elbows rather than relying on shoulder and pelvis. The shortening of the flexor muscles of this runner imposes this generalized semi-flexed posture. The weakness of the extensor muscles precludes antagonistic balancing of the shortened flexors.

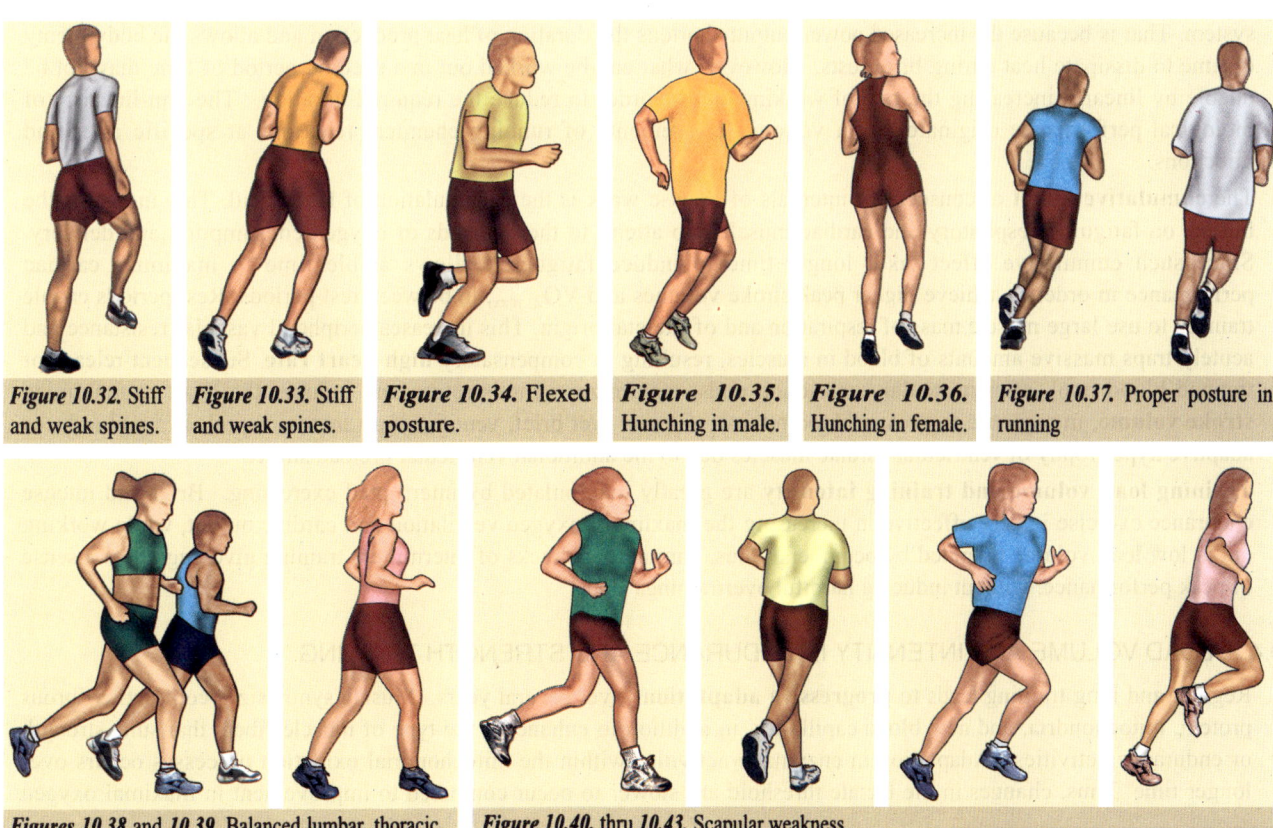

Figure 10.32. Stiff and weak spines.
Figure 10.33. Stiff and weak spines.
Figure 10.34. Flexed posture.
Figure 10.35. Hunching in male.
Figure 10.36. Hunching in female.
Figure 10.37. Proper posture in running

Figures 10.38 and *10.39.* Balanced lumbar, thoracic, and cervical curvatures.
Figure 10.40. thru *10.43.* Scapular weakness.

- *Figures 10.35* and *10.36* present two runners with **hunched upper back** that forces the head to displace forwards during running, shifting the center of gravity forwards. Weight training beside running offers theses runners the advantage of balance and flexibility, in addition to their proper bodyweight. Of course, weight training does not rectify bony deformities, yet it improves the muscular conditions and enables the individual to control his or her posture to greater extent.
- *Figure 10.37* presents a couple who managed to maintain **graceful posture** and are able to keep their entire body symmetrically balanced around straight line, with proper curvatures at the neck, chest, and lumbar regions.

10.3.11. EFFECT OF REGULAR AND BALANCED ACTIVITIES ON RUNNING

Regular and balanced activities help maintain proper body proportions in these five young female runners and demonstrate the value of flexibility, proper body weight, and strength on the mechanism of running.
- *Figures 10.38* and *10.39* show **well built and trained** female runners. Their proper shoulder training enables them to rotate the shoulders and relax the scapular muscles in proper balance. The two runners maintain proper body curvatures, at ease during running.
- *Figures 10.40* thru *10.43* show two females compensating for **weak shoulders** by shrugging them (narrow space between shoulders and neck) and losing the smooth concavity of the lower back despite their general level of higher fitness.

10.4. TRAINING FOR ENDURANCE AND STRENGTH

10.4.1. INTERMITTENT PHYSICAL WORK

- Repeated **intervals of brief and hard physical work** have become the standard of modern strength training. Brevity allow for regeneration of new influx of nutrients. The high intensity of work stimulates adaptation to higher power output. It seems that all strong animals have to resort to brief and intense actions in order to maintain strength and avoid burning out. Interrupted work maintains lactate accumulation below threshold, for longer duration of training, than with long periods of work without rest.
- Despite the **nonlinear interdependence** of performance variables, *Figures 10.1* and *10.5*, humans can endure lengthy physical work, if heart rate and oxygen consumption are kept under control below maximum. Performing double the amount of the same physical work throws the heart rate and ventilation effort out of control. This induces fatigue in much less than the anticipated in half the time, taken in performing half the amount of work. Lactate accumulation is thus not linearly related to heart rate, VO_{2max}, and amount of physical work.
- Intermittent exercise allows a **higher volume of intense work** due to reduced physiological strain on biological system. That is because the increased power output shortens the duration of heat production and allows the body plenty of time to dissipate heat during brief rests. However, what can be worked out in a specific period of time may not be doable by linearly increasing the rate of working out, in order to reduce the required duration. The non-linearity of biological performance originates from various requirements of running chemical reactions at specific rates and directions.
- The **cumulative effect** of consecutive intervals of intense work is the accumulation of lactic acid. This increases the burden on fatiguing respiratory and cardiac muscles, to attend to the demands of oxygen consumption and delivery. Since such cumulative effect takes longer time to induce fatigue, it allows amble time to maximize cardiac performance in order to achieve higher peak stroke volumes and $VO_{2\ max}$, in between rest periods. Rest periods enable trainees to use large muscle mass of respiration and of skeletal origin. This increases peripheral vascular resistance and acutely traps massive amounts of blood in muscles, resulting in compensatory **high heart rate**. Subsequent release of trapped blood pool, after muscular contraction ends, maximizes venous return and induces the heart to maximize **stroke volume**, in response to greater blood return. Greater, yet brief, venous return increases preload [2] and induces adaptive hypertrophy of ventricular cardiac muscles due to the additional ventricular preload stretch.
- **Training load volume and training intensity** are greatly manipulated by interrupted exercising. Brief and intense endurance exercise is very effective in increasing the maximum oxygen ventilation and cardiac output, while working out at low load volume tolerated by beginners. Thus, stimulating shocks of intermittent training give beginners a sense of peak performance, without inducing harmful overtraining.

10.4.2. LOAD VOLUME AND INTENSITY IN ENDURANCE AND STRENGTH TRAINING

- Regular and long training leads to **progressive adaptations** over several years. Muscle synthesizes contractile fibrous protein, mitochondria, and new blood capillaries, in addition to enhancing the type of muscle fibers that suits strength or endurance activities. Adaptation in enzymatic activities within the mitochondrial oxidation processes occurs over longer time. Thus, changes in the lactate threshold are slower to occur compared to improvement in maximal oxygen

---

[2] Preload, in heart physiology, refers to the stretch of the walls of the ventricles before commencing pumping out blood. That is before systole begins. It signifies pre-systolic inter-ventricular pressure.

consumption. Thus, the trainee's ability to maximize ventilation occurs faster than enduring protracted physical work, despite the improved oxygen consumption.

o While **interrupted work** improves maximal ventilation and cardiac output, that are critical to improving physical strength, **continuous work** improves mitochondrial density and activity, and favors slow switching muscle fibers. A combination of interrupted and continuous work is necessary to enhance strength and endurance. There is an optimum mix, of strength and endurance, that suits various activities, *Figure 10.44*. Top endurance athletes may enhance their performance by a fine touch of strength training that improves weak links; yet, continuous exercising is more crucial to endurance athletes than to others. In addition, elite strength athletes benefit from endurance training by enhancing their recovery during peak levels of intense training, yet intermittent exercising is similarly more crucial to strength athletes than others.

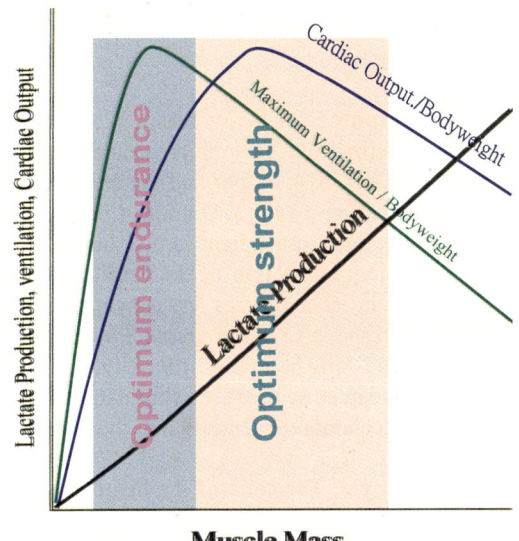

Figure 10.44. Effect of muscle mass on strength and endurance.

o **Off-season and contest workout.** During off–season, training proceeds at lower intensity and higher volume, with periodic brief sessions of high intensity. Long exposure to high intensity training increases lactate concentrations, sympathetic stress, and tissue injury, which all culminate in overtraining and failure. Pre-contest training differs from off-season training in the distribution of load volume and intensity. Highly intense training is carefully introduced and monitored by heart rate, quality of performance of skilled technique, and progress curve. Random introduction of intense training is serious business that may put an end to athletic careers.

10.5. ADAPTATION TO EXERCISE

10.5.1. HEART ADAPTATION

o **Heart rate.** Exercise intensity is best assessed by heart rate. Higher exercise intensity causes higher heart rate. Variation of heart rate with exercise intensity is attributed to neural control of the cardiac output in response to the pooling of blood in intensely working muscles. Thus, heart rate variation is an index of muscular trapping neurocardiac regulation of blood, healthy vascular sensors of blood pressure, healthy cardiovascular regulatory center, and healthy.

o **Variation in heart rate.** Maximal heart rate depends on the drop in venous return during muscular contraction.
   i. Activities that is restricted to isolated muscles affect heart rate less than in whole body activities.
   ii. Training improves neural feedback mechanism and causes higher heart rate on performing isolated activities. Endurance trained hearts do not beat faster or powerfully at maximum intensities and thus can maintain lower lactate accumulation.
   iii. Since heart regulation is central, it is affected by environmental factors (such as heat, humidity, noise, and light) and on personal state of mind. Higher temperature increases heart rate in order to enhance heat dissipation from the skin surface. Increased humidity decreases evaporation from the skin and increases core temperature.
   iv. The neural control of heart rate is balanced by stimulation from the sympathetic and parasympathetic autonomic nervous system, via the sinoatrial node on the right atrium. Parasympathetic stimulation slows down the rate, while sympathetic stimulation increases it. Without neural control, intrinsic heart rate is about 60/min. Untrained folks experience constant sympathetic stimulation that speeds the heart form 60/min to 75/min. Training reduces sympathetic stimulation at rest, resulting in a slower resting heart rate.
   v. The initiation of exercise results in withdrawal of the parasympathetic stimulation and increase in sympathetic stimulation, in proportion to the intensity of exercise, resulting in increased heart rate.

o **Heart endurance.** The heart muscle is designed to contract automatically, rhythmically, and continuously, for life. It is rich in capillaries and in cellular mitochondria. Thus, the heart can both extract a reliable delivery of oxygen from the circulation and process a reliable delivery of fat, lactate, and glucose, for energy production. About 25% of the human heart cell volume consists of mitochondria, compared to about 5% of the skeletal muscle cell volume.

o **Stroke volume.** Cardiac muscles hypertrophy with resistance training. This results on increase in the stroke volume with training. This is the blood volume ejected from the left ventricle with each heartbeat, which is about 70 ml during rest. Cardiac hypertrophy exists during rest as well as during exercise, in trained athletes. It causes heart rate to drop during rest below 70/min, after few months of training. Since cardiac output (5 liters/min) is the product of heart rate and stroke volume, higher stroke volume (over 70 ml) dominates during rest, and increases further during exercise.

Thus, heart rate is more responsive to exercise level than stroke volume. Training thus increases the quantity of work performed by the muscles by enhancing both cardiac mass and neural control, in order to deliver more blood to working muscles.

o **Cardiac output.** Exercise increases heart rate if large enough muscle mass is worked out. It also increases stroke volume by strong hypertrophic ventricle. Thus, cardiac output increases in response to exercise, in order to increase oxygen delivery, by a bigger and faster cardiac pump. Cessation of training returns both heart rate and stroke volume towards pre-training values. Untrained people suffer **dizzy spells** when cardiac output fails to nourish the brain, during heavy lifting. Such insufficient cardiac output can be caused by the following:
  i. Insufficient adaptation of the cardiac muscle. This can be demonstrated by the lesser muscle hypertrophy, less mitochondrial density, or less enzymatic activity within the mitochondria.
  ii. Poorly responsive blood pressure sensors, blood gases sensors, and feedback control of cardiovascular system, as in old age, long periods of inactivity, and arteriosclerotic vascular diseases.
  iii. Poorly adapted sympathetic stimulation of the cardiac rate of contraction and the force of contraction.
  iv. Imbalance ionic concentration of the blood, as in water intoxication, dehydration, and hypoglycemia.

o **Cardiac muscle.** The cells of the heart muscle are geared for endurance work. They differ from skeletal muscle in their ability to contract spontaneously and rhythmically, even without external nerve control. They are densely populated with mitochondria, have shorter diffusion distances, and rich in circulation. Their enzymatic activity is also adapted to low power output aerobic work, for whole life duration. Exercise affects the new growth of muscle fibers that causes ventricular hypertrophy and increases stroke volume. Though ventricular hypertrophy is also encountered in advanced heart failure, exercise hypertrophy of the heart presents without the high peripheral vascular resistance of heart failure. The enhanced sympathetic regulation of peripheral vascular resistance, due to exercise, prevents the high preload and high after-load[3] encountered of heart failure.

10.5.2. SKELETAL MUSCLE ADAPTATION

o **Response.** Skeletal muscle reacts to progressive increase in energy expenditure by definitive changes that aim to restore normal physiological processes or homeostasis. Muscle cells increase protein synthesis in order to convert more chemical energy into kinetic energy, by the contractile proteins: actin and myosin. Increased contractile elements require more mitochondria in order to increase ATP replenishment rate and biodegrade Pyruvates, at higher rates, through the Tricarboxylic acid cycle.

o **Limitation on enhancement.** However, if increasing contractile protein and mitochondrial density is without limits, one should be able to enhance both strength and endurance indefinitely. The main reason for not being able to reach that hypothetical state is, most probably, due to the thermal limitation of dealing with high power output. Expending energy for long time (endurance) and at higher rates (strength) is thermally impossible, since chemical reactions are very sensitive to temperature variation. Chemical reactions occur at the electronic level of the atom. Therfore, they are affected by temperature variation. Thus, optimum muscle endurance and maximum muscle strength are mutually exclusive. The hypothesis of "mitochondrial dilution" with respect to contractile protein hypertrophy, as a cause for limitation of developing strength, can be easily refuted by the fact that little amount of mitochondria could exhibit higher level of enzymatic activities.

o **Glycolysis.** Strength training operates at greater anaerobic glycolysis. That provides high power output in the absence of oxygen by generating ATP and lactate molecules from degradation of glucose. Endurance training leads to greater oxidation of pyruvates in the mitochondria. The cytoplasmic pyruvates enter the effective aerobic oxidation in the mitochondrial citric acid cycle and produce plentiful of ATP supply, but at slower rate than anaerobic glycolysis. Optimization of energy expenditure, therefore, rests on whether ATP is obtained by fast anaerobic degradation of glucose to lactate or the slow aerobic degradation of glucose, fat, and protein, into carbon dioxide and water.

o **Muscle mass.** There must be a minimum muscle mass for expending minimally required energy for optimally desired performance. Such minimum muscle mass should produce the desired power output, remove byproducts, replenish resources, and maintain basic vital function. There also should be a minimum muscle mass for the specific working part of the body, in various activities, that requires special and extensive training in order to perform special skills at high performance. Strength training in endurance athletes enhances such basic muscle mass in order to maintain functional mobility and avert the development of deformities. These are caused by unattended wasting of vital muscular support. However, excessive weight training leads to increase in muscle mass and decline in endurance. That is because more oxygen demand is imposed on the heart pump by the extra weight, in addition to the extra lactate production. In Bodybuilders, strength training can tremendously enhance both strength and endurance, but only for isolated muscles. Such accomplishment occurs at the expense of total body strength and endurance. Bodybuilders spend most of their load volume in training small percentage of whole body muscle mass. Thus, their cardiac output is no longer a limiting variable in delivering adequate oxygen to the isolated working muscles. Adding all isolated

---

[3] After load, in heart physiology, refers to the systemic pressure encountered by ejected blood, during the systole. It signifies the rule of systemic peripheral resistance in maintaining systemic blood pressure.

muscles together, in multi-joint exercises, causes easy fatigue in Bodybuilders, during lifting comparable heavy weight from the floor.

- **Muscular balance.** Strength training is the magic remedy after injuries, surgery, or when dealing with personal deficits of muscular vigor. Weight training stimulates muscle growth and control, and offers great hopes for motivated athletes with specific problems. Promoting strength during a learning period helps acquiring new techniques and ingrains new skills into the neuromuscular system. Beginners and young athletes benefit most from combined strength and endurance training. In addition, beginners need the assuring self-esteem that comes with extra strength and stamina. In different sport activities, working muscles are more crucial to performance than whole muscle mass. For example, Weightlifters perform better Snatch with stronger arms, and better Clean and Jerk with stronger shoulders, back, and legs. Small-muscle sports benefit greatly from strengthening working muscles by weight training, since whole bodyweight is not greatly stressed. The most beneficiary from strength training are women, most of whom can revolutionize their level of strength and fitness by strengthening the upper body.

- **Adaptation in the type of muscle fiber.** The mixed combination of slow (red cytochrome and myoglobin pigment) and fast (white) muscle fibers, in mammals, serves distinctive specialized functions in the body. Low power output processes, such as maintaining posture and endurance activities, require slow twitching fibers in order to endure longer duration of energy expenditure, at low lactate buildup. High power output processes, such as heavy lifting, sprinting, and other vigorous activities, require fast twitching muscles in order to generate greater forces in short intervals. Training enhances the sort of muscle fibers favored in such activities, while the less favored muscle fiber type atrophies.

- **Muscle strength.** Strength is determined in part by the muscle size, which in turn is determined by the number of fibers per unit area across the muscle length. Heavy and sustained physical work stimulates muscle fibers to multiply by binary division in order to generate new fibers. This process of new cell formation is called "hyperplasia". That is evidenced by the fact that average fiber size, judged by cross section area in biopsy slides, is almost constant in trained and untrained people. The whole muscle size is larger in strength-trained than in untrained. High muscle tension might knock down the weak muscle fibers, thus initiates new growth process, of higher number of fibers that can stand high tension. This may take place within the primitive stem cells. Alternatively, it might work by means of different mechanism of regulating the new growth of contractile muscle protein. Stimulating the chemical catalysts along the protein synthesis process, by high work tension, might alter genetic expression in response to strength training. That may explain why some people develop large muscle-mass faster than others do, under similar training conditions. Enlarged average fiber size, if at all, may be explained by decline in the number of weak fibers and growth of new fibers of average size, instead of the below average, weak ones. New growth of cells is not alien to connective tissues such as muscles, skin, bone, and nerves. At low load volume, muscle generates force by regulating recruitment of a constant pool of muscle fibers, without the need to generate new fibers. The nature of tension stimulus also impacts muscle strength and size. Slow, heavy, and eccentric resistance (Bodybuilding training) enhances new growth, than fast and concentric resistance. That is why Weightlifters have to perform slow and heavy Squat, Deadlift, Goodmorning, and arm exercises, in order to enhance their high speed Olympic lifting. Training solely by Olympic exercises is restricted to pre-contest periods. The long learned lesson since the 1950's is that progressive increase in workout load volume and intensity, over few months, is crucial to promoting muscle strength and mass. Progressive muscular tension might stimulate dormant genetic features in contractile muscle fibers. These fibers regenerate thicker and stronger fibrous protein. Alternatively, it might stimulate stem cells to differentiate into new muscle cells in order to replace damaged cells, as in the cases of continuous growth of hair, skin, bone, and nerves.

- **Muscle cells.** Skeletal muscle cells are connective tissue cells that are long, spindle shaped, and attaches to tendons at both ends, by means of their connective tissue coverings. These can span the long distance between two major joints in the body. Different muscle cells are enmeshed in a network of connective tissue that transmits forces between the fibers and the tendons. The cells are separated from surroundings by highly functional cell membrane. That controls inflow and outflow of nutrients, in addition to chemical (hormonal and ionic concentration) and electrical signals. Cell membranes give muscle cells distinctive role in biological system and their ability to adapt to physical activities. For example, excessive drinking during training may dilute blood concentrations of ions and causes muscle membranes to fail to regulate sodium and potassium traffic, resulting in decline in performance during exercises. In addition, warming up help adjust blood concentration of ions by increasing renal flow and filtration of excessive volumes of fluid, resulting in ameliorating milieu surrounding muscle membrane. Muscle membrane encloses the cytosol, the fluid matrix of the cell that encompasses networks of protein synthesis reticulum, granules, contractile protein, and the nucleus. The contractile proteins, **actin** and **myosin**, are arranged in interlacing threads, like the cylinders and pistons of combustion automotive engines. Within the cytosol are embedded various types of cellular elements, the most important of which are the mitochondria, which are the powerhouse of the cell. Mitochondria host the oxidation processes of carbohydrates, fats, and proteins and generate the chemical energy that is stored on ATP molecules. The byproducts of oxidation (water, carbon dioxide, various organic acids, and heat), each play a role in the homeostasis of the body. Exercise shifts ionic concentration of the plasma towards acidosis by the carbon dioxide generated by the mitochondrial oxidation. Acidosis influences muscular contraction through the rate of diffusion of calcium, from the sarcoplasmic reticulum (tubular structure within the muscle cell) and is influenced by the rate of ventilation. The function of muscle cells is most affected by vascular capillaries and nerve endings. Exercise increases capillary density around working muscle fibers and thus enhances delivery of nutrients and removal of byproducts. Exercise also enhances sympathetic nerve control of vascular capillaries, in order to retain sufficient circulation for working muscles and preclude pooling of blood within inactive organs.

- **Brain control over muscles.** Motor brain centers control muscles by selective recruitment of muscle units for various levels of force. This is inducted by firing electric signals from central neurons[4]. These signals reach the spinal cord neurons, through long nerve tracts in the spinal cord. In the spinal cord, the long nerve tracts branch and synapse with many lower motor neurons. The motor unit consists of a lower motor neuron; afferent (returning) and efferent (exiting) nerve axes, in addition to the muscle innervated by these nerve axes. Although the lower motor neurons are the final gateway for executing recruitment signals from the brain, terminal muscle fibers can decline recruitment if neuromuscular transmitters are depleted, lactate accumulation exceeds threshold, or the muscle fiber is already depolarized (maximally stimulated). A single muscle can consist of many motor units. Each motor unit contains thousands of fibers of the same twitch type. Mixed types of motor units (fast or slow) may exit in the same muscle. Thus, muscles are heterogeneous in muscle fiber type, while motor units are homogeneous, in affecting the same type of muscle fibers. Greater forces of resistance require recruitment of larger muscle units. The instantaneity of resistance is also managed by selecting among fast and slow muscle fiber type, through their designated central neurons. The intensity of contraction of muscle units is further regulated by the frequency of firing of the motor neuron. More frequent firing increases the duration of muscular contraction and hence increases force. In addition to the higher control by the brain, muscles rely on muscle spindles and ligament ganglions to regulate reflex reactions to motor activities, through the spinal lower motor neurons. The reflex muscle spindles are additionally regulated by the extrapyramidal system, through the gamma spinal neurons and nerves. This reflects the effects of sleep, rest, motion, and mediation on neuromuscular regulation. Specific training modifies different aspects of brain control over muscles. Strength training modifies recruitment synchrony and frequency of brain firing, in addition to enhancing specific muscle fiber type and promoting new growth of muscle fibers. Put simply, training enhances brain and muscle function and structure in order to better performance.

10.5.3. INCREASED MAXIMAL OXYGEN CONSUMPTION

- **Oxygen energy.** Oxygen is a vital chemical substance that interacts with hydrogen and produces energy within living cells. The interaction energy transfers the chemical energy of the food ingredients into universal energy transport molecules, the ATP. The rate of oxygen consumption is a realistic measure of overall cellular energy expenditure. It thus increases with activity. Oxygen delivery from the lungs to remote cells depends on cardiac output, local arterial capillaries of the working muscles, oxygen carrying capacity of the blood, and sympathetic regulation of circulation. Under normal physiological conditions, oxygen is efficiently utilized by cellular mitochondria as soon as it is delivered. Impedance of mitochondria enzymatic oxidations results from fever, accumulation of excessive byproducts as in overtraining, or other external noxious insults.

- **Oxygen delivery.** Training increases maximal stroke volume of the heart and hence increases cardiac output and oxygen delivery. Yet, this enhancement plateaus after few months. That is because the enhanced coronary capillaries to the enlarged heart muscles maximize. Further heart enlargement is curtailed by limited new growth of arterial coronary capillaries. Thus, further advanced training would not enhance oxygen delivery beyond that plateau. On the other hand, cessation or reduction of physical activity reverses the gained enhancement of cardiac output and oxygen delivery.

- **Neural budgeting.** Training enhances selective perfusion of working muscles in order to grab a higher share of the limited cardiac delivery of oxygen. Exercises that involve simultaneous use of major muscle group (such as running, Weightlifting, and Plyometrics) enhance highly adapted sympathetic control of arterial circulation. This budgets such limited availability of cardiac oxygen delivery among the major muscle groups. People unaccustomed to whole body training find such activities daunting. Dizzy spells and cardiac angina results from poor budgeting of circulation by a central nervous system that is unaccustomed to high oxygen demands by working muscles. In untrained people, the limited cardiac output is squandered among needy and not so needy tissues, resulting in oxygen deprivation of vital organs, such as the brain and heart. Training results in more muscles being able to obtain adequate oxygen supply, simultaneously without jeopardizing vital circulation.

- **Cellular utilization.** Cells can enhance their ability to utilize oxygen by growing new mitochondria, possessing oxidative enzymes with higher activity to biodegrade larger amounts of substrates at higher rates, or by enhancing diffusion processes. Endurance training enhances oxidation capacity up to three time that of untrained people, through the three mechanisms.

- **Measurement of maximal oxygen consumption.** VO_{2max} is measured at sea level during activities that involve major muscles such as treadmill walking or running. Steady pace activity eliminates confounding variables such as bodyweight, muscle mass, or agility, thus permits better estimation of cellular consumption of oxygen. Oxygen measurements are performed through a breathing device. This uses calibrated system of sensors to oxygen

---

[4] Central neurons are those in the brain cerebrum, also called Upper Neurons. Spinal neurons are located in the spinal cord, also called Lower Neurons. Both types of neurons are part of the central nervous system.

consumption. The device collects air expired by the person versus exercise intensity (speed of running or incline of platform of treadmill). Curve maximum determines peak oxygen consumption, which ranges from 2.5 liters/min to six liters/min.

10.5.4. LACTATE THRESHOLD

o **Anaerobic energy production.** Glucose is foodstuff that can supply energy, in the absence of oxygen, in order to fulfill the immediate need of swift power production for muscular activity. Glucose is a byproduct of the degradation of carbohydrates by the gastrointestinal tract and liver. Glucose can also be synthesized by the liver or kidneys from the carbon atoms of fats and proteins. It is taken up by cells and stored as glycogen, or utilized in energy production. Extended anaerobic activities result in the accumulation of lactic acid in blood. Lactates accumulate because they are produced, from the breakdown of glucose during anaerobic glycolysis, faster than they are eliminated from working cell. Lactate molecules contain three carbon atoms that originated from the breakdown of the six carbon atoms of glucose molecule. Thus, two lactic acid molecules are produced by the break down of one glucose molecule, with net energy production of two molecules of ATP. If mitochondrial oxidation were available, the lactate would not form from pyruvate. Instead, pyruvic acids will be oxidized into carbon dioxide and water, resulting in a net of 36 molecules of ATP produced by aerobic burning of a molecule of glucose.

o **Aerobic enhancement.** Accumulated lactic acid increases the acidity of the medium and inhibits performance. Training delays accumulation of lactates by increasing vascular capillary and mitochondrial densities in addition to increasing cardiac output, ventilation effort, and, metabolism of fatty acid. The increased capacity of the cellular powerhouse, due to training, allows more oxidation of Pyruvate via the citric acid cycle. This takes place in the mitochondria of the cells and results in reduced lactate accumulation and increased ATP production. Endurance athletes burn more fat and less carbohydrates by aerobic oxidation and thus accumulate less lactate. Aerobic cellular oxidation continues improving by training, even after maximum oxygen delivery has long reached plateau. That is because cellular oxidation is limited by the adaptation of total muscle mass, while oxygen delivery is limited by the cardiac muscle adaptation.

o **The aerobic-anaerobic switch.** The forking of the pathways of energy production by muscles, between aerobic (by converting glucose and other foodstuff into carbon dioxide, water, heat, and ATP) or anaerobic (by converting only glucose into lactate) is determined by a hierarchy of events. The activity of enzyme complex PDH[5] (Pyruvate dehydrogenase complex or PDH complex) determines the rate of utilization of Pyruvate, from the cytosol into the mitochondrial powerhouse, and its entry into the aerobic respiratory engine of the cell. Accumulated Pyruvates, in the cytosol, are converted by the cytosol enzyme "Lactate dehydrogenase" into lactates. These diffuse outside the cell and alter the acidity of extracellular fluids. The net power output by an entire muscle determines whether the diffusing lactates suffice causing muscular fatigue of adjacent and remote fibers. The liver and kidneys take up lactate from the blood and utilize them in gluconeogenesis. Thus, the mode of energy production is determined by a chemical reaction that is driven, in directions of either aerobic or anaerobic, by the activity of PDH complex.

o **Measuring the blood Lactate accumulation.** Six successive samples of blood are withdrawn during exercise and are analyzed chemically for lactate. These successive blood samples correspond to six increasing levels of exercise intensity, for constant duration. The threshold of lactate is interpreted by the peaking of the lactate-exercise intensity curve. Such interpretation is bounded by the tempo of exercise and the level of oxygen consumption. It should only serve as a relative measure for the conditions of the test.

10.5.5. EFFICIENCY OF PERFORMANCE

o **Integration of systems.** Optimum performance is the ultimate goal of integrating internal physiological processes to do most work at minimal expense. Yet, the number of variables that plays such integration is daunting. The main index of assessing the interplay of these variables is the power output by the whole body during the execution of physical work.

o **High power output exercises** refer to whole body **exercises**. These refine neural integration of major body components and enhance overall performance, without great improvement of local and isolated muscles. Neural control synchronizes the individual roles of muscle fibers of various types, sizes, and mechanical relationship, in order to generate great force in brief duration. Many people do not appreciate the benefits of such activities, since these require years of training and produce vaguely noticed physical changes. Weightlifters are criticized for having weak chest, less defined muscles, compared to Bodybuilders, yet they perform whole body activities for longer years with higher mobility. The greatest assets of high power activities lie in the neural synchrony of vital biological processes and not in the size or definition of muscles.

o **Low power output exercises** refer to exercises of isolated muscles. These refine the neural control of energy resources by alternating the burden among muscle groups. Such isolated recruitment allows recuperation and excitation of different muscle groups to proceed simultaneously. This precludes synchronized recruitment of major muscle groups. Endurance athletes train hard to eliminate any unnecessary body fat and sharpen the most effective muscles used in

---

[5] PDH complex comprises of TPP, Lipoic acid, CoA, FAD, NAD, and Pyruvic acid dehydrogenase. It exists in all mitochondriated cells. *See Table 17.3, Chaper 17.*

their sort of activities, in order to enhance oxygen consumption and reduce lactate accumulation. The contradictory relationship between low and high power activities stems from the fact that high power activity produces too much heat, in shorter duration. Thus, it requires more fluid volume to dissipate heat. On the other hand, low power activity produces heat at lower rate and requires low muscle mass with higher respiratory capacity, in order to maintain minimum byproducts. The recruitment of low muscle mass, in partial training, increases the relative capillary density and thus improves both oxygen delivery and waste removal, in the active muscles.

- **Technical skills**. These learned skills, most probably, occupy specific physical areas in the brain. This explains the long-term memory and ability to further enhance previously acquired skills, even after many years away from training. Ingraining early life skills requires lengthy, regular, and constant modification of behavior in order to override the individual's perception of specific activities. Since memorization of motor skills is modified by other brain activities, such as emotions, cognition, and arousal, many people cannot acquire specific new motor skills after certain age. Emotions may influence the person, even without the person awareness, and causes him or her to avoid specific portions of training that are crucial to enhancing performance. Suppression of such emotional interference with decision-making is best done at younger age. Cognition also works against refining performance in older age, when individuals seek interpretation for every detail and mostly would settle on the simplest interpretation that suits his or her perception. Younger trainees take older mentors at their word, and substitute their cognitive decisions for their own, thus can easily acquire complex performance and seek interpretation years later. Arousal also impacts skill acquisition at various ages. People who are trained at younger age are easily stimulated during exercise than those started later.

- **Fatigue**. This is caused by diminished fuel supply (carbohydrate depletion), increased accumulation of byproducts (lactate buildup), degeneration of active muscle fibers (high intensity training and high load volume), depletion of neurotransmitters, and suppression of hormonal regulation. Fatigue is delayed by various biological mechanisms. Chemically, muscles delay fatigue by switching between immediate fuel usage of carbohydrates by anaerobic glycolysis and delayed fuel usage of fatty acids by aerobic oxidation. This prevents acute accumulation of lactate. Physiologically, muscles switch between slow and fast twitching fibers, for different levels of muscular tension. This spares large groups of fibers from being activated unnecessarily. The variable levels of recruitment of muscle fibers, of various sizes and numbers, prevent unnecessary energy waste. Yet, the most important factor in delaying fatigue may lie in the autonomic regulation of physiological functions during activity. The sympathetic regulation of blood flow in peripheral blood vessels and of heart beating budgets the vital energy resources of the body for optimum performance. Training adds to all innate mechanisms the element of skillful use of proper muscles, at optimum times, in order to generate effective force with minimum waste of energy.

10.6. EFFECTS OF AGE ON STRENGTH AND ENDURANCE

10.6.1. TRAINING VOLUME AND PHYSICAL DECLINE WITH AGE
Aging influences physical performance through the decline of both adequate training volume and physical health. The most affected organs are the connective tissues[6] that deteriorate with cumulative inactivity and higher intake of food. Vascular, neural, and musculoskeletal tissues undergo aging changes more than others do. The decline in neural recruitment of muscles is either due to decline in the drive of the central nervous system that is occupied by many other interests, or due to vascular oxygen deprivation of the brain. This reduces ability to perform high intensity training and reduces maximal power output with age. Brief high-intensity training at older age can still increase power output, in comparison to sedentary population, by enhancing neural and vascular control.

10.6.2. MUSCLE MASS REDUCTION WITH AGE
Inactivity of old age wastes muscle mass and drags the entire health down the path of ailment. Muscles transform chemical energy into kinetic energy, while the rest of the body can only transform chemical energy into heat. Muscles waste by losing fibers, contractile force, and glycogen storage. Reduction in muscle mass with inactivity can be confirmed with reduced levels of creatinine excretion in urine. Since muscles control circulation through the pumping action of heart and the constriction and dilation of blood vessels, their wasting also reduces cardiac stroke volume, and maximal oxygen consumption. The reduced oxygen delivery, due to inactivity, diminishes both capillary and mitochondrial densities that were enhanced by training. This leads to faster accumulation of lactate and easy fatigability.

10.6.3. EFFECTS OF AGE ON TRAINING
- Strength training of old people can reverse the wasting of **muscle mass** to great extent and can ameliorate many of the consequences of losing active tissues. Late training can, at least, partially preserve muscle mass and slow aging. Vibrant musculature at old age enables the individual to tolerate fluctuations in the environmental elements and enhances mobility. With adequate degree of mobility, the heart, lungs, and kidney can function effectively and maintain normal homeostasis, which is essential for brain normalcy and mental health.

---

[6] Connective tissues refer to biological entities such as blood vessels, nerves, bones, muscles, ligaments, and tendons.

o **Cardiac stroke volume** can improve significantly by strength training, but not the maximum heart rate. The former depends on cardiac hypertrophy gained from strength training, while the latter is determined by neural control that is not amenable to strength training at old age. The inevitability of reduced reactive maximum heart rate by aging diminishes maximum cardiac output and maximum ventilatory volume. Reactive maximum heart rate declines from 190 bpm (beat per minute), in young age, down to 160 bpm, or so, in old age. This is attributed to either loss of sensitivity to sympathetic stimulation or to inadequate central neural stimulation of the heart, during maximal power production. Changes in the heart conduction system may affect regularity of beating, but not maximal beating, thus produces arrhythmias. Training can ameliorate cardiac output decline by enhancing stroke volume and improving general vascular conditions. This is achieved by enhancing vascular elasticity, patency, and capillary density. Training enlarges cardiac muscles of aged people compared to sedentary ones. In addition, burning body fat reduces arterial wall deposition of fat. That maintains vibrant elastic arterial walls and reduces peripheral vascular resistance, in comparison to untrained aged people. Flexible arterial walls reduce cardiac effort to pump maximal volumes during systoles. In addition, compliant arterial walls generate recoil energy, during diastole that enhances further pumping of arterial blood through the coronary, cerebral, and peripheral arteries.

o **Cellular respiration** also improves with training at old age, by slowing the decline in mitochondrial loss and increasing capillary density. Few months of vigorous training, results in clinical evidence of improvement in cellular respiration in sedentary people. This can be assessed by measuring the byproducts of the citric acid cycle, of cellular mitochondria. An example of these byproducts is the enzyme Citrate synthetase, which catalyzes condensation of the 4-carbon oxaloacetic acid with the 2-carbon acetyl coenzyme-A in order to produce citric acid. Acetyl coenzyme-A carries the end products of carbohydrates, fats, and proteins into the citric acid cycle that produces energy from aerobic oxidation. The improved oxygen delivery, by training, preserves mitochondrial integrity by reducing accumulation of byproducts of metabolism. These are Pyruvate, aminoacids, and fatty acids, which all must convert to acetyl coenzyme-A, through complex chemical process, in order to enter the citric acid cycle. In addition, the improved oxygen delivery significantly increases capillary circulation to working muscles in aged people and hence improves neuromuscular control and muscle strength.

o Improvement in **cerebral circulation** by training enhances coordination, by allowing better recruitment of skeletal muscles. This in itself is crucial to the ambulance of old people. Thus, old persons who can train at the same load volume and intensity, as a younger adult, should be capable of performing similarly.

o Strength training is highly effective in maintaining **muscular strength** throughout life by increasing muscle mass and neural control. Aside from its peripheral effects on the body, strength training stimulates the hypothalamic regulation of growth hormone and gonadotropin, which greatly affect mood, motivation, and cognition. Training sparks life into the mind and body by engaging in stimulating activities.

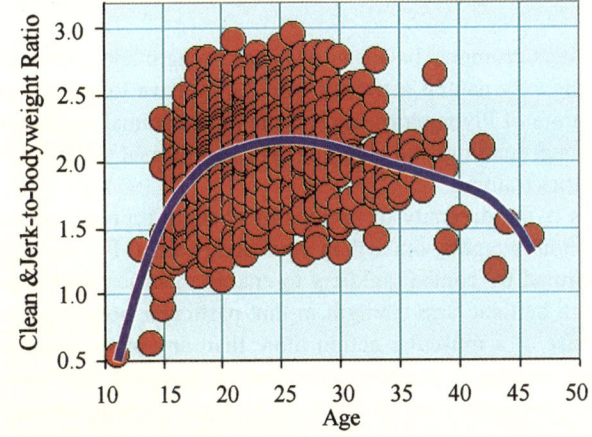

Figure 10.45. Relative strength of men in the Clean and Jerk, from 1999 World Championship for 1014 lifters.

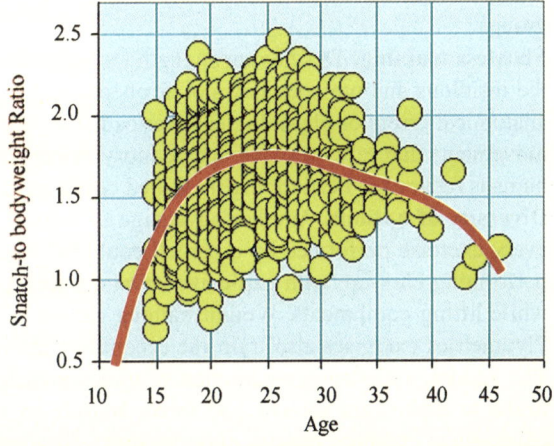

Figure 10.46. Relative strength of men in the Snatch, from 1999 World Championship for 1014 lifters.

o The data from 1999 world championship, shown in *Figures 10.45* thru *10.48*, demonstrate the following trends in relative strength[7].
  i. Relative strength increases, almost, linearly with age, under the age of twenty.
  ii. The rate of increase in relative strength diminishes after the age of twenty, and changes to decrease in relative strength after the age of twenty five, for both male and female Weightlifters.
  iii. Maximum strength occurs at the age of twenty-five, for both male and female Weightlifters.
  iv. The decline in relative strength after the age of forty-five cannot be justified from these data, since the number of people practicing Weightlifting declines in this age group, due to factors other than age.

---

[7] Source: International Weightlifting Federation, IWF. http://www.iwf.net.

ENDURANCE VERSUS STRENGTH

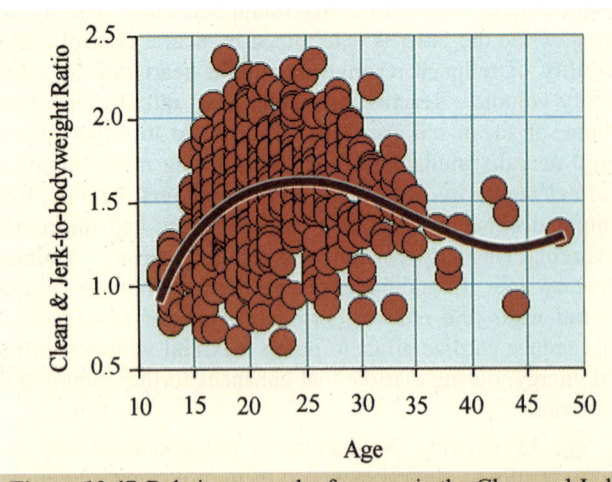

Figure 10.47. Relative strength of women in the Clean and Jerk, from 1999 World Championship for 529 lifters.

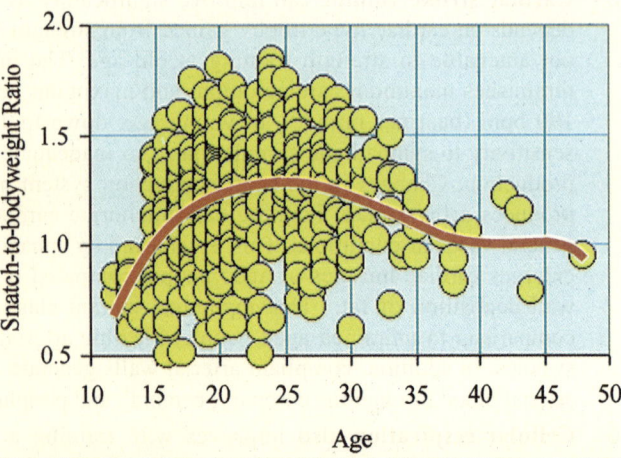

Figure 10.48. Relative strength of women in the Snatch, from 1999 World Championship for 529 lifters.

o   Training modality favors the **type of muscle twitch** that suits its performance. Thus, loss of fast twitch fibers by endurance training is attributed to atrophy and disuse of these fibers. There is no conversion among fiber types, since each has its own neural circuit and central control. There is, however, general loss of number of fibers by aging and inactivity. Aging may play role in muscle loss by altering hormonal control, if not through genetic expression.

10.7. PLYOMETRICS

10.7.1. GENERAL FEATURES

o   **Strength training.** Plyometrics are natural strength training activities that incorporate major muscle groups in entertaining and playful training. Common Plyometrics exercises, such as jumping, sprinting, and hopping, utilize bodily inertial energy to generate muscular resistance. Such activities are superior to weight training in enhancing motor skill, in real life situation with minimal planning effort. The improved ability to control speed, acceleration, and momentum of the whole body by Plyometrics training, outmatches any other activity in strengthening relevant muscle groups.

o   **Flawless training.** Developing strength through natural activities promotes balanced physical strength and overcomes the insidious and ominous flaws of erroneous technical training. By natural activities, you do not have to bother with anatomical errors or physiological overload. The "natural" feature of Plyometrics triggers the innate animal instincts of movements that rely on visual and auditory dynamics of jumping, running, and climbing. These universal skills among humans reduce the need for highly skilled coaching in Plyometrics training.

o   **Diversity of options.** Another advantage of natural activities is the diversity of options of strength training. Almost every exercise performed by a barbell could be executed without weights, other than your bodyweight. For example, performing chin-up, with explosive upward pulling, is performed by combat soldiers to enable them to climb ropes while lifting equipments. Weight training cannot achieve such ballistic arm strength in that particular body position. Plyometrics exercises also train the eccentric contraction phase of a muscular action more than any other activities. The sudden and strong contraction of major muscles, during landing in jumping, sprinting, or hopping, sets strong brake to downward motion and forces muscle to resist the enormous inertial forces. The high intensity eccentric contraction enlarges muscle mass in short duration and enhances neural recruitment, in relatively short duration compared to weight training. The latter depends mostly on concentric contraction.

10.7.2. PLYOMETRICS EXERCISES
The following are examples of Plyometrics exercises that strengthen lower body and upper body.

o   **Drop jumping.** This exercise involves the athlete dropping to the ground from a raised platform or box, and then immediately jumping up. The drop down is resisted by eccentric Quadriceps and Gluteal contraction. The vigorous upward drive is inducted by concentric contraction of the same muscles. Both motions affect spinal erectors and scapular muscles that stabilize the upper body during jumping. The exercise can be intensified by increasing the height of drop and jumping upwards sooner after dropping down.

o   **Bounding and hurdling.** This exercise involves vigorous leaping forwards and upwards, by either two-legged or one-legged bounds, to bring the body airborne. It can be performed on a horizontal flat surface or an uphill incline. It can be performed by jumping over hurdles, in order to enhance vertical drive and visual coordination.

- **Two-foot hop.** This is simple and very effective exercise in strengthening the most essential muscles of posture of the lower legs. In place hopping up and down tones the ankles, calves, and spines. This very effective warm-up exercise fosters sympathetic stimulation. Recall that only sympathetic neural control that maintains blood flow to the brain and upper body during standing, running, hopping, or jumping. Without such active nervous control, blood pressure tumbles to very low value that is incompatible with maintaining upright posture.
- **Rim jumps.** Jumping high to touch elevated rims, such as basketball rims, strengthen the fast twitching components of the lower legs. The cardiovascular system work hard to initiate the jump. In addition, the accessory respiratory muscles are vigorously activated during the jump. Higher and vigorous jumps intensify the muscular resistance. Rim jumps engage the upper body in jumping.
- **Box to box jumps.** This is performed by jumping from the ground to the top of one box, stepping off to the ground, then jumping again to the top of the other box. The cycle is repeated by turning around, executing the jumping, and stepping down with the other leg. This exercise works the eccentric and concentric contraction of the Quadriceps and Glutei.
- **Zig zags and side-to-side hop.** This is executed by side hopping, back and forth, over a straight marker, such as a rope or a line in the ground. The lateral hopping enhances the lateral spinal muscles and oblique abdominal muscles, in addition to the leg muscles.
- **Sprints.** These strengthen the Gastrocnemius, Hamstrings, and Quadriceps, in addition to the scapular and spinal muscles. Sprints can quickly and easily tone the leg muscles and improve the cardiovascular and pulmonary function. Their danger lies in the speed and force of resistance. This danger mandates thorough slow increase in the intensity of sprinting in addition to prior weight training to ensure knee, hip, and spinal stability.
- **Pushups and hand-claps.** Pushups, with a handclap in between in the way up, strengthen the Triceps, Deltoids, and Pectoral muscles. This can effectively enhance chest, shoulder, and arm sizes. The change in the direction of upper arms determines whether the chest or shoulder muscles carry the burden of resistance.
- **Asymmetric Squat.** Squatting while leaning on one leg more than the other, then alternating the leaning enhances the control and strength of Quadriceps and the lateral spinal muscles. The supporting foot falls under the body while the other foot moves off-center. The depth and tempo of descent control the intensity of squatting. This exercise can be as effective as squatting with heavy weight.

10.8. HIGHLIGHTS OF CHAPTER TEN

1. The greatest assets of high power activities lie in the neural **synchrony of vital biological processes** and not in the size or definition of muscles. The ability of the biological system of organs to persevere for minutes and hours, expending energy and generating forces, depends on inherent capacity of **managing energy resources** as well as on the acquired skills and adaptation to nurturing activities.
2. **Maximum endurance and maximum strength are mutually exclusive** since each tackles the rate of expending of one, and only one, thing that is energy. We have to choose our desired combination of strength and endurance. Running for longest distances precludes us from lifting heaviest weights. All physical activities have various **proportions of endurance and strength**. Minimal endurance lowers the threshold for physical and mental fatigue during activity and prolongs recuperation from stressful activities. In addition, minimal strength destabilizes the coherence of the framework of the system and undermines the pumping power of the heart and the respiratory effort of the chest and diaphragm. There is an **optimum mix of strength and endurance** that suits various activities. Top endurance athletes may enhance their performance by a fine touch of strength training that improves weak links, yet continuous exercising is more crucial to endurance athletes than others
3. Despite the complexity of the interplay of great number of variables involved in energy regulation, few fundamental variables greatly impact the effect of endurance and strength training on our biological system. At least four variables, each relates to one of the four basic entities of the biological system, can be clearly studied for enhancement and evaluation of physical performance. The four variables are
    i. **Maximum oxygen consumption (ventilation).**
    ii. **Maximum cardiac output (delivery).**
    iii. **Maximum lactate accumulation (metabolism).**
    iv. **Mechanical efficiency (muscle mass).**
4. All conventional burning involves **oxygen and hydrogen**. In addition, all produces carbon dioxide and water plus thermal energy. In its primitive nature, **thermal energy amounts for change of volume** of mater and, therefore, a significant portion of thermal energy is converted into kinetic energy. That is motion. The change of volume of hot water in steam turbine drives its blades. The change of volume of burning gasoline in automobile engines drives its wheels. The change of volume of muscle proteins by energy expenditure causes its fibrous protein to slide and generate muscular force.

5. **Running** constitutes the basic sort of aerobic activity that lubricates the engine of life. The simplicity, accessibility, and effectiveness of running, on controlling energy expenditure, make running a common remedy for many maladies. This is attributed to the process of moving large muscle mass, consuming large volumes of oxygen, and imposing heavy demands on the heart capacity.

6. Training also modifies **genetic expression of protein synthesis**. Thus, new muscle fibers are generated and new enzymes with higher activities are produced. The growth in the smooth muscle fibers is expressed in thicker heart muscles, new blood capillaries, and more compliant and flexible vascular arterial network. The growth in skeletal muscle mass is expressed in bigger and stronger muscles, heavier bones, and improved recruitment. The growth in enzymatic capacity is demonstrated by microscopic changes in cellular elements with higher densities of mitochondria and contractile muscle protein. Regular and long training leads to **progressive adaptation** over several years. Muscle synthesizes contractile fibrous protein, mitochondria, and new blood capillaries, in addition to enhancing the type of muscle fibers that suits strength or endurance activities

7. Relative strength is defined as the ratio of the maximum lift to the bodyweight of the lifter. Relative strength is inversely and linearly proportional to bodyweight. **Optimum body weight for male Weightlifters falls within the range of 65 to 75 kg.** Up to 80 kg bodyweight, top Weightlifters can lift 2.8 times their bodyweight, in the Clean and Jerk lift, and 1.8 times their bodyweight, in the Snatch lift. Over 110 kg bodyweight, drastic decline in relative strength is the rule.

8. Repeated intervals of **brief and hard physical work** have become the standard of modern strength training. Brevity allow for regeneration of new influx of nutrients. The high intensity of work stimulates adaptation to higher power output. It seems that all strong animals have to resort to brief and intense actions, in order to maintain strength and avoid burning out. Interrupted work maintains lactate accumulation below threshold for longer duration of training, than with long periods of work without rest. While interrupted work improves maximal ventilation and cardiac output, that are critical to improving physical strength, **continuous work** improves mitochondrial density and activity and favors slow switching muscle fibers. A combination of interrupted and continuous work is necessary to enhance strength and endurance.

9. The neural control of heart rate is balanced by stimulation from the sympathetic and parasympathetic autonomic nervous system, via the sinoatrial node on the right atrium. Parasympathetic stimulation slows down the rate, while sympathetic stimulation increases it. Without neural control, intrinsic heart rate is about 60/min. **Untrained folks experience constant sympathetic stimulation that speeds the heart form 60/min to 75/min.** Training reduces sympathetic stimulation at rest, resulting in a slower resting heart rate.

10. **Dizzy spells** and cardiac angina results from poor budgeting of circulation by a central nervous system that is unaccustomed to high oxygen demands by working muscles. In untrained people, the limited cardiac output is squandered among needy and not so needy tissues resulting in oxygen deprivation of vital organs, such as the brain and heart. Training results in more muscles being able to obtain adequate oxygen supply simultaneously without jeopardizing vital circulation.

11. **Endurance athletes burn more fat** and less carbohydrates by aerobic oxidation and thus accumulate less lactate. Aerobic cellular oxidation continues improving by training, even after maximum oxygen delivery has long reached plateau. That is because cellular oxidation is limited by the adaptation of total muscle mass, while oxygen delivery is limited by the cardiac muscle adaptation.

12. The activity of **enzyme complex PDH** (Pyruvate dehydrogenase complex or PDH complex) determines the rate of utilization of Pyruvate, from the cytosol into the mitochondrial powerhouse, and its entry into the aerobic respiratory engine of the cell. Accumulated Pyruvates, in the cytosol, are converted by the cytosol enzyme "Lactate dehydrogenase" into lactates. These diffuse outside the cell and alter the acidity of extracellular fluids.

Chapter 11 Axial Training versus Peripheral Training

11.1. AXIAL TRAINING VERSUS PERIPHERAL TRAINING

11.1.1. DEFINITIONS

o **Axial training** can be defined as exercise activities that simultaneously involve muscles proximal to the spines, the pelvic, and the shoulder girdles. These exercises engage both pelvic and shoulder girdles in simultaneous execution of resistance. Thus, axial training enhances the muscles that directly or closely act on the vertebral column, *Figure 11.1*. Major axial muscles are the Trapezius, the Erector spinae, the Glutei, the Hamstrings, the Deltoids, the Pectoralis, the Iliopsoas, and the Quadriceps. Examples of such exercises are the Clean and Jerk, Snatch, Pulls, Deadlift, Goodmorning, and Squat.

o **Peripheral training** may be defined as exercise activities that work out distal muscles and that engage one girdle but not the other, during execution of resistance. Thus, peripheral training enhances the muscles that act on the joints that are farther peripheral from the vertebral column. The major distal muscles are the Biceps brachii, the Triceps, the muscles of forearms, and the muscles of the lower legs. Examples of peripheral exercises are Biceps Curls, Triceps Extension, Wrist Curls, Cable Rowing, and Calf Exercises.

o The **combination of axial and peripheral exercises** distinguishes athletic sport from purposeless, casual training. Axial training requires self-motivation and serious minded individual who can comprehend the integral components of fitness.

o The most notorious side effects of sole peripheral training are **postural deformities,** which cannot be reversed even by the best fitness program on Earth. The majority of people frequenting public gyms incur postural deformities from imbalanced mix of axial and peripheral activities. The most common postural deformities due to such poor mix are:

  i. Lack of proportion of muscle strength, size, and coordination, between upper and lower body.
  ii. Inflexible, weak, and wasted back muscles.
  iii. Wasted limb muscles, due to inadequate differential load volume of limb training.
  iv. Truncal obesity, due to inadequate overall mobility.
  v. Abnormal body curvatures, due to long shrunk ligaments and imbalanced, wasted muscles.
  vi. Limited range of motion, due to imbalanced muscular antagonism in unaccustomed extremes of motion.

o In *Figure 11.2*, the apparent difference between the posture of the child and that of Hitler demonstrates the effects of life activities on acquiring musculoskeletal imbalance. The child can easily and comfortably maintains his head on vertical line over his feet that are kept together. The child can also

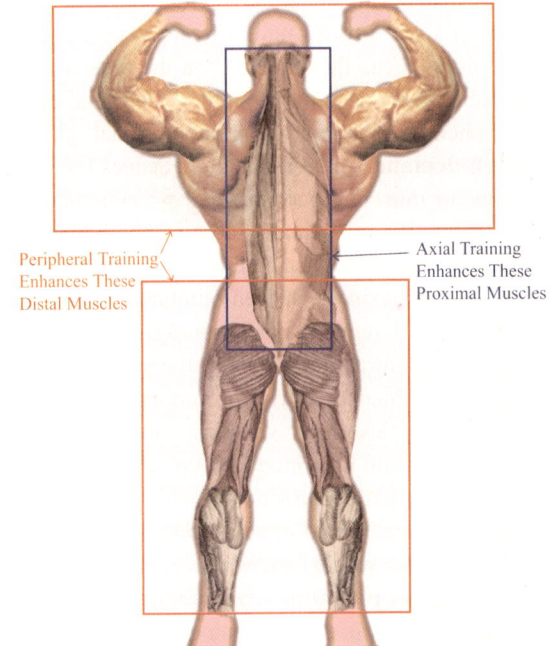

Figure 11.1. Major axial and peripheral muscles.

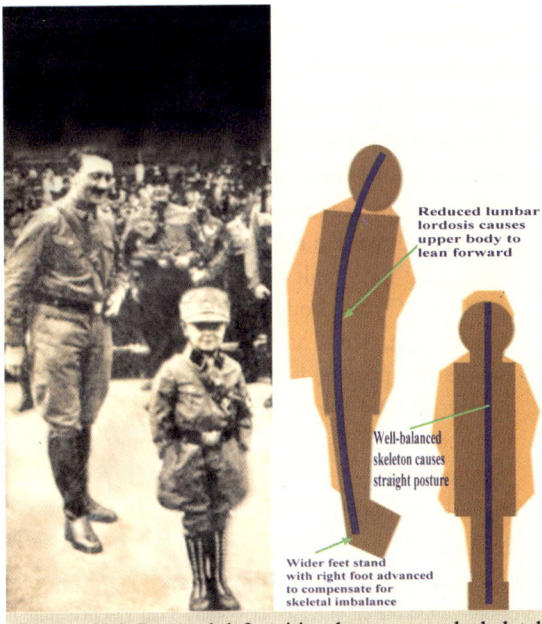

Figure 11.2. Postural deformities due to musculoskeletal imbalance.

maintain well-thrust chest, as evidenced from his backwards thrown shoulders. On the other hand, the infamous dictator cannot keep his head vertically over his feet. The forward thrown shoulders and the caving chest are due to scapular imbalance and thoracic kyphosis, despite the filling enhancement of the military uniform. In addition, the rounding of the lower back is apparent from the posterior displacement of the belt region that is closing the gap between the arm and the body, in the oblique view.

11.1.2. DIFFICULTIES WITH AXIAL TRAINING
The major difficulties in incorporating axial exercises in proper proportion, in daily, training are as follows.
- **Delayed gain.** Physical gains from axial training are deeper than superficial muscles. Therefore, changes in the outer contour of the trainee require long training, before bulging of muscles and exaggeration of body's curvatures become apparent. The muscles that benefit most, from axial training, are back muscles, and deep layers of muscles surrounding the shoulders and pelvis. Those are difficult to observe in front view mirrors.
- **Soreness.** The frequent and intense soreness following axial training frightens many people away from such activities, particularly when many new commercial gym equipments promise to fulfill similar role with less pain. Long and annoying soreness following axial training is due to long inactivity of those muscles, besides the greater production of lactic acid during major muscle training.
- **Out of sight out of mind.** The apparent irrelevance of deeper muscles, to immediate mechanical function, leads many people to focus their training on the muscle they feel doing the work. The Biceps is an example of such superficial muscles that does much less than the spinal erector muscles. Yet, many people spend most of their time training such peripheral muscles and little time of spinal, gluteal, or thigh muscles.
- **High demand.** Axial training challenges the cardiovascular, pulmonary, and neural systems. The slightest contraction of major muscle groups disrupts systemic and cellular functions and causes many people to worry about wrongdoing. With regular axial training, the sympathetic system adapts by budgeting blood flow and muscular recruitment in a manner that permits smooth transition from regular to vigorous activities. Many symptoms of poor conditioning, such as sudden dizziness, sudden numbness of limbs, diminished peak strength, and incoordination, disappear shortly after few days of regular axial training. These symptoms are caused by a sequence of events that result from major muscular contraction. As muscular contraction begins, the veins surrounding the contracting muscles are compressed causing sudden brief rise in venous return. As the contraction continues, the arterial blood is trapped within the muscles by arteriolar valvular contraction[1], causing sudden drop in cardiac return and hike in heart rate. The respiratory rate also increases voluntarily, compounding the dynamics of ventilation and perfusion, during the brief major muscular contraction. Enduring such major systemic alteration is easy on young trainees. Adult beginners require longer period of adjustment since their sensors for variation in blood pressure and blood chemicals are slower in adapting to whole bodywork.
- **Difficulty in planning.** Evaluating your gains from axial training is best achieved by progressing in lifting from the floor. Changes in muscle contours and size due to axial training are misleading, since deep muscle layers do not bulge to the surface of the skin as quickly as superficial muscles. Your sense of being able to maintain erect spines, while performing axial exercises, tells you that deeper muscles are working better on the skeleton and that resistance does not cause your skeleton to crumble. For example, moving the bar from the floor, during the Clean, Deadlift, or Bent-Over Row, causes untrained people to cave their chest, round back, and drop shoulders. With axial training, you can maintain solid alignments of the chest, back, and shoulders while resisting maximal forces. Therefore, the rule of thumb in planning is including systemic and regular portion of axial exercises into your daily workout, based on weekly cyclic routine. This practice should continue even if you do not notice changes in size or definition of muscles. You would not be able to assess early gains in deep para-vertebral, spinal erectors, shoulder rotators, hip adductors and abductors, or Hamstrings, by looking in a front view mirror.
- **Difficulty in performing.** Performing axial exercises is technically challenging. The trainee has to master the skill of breaking down the motion into its basic dynamic elements. Most axial exercises require rationing of the limited power output by the whole body. When you perform the Deadlift, Clean & Jerk, Snatch, or Squat, you must move only a portion of your body by concentric isotonic contraction, while maintaining the rest of the body with isometric contraction. Thus, as the bar is lifted from the floor up, to the thigh level, only the lower body moves by extension, while the upper body assumes tight fixation. The pattern is reversed above the thigh level. Fixing a portion of the body, while moving the other portion, diverts most of the cardiac output to the moving parts and spares the fixed part to subsequent tasks. Moving both upper and lower body, simultaneously, causes failure of both parts. Yet, the most challenging task is to compile body dynamics, with weight dynamics, in timely fashion. This requires weeks or months in order to learn how to automate the execution of motion with ease, through adaptive reflexes.

---

[1] Recent discovery suggests that there is a physiologic, nitric oxide-dependent vasodilator tone that is essential for the regulation of blood flow and pressure within the cardiovascular system. That vascular tone is maintained through the physical activation of endothelial cells by pulsatile blood flow and shear stress on the vascular walls. S. Moncada and A. Higgs. **The L-Arginine-Nitric Oxide Pathway**, N. Engl. J. Med., December 30, 1993; 329(27): 2002 - 2012.

o **Unpopular exercises.** The predominant perception that heavy lifting causes back and knee injuries discourages many people from attempting to train major muscle groups. Resorting to machines, benches, and aiding devices predispose to more injuries than freestyle lifting, on your own feet, back, and shoulders. The knees and back weaken by dismissal of axial training or inadequate training. Regular and adequate axial training enhances mobility of major joints. It should be performed regardless of its unpopular appeal.

11.1.3. POPULARITY OF PERIPHERAL TRAINING

o **Superficial muscles.** Peripheral training is so popular because it targets muscles that are easily visible, moving under the skin. Most people like to see their arms, chest, and legs enlarged in size and strength and most know the simplest exercises that can achieve that goal. Peripheral exercises enhance the immediate contact with resistance such as hand griping of barbell or pushing against the floor during lifting. While axial muscles generate most of the momentum and power required to move body inertia, peripheral muscles transmit that momentum and power to external resistance. Thus, peripheral training is a fundamental part of athletic training and serves as a link between the major power producers and the final beneficiaries of the produced power.

o **Peripheral training in Weightlifting.** Many Olympic athletes have developed their personal tricks of developing outstanding peripheral muscles in order to enhance axial performance. Developing strong arms, shoulders, abdomen, and chest muscles helps many Olympic Weightlifters to breakthrough long plateau of performance. However, combining small and frequent doses of peripheral exercises, amidst axial exercises, is more productive to sports athletes than spending entire sessions training peripherally. Isolated peripheral training, for long periods of time, aggravates inflexibility and limits the range of motion. That is the reason why many Weightlifters refrain from sole limbs or chest exercises in order to master better lifting technique, *Figures* **11.3** thru **11.6**. Most successful Weightlifters find that strengthening arms and shoulders with Weightlifting exercises (such as the Military Clean and Military Shoulder Press, after the Clean) are superior to Biceps Curls or seated Shoulder Press. If the technique of execution of exercise is closer to the practiced sport then it results in less interference with performance.

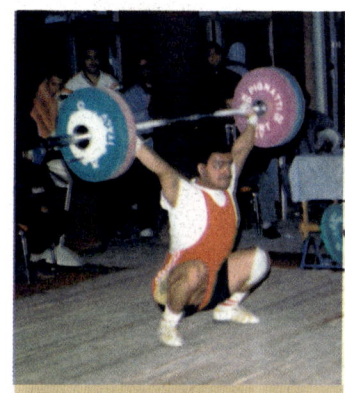

Figure 11.3. A lifter barely able to support a Snatch lift.

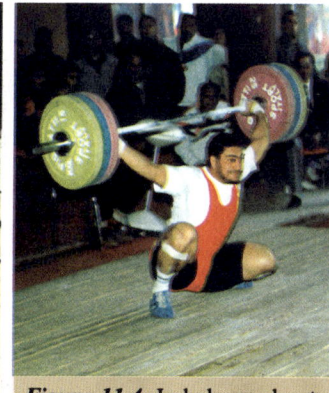

Figure 11.4. Imbalance due to inadequate puling.

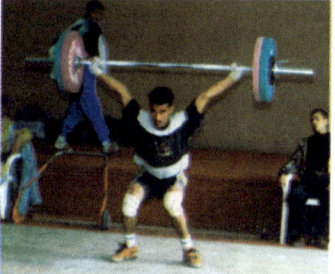

Figure 11.5. Extreme weakness of the limbs does not preclude the lifter from mobilizing more than his bodyweight in a successful Snatch lift.

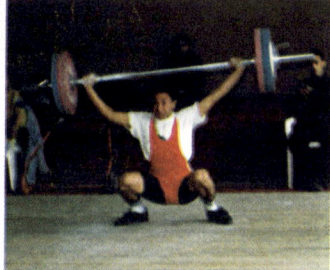

Figure 11.6. The effect of weak arms on the Snatch support.

o **Interdependence of axial and peripheral muscles.** For common people, peripheral training offers small doses of hope of building small pieces, little by little, in order to pull out of sedentary living and revitalize weak muscles. One can easily determine to alter his or her body composition by persistent peripheral training. When supplemented with few minutes of running, Plyometrics, or whole body exercises, on daily basis, improvement follows in endurance, strength, and flexibility, aside from adjustment in bodyweight and body fat. That is because fitness components and performance are interdependent.

o It is well known in neurology that peripheral distal muscle weakness is best explained by abnormal innervation, while proximal muscle weakness best explained by abnormal muscle conditions. In training, the same principle is paralleled by similar logic. Training distal muscles improves neural control of motor skill particularly during heavy resistance. *Figures* **11.3** thru **11.6** show the loss of neural control even after maximal peak power was generated to snatch heavy weights. Training proximal muscles improves muscle conditions in terms of size, circulation, strength, and effect on the skeleton.

o *Figures* **11.7** and **11.8** present an Olympic lifter, Abu Kalila, from the Los Angeles Olympic games of 1984 who utilized Bodybuilding effectively to excel in Weightlifting. The author grabbed Abu Kalila from the Bodybuilding room, introduced him to the Weightlifting team, and convinced him with the better future of practicing a technical sport. He has developed his secretive plans of exercises that widened his shoulders and chest, enlarged his arms, and trimmed his waist. With background in agricultural products, Abu Kalila relied heavily on diary products, proteins, and fruits to maintain lean body. The only drug he ever used was Indomethacin injections for knee and back pain, after few years of weight training. No other athlete, the author has known, has the intuition that led him to success as Abu Kalila.

11 AXIAL TRAINING VERSUS PERIPHERAL TRAINING

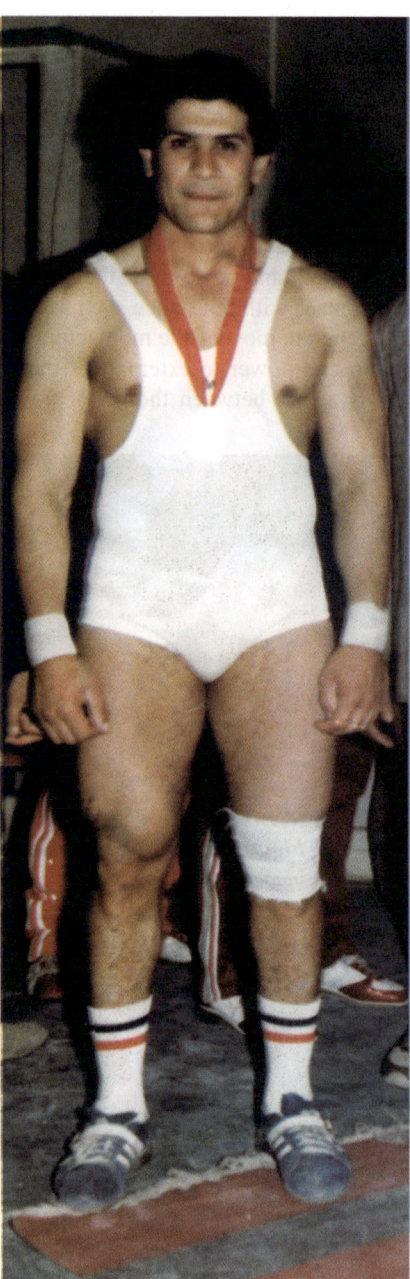
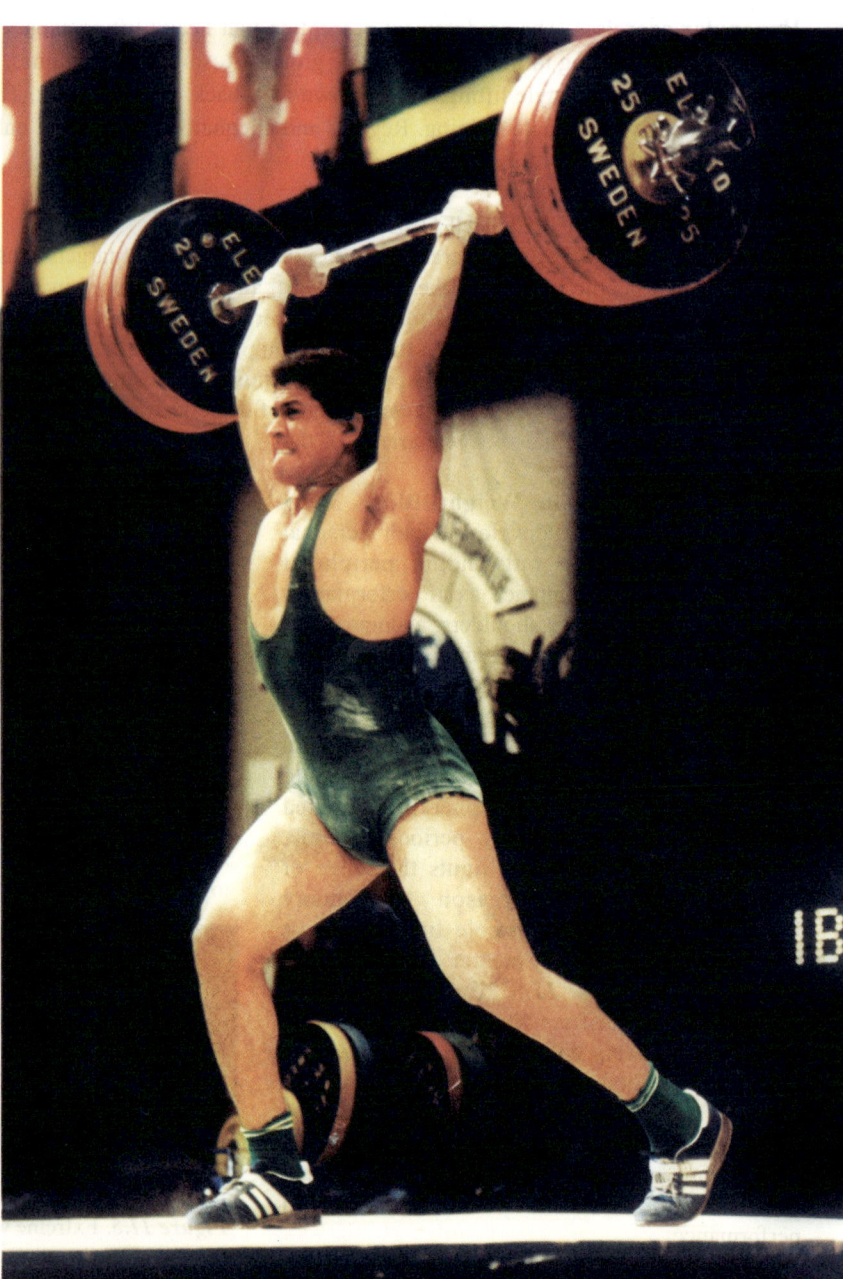

Figure 11.7 *Figure 11.8*
Ibrahim Abu Kalila, Los Angeles Olympic games, 1984, 5th position in the 82.5 kg class, and Barcelona Olympic games, 1988, from Egypt.
Biography: (1) Born 1952, Alexandria, Egypt, to a family that traded in dairy products. Has four brothers, all of them trained with weights, and all had surpassed others. Yet, he is the only one who persevered to the top Olympic games. Finished his vocational high school in agricultural technology. (2) Started weight training in a nearby mediocre gym, following the example of his two older brothers. His weight training years extended over three years, from 1969 to 1972. His weight training method might have excelled him to the top. He trained light, with supersets, with very diverse exercises, and with great emphasis on the arms and upper back. (3) His father's dependence on his five sons to run the twenty-four hour business put him in the workforce at very early age. Thus, he matured economically and business-wise, before all of us did. (4) In the year 1972, the author was the only team member in the Weightlifting group in that town that has advanced college education. The constant bragging of the team coach about the author's success, in the College of Engineering and in Weightlifting training, made many gym members aspire to the author's example. Abu Kalila was one of many who took the author's advice very seriously, despite of his stubborn and opinionated personality. (5) He converted to Weightlifting for a simple reason, that is, there were a group of people that meet and train in that remote room of the gym, three days every week, for many years, consistently. This strong family bonding atmosphere attracted that young man to train, listen, and learn. Few years latter, he traveled allover the world, because of that perfect choice he had made by joining a serious group of people. The author pursued his dream in medical education and engineering research from 1969 thru 1983, when Abu Kalila, had started, developed, excelled, and roamed the Earth, competing in Weightlifting. (6) His body posture has changed from a Bodybuilder who wants to show his muscular definition, wing his Latissimus dorsi, and bulge his veins, into a lifters with sedated, relaxed posture, yet, awesome and agile Weightlifter. Axial training had altered his musculoskeletal distribution into more dynamic and functional physique. (7) Along with training and his family occupation, he studied the law and graduated as a lawyer.

AXIAL TRAINING VERSUS PERIPHERAL TRAINING

He realized that low intensity and high volume peripheral training could alter body anatomy very effectively and could lead, in the end, to great axial strength. He worked hard and long to get his Latissimus dorsi to bulge on both sides, his rams to develop massive muscles from the wrist to the Deltoid, and his abdomen to develop the striation of Bodybuilders. His personal secret was simple and rich diet. As a son of a farmer, he relied on fruits as a source of carbohydrates, fish and chicken for protein, and milk and yogurt for calcium.

11.1.4. AXIAL VERSUS PERIPHERAL TRAINING

A comparison between axial training and peripheral training is summarized in *Table 11.1*.

Table 11.1. Comparison between axial training and peripheral training.

FEATURES	AXIAL TRAINING	PERIPHERAL TRAINING
Function	o Works out muscles proximal to the spines, pelvic, and shoulder girdles. o Involves both pelvic and shoulder girdles in simultaneous execution of resistance.	o Muscles acting on the joints that are farther peripheral from the spines. o Involves mostly one girdle during the execution of resistance.
Muscles	o Trapezius, the Erector spinae, the Glutei, the Hamstrings, the Deltoids, the Pectoralis, the Iliopsoas, and the Quadriceps. o Builds major muscles that possess multiple pinnation and multiple origins and insertion thus enables the body to exert maximal force utilizing many joints.	o Biceps brachii, the Triceps, the muscles of forearms, and the muscles of the lower legs. o Muscles with simple pinnation that performs fine motion, at low power output.
Exercises	o Clean and Jerk, Power Clean, Hang Clean, Military Clean. o Snatch, Overhead Squat, Power Snatch, Military Snatch, Hang Snatch. o Pulls form the floor with various grips and heights. o Deadlift, Stiff-legged Deadlift. o Goodmorning, Jump Goodmorning. o Bent-Over row. o Squat; Back Squat, Front Squat, Half Squat, and Jump Squat.	o Biceps curls, Hammer Curls, One-hand exercises, Wrist curls. o Triceps extension, Wrist extension. Cable rowing, Cable Pulldown o Leg extension, Leg Curls o Calf exercises, o Bench Press, Inclined Press, Flyes, o Declined Press.
Advantages	o Regular axial training causes the sympathetic system to adapt by budgeting blood flow and muscular recruitment. o The respiratory rate increases voluntarily, compounding the dynamics of ventilation and perfusion. o Conditions the major links between skeletal elements across major joints. Working major muscles, simultaneously, helps mineralization of the skeleton thus more calcium and phosphate are deposited into the bones. o Increased capacity for prolonged and powerful work. Calcium mediates muscular contraction, cardiac rhythm, and neuromuscular regulation.	o Involves submaximal muscle mass and thus does not require peak cardiac output. o Allows low intensity training to proceed for longer duration. This helps many people sculpture their body in any manner they wish. o Stimulates elements of the central cardiovascular and pulmonary regulation system but would not integrate such elements in orchestrated whole activity.
Disadvantages	o Gains are deeper than superficial muscles. Changes in the outer contour of the trainee require long training. o Frequent and intense soreness frightens many people away from such activities. Soreness is due to the greater production of lactic acid during major muscle training. o Challenges the cardiovascular, pulmonary, and neural systems. o Most axial exercises require rationing of the limited power output by the whole body. o Symptoms of poor conditioning are sudden dizziness, sudden numbness of limbs, diminished peak strength, and incoordination; disappear shortly after few days of regular axial training. o Technically challenging, requires weeks or months in order to learn how to automate the execution of motion. The trainee has to master the skill of breaking down motion into its basic dynamic elements.	o Common postural deformities due to lack of proportion between upper and lower body, abnormal body curvatures, and limited range of motion. o Resorting to machines, benches, and aiding devices predispose to more injuries o Peripheral training alone hinders the reactive response of heart and lung for vigorous activity. o Develops inflexible shoulders, upper and lower back, and legs, because of the lack of combined training of both girdles, each and every training session.

AXIAL TRAINING VERSUS PERIPHERAL TRAINING

11.2. EFFECT OF TRAINING EMPHASIS ON BODY COMPOSITION

11.2.1. MINERAL DEPOT

o Axial exercises condition the major links between skeletal elements across major joints. Working major muscles, simultaneously, fosters **mineralization** of the skeleton. Thus, more calcium and phosphate are deposited into the bones. The metabolism of the liver, kidneys, and intestines adapts to axial training by producing more vitamin-D, enhancing intestinal absorption of calcium, and depositing calcium and phosphate from the blood into the bones.

o The increased bone density, with axial exercise, amounts to increased capacity for prolonged and powerful work. That is because calcium mediates muscular contraction, cardiac rhythm, and neuromuscular regulation, in addition to many major chemical mediation in the body. Phosphate carries **chemical energy** on the ATP, ADP, and AMP molecules, as well as on other energy transport molecules.

o The regulation of blood content of calcium and phosphate is conducted by the **parathyroid hormone**. This affects the synthesis of vitamin-D by the liver and kidney, mediates the absorption of these minerals from the intestine, resorption and excretion by the kidney, as well as deposition and release from bones.

o The **thyroid gland** plays crucial role in the cellular metabolism of all these players (liver, kidney, parathyroid, intestine, and bone). Axial exercise, more than peripheral exercise, enhances systemic delivery of nutrients and removal of byproducts, from major muscle groups. This signifies its role in enhancing hormonal regulation of mineral content and improving cellular metabolism of the hormone producing glands (thyroid and parathyroid) and the hormone affected organs (bone, kidney, liver, intestine).

o To these immediate and short term hormonal processes, axial training also affects the secretion of growth hormone by the **pituitary gland** more than peripheral training. The growth hormone controls the development of the ossification centers and trends of bone deposition. On the long term, growth hormone delineates the general appearance of the skeletal posture. Growth hormone acts on the receptors of the active bones. These receptors are better prepared by axial training to welcome the influence of growth hormone, more readily than by peripheral training. Thus, the hunching of back, wasting of pelvic and leg bones, encountered in peripheral training addicts, could be easily attributed to the diminished effect of growth hormone on those location, where both exercise intensity and volume were inadequate for proper growth.

o *Figures 11.7* and *11.8* demonstrate the toughness of the musculoskeletal frame, with lower muscle mass, compared to Bodybuilders. Weightlifters develop condensed musculature, in body distribution that optimally performs antigravity resistance.

11.2.2. RATIONING DEMANDS

o As the mineral depot of the human body increases, more energy could be utilized in changing bodyweight composition. That is because minerals, particularly Calcium and Phosphate, play essential role in carrying and transferring energy in all biochemical reactions.

o Training peripheral muscles, for long, would not produce great increase in bone density. Peripheral exercises do not produce higher amounts of lactates, do not require maximum cardiac output, and do not demand maximal oxygen consumption. Thus, the body fulfills peripheral demands by reducing access to resources to inactive muscles, while availing resources to the small mass of peripheral muscles. A Bodybuilder might develop heavy bones in the arms or chest, but not in the axial skeleton that accounts for most of mineral depot.

o On the other hand, axial training requires maximum ventilation, delivery, and metabolism. The lightest weights, lifted axially, impose greater demand on the entire body to enhance adaptation and thus effectively impact body composition.

o The mode of training affects rationing of energy demands through the central nervous system and its sympathetic outflow to the cardiovascular system. In athletes, sympathetic stimulation on the heart diminishes during rest, resulting in lower heart rate. The cardiac response to sympathetic stimulation during activity becomes more gauged and controllable by the enlarged cardiac muscle that can easily respond to stimulation, in steady and strong reaction. Sympathetic control of the vascular network is crucial in directing the flow of traffic of nutrients to active and vital organs, while maintaining adequate pressure and flow within the network[2].

o Axial training affects the regulation of the entire arterial and arteriolar network, during working out, thus will ensure robust integration of nervous and vascular control. In comparison to axial training, peripheral training targets partial segments of the vascular networks and omits the rest of the body.

o People with diseased neurovascular control do not have the luxury of enjoying comfortable standing or walking, let alone exercising. Atherosclerosis and other hyaline degenerative diseases of the arterial and arteriolar walls interfere with sympathetic vascular regulation and impede rationing of energy demands during exercises.

---

[2] While the release of Nitric Oxide explains vasodilation and regulation of blood flow during exercise, yet sympathetic nervous regulation is still a plausible mechanism in preventing postural hypotension, during upright posture and without any exercise. That is because, if the rush of blood towards gravity dependent blood vessels causes more vasodilation, then shock would ensue due to severe hypotension.

11.2.3. WATER CONTENT
Water comprises 60% of bodyweight and is stored in multiple compartments within the body. Cells contain about 60% of total water content in intracellular fluid, while the remaining 40% lie outside the cells, in extracellular fluid; 30% in the interstitial space and 8% in blood vessels. Water regulation results in balance between intake and losses. The main compartment that is influenced by training is the extracellular fluid compartment. The various fluid compartments, affected by axial training, are as follows.
- o **Waist size.** The abdominal cavity can hold greater amounts of water under various conditions. Such conditions are: excessive and frequent water intake or food intake, diminished absorption, large amounts of excretion by the liver and the pancreas during digestion, or by the greater increase in the size of guts and surrounding tissue such as the greater omentum. Axial training challenges the delivery and respiratory system to circulate extracellular fluids, particularly in the waist region. This effort links the circulation of the lower limbs with the systemic fluid pool and thus allows room for diaphragmatic excursion. Thus, the kidneys and the intestines work harder during axial training in order to maintain fluid balance at optimum concentration, suitable for whole bodywork. The greater beneficiary from axial training is the spinal cord. Since mobilizing fluids from the waist, and lower limbs, and throwing them into systemic circulation at higher rates, during axial training, enhances spinal cord circulation. Recall that the spinal cord resides in a sanctuary location within the spinal canal, is long extension of the central nervous system, and it drives its blood supply from many small arteries along the vertebral column. Thus, removing waist congestion and enhancing lower leg circulation, simultaneously during whole bodywork, improves spinal control of motor function.
- o **Intravascular fluid.** The vascular content of water differs from the rest of extracellular water content in that vascular fluid is moving and exerting higher pressure. Exercise affects the "give and take" process between the heart pump and the body. Arteries benefit from axial training, during whole body involvement, by maintaining regular compliance with pulsating arterial system that is loaded with greater stroke volumes of blood. Maintaining regular and vigorous arterial pulsation of the whole body reduces plaque deposition and enhances sympathetic control (also, see footnote, on Nitric Oxide generation by capillary pulsation). Thus, axial exercises improve arterial blood flow and prevent turbulences that result from rigid, atherosclerotic, and noncompliant arteries. Venous circulation also benefits from axial training more than peripheral training, since veins depend on gravity and adjacent muscular contractions to propel blood back to the heart. In addition, since axial exercises, in particular, challenge the cardiovascular and central nervous systems, more than peripheral exercises, therefore, they facilitate not only the renal control on water balance, but also the skin perspiration and respiratory expiration of water vapor. That is because water excretion by the kidneys is regulated by the antidiuretic hormone that is secreted by the pituitary gland, in conjunction with the Aldosterone hormone that is secreted by the adrenal gland cortex. This signifies the role of the central nervous system and the cardiovascular system in producing and delivering hormones that control body water content.
- o **Interstitial fluid.** This fluid compartment forms by diffusion from the arterial capillaries that delivers nutrients to cells, in addition to the fluid excreted by cells that returns back to systemic circulation. Interstitial fluid is destined to join systemic circulation via two routes: venous and lymphatic channels. Axial exercise empties the venous pool more effectively than peripheral exercise thus creates greater diffusion gradient between the interstitial space and the venous space, encouraging faster circulation of interstitial contents. This refreshes the milieu of surrounding cells and improves cellular existence. The effect on the entire body is the absence of swelling and of accumulation of intercellular fluids plus enhanced cellular metabolism.

11.2.4. FAT CONTENT
- o Fat deposits in selective locations in the body, where the subcutaneous compartment permits deposition, and the body activity leaves deposited fat undisturbed. Fat deposition also prefers location where inflammation and healing processes are more active. The liver is a common site for fatty swelling in obese people. The arterial walls develop fatty plaques as early as the third decade of life, two decades before arteriosclerosis presents clinically. Internal organs such as kidneys, mesenteries, and intestines also attract fat deposition.
- o Axial training induces more deeper and global effects than peripheral training in mobilizing fat deposits. This sort of training hikes both heart rate and cardiac output to maximum, and effectively engages major muscles. These tremendously increase the flow gradient of blood in most of the circulatory network. Thus, internal fats move earlier than subcutaneous fat, as a result of the acutely changing internal flow of fluids.
- o Subcutaneous fat mobilization depends on fuel availability. If fewer carbohydrates are available, fat depot is tapped into and fat is converted into fatty acids and glycerol. Fatty acids are taken up by muscle cells, converted into acetyl coenzyme-A and consumed aerobically in the mitochondria, within the citric acid cycle. The glycerol portion, of broken down fat, is utilized mainly by the liver in the pathway of gluconeogenesis to synthesize glucose. The switch from carbohydrate fuel to fat fuel is triggered by the drop of blood glucose, through the action of Glucagon hormone

released by the pancreas. The fat cells react to the Glucagon signal by breaking down neutral fat by a Lipase enzyme. Thus, the availability and activity of the Lipase enzyme impact fat breakdown and oxidation. Other hormones that modulate the action of the Lipase enzyme are the Adrenalin, Cortisol, Growth hormone, and Thyroxin.

o Peripheral exercises can alter local fat deposition, as in exercising the abdominal and gluteal muscles. The main disadvantages of peripheral training, in body fat reduction, are the need for long and tedious training in order to shed down calories. This is accomplished at the expense of the musculoskeletal balance due to isolated partial training of individual muscles. Axial exercises work the whole body and reduce the effort required in planning musculoskeletal anatomical balance. In addition, axial exercises burn calories utilizing major muscles that are capable of expending maximal energy.

11.2.5. PROTEIN CONTENT

o The food intake of proteins is degraded in the intestinal tract into amino acids that are then absorbed in the small intestines. From the small intestine, amino acids travel through the portal vein and end into the systemic circulation, after transiting the liver. This route differs from that of ingested fat, which initially skips the liver via the lymphatic system. Ingested fats reach the heart through the thoracic duct and superior vena cava, instead of the portal vein and inferior vena cava, as do the amino acids and carbohydrates.

o The body can synthesize various nonessential amino acids from the limited number of amino acids ingested daily. In humans, nine essential amino acids have to be supplied from food intake, since these cannot be synthesized by the body[3]. The synthesis of amino acids, from other amino acids, provides adequate pool of amino acids for the synthesis of complex proteins.

o Protein synthesis is achieved by the combined functions of the nucleus and cytoplasm of cells. In the cell nucleus, the DNA transcribes template for protein buildup from ribonucleic acids, RNA. In the cytoplasm, the messenger RNA templates are translated into series of amino acids in peptide chains.

o Exercise enhances protein synthesis of new muscle fibers. It thus diverts the excess amino acids, from being consumed as fuel source, into the synthesis of new muscle protein. Inactivity causes amino acids to convert to fat and stored in fat cells. In the absence of Glucose, aminoacids can be used by liver and kidneys in the gluconeogenesis of glucose.[4] The signaling communication between genetic DNA and muscle workout might take place through the nitric oxide synthase expression.[5]

o Axial training builds major muscles that possess multiple pinnation and multiple origins and insertion thus enables the body to exert maximal force utilizing many joints. Examples of these major muscles, worked out simultaneously by axial training, are the Spinal erectors, Glutei, Quadriceps, Trapezius, Deltoid, Calves, and Triceps, all of which work closely on the axial bones and their immediate proximal attached appendices.

o While peripheral training also undoubtedly targets these muscle groups, neither the load intensity, nor the load volume achieved by peripheral training comes close to those of axial training. Axial training hits most of these muscle groups in single bouts of workout. The Power Clean for example works out the Quadriceps, Glutei, Spinal erectors, Trapezius, Triceps, and Deltoid in quite few seconds, while peripheral training would require at least three different exercises to accomplish the same effect.

11.3. EFFECT OF TRAINING EMPHASIS ON CARDIOVASCULAR FUNCTION

11.3.1. HEART AND LUNG RACING

o The net effect of any exercise fitness plan is best assessed by its impact on cardiovascular performance. The central pump of the cardiovascular system is the heart that benefits significantly from axial training. The heart develops more power by producing contractile tissue, in addition to resetting its neuromuscular sensors in response to the sympathetic stimulation. The left ventricular wall thickens with vigorous training and the resting heart rate drops below 70 beat per minute.

o At peak axial exercise, the heart and respiration race to deliver maximum cardiac output and maximum oxygen extraction. The limiting factor, in reaching peak muscular strength, occurs when cardiac ejection rate exceeds oxygen extraction rate. At this point, arterial blood fails to grab more oxygen from the lungs, despite the increased cardiac output. Thus, muscle cells are forced to cease energy production due to the limited oxygen delivery.

o Regular and adequate axial training pushes that limiting factor to higher levels of cardiac outputs, before oxygen

---

[3] Protein is broken down by digestion into twenty-two amino acids. The following nine are essential amino acids: histidine, isoleucine, leucine, lysine, methionine, phenylalanine, threonine, tryptophan, and valine. Source: **"Review of physiological chemistry"**, by Harold A. Harper, 15th edition, Los Altos, California, 1975.

[4] The carbon skeleton of amino acids goes into the formation of new glucose or fat molecules. The amine group of aminoacids is carried by amino acid arginine to the formation of urea that is excreted by kidneys. Arginine can release nitric oxide gas by the action of a synthase enzyme. The gas relaxes smooth muscles and regulates blood flow.

[5] "Nitric oxide production and NO synthase gene expression contribute to vascular regulation during exercise." By Shen W, et al. Med Science Sports Exercise 1995 Aug; 27(8): 1125-34.

saturation of arterial blood reaches maximum. The mechanism for setting such higher threshold, for cardiopulmonary limitation of peak power, is through sympathetic opening of inactive pulmonary vascular bed. This new vascular circuitry allows greater surface area for gas exchange. On the cellular end, the excessive production of lactates, during peak exercise, alters the ionic composition of blood and increases the rate of extraction of oxygen by the cells. This also increases the rate of hemoglobin binding of oxygen at the pulmonary vascular-alveolar interface.
o Peripheral training alone hinders the reactive response of heart and lung for vigorous activity. Untrained people perspire excessively and run out of breath with minimal multi-joint exercises, due to the sluggish conditioning of the sympathetic regulation of heart and lung. Regular training, with properly managed load volume and intensity, enhances the tolerance to vigorous training. The signs of inadequate sympathetic regulation of the heart and lung, other than excessive perspiration, are excessive dryness or fluid excretion in the upper respiratory tract, dizziness, hyperventilation, arrhythmias, or palpitation.

11.3.2. SUBMAXIMAL CARDIAC POWER OUTPUT
o Peripheral training involves submaximal muscle mass and thus does not require peak cardiac output. Working out the chest or arms, for example, can be performed by rationing limited cardiac output to the working muscles, while reducing blood flow to other muscles, by isometric contraction. Isometric contraction hardens muscles, in motionless state, and thus increases peripheral vascular resistance that leads to reduction in blood flow. The increase in resistance causes increase in pressure and reduction in flow rate according to Ohm's law, $V = IR$, where V is the potential or pressure, R the resistance, and I the current or flow rate.
o The submaximal cardiac work during peripheral training is two-edged weapon. It allows achieving high volume of training before reaching cardiac fatigue, by allowing low intensity training to proceed for longer duration. This helps many people sculpture their body in any manner they wish, in order to fit the sport of their interest. The negative side of working out at submaximal cardiac ejection for long time, by peripheral training, is the loss of ability to condition the heart and lung to accommodate high power output.
o Many people, in the third decade of life and beyond, find axial training extremely taxing. When not performed regularly and adequately at earlier age, axial training upsets the vascular sensors of pressure and blood gases and causes dizziness, long recovery time, and protracted soreness. After few years of training intermission, the sympathetic nervous system might be thrown into chaos, in reaction to few sets of axial exercise.
o The cardiac enzymes adapt to axial training by enhancing aerobic oxidation of lactates. Thus, though the cardiac muscle enlarges, its peak force increases, and its lactate production increases, yet lactates do not accumulate excessively below certain threshold. That threshold of maximum lactate accumulation is elevated by axial training. Without such major muscle work of axial training, the cardiac muscle may not encounter such challenging resistance and stimulation to produce high power output.

11.3.3. ORCHESTRATED CENTRAL DELIVERY
o The vascular network of the cardiovascular system benefits from axial training in three ways, as follows.
  i. New blood capillaries grow around the newly grown cardiac muscle fibers. These are stimulated by the vigorous impulsive forces applied on the ventricular walls, during heavy workout. Thus, the cardiac muscle develops enhanced cellular nutrition and removal of byproducts.
  ii. The neural control of the vascular system improves dramatically, both centrally through vascular control center in the medulla oblongata, as well as peripherally, at the neuromuscular junctions of arterioles.
  iii. Finally, the walls of the blood vessels develop active smooth muscles and rid of fat deposits that narrow and harden the vessels. These three adaptive changes, due to axial training, result from the action of major muscle groups and the enhanced cardiopulmonary work of axial training.
o The distinctive difference in effect, between peripheral and axial training, on fitness is attributed to the way the human brain conducts business. You can determine by choice which exercise you would pick for execution, yet you have no much choice on overriding the cardiovascular and pulmonary integration. All you can do is to force your respiration to endure for the longest possible duration, until the carbon dioxide accumulates and takes control over the respiratory center against your will.
o Your goal, therefore, should be directed towards enhancing the innate mechanism of integration on which your immediate volitional power has little control, but your long term planning can significantly make impact. Peripheral training will stimulate elements of the central cardiovascular and pulmonary regulation system but would not integrate such elements in orchestrated whole activity.

11.4. EFFECT OF TRAINING EMPHASIS ON MUSCULOSKELETAL FUNCTIONS

11.4.1. STRENGTH
o **Force and resistance.** Conventionally, force is defined as the action imparted on external objects by the athlete, while resistance is defined as the reaction of joints to external forces. If forces exceed the ability of tissues to resist, pathology ensues, as follows.

11 AXIAL TRAINING VERSUS PERIPHERAL TRAINING

i. In strength training, care must be taken to maintain forces below the maximum level of resistance. Thus, forces should be kept below the threshold of disrupting internal structures. The common mean of applying this rule is entirely empirical, yet effective. First, you should not execute **sudden resistance** to new weights. This may trigger acute trauma and damage to structures. Second, you should not perform resistance with **unfamiliar** or newly invented technique, unless you understand the applied anatomy of your invention. Technique that breach anatomical bounds may injure joints, ligaments, tendons, muscles, or even bones.

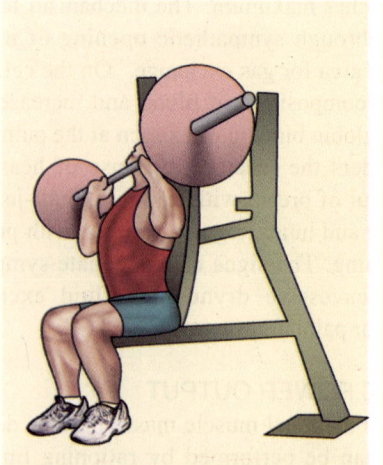 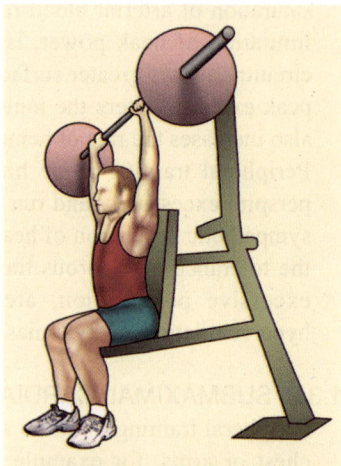

Figure 11.9. Shoulder Press, Start Position with upright torso.

Figure 11.10. Shoulder Press, standalone, unsupported back.

ii. The best example of this rule (of maintaining force below resistance) is the seated Shoulder Press exercise, *Figures 11.9* and *11.10*. Seated Shoulder Press should be performed with the torso in upright position, without the support of the vertical backboard of the designated seat. Leaning backwards against the back support, while pressing, deforms the upper back vertebras and stiffens the shoulder joint. The upright, free seating position, strengthens the hip flexors and the upper back erectors. That maintains normal curvatures at the lumbar, thoracic, and cervical regions. That is because, the force of resistance during seated Shoulder Press travels along the posterior joints of the vertebral joints. When these spinal joints are positioned vertically under the barbell, the balance of forces of resistance will prevent extreme tension on the back of the spines and extreme compression on the front of the spines.

iii. Furthermore, the upright back posture in the Seated Shoulder Press **balances the actions** of the posterior and anterior rotator cuff muscles. These are the Supraspinatus and Subscapularis, respectively. With balanced rotator cuff muscles, your shoulder will not freeze in limited range of motion. You can test the effect of this exercise on shoulder flexibility by front squatting deeply and squatting while lifting overhead weight. If the rotator cuff muscles are balanced then your arms should comfortably support the front Squat and overhead weight. If the Subscapularis is short and tight, due to faulty shoulder exercises or lack of it, then you will have trouble performing that posture.

o **Structural changes.** Axial training imposes significant strain on the major ligaments, cartilages, and bones, thus prepares the body for extreme conditions, as follows.
  i. Over the years, these major mechanical support elements withstand the imposed strain by gaining more structural elastic fibers, cartilaginous, and osseous matrix. The long, slow, and symmetric alteration in musculoskeletal elements lends great help to performing vigorous physical activities, without acute stain, sprain, or rupture of soft tissue elements.
  ii. Peripheral training jeopardizes the buildup of such structural support system, by inadequate and asymmetric straining of dispersed locations in the body. Bodybuilders with huge and strong shoulders may develop arthritic shoulder joint due to excessive overloading, while their lower back and legs are undertrained and inflexible. Diversification of training emphasis ensures symmetric and adequate buildup of structural strength and helps prevent weak and inflexible joints.

o **Mode of muscle contraction.** Axial exercises such as Squat, Clean and Jerk, Snatch, Deadlift, and Goodmorning provide the greatest load volume of eccentric and concentric contraction training of the axial muscles, as follows.
  i. The slow descent, during squatting, gives great sense of strength to the back erectors. These work like brakes, preventing the bodyweight and the barbell from tumbling to the ground.
  ii. The Goodmorning exercise exerts similar effect on the Hamstrings.
  iii. The floor lifts maximize concentric contraction, from minimal recruitment to peak contraction, followed by significant relaxation. These extremes of muscular work stimulate musculoskeletal structures to withstand extremes of virtual forces.[6]
  iv. Although peripheral exercises offer similar combination of muscular contraction, they lack both the maximal systemic influence and maximal muscle mass recruitment. Biceps curls and Bench Press, for example, work both concentric and eccentric contraction but operate at submaximal cardiac output, submaximal sympathetic stimulation, and partial muscle mass recruitment. Performing Biceps curls and Bench Press, without at least one axial exercise such as Deadlift, Squat, or Clean, results in imbalance of the musculoskeletal system. That is

---

[6] Virtual forces result from kinetic motion. For example, you may sense greater forces on the knees during running than during walking or standing.

because the strong peripheral limbs will lack axial structural support, and hence their actions will produce severe and traumatic reactions in the weaker axial frame.

11.4.2. ENDURANCE

o **Endurance kinetics.** Endurance is characteristic of systemic unison of producing power, at low and regular rate, for long duration.
  i. The ingredients of endurance are the abundance of cellular respiratory organelles (mitochondria), the abundance of muscle fuel (carbohydrate, amino acids, and fatty acids), and the abundance of catalytic agents for aerobic oxidation. These catalysts are: calcium, thiamine pyrophosphate, lipoic acid, coenzyme–A, FAD, NAD, and dehydrogenase enzymes. These catalyze the removal of carbon dioxide from pyruvic acid and its conversion to the active compound "acetyl coenzyme–A".
  ii. Though muscle fuel is provided by food intake, or stored fat or glycogen, yet its conversion into useable fuel requires chemical reactions that are catalyzed by many enzymes, in addition to calcium and phosphate ions, through hormonal regulation.
  iii. Skeletal bone maintains blood concentration of calcium and phosphate, under the control of the parathyroid and thyroid hormonal regulation. Axial training intensifies the traffic of mineral ions between the blood and bone such that high rate of bone restructuring and strengthening is ongoing, simultaneously with high rate of energy production, within the major muscle mass acting on the skeletal bone.
  iv. Your short-term endurance might be limited by your threshold of maximal lactate accumulation that is capable of inducing fatigue and inaction. Yet, your long-term endurance depends mainly on the hormonal maintenance of steady blood homeostasis[7]. Strong bones are great assets to the stability of blood homeostasis and are acquired by axial training, good nutrition, proper rest, and abstinence from destructive habits.
  v. Marathon runners demonstrate the validity of the hypothesis that heavy bones of males attribute to their higher strength at endurance marathons, *Figure 11.11.*

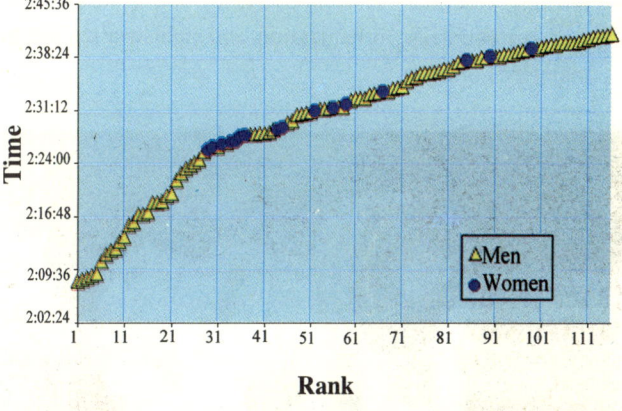

Figure 11.11. Results of the New York city marathon show the dominance of men in marathon running. First women ranked at 29th position. First male ran 26 miles in 2:08:07 hour. First female ran the same distance in 2:25:56 hours.

o **Brain coding**. Enhancing endurance is better achieved by performing activities similar to the kind of sport that is practiced. Thus, training on running enhances endurance during similar activities, but not across different disciplines. The same can be said about Weightlifting. Building strong and big muscles by peripheral training requires long time to translate to endurance or strength, in Weightlifting. The main reason for the lack of reciprocity of skills across different activities is attributed to neural adaptation. As a newly learned language occupies distinctive physical area on the cerebrum, motor skills might also be handled similarly by the brain.

o **Chronic fatigue.** Endurance training is a basic component of any successful planning, as follows.
  i. Strength training relies on the aerobic oxidation phase for regeneration of the consumed ATP molecules and the production of substrates for protein synthesis. Therefore, getting strong and staying strong requires adequate endurance training to enhance recovery.
  ii. Young competitive Weightlifters can train two or three times per day, and feel good and healthy each time. This is a sign of strong bones and great ability of their system to supply nutrients, remove byproducts, and generate lost tissues and enzymes. Athletes with low endurance require days or weeks to recuperate before returning to training.
  iii. Beside the higher strength and endurance of males over females, gained by developing heavy bones in endurance marathons, males also suffer less from chronic fatigue, compared to females. Most probably, axial training may ameliorate chronic fatigue in females, and untrained people, by stacking greater amounts of minerals in the bones, thus allowing long and stable blood homeostasis and hence higher stamina.

---

[7] Homeostasis refers to the ability of an organism or a cell to maintain internal equilibrium by adjusting its physiological processes through addition or removal of ions, such that biochemical reactions maintain designated range of function.

11 AXIAL TRAINING VERSUS PERIPHERAL TRAINING

11.4.3. FLEXIBILITY

o **Strength and motion.** Flexibility is crucial to performance since the strongest muscle would not finalize motion unless joints comply with fullest range of flexibility. Peripheral training is notorious in undermining flexibility since exercises are executed in bits and pieces and across few joints, without regard to whole body performance. Many Bodybuilders cannot flex the shoulders in the Front Squat of the Clean because of the diminished flexibility of the shoulder and lower back. Overhead squatting is formidable to all athletes, but Weightlifters. Those train pelvic and shoulder girdles simultaneously and regularly. The author recalls an incident when a guy in the gym, who never trained on any sport, was able to join an ongoing session of Weightlifting and execute the Deadlift with 500-pound barbell. He weighed about 250 pounds. Yet, he was not able to perform the Clean or the Snatch with a 100-pound barbell, due to stiff shoulders, back, and legs. In *Figure 11.12,* an Egyptian Weightlifters can squat as deep as anatomy can tolerate, simultaneously, with flexing his shoulders and supporting a 167.5 kg barbell. In *Figure 11.13,* the same lifter is hyperextending his lower back and excessively thrusting his chest, simultaneously with widely sprung legs, under 175 kg. Therefore, the combination of strength and full range of motion is attainable with regular Weightlifting training. The Weightlifter shown in those two figures was trained by his brother, ex-Weightlifter, both had limited access to modern scientific Weightlifting. Their only exposure to information was through living in the seaport city of Port Said, where major international sea trade takes place. It is interesting to note that before the Radio and TV era, sports flourished mostly in costal towns, where inhabitants have greater opportunities for entertainment and exposure to foreign cultures. Inner cities, far away from the sea, did not catch up with global trends in sport and indulged heavily in farming and other survival activities that secure basic living commodities. On the other side of the world, in the western countries, urbanization and industrialization are doing away with strength and flexibility in the populace majority.

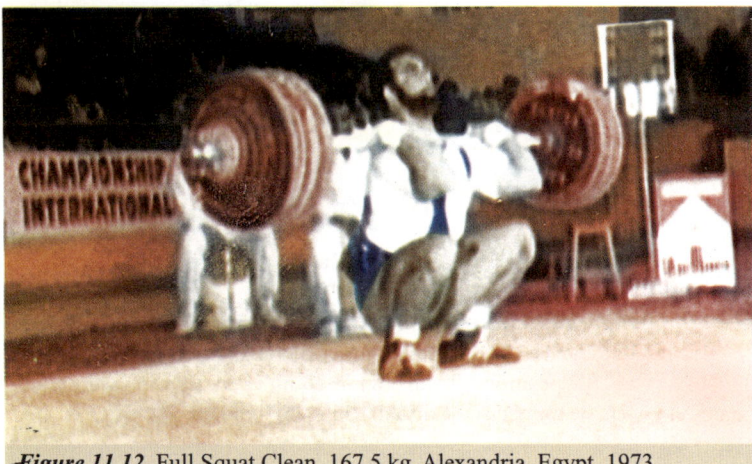

Figure 11.12. Full Squat Clean, 167.5 kg. Alexandria, Egypt, 1973.

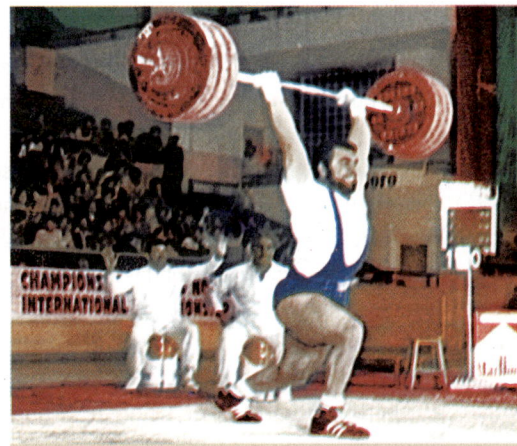

Figure 11.13. Full Extension Jerk, 175 kg. Alexandria, Egypt, 1973

o **Maintaining flexibility.** The main ingredients to flexibility are regular and adequate stretching of joints to full range, regular and adequate balanced strengthening of muscles around joints, and regular and adequate training in proper range of motion, as follows.

  i. Stretching alone prepare muscles, ligaments, and tendons for resistance training by modifying the neural perception and control of joints. You should not try lifting weights without prior stretching, in the form executing the same motion of lifting in full range without weight. This allows your mind to prepare the strategy of executing the proper technique. In *Figure 11.14,* the lifter tackled the Snatch lift of 115 kg with inadequate stretching. The outcome of rigid, incompliant major joints is very apparent. The lifter failed to pull adequately, to extend arms, to hyperextend lower back, or to stabilize his pelvis. In *Figure 11.15,* the same lifter, in competition, was able to lift 125 kg, with adequate flexibility. Thus, stretching is very crucial to neuromuscular performance.

  ii. Strengthening exercises are performed at slower rate, with progressive weights. These extend stretching beyond negative resistance to concentric contraction. Strengthening knock down weak and fragile muscle fibers and replaces them with stronger ones. It is not true that strengthening and flexibility are mutually exclusive, *Figures 11.16* thru *11.18*. Strengthening only leads to stiffness when training is limited to restricted range of motion.

  iii. Training on sport-like activities generates dynamic virtual forces that exceed Bodybuilding strength training. In strong athletes, many inflexible joints can perform better at heavy resistance, such as during the Power Clean and Power Snatch.

AXIAL TRAINING VERSUS PERIPHERAL TRAINING

Ibrahim Abu Kalila
(Courtesy of Ibrahim S. A. G. Abu Kalila and Dr. Salah F. El-Hewie).

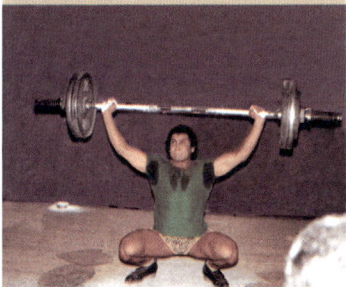

Figure 11.14. Incomplete Snatch lift in training, 115 kg, Alexandria, Egypt, *1973*. This lift shows inflexible elbows, shoulders, back, hips, and knees. Inflexibility is due to recent conversion from Bodybuilding to Weightlifting. Note the imbalance between shoulder and pelvic girdles. Note also the dismal condition of the gym.

It will take this lifter eleven years to be able to stabilize his shoulders in full Squat overhead lifting. His reflexes will only adapt to regular and progressive axial training. The cardinal reflex is that of lower back hyperextension, when the knees and hips flex and the shoulders elevate and abduct.

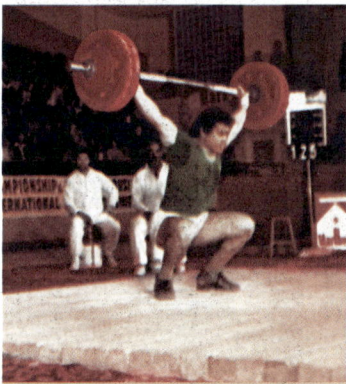

Figure 11.15. Complete Snatch lift in contest, 125 kg. This lift shows enhanced flexibility. Alexandria, Egypt, 1973. The shoulder-back-pelvis is still tight. Now, the lifter has advanced to state level. Note the signs of Marlboro sponsorship. As a novice champion, he relies heavily on his rams and shoulders, with less reliance on thighs, hips, and lower back. These will develop in a decade of hard training.

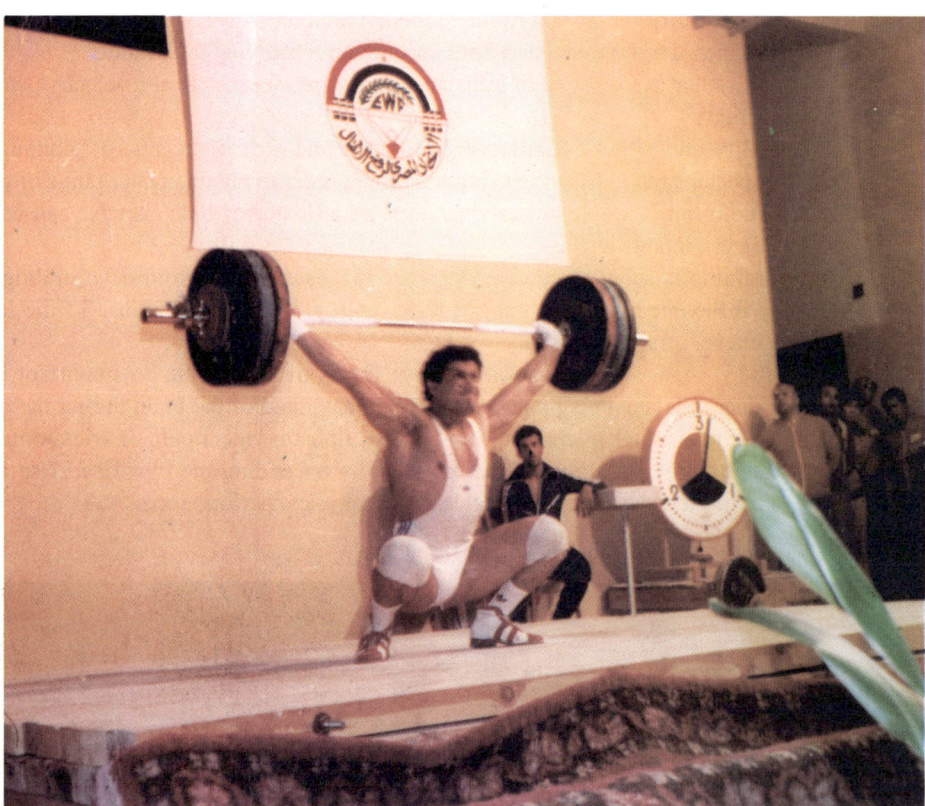

Figure 11.16. Complete Snatch lift in contest, 147.5 kg. Now, the entire axial spines, shoulders, and pelvis are in full coordination. The two wrapped knees hint to over training.

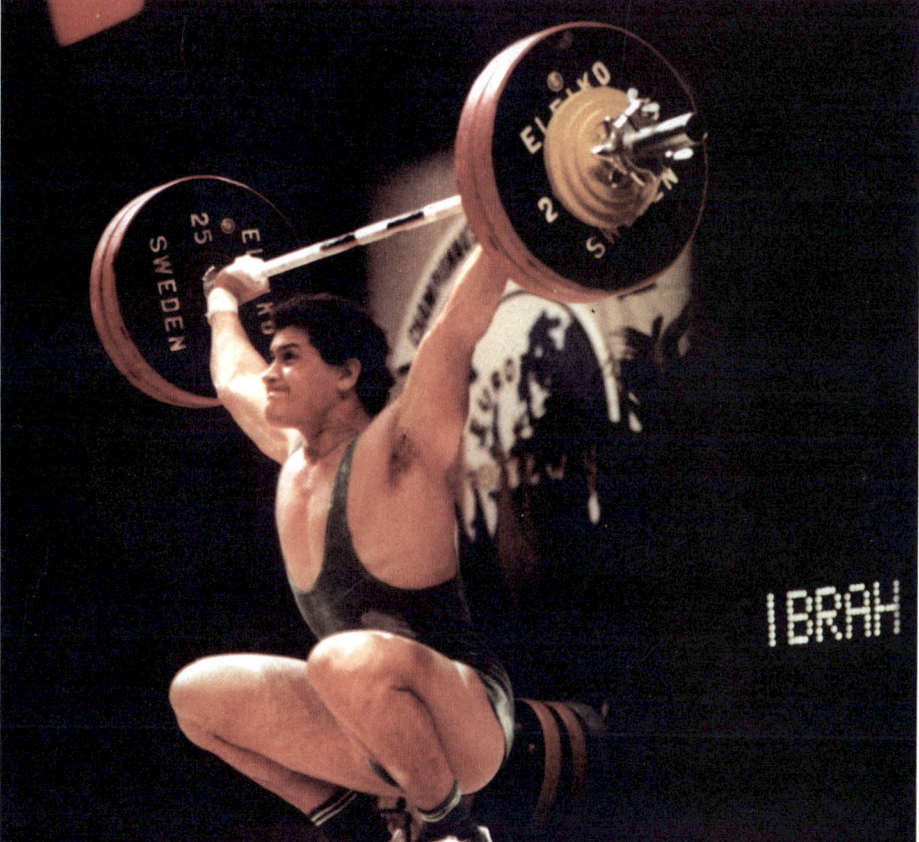

Figure 11.17. Exquisite flexibility, coordination, and agility. Snatch of 150 kg, Los Angeles Olympic games, 1984. The absence of knee wraps and waist belts attest to the well planned program this lifter had undergone. The erect lower back during Full Squat, properly placed feet, thrust chest, and elevated and abducted shoulders, all are the outcome of sixteen years of serious peripheral and axial training.

11 AXIAL TRAINING VERSUS PERIPHERAL TRAINING

o **Causes of inflexibility.** These can reside in the dynamic imbalance of muscular recruitment, short and rigid ligaments, or deformed bones. The following is a brief account on remedying inflexibility.
   i. Inflexibility that is attributed to imbalanced joints may benefit from selective strength training of the weak aspect of these joints.
   ii. Inflexibility due to long duration of shortened and stiff ligaments, or tendons, are difficult to cure and might require special stretching and relaxing training in order to regain greater range of motion.
   iii. If bone deformities are the underlying cause of inflexibility then exercise can only maintain current state, without further deterioration.
   iv. Axial training is suburb is preventing major muscle masses from deteriorating insidiously. Many Bodybuilders develop inflexible shoulders, upper and lower back, and legs, because of the lack of combined training of both girdles in every training session.
   v. Relaxation, yoga, and meditation increase levels of Melatonin, an important hormone that promotes deep and restful sleep. Melatonin is produced by the pineal gland of the brain during the darkness of night. Overnight urine samples contain higher concentration of 6-sulphatoxymelatonin, a Melatonin breakdown product. Melatonin increases body warmth and relaxes muscles by overriding the overtone of spinal motoneurons. This allows the person to master control of his muscles during physical performance.

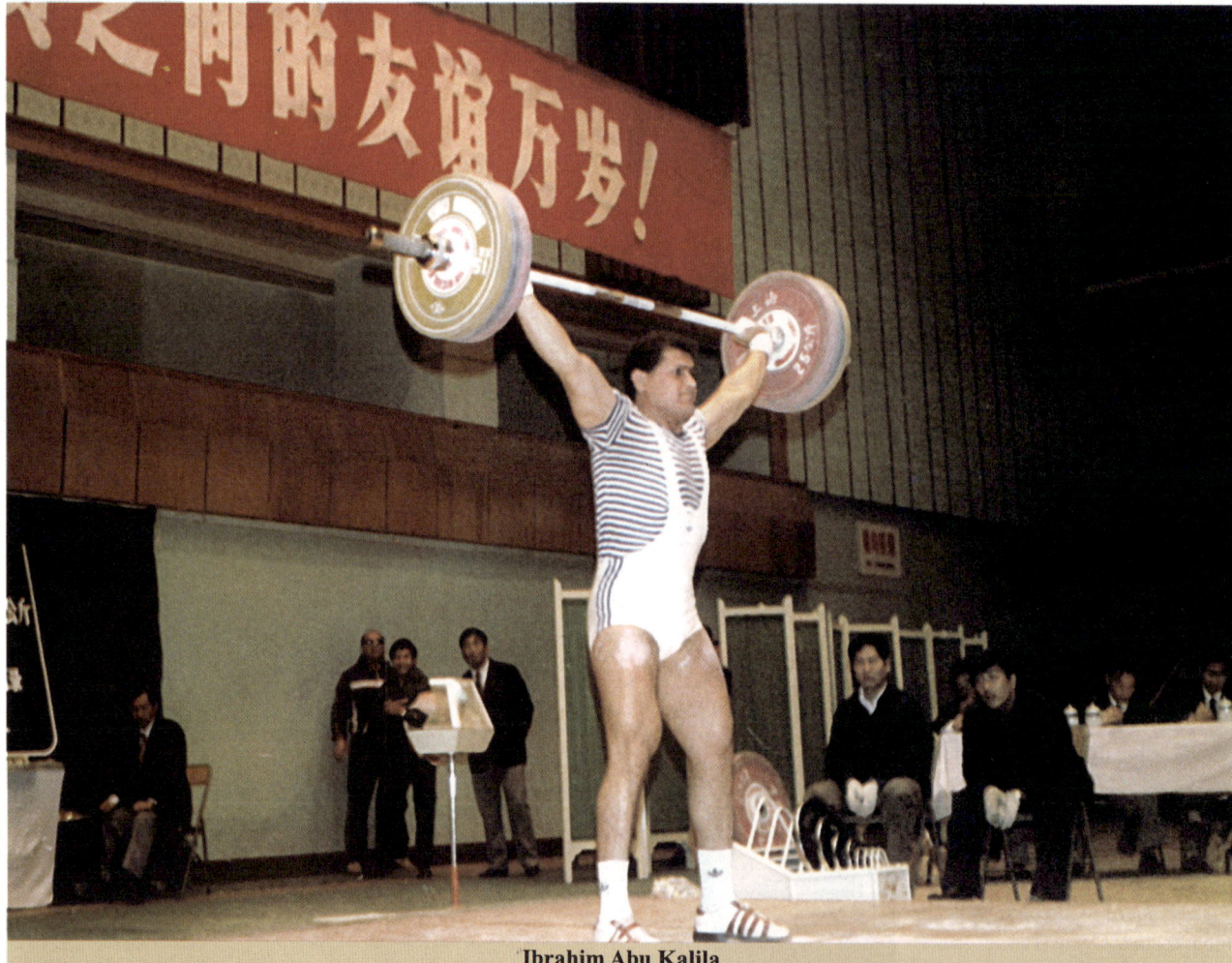

Ibrahim Abu Kalila

Figure 11.18. Complete Snatch lift in contest, 153 kg. It took fifteen years of hard work to get that far. Axial training fosters the thighs, spinal erectors, shoulders, and arms to perform such freestyle heavy lift. The speed of lifting such heavy weight requires more than just strong muscles. It requires well adapted reflexes. The balance of muscular forces is critical in Full Squat Overhead Snatch. Very long and consistent training is required to balance the scapular forces with the lower body forces, around flexible and strong spines.

11.5. EFFECT OF TRAINING EMPHASIS ON POWER OUTPUT

Muscular power output during physical activities is determined by the combination of the viability and strength of the muscles, the adequacy of the neural control over muscles and other systems, and, most importantly, the will and skill of the person. These essential elements interplay as follows.

AXIAL TRAINING VERSUS PERIPHERAL TRAINING

11.5.1. INVOLUNTARY CONTROL
Performing axial exercises by unaccustomed people induces hyperventilation, perspiration, and excessive palpitation. Even strong and well-built Bodybuilders experience such sympathetic hyperactivity when performing axial exercises, anew. Weightlifters master the skill of meditated relaxation prior to peaking muscular contraction. Weightlifters can impose complete silence of neuromuscular activity, immediately preceding maximal storming recruitment of fiber contraction. Such learned skill of neuromuscular control is well known to many people. Those have long learned various ways of control of movements of involuntary muscles, such as those of the pupils, ears, and of hair papilla. This autonomic regulation of motor activity affects muscular power output through the modulation of the cardiovascular, cardiopulmonary, and neuromuscular responses. The anatomic proof that meditation can alter muscular power output resides in the presence of alpha and gamma motor nerve fibers that control neuromuscular control. The alpha fibers convey voluntary brain signals and reflex signals to the contracting muscle, whereas the gamma nerve fibers convey the involuntary brain signals to muscle spindles of the contracting muscles. Thus, higher brain functions, other than mere voluntary motor decision, can alter muscular strength. Loss of self-esteem and anxiety are examples of such brain stresses that affect performance negatively.

11.5.2. FEEDBACK REGULATION OF AXIAL MUSCLES
Learning how to orchestrate motor control, in order to maximize power production, is promoted by axial training. This sort of training synchronizes major working muscles in performing complex tasks. Many people experience sudden loss of voluntary control of a limb or a major muscle group due to various reasons such as overtraining, chronic insomnia, fasting, alcohol and smoking, or due to unaccustomed activities. The integrity of the motor units, and the central system that incorporate such motor units, determines the status of voluntary control. Axial training enhances such integrity by promoting new formation of muscle fibers, blood capillaries, and nerve fibers in the axial locations, where control of the musculoskeletal stability is pivotal. Animals, for example dogs, can twist their body and land on their four legs, when dropped, in upside down position to the ground, from appropriate heights. This axial equilibrium is controlled by the vestibular apparatus of the inner ears, in conjunction with the neuromuscular regulation of the central nervous system. These receive signals from the proprioception sensors located along the major joints in the neck, back, pelvis, and legs. Thus, even if you have developed large and strong muscles by peripheral training, you will need axial training to enhance the weak links between proprioceptors, the vestibular sensors, and the brain central control.

11.5.3. GUIDING THE FIRE
In the end, the whole purpose of physiological control of the body is to determine how much fire is needed to produce desired power output. Thus, the respiratory center works, with both voluntary and involuntary brain centers, to regulate oxygen delivery and carbon dioxide removal. The cardiovascular center is mainly commanded by the involuntary brain control and only reports to voluntary cessation of physical operation. Axial training promotes and refines the manner of where and when such "physiological fire" should take place. You might already experienced strange sensation when you try to perform new activities, or after long period without practice. Even the eight hours of night-sleep may require little refreshment, of the brain and memory, about the best way to go around a new day of activity. The delusion of gaining great motor skill from peripheral training dominates most weight training activities. As soon as people start seeing muscles growing, blood vessels bulging under skin, and strength enhanced by peripheral training, they content themselves with the easy and sure gain of individual and free activity, without the tutelage of a coach. Yet, experience has shown the great importance of complex activities, such as running, freestyle lifting, Plyometrics, swimming, and yoga, in improving the system as a whole, not just piece by piece. My early life experience was with fellows who perfected arm strengthening and bulking huge chest and leg muscles, yet were unable to Squat or breathe properly during unaccustomed activities.

11.5.4. RATIONING YOUR EMOTION
Axial training is a learning experience of the control of mind over the body. Instead of being hyped with stimulating energy, prior to executing tough peripheral exercises, you will learn to silence such stimulating hype during axial exercises. Axial exercises demand a sequence of consecutive decisions to be made, voluntarily and involuntarily, during a snap of fractions of a second. Each decision requires specific level of stimulation in order to attain graceful execution of motion. In *Figure 11.19*, the lifter was able to perform strong pull and deep squat but failed to tighten his

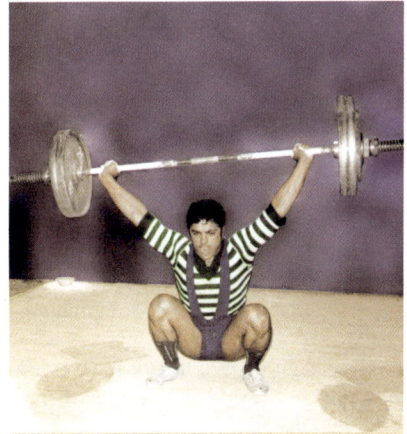

Figure 11.19. Full Squat Snatch. Alexandria, Egypt, 1974, 122.5 kg.

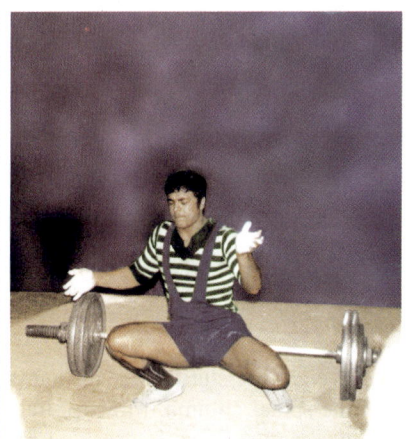

Figure 11.20. Failed Snatch and forward escape. Alexandria, Egypt, 1974, 122.5 kg.

11. AXIAL TRAINING VERSUS PERIPHERAL TRAINING

back and thrust chest. The result was imbalance by placing the barbell center of mass away, in front of the feet balls. In *Figure 11.20,* after losing control, the lifter was able to bail out by dropping the bar from behind the body. The main reason for failure, in this lifter, was poor rationing of emotion. The aggressive pull and dangerously deep overhead squat was not followed by adequate alertness.

Coaches have to teach trainees the skill of relaxation and the habit of focusing on sequential execution of events. This lends each portion of the execution mechanism its maximal delivery of power. You cannot be hyped up when you lift Power Clean, for example. In such complex motion, you must execute phases of activities that require very slow motion with maximal muscular contraction, before your body and the bar accumulate adequate momentum to initiate a ballistic course of motion.

11.6. EFFECT OF TRAINING EMPHASIS ON SPEED

11.6.1. MENTAL WILL
Enduring fast pace activity, for long duration, requires overcoming lack of motivation, distraction, or apprehension from unaccustomed course of events. Axial training invigorates imagination and lends a sense of purposeful involvement in playful activity thus reduces distraction and apprehension. Performing axial activities such as running, Plyometrics, or Weightlifting advances the knowledge of the expected course of events, when performing specific actions. Weightlifters are perfect examples that demonstrate the significance of knowing how the body behaves at extremes of strain. Embarking on such dangerous venture of Weightlifting is made safe by progressive and gradual increase of speed during lifting. The learned lesions from Weightlifting are very rich in substance and cannot be mastered without practice and constant development.

11.6.2. DYNAMICS OF MOVING MASS
o   Speeding body matter energizes each part of the body, according to its mass density and its relation to the center of mass of the whole body. Thus, swinging an arm at fast pace could generate more resistance energy at the shoulder than during weight training. Most injuries to musculoskeletal structures result from mismanaging speedy motion. This applies to warming up with exercises that are irrelevant to the core exercises, in terms of speed. It also applies to executing exercises in improper sequence. Accounting for the effect of speed in increasing forces, by changing momentum, should be an essential element of training.

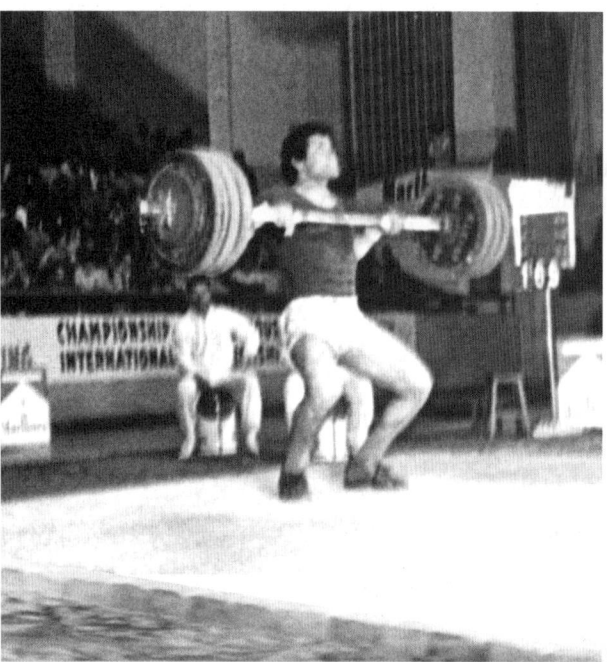 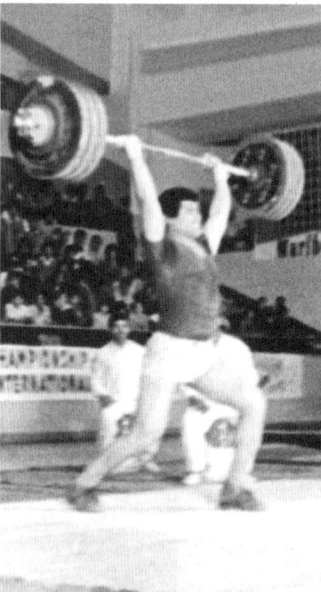 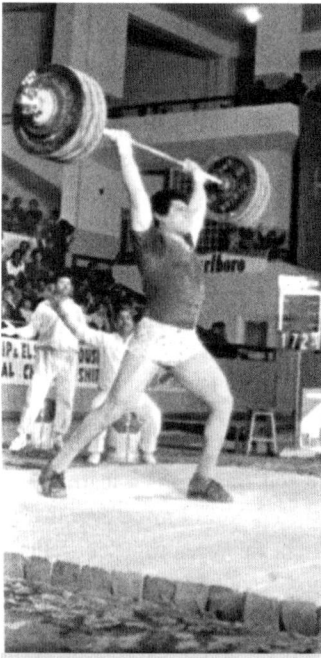

Figure 11.21. Clean pull with strong shoulder transverse adduction and extension, to chest high level. Alexandria, Egypt, 1973, in training, 165 kg.

Figure 11.22. Failed Jerk lift due to lax low back. Alexandria, Egypt, 1973, in training, 172.5 kg.

Figure 11.23. Successful Jerk lift. Alexandria, Egypt, 1973, in training, 172.5 kg.

o   Weightlifters utilize the distinctive body design of two heavy masses; skull and pelvis, at the ends of the skeletal lever; the spinal column. Moving such body design around the center of the lever- the lower back- generates great angular momentum. This is executed by throwing the head backwards and thrusting the pelvis forwards, while maintaining tight spines and pivoting on the feet balls. For lay people, such body motion is frightening, even without external weights. Yet, axial training does not only enhance the strength of muscles that support this extreme extension, but it also enforces the control on timing of motion, without exceeding structural limits. In *Figure 11.21,* the lifter is utilizing the head's backward retreat and pelvic thrust under the bar, in aggressive Clean Pull. The timing of the pull, body torque, and dipping are gained by regular and serious training. In *Figure 11.22,* the lifter failed to thrust his chest forwards, failed to hyperextend his back, and failed to thrust the rear leg backwards. The result was imbalance and failure. . In *Figure 11.23,* after rectified those three mistakes, the lifter and was able to achieve successful lift.

o Executing such extremes of motion cannot be performed on part-time or casual basis. In fact, few days of intermission of training can result in intolerance to strongly impulsive movements. The top ranking Weightlifters can easily incur acute trauma to the lower back muscles, when they experience overconfidence or ignore the essentials of Weightlifting. Most such acute injuries are strains to muscles and ligaments that support the spines, and rarely affect the spinal discs or joints.

11.6.3. MUSCULAR EFFECTS

Fast physical actions are effectively executed not by large and strong muscles but rather by fast twitching and highly recruited muscle fibers. These are enhanced by similar activities of fast and vigorous movements, in training. As the muscles develop adequate neural control for vigorous movements, the associated connective tissues also develop higher tensile strength. In addition, the supporting bone is also enforced by mineral deposition, on long period of training. The general characteristics of these processes of structural adaptation to momentum changes are the distribution of tensile strength of soft tissues and bone density according to axial stresses, from the feet to the skull, *Figures 11.24* thru *11.26*. Although the lower body generates most of the momentum that speeds lifting, yet scapular muscles are crucial to transferring, supporting, and balancing speedy movements.

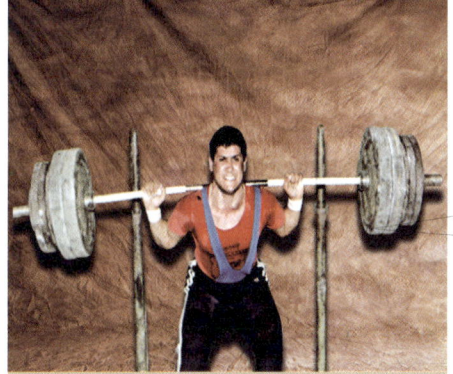
Figure 11.24. Heavy Back Squat is the last axial training in most Weightlifting sessions. It is a basic strengthening exercise for the thighs, hips, and spines. Above all, it conditions the heart and nervous system to tolerate great resistance.

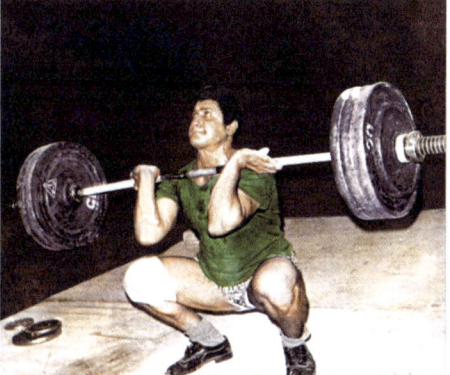
Figure 11.25. Full Squat Clean requires both strong legs and scapular muscles. Abu Kalila was able to lift this 155 kg Clean after two years of training, at bodyweight 88 kg and age 23. His prior Bodybuilding training required him to work harder on skipped axial elements.

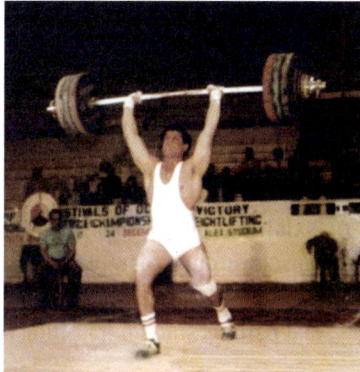
Figure 11.26. Strong muscles alone do not guarantee perfect performance. Inflexible shoulders and fatigued lower back are very apparent in this stiffed jerk performance and during the long travel, from floor to overheads.

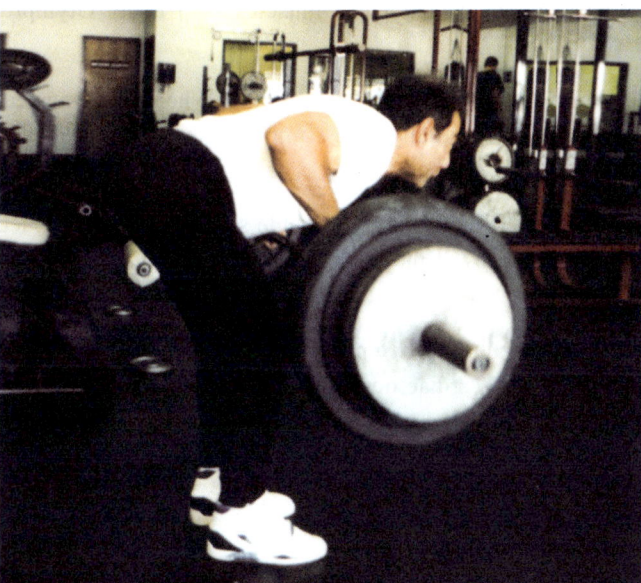
Figure 11.27. Bent-over row with fully straightened lower back, in horizontal position

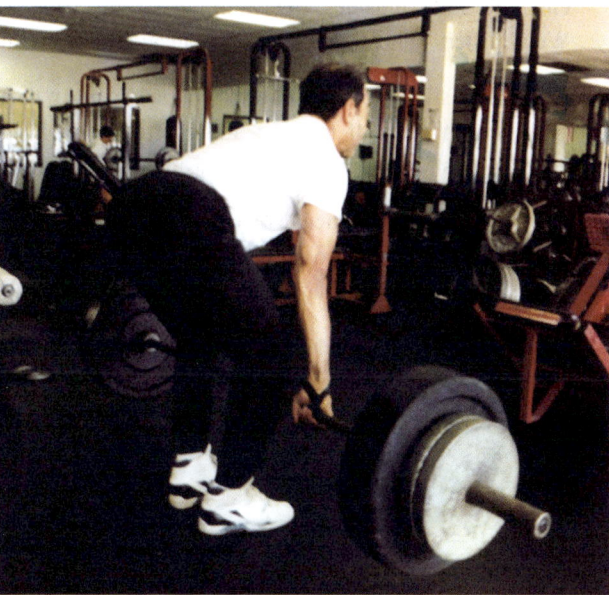
Figure 11.28. Bent-over and row with oblique back.

11 AXIAL TRAINING VERSUS PERIPHERAL TRAINING

Weightlifters perfect scapular strengthening in the ballistic mode of contraction. *Figures 11.27* and *11.28* show the difference between executing the "Bent-over and row" by a Weightlifter, compared to Bodybuilding style, *Figure 6.6,* Chapter Six. As the bar is pulled upwards, the lower back is kept strictly horizontal and arched inwards. The back can assume oblique position during lowering the weight, not during elevating it. The regular and frequent performance of this version, of Bent-over and row, is alternated with the Pulls and Deadlifts. The motion of this kind of Bent-over and row proceeds in ballistic manner upwards, and in eccentric slow motion downwards. Its main purpose is strengthening the middle Trapezius muscles. In addition, the back erectors, Hamstrings, Latissimus dorsi, Teres, and long head of Triceps are also activated. Yet, the most important aspect of ballistic Bent-over and row, with strict horizontal back, is the axial strengthening under impulsive forces. This is paramount to strengthening safe, ballistic lifting.

11.7. HIGHLIGHTS OF CHAPTER ELEVEN

1. **Axial training** can be defined as exercise activities that simultaneously involve muscles proximal to the spines, the pelvic, and the shoulder girdles. These exercises engage both pelvic and shoulder girdles in simultaneous execution of resistance. Thus, axial training enhances the muscles that directly or closely act on the vertebral column, *Figure 11.1*. Major axial muscles are the Trapezius, the Erector spinae, the Glutei, the Hamstrings, the Deltoids, the Pectoralis, the Iliopsoas, and the Quadriceps. Examples of such exercises are the Clean and Jerk, Snatch, Pulls, Deadlift, Goodmorning, and Squat.

2. Peripheral training may be defined as exercise activities that work out distal **muscles and involve mostly one girdle but not the other,** during execution of resistance. Thus, peripheral training enhances the muscles that act on the joints that are farther peripheral from the vertebral column.

3. Physical gains from axial training are **deeper than superficial muscles**. Therefore, changes in the outer contour of the trainee require long training, before bulging of muscles and exaggeration of body's curvatures become apparent.

4. Axial training **challenges the cardiovascular, pulmonary, and neural systems.** The slightest contraction of major muscle groups disrupts systemic and cellular functions and causes many people to worry about wrongdoing. With regular axial training, the sympathetic system adapts by budgeting blood flow and muscular recruitment in a manner that permits smooth transition from regular to vigorous activities

5. The rule of thumb in planning is including **systemic and regular portion of axial exercises** into your daily workout, based on weekly cyclic routine. This practice should continue even if you do not notice changes in size or definition of muscles. You would not be able to assess early gains in deep para-vertebral, spinal erectors, shoulder rotators, hip adductors and abductors, or Hamstrings by looking in front view mirror.

6. Many Olympic athletes have developed their **personal tricks** of developing outstanding peripheral muscles in order to enhance axial muscles. Developing strong arms, shoulders, abdomen, and chest muscles help many Olympic Weightlifters to breakthrough long plateau of performance.

7. One can easily determine to alter his or her **body composition** by persistent peripheral training. When supplemented with few minutes of running, Plyometrics, or whole body exercises, on daily basis, improvement follows in the endurance, strength, and flexibility, aside from adjustment in bodyweight and body fat.

8. People with **diseased neurovascular control** do not have the luxury of enjoying comfortable standing or walking, let alone exercising. Atherosclerosis and other hyaline degenerative diseases of the arterial and arteriolar walls interfere with sympathetic vascular regulation and impede rationing of energy demands during exercises.

9. Peripheral training involves **submaximal muscle mass and thus does not require peak cardiac output**. Working out the chest or arms, for example, can be performed by rationing limited cardiac output to the working muscles, while reducing blood flow to other muscles by isometric contraction.

Chapter 12 Making Training Choices

12.1. SETTING GOALS

12.1.1. EXPOSURE AND INDIVIDUAL CIRCUMSTANCES

o   Embarking on the right training program depends on many factors. Some of these factors are optional choices made by the individual, while others are imposed by permanent circumstances.

o   Among the optional factors that guide training choices are: athletic ambition and drive to endure experimentation, training for health and fitness or for competition, and education and effort to advance repertoire of knowledge. The drive to venture into systemic and long entertaining activity that does not return immediate material gain is, most probably, an innate human drive. The benefit gained from training, in the form of improved health and fitness, cannot explain the motivation of the already young and healthy adults, those indulge in strenuous and demanding physical training. In addition, people with less educational background always excel better in training than those with advanced education. The main reason in such trend is, most probably, the desire of the deprived to compensate for lost opportunities to better their life.

o   Imposed factors are beyond the control of the person such as age, level of previous training, personal limitation such as diseases and deformities, and timely access to proper training knowledge.

o   Setting clear and enduring personal goals depends on your vision during various phases of life. Whatever has shaped your perception of issues, will undoubtedly impact your choices. Nobody will coerce you to get out and engage in motivating training but your own mindset of believes. Your earliest exposure to strength sport and active lifestyle, guides you through the initial choices of strength training.

o   From my personal experience, I discovered Weightlifting by mere accident and fell in love with it since then. When many of my high school fellows were squandering their leisure time in vanities, I trained seriously and passionately. My first exposure to Weightlifting, though, was not very pleasant. As naïve novice to sport, I was displeased with the dismal conditions of Weightlifting gyms (dens is better wording), the sloppy and inexpensive clothes of the lifters, and the screaming and grunting during lifting. Yet, in those dismal training dens, I met a coach with graduate education in engineering and physical training from East Germany who had convincingly altered my misperceptions of Weightlifting. I struggled for some time with the neat pictures of Bodybuilders, and what they stand for, versus the persuasive reasoning of the Weightlifting coach, *Figures 12.1* thru *12.5*.

12.1.2. DISCOVERY CONQUEST

From my personal experience, other fellows had started with me and gone through the same experience of exposure, yet after few years, each individual followed different course. Many resorted to sport in their leisure time and dismissed it during the school season. Others never appreciated the role of sport in shaping the personal repertoire of accomplishments. All, including myself, never appreciated the cumulative effects of regular and dedicated training. That cannot be gained in haste, cannot be reclaimed after long intermission, and that distinguishes athletes from others, for lifelong duration. I have committed myself to training with intuitive passion that was devoid of any material health or fitness gains. Training was crucial to my psychic balance than to my physical fitness. Among my fellow trainees, some educated and many uneducated, the common impetus to enduring training and committing time and resources, away from other essentials of surviving in society, was the keen sense of discovery. There was challenging conquest in discovering how to compete and beat other strong and accomplished athletes, with just sticking around and working out like others. Of course, there are many other fields in life that await our dearest efforts to discover and conquer. Yet, Weightlifting was one of the greatest conquests, at least for me. None of Newton's laws of mechanics would have gotten my attention, without learning in practice, how mass, distance, and time constitute the basics of existence. In addition, the greatest two mathematicians, Isaac Newton and Archimedes, both had developed their understanding of nature by appreciation and practical observation of real natural events.

12 MAKING TRAINING CHOICES

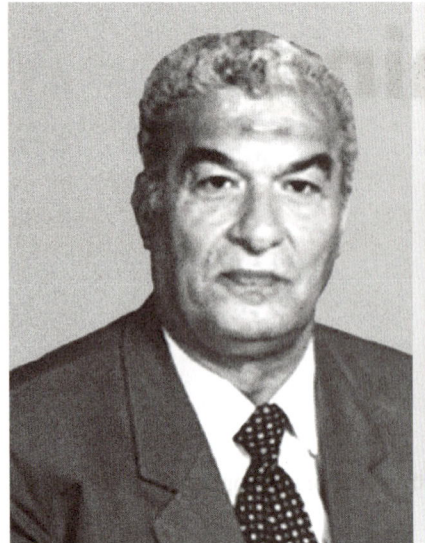

Figure 12.1.

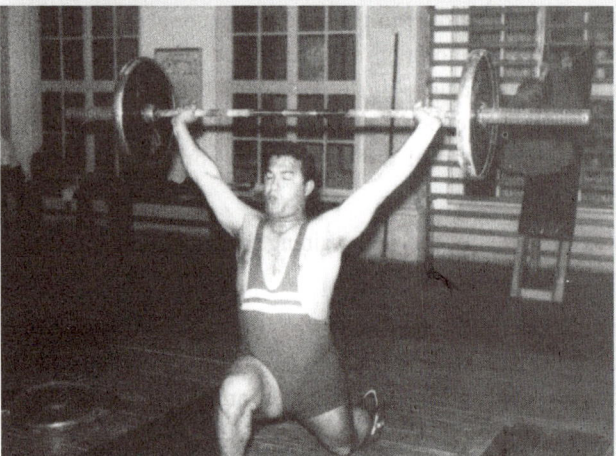

Figure 12.2.

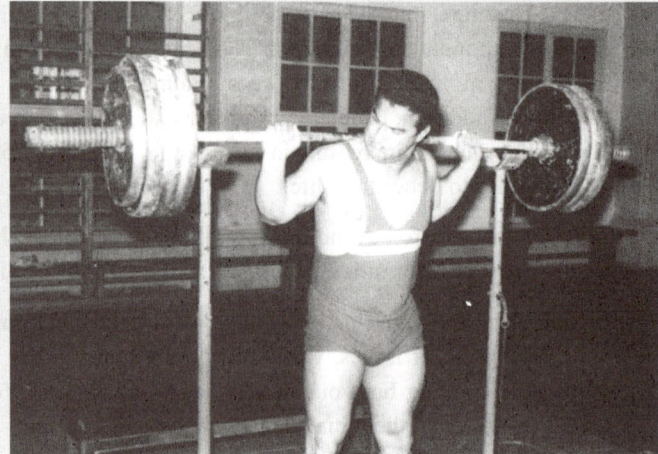

Figure 12.3.   *Figure 12.4.*

Figure 12.1. Mohammad Al-Kassabany.
No other man, I have known, has devoted his life to learning and teaching Weightlifting as this mentor. His passion to this sport surpassed all his other social and professional commitments. He committed himself to training from the age of 34, through his retirement, as a bank executive. As an agricultural engineer and economist, he added long needed "class" to this impoverished sport. He was the first coach to use pencil and paper to document events, in a sport dominated by illiterate followers. He showed up three days every week, at 2:00 pm, and ran the training session until 5:00 or 6:00 pm, for all the years I knew him (1967-1984). From the dusty training rooms, to the lecturing classes about Weightlifting, to the offices of Club managers, he spared no effort to make the sport known, even to the deaf ears and the indifferent politicians. His passionate commitment contributed to the success of all his five children who joined colleges and graduated in different disciplines. None of his children got involved in any sport activity.

Figure 12.2. In 1966, Al-Kassabany was sent to East Germany to pursue higher academic training in Weightlifting. The socialist government of Gamal Abdel Nasser had sponsored aggressive educational and sport programs in cooperation with the eastern communist bloc. His one-year academic training, in Leipzig, East Germany, had polished his entire training methodology. He returned to Egypt with strong belief in axial training and the effective and predictable course of progressive incremental resistance training. In this photo, he was studying the breakdown of the overhead Jerk style, which he will teach others, for many years later.

Figure 12.3. Although, he trained mainly on the old and obsolete leg lunging technique, he was the first to introduce and insist on the Full-Squat lifting technique. This photo is a part of comparative research on the difference between Full-Squat Snatch and Leg-Spring Snatch. It was conclusive from his research that Leg-Spring will never lead to farther progress in Weightlifting. He never attempted to teach his trainees this cumbersome form of freestyle lifting.

Figure 12.4. In this photo, of 175 kg Back Squat, he developed solid belief that Back Squat is an essential component of training for Weightlifting and that the Squat has to fall at the end of training sessions, after the core Olympic lifts.

MAKING TRAINING CHOICES 12

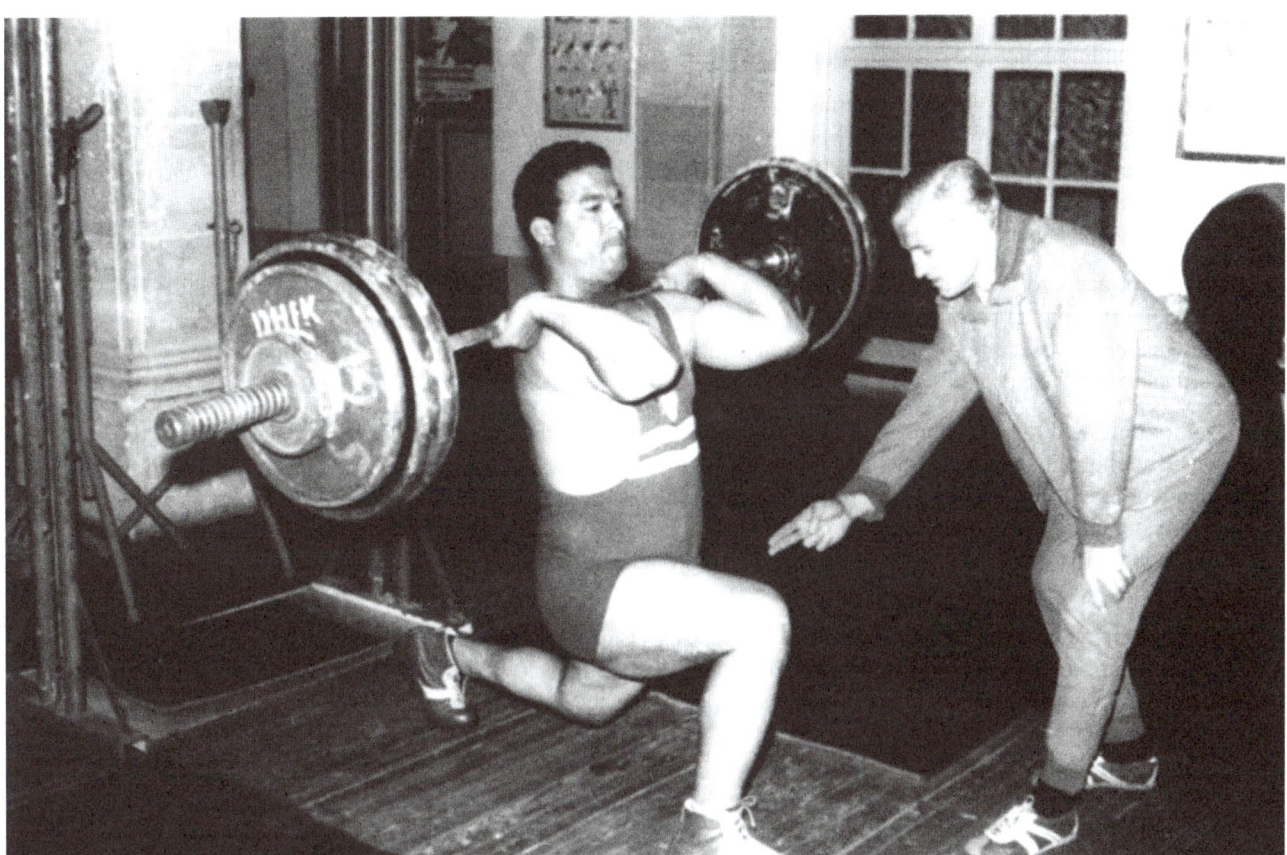

Figure 12.5. The East German coach and professor, and the Egyptian coach-in-training, are analyzing the split-leg Clean and Jerk in 130 kg barbell, in the year 1966.

o Although this lifting style will never be taught again to beginners, it was never thought, in 1966, that the world will soon change beyond return. Here, the lifter learns to shelve the bar on well flexed shoulders and thrust chest, support the front leg on full foot-to-ground contact, and maintain the rear foot on the metatarsal heads of the toes.
o The drawbacks of this obsolete style of lifting are as follows:
   i. It translates the center of mass of the lifter horizontally, thus wastes significant effort in spread lunging the feet.
   ii. It is entirely asymmetric. Thus, the shoulder on the side of the rear leg will develop greater strength than the other shoulder. In addition, the spines and hips will endure long and intense asymmetric imbalance.
   iii. The sprung legs prohibit deep descent under the bar. Even if the lifter is very flexible and strong, lifting with one leg flexed and the other extended is never an effective way of maximizing muscular power.
   iv. The short longevity of the lifters of this style is due to asymmetric strains and demands of vigorous whole body
o The advantages of leg spring lifting are:
   i. It does not need long and heavy leg training, since knee bending is limited.
   ii. It suits old and inflexible athletes, who lack spinal, pelvic, and shoulder flexibility.
   iii. Its spectacular outlook impresses others and makes the lifter feel accomplishing something outstanding.
o In the 1960's, the preoccupation with enhancing the old technique of lifting, through adjusting feet stance, hand gripping, and body posture, was overturned by the new invention of full squatting, after pulling from the floor. In addition, the eastern bloc cared less for nutritional guidelines and caloric balance. Nutrition was left to the discretion of trainees. Moreover, the eastern bloc coaches did not appreciate the consequences of gaining weight on prospective health issues. The only concern was developing strength, competing in weight class, and winning contests. That may be explained in the context of the shortage in living necessities in the communist bloc, the absence of fast food industry, and immense need to win contests in order to survive in an impoverished society.

12.1.3. APPEARANCE AND FITNESS

o Having been introduced to the world of Weightlifting, been motivated to pursue ambitious goals, and been comforted with your ability to attain your goals, you should settle the conflict of appearance versus fitness, as early as you can, such that you proceed without doubts about training.
o Bodybuilding training is essential for any strength training. It should blend smoothly into any strength training. Yet, the overwhelming propaganda about the commercial methods of Bodybuilding makes modern Bodybuilding jocular activity. Engaging in muscular enlarging and sculpturing with weights, without putting performance to test, is ridiculous. Once joints freeze in restricted range of motion, it is almost impossible to undo long-term calcification and

shortening of soft tissue. Sole Bodybuilding training impairs natural reflexes of flexion and extension. These are crucial to bending joints and enhancing performance.

o On the other hand, sport activity alone favors major working muscles, thus leaves many supporting muscles lacking in strength. Therefore, a proper mix between Bodybuilding and Weightlifting is judicious. In sport activity, you can compensate for lagging components of the technique by relying on stronger components to finalize the technique. In Bodybuilding you can tide lagging muscles to catch up in strength and participate vigorously in sport activity, or at least, stimulate weak muscular components of the body.

o Many sport achievers debate the usefulness of isolated muscle training, and rightfully claim that overtraining or inadequate training are more responsible for lagging muscles than the neglect of individual components, per se. In the end, whether you settle on peripheral Bodybuilding or axial Weightlifting training, your appearance will change in accordance with the extent of your activity.

o Axial training will impose characteristic curvatures on your backbone, your shoulders and chest, and on the way you walk. Bodybuilding will bulge those muscles that you chose to train hard and long. Yet, with incoherent strengthening, you will regret disregarding balancing the proportion of your body and the inability of each portion to function is harmony with others. Bodybuilders walk with huge and still upper body, seriously straining slim and weak waist. Bouncing massive upper body, on knees that are not trained for impulsive forces, induces premature knee and hip injuries.

o Thus, casting your body into an iron clad of muscles is all what you get from muscular appearance, gained by Bodybuilding alone. You should can take advantage of such muscle building capabilities of Bodybuilding routines and utilize such muscle gain in excelling in sport. This can be achieved by inserting axial exercises in training on regular basis.

12.1.4. POWER AND STRENGTH

Strength gained by "**controlled high-tension lifting**" is not all what you need from strength training. Such narrow definition of powerful strength of muscle groups is detrimental to most sport activities. Powerful strength is a hindrance, if fails to act along the normal range of motion of joints, or to respond to the tempo of real living activities. Weight training activities are not a substitute for whole body performance. In order to develop useful physical strength, you should consider the following issues.

o Enhancing physical strength should spare the **bodyweight** from hiking beyond control. Excessive increase in bodyweight is difficult to reverse and predispose to serious health problems. These would do away with any benefit gained from strength training.

o Enhancing physical strength should render the **joints responsive to individual needs**. Imbalanced strengthening causes weakness of neglected muscles. Weak muscles predispose to injuries. Injuries require time to heal and result in stiffness. Stiffness aggravates weakness. Thus, the vicious cycle keeps worsening due to muscular imbalance.

o Your best route, in choosing the kind of strength training that results in useful physical strength, is **resisting temptation.** Tempting modern gym machines and fitness advertisement do not enhance great training planning, unless you advance your critique skills in spotting deceptive intruders.

o Useful physical strength should constitute gain in **functional performance**, not just athletic appearance. The latter is relative, subjective, and deceptive. You might think that tight belly and large arms are the ultimate goal in appearing fit. Thus, you may entirely omit the fact that you walk on this planet on legs, supported by spines, like all vertebrate mammals. On the other hand, functional performance is easy to gauge by running, walking, sitting on or getting up from the ground, without aid. These simple activities require useful strength, flexibility, and muscular balance.

o The major problem, with choosing proper strength enhancement regimen, is the **preoccupation with few facets** of fitness that appeal to individual's psyche. Such bias shapes the entire realm of strength training and discourages many folks from engaging in the right regimens and resort to routines that are appeal to them. Take the example of the exercise of Bench Press that emphasizes strengthening the chest muscles. If you cannot perform front Squat with the same weight used in Bench Press, or heavier, that means that your shoulders fail to deliver power in that awkward position, of front Squat. That is because you did not train in that range of motion. In addition, if you cannot lift your Bench Press weight freely from the floor, to an arm stretch overhead, that means your axial muscles are seriously neglected. Not too many weight trainees opt to enhance axial and shoulder muscles, along with the Bench Press. Again, putting all the weights of the gym behind your shoulders, and dipping in Squat, would not benefit your strength in activities that require full range of motion and agility. Your Weightlifting fellows learn the progressive and patient ways to performing powerful actions at extremes of range of motion. Thus, do not be fooled with the wattage output of the Deadlift, Bench Press, and Squat, since greatest wattage has little to do with how this wattage is outputted, or how neural mechanism is used in its regulation.

MAKING TRAINING CHOICES 12

12.2. AGE CONSIDERATION

12.2.1. PHYSIOLOGICAL CONSIDERATION
Dramatic and substantial physical changes occur during adolescence as a result of physical activity. Yet, training prior to puberty leaves many permanent signatures on the musculoskeletal shape and function. As age progresses, weak links develop and may interfere with whole body performance, particularly, if the trainees is unfamiliar with issues of anatomical imbalance. Further age progress impairs vital systems, other than the musculoskeletal, and interferes with regulation and control of performance. The fact however is that, muscle growth and strength development continue throughout life. It seems that keeping close watch on various organs, such that they perform within the proper physiological domain, might help promote fitness beyond expectation, at any age.

12.2.2. EARLY START
Under the age of ten, weight training should emphasize on the playful aspect of performance of proper technique with comfortably light weights. The growth centers of bone remain active until the early twenties[1]. Thus, early training should focus on neural development and maintaining full range of motion of the soft tissue. Many children of modern societies develop limited knees, hip, back, and shoulder flexibility due to limited activity of urban lifestyle. Full squatting during lifting and high coordination motion are the basic skills that youngsters should master, while their bones are growing and reshaping. The peak muscular power output would not be reached prior full development of the HPA axis (Hypophyseal-Pituitary-Adrenal axis). This controls corticosteroid hormone production by the adrenal glands and the subsequent production of testosterone and growth hormone. Most probably, early starters may develop maximum strength, completely and solely, by axial training and whole body exercises than by Bodybuilding training. Most probably also, Bodybuilding is effective only at advanced age, when the whole muscle system is left to disproportionate wasting and decline of various muscles. Youngsters develop proportionate body parts with whole body axial training, due to the activation of hormone receptors allover the body, during adolescence, unlike adults with plateaued responsiveness to hormonal stimulation.

12.2.3. QUEST FOR POWER
Juvenile Weightlifting has gaining popularity in cultures, where old and retired Weightlifters are actively spreading the sport. It is entirely alien to cultures that rely solely on institutional education, such as the western developed nations.
In Alexandria, Egypt, there are remains of the Ottoman Empire and British colonies, from the era of dominance in Weightlifting. The following figures demonstrate the overzealous efforts to spread this old sport of power.

o *Figure 12.6* shows an 8-year old child performing the classic Clean in a colorful barbell. Perfecting the start position, hand gripping, shoulder flexion, and back erection is greatest accomplishment in this age group. These skills are learned easily and last for the rest of the child's life. The child in the back, with the blue costume is taking pride in his athletic look and is getting ready to perform the same lift. Adults surround the platform, watching and cheering the great progress of their fellow youngsters.

o *Figure 12.7* shows a private lesson in the Power Clean between the father and his son. The father is as excited at his youngster. Power Clean in this single-piece dumbbell strains the wrists, elbows, and shoulders, yet the father is insisting on harder training in order to gain more benefits from such rough training. Note that the child cannot flip the elbows into high flexion as in *Figure 12.6*, due to the lack of spinning of the dumbbell.

o At the age of 12, *Figure 12.8*, the same child is now Snatching 55 kg and can squat fully and fast, though his skeleton is not yet well developed. His pelvic and shoulder bones are working hard to support this extreme posture for a 12-year old.

o In *Figure 12.9*, the lower back cannot tolerate full extension is asymmetric leg spring and the child has to exaggerate the upper back curvature to support the jerk of 65 kg. In the next few years, this child will concentrate on the basic axial lifts, Clean, Snatch, Pulls of the Clean and Snatch, Deadlift, and Squat, in order to maintain whole body performance. When weakness is suspected in some aspect of performance, his father, and coach in the same time, will focus on the training volume and exercise intensity to remedy weakness. I doubt that he would resort to any Bodybuilding assistance, since the son and father are descendents of a culture that is well familiar with natural course of progress in Weightlifting.

o *Figures 12.10* thru *12.13* demonstrate the invaluable nurturing aspect of Weightlifting to impoverished children. The fun and complexity of performing highly challenging lifting provide child trainees a sense of great hope. Instead of growing up cynical about a society that has abandoned them, they discover the real strength within their mind and body. Young girls are no less than boys in acquiring strength and performing complex technical lifting.

---

[1] Growth centers of bone, known as ossification centers, are active spots in bones that are responsible for bone growth during the early years of physical development. These centers are regulated by hormones, such as growth hormone, testosterone, and thyroxin. Ossification centers have definitive anatomical locations and chronological course of maturity.

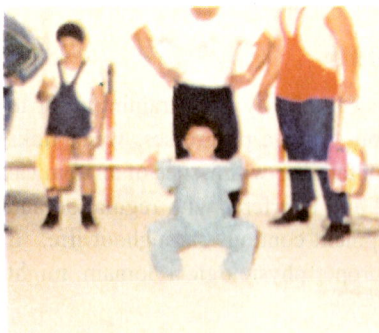
Figure 12.6. Classical Clean at the 8-year of age.

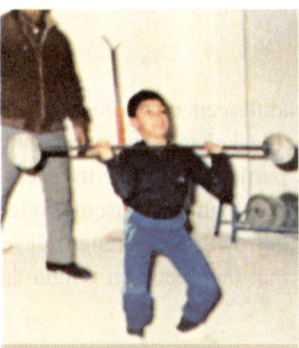
Figure 12.7. Power Clean of 20 kg at 9-year age.

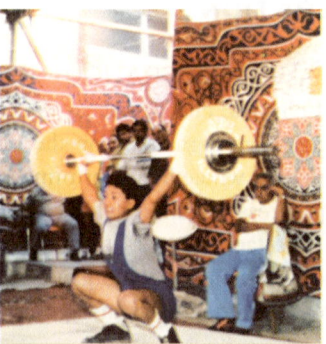
Figure 12.8. Snatch of 55 kg at 12-year age.

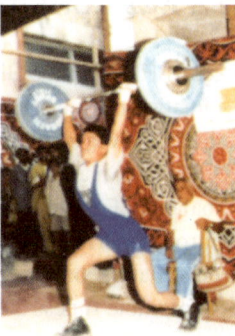
Figure 12.9. Jerk of 65 kg at 12-year age

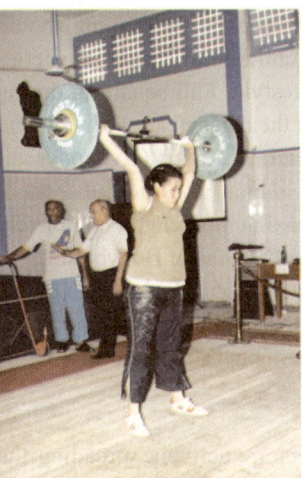

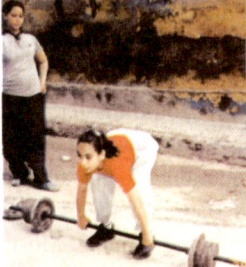
Figure 12.11. Training on Weightlifting on the street is the only activity these girls can do under the supervision of a well trained neighbor.

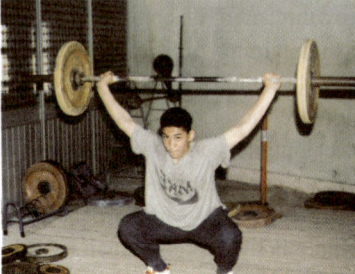
Figure 12.12. Early start is crucial for this boy to excel in Weightlifting. He will go through fifteen years, or so, to reach top performance. His axial curves will develop to match the task of lifting in Full Squat.

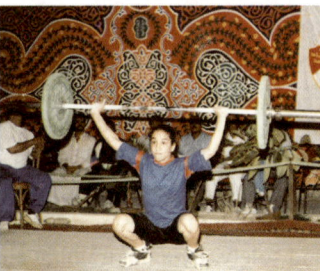
Figure 12.13. This girl is no less powerful than boys counterpart are. Although her left arm buckled in the Snatch, she will soon work on a remedy for her shortcoming.

Figure 12.10. (Above left) Training girls on Weightlifting is empowering to their self-esteem. It emphasizes their vital and equal role in society. The beginner girl, with noticeable body disproportions, will soon revolutionize her physical appearance with consistent training and invigorating social and coaching environment.

12.2.4. QUEST FOR HEIGHT

Juvenile gymnastics is more common than Weightlifting, yet both confront the same challenges of great needs for resources and public awareness. The common denominator in both sports is the need for muscular control and strength. **Strength training** of child gymnasts emphasizes strengthening the major axial extensors and flexors of whole body motion. The extensors erect the vertebral axis and transmit forces to and from the limbs. The flexors support the visceral contents of the abdomen and chest, facilitating respiration and circulation. In all sports activity, these muscles capture the focus of attention in promoting physical performance, as follows.

12.2.4.1. Hip Flexors And Abdominal Muscles

These axial flexors support the joints between the thighs and the pelvis and between the pelvis and chest, as follows.

- o The **hip flexors**, mainly the Iliopsoas, pull the pelvis, from the front downwards toward the femurs, during standing. They oppose the downward pull of the Hamstrings on the pelvis, from behind the hips. The balance of front and back pulls, on the pelvis, maintains as a horizontal platform that supports the upright posture of the vertebral axis. The hip flexors act intensely during squatting to prevent the backward fall of the body. Strong hip flexor contraction helps erect the lumbar region of the lower back during full squatting thus prevents disc herniation.

- o The **abdominal muscles** maintain high abdominal tone thus prevent accumulation of gases, fluids, and intestinal contents from stagnation along the 20 feet long small intestines and the tortuous and large intestines. Abdominal muscles are crucial to vigorous respiration in containing visceral guts and preventing herniation through the weaker spots of the abdominal wall.

- o **Unaided exercises of axial flexors.** Concentric contraction of these muscles is performed by raising the legs during lying down. Leg raising contracts the Iliopsoas muscles, in front of the hips. In addition, raising the buttocks contract the abdominal rectus, on the sides of the central front line of the belly, *Figure 12.14*. Heavier trainees need to anchor their upper body, by holding weights in the hands or gripping the sides of the bench. Lowering the lower body slowly increases eccentric contraction and produces soreness quickly. Highly toned abdominal muscles and hip flexors are paramount in enhancing circulation and respiration and, consequently, whole body performance. If you cannot move your buttocks upwards away from the ground, while keeping your upper body anchored to the bench or a surrounding fixed object (such as the legs of a partner), you have to work hard on the upper body and abdomen in order to accomplish progress in whole performance.

o Reverse bridging, *Figure 12.15,* works the abdominal rectus and hip flexors by eccentric contraction, but requires flexible back joints. Though one type of exercise suffices to attain strength of these body flexors, gymnasts prefer the diversity of neuromuscular control that promotes natural performance, when executing the complex technical motion of *Figures 12.27* thru *12.29.* In both *Figures 12.14* and *12.15,* no external weights are used, yet resistance can be greatly altered by changing the speed of raising the lower body, on the fixed upper body, or lowering the upper body on the fixed lower body. Without weights, longer duration of resistance can be endured and slow twitching muscle fibers participate more in the activity.

o The combined effects of vertebral flexion, *Figure 12.14,* and vertebral extension, *Figure 12.15,* ensure highly mobile spinal and hip joints and provide the gymnast utmost control of flexible joints. The natural performance of exercises, similar to sport activity, ingrains the neuromuscular control of body parts and facilitates the perfection of the skill. The 9-year old gymnast in these figures practices over five hours daily, spread on eight hours of gym stay. After regular and progressive incremental strength training, she can tolerate the stress of a long day of workout beside her school hours.

o **Eccentric exercises of axial flexors.** Weight training with 10 kg plate enhances strength and endurance in optimal proportion.

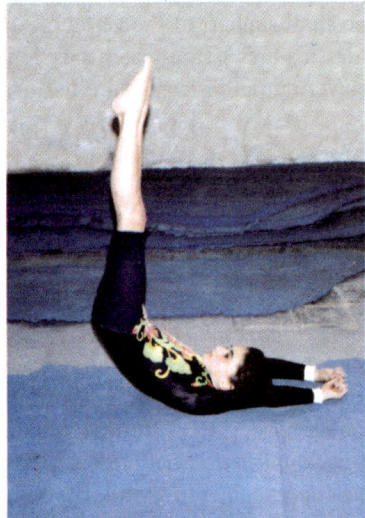

Figure 12.14. Abdominal muscles bring the pelvic bones closer to the chest whereas hip flexors bring the thighs closer to the abdomen. Raising the buttocks above ground works abdominal muscles perfectly.

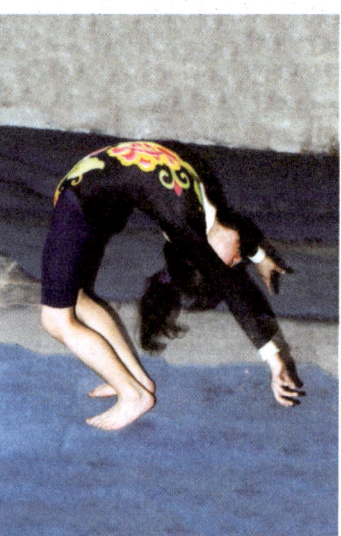

Figure 12.15. The same axial flexors, abdominal muscles, and hip flexors work out by eccentric contraction during reverse bridging. Eccentric contraction is superior to concentric contraction in developing muscular strength, in short time.

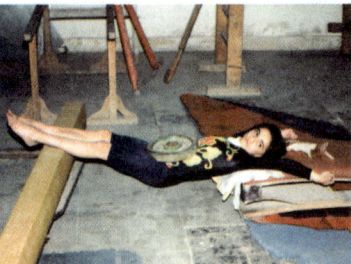

Figure 12.16. Abdominal eccentric contraction. Putting 10 kg plate on the belly of a 9-year old gymnast stimulates abdominal muscles to resist abdominal collapse.

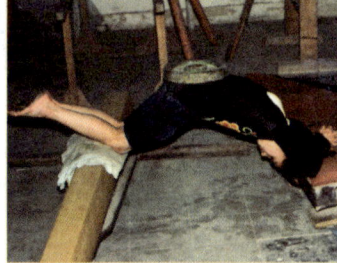

Figure 12.17. Exercising the hip flexors and abdominal muscles by eccentric contraction. Adding extra weight of 10 kg increases the eccentric contraction that prevents the body from caving in.

Figure 12.16 shows abdominal strengthening with pure eccentric contractions. The abdominal muscles resist the external weight, without moving the chest cage closer to the pelvis. Putting external weights, directly on the abdomen, is a serious matter that should not be practiced before many months of training. That is to ensure that the abdominal muscles are reactive enough to resist the external weight and prevent any vascular rupture. In young athletes, arteries are elastic and compliant, but not in adults and older athletes, where severe internal bleeding can result from external pressure. The advantage of putting external weight on the abdomen is the direct stimulation of a resilient muscle that is hard to train with mere eccentric and concentric contraction. Resisting direct external weight also stimulates the diaphragm to resist externally applied pressure, thus strengthens the diaphragmatic muscles.

o In *Figure 12.17*, the Iliopsoas (hip flexor) are strengthened by eccentric contraction with 10 kg plate put on the lumbar region and buttocks. Also, reverse bridging, *Figure 12.15,* greatly strengthens the Iliopsoas by eccentric contraction, which enhances neuromuscular control to greater extent. Eccentric contraction isolates the individual muscles and stimulates the higher recognition of its action. There is definite, yet unclear difference, between exercising muscle with isometric versus isotonic contraction.[2] Isotonic contraction increases muscular strength through regulating recruitment control, while isometric contraction increases strength through increasing muscle size.

---

[2] Eccentric and concentric contractions are isotonic since muscular tone remains constant while the length of the fibers change.

12 MAKING TRAINING CHOICES

12.2.4.2. Exercising Axial Extensors

o These muscles erect the vertebral column and provide stability to the spinal tunnel that hosts the spinal cord. The spinal cord is an extension of the central nervous system. It performs very vital function of neural control over sensation and motor regulation of the whole body, below the skull. The muscular support of the axial extensors, during low stress situation, provides postural support of the vertebras during rest, sleep, walking, and sitting. Active muscular support during vigorous activities requires both greater muscle mass and greater neural control of recruitment. During high endurance activity, low power output processes are performed by slow twitch muscle fibers and low recruitment level.

o The spinal erectors differ, from the rest of the major muscle groups of the body, in their high pinnation anatomy and richness in tendinous contents. Stretching the spinal erectors, prior to any resistance training, is vital to the stimulation of neural control. Even few back bends, prior to starting exercise, can prevent serious back injuries. Spinal stretching is the main thrust in yoga training. It enhances mobility and relieves posttraumatic inflammation caused by resistance training.

o Progressive and gradual stretching, *Figures 12.18* thru *12.23*, using external weight to increase the range of motion of the spinal joints, should not be performed without full body warm-up and thorough understanding of the seriousness of inducing disc herniation. In young children, the paravertebral structures are more elastic than in adults and intervertebral discs occupy roomier spaces, thus are less vulnerable to herniation. Older athletes have to understand the risks of rounding the lower back under external pressure. Back stretching has to stop immediately if any discomfort or sudden pain occurs. The best approach is to monitor the progress in stretch, over many weeks, by measuring the distance of forward reaching of the hands towards the feet.

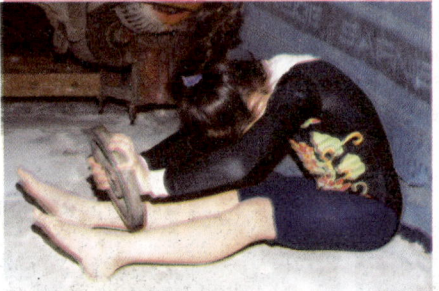

Figure 12.18. Back stretching sometimes needs little weight to force ligaments to comply. A plate of 10 kg can lend some support to stretching which has to proceed very slowly.

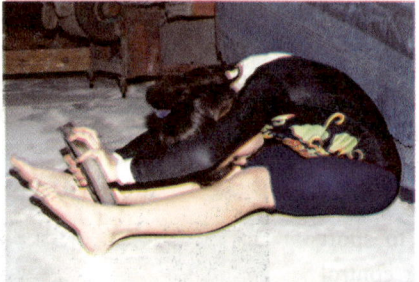

Figure 12.19. In young children, it is possible to achieve this stretchability of the back. Older athletes may not be able to equally combine spinal strength and stretchability

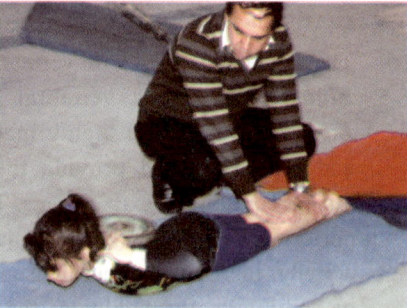

Figure 12.20. The father is taking his turn to motivate his daughter gymnast performs back raises with 10 kg plate. This will balance axial flexors (next figure) and extensors (this figure).

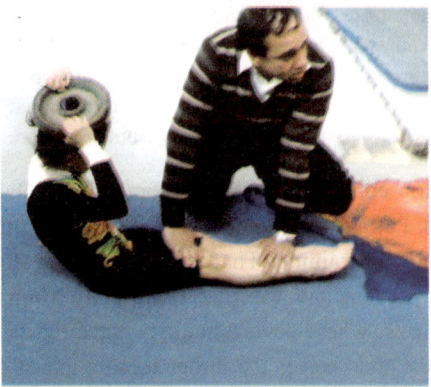

Figure 12.21. The Hip flexors and abdominal rectus work harder during resisting weighed sit-ups.

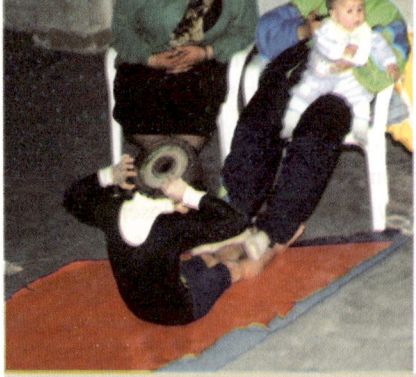
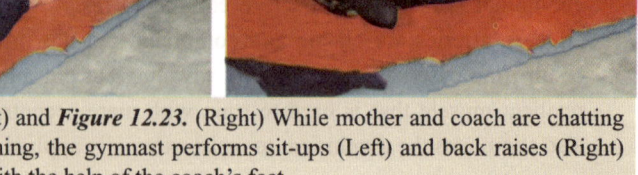

Figure 12.22. (Left) and *Figure 12.23.* (Right) While mother and coach are chatting and the baby watching, the gymnast performs sit-ups (Left) and back raises (Right) with 10 kg plate, with the help of the coach's feet.

o Back raises with weights, *Figure 12.20,* strengthen the muscles of the back and increases both strength and size of the spinal erectors, from the back of the skull down to the lumber region. Fixing the legs, during back raises, extends the strengthening to the Glutei and Hamstrings. Working out the Hamstrings and the spinal erectors, simultaneously, promotes their proportionate strength and ability to concert back extension in many sports activity, such as that of *Figure 12.27.* Concerted back extension in that complex motion can prove very invaluable to efficient performance. In *Figures 12.21* and *12.22*, the opponents of the Hamstrings and spinal erectors are exercised, in alteration with the latter two. The hip flexors and abdominal rectus should be treated equally, and in the same session, in order to maintain balanced spinal axis. This assisting strengthening makes the whole motion, of **Figures 12.27** thru **12.29**, remarkably less taxing.

o The effort spent on whole sport's activity, in conjunction with training isolated regions of the body, is what makes athletes perform extraordinary activity, with apparently remarkable ease. The hard work of long hours of daily conditioning ingrains the skill of mind-over-body control and facilitates the compliance of the body to mental demands. The visual appreciation of what different muscles can do, when required to act, lends the athlete self-esteem in his or her ability to know his or her best assets. In addition, the sensory appreciation, of how muscles listen to resistance calls, gives the person confidence in initiating and finalizing complex technical protocols. Having performed another round of whole sport's exercises, the gymnast and her coach will assess the source of difficulty with the whole technique, in order to identify the underlying anatomical causes of difficulty. When axial erectors and flexors are suspected to be the source of weakness, the coach decides to increase the load volume, by adding more sets of sit-ups and back raises with weight.

o Assessing the need for additional training volume of axial flexors and extensors is done by mere guessing, suspecting relevant technical weakness, or desire to control bodyweight. In many instances, it is difficult to interpret the anatomical flaws of technical performance and the coach has to work around the troubled region. In **Figures 12.24** thru **12.26,** the coach suspects relative weakness of the spinal erectors, with respect to the flexors, since the child maintain exaggerated convex back, in **Figures 12.24** and **12.26,** and straight back, in **Figure 12.25**. Adding more exercises for the spinal erectors and flexors would supposedly help the child gymnast overcome the higher tone of the axial flexors and impose more extension on the back.

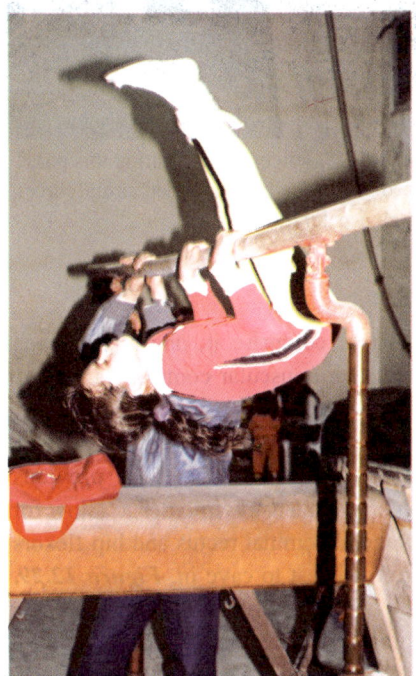
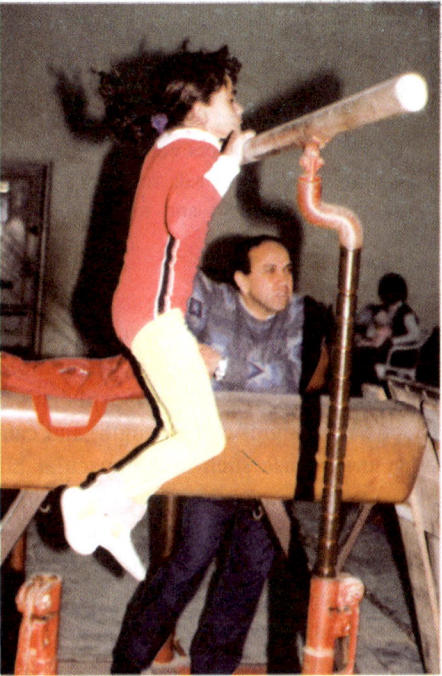
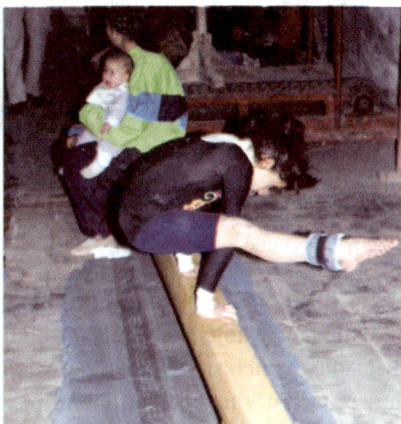

Figure 12.24. (Left) Chin-ups in this position work out abdomen; hip flexors, back muscles, and both arm flexors and extensors.
Figure 12.25. (Middle) Vertical chin-ups work out the Latissimus dorsi and arms muscles.
Figure 12.26. (Above) Strengthening of combined axial flexors and extensors.

12.2.4.3. Shoulder Strengthening In Children

o The second major task, after axial training of the pelvis and torso, is shoulder strengthening. Adequate shoulder control promotes the compliance of the child with progressive training demands. The avid wasting of shoulder muscles, due to lack of training, is attributed to their lack of daily participation in resistance activity such as walking or climbing. Thus, regular and constant inclusion of shoulder exercises must be an integral part of modern training.

o Shoulder exercises must target the four directions of the shoulder joint. Exercising the chest supports the front of the shoulder, the back supports the back of the shoulder, and the Deltoids and Trapezius support the outer and upper sides of the joint. The chest and the back -Pectoralis major and Latissimus dorsi- work together to support the lower side of the shoulder ball. The Chin-ups, **Figure 12.24,** group many major muscles together, in addition to the back of the shoulders. This trend is superior to peripheral training that aims to exercise weak muscles with dumbbells, cables, or barbells, since high performance depend on concerting groups of muscles, not just isolated muscles. While the child is exercising the arms and back, with the shoulder linking the two, the father of the child is reminding her of her lax back that needs more erection. Thus, the child gymnast develops the skill of rationing her focus of attention to specific goals, while maintaining vigilant peripheral attention to other crucial body parts. That might hinder performance if not included properly in the whole motion.

o In **Figure 12.25**, upright Chin-ups focus on the arm and back muscles, giving the lower body a break. Performing

Chin-ups by children, helps maintain the musculature of the arms and back that waste avidly in all modern women and most men. Every success in gymnastics depends on the strength and endurance of hand gripping. This exercise increases the reserve strength of the finger flexors by practicing slight loosening and tightening of the handgrips, during chin-ups. In *Figure 12.24,* the wrist flexors are exercised by bending the wrist during gripping the bar. In *Figure 12.25,* the digital flexors are exercised by loosening and tightening the fingers on the bar. The Serratus anterior and anterior chest muscles are exercised in *Figure 12.26,* in combination with back extensors and hip flexors. Again, the wrist is the main beneficiary of this whole body workout. Both wrist and digital flexors and extensors concert the body balance, while the shoulders link the torso to the arms, with particular strengthening of the scapular and chest muscles (Serratus anterior and Pectoralis major).

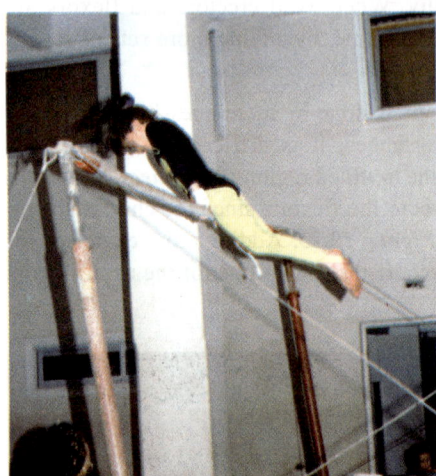
Figure 12.27. Axial body extension is crucial in generating the momentum required to produce the centrifugal force for rotating the body around a fixed center.

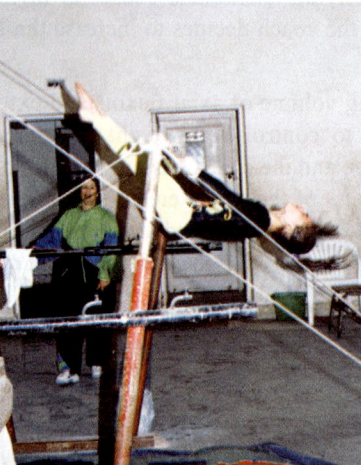
Figure 12.28. Flexors concert with extensors, during peak resistance, against bodyweight and inertia of accelerated body.

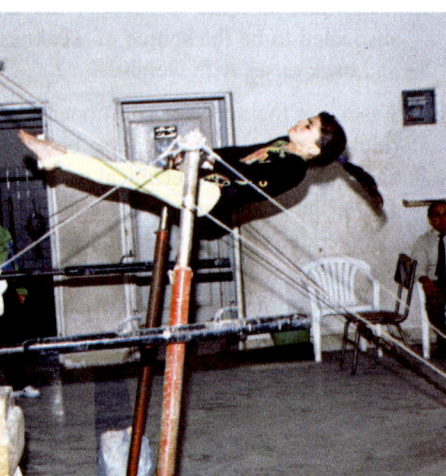
Figure 12.29. Forces created during this phase exceed bodyweight by the added virtual forces of high acceleration.

12.2.4.4. Whole Performance And Regional Participation
In analyzing whole body motion and trying to identify the anatomical components that comprise it, one might reach misleading conclusion due to the nonlinear behavior of the circulation, respiration, and neuromuscular control. As will be shown later in this chapter, mere muscular weakness is not the only explanation of failed performance. Neuromuscular control could override specific muscles, despite their significant strength, and cause mechanical failure. Both, inadequate group training of muscles, and overtraining, may cause such neuromuscular hindrance of performance. The previous strength training activities will not pay back before few days of rest and reduction in exercise intensity, in order to allow for recuperation. During the performance of *Figures 12.27* thru *12.29,* the coach suspects the abdominal rectus and hip flexors to cause the pelvis to drop, in *Figure 12.28,* and the middle back retractors to cause the chest to cave in, *Figure 12.29.* Both suspected weak regions became apparent during the fast dynamic performance, where excessive forces are generated by the centrifugal acceleration of the body around the wrists. Few months of training, of axial flexors and scapular retractors, may streamline the performance of the gymnast. This is judged by the triangle between the arms, torso, and legs, in *Figure 12.28.* This triangle should shrink to straight line slit. The collapsing chest, in *Figure 12.29,* may thrust forwards, lending the arms more strength from the back retractors of the scapulas, mid Trapezius fibers, Rhomboids, and Serratus anterior.

12.2.5. STARTING IN LATE ADOLESCENCE
After the age of sixteen, weight training may proceed into full gear, year after year, until the age of twenty-one. The best years of maximal growth in strength are between the ages of eighteen and twenty-four. In this age group, great emphasis should be put on musculoskeletal foundation. The thighs, back, and shoulders should be the focus of attention. Later, in the twenties of age, it would be very difficult to reverse wasting in these major regions. I have not saw anybody that passed this window of age, with weakness of the thighs, back, or shoulders, that was able to reclaim peak strength, had he or she have started earlier. The fact that many Bodybuilders can bulk massive muscles in these three regions, even late in their twenties, overlooks the robust neural control of muscles that are strengthened proportionally, under the age of twenty-four. The back erectors are notorious in resisting strength training, late in the twenties of age, if not trained early. That is because the geometrical dimensions of the knee, hip, vertebras, and shoulder bones reach their permanent maximal values by the age of twenty-four. This signifies the role of training, prior to that age, on axial joints that support any added muscle mass, after that age. The mobility of the ball and socket joints, of shoulders and hips, is affected, for the entire life, by the nature of training of this window of age.

12.2.6. FUNDAMENTALS VERSUS DETAILS OF WORKOUT

o   The major task in training adolescents should be directed towards the three fundamental regions of the body, without getting distracted in the minute details of the whole body. The **thighs, back, and shoulders** should be trained to move strongly and fully, along the normal range of motion of childhood.

o   No attempt should be made that limits the **range of motion,** such as implementing alternative days of working different body parts. Limited range of motion exercises, such as one-hand dumbbell Press or Biceps Curls, Bench Press, Squat, or Cable Rowing, should be combined with whole body exercises, in the same working session. Traumatic dose of shoulder, back, leg, or chest training, without including whole body exercises, in the same day, limits your performance. This incoherent strengthening localizes inflammation and rigidity in isolated body regions.

o   Even the lightest intensity of **whole body training** will serve the purpose of keeping axial muscles robust and ready to integrate peripheral muscles. The golden rule of combining peripheral and axial training is that minimal inclusion, of either, is superior to total exclusion of either of the two. You can perform, on daily basis, three sets of Power Clean or Power Snatch, and three sets of heavy Pull for the Clean or the Snatch, in order to assist peripheral training in just few extra minutes.

o   *Figure 12.30* shows a lifter caught in the transition, from the old styles of lifting by leg springing (*Figures 12.2, 12.3, & 12.5*) to the new style of front squatting. The old lifting style predisposed to stiffness in the shoulder and pelvic muscles that hindered mobility in significant range of motion. Lifters had to move the barbell as high as the mid-torso, in order to spring under the bar and catch the lift. After converting to the new style of front squatting, this lifter was frustrated with his inflexible shoulders, back, and hips. He still lifts too high, before he can dip under the bar, and finds it very hard to ascend from deep squatting. His worst nightmare will come after ascending and beginning the Overhead Jerk. Attempting to mass muscles on the arms and shoulders, after that long course of training, was formidable on that lifter. He thought that change of lifting style would get easier, as days go by, and it did not. The front Squat with heavy weight, followed by the Jerk, in the same breath, never gets easier when harmonious musculoskeletal, cardiopulmonary, and neurovascular systems are not adapted to such notoriously taxing lift.

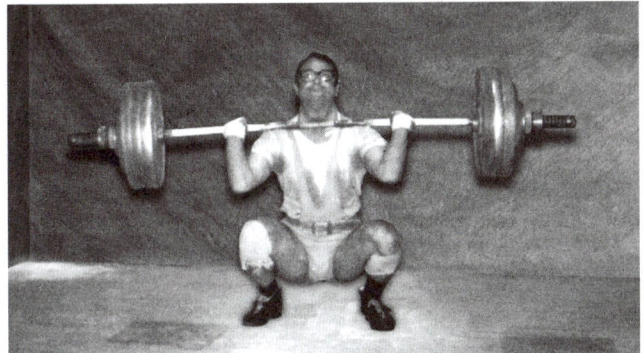

Figure 12.30. Learning the new technique of front squatting under the Clean lift is tough on this convert from old styles of leg-spring lifting. His shoulders can hardly flex under 165 kg Clean, in the 90 kg class. Note the stainless steel plates and poor training condition of 1970's, Egypt. The poor development of arms and shoulder of old Weightlifting generation makes front squatting more taxing.

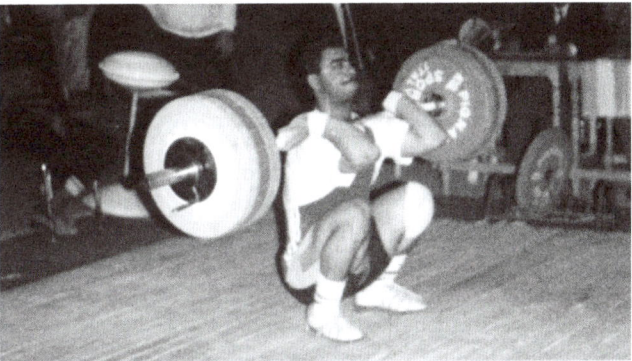

Figure 12.31. Clean of 160 kg in year 1995, Egypt. The new generation of Weightlifters has no trouble squatting deep and fully flexing shoulders. Note the colorful milieu, rubber plates, and enthusiastic spectators. Modern lifters are well built than older generations.

o   Twenty years later, his counterpart, in *Figure 12.31,* can dip in front Squat, with buttocks abutting the backs of his heels and abdomen squeezed on the thighs. Modern Weightlifters develop larger arms and shoulder in addition to flexibility of wrist, elbows, shoulders, back, hips, and knees. That lifter will ascend from that deep and, apparently, unbalanced Squat and jerk the weight overheads, with less trouble compared to the 1970's lifter of *Figure 12.30*.

o   Keep in mind that **peripheral training** plays important role, when **intertwined with axial training**. It helps various muscles compensate in the concerted effort of long and heavy resistance, from the floor overheads. However, the way that peripheral exercises are intertwined with axial exercises is very individual in nature and is subjected to a lot of experimentation. Whether to lift heavy for less repetition, or hike the volume with light lifting, is a matter of experimental trials. The determining factors are nutrition, rest, and managing intervals between high intensity sessions. If muscles are allowed to grow and rest, in such a manner as not to interfere with neuromuscular performance, then axial training can benefit from peripheral training, and both may lead to progress. However, a sore chest, Biceps, or knee may interfere with axial training and hinder progress, as compared to axial training alone. Thus, the key index, of proper intertwining of peripheral and axial exercise, is to keep close attention on the volume and intensity of axial exercises. If peripheral training assists in progressive increase in volume and intensity of axial exercises, over few months of training, then planning should continue along that course. If intention is to concentrate solely on peripheral training, until adequate muscle mass is achieved, then proportionate volume and intensity should be applied in exercising the legs, back, and shoulders, in order to avoid muscle wasting and freezing of joints.

12.2.7. STARTING IN THE TWENTIES
The cumulative effects of all previous life activities determine the outcome of late starters. Smart trainees have to make up for the lost years by vigilant inquisition and understanding how to reclaim lost muscular balance. The major exercises that expedite such reclamation of balance are **whole body exercises** such as Front Squat, Overhead Press with Squat dipping, Snatch and Clean from the hang, and Deadlift and Pulls. The major task of this age group is different from earlier age groups. Balancing upper and lower body, on a tremulous and weak back, is high priority. No promise can be made that back strength may reach the peak of early starters. Since early starters developed bony and cartilaginous structures that adapted to strength training, thus, adding more muscle mass and strength is not as hard as in older groups with lesser skeletal development.

12.2.8. STIMULATING APPROACHES

o   It must be borne in mind that the key for developing strength is very individual, since many athletes have found ways for breaking barriers that have not been broken by many predecessors. The ingredients for such personal experimentation are: training time, distribution of training volume and the profile of intense training over weeks and months duration, the daily intertwining of axial and peripheral exercises, and, finally, nutrition and rest.

o   If strength is promoted along the whole range of motion of major muscles and simultaneous usage of major muscles is implemented, there should be no limitation on reclaiming balance and strength. *Figures 12.32* and *12.33* present the old trend of thoughts that dominated strength training during the first half of the last century. Strength training was mainly axial strengthening with ballistic muscular contraction. We never thought about eccentric contraction as a way of massing muscles. The dominant belief was that mental concentration could make smaller muscles work effectively. The Snatch lift, in *Figure 12.32,* was executed at high speed and high pull, in contrast to today's low pull. The high pull permitted inflexible joints to function in their tolerated range of motion. Today, lifters are confident that joints can function with great capacity, in full range of motion, as long as gradual and progressive training is carried out.

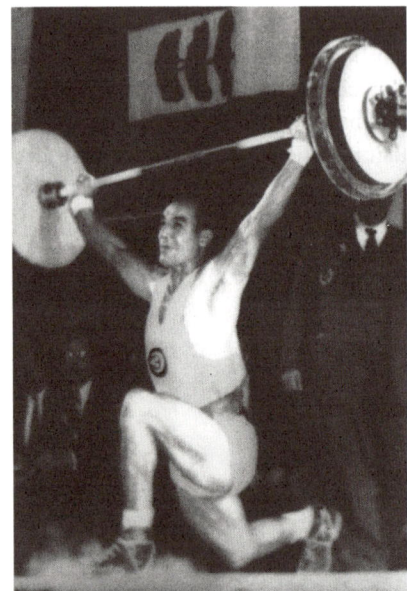

Figure 12.32. **Kamal Mahgoob**, of Egypt. Spectacular Snatch of 97.5 kg with leg spring. Note the poor muscular development despite the high performance of ballistic lifting. Paris. France 1951.

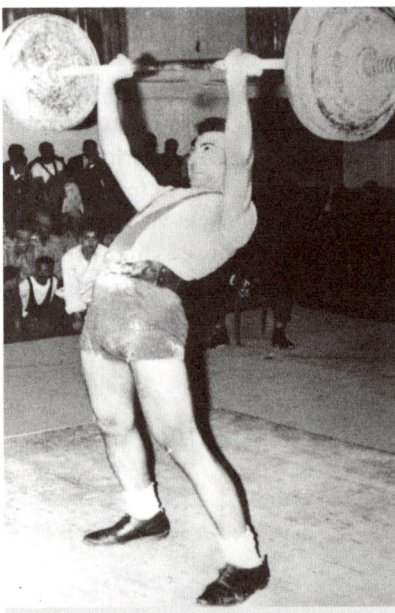

Figure 12.33. The author in the Clean and Press lift of 110 kg. The Press was the first lift in Weightlifting competition, prior to its cancellation in 1972. Note the exquisite back hyperextension under heavy weight. Alexandria. Egypt. 1971.

o   The Press lift, in *Figure 12.33,* is best likened to today's inclined Bench Press, while standing on both feet. By today's standards, the techniques in *Figures 12.32* and *12.33* are risky propositions. Such phase of thinking through advancing the method of lifting have led to the current lifting style of relying on both shoulder and pelvic girdles, instead of the old style of reliance on back and hip muscles.

o   The issues of particular interest in the third decade of life, beside physical changes in the body, are social in nature. Young adults face the challenge of forming a family and finding the right employment to support themselves. This diverts most of the individual's attention to concerns outside the realm of training. The lifter in *Figure 12.30* was the hope of an entire nation, in his teens, as a clean-cut athlete with modest education and personal appeal, yet he spent his best years during the time of turmoil in Weightlifting.

o   By the time Weightlifters have settled on the best technique of lifting, by dipping under the bar in full Squat, instead of springing by the legs, that lifter had advanced into his twenties, with the mind of the past. Transferring the assets of leg springing in Weightlifting to full squatting was mere hindrance. For such technical transfer to succeed, a full decade of strengthening and refining reflexes would be required to alter the anatomical and physiological makeup of the lifter.

o Without extensive peripheral training and reconditioning the upper body to adapt to the new lifting style, progress was impossible. The only factor he was able to control was gaining more bodyweight, in order to increase the Clean from 140 kg into 170, and the Snatch from 110 kg up to 135 kg. None of these records got him beyond local competition level.

12.2.9. PERMANENT PHYSICAL CHANGES

o Weightlifters, in particular, recognize the clear and evident fact that each person has a very specific maximum of strength in certain lifting modes. We know that we can enhance the high-tension controlled lifts, such as the Bench Press, Squat, or Deadlift, by progressive and regular training at proper volume and intensity. Yet, we have very little understanding of why lifters cannot exceed specific maximal limits, for long time, or why others differ in that maximum. I know my ways around the Squat, Shoulder Press, and Goodmorning and can perform Goodmorning, with jump with 140 kg on short notice, yet whole body free lifts require full integration of all fitness components, not just the strength factor.

o Early-life axial-training undoubtedly leaves life-long changes in the body that affect locomotion and strength related activities. In *Figures 12.34* and *12.35,* after 25 years of

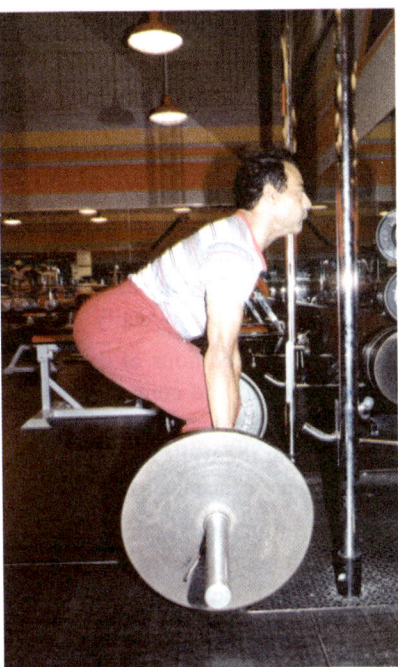

Figure 12.34. Maintaining straight upper back and concave lower back during all phases of lifting is best learned during adolescence. This habit will stay for the rest of life.

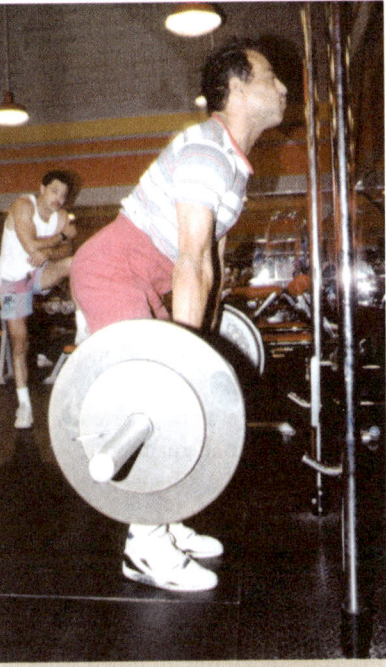

Figure 12.35. As pulling proceed, the lifter enhances lower back lordosis and chest thrusting. This will effectively utilize the Hamstring torque of the torso.

Weightlifting and in my early forties, I can unconsciously perform the **technique** ingrained in my mind all these years. That attracts the attention of close encounters in the training room. The characteristic permanent changes due to axial training are the strong and concave lumbar region that links the pelvis to the axial skeleton. The ingrained scapular balance, during equalizing the weight, maintains elevated shoulders and forward and upward thrust chest.

o In addition to anatomical changes during the early years of axial training, **physiological changes** occur in the ability to control muscles by enhancing motor unit reflex. This is evident in *Figures 12.34* and *12.35,* where intense stretching of the arms and Hamstrings is initiated unconsciously, prior to employing explosive ballistic force. This will easily drive the bar to the shoulder level. The ability to perform pre-stretching of the working muscles enhances muscle spindle activation of AHC[3] motor neurons. This amplifies the higher brain signals and recruit muscle fibers more effectively. Learning and mastering this skill of pre-stretching, before storming with peak force of contraction, explains how Weightlifters exceed all expectation when it comes to muscular power production, as follows.

  i. The pre-stretched **Biceps** anchors the shoulder ball snuggly into its socket and thus enables the cuff rotators to maintain shoulder integrity during peak torque of lifting the barbell, from the lower chest level to the shoulder level.

  ii. The pre-stretched Hamstrings also vigorously torques the pelvis on the hip joints, while maintaining knee antagonism to the **Quadriceps.**

  iii. The same pre-stretch principle applies to the **scapular muscles.** The Trapezius, Rhomboids, and Serratus muscles are pre-stretched by maintaining elevated shoulders and thrust chest thus allowing the Trapezius to vigorously shrug the shoulders, during the explosive ballistic phase.

o Regular training ingrains such anatomical and physiological changes in the mind of the young. These changes help maintaining proper body curvatures and implementing proper muscular control. These are more important than bulking muscles, with limited skill on how to put them into useful action, let alone misusing them in serious traumatic injuries to the vertebras and joints. The most common injuries in weight training are caused by the strong pull of large muscles

---

[3] Anterior Horn Cells are neurons in the anterior horn of the spinal cords that operate as lower motor neurons of peripheral muscles. The lateral and posterior horns of the spinal cord convey sensation and proprioception signals. The alpha neurons of AHC regulate voluntary and reflex neuromuscular contraction. The gamma neurons of the AHC regulate involuntary (extra-pyramidal) control of the brain on the spindles of the muscles.

12 MAKING TRAINING CHOICES

against weak antagonism of neglected muscles. This is very evident in spinal disc injuries due to imbalanced spinal erectors against Iliopsoas and abdominal muscles.

12.2.10. STARTING IN THE THIRTIES

o Training for strength in the thirties of age has specific aspects that affect choice making. By this age, the trainee has mostly settled his concerns regarding forming a family and securing a source of income. In addition, body growth has reached peak maturity. Starting anew, without any previous training, makes choices quite limited. The person should reduce his routine to the simplest possible in order to bring all body systems to work in concert.

o Peak strength is attainable in few years of training. The habits of utmost importance, in this age group, are warming up and progressive increase in intensity. Both tasks prevent inflexibility of muscles that have long been neglected. Peripheral training should comprise of small number of exercises and repetition per sets of exercises, and with progressively intense load. This can enhance strength and size of muscles in few months. The Highest percentage of daily exercise should entail lifting from the floor.

o Definite progress can be attained if legs, axial back, and shoulders are trained every training session, for at least four days per week. There is little chance to undo risky practice in this age group. Disproportionate Bodybuilding of upper body, with respect to lower body, is notoriously difficult to rectify.

o The major unknowns in this age group are the conditions of the cardiovascular and musculoskeletal systems. If the heart pump is structurally and functionally sound and compliant with physical activity, one has to worry about the vascular network of arteries and veins. Progressive incremental strength training should be supplemented with aerobic component adequate to lower fat deposits along the walls of the arteries. Aerobic exercises ensure access of adequate oxygen and nutrients to cells during activity thus reduce the harmful effects of accumulation of anaerobic byproducts.

o Fats do not burn anaerobically and have to wait until vigorous exercise ceases, before gaining access to aerobic energy production if, and only if, carbohydrates are not adequate for fueling. Lack of aerobic exercises causes inflammation of connective tissues (these are muscles, nerves, bones, vessels, and fibrous tissues), which is proven detrimental to mobility and survival.

o The golden rule of progressing, in the thirties, is starting all exercises with very light weights (under 40% of 1RM) and performing few sets of warming up prior to all exercises. Getting each joint and muscle group accustomed to the intended exercise should ingrain new memory of motor skill and should encourage the person to proceed after testing the new grounds. The most apprehending exercise, such as the Front Squat or Overhead Squat, can be executed with relief, if this simple trick is implemented. Hitting it hard and heavy from the start may lead to failure and discouragement.

12.3. FITNESS CONSIDERATION

o The choices to make, based on your desired level of fitness, range from various proportions of aerobic and anaerobic activities, and various mix of peripheral and axial exercises. Finding the right routine depends on your state of strength and endurance. In this realm of wide spectrum of choices, fitness can be defined as the **optimum combination** of aerobic, anaerobic, peripheral, and axial activities. The optimum mix of strength and endurance determines your energy utilization efficiency. Strength training maintains the minimum muscle mass required for endurance performance. It stimulates growth of new muscle fibers of the twitch rate needed for the kind of strength training you practice. On the other hand, endurance training hastens recovery from the aftereffects of vigorous activity by enhancing the enzymes of cellular aerobic respiration.

o Fitness consideration emphasizes **systemic, rather than local conditioning**. Thus, axial exercising should dominate strength-training portion of your routine. If you are not distracted by exercising individual muscles then you can engage major muscle groups in universal exercises such as the Clean, Snatch, Chin-ups, parallel bar dips, Squat, and running. These freestyle activities target major flexors and extensors.

o If your **bodyweight** falls above average norms then axial training has to comprise high percentage of your workout and aerobic activity[4] comprises greater portion of those axial exercises. On the other hand, if your bodyweight is below or at average norms then peripheral exercises can expedite strengthening of those parts that lag behind during axial training. For example, arms and shoulders peripheral exercises make significant difference in the performance of Weightlifters with average bodyweight, since their body inertia is lower than heavier lifters.

o The most remarkable fact about fitness enhancement by training is that **significant improvement** in strength, endurance, and general health is felt within weeks of training. These continue to improve with regular training. Your ability to tolerate extremes of stresses is greatly enhanced by training. Adding more muscle mass, by strength training,

---

[4] Aerobic activity does not refer solely to the commonly familiar aerobic exercises without weight. Any protracted exercise, with or without weight, will have an aerobic component to it. Thus, the aerobic feature refers to activities that are not brief and intense, but rather long and allowing relatively easy breathing.

makes you tolerate changes in weather, daily work activity, and mental stresses, in addition to vigorous activities. Adding more stamina, by endurance training, helps you recuperate faster from demanding work and resume activities with minimal decline in performance.

o The one factor you have to remember is that you are budgeting your energy in various ways. Massing too much **muscles and bodyweight** diverts energy from kinetic form of mobility into potential energy. Potential energy maintains the large body from crumbling and falls, muscular wasting, or inadequate delivery of nutrients and oxygen and removal of byproducts. Optimum muscle mass does not have to be huge. You can get by, with great performance, with just strengthening thighs, axial back, and shoulders. In addition, you hinder your performance if only arms are massive while legs are slender. On the other hand, very low bodyweight fails to provide adequate force to meet daily demands, such as lifting grocery, opening jammed doors, lifting a child, or moving furniture around the house.

o If you are sure that you are a good planner and executor then peripheral training is your best artistic tools to shape your body, the way you want. All you need is to study and learn **mechanics of various exercises** and then plan to maintain overall balance of function and size. Thus, if you worked hard on the arms by various sculpturing exercises then you need to test how the arms perform in the Front Squat or the Power Clean. Three sets of major axial exercises should test your art of planning balancing muscular strengthening. If the trained arms interfere with axial exercises, then you should examine the causes of interference, such as disproportionately weak shoulder or imbalanced scapular muscles. Another example is the peripheral exercising of the legs. Including three peripheral leg exercises in one session, and skimping on other body parts, intensely stresses the legs and interferes with walking and running. Thus, proper planning of peripheral training should not follow the commercial advertised routines of fitness, but rather your own fitness consideration.

o There may come a moment when you discover the **definitive weak links** in your body that deserve your highest attention. Abdominal, leg, back, chest, and shoulders, are greatest links to fitness and their concerted work enhances performance. Their importance stems from the fact that they support blood flow and neural control to all body systems. On deciding, on the proportions of aerobic versus anaerobic exercises and axial versus peripheral exercises, you should bear in mind balancing the profile of these five great links of the body, as follows.

   i. **Weak legs** demand constant inclusion of leg exercises in daily workout, not just acute sparse intense exercises. Strengthening the legs requires many months and has to proceed steadily and firmly.

   ii. **Unconditioned abdomen** upsets the entire body. The abdomen works as a reservoir for ventilation and circulation. Strong abdominal muscles enhance cardiac return and respiratory excursions during vigorous activity, in addition to facilitating easy circulation and ventilation during endurance work. You should not divert all your attention to gaining strength if your belly is bulging in front of you. Increasing axial and aerobic portions of your exercises reclaims abdominal fitness and breaks the cycle of decline in health, due to hampered circulation and ventilation. Remember that, animals with high-pressure vascular system, such as mammals, require a shock-absorbing reservoir in order to sustain pressure gradients on different regions of the body. The abdomen functions as such dampening reservoir. If the abdomen were a rigid container, then serious intravascular turbulence would ensue. That is the case in people with weak abdominal wall. In this case, intraabdominal contents cannot be contained efficiently with toned muscular wall. These people suffer from circulatory problems due to poor abdominal compliance with breathing, circulation, and heart pumping. Plants do not need such shock-absorbing reservoir, since they live on low-pressure fluid circulation.

   iii. As with the legs, **weak back** requires daily insertion of back strengthening exercises, in small doses and for long duration. The axial back muscles are very tendinous and act on joints supported by heavy network of ligaments. These require many months of training to show improvement in strength. Back weakness is quick to protest and forces many people to cease lifting.

   iv. The importance of **chest strengthening**, is not only enhancing breathing, but also stabilizing the shoulders. During Bench Press, or any one-hand Press in the lying position, the scapulas have to be supported by the Serratus anterior muscles. These are the muscles that help keep the shoulder elevated during any lifting and prevent the collapse of the clavicle on the major vessels outlet, at the neck and shoulder area. Thus, bench-pressing also helps freestyle lifting.

   v. Finally, the **shoulder** issues are also crucial in your fitness consideration. Recall that having bulging and strong shoulders is a cardinal sign of fitness. Shoulders are the most beneficiaries of peripheral training. There are so many Bodybuilding exercises that can shape your shoulders to your best ability. Including one or two shoulder exercises into your daily routine enhances its effectiveness.

12 MAKING TRAINING CHOICES

12.4. GENDER CONSIDERATION

o Fortunately, modern women are more aware of their right to equality with men, at least in developed countries. This has led many women to venture the uncharted territories of sport. Weight training and aerobic activities are witnessing greater **participation of women**. Training for fitness and competition may reverse many trends in diseases that afflict women. In particular, osteoporosis, obesity, diabetes, hypertension, and cardiovascular disease, are few to mention.

o Strength training is not new to women throughout history. In many rural communities, throughout the globe, women perform heavy and tedious physical work that contributes to strong and fit women's physique. The **hormonal changes** in women causes loss of minerals during menses, as well as in between menses, due to the action of progesterone on relaxing muscles, ligaments, and tendons. This causes thinning of bone. Osteoporosis begins in the third decade of women's life. It can be slowed down or even prevented by exercise, calcium intake, and vitamin D.

o Peripheral exercises give women great hope in overcoming selective weakness of long neglected upper body. Axial exercises enhance major links along the vertebral axis. If social and cultural progress is made in equating girls with boys in their rights to build better future, then girls may be able to engage in **strength training prior to the age of 16**, when skeletal changes actively take place. The well-known fact in competitive Weightlifting is that the minimum duration of training for young adolescents to reach peak performance is five to eight years, prior to the age window of 23 to 25 years. In the early teens, axial training alone offers significant permanent skeletal changes.

o The most important gain from axial training is enlarging the **shoulder and the upper body** in relation to the pelvic dimensions. Unlike men, women have to include higher proportion of upper body exercises than men. Balancing the upper body extensors and flexors is best done by keeping close watch on the cycle of these exercises: Shoulder Press, inclined Bench Press, Bench Press, Bend-Over Row, Chin-ups, and parallel bar dip. At least two of these six exercises should be included in the assisting portion of daily training.

o In the late teens and early twenties, a **fixed core of axial exercises** should be maintained in the form of 4 to 6 whole body exercises. This is to be complemented with assisting exercises of the weak links. Aerobic exercises help in assessing the right proportions between peripheral and axial exercises. In this age group, many parts of woman's body fall in disproportion, if training is interrupted for weeks at a time. The vertebral axis, pelvic, and shoulder bones need not only participate in every training session, but also receive the adequate load volume and intensity, in progressive incremental manner, in order to enhance strength.

12.5. AVAILABILITY ISSUES

o This is the most common excuse for not engaging in regular training given by parents of interested children and adults. A serious training session requires an hour and half per day, for 3 to 7 days per week. The benefits gained from such investment will affect every aspect of your life. The most significant benefit is learning the practical basis of anatomy, physiology, and behavior. The material benefit is the comfort you will find in performing basic living needs such as eating, digesting, breathing, moving, sleeping, and reproduction, by virtue of enhancing **health and strength**.

o Thus, making training a top priority is both reasonable and intelligent. Many times you may hurry getting into and out of the gym, yet to discover that shorter and serious training sessions are the best you have done. In a matter of **thirty minutes** you can warm up, perform few parallel bar dips and chin-ups, and few sets of exercises for the back, legs, and shoulders. That is almost a whole body workout. Yet, if you skip those thirty minutes of basic training altogether, your health slips down the paths of wasting, debility, and diverse and ambiguous ailments and complaints. A brief workout can be easily planned as follows.

   i. The **fundamental exercises** for brief sessions should include some of the floor lifts: the Clean, the Snatch, the Deadlift, Bent-over rows, and Pulls from the floor. These work out the immediate muscles of the vertebral axis.
   ii. Second in importance, are the fundamental **assisting exercises** that hike the training volume in few sets and that may require benches, machines, or other devices. These are the Squat, Goodmorning, Shoulder Press, Bench Press, and cable rowing.
   iii. Third in importance, are exercises that work out muscles that are little **farther away from the axis**. These are the Biceps Curls, Triceps extension, forearms exercises, seated leg extension and seated leg curls, Calf exercises, and abdominal exercises.
   iv. **Aerobic exercises** must complement brief sessions, even in 5 to 10 minutes of nonstop running, jugging, brisk walking, or Calisthenics. These prevent injuries and help in continuing activity.

o When training time is not restricting, the trainee can reduce axial component to few fundamental exercises (such as the Clean or Snatch, the Deadlift or Pulls, the Jerks or the Shoulder Press) and expand the **peripheral exercises**. These tide the weak body parts over lagging levels. The total volume of training can then compose of around 60% of peak intensity, with larger number of exercises targeting different parts of the body.

o The fear of designating an entire session to a **single body region** (arms and shoulders, chest and abdomen, or lower legs and back) is that, performance will greatly decline if whole body exercises are not inserted into daily sessions. Achieving large muscle mass and strength in assisted exercises is deceiving, in regarding to whole body activities. Since neuromuscular adaptation and control evolve on daily basis, therefore, daily activities should include whole body performance.

o Experienced Weightlifters can utilize split daily sessions, of peripheral exercises, in one session, and axial exercises, in the other session, of the same day. This **daily split double-sessions** require that axial exercises, either performed at lighter intensity, or progressed from very light to average intensity. High intensity axial training has to be performed in the session prior to the peripheral training session, in order to avoid interference with flexibility and coordination.

o Availability of training time can become a great asset when the athlete can remedy all **weak links of strength and coordination**. The slightest muscles, such as the wrist extensors and flexors, can make significant difference in strength training. Conditioning the wrists requires only few minutes of daily wrist curls and reverse curls exercises. In addition, steady and regular inclusion of even four sets of Squat, Pull, and Shoulder Press, on daily basis, can add up to remarkable progress in axial performance.

12.6. BODYWEIGHT ISSUES

o Muscles grow in size over few months duration by **progressive increase in resistance.** At least an hour per day of resistance exercise is needed for beginners to develop muscle growth. Minimal groups of exercise that alter bodyweight consist of three or more groups of various modes of exercising. Each group is performed in three to eight sets. Sets are separated by a brief break of less than three minutes. The magnitude of resistance should allow smooth, full range of motion, but not so light that can be repeated over fifteen times per set. Such discrete mode, of resisting and taking breaks, is called "interval training". Although breaks separate sets apart, repetitions are separated by reversal of contraction, from eccentric to concentric, thus allowing muscle fibers to alternate recruitment. The rationale for resting between sets is to allow aerobic energy utilization to clean up the byproducts of the anaerobic activity.

Proceeding with strength training without breaks predisposes to chronic and protracted aftereffects. Protracted activities, such as long distance running and aerobics, do not increase muscle mass, yet increase muscle ability to endure for long, at lower energy utilization.

o Building stronger and bigger muscles is desirable as long as joints can maintain full range of motion. The misperception that large muscles essentially limit the range of motion stems from the long tradition of developing muscles by exercises of limited range of motion, such as in Bodybuilding and Powerlifting routines. The huge thighs and abdomen did not prevent the lifter in Figures 12.36 and 12.37, from squatting fully and fast, under heavy weight.

o It is evident that shortening of ligaments and tendons in Powerlifters and Bodybuilders is attributed to the practice of lifting on benches, from racks, and with the aid of machines. Strengthening by whole body exercises promote joint mobility in the extremes of motion.

o Without adequate whole body training, the 19-year old heavy Weightlifter, in Figures 12.38 and 12.39, cannot Squat as deep as his counterpart in Figure 12.37, and

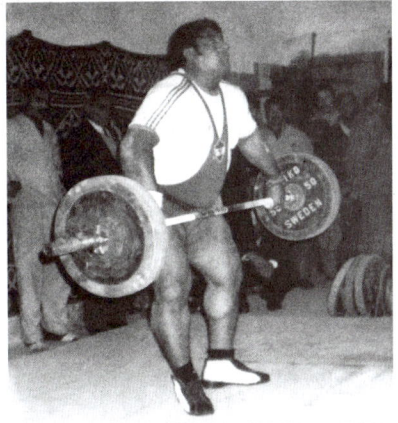

Figure 12.36. Pulling 150 kg in the Snatch is mostly achieved by axial muscles. The arms work as fixed levers that transfer axial forces to the bar. Cairo, Egypt, 1974.

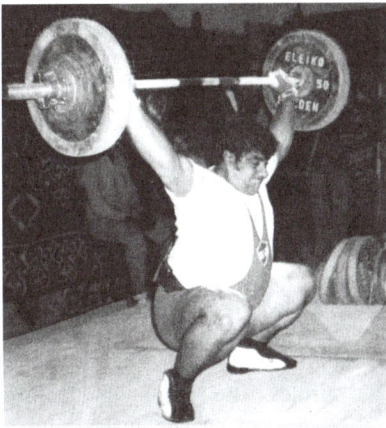

Figure 12.37. Full Squat Snatch of 150 kg by an overweight lifter is possible by regular and progressive training. Cairo, Egypt, 1974.

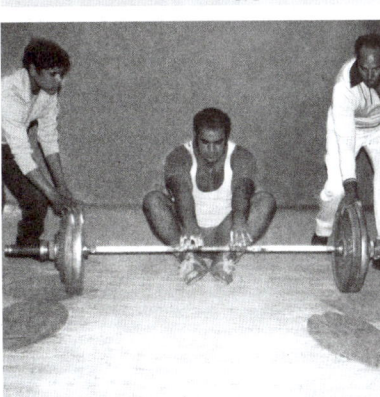

Figure 12.38. A 19-year old heavy weight lifter fails in snatching 120 kg due to very tight and massive muscles.

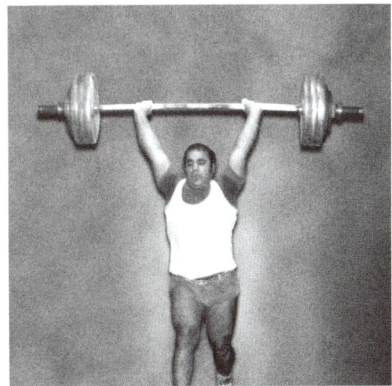

Figure 12.39. Though he was able to Clean and Jerk 160 kg, he relied totally on his strength, not his technique.

cannot spring his legs wide enough to ease his jerking of 160 kg. Both heavy lifters incurred diabetes mellitus in their thirties. The course of developing diabetes in heavy athletes seems to be very predictable unless serious weight reduction in carried out early in life.

o In the process of building large and strong muscles, one should not overlook the two main issues of losing **control on bodyweight** and **joint flexibility**. Both of these issues undermine one's mobility and health. Once your mobility is restricted, you start avoiding many essential exercises such as the full Squat, freestyle lifting from the floor, and standing weight exercises. These three basic activities strengthen average people beyond the norms of physical strength of general population. Inability to resist weights while standing and squatting freely, without aid, sets the chain reaction of wasting of thighs, Glutei, and back erectors. Thus, the skeletal axis wastes away with immobility. In all cases of body overweight and joint inflexibility, the underlying causes are preventable. Slight modification in exercise planning, of implementing full range of motion during strength resisting, and watching intake of calories, suffices preventing the two problems.

12.7. MUSCULAR IMBALANCE

12.7.1. SHOULDER AND PELVIS IMBALANCE

Weightlifters with **short stature and wide** frame perform efficiently in freestyle lifting. These lifters utilize the shoulders and pelvis optimally to generate torque by torso leverage. Though one may believe that long stature should generate greater torque, yet it should be emphasized that torque is generated by the axial muscles of the torso and legs, not the peripheral limbs. The tensile strength of the lumbar structures is the crucial limiting factor for maximal torque generation. That is because all remote forces, at the hands and feet, must balance around the lumbar joints. Thus, short and wide stature possesses greater strength of the lumbar region and reduces the torque required to move the remote limbs. The following examples support this argument.

o Strength and flexibility are crucial to the coordination of complex motion. In *Figure 12.40*, a lifter with adequate shoulder, back, and leg flexibility, snatches 95 kg. Muscular balance, of the shoulder girdle with the pelvic girdle, is perfectly executed around the lower back. The lifter uses his head and hips as adjustors for such balance. Without great shoulder and knee flexibility, balance cannot be maintained with such perfection.

o In *Figure 12.41*, another lifter with relatively inflexible shoulders fails to balance the 110 kg barbell over the two girdles. The rigid shoulders throw the lower back into spastic inflexibility, causing the bar to fall in front of the shoulders. The lift failed and the bar fell to the floor, from the front. In *Figure 12.42*, his second trial of 110 kg succeeded, by squatting deeper, with the buttocks seated on the heels and the belly on the thighs. Yet, his rigid shoulders are also preventing secure balance of the head and hips. The third trial of 115 kg Snatch, *Figure 12.43*, succeeded remarkably owing to the exaggerated back concavity and strong and deep Squat.

o *Figures 12.41* thru *12.43* demonstrate the disproportionate weakness of the upper body, with respect to the lower body. Note that, in these figures, the head is retreating backwards, relative to the previous figure. If the shoulders and arms were little stronger, the lifter would be able to perform the

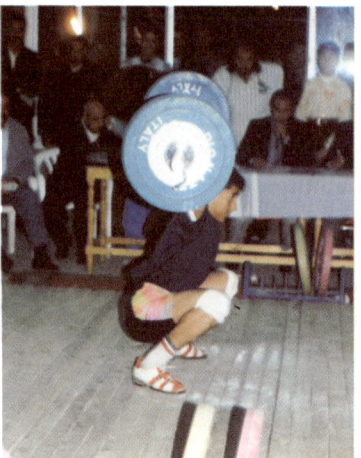

Figure 12.40. Strong and robust Snatch of 95 kg. The bar is balanced over the back of the upper chest.

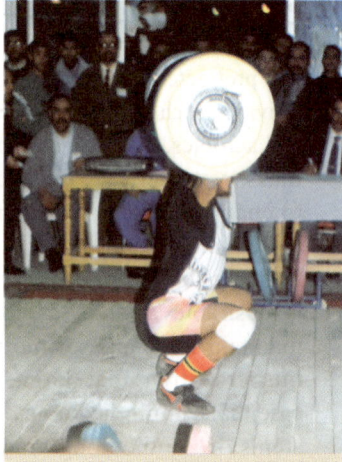

Figure 12.41. Incomplete Snatch of 110 kg. The bar falls short of vertical over the back of the upper chest.

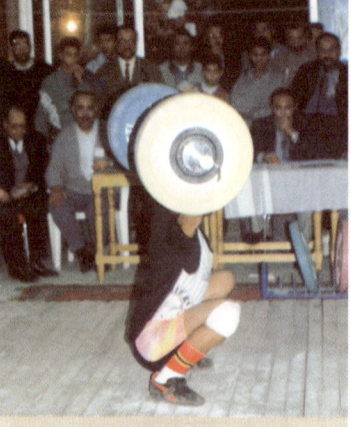

Figure 12.42. Deep Squatting in 110 kg Snatch, with lax lumbar spinal erectors.

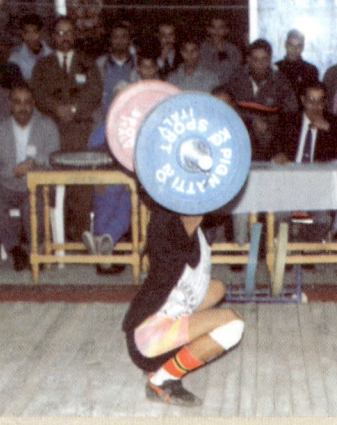

Figure 12.43. Deep Squat in 115 kg Snatch with actively erect lower spines.

alance of *Figure 12.40*, with slanted back and strongly contracting Trapezius. Depending heavily on deep squatting is an indication that the upper body cannot pull higher and stronger. This forces the lifter to dip earlier in the lift. Recovering from the deep Squat depends on the strength of the shoulder and pelvic girdles, the linking spinal erectors, and the cardiac reserve.

o   Remedial approaches for inflexible shoulders and spines have to include **whole body strength**, not merely strengthening individual muscles. For example, though the previous lifter has problem balancing the overhead weight, he might have weak pull or other hidden scapular imbalance. The cardiovascular and pulmonary functions also deserve great attention, in view of whole body strengthening. The most reliable index of progress, in resolving this imbalance, is the differential load volume of the Snatch training. Increase in load volume parallels increase in general strength.

o   **Upper body strengthening:** Peripheral training of the upper body benefits this group of lifters since their bodyweight cannot generate greater momentum, even with exaggerated bouncing of the torso and head over the feet balls, hips, and knees. Taking advantage of the shorter spans of levers between the joints, stronger arms and shoulders make significant difference is increasing muscle-to-bone efficiency of mechanical work. Yet, peripheral training is counterproductive, if not planned to balance the shoulders in all directions. The Deltoids are just partial effectors of the shoulders. The whole shoulder effectors are the Trapezius, Deltoids, Pectoral muscles, Latissimus dorsi, Teres major and minor, Serratus anterior, front neck vertebral muscles, and most importantly the scapular muscles (Supraspinatus, Infraspinatus, Subscapularis, Rhomboids, and Levator scapulae). These muscles transfer forces from the axis of the body to the arms. These make the widest variation in performance among individual lifters. Pinpointing weak links, in shoulder strengthening, is quite challenging. It requires good deal of understanding applied anatomy.

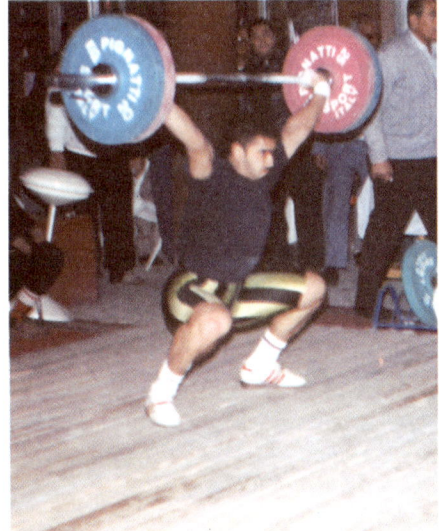

Figure 12.44. Strong well-belt lifter can Snatch 115 kg with high pull. His long torso stretches upward travel and makes it hard to squat deeper and recover without failure.

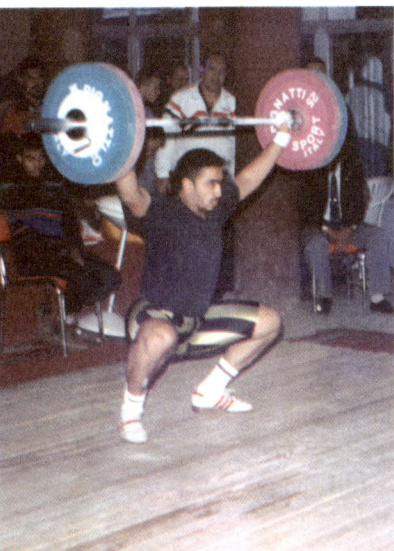

Figure 12.45. Inability to squat deeply under 125 kg Snatch caused the shoulders and elbows to buckles and defaulted the Snatch.

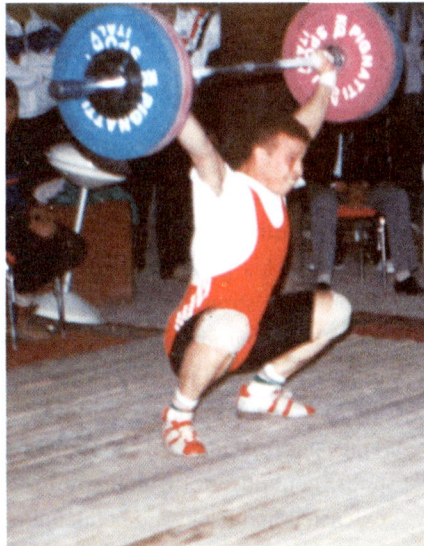

Figure 12.46. A tall lifter with strong legs compensates for his disadvantageous height and weaker arms with deep squatting, under 120 kg Snatch.

12.7.2. TORSO IMBALANCE

Weightlifters with long stature and narrow frame confront the challenge of generating adequate torque and maintaining balance, at the end of ballistic motion. These lifters have to advance the essential needs of whole body performance. These involve strong and flexible legs and spines, in addition to strong and balanced scapular muscles. Peripheral training might assist in advancing these needs. Yet, axial training is paramount for developing high neuromuscular control. The following examples support this argument.

o   The lifter in *Figure 12.44* has long stature and narrow shoulders. He can snatch 115 kg, with remarkable ease, and with high Squat. As the weight increases to 125 kg, *Figure 12.45*, the high Squat hinders the Snatch. The shoulder strength cannot help much with this weight, unless deep Squat is executed. His elbows buckled and the Snatch was defaulted. Tall lifters compensate with wide hand gripping of the bar in order to cut short the vertical travel. This lifter worked hard and long on his arms and muscle mass, yet overlooked flexibility. Neither his shoulders are able to bounce backwards (in order to balance the bar in posterior vertical plane over the body center of mass), nor is his back flexible to tolerate chest thrusting. In *Figure 12.45*, the chest is retreating backwards due the weak detraction of the scapulas (by weak Serratus anterior) and weak spinal erections. Such weakness is relative to the magnitude of great torque, generated by the back of this tall lifter.

o   The lifter in *Figure 12.46* has the same height as the previous lifter, but his strong spinal erection, scapular retraction, and leg flexibility is compensating his weak arms and his disadvantageous long stature. Note the full contact of the thighs with the calves. The abdomen is kept tight by the action of chest thrusting and diaphragmatic elevation. The previous lifter was able to tighten his abdomen, in *Figure 12.44,* when he executed chest thrusting, yet forgot to do the same thing in *Figure 12.45*. The poor tightening of the abdomen while lifting is a sign of a triad of flaws in the technique. These are: lax back erection, poor chest trusting, and poor Trapezius shrugging. This triad causes the upper body to buckle under resistance, causing the abdomen to trap most of the blood pool and reduce maximum cardiac output. The lifter of *Figure 12.46* is able to create chest inflation and abdomen deflation thus maximizing his cardiac output to peak performance.

12.7.3. IMBALANCE DUE TO BODY DISPROPORTION

The temptation of developing greater muscle mass, prior to engaging in Weightlifting programs, has benefited many lifters, particularly, those started training at late teens. Beyond that age, it is very difficult to reverse chronic stiffness and weakness of linking joints. The main disadvantage of starting with Bodybuilding training is the development of disproportion peripheral and axial muscles. The following two examples of ex-Bodybuilders foster this argument.

o   The lifter in *Figure 12.47* converted from Bodybuilding to Weightlifting and was able to overcome his greatest disadvantage, of being tall, by building strong legs, arms, and back. However, this 135 kg barbell has a long way to travel in this lifter's Snatch. His lack of experience is shown in the loss of chest thrusting, pulling with the upper Trapezius instead of the scapula retractors, and poor generation of momentum by full body extension and backward bouncing on the feet balls. Thus, strong muscles, with poor technique, delay the progress in Weightlifting. Bodybuilding training has enhanced muscular mass in this lifter, yet the disproportionate strength of the scapular

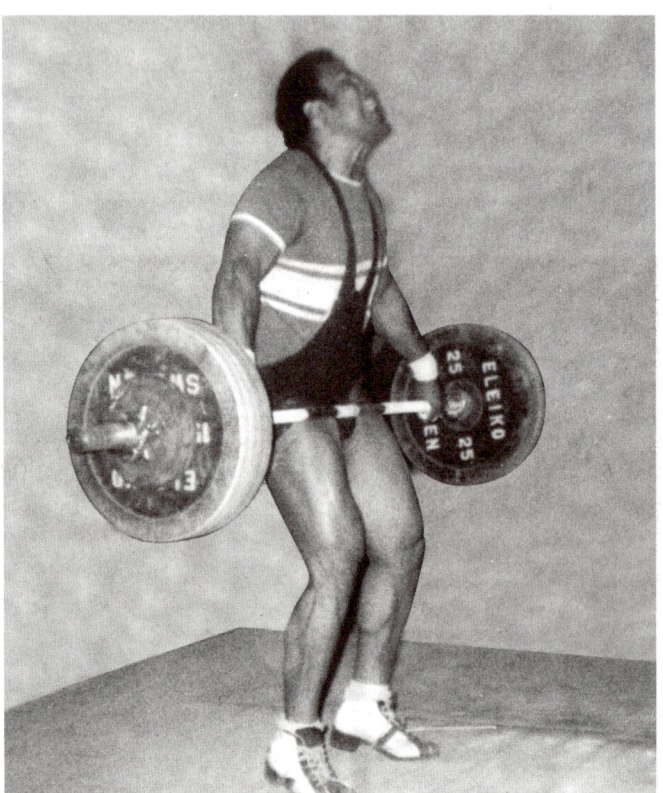

Figure 12.47. Tall lifters benefit greatly from developing greater muscle mass to compensate for their inability to bounce head and torso, as do shorter lifters. This lifter exerts much effort in Snatch 135 kg, than shorter lifters.

and spinal muscles, compared to the leg muscles, led this lifter to rely on the less effective muscles of arms. His counterpart, Weightlifters from the start, can effectively deploy scapular and spinal forces to execute the Snatch Pull, with maximal spinal torque.

o   The Olympic lifter, Abu-Kalila, in *Figures 12.48* and *12.49,* is shorter than the previous lifter and had practiced Bodybuilding from the age of 16 until 18, prior to converting to Weightlifting. His short stature and wide shoulders, in addition to well-refined technique, helped him excel in Weightlifting to the fifth rank in the 82.5 class, Los Angeles Olympic games of 1984. In this *Figure 12.48*, he was able to Clean and Jerk 172.5 kg, mostly with great muscular strength and less technical superiority than in *Figure 12.49*, ten years latter. Most highly ranking Weightlifters grow up as Weightlifters from the start and utilize modern simple routine. In preparation for contest, they perform split daily double-sessions and train up to 6 days weekly. This regimen develop huge thigh, back erectors, shoulder and arms muscles through the simple routines of the axial exercise of Clean, Snatch, Jerk, Squat, and Deadlift, in addition to one-hand dumbbell Presses. The load volume and intensity of training are the crucial factors in shaping the anatomical features of modern Weightlifters. Such specific and selective exercise program prevents the flaws in performance observed in *Figures 12.47* and *12.48*.

MAKING TRAINING CHOICES

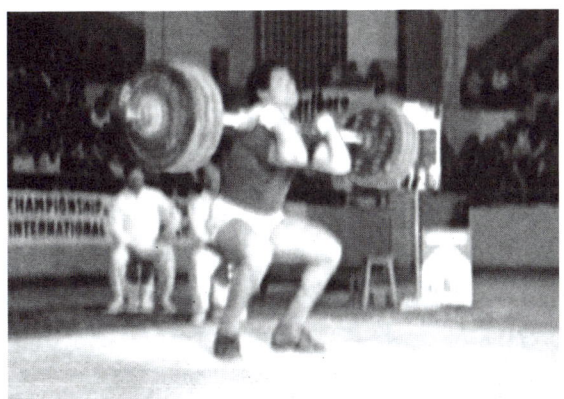

Figure 12.48. Ibrahim Abu-Kalila performing very high pull in the Clean of 172.5 kg, with awesome strong arms, relying heavily on his strong scapular and arm muscles. Alexandria, Egypt, 1974.

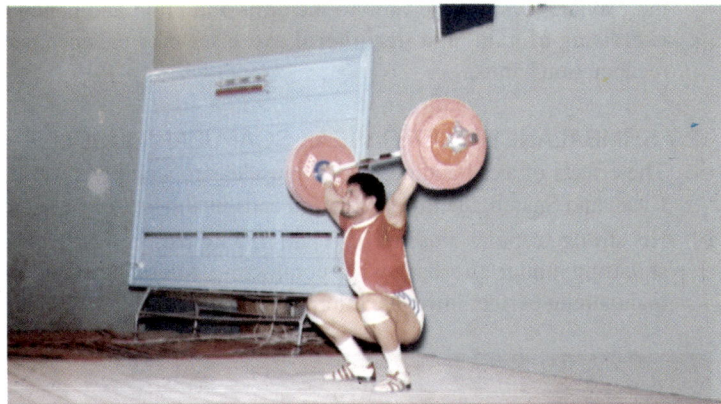

Figure 12.49. Ten years later, in 1984, Ibrahim Abu-Kalila has advanced in the Snatch of 140 kg. He will lift 150 kg in Snatch, in the weight class 82.5 kg, in Los Angeles Olympic Games, 1984.

12.7.4. IMBALANCE DUE TO WEAK ARMS AND SHOULDERS

Though developing strong and massive muscles, by sole Bodybuilding exercises and prior to Weightlifting, leaves the signature of stiffness of joints and weak links, yet the other option, of sole Weightlifting training, leads to other disadvantages. Skipping peripheral training by Weightlifters causes serious imbalance problems due to weak arms, chest, and shoulders, as follows.

o The lifter, in *Figures 12.50* and *12.51*, seems to have dismissed arm and shoulder training for quite long time. His weak pull in the Clean ends with the bar arriving too short, in its route to the shoulders. The weak shoulder and scapular muscles caused the right shoulder to drop and incapacitate the lifter, *Figure 12.50*. The same shoulder and arm buckle in the Snatch, *Figure 12.51*. Solving the problems of muscular imbalance requires tedious and patient planning. This includes managing volume and intensity, in addition to managing rest, nutrition, and relaxation. Consistent and regular insertion of shoulder and arms exercise, along with Weightlifting exercises, may pull this lifter out of this imbalance dilemma. These foster muscle strength without undermining the flexibility and coordination needed in full range of motion of sports activity.

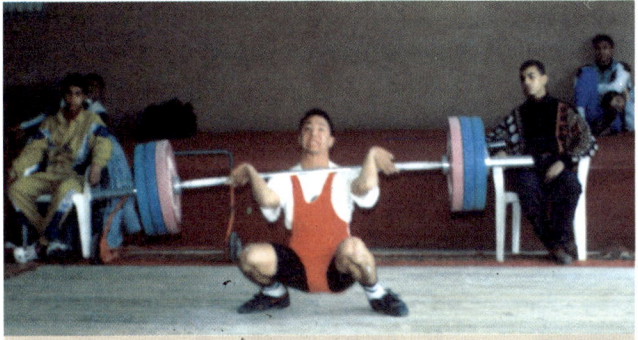

Figure 12.50. Muscular imbalance is very common in Weightlifters with weak arms and shoulders. In full squatting with 135 Clean, the bar is crushing the chest.

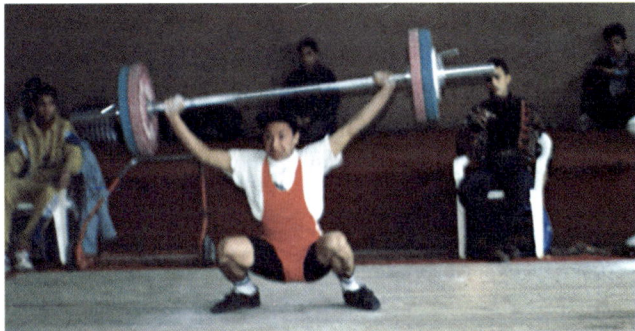

Figure 12.51. The apparently weak arms and shoulders become more apparent in overhead Snatch of 105 kg.

o Recommended exercises that can solve this sort of muscular imbalance are **axial exercises**, such as the military and Power Clean and Snatch, full Squat, Hang Clean and Snatch. In addition, the problematic shoulder and arm should be strengthened by **peripheral exercises** such as Biceps and wrist curls, Triceps extension, and one-hand dumbbell Shoulder Presses. Two or three of these exercises should be inserted in daily training sessions, in alteration and in excess of his regular training program.

o The rationale for combining axial and peripheral exercises, in dealing with muscular imbalance, stems from the multiple facets of imbalance. Strong axial muscles would have helped this lifter pull higher and stronger and, in the same time, maintain stable feet stance during the ascent and descent phases, as is the case in *Figure 12.48*. Axial strengthening enables the lifter execute the Pull, descend, and then ascend, on the exact feet stances he begins with. Strong peripheral muscles finalize the support of the bar on the shoulders, in the Clean, and overheads, in the Snatch. The strong shoulders and arms helped the lifter in *Figure 12.48* maintain both hands closer to the neck and chin, thus facilitating the major blood flow under the clavicles to the arms and brain. In contrast, the weak arms and shoulders of the lifter in *Figures 12.50* and *12.51,* caused his hands and arms to drop downwards, away from the neck, thus causing

12 MAKING TRAINING CHOICES

the clavicles restrict the flow to the arms and brain and hence the loss of legs and arms coordination. The **combined exercising of axial and peripheral exercises** may enhance performance, after few months of training and disciplined recuperation habits.

12.7.5. IMBALANCE DUE TO WEAK SCAPULAR MUSCLES

o The effects of axial and peripheral muscles are well demonstrated in the lifter of *Figures 12.52* and *12.53*. In both, the Clean and Snatch, the lifter starts and ends in almost the same location of initial feet stance.

o His strong scapular muscles help pull 135 kg bar, in the Snatch, very close to his chest and high enough to enable him squatting under the bar, with comforting tolerance. Getting the scapular muscles to perform that well, while maintaining perfect lower back lordosis, is the ultimate goal of axial and peripheral training.

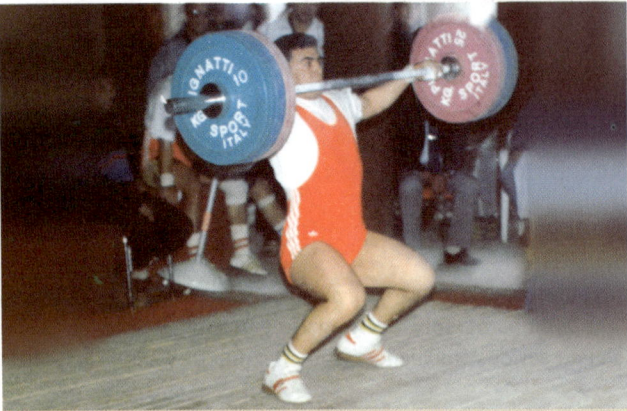

Figure 12.52. Heavy and tall lifters can still perform the full Squat Snatch. The strong axial erection of the Hamstrings, spinal erectors, and Trapezius assist the bar ascent, while the strong pelvis assist body descent, in 135 kg Snatch.

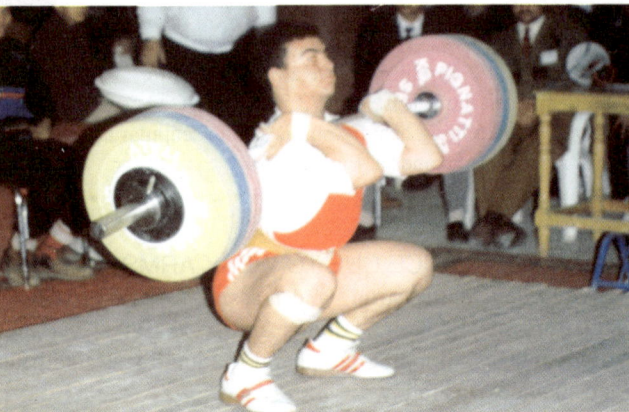

Figure 12.53. Note the difference between this lifter and the lifter in *Figure 12.61*. This lifter cannot keep closed handgrips with extended wrist, cannot dip into full Squat, and has very active back erection, under 160 kg Clean.

o In the Clean, *Figure 12.53,* the strength of the scapular and shoulder muscles is very evident in flexing the shoulders and elevating the elbows under 160 kg barbell, in full Squat. The hands, the bar, and the shoulders are all kept closer to the neck and chin, with the strong action of front vertebral cervical muscles, the Trapezius, and the Deltoids. The vertebral cervical muscles are invisible from outside, since they are located behind the neck vessels and on the front of the vertebral bodies and transverse processes. The strong shelving of the bar on the shoulders and hands, closer to the neck, enabled this lifter to maintain adequate circulation to the arms and brain, thus facilitates motor balance.

o Training on the shoulder shelving of the bar, in the full Squat Clean, is a well known habit in Weightlifting. That is totally unimaginable to outsiders, who fear letting a heavy bar pressing the vital blood vessels at the root of the neck. With regular Weightlifting training, the muscles that elevate the clavicles, the ribs of the chest cage, and the sternum, all, get stronger and hypertrophy by strength resistance, thus support shelving the bar on the top of the joint of the clavicles and sternum.

12.7.6. RECTIFYING SHOULDER IMBALANCE

Shoulder imbalance becomes evident under resistance. The most common shoulder imbalance is the inability to flex the shoulders and elevate the elbows under resistance, during full Squat. Weak shoulder flexion results from short and tense Subscapularis and Pectoralis muscles that oppose the action of weak Supraspinatus and front Deltoids. This imbalance can be rectifies as in the following four figures.

o In *Figures 12.54* thru *12.57,* the lifter is working on bar shelving skill. In the beginning, the bar lands too far in front of the body and the lifter has to lean forwards to catch the bar. That is because

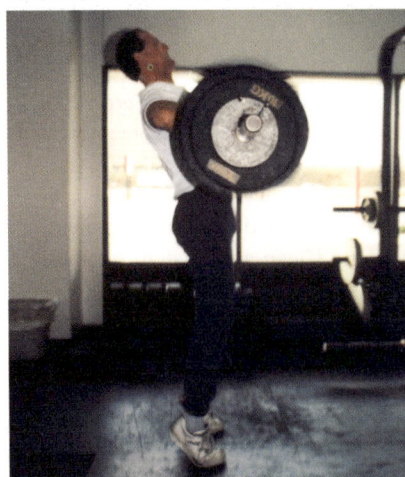

Figure 12.54. Training on head retreat and pelvic thrust, in the Clean Pull, enhances momentum generation. Courtesy of Nathan A. Lindeburg, Denver, Colorado, USA, 1993.

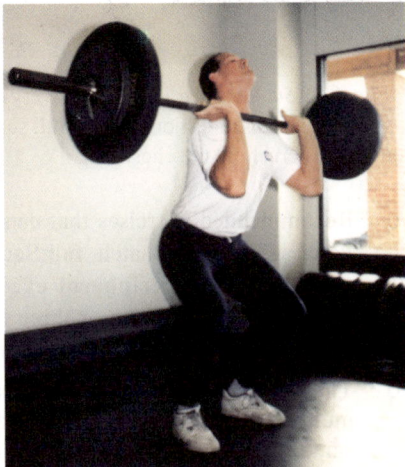

Figure 12.55. Shoulder flexion and elbow elevation take long training to achieve adequate balance between the Supraspinatus, Deltoids, and Subscapularis muscles.

- the pull, prior to shelving, did not generate sufficient body momentum.
- o With proper generation of momentum, the bar can comfortably be shelved as in *Figure 12.56*. Here, the hands, the bar, and the shoulders, all, concert supporting the bar, away from obstructing the space under the clavicles, where vital structure pass through.
- o As the Squat deepens, in *Figure 12.57*, the scapulas have completely been separated from the chest cage, compared to the dropped elbows in *Figure 12.55*. The muscles that maintain the scapulas steady and under traction, away from the chest cage, are the Serratus anterior muscles, which drive their origin from the front of the ribs. These muscles tighten when the chest is thrust forwards and upwards.
- o In these four figures, the lifter is refining the skill of spreading the scapulas away from the chest cage, and thrusting the

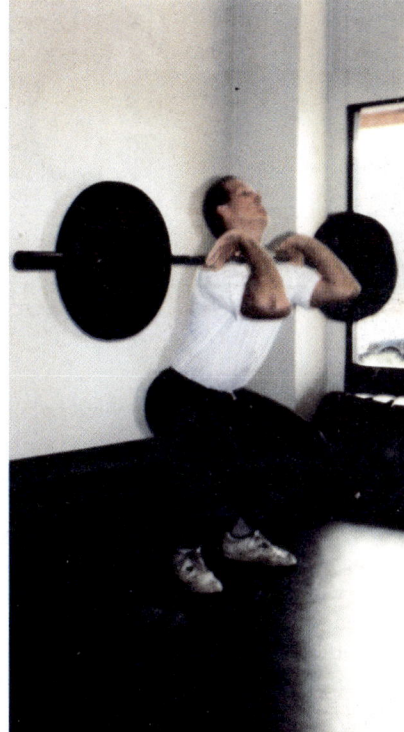

Figure 12.56. Full shoulder flexion and elbow elevation is attainable by balancing shoulder muscles.

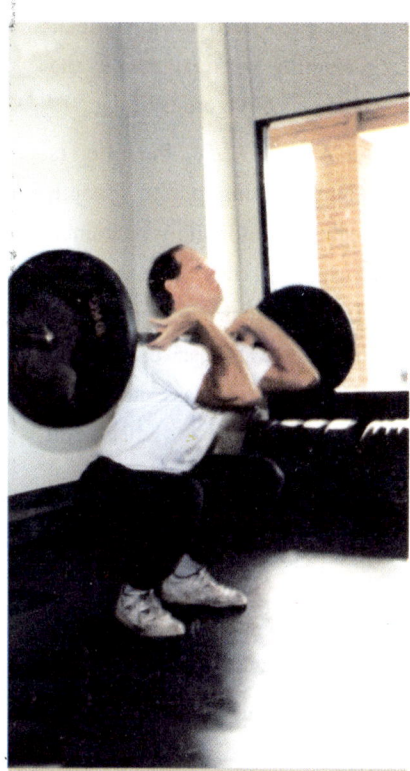

Figure 12.57. Descending in full Squat compromises the chest thrusting, in tall lifters, and requires constant reminding.

chest in order to rotate the shoulders in full flexion, and elevate the elbows. This skill is formidable to Bodybuilders and Powerlifters, since it requires not just shoulder flexibility but also the practice on moving the entire shoulder complex. This comprises of the scapulas, the clavicles, and the humerus. Practice of full Squat Clean helps approximate the shoulders and upper arms to the neck, with fully flexed elbows. Getting comfortable with this positioning of the bar, in front Squatting, is a
- o sign of developing well conditioned axial muscles and ligaments that can lift the chest cage, shoulders, and the external weight, during the extremely demanding front Squat position.

  Many well-trained Weightlifters learn the hard way that developing strong and proper front Squat requires persistent training. Starting with the lightest weight on the shoulders, and proceeding with the front Squat warms up the deep front vertebral neck muscles. This facilitates performing subsequent heavier sets of front Squat. The development of strong combination of front Deltoid contraction, scapular traction, chest thrusting, and neck extension, reduces the stressful feeling during deep front Squat with heavy weights. In *Figure 12.57*, the lifter has developed good control on relaxing the Triceps and wrist and finger flexors,
- o in order to allow the elbow to bend fully, and the shoulders to flex, in the manner shown in the figure. This elbow position secures shelving of the bar in the horizontal ditch formed by the Deltoids, Claviculomandibular joints, and the palms of hands.

  New comers need few weeks of coaching to grasp the relaxing techniques of the arms and scapulas that allow them to assume the position in **Figure 12.57**. The most common habits in beginners, learning front Squat, are: raising the heels, lowering the elbows, and maintaining straight back, instead of concave and strong back. The three habits are attributed to poor stretchability of the Achilles tendons, Quadriceps tendons, Triceps tendons, and wrist flexors. These structures will be targeted for strengthening, stretching, and coordination by front squatting.

12.7.7. GREATEST WEIGHTLIFTING ASSETS

- o The introduction of Squat in Olympic lifting, in the 1960's, as an alternative to leg lunging or springing, has altered the foundation of lifting mechanics. In the past, lifting was performed by generating momentum with stiff and slender limbs, *Figures 12.3, 12.5*, and *12.32*.
- o Today, Weightlifters have adopted training doctrine that bulks large leg, pelvic, and spinal muscles. These are the modern producers of momentum during freestyle lifting, *Figures 12.58* thru *12.61*.
- o Modern Weightlifters possess their greatest assets in their strong and flexible thighs, spinal erectors, and the shoulders. These three groups of muscles work on the two girdles, shoulder and pelvis, and the spinal axis. Their strength would

12 MAKING TRAINING CHOICES

not be as effective without their flexibility, when required by the demands of vigorous lifting.

o In *Figure 12.58,* the lifter is demonstrating perfect Snatch technique utilizing well trained thighs, spinal erectors, and shoulders. These axial strength enabled the lifter reduce horizontal displacement to minimum. This is evident from maintaining heels, wrists, and lumbar spines in one vertical plane, and by placing the bar over mid-thighs in, *Figure 12.59*. In addition, axial strength increased vertical displacement to maximum. This is evident from the straight arms and concave lower back.

o The imbalanced Snatch, in *Figure 12.60,* was caused by wide handgrips and wide feet stance. The relatively weak upper body undermined the neuromuscular balance and forced the lifter to dip under the bar by squatting, before the inertial energy of the bar was equalized by the adequate vertical pull.

o *Figure 12.61* shows similar problem, where the 160 kg was clearly, pulled strongly and shelved snuggly to the shoulders, but the back erectors failed to assume adequate lumbar concavity. Note that his lower back is still actively erect and the lifter was able to ascend and complete the Jerk.

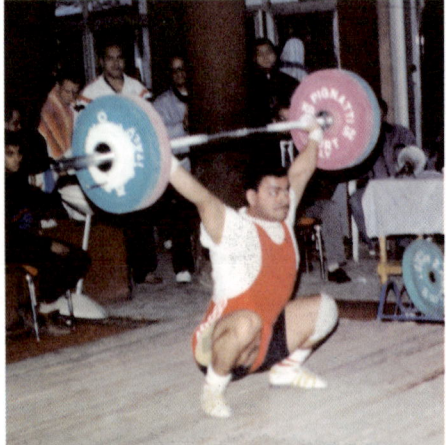

Figure 12.58. This lifter started his Snatch with 125 kg then increased the weight by 10 kg increments, to 135kg and 145 kg. His strong muscular development delineates the sharp curves of the chest thrusting, over the sucked abdomen, and back concavity, over the perfectly balanced pelvis.

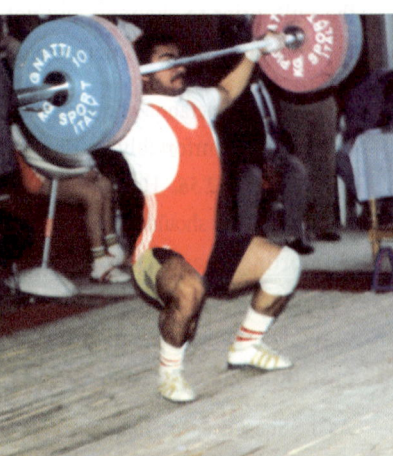

Figure 12.59. The 135 kg bar is kept vertically over the thrust chest cage by the strong pull of the Hamstrings, spinal erectors, and Trapezius. The tightly concaved lower back demonstrates the active state of "fight" prior to Full Squat.

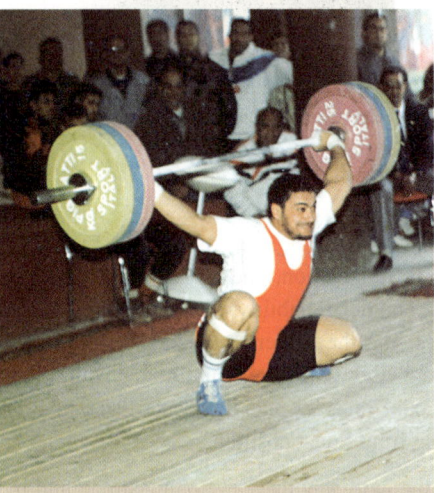

Figure 12.60. The unfortunate decision of widening the handgrips to maximum weakened the Trapezius resistance. The pelvis descended fairly low, but the shoulders buckled, under 145 kg Snatch.

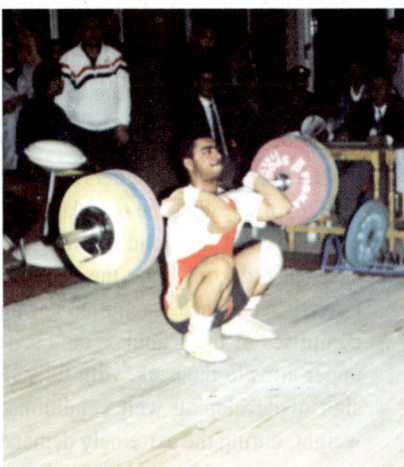

Figure 12.61. Modern Weightlifters can recover from this formidable full flexion position, under 160 kg Clean. Developing such full range of motion of shoulders, elbows, wrists, hips, and knees is a fundamental goal in Weightlifting.

o The combined strength and flexibility of this lifter are well demonstrated in fully flexed knees, hips, shoulders, and elbows, in addition to his remarkable recuperation from the drastically strenuous Snatch of 145 kg, in *Figure 12.60,* to the execution of the 160 kg Clean, few hours later, in *Figure 12.61*. The upper-to-lower body disproportion is common in Weightlifters, due to the high demand of regular training and the limited time availability of most Weightlifters. Those have other living necessities to attend to, besides amateur training.

12.7.8. MAXIMUM STRENGTH WITH MINIMUM MUSCLE MASS

o The old school of Weightlifting had long adhered to the belief that muscular strength has little to do with muscle size and, that lifters can be very strong, yet very skinny.

o The lifter in *Figures 12.62* thru *12.65* is as a bona fide witness for the common dismissal of peripheral training, in Weightlifting. His mere reliance on axial training is apparent in the lack of impressive muscular definition and limited range of motion of the scapulas and spinal column. The absence of large muscle mass led to the limited range of

MAKING TRAINING CHOICES

motion, due to the limited muscular strength along that range. Limitation of the range of motion also occurs with developing large muscles by Bodybuilding training alone.

o In *Figure 12.62,* the limited scapular flexibility undermines the chest thrusting, causing the Snatch pull to weaken and significantly compress the lifter to the floor, *Figure 12.63*. In *Figure 12.64,* the lifter is relying heavily on the axial muscles (Trapezius, Spinal erectors, Hamstrings, and Calves) in order to pull the 152.5 kg Clean, as high as he could. His relatively thin arms and shoulders weaken the pull and cause him to spring wide and deep, in order to jerk the weight, and almost missed, *Figure 12.65.*

o Both the disproportion in body strength and inflexibility, in this lifter, can be rectified with regular and frequent added doses of peripheral exercises. These remedy the weak links and stretch the stiffed joints. The only constraint, in most of these cases, is the time availability. Note that most Weightlifters do not gain substantial financial support from mere training. Most of them have to sacrifice not only with the money and time, but also with losing great opportunities of employment and social betterment due to their passionate dedication to the sport of bumping iron.

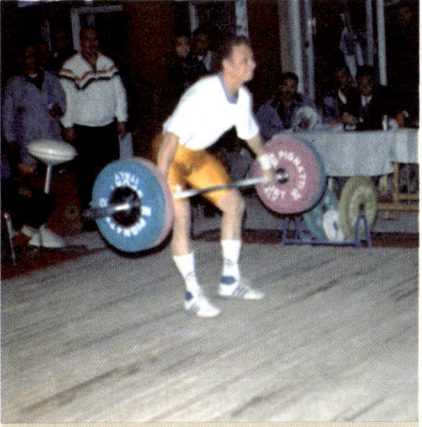

Figure 12.62. Tall and light lifters can develop strength and flexibility comparable to that of shorter lifters. This lifter can lean forwards and utilize the Hamstring pull on the upper phase of Snatch of 120 kg. Shorter lifters can exceed this angle of forward bending, due to the shorter torso.

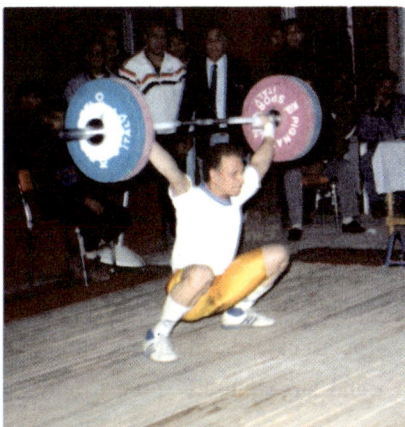

Figure 12.63. Despite his extreme undersized muscle mass, he can still dip in full Squat under 125 kg Snatch, in remarkable coordination and strength, and still maintain erect back. The downward and forward advancing of the pelvis makes chest thrusting very taxing.

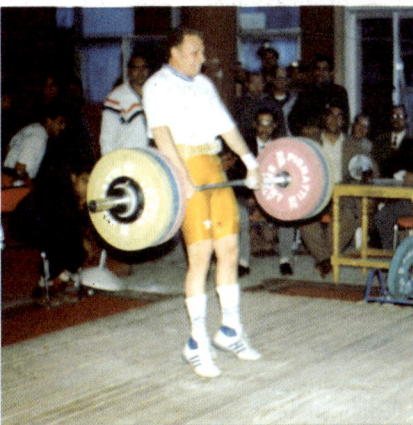

Figure 12.64. The disadvantage of being tall and thin can only be compensated by perfecting the technique of full extending the body on the feet balls, while keeping straight and solid elbows. This generates backward momentum that accelerates this 152.5 kg barbell, from the level of the groin to the waist level.

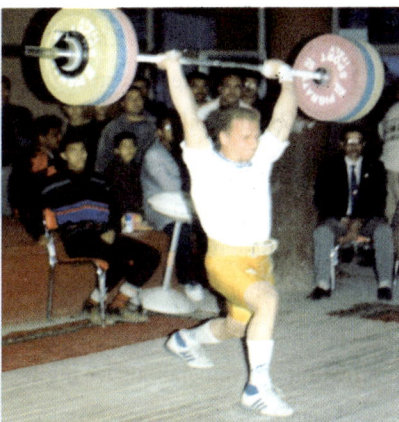

Figure 12.65. Remarkable success in the Clean and Jerk of 152.5 kg despite the poor chest thrusting, the poor back erection, and the limited range of motion of the shoulders. The wide and low leg spring compensated for his disadvantages.

o The fact that competitive training is, in it self, a substantial accomplishment in life, is not directly transparent to needy young lifters. The lifter in *Figures 12.38* and *12.39* for example, was able to smash all national records in all age groups, but was forced to abandon Weightlifting for dire financial needs. Few years latter, his heavy bodyweight caused him to suffer from diabetes, sickness, and disability.

12.7.9. DEALING WITH LONG LIMBED LIFTERS

o People with long limbs confront specific problems in producing joint torque and maintaining muscular strength. The weak conversion of muscular forces to bone leverage makes training and physical activity more daunting, compared to people with short limbs. This discourages the majority of people with long limbs from participating in **strength training**. Inadequate training or inactivity is more detrimental to the strength of these folks than others, since they need stronger muscles to accomplish the same tasks others can perform with relative ease.

o Strength training for sport activity is founded on a cardinal rule that flexibility and strength are inseparable. This opposes, at least apparently, the common belief among physical therapists that strong muscles tighten joints and do away with flexibility. The apparent paradox between strength and flexibility is easily eliminated by realizing the need for active neuromuscular control in sport activity.

12 MAKING TRAINING CHOICES

o Thus, strong muscles can only restrict mobility if joints were not strengthened, from the beginning, by full range of motion resistance. The example in *Figures 12.38* and *12.39,* demonstrates the restricting effects of large and strong muscles on joint flexibility. In that case, the trainee had strong and large muscles prior to any training, and did not build those muscles with full range of motion resistance. On the other hand, the lifters in *Figures 12.37* and *12.61* have significant leg, pelvis, and back flexibility despite the large muscular mass.

o The lifter in *Figures 12.66* thru *12.69* demonstrates his struggle with poor flexibility, despite his average bodyweight and muscle mass. His long arm and leg bones compromise the flexibility of elbows, shoulders, hips, knees, and ankles. That is because executing flexible movements, under high resistance, requires great muscle-to-bone conversion of force. The signs of poor flexibility, in that lifter, are the Achilles stiffness and

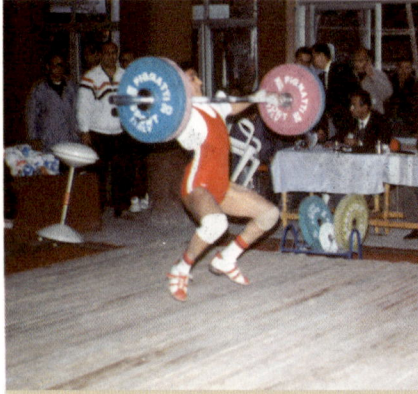

Figure 12.66. Pulling the bar closer to the body enables this lifter with relatively weak arms to Snatch 115 kg. Any departure of the bar away from the body increases the forward-downward torque of the weight on the body.

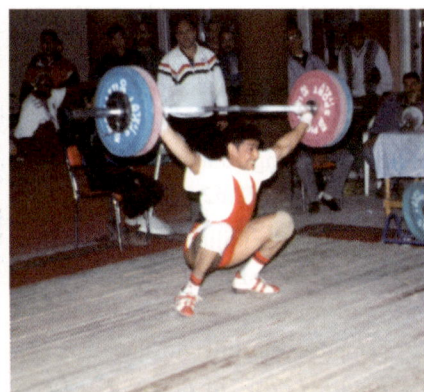

Figure 12.67. Relatively weak arms and shoulders are common causes of failure in the Snatch. This 120 kg Snatch would fail due to inadequate shoulder support. The imbalanced shoulders caused lack of attention to proper feet stance.

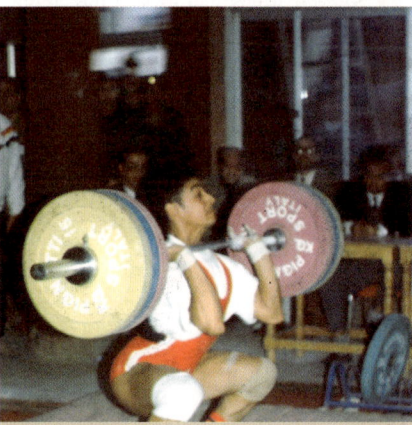

Figure 12.68. In the Clean, the relatively weak arms and shoulders hinder the flexion of the shoulders and cause the elbows to drop down, in this 145 kg Clean.

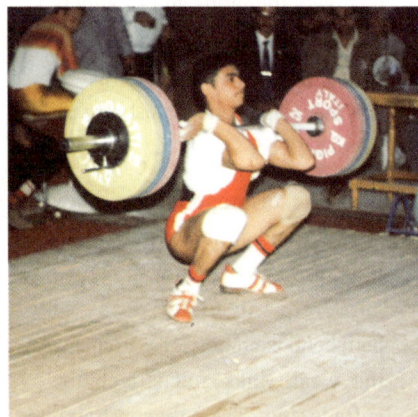

Figure 12.69. With deeper Squat, the shoulders are getting some help and can elevate the elbows, in 150 kg Clean. Note the bar is well seated on the shoulders.

Quadriceps imbalance (poor right foot positioning in all figures), the shoulder imbalance, *Figure 12.67,* and the poor shoulder flexion, *Figure 12.68*. Long and dedicated training can compensate for disadvantageous leverage configuration of the long bones.

o In this category of people with long limbs, peripheral exercises combined with axial exercise can accomplish great development. Emphasis should be on ligamentous strengthening with controlled high-tension movement. The following exercises could remedy inflexibility issues in these lifters.
  i. **Scapular balancing** by Cable rowing, Stiff-legged Deadlift, Shoulder Shrugs, One-hand Dumbbell Press in various inclinations.
  ii. **Spinal balancing** by Jump Goodmorning, Jump Squat, Front Squat, Overhead Squat, and Bent-Over Row.
  III. **Leg balancing** by Weighted Stepping, Weighted hopping, Half Squat, and Stretching.

12.7.10. WEIGHTLIFTING TRAINING, FROM START TO END

Making the choice of Weightlifting training, from early adolescence, has helped those with close relatives, familiar with this sort of training. From the early years, the child plays with the technique of execution. Most probably, those young Weightlifters develop privileged strong axial musculoskeletal structures that enable them exceed all expectation, in lifting strength and performance. These lifters mostly rely on classical Olympic exercises and meditative techniques of rest, massage, and relaxation. The following four figures demonstrate the features of training on Weightlifting, from adolescence and up.

MAKING TRAINING CHOICES

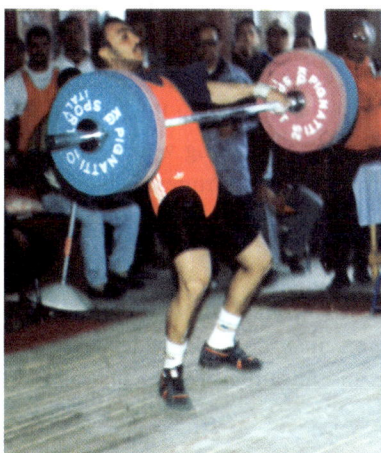

Figure 12.70. Modern Weightlifters are lighter and stronger. The Snatch of 135 kg is executed with the body momentum generated by the axial erectors (Trapezius, Spinal erectors, Glutei, and Hamstrings).

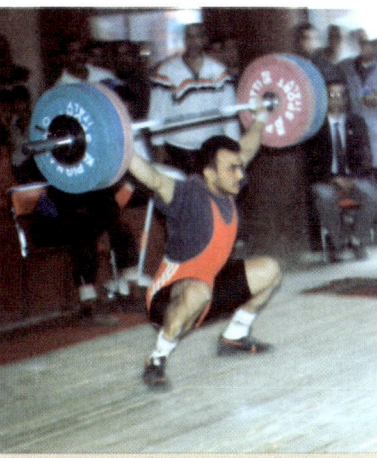

Figure 12.71. Proper body proportions help this lifter (class 82 kg) to lift 140 kg, Snatch, and balance the weight with erect back, thrust chest, tight abdomen, and elevated shoulders. He still has a room for deeper Squatting.

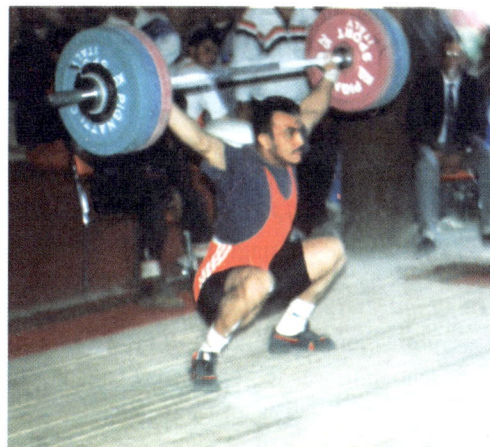

Figure 12.72. Snatch of 142.5 kg is executed with the exact perfect performance of 140 kg. Notice the precise curves, stance, and handgrips, as in previous figure. This lifter is a second generation in a family of Weightlifters.

o *Figures 12.70* thru *12.73* show a lifter with short stature, compared to the previous lifter, that was able to add more than 20 kg in the Snatch, and 10 kg in the Clean, over the previous lifter's maximum. The short arms and legs of this lifter gave him greater advantage is balancing the shoulders and the feet stance, throughout his lifting. Both lifters, however, have benefited greatly from axial training by enhancing their ability to mobilize the entire body mass, into full extension over the feet balls, and gauge the timing of dipping under the bar that far exceeds their bodyweight. Note that with those slim arms, relative to Bodybuilding standards, both lifters were able to accelerate such heavy weight to overhead reach, without any aiding tools. The virtual dynamic forces, generated by acceleration of both the bodyweight and the weight of the barbell, compound the effect of resistance strengthening of the major supporting ligaments, tendons, muscles, and bones. Weightlifters develop proper distribution of bone density and tensile strength, in an ascending pattern, from the toes to the skull, owing to the performance of whole balanced lifting. None of these lifters would have been able to extend flexibility to overhead lifting had they content themselves with Powerlifting exercises, of the Squat, Bench Press, and Deadlift.

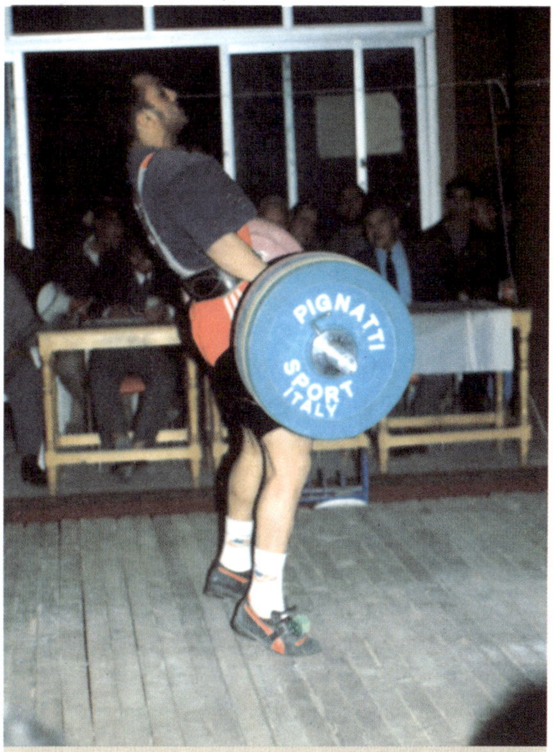

Figure 12.73. The Clean pull is also aided by whole body extension, prior to any arm bending. Bouncing the entire body backwards, on the feet balls, generates enough momentum to move this 160 kg barbell to the waist height.

o It may be naïve to draw conclusion about the dynamics of lifting by just analyzing the mechanics and anatomy of performance, since physical strength is a culmination of psychological and physiological interplay of events. The best strength-training program would not overcome many psychological issues that affect performance. The psychic makeup of Weightlifters could sometimes be traced back to extended generations of family members.

o From my own personal experience, some lifters in the prime of their strength lose interest in competition, altogether, when crucial social conflicts occupy their mind. For example, Mahgoob, the lifter in *Figure 12.32* (year 1951) had great fame by competing in Weightlifting as a national champion, in times when social fame meant job security. His passion to Weightlifting continued to his old age. On the other hand, the lifter in *Figure 12.38*, Safa, flunked Weightlifting altogether to earn living in various menial jobs. Abu Kalila, *Figures 12.48* and *12.49*, had his entire life changed, for good, by engaging in Weightlifting. I have convinced him, from day one, to advance his education, from the vocational trade to college. In the ten years he struggled to finish high school and obtain a law degree form the University of Alexandria, he was content and happy to lift weights. After his graduation and his Olympic accomplishment of 1984 games, other life affairs had drifted him away from sport. The heavyweight lifter, in *Figures 12.36* and *12.37,* was a school teacher, with background in theology, his main impetus to training was the religious belief that excelling is sport is a religious duty, to set good role model for the young people he nurtures. The last lifter, Kareem, *Figure 12.70*, was born to two brothers who dedicated their life to Weightlifting. His childhood play and fun was around the single room gym, in the ghettos of Alexandria, Egypt.

o   *Figures 12.74* thru *12.78* and *12.81* show glimpses of the life of a Weightlifter who made this sport his passion, profession, and future. Lifting weights in a big city was a way to build social relationships and find a better job. When schooling was too expensive, tedious, and long, Weightlifting was fun, nurturing, and rewarding for the man in these figures, as well as for many others

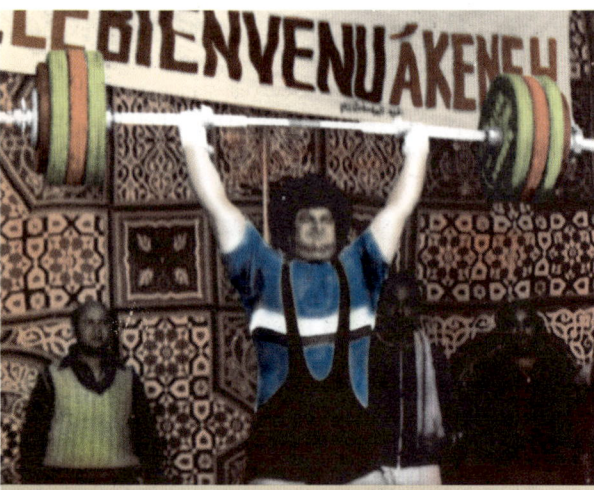 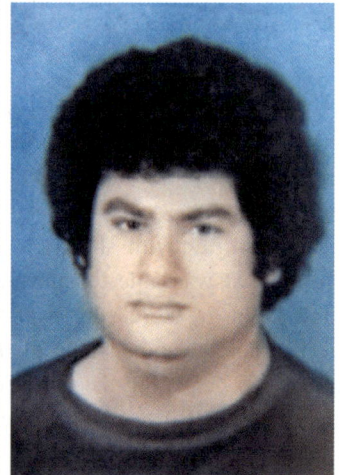 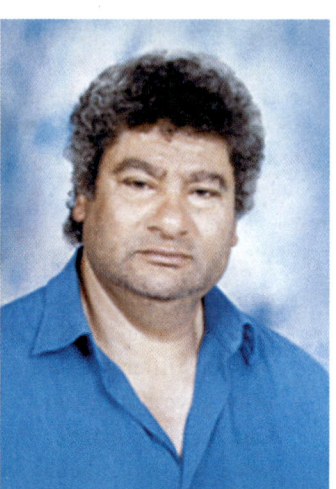

Figure 12.74.   *Figure 12.75.*   *Figure 12.76.*

Figure 12.74. Gaber Hafez

He is Egyptian icon in Weightlifting of modern times. Although he has never won an advanced Olympic medal, yet he revived the sport for over forty years. After the end of the greatest Egyptian triumphs in Weightlifting in 1951, Gaber tried tirelessly to reclaim past glory. The author grew up when Gaber Hafez was the only champion in Weightlifting, in Egypt. He was the first generation to adopt the Full Squat during lifting. That will take another three decades, before an avalanche of newly born young people will follow the example of Gaber Hafez. His biggest obstacles were lack of education and poor socioeconomic status. That repelled highly qualified coaches to bid on bettering his career. Thus, he stuck with sympathetic coaches, whose technical resources were no greater than his. He managed his own training program and used his coaches as paternal stimulating figures. Al-Kassabany, *Figures 12.1* thru *12.5*, was one of those skilled coaches who declined to associate with Gaber, and preferred to train brand-new generation of young people. Al-Kassabany's first success was Abu-Kalila that snatched the national attention away from Gaber and proved the correctness of Al-Kassabany's prophecy. In addition to his personal predicament, revolutionary advances were being made by the communist bloc in scientific training. Had he learned about nutritional science or had the financial resources to eat healthy food, he might have climbed to the top of international Weightlifting. His main diet was sugar cane molasses and carbohydrate rich food.

Figure 12.75, from 1964 until 1988, his name and pictures associated with Weightlifting in all media news, in Egypt. He had traveled allover the world, representing Egypt as a top Weightlifter. His great sense of humor and affectionate personality earned him the lifetime position of National Weightlifting Coach, *Figure 12.76*. Despite his limited intellectual resources, he can, effectively and ingeniously compensate for such shortcomings with his experience in training, failure-prevention, contest psychology, and interpersonal relationship. His limited educational background was a plus in some other ways. He never knew or understood the concept of anabolic steroids. The only drug that he used to inject his trainees with Vitamin B-complex. He carried the injection kits and a supply of ampules in his room and practiced the injection by himself, for the purpose of showing his bonding and caring about his trainees. Although he traveled allover the world as a national Weightlifting champion, he only mastered few foreign words such as "Thank you", "mercee", "cpa-cipa", and "dunkea", which he used, altogether, whenever he met a foreigner. He jocularly, but seriously, stated that all foreigners understand the same foreign language. His simplistic views about life made him content with living, competing, and training in very dismal economic environment.

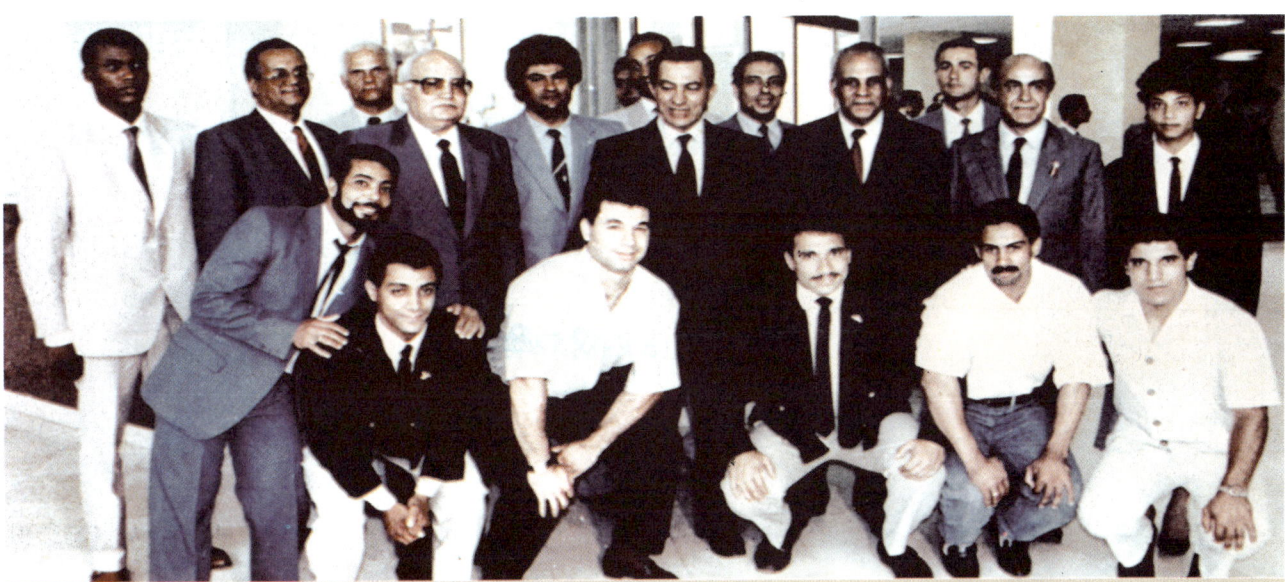

Figure 12.77. Gaber Hafez standing behind, to the right of the President of Egypt, Hosni Mubarak. The forty years of Weightlifting training, coaching, and representing the country in international contests, had earned him this privileged moment. He started Weightlifting in the army, when Gamal Abdel Nasser brought the soviet experts to train and modernize the Egyptian military. After the 1967 war, athletes were kicked out of the army, and many, including Gaber Hafez, had to seek other employments, in grim economic environment. That was a career blow to this young and ambitious Weightlifter. In fact, like many other athletes with no education, Gaber did not made any attempt to explore the world beyond Weightlifting. It became his passion and source of income, fame, and social life. His content with financial and intellectual deprivation earned him this association with the president of the country. Many others who had pursued academic prosperity had never enjoyed such fun and pleasure or even enriched their life, as did this dedicated and simple man.

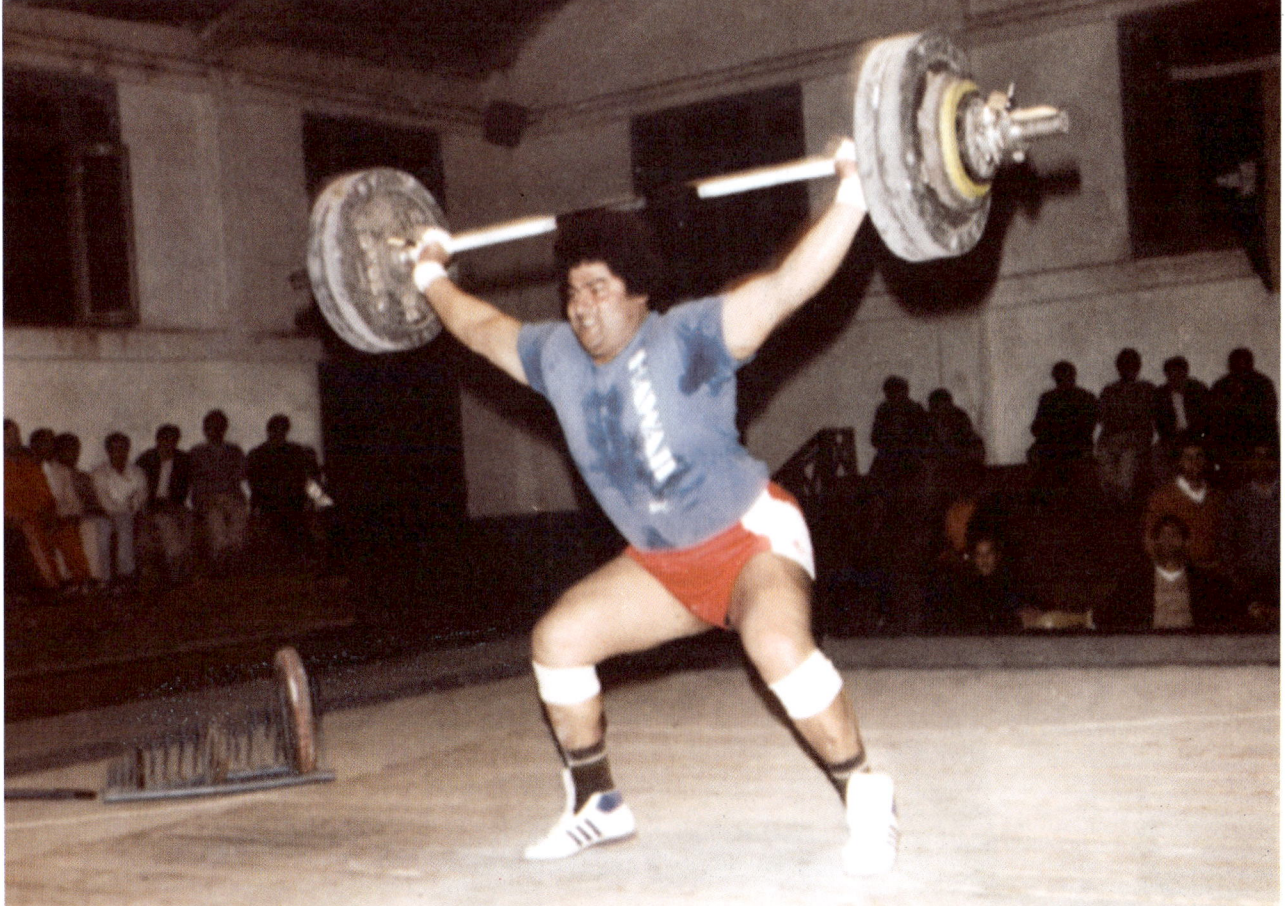

Figure 12.78. Too many years of training on Weightlifting had led to this stiffed body posture. The lack of adequate and proper stretch had caused this dedicated Weightlifter to lose flexibility, in almost all his joints. The below-knee bandages cannot explain any reasonable anatomical cause of pain other than stiff tendons and ligaments, or peripheral arterial compromise. Alexandria, Egypt (1973). Compare the technique of *Figures 12.79* and *12.80* (year 2002) of full Squat and flexibility, with the 1973 technique, above.

12 MAKING TRAINING CHOICES

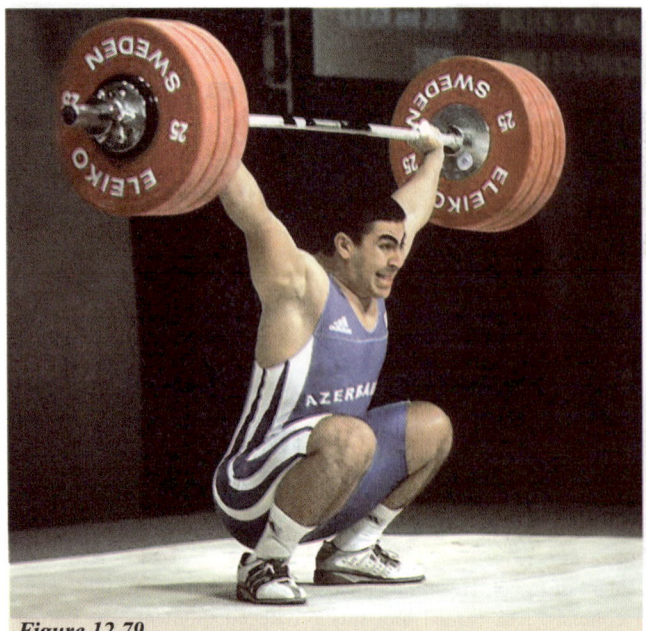

Figure 12.79.
Nizami Pashaev, from Azerbaijan, born 1981, BW 92.65 kg, Snatch 177.5 kg, C & J 215.0 kg. 2002 World Championships, November 18 – 26. Warsaw, Poland.

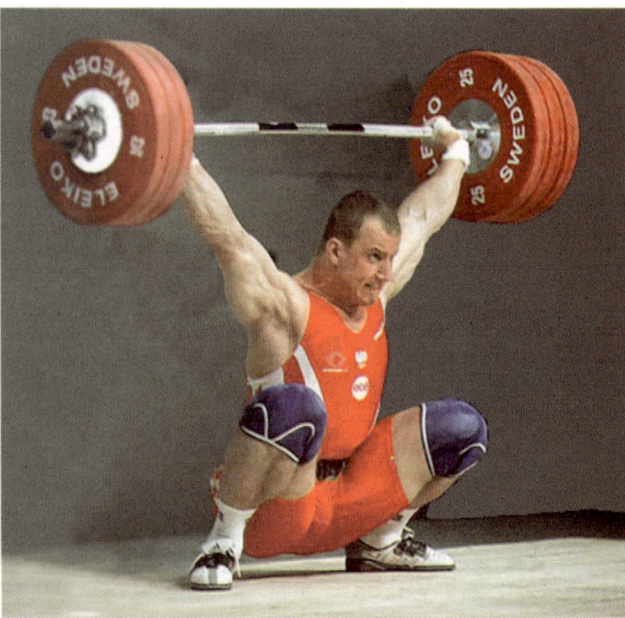

Figure 12.80.
Dolega, Marcin, from Poland, born 1982, BW: 104.05 kg, Snatch: 192.5 kg, C & J: 220.0 kg. 2002 World Championships, November 18 – 26. Warsaw, Poland

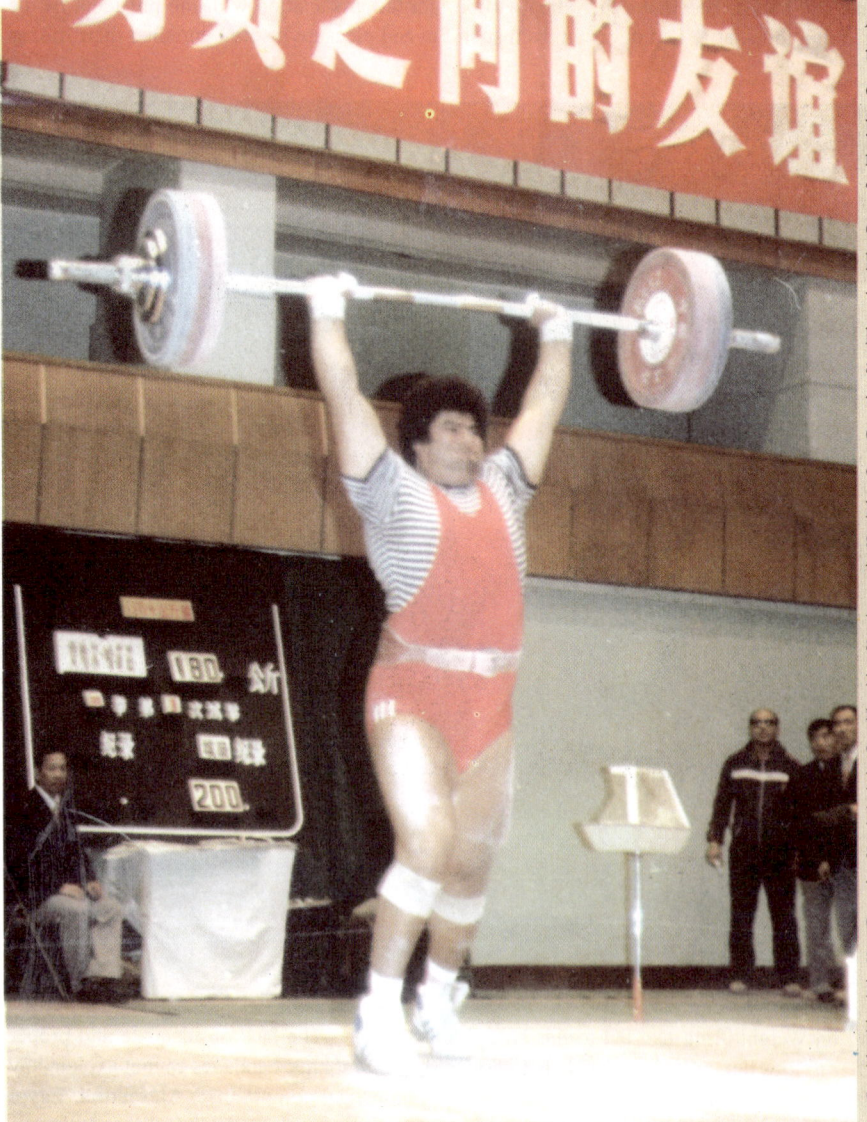

Figure 12.81. Although lifting 180 kg in the Clean and Jerk, in Superheavy weight class, is not a great deal, internationally, yet the story of struggle behind it is noteworthy.

This lifter had trained mainly on axial exercises. Most of his training was with heavy weights. His main assisting exercises were the one-hand dumbbell Presses, push-ups upside down against the wall, and weighed abdominals. His core training followed the Russian model. The Clean and Jerk and the Snatch were the core of his training sessions. These were performed in different style in different sessions. Each lift was assisted, in exercise, by its Pull, Press, and Squat version.

Although he performed sufficient massage and used hot saunas on weekly basis, he never stretched enough or properly. His muscles were tight and overtrained, most of the times. The two bandages below the knees hint to his stress.

His opinionated self-coaching style, in addition to his lack of education, led him to repeat the same mistakes and shun any effort to change his training method. Although such self confidence and determination had limited his options of international rising, yet it made him succeed in very rivalrous community of competing coaches, managers, and opponents.

Chapter 13: Managing Load Volume and Intensity

13.1. PROGRESSIVE STRENGTH TRAINING

13.1.1. SOURCE OF INFORMATION

In order to enhance physical strength, training must proceed in progressive increments of increase in resistance. Though the rate of such progression varies from one individual to another, there are universal features that apply to all people. Beginners of weight training will probably make progress no matter what they do, as long as they train regularly, frequently, and consistently. The best example for natural progress is seen in farmers and factory workers. However, after some time, the absence of documented and thoughtful planning leads to either over training, inadequate stimulation of muscular growth, or muscular imbalance. The widespread musculoskeletal deformities among non-athlete lifters, such as the previously mentioned groups, attest to the importance of planning balanced training. **Reliable planning for strength training** should enable trainees to intensify their workouts, maintain high load volume, prevent muscular imbalance due to poorly distributed load volume over participating chains of muscles and joints, and, most significantly, achieve realistic goals in appropriate time frame.

The task of gathering information about the best suitable planning for an individual is hampered by the many contradicting approaches to strength training. Most approaches are based on **individual and empirical experience**. In this book, the author relied on his 40 years of Olympic training, in addition to his medical and engineering backgrounds. The author has used diary notes along these years and compared them with other's experience. Therefore, beginners should follow training programs used by experienced lifters. Advanced individuals do not necessarily work out harder, since they already developed good grasp on the scope of recuperation and resistance.

Recuperation takes place between workouts. If the body has not fully recovered between workouts, overtraining can ensue. This is, most probably, the most common drawback of **mismanaging weight training**. Experience and knowledge of managing volume and intensity of weight training are passed from older generation of lifters to offspring. In agricultural communities, farmers gain such knowledge from the close social settings of big and coherent families. The case is different in costal cities. Here, proliferation of information flourishes through the great traffic of travelers, from diverse parts of the world. Presently, the Internet plays great role in disseminating information.

13.1.2. SETS, REPETITION, INTENSITY, AND VOLUME

A **set** of exercise group is defined as the starting and ending of an exercise without long pause. Pauses between sets range from 1.5 minutes to 3 minutes. Performing one set of exercise elicits slightly greater strength gain. Additional sets should be performed in order to improve such gain. The optimal number of sets, per exercise group, is between two and five sets. The reason for the multiple-set routine is to accommodate for neuromuscular, cardiopulmonary, and cardiovascular adaptation. These require a total net of high physical work in order to produce significant changes in structures.

A set of exercise may comprise of multiple repetition, of a cycle of concentric and eccentric muscular contractions. The number of cycles per set constitutes "**repetition**". Also, the magnitude of resistance, during each cycle, constitutes the "**intensity**" of that set. The net intensity of an exercise group is the **product of number of sets, repetition, and magnitude of resistance**. This determines the extent of physical work by muscles and heart, in that exercise.

There are limits on trying to manipulate the net physical work of exercise, by merely increasing or decreasing the number of sets, repetition, or intensity. The daily and weekly sum, of all differential work of various exercises, determines daily and weekly load volumes, respectively. Therefore, in addition to counting the net load volumes, different muscle groups require specific **allotment differentials** of daily and weekly volumes. For example, by training each muscle group every four days, instead of every three days, the number of exercises or sets may be increased, or the magnitude of resistance may be increased. This compensates for differential load volume per muscle group. However, managing these four components (intensity, number of sets, repetition, and volume) is bounded by the complex process of **physiological recuperation**. Intensity of resistance is crucial to advancing physical strength.

13.1.4. EXERCISE INTENSITY

Increasing weekly load-volume, or session load-volume, with **low intensity resistance**, serves different purpose, other than developing strength. That is enhancing aerobic oxidation by muscles, and depleting fuel depots. Additional sets yield less progress in strength, to a point of diminishing return. Therefore, individuals accustomed to a high volume, low intensity training confront real challenge when switching to high intensity programs. It may take months before these individuals adapt to progressively intense training. Increasing resistance stimulates anaerobic oxidation and enhances the population of strong muscle fibers, in the place of the fragile and weak ones. Furthermore, resistance should be increased progressively in order to foster physiological changes for strength. A progressive intensity program seems to be the key factor in strength development, and consequently enlarging muscle mass.

Although intense resistance does not consume body fat, at least immediately and during exercise, it requires active, after-exercise, cycling of byproducts and replenishing consumed substrates. In fact, anaerobic activity utilizes only less than 5% of the energy available for fast **fuel supply**. However, the high magnitude of power output, during intense resistance, conditions the integration of many systems in response to high demands of physical work. Thus, the essence of physical strength is doing the most, within the least number of sets and exercises. This involves performing as many repetitions as possible with heavy resistance, within the repetition range of the workout set, one repetition short of failure, without compromising exercise technique.

13.1.5. RECUPERATIVE INTERVALS

Higher numbers of exercise repetition, per set, operate by aerobics oxidation of fuel. These burn more calories than grow more muscle mass, as in endurance exercise. The reverse is true in strength training, where more rest is needed between sets, repetitions, and sessions, in order to foster **growth of muscles**. Rest decreases traumatic effects of vigorous muscular work. Since strength training emphasizes whole body strength, therefore, there is no need to divide the body into as many muscle groups, when planning strength-training program. Three or four muscle groups suffice better management of load volume per major muscular groups. Recuperative intervals between intense training sessions are typically 12-24 hours.

Each muscle group can be strengthened with **greater frequency,** more than just once a week. Daily double training sessions can be designed to engage various muscle groups, within closely watched differential load volume, for each group. However, such short recuperative regimen necessitates greater individual flexibility, in abandoning fixed number of sets and repetition, and adhering closely to total and differential load volume.

13.1.6. PERIODIZATION OF LOAD VOLUME

Resistance load volume has more impact on **power output** than muscular strength. That is because, power output depends more on systemic integration than strength of local muscles alone. In addition, high monthly load-volume advances systemic processes by availing greater oxygen delivery and cardiac stroke volume to cellular demands. This is the rationale of performing multiple sets in Olympic weightlifting. Multiple sets enhance the neuromuscular adaptation and power output, required for freestyle lifting. Yet, the cost of these accomplishments is abbreviating the number of exercise groups and exercise repetition, in daily sessions.

Though progressive intensity training is the prescribed method of developing strength, it does not amount to indefinite, constant, and linear progression. It should accommodate the inherent relative changes at the different phases of life. In other words, you will be climbing the same hills, and descending the same valleys, over and over, many times through your life. That is described as "**periodization**". This consists of cycles of periods of progressive, weekly load volume. A period involves cycles of progressively intense exercises, added weekly. As the number of sets increases, the number of repetition decreases, with heavier resistance than previous sets. A cycle may last weeks. It can be made up of several intricate cycles, growing progressively longer each successive cycle. After six to twelve weeks, a period may lead to contest. Subsequent periods should start with higher volume baseline.

The final results of managing load volume and intensity are judged by reducing burning of contractile tissues and enhancing their strength and mass. In other words, maximizing a **good mix of endurance and strength** is the ultimate goal of wise management of strength training. Lack of understanding, of the relationship between resistance and physiologic adaptation, leads to poor mix, such as reaching plateau in endurance level, because of decline in basic strength, or reaching plateau in power output, due to sluggish recuperative endurance.

13.2. PHYSICAL OVERTRAINING

13.2.1. CAUSES OF OVERTRAINING

Overtraining can be defined as a shift in metabolism towards the catabolic side. Such shift is caused by exerting **physical work** in excess of the body's ability to regenerate consumed energy molecules and re-synthesize essential cellular components necessary for anabolism. Catabolic shift might occur in vital organs such as the heart or the nervous system. Thus, while muscles might be spared of catabolic changes, the entire body might feel the ill effects of the heart and nerves. It must be remembered that all physiological processes operate by biochemical reactions that consume substrates and require catalysts, and are regulated by multiple systemic hormones and ionic changes. Thus, overtraining can be viewed as either depletion of essential biochemical substrates or catalysts, or excess production of byproducts. In either case, the alteration in the rate of biochemical reactions results in the general clinical condition of overtraining. **Nutrition** plays important role in overtraining. The depletion of minerals and vitamins are of particular concern in western societies. Protein and carbohydrate deficiency or imbalance intake are common causes in developing societies. **Rest and sleep** are also essential in maintaining adequate recuperation of vital organs.

Whatever the cause of overtraining may be, the final outcome is that **progress in strength training is hampered** by the lack of anabolic shift of cellular metabolism. The clinical manifestation of overtraining scans a wide spectrum, from mild fatigue, brief and extreme exhaustion, to protracted weariness. Trainees can still make progress, though overtrained, but not at the expected performance as if they were not overtrained. The quick recognition and management of overtraining can prevent its chronic and grave consequences.

13.2.2. MANAGING OVERTRAINING

o **Causes of overtraining:** Acute overtraining may be caused by local insults such as exhaustion of muscles due to high load volume, or by acute neuromuscular upset due to injury to tough structures, such as cartilages, ligaments, tendons, or bones. Acute exhaustion can also be caused by systemic disturbances such as high total load volume, sympathetic hyperactivity (insomnia, caffeine, or smoking), or disturbed circadian cycle. Chronic overtraining can be caused by muscle weakness due to improper planning of load volume, poor nutrition, or lack of rest. It can also be caused by overuse injury (of knees, hips, shoulders, spines, elbows, or writs) or hormonal disturbances.

o **Clinical signs of overtraining:** These result from either abnormal nervous stimulation or abnormal response of tissue to nervous stimulation. The fact that neurons, nerves, and their communication with other tissues, are most sensitive to overtraining is attributed to the high demands of the nervous system to oxygen and glucose. The autonomic nervous system manifests the cardinal signs of overtraining, since autonomic nerves are longer and thinner than somatic nerves. The autonomic nervous system consists of sympathetic and parasympathetic nervous system. These manifest signs of overtraining as follows, *Table 13.1*.

Table 13.1. Signs of Overtraining.

Sympathetic hyperactivity	Parasympathetic hyperactivity
Cardiovascular	Cardiovascular:
• Increased resting heart rate > 75 bpm.	• Decreased resting heart rate
• Increased resting blood pressure.	• Faster return of heart rate to resting value after exercise
• Decreased cardiac stroke volume.	Central nervous system
Central nervous system	• Decreased sports performance
• Increased irritability and depression	• Decreased desire to exercise
• Increased appetite	• Depression, fatigue
• Insomnia and anxiety	• Psychomotor retardation
Neuromuscular	Cellular metabolism
• Increased incidence of injury	• Decreased blood lactate concentrations during submaximal and maximal exercise
• Decreased maximal blood lactate concentrations	• Decreased vigor
Cellular metabolism	
• Slower recovery after exercise	
• Weight loss	
• Increased incidence of infection	
• Muscle soreness	

o **Remedial approach to overtraining:** This comprises of taking mini break periods, occasional changes in routine in order to avoid boredom, long recovery period, or modifications to the intensity-volume plan of workout. Also, modification of exercise picking can dramatically resolve overtraining. For example, cross training between endurance and strength can be counterproductive if the athlete fails to understand that the two are mutually exclusive in maxima. Exercise picking should follow similar metabolic pathways and motor skills needed for that particular sport.

13.3. PERIODIZATION OF LOAD INTENSITY AND VOLUME

13.3.1. POWERLIFTING PERIODIZATION

Powerlifters emphasize strengthening major muscle groups in few and simple movements. The following is an example of progressive strength training for Powerlifters, for a period of eight-week cycle. It consists of three, core Powerlifting exercises (Back Squat, Bench Press, Deadlift) and twelve assisting exercise, *Tables 13.2* and *13.3*. The following are the common features of training periods of Powerlifting.

Table 13.2. Progressive relationship between intensity and exercise repetition.

Week	Repetition	Percentage of 1RM
1	12	60
2	10	65
3	8	70
4	6	75
5	5	80
6	4	85
7	3	90
8	2	95

o   Powerlifting training requires longer recuperative intervals. The training sessions emphasize strengthening the components on of one core lift. Thus, sessions cycle among Squat day, Bench day, and Deadlift day.
o   Exercise **sets** remain constant at three sets per exercise group.
o   **Repetitions** per sets cycle every eight weeks, by dropping one or two reps weekly, from twelve reps/set down to two reps/set.
o   The **percentage of maximum** one-repetition intensity, of a particular exercise, rises from 60% 1RM to 95%, over eight weeks, by 5% increment/week.
o   Each session comprises of one core Powerlifting exercise assisted by five auxiliary exercises.
o   The **Squat day** comprises of the Back Squat, exercises for the thigh extensors and flexors, calf, and hip flexors.
o   The **Bench Press day** comprises of the Bench Press, exercises of the shoulders, and Triceps exercises.
o   The **Deadlift day** comprises of the Deadlift, back exercises, Biceps brachii curls, and abdominal strengthening.

Table 13.3. Core Powerlifting exercises and assisting exercise of a basic Powerlifting period of eight weeks period. Repetitions vary according to *Table 13.2*, above.

		Squat Day		Bench Press Day		Deadlift Day	
		Exercise	Sets x Reps	Exercise	Sets x Reps	Exercise	Sets x Reps
Core		Squat	3 x 12-2	Bench press	3 x 12-2	Deadlift	3 x 12-2
Assistance Exercises		Leg Press	3 x 8-12	Incline Bench Press	3 x 8-12	Power Cleans	3 x 2-5
		Leg Curl	3 x 8-12	Parallel Dips	3 x 8-12	Cable Row	3 x 8-12
		Leg Extensions	3 x 8-12	Shoulder Press	3 x 8-12	Stiff Leg Deadlift	3 x 8-12
		Calf Raise	3 x 8-12	Lateral Raise	3 x 8-12	Arm Curls	3 x 8-12
		Incline Sit-ups	3 x 20-30	Triceps Extension	3 x 8-12	Crunches	3 x 30-50

13.3.2. CRITIQUE ON THE PERIODIZATION OF POWERLIFTING

The previous method of Powerlifting training has major flaws and complies with no known expert professional planning. It is a **haphazard way of massing muscles** that compromises flexibility and predisposes to injury. It is practiced by the newly invented sport of Powerlifting. Its flaws may be summarized as follows.
o   Training one anatomical region of the body in separate sessions causes muscular imbalance. It allows muscles to grow in size and strength but lacks coordination or high recruitment.
o   It lacks full range of motion, since most exercises are machine bound or executed for short travel distance. Full travel distance equals full height of the individual, plus the length of the forearms.
o   It comprises of too many repetitions per sets or controlled high-tension and low speed motion. This mostly promotes the slow twitch fibers and compromises neuromuscular coordination.

13.3.3. WEIGHTLIFTING PERIODIZATION

Managing load-volume and intensity in Weightlifting is more problematic. It must account for form and strength. It also have been enhanced and refined for over a century of global human effort. The reliability of periodization of volume and intensity, in Weightlifting, is well manifested in Olympic game records that do not cease to climb, game after game. The rest of this chapter entails a description of a four-month training plan that was implemented since 1974 by Egyptian Weightlifting training planners. The plan was composed and enhanced after many probing research and development efforts and borrowed major features from Romanian, Bulgarian, and Polish Olympic training plans, as discussed in Chapter 12 and in Section 13.5, below.

13.3.3.1. Number Of Daily Lifts

Modern Weightlifters can train eight sessions per week, spread over five days. The two off-training days are usually not consecutive. The five workout days are split into three days of double split-sessions and two days of single sessions. Thus, in a four-month period, the lifter trains twenty days, every month, as follows, *Table 13.4*.

MANAGING LOAD VOLUME AND INTENSITY

Table 13.4. The number of lifts over the Four-month period of progressive strength training for Weightlifting. Exercise differentials are listed in *Table 13.5,* below.

Day Number	\multicolumn{20}{c	}{Total Daily Number of Sets}	Monthly No. of Sets
	1	2	3	4	5	6	7	8	9	10	11	12	13	14	15	16	17	18	19	20	
First Month	129	127	127	87	124	124	105	97	78	150	94	88	110	81	87	148	88	118	81	121	2164
Second Month	126	114	114	78	92	112	96	100	70	137	122	96	106	76	76	166	104	102	66	114	2067
Third Month	122	98	106	78	79	114	74	120	76	136	114	76	112	70	78	106	100	114	76	124	1973
Contest Month	103	107	129	87	144	94	110	134	86	114	114	90	137	78	52	54	51				1684

o The beginning of the period starts with low intensity and higher number of sets. In the first month, the lifter executes about 2164 lifts, over 60% 1RM, *Figure 13.1*.

o The 100 kg 1RM, for all exercises, is adopted in order to render **planning applicable to the individual needs.** For example, if your maximum in certain lifts are 200 and 300, kilograms or pounds, you can multiply the differentials by 2 and 3, respectively, in order to obtain the projected load volume for your plan.

o The consecutive three months will see drop in the total number of lifts to 2067, 1973, and 1684 per month, respectively. The fourth month precedes the contest date and starts with highest volume that tapers downwards to lowest volume, days before the contest, *Figure 13.1*.

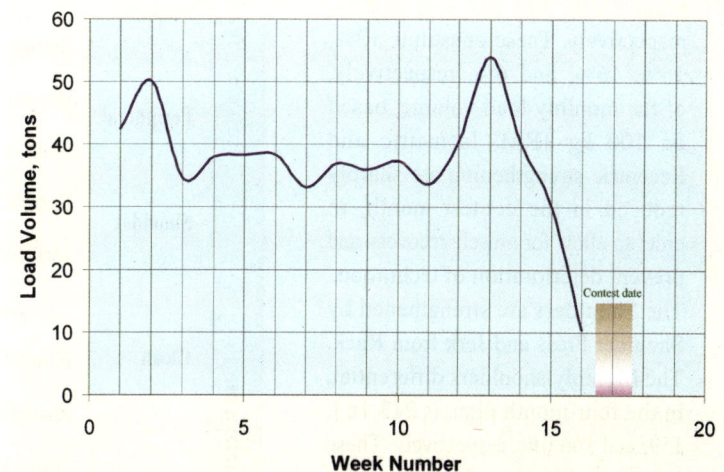

Figure 13.1. Four-month weekly load volume based on 100 kg 1RM in all fifteen basic Weightlifting lifts.

o The maximum number of lifts per day is under 190, of 60% 1RM. The minimum daily number of lifts is 51, the last day before competition.

o The contest month comprises of only 17 training session, instead of the regular 20.

o The week before the last week, in the contest month, comprises of four training days, while the last week of only three training days, of single session each.

13.3.3.2. Monthly Exercise-Differentials

Weightlifting exercises, for professional training, consist of six core exercises and their assisting nine auxiliary exercises. The distribution of exercise differentials of the monthly total lifts, presented in *Table 13.5*, is as follows.

o The **Clean lift** is performed in three different styles. These are: Classic Clean, Hang Clean, and Power Clean and Jerk. The Monthly Clean differential, in the four-month plan, is 430, 401, 392, and 373 lifts, respectively. The volume percentage of the Clean-differentials is 18%, 17%, 18%, and 21%, respectively, of the total monthly load volume. This is based solely on 100 kg 1RM in all lifts. This is a very empirical approximation of the proportion of the Clean lift to whole training volume.

o The **Snatch lift** is performed in three different styles. These are: Hang Snatch, Power Snatch, and Snatch Classic. The Monthly Snatch differential, in the four-month plan, is 434, 412, 368, and 376 lifts, respectively. These are also broken down into their subgroup lifts, in *Table 13.5*. The volume percentage of the Snatch differential is 19%, 19%, 18%, and 21%, respectively, of the total monthly load volume, of the four-month period. This is also based solely on 100 kg 1RM in all lifts.

o The **spinal erectors** are strengthened by various back exercises such as the Deadlift, Goodmorning, Jump Goodmorning, and Jump Deadlift. The Monthly back differential, in the four-month plan, is 292, 256, 256, and 224 lifts, respectively. These constitute 12% to 16% of load volume, based on 100 kg 1RM.

o The **legs** are strengthened by Back Squat and Front Squat. The Monthly leg differential, in the four-month plan, is 348, 342, 312, and 253 lifts, respectively. These constitute 16%, 18%, 17%, and 16%, respectively, of the total monthly load volume. This is also based solely on 100 kg 1RM in all lifts. Leg strengthening is thus a major strengthening component of training for Weightlifting during periodization.

13 MANAGING LOAD VOLUME AND INTENSITY

o The **scapular muscles** are strengthened by Clean Pull and Snatch Pull. The Monthly scapular muscles differential, in the four-month plan, is 193, 188, 198, and 204 lifts, respectively. These constitute 9%, 10%, 11%, and 13%, respectively, of the monthly load volume, based on 100 kg 1RM.

o The **Upper peripherals** are strengthened by Eccentric and Isometric Clean Pull or Snatch Pull. The Monthly arms differential, in the four-month plan, is 216, 300, 288, and 76 lifts, respectively. These constitute 12%, 16%, 16%, and 6%, respectively, of the monthly load volume, based on 100 kg 1RM. Isometric and Eccentric strengthening are sharply reduced in the contest month, in order to allow for muscle recovery and prevent deterioration of technique.

o The **Shoulders** are strengthened by Shoulder Press and Jerk from Rack. The Monthly shoulders differential, in the four-month plan, is 213, 168, 159, and 166 lifts, respectively. These constitute 9%, 8%, 7%, and 10%, respectively, of the monthly load volume, based on 100 kg 1RM.

o The weekly differentials of lifts are listed in **Table 13.6**. These are compiled from **Table 13.4**.

Table 13.5. Monthly Weightlifting **Exercise-Differentials** of load volume and number of lifts.

Exercise emphasis	Anatomic Region	Exercises	1st Month Set No	1st Month % of Volume	2nd Month Set No	2nd Month % of Volume	3rd Month Set No	3rd Month % of Volume	Contest Month Set No	Contest Month % of Volume
Assisting Exercises	Low Back	Back Exercise	292	16	256	12	256	14	224	14
	Legs	Back Squat	156	7	150	8	162	9	129	8
		Front Squat	192	9	192	10	150	8	124	8
	Scapular	Clean Pull	88	4	92	5	102	6	89	6
		Snatch Pull	105	5	96	5	96	5	115	7
	Peripheral	Eccentric	72	4	108	6	108	6	36	3
		Isometric Clean Pull	144	8	192	10	180	10	40	3
	Shoulder	Shoulder Press	132	5	92	4	96	4	102	6
		Jerk from Rack	81	4	76	4	63	3	64	4
Core Exercises	Clean	Classic Clean	174	7	161	6	176	8	162	9
		Hang Clean	136	6	112	5	104	5	72	4
		Power Clean and Jerk	120	5	128	6	112	5	139	8
	Snatch	Hang Snatch	140	6	124	5	96	5	91	5
		Power Snatch	136	6	120	6	96	5	139	8
		Snatch Classic	158	7	168	8	176	8	146	8
Total Monthly Number of Sets			2164		2067		1973		1684	

Table 13.6. Weekly total number of lifts

No. of lifts	594	554	460	556	524	515	476	552	450	520	385	520	570	538	419	157
Week	1	2	3	4	5	6	7	8	9	10	11	12	13	14	15	16

13.4. DETAILS OF A FOUR-MONTH PERIOD FOR WEIGHTLIFTING TRAINING

13.4.1. FIRST-MONTH DAILY EXERCISE-DIFFERENTIALS

The first month, of the four-month period of progressive resistance training comprises of 32 training session, spread over the four weeks of the month, *Table 13.7*.

o Each week comprises of eight sessions, performed in consecutive daily sequence of 2-1-0-2-1-2-0.[1]

o The double-session day comprises of morning and evening sessions, each session lasts 90 minutes. Two nonconsecutive days are taken off training. In this month, the third and seventh day of each week are taken off.

o **FIFTEEN** exercises are performed throughout the all four months of the period. In the first month, each exercise is executed 70 to 300 times, with weights over 60% 1RM.

o The combined daily sets of all exercises varies from 78 to 129, being higher at the beginning of the month and lower at the end, with weekly fluctuation in the number of sets.

o Among the fifteen exercises, only four to six exercises are executed daily. Exercise picking is based on balancing a core Olympic lift with its assisting exercises. The rationale for basing training around a core Olympic lift is that the full range of motion of freestyle lifting enhances the balance of the **scapular-spinal-pelvic** chain of musculoskeletal dynamics.

---

[1] The numbers in the formula 2-1-0-2-1-0 refer to the number of training sessions in each of the seven days of the week.

MANAGING LOAD VOLUME AND INTENSITY

Table 13.7. Total daily exercise sets during the **First Month,** of the four-month training cycle

	Week 1					Week 2					Week 3					Week 4					Total Exercise sets
Sessions / Day	2	1	2	1	2	2	1	2	1	2	2	1	2	1	2	2	1	2	1	2	
Day Number	1	2	3	4	5	6	7	8	9	10	11	12	13	14	15	16	17	18	19	20	
Exercises								Exercise sets													
Snatch Classic	24		24		16		24		14			21		14			21				158
Power Snatch		24		24		24					16		24		24						136
Hang Snatch		24						16	24	24					12			24		16	140
Snatch Pull			15		15			15	12			12		12			12			12	105
Classic Clean			16		24			16	24			14		21	24		14			21	174
Power Clean and Jerk	24		24			24				8			24				16				120
Hang Clean		24			24		24			16					24			24			136
Clean Pull	15		15		12			12		4			12		6			12			88
Jerk from Rack		15			12	12			12		12			6		12					81
Front Squat	18		24		24			18		24			24		24				24	12	192
Back Squat			24	30			6			24			24		24			24			156
Shoulder Press	16		16			16		12			12		12			12		12		24	132
Isometric Clean Pull		54							54							36					144
Eccentric							36				36										72
Back Exercise	32		32			32		32			32		32			32		32		36	292
Total Daily sets	129	127	127	87	124	124	105	97	78	150	94	88	110	81	87	148	88	118	81	121	2164

13.4.2. FIRST-WEEK DAILY EXERCISE-DIFFERENTIALS

Table 13.7.1 shows the breakdown of load volume and intensity, during the first week of the first month, of the four-month period.

o   The double-session days comprise of five to six exercises while the single-session days comprise of only four exercises.

o   Resistance starts from 60% 1RM and increases to 80% or 90%, in some exercises.

o   The net total weekly lifts are 594, the highest among the sixteen weeks of the period.

o   The daily number of exercises follows the formula 6-4-6-4-5.[2]

o   The net weekly load volume is **42.48 tons,** based on a 100 kg-1RM in all lifts.

o   The increase of resistance occurs every two sets, in most cases. That means that the barbell is loaded with additional plates every other set, in most cases.

o   Exercise sequence is important in smoothing the performance of technique and preventing injuries due to fatigued links, along the lifting chain of muscles and joints. For example, the Shoulder Press is a warm-up for the Snatch. Also, the Back Squat should end the session or precedes back exercises, but should NOT precede complex Olympic lifts. The Snatch precedes the Clean because of the need for full shoulder motion.

---

[2] The numbers in the formula 6-4-6-4-6 refer to the number of exercise groups per each of the five training days of the week.

13 MANAGING LOAD VOLUME AND INTENSITY

Table 13.7.1. Daily exercise sequence, sets, repetition, and percentage of 1RM during the **First Week** of the first month.

WEIGHTLIFTING EXERCISES	Time of day	100 kg-1RM Daily Volume Differential, kg	Sequence	Sets x Percentage x Repetitions[3]				100 kg-1RM Exercise Volume Differential, kg
Shoulder Press	AM	Day 1 10050	1	2 x 60 x 4	2 x 70 x 4			1040
Snatch Classic	AM		2	2 x 60 x 3	2 x 70 x 3	2 x 80 x 2	2 x 85 x 1	1270
Front Squat			3	2 x 70 x 5	2 x 80 x 5	2 x 90 x 3		2040
Power Clean and Jerk	PM		4	2 x 60 x 3	2 x 70 x 3	2 x 80 x 2		1100
Clean Pull			5	1 x 70 x 3	2 x 80 x 3	2 x 90 x 3	2 x 85 x 1	1400
Back Exercise			6	4 x 100 x 8				3200
Hang Snatch	AM	Day 2 9470	1	3 x 60 x 3	3 x 70 x 3	2 x 80 x 2		1490
Hang Clean			2	2 x 60 x 3	3 x 70 x 3	3 x 80 x 2		1470
Jerk from Rack			3	3 x 70 x 3	2 x 80 x 3			1110
Isometric Clean Pull			4	3 x 100 x 9	3 x 100 x 9			5400
Shoulder Press	AM	Day 4 9920	1	2 x 60 x 4	2 x 70 x 4			1040
Power Snatch			2	3 x 60 x 3	2 x 70 x 3	3 x 80 x 2		1440
Snatch Pull			3	1 x 70 x 3	2 x 80 x 3	2 x 90 x 3		1230
Classic Clean			4	2 x 60 x 3	3 x 70 x 2	2 x 80 x 2	1 x 85 x 2	1270
Back Squat	PM		5	2 x 70 x 4	2 x 80 x 4	2 x 90 x 3		1740
Back Exercise			6	4 x 100 x 8				3200
Snatch Classic	AM	Day 5 6120	1	3 x 60 x 3	3 x 70 x 3	2 x 75 x 2		1470
Power Clean and Jerk			2	2 x 60 x 3	3 x 70 x 3	3 x 80 x 2		1470
Clean Pull			3	1 x 70 x 3	2 x 80 x 3	2 x 90 x 3		1230
Back Squat			4	2 x 61 x 5	2 x 70 x 5	2 x 80 x 4		1950
Snatch Classic	AM	Day 6 6920	1	2 x 60 x 3	3 x 70 x 3	3 x 80 x 2		1470
Snatch Pull			2	2 x 70 x 3	2 x 80 x 3	1 x 90 x 3		1170
Back Squat			3	2 x 60 x 5	2 x 70 x 5	2 x 80 x 4		1940
Classic Clean	PM		4	2 x 60 x 3	3 x 70 x 3	3 x 75 x 2		1440
Jerk from Rack			5	2 x 70 x 3	2 x 80 x 3			900
Total of 100 kg-1RM, kg =								**42480**

13.4.3. SECOND-WEEK DAILY EXERCISE-DIFFERENTIALS

Table 13.7.2 shows the breakdown of load volume and intensity, during the second week of the first month, of the four-month period.

o   This week follows the same trends of the previous week, with difference in the number of lifts and load volume.
o   The net weekly lifts are 554, of 60% 1RM or higher.
o   The daily number of exercises follows the formula 6-4-6-4-6. Thus, the last day adds an extra exercise to the morning session.
o   The net weekly load volume is **50.10 tons** based on a 100 kg-1RM in all lifts. This is the highest volume in the first three months of the period, *Figure 13.1*.

---

[3] The formulas in the columns, of "Sets x Percentage x Repetitions", describe the number of exercise sets to be executed, with the same load of a barbell, and the numbers of repetitions per set. The increase in the barbell load is accounted for in following columns.

Table 13.7.2. Daily exercise sequence, sets, repetition, and percentage of 1RM during the **Second Week** of the first month.

WEIGHTLIFTING EXERCISES	Time of day	100 kg-1RM Daily Volume Differential, kg	Sequence	Sets x Percentage x Repetitions				100 kg-1RM Exercise Volume Differential, kg
Shoulder Press	AM	Day 1 9870	1	4 x 60 x 3	2 x 70 x 4			1280
Snatch Classic			2	2 x 60 x 3	2 x 70 x 3	2 x 80 x 2	2 x 90 x 1	1280
Front Squat			3	2 x 70 x 5	2 x 80 x 4	2 x 90 x 3		1880
Hang Clean			4	2 x 60 x 3	2 x 70 x 3	2 x 80 x 2	2 x 85 x 1	1270
Clean Pull	PM		5	1 x 70 x 3	2 x 80 x 3	1 x 90 x 3		960
Back Exercise			6	4 x 100 x 8				3200
Power Snatch	AM	Day 2 6900	1	2 x 60 x 3	2 x 70 x 3	2 x 80 x 2	2 x 85 x 2	1440
Power Clean and Jerk			2	2 x 60 x 3	2 x 70 x 3	2 x 80 x 2	2 x 85 x 2	1440
Jerk from Rack			3	1 x 70 x 3	2 x 80 x 3	1 x 90 x 3		960
Eccentric			4	3 x 80 x 6	3 x 90 x 6			3060
Shoulder Press	AM	Day 4 9880	1	1 x 60 x 4	1 x 70 x 3	2 x 80 x 3		930
Hang Snatch			2	2 x 60 x 3	2 x 70 x 3	2 x 80 x 2	2 x 90 x 2	1460
Snatch Pull			3	1 x 70 x 3	2 x 80 x 3	2 x 90 x 3		1230
Classic Clean			4	2 x 60 x 3	2 x 70 x 3	2 x 80 x 2	2 x 90 x 1	1280
Back Squat	PM		5	2 x 80 x 4	2 x 90 x 3	2 x 100 x 3		1780
Back Exercise			6	4 x 100 x 8				3200
Snatch Classic	AM	Day 5 5710	1	3 x 60 x 3	3 x 70 x 2	2 x 80 x 2		1280
Hang Clean			2	2 x 60 x 3	2 x 70 x 3	2 x 80 x 2	2 x 90 x 2	1460
Clean Pull			3	1 x 80 x 3	2 x 90 x 3	1 x 100 x 2		980
Front Squat			4	1 x 70 x 5	1 x 80 x 4	2 x 90 x 4	2 x 100 x 3	1990
Classic Clean	AM	Day 6 17740	1	3 x 60 x 3	3 x 70 x 3	2 x 80 x 3		1650
Jerk from Rack			2	1 x 70 x 3	2 x 80 x 3	1 x 90 x 2		870
Back Squat			3	2 x 70 x 5	2 x 80 x 40	2 x 90 x 3		7640
Isometric Clean Pull			4	6 x 100 x 9				5400
Hang Snatch	PM		5	3 x 60 x 3	3 x 70 x 2	2 x 80 x 2		1280
Snatch Pull			6	2 x 70 x 3	2 x 80 x 3			900
Total of 100 kg-1RM, kg =								50100

13.4.5. THIRD-WEEK DAILY EXERCISE-DIFFERENTIALS

Table 13.7.3 shows the breakdown of load volume and intensity, during the third week of the first month, of the four-month period.

o This week also follows the same of trends of the previous week, with some differences.
o The net weekly lifts are 460, of 60% 1RM or higher.
o The daily number of exercises follows the formula 6-4-6-4-5.
o The net weekly load volume is **34.65 tons**, based on a 100 kg-1RM in all lifts. This is a significant drop in weekly volume after the high volume of second week.

13 MANAGING LOAD VOLUME AND INTENSITY

Table 13.7.3. Daily exercise sequence, sets, repetition, and percentage of 1RM during the **Third Week** of the first month.

WEIGHTLIFTING EXERCISES	Time of day	100 kg-1RM Daily Volume Differential, kg	Sequence	Sets x Percentage x Repetitions				100 kg-1RM Exercise Volume Differential, kg
Shoulder Press	AM	Day 1 9550	1	2 x 60 x 4	1 x 70 x 3	1 x 30 x 3		780
Classic Snatch	AM		2	2 x 60 x 3	3 x 70 x 3	2 x 80 x 2		1400
Front Squat			3	2 x 70 x 5	2 x 80 x 3	2 x 90 x 3	1 x 90 x 1	1720
Power Clean and Jerk			4	2 x 60 x 3	3 x 70 x 3	2 x 80 x 2		1490
Clean Pull	PM		5	1 x 70 x 3	2 x 80 x 3	1 x 90 x 3	1 x 90 x 2	960
Back Exercise			6	4 x 100 x 8				3200
Hang Snatch	AM	Day 2 5085	1	2 x 60 x 3	3 x 70 x 3	3 x 80 x 3		1710
Hang Clean			2	2 x 60 x 3	3 x 70 x 3	2 x 80 x 2		1400
Jerk from Rack			3	1 x 75 x 3	1 x 85 x 2	2 x 95 x 2	1 x 90 x 1	775
Eccentric			4	2 x 100 x 6				1200
Shoulder Press	AM	Day 4 8855	1	2 x 65 x 4	1 x 75 x 3	1 x 85 x 2		915
Classic Clean			2	2 x 60 x 2	2 x 70 x 2	2 x 80 x 1		770
Back Squat			3	2 x 70 x 4	2 x 80 x 4	2 x 90 x 4	1 x 90 x 1	1920
Power Snatch			4	2 x 60 x 2	3 x 70 x 2	2 x 80 x 2		1070
Snatch Pull	PM		5	1 x 80 x 3	2 x 90 x 3	1 x 100 x 2	1 x 90 x 1	980
Back Exercise			6	4 x 100 x 8				3200
Classic Snatch	AM	Day 5 5400	1	2 x 60 x 3	3 x 70 x 3	2 x 80 x 2		1310
Classic Clean and Jerk			2	2 x 60 x 3	2 x 70 x 3	3 x 80 x 2		1430
Clean Pull			3	1 x 80 x 3	2 x 90 x 3	1 x 100 x 3	1 x 85 x 2	1080
Front Squat			4	2 x 80 x 4	2 x 90 x 3	2 x 100 x 2		1580
Power Snatch	AM	Day 6 5760	1	3 x 60 x 3	3 x 70 x 3	2 x 80 x 2		1490
Snatch Pull			2	1 x 70 x 3	1 x 80 x 3	2 x 90 x 3		990
Back Exercise			3	2 x 80 x 4	2 x 90 x 4	1 x 100 x 3		1660
Classic Clean	PM		4	2 x 60 x 3	3 x 70 x 2	2 x 80 x 2		1100
Jerk from Rack			5	1 x 80 x 3	1 x 90 x 2	1 x 100 x 1		520
Total of 100 kg-1RM, kg =								**34650**

13.4.6. FOURTH-WEEK DAILY EXERCISE-DIFFERENTIALS

Table 13.7.4 shows the breakdown of load volume and intensity, during the fourth week of the first month, of the four-month period.

o This week also follows some of the trends of previous weeks, with some differences.
o The number of lifts has increased once again by 96 lifts. The net weekly lifts are 556, of 60% 1RM or higher.
o The net weekly load volume is **38.02 tons**, based on a 100 kg-1RM in all lifts. This is a gradual increase in weekly volume over the third week. The volume increase was achieved through increase in number of sets and not through intensifying lifting.
o Thus, The daily number of exercises follows the formula 6-4-6-4-6, as is the case of the second week.

Table 13.7.4. Daily exercise sequence, sets, repetition, and percentage of 1RM during the **Fourth Week** of the first month.

WEIGHTLIFTING EXERCISES	Time of day	100 kg-1RM Daily Volume Differential, kg	Sequence	Sets x Percentage x Repetitions					100 kg-1RM Exercise Volume Differential, kg
Shoulder Press	AM	Day 1 8636	1	1 x 60 x 3	2 x 70 x 3	1 x 80 x 3			840
Snatch Classic	AM		2	2 x 60 x 2	2 x 60 x 2	1 x 80 x 2	1 x 90 x 1	1 x 95 x 1	826
Front Squat			3	2 x 70 x 4	2 x 70 x 4	2 x 90 x 3			1660
Hang Clean			4	2 x 60 x 3	2 x 70 x 2	2 x 80 x 2	1 x 85 x 2		1130
Clean Pull	PM		5	1 x 80 x 3	2 x 90 x 3	1 x 100 x 2			980
Back Exercise			6	4 x 100 x 8					3200
Power Snatch	AM	Day 2 8720	1	3 x 60 x 3	3 x 70 x 3	2 x 80 x 2			1490
Power Clean and Jerk			2	2 x 60 x 2	3 x 70 x 2	2 x 80 x 1	1 x 90 x 1		1120
Jerk from Rack			3	1 x 60 x 3	1 x 70 x 3	2 x 80 x 2			710
Isometric Clean Pull			4	6 x 100 x 9					5400
Shoulder Press	AM	Day 4 9176	1	1 x 60 x 3	1 x 70 x 2	1 x 80 x 2	1 x 85 x 2		650
Hang Snatch			2	3 x 60 x 3	3 x 70 x 3	2 x 80 x 2			1490
Snatch Pull			3	1 x 80 x 3	2 x 90 x 3	1 x 100 x 2			980
Classic Clean			4	1 x 60 x 2	3 x 70 x 3	2 x 80 x 1	1 x 90 x 1	1 x 95 x 1	1096
Back Squat	PM		5	1 x 70 x 4	2 x 80 x 4	2 x 90 x 3	1 x 100 x 3		1760
Back Exercise			6	4 x 100 x 8					3200
Snatch Classic	AM	Day 5 5060	1	2 x 60 x 3	2 x 70 x 3	2 x 80 x 2	1 x 85 x 2		1270
Hang Clean			2	2 x 60 x 3	2 x 70 x 2	2 x 80 x 2	2 x 90 x 1		1140
Clean Pull			3	1 x 70 x 3	1 x 80 x 3	2 x 90 x 3			990
Front Squat			4	1 x 70 x 4	2 x 80 x 4	2 x 90 x 3	1 x 100 x 2		1660
Hang Snatch	AM	Day 6 6426	1	2 x 60 x 2	3 x 70 x 2	2 x 80 x 2	1 x 90 x 1		1070
Snatch Pull			2	2 x 70 x 3	2 x 80 x 3				900
Back Squat			3	2 x 80 x 4	2 x 80 x 3	2 x 90 x 4			1840
Classic Clean			4	1 x 60 x 3	2 x 70 x 2	2 x 80 x 2	2 x 85 x 1		950
Jerk from Rack	PM		5	1 x 60 x 3	2 x 70 x 3	1 x 80 x 3			840
Eccentric			6	2 x 60 x 2	2 x 60 x 2	1 x 80 x 2	1 x 90 x 1	1 x 95 x 1	826
Total of 100 kg-1RM, kg =									38018

13.4.7. SECOND-MONTH DAILY EXERCISE-DIFFERENTIALS

The second month, of the four-month period of progressive resistance training comprises of 32 training session, spread over the four weeks of the month, **Table 13.8.**

o Weekly sessions are organized as the first month of the period.
o Double-session days alternate with single session days.
o Also, the number of exercises in each week alternates between 6-4-6-4-5 and 6-4-6-4-6.
o The fifteen essential exercises are executed 76 to 256 times, with weights over 60% 1RM.
o There is net drop of 97 sets from the previous month.
o Also, among the fifteen exercise, only four to six exercises are executed daily. Exercise picking is based on balancing a core Olympic lift with its assisting exercises.

Table 13.8. Total daily exercise sets during the **Second Month,** of the four-month training cycle.

	Week 1					Week 2					Week 3					Week 4					Total Exercise sets
Sessions / Day	2	1	2	1	2	2	1	2	1	2	2	1	2	1	2	2	1	2	1	2	
Day Number	1	2	3	4	5	6	7	8	9	10	11	12	13	14	15	16	17	18	19	20	
Exercises									Exercise sets												
Snatch Classic	16		24		16		24			24			24		16			24			168
Power Snatch		24		24		24						16		16	16						120
Hang Snatch		24					16		16		24			12		16		16			124
Snatch Pull		12		12			12		12		12		12		12				12		96
Classic Clean		16		24			16		1		16		24	24		16			24		161
Power Clean and Jerk	24		24		24			24		16			16								128
Hang Clean		24			16		16				24			16			16				112
Clean Pull	12		12		12		12		12			12		12	0		8				92
Jerk from Rack		6		8		12			12		12		6		12				8		76
Front Squat	30		18		24		18		18			24		42			18				192
Back Squat		18		24		12		24			18		18		18			18			150
Shoulder Press	12		12			12		12			12		12		12		8				92
Isometric Clean Pull	60									72				60							192
Eccentric				36				36									36				108
Back Exercise	32	32			32	32				32	32			32			32				256
Total Daily sets	126	114	114	78	92	112	96	100	70	137	122	96	106	76	76	166	104	102	66	114	2067

13.4.8. FIFTH- WEEK DAILY EXERCISE-DIFFERENTIALS

Table 13.8.1 shows the breakdown of load volume and intensity, during the first week of the second month, of the four-month period.

o The double-session days comprise of 5 to 6 exercises while the single-session days comprise of only four exercises.
o Resistance starts from 60% 1RM and increases to 80 or 90, in some exercises.
o The net total weekly lifts are 524.
o The daily number of exercises follows the formula 6-4-6-4-5.
o The net weekly load volume is **38.22 tons,** based on a 100 kg-1RM in all lifts.
o The increase of resistance occurs after 2 sets, in most cases.

MANAGING LOAD VOLUME AND INTENSITY

Table 13.8.1. Daily exercise sequence, sets, repetition, and percentage of 1RM during the **First Week** of the second

WEIGHTLIFTING EXERCISES	Time of day	100 kg-1RM Daily Volume Differential, kg	Sequence	Sets x Percentage x Repetitions					100 kg-1RM Exercise Volume Differential, kg
Shoulder Press	AM	Day 1 8896	1	1 x 60 x 3	2 x 70 x 3	1 x 80 x 2			760
Classic Snatch	AM		2	2 x 60 x 2	2 x 70 x 2	3 x 80 x 2	1 x 90 x 1		996
Front Squat			3	1 x 60 x 5	2 x 70 x 5	3 x 70 x 5			1740
Classic Clean and Jerk			4	2 x 60 x 3	2 x 70 x 3	2 x 80 x 2	2 x 90 x 1		1180
Clean Pull	PM		5	2 x 80 x 3	2 x 90 x 3				1020
Back Exercise			6	4 x 100 x 8					3200
Hang Snatch	AM	Day 2 6950	1	2 x 60 x 3	3 x 70 x 3	3 x 80 x 2			1650
Hang Clean			2	3 x 60 x 3	3 x 70 x 2	2 x 80 x 2			970
Jerk from Rack			3	1 x 70 x 2	1 x 80 x 2	1 x 90 x 2			730
Isometric Clean Pull			4	5 x 100 x 12					3600
Shoulder Press	AM	Day 4 8371	1	1 x 60 x 3	1 x 70 x 3	1 x 80 x 2	1 x 90 x 2		620
Classic Clean and Jerk	AM		2	2 x 60 x 2	2 x 70 x 2	2 x 80 x 2	1 x 90 x 1		960
Back Squat			3	2 x 80 x 3	2 x 90 x 3	1 x 100 x 2	1 x 110 x 1	1 x 95 x 1	1335
Power Snatch			4	1 x 60 x 3	2 x 70 x 2	3 x 80 x 2	2 x 90 x 1		1236
Snatch Pull	PM		5	2 x 8 x 3	2 x 90 x 3				1020
Back Exercise			6	4 x 100 x 8					3200
Classic Snatch	AM	Day 5 4676	1	2 x 60 x 3	2 x 70 x 3	2 x 80 x 2	2 x 85 x 2		1470
Power Clean and Jerk	AM		2	2 x 60 x 3	3 x 70 x 2	3 x 80 x 2			1026
Clean Pull			3	2 x 90 x 3	1 x 100 x 2	1 x 110 x 2			960
Front Squat			4	2 x 80 x 3	2 x 90 x 3	1 x 100 x 2	1 x 110 x 1		1220
Power Snatch	AM	Day 6 9330	1	1 x 60 x 3	2 x 70 x 3	2 x 80 x 2	2 x 90 x 1		1010
Snatch Pull	AM		2	1 x 80 x 3	1 x 90 x 3	1 x 100 x 3	1 x 110 x 2	1 x 95 x 1	620
Back Squat			3	2 x 70 x 4	2 x 80 x 4	2 x 90 x 4			1240
Classic Clean and Jerk	PM		4	2 x 80 x 2	1 x 90 x 2	1 x 100 x 1			1020
Jerk from Rack			5	1 x 60 x 3	2 x 70 x 3	1 x 80 x 2			4500
Total of 100 kg-1RM, kg =									38223

13 MANAGING LOAD VOLUME AND INTENSITY

13.4.9. SIXTH-WEEK DAILY EXERCISE-DIFFERENTIALS
Table 13.8.2 shows the breakdown of load volume and intensity, during the second week of the second month, of the four-month period.
o   This week follows the same trends of the previous week, with difference in the number of lifts and load volume.
o   The net weekly lifts are 515, of 60% 1RM or higher.
o   The daily number of exercises follows the formula 6-4-6-4-6. Thus, the last day adds an extra exercise to the morning session.
o   The net weekly load volume is **38.22 tons** based on a 100 kg-1RM in all lifts. This is a week of buildup and maintenance, rather than stimulation, *Figure 13.1*.

Table 13.8.2. Daily exercise sequence, sets, repetition, and percentage of 1RM during the **Second Week** of the second month.

WEIGHTLIFTING EXERCISES	Time of day	100 kg-1RM Daily Volume Differential, kg	Sequence	Sets x Percentage x Repetitions				100 kg-1RM Exercise Volume Differential, kg
Shoulder Press	AM	Day 1 8896	1	1 x 60 x 3	2 x 70 x 3	1 x 80 x 2	1 x 95 x 1	760
Snatch Classic	AM		2	1 x 60 x 2	2 x 70 x 2	2 x 80 x 2		996
Front Squat			3	2 x 70 x 4	2 x 80 x 4	2 x 90 x 3		1740
Hang Clean			4	2 x 60 x 2	2 x 70 x 2	3 x 80 x 2		1180
Clean Pull	PM		5	2 x 80 x 3	2 x 90 x 3			1020
Back Exercise			6	4 x 100 x 8				3200
Power Snatch	AM	Day 2 6950	1	2 x 60 x 3	3 x 70 x 3	2 x 80 x 2		1650
Power Clean and Jerk	AM		2	2 x 60 x 3	2 x 70 x 2	2 x 80 x 1		970
Jerk from Rack			3	1 x 70 x 3	1 x 80 x 2	2 x 90 x 2		730
Eccentric			4	6 x 100 x 6				3600
Shoulder Press	AM	Day 4 8371	1	1 x 70 x 3	2 x 80 x 2	1 x 90 x 1		620
Classic Clean	AM		2	1 x 60 x 3	2 x 70 x 2	2 x 80 x 2		960
Back Squat			3	2 x 80 x 3	2 x 90 x 3	1 x 100 x 2	1 x 95 x 1	1335
Hang Snatch			4	2 x 60 x 3	2 x 70 x 2	2 x 80 x 2		1236
Snatch Pull	PM		5	2 x 80 x 3	2 x 90 x 3			1020
Back Exercise			6	4 x 100 x 8				3200
Snatch Classic	AM	Day 5 4676	1	2 x 60 x 3	3 x 70 x 3	3 x 80 x 2	1 x 95 x 1	1470
Hang Clean	AM		2	2 x 60 x 2	2 x 70 x 2	2 x 80 x 2		1026
Clean Pull			3	2 x 90 x 3	1 x 100 x 2	1 x 110 x 2		960
Front Squat			4	2 x 80 x 3	2 x 90 x 3	2 x 100 x 1		1220
Classic Clean	AM	Day 6 9330	1	2 x 60 x 2	2 x 70 x 2	2 x 80 x 2		1010
Jerk from Rack	AM		2	1 x 80 x 2	2 x 90 x 2	1 x 100 x 1		620
Back Squat			3	2 x 80 x 3	2 x 90 x 2	2 x 100 x 2		1240
Hang Snatch			4	2 x 60 x 2	2 x 70 x 2	2 x 80 x 2		1020
Snatch Pull	PM		5	2 x 90 x 3	2 x 100 x 2			940
Isometric Clean Pull			6	5 x 100 x 9				4500
Total of 100 kg-1RM, kg =								38223

MANAGING LOAD VOLUME AND INTENSITY 13

13.4.10. SEVENTH-WEEK DAILY EXERCISE-DIFFERENTIALS

Table 13.8.3 shows the breakdown of load volume and intensity, during the third week of the second month, of the four-month period.

o   This week also follows the some of trends of the previous week, with some differences.
o   The net weekly lifts are 476, of 60% 1RM or higher.
o   The daily number of exercises follows the formula 6-4-6-4-5.
o   The net weekly load volume is **33.15 tons**, based on a 100 kg-1RM in all lifts. This is one of few low volume weeks throughout the period.

Table 13.8.3. Daily exercise sequence, sets, repetition, and percentage of 1RM during the **Third Week** of the second month.

WEIGHTLIFTING EXERCISES	Time of day	100 kg-1RM Daily Volume Differential, kg	Sequence	Sets x Percentage x Repetitions					100 kg-1RM Exercise Volume Differential, kg
Shoulder Press	AM	Day 1 8245	1	1 x 60 x 3	2 x 70 x 3	1 x 80 x 2			760
Classic Snatch	AM		2	2 x 60 x 3	2 x 70 x 2	2 x 80 x 2	2 x 90 x 1		1140
Front Squat	AM		3	2 x 80 x 3	2 x 90 x 3	2 x 100 x 2			1420
Hang Clean	AM		4	2 x 60 x 2	2 x 70 x 2	1 x 90 x 1	1 x 95 x 1		705
Clean Pull	PM		5	2 x 80 x 3	2 x 90 x 3				1020
Back Exercise	PM		6	4 x 100 x 8					3200
Hang Snatch	AM	Day 2 5630	1	2 x 60 x 3	2 x 70 x 3	2 x 80 x 2	2 x 85 x 2		1440
Hang Clean	AM		2	2 x 60 x 3	2 x 70 x 2	2 x 80 x 2	2 x 85 x 2		1300
Jerk from Rack	AM		3	1 x 70 x 3	1 x 80 x 2	2 x 90 x 2			730
Eccentric	AM		4	3 x 120 x 6					2160
Shoulder Press	AM	Day 4 8617	1	1 x 60 x 3	1 x 70 x 3	1 x 80 x 2	1 x 85 x 2		720
Classic Clean	AM		2	2 x 60 x 3	2 x 70 x 2	2 x 80 x 2	1 x 90 x 1		1146
Back Squat	AM		3	1 x 70 x 3	2 x 80 x 3	3 x 90 x 3		1 x 95 x 1	1500
Power Snatch	AM		4	2 x 60 x 2	2 x 70 x 2	2 x 80 x 2	1 x 90 x 1		1031
Snatch Pull	PM		5	2 x 80 x 3	2 x 90 x 3			1 x 100 x 1	1020
Back Exercise	PM		6	4 x 100 x 8					3200
Classic Snatch	AM	Day 5 6338	1	2 x 60 x 3	2 x 70 x 2	3 x 80 x 2	3 x 80 x 2		1687
Classic Clean and Jerk	AM		2	2 x 60 x 2	2 x 70 x 2	2 x 80 x 2	2 x 80 x 2	1 x 85 x 2	1341
Clean Pull	AM		3	1 x 90 x 3	2 x 100 x 2			2 x 90 x 1	670
Front Squat	AM		4	2 x 70 x 4	2 x 80 x 4	2 x 90 x 4	2 x 90 x 4		2640
Classic Clean	AM	Day 6 4275	1	2 x 60 x 3	3 x 70 x 2	3 x 80 x 2			1260
Jerk from Rack	AM		2	1 x 90 x 2	1 x 100 x 1	1 x 110 x 1			390
Back Squat	AM		3	1 x 80 x 2	2 x 90 x 2	1 x 100 x 1	1 x 115 x 1		735
Power Snatch	PM		4	2 x 60 x 2	2 x 70 x 2	2 x 80 x 2	2 x 90 x 1		1020
Snatch Pull	PM		5	1 x 90 x 3	2 x 100 x 3				870
							Total of 100 kg-1RM, kg =		33105

MANAGING LOAD VOLUME AND INTENSITY

13.4.11. EIGHTH-WEEK DAILY EXERCISE-DIFFERENTIALS

Table 13.8.4 shows the breakdown of load volume and intensity, during the fourth week of the second month, of the four-month period.

o   This week also follows the same of trends of the previous week, with some differences.
o   The net weekly lifts are 552, of 60% 1RM or higher.
o   The daily number of exercises follows the formula 6-4-6-4-6.
o   The net weekly load volume is **36.89 tons,** based on a 100 kg-1RM in all lifts.

Table 13.8.4. Daily exercise sequence, sets, repetition, and percentage of 1RM during the **Fourth Week** of the second month.

WEIGHTLIFTING EXERCISES	Time of day	100 kg-1RM Daily Volume Differential, kg	Sequence	Sets x Percentage x Repetitions					100 kg-1RM Exercise Volume Differential, kg
Shoulder Press	AM	Day 1 8716	1	2 x 70 x 3	1 x 80 x 3	1 x 85 x 2	2 x 90 x 1		830
Snatch Classic			2	2 x 60 x 2	2 x 70 x 2	2 x 80 x 2	1 x 110 x 1	1 x 95 x 1	1116
Front Squat			3	1 x 80 x 3	2 x 90 x 3	2 x 100 x 2	2 x 90 x 2		1290
Hang Clean	PM		4	2 x 65 x 2	2 x 70 x 2	2 x 90 x 2			1260
Clean Pull			5	2 x 80 x 3	2 x 90 x 3				1020
Back Exercise			6	4 x 100 x 8					3200
Power Snatch	AM	Day 2 5750	1	2 x 60 x 2	2 x 70 x 2	3 x 80 x 2	1 x 85 x 2		1170
Power Clean and Jerk			2	2 x 60 x 2	2 x 70 x 2	2 x 80 x 2	2 x 85 x 1		1010
Jerk from Rack			3	1 x 60 x 3	1 x 70 x 3	2 x 80 x 3			870
Isometric Clean Pull			4	3 x 100 x 9					2700
Shoulder Press	AM	Day 4 8297	1	1 x 60 x 3	1 x 70 x 3	1 x 80 x 2	1 x 90 x 1		640
Classic Clean			2	2 x 60 x 2	2 x 70 x 2	2 x 80 x 2	2 x 90 x 1	1 x 95 x 1	1116
Back Squat			3	1 x 80 x 3	2 x 90 x 3	2 x 100 x 2	1 x 110 x 1		1290
Hang Snatch	PM		4	2 x 60 x 2	2 x 70 x 2	2 x 80 x 2	1 x 90 x 1	1 x 100 x 1	1031
Snatch Pull			5	2 x 80 x 3	2 x 90 x 3				1020
Back Exercise			6	4 x 100 x 8					3200
Snatch Classic	AM	Day 5 4425	1	2 x 60 x 3	3 x 70 x 3	3 x 80 x 2			1470
Hang Clean			2	2 x 60 x 2	2 x 70 x 2	2 x 80 x 2			840
Clean Pull			3	2 x 90 x 2	1 x 100 x 2	1 x 115 x 1			675
Front Squat			4	2 x 70 x 3	2 x 80 x 3	2 x 90 x 3			1440
Hang Snatch	AM	Day 6 9700	1	2 x 60 x 2	2 x 70 x 2	2 x 80 x 2	2 x 90 x 2		1200
Snatch Pull			2	1 x 80 x 3	2 x 90 x 3	1 x 110 x 1			890
Back Squat			3	2 x 70 x 3	2 x 80 x 3	2 x 90 x 3			1440
Classic Clean			4	2 x 60 x 3	2 x 70 x 3	2 x 80 x 2	2 x 85 x 1		1270
Jerk from Rack	PM		5	1 x 70 x 2	1 x 80 x 2	1 x 90 x 2	1 x 100 x 1		580
Eccentric			6	6 x 120 x 6					4320
				Total of 100 kg-1RM, kg =					36888

13.4.12. THIRD-MONTH DAILY EXERCISE-DIFFERENTIALS

The third month, of the four-month period of progressive resistance training comprises of 32 training session, spread over the four weeks of the month, *Table 13.9*.

o Each week comprises of 8 sessions that are performed in consecutive daily sequence of 2-1-0-2-1-2-0.
o The double-session days comprise of morning and evening sessions, each session lasts 90 minutes.
o Two nonconsecutive days are taken off training. Also, in this month the third and seventh day of each week are taken off.
o Each of the fifteen exercises is executed 63 to 256 times, with weights over 60% 1RM. The combined daily sets of all exercises vary from 70 to 136 lifts.
o Among the fifteen exercises, only five to seven exercises are executed daily.
o Exercise picking is also based on balancing a core Olympic lift with its assisting exercises.

Table 13.9. Total daily exercise sets during the **Third Month**, of the four-month training cycle.

	Week 1					Week 2					Week 3					Week 4					Total Exercise sets
Sessions / Day	2	1	2	1	2	2	1	2	1	2	2	1	2	1	2	2	1	2	1	2	
Day Number	1	2	3	4	5	6	7	8	9	10	11	12	13	14	15	16	17	18	19	20	
Exercises									Exercise sets												
Classic Snatch	24		24		16		24		24			24				16			24		176
Power Snatch		16		16		16						16		16		16					96
Hang Snatch		16					16		16		16							16		16	96
Snatch Pull			12		12		12		12			12		12				12		12	96
Classic Clean and Jerk		16		24			24		24			16		24				24		24	176
Power Clean and Jerk	24		24				16				16			16			16				112
Hang Clean		16				24		16			16			16			16				104
Clean Pull	12			12		12			12		12			12		12	0		18		102
Jerk from Rack		6			9		6				6		8			8		8		12	63
Front Squat	18			18		18			24		18			18			18		18		150
Back Squat			18		18			24		18			24		18			18		24	162
Shoulder Press	12		12			12		12			12		12			12		12			96
Isometric Clean Pull			60							60							60				180
Eccentric							36						36							36	108
Back Exercise	32			32		32		32			32		32			32		32			256
Total Daily sets	122	98	106	78	79	114	74	120	76	136	114	76	112	70	78	106	100	114	76	124	1973

13 MANAGING LOAD VOLUME AND INTENSITY

13.4.13. NINTH- WEEK DAILY EXERCISE-DIFFERENTIALS
Table 13.9.1 shows the breakdown of load volume and intensity, during the first week of the third month, of the four-month period.
o The double-session days comprise of 5 to 6 exercises while the single-session days comprise of only four exercises.
o Resistance starts from 60% 1RM and increases to 80 or 95, in some exercises.
o The net total weekly lifts are 483.
o The daily number of exercises follows the formula 6-4-6-4-5.
o The net weekly load volume is **35.99 tons,** based on a 100 kg-1RM in all lifts.
o The increase of resistance occurs every two sets, in most cases.

Table 13.9.1. Daily exercise sequence, sets, repetition, and percentage of 1RM during the **First Week** of the third month.

WEIGHTLIFTING EXERCISES	Time of day	100 kg-1RM Daily Volume Differential, kg	Sequence	Sets x Percentage x Repetitions					100 kg-1RM Exercise Volume Differential, kg
Shoulder Press			1	2 x 60 x 3	1 x 70 x 3	1 x 80 x 2			730
Classic Snatch	AM		2	2 x 60 x 3	2 x 70 x 3	2 x 80 x 2	2 x 90 x 1		1280
Front Squat		Day 1	3	2 x 80 x 3	2 x 90 x 3	3 x 100 x 5			2520
Classic Clean and Jerk		9640	4	2 x 60 x 3	2 x 70 x 2	2 x 80 x 2	2 x 85 x 1		1130
Clean Pull	PM		5	1 x 90 x 3	2 x 100 x 2	1 x 110 x 1			780
Back Exercise			6	4 x 100 x 8					3200
Hang Snatch			1	2 x 60 x 2	2 x 70 x 2	2 x 80 x 2	2 x 85 x 2		1180
Hang Clean	AM	Day 2	2	2 x 60 x 2	2 x 70 x 2	2 x 80 x 2	1 x 90 x 1	1 x 95 x 1	1026
Jerk from Rack		7246	3	1 x 80 x 2	1 x 90 x 2	1 x 100 x 2			540
Isometric Clean Pull			4	5 x 100 x 9					4500
Shoulder Press			1	2 x 60 x 3	1 x 70 x 3	1 x 80 x 2			730
Classic Clean and Jerk	AM		2	2 x 60 x 2	2 x 70 x 2	2 x 80 x 2	1 x 90 x 1	1 x 95 x 1	1026
Back Squat		Day 4	3	2 x 70 x 3	2 x 80 x 3	2 x 90 x 3			1440
Power Snatch		8562	4	2 x 60 x 3	2 x 70 x 2	2 x 80 x 2	1 x 90 x 1	1 x 95 x 1	1146
Snatch Pull	PM		5	2 x 80 x 3	2 x 90 x 3				1020
Back Exercise			6	4 x 100 x 8					3200
Classic Snatch			1	2 x 60 x 3	2 x 70 x 3	2 x 80 x 2	2 x 85 x 2		1440
Power Clean and Jerk	AM	Day 5	2	2 x 60 x 3	2 x 70 x 2	2 x 80 x 2	2 x 85 x 2		1300
Clean Pull		5330	3	2 x 80 x 3	2 x 90 x 3				1020
Front Squat			4	3 x 80 x 3	2 x 90 x 3	1 x 100 x 2	1 x 110 x 1		1570
Power Snatch			1	2 x 60 x 3	2 x 70 x 3	2 x 80 x 2	2 x 90 x 1	1 x 95 x 1	1376
Snatch Pull	AM		2	1 x 90 x 3	1 x 100 x 2	2 x 110 x 1	1 x 115 x 1		805
Back Squat		Day 6	3	2 x 80 x 3	2 x 90 x 3	1 x 100 x 2			1220
Classic Clean and Jerk	PM	5211	4	2 x 60 x 3	3 x 70 x 2	3 x 80 x 2			1260
Jerk from Rack			5	1 x 70 x 3	1 x 80 x 2	1 x 90 x 2			550
Total of 100 kg-1RM, kg =									**35989**

13.4.14. TENTH-WEEK DAILY EXERCISE-DIFFERENTIALS

Table 13.9.2 shows the breakdown of load volume and intensity, during the second week of the third month, of the four-month period.

o   This week follows the same trends of the previous week, with difference in the number of lifts and load volume.
o   The net weekly lifts are 520, of 60% 1RM or higher.
o   The daily number of exercises follows the formula 6-4-6-4-6.
o   The net weekly load volume is **37.28 tons**, based on a 100 kg-1RM in all lifts.

Table 13.9.2. Daily exercise sequence, sets, repetition, and percentage of 1RM during the **Second Week** of the third month.

WEIGHTLIFTING EXERCISES	Time of day	100 kg-1RM Daily Volume Differential, kg	Sequence	Sets x Percentage x Repetitions					100 kg-1RM Exercise Volume Differential, kg
Shoulder Press	AM	Day 1 8636	1	1 x 60 x 3	1 x 70 x 3	1 x 80 x 3	1 x 90 x 1		720
Snatch Classic			2	2 x 60 x 2	2 x 70 x 2	2 x 80 x 2	1 x 90 x 1	1 x 95 x 1	1026
Front Squat			3	2 x 70 x 3	2 x 80 x 3	2 x 90 x 3			1440
Hang Clean			4	2 x 60 x 3	2 x 70 x 3	2 x 80 x 2	1 x 85 x 2		1270
Clean Pull	PM		5	1 x 90 x 3	2 x 100 x 3	1 x 110 x 1			980
Back Exercise			6	4 x 100 x 8					3200
Power Snatch	AM	Day 2 5300	1	3 x 60 x 3	2 x 70 x 2	2 x 80 x 2	2 x 85 x 2		1480
Power Clean and Jerk			2	2 x 60 x 2	2 x 70 x 2	3 x 80 x 2	1 x 90 x 2		1180
Jerk from Rack			3	1 x 90 x 3	1 x 100 x 1	1 x 110 x 1			480
Eccentric			4	3 x 120 x 6					2160
Shoulder Press	AM	Day 4 8150	1	1 x 60 x 3	1 x 70 x 2	1 x 80 x 2			480
Classic Clean			2	2 x 60 x 3	3 x 70 x 2	2 x 80 x 2	1 x 90 x 2		1280
Back Squat			3	2 x 70 x 4	2 x 80 x 2	1 x 90 x 4			1240
Hang Snatch			4	2 x 60 x 2	2 x 70 x 2	2 x 80 x 2	1 x 90 x 1		930
Snatch Pull	PM		5	2 x 80 x 3	2 x 90 x 3				1020
Back Exercise			6	4 x 100 x 8					3200
Snatch Classic	AM	Day 5 5256	1	2 x 60 x 3	3 x 70 x 2	3 x 80 x 2			1260
Hang Clean			2	2 x 60 x 3	2 x 70 x 2	3 x 80 x 2	1 x 90 x 2	1 x 95 x 1	1396
Clean Pull			3	2 x 80 x 3	2 x 90 x 3				1020
Front Squat			4	2 x 80 x 4	2 x 90 x 3	2 x 100 x 2			1580
Classic Clean	AM	Day 6 9936	1	2 x 60 x 3	2 x 70 x 3	2 x 80 x 2	2 x 85 x 2		1440
Jerk from Rack			2	1 x 70 x 2	1 x 80 x 2	2 x 90 x 2			660
Back Squat			3	2 x 80 x 3	2 x 90 x 3	1 x 100 x 2	1 x 110 x 1		1330
Hang Snatch			4	2 x 60 x 2	2 x 70 x 2	2 x 80 x 2	1 x 90 x 1	1 x 95 x 1	1026
Snatch Pull	PM		5	1 x 80 x 3	2 x 90 x 3	1 x 100 x 2			980
Isometric Clean Pull			6	5 x 100 x 9					4500
Total of 100 kg-1RM, kg =									**37278**

13.4.15. ELEVENTH-WEEK DAILY EXERCISE-DIFFERENTIALS

Table 13.9.3 shows the breakdown of load volume and intensity, during the third week of the third month, of the four-month period.
o   This week also follows the same of trends of the previous week, with some differences.
o   The net weekly lifts are 385, of 60% 1RM or higher.
o   The daily number of exercises follows the formula 6-4-6-4-5.
o   The net weekly load volume is **33.67 tons**, based on a 100 kg-1RM in all lifts. This is also one of few low volume weeks throughout the period.

Table 13.9.3. Daily exercise sequence, sets, repetition, and percentage of 1RM during the **Third Week** of the third month.

WEIGHTLIFTING EXERCISES	Time of day	100 kg-1RM Daily Volume Differential, kg	Sequence	Sets x Percentage x Repetitions					100 kg-1RM Exercise Volume Differential, kg
Shoulder Press	AM	Day 1 8736	1	1 x 60 x 3	1 x 70 x 3	1 x 80 x 2	1 x 85 x 2		720
Classic Snatch	AM		2	2 x 60 x 3	2 x 70 x 2	2 x 80 x 2	2 x 90 x 1		1140
Front Squat			3	2 x 70 x 4	2 x 80 x 4	2 x 90 x 3			1740
Power Clean and Jerk			4	2 x 60 x 2	2 x 70 x 2	2 x 80 x 2	1 x 90 x 1	1 x 95 x 1	1026
Clean Pull	PM		5	1 x 80 x 3	1 x 90 x 3	2 x 100 x 2			910
Back Exercise			6	4 x 100 x 8					3200
Hang Snatch	AM	Day 2 5010	1	2 x 60 x 2	2 x 70 x 2	2 x 80 x 2	2 x 85 x 2		1180
Hang Clean			2	2 x 60 x 2	3 x 70 x 2	2 x 80 x 2	1 x 85 x 2		1150
Jerk from Rack			3	2 x 80 x 2	2 x 90 x 2	2 x 100 x 1			880
Isometric			4	3 x 100 x 6					1800
Shoulder Press	AM	Day 4 8816	1	2 x 60 x 3	2 x 70 x 3				780
Classic Clean			2	2 x 60 x 2	2 x 70 x 2	2 x 80 x 2	2 x 90 x 1	1 x 95 x 1	1116
Back Squat			3	2 x 70 x 4	2 x 80 x 4	2 x 90 x 4			1920
Power Snatch			4	2 x 60 x 2	2 x 70 x 2	2 x 80 x 2	2 x 90 x 1		1020
Snatch Pull	PM		5	1 x 80 x 3	2 x 90 x 3				780
Back Exercise			6	4 x 100 x 8					3200
Classic Snatch	AM	Day 5 5500	1	2 x 60 x 3	3 x 70 x 3	3 x 80 x 2	2 x 85 x 2		1810
Classic Clean and Jerk			2	2 x 60 x 2	2 x 70 x 2	2 x 80 x 2	2 x 90 x 1		1020
Clean Pull			3	1 x 80 x 3	3 x 90 x 3	1 x 100 x 2			1250
Front Squat			4	2 x 80 x 3	2 x 90 x 3	2 x 100 x 2			1420
Power Snatch	AM	Day 6 5610	1	2 x 60 x 2	2 x 70 x 2	3 x 80 x 2			1000
Snatch Pull			2	3 x 90 x 3	1 x 100 x 3				1110
Back Squat			3	1 x 70 x 3	2 x 80 x 3	2 x 90 x 3	1 x 100 x 2		1430
Classic Clean	PM		4	2 x 60 x 3	3 x 70 x 3	3 x 80 x 2			1470
Jerk from Rack			5	2 x 80 x 2	1 x 90 x 2	1 x 100 x 1			600
Total of 100 kg-1RM, kg =									**33672**

13.4.16. TWELFTH-WEEK DAILY EXERCISE-DIFFERENTIALS

Table 13.9.4 shows the breakdown of load volume and intensity, during the fourth week of the third month, of the four-month period.
o   This week also follows the same of trends of the previous week, with some differences.
o   The net weekly lifts are 520, of 60% 1RM or higher.
o   The daily number of exercises follows the formula 6-4-6-4-6.
o   The net weekly load volume is **40.49 tons**, based on a 100 kg-1RM in all lifts. This in the beginning of maximizing intensity for the month of competition.

Table 13.9.4. Daily exercise sequence, sets, repetition, and percentage of 1RM during the **Fourth Week** of the third month.

WEIGHTLIFTING EXERCISES	Time of day	100 kg-1RM Daily Volume Differential, kg	Sequence	Sets x Percentage x Repetitions					100 kg-1RM Exercise Volume Differential, kg
Shoulder Press	AM	Day 1 8415	1	1 x 60 x 3	2 x 70 x 3	1 x 80 x 2			760
Snatch Classic			2	1 x 60 x 3	2 x 70 x 2	2 x 80 x 2	2 x 90 x 1	1 x 95 x 1	1055
Front Squat			3	2 x 70 x 4	2 x 80 x 3	2 x 90 x 3			1580
Hang Clean			4	2 x 60 x 2	2 x 70 x 3	2 x 80 x 2			980
Clean Pull	PM		5	2 x 80 x 3	2 x 90 x 2				840
Back Exercise			6	4 x 100 x 8					3200
Power Snatch	AM	Day 2 6195	1	2 x 60 x 2	2 x 70 x 2	2 x 85 x 1			690
Power Clean and Jerk			2	2 x 60 x 2	2 x 70 x 2	1 x 90 x 1	95 x 1 x		705
Jerk from Rack			3	1 x 70 x 2	1 x 80 x 2				300
Isometric Clean Pull			4	5 x 100 x 9					4500
Shoulder Press	AM	Day 4 8640	1	2 x 60 x 3	2 x 70 x 3				780
Classic Clean			2	2 x 60 x 3	2 x 70 x 2	2 x 80 x 2	1 x 90 x 1		1050
Back Squat			3	1 x 80 x 3	2 x 90 x 3	2 x 100 x 2	1 x 110 x 1		1290
Hang Snatch			4	2 x 60 x 2	3 x 70 x 2	2 x 80 x 2	2 x 90 x 2		1340
Snatch Pull	PM		5	1 x 80 x 3	2 x 90 x 3	1 x 100 x 2			980
Back Exercise			6	4 x 100 x 8					3200
Snatch Classic	AM	Day 5 5755	1	2 x 60 x 3	3 x 70 x 3	3 x 80 x 2			1470
Hang Clean			2	2 x 60 x 3	2 x 70 x 2	2 x 80 x 2	2 x 85 x 2		1300
Clean Pull			3	3 x 90 x 3	2 x 100 x 2	1 x 115 x 1			1325
Front Squat			4	3 x 80 x 3	2 x 90 x 3	2 x 100 x 2			1660
Hang Snatch	AM	Day 6 11480	1	2 x 60 x 3	2 x 70 x 2	2 x 80 x 2	2 x 85 x 1		1130
Snatch Pull			2	1 x 80 x 2	2 x 90 x 2	1 x 100 x 1			620
Back Squat			3	2 x 70 x 4	7 x 80 x 4	2 x 90 x 4			3520
Classic Clean			4	2 x 60 x 2	2 x 70 x 2	2 x 80 x 2	2 x 90 x 2		1200
Jerk from Rack	PM		5	1 x 80 x 3	3 x 90 x 3				1050
Eccentric			6	6 x 110 x 6					3960
				Total of 100 kg-1RM, kg =					**40485**

MANAGING LOAD VOLUME AND INTENSITY

13.4.17. PRE-CONTEST-MONTH DAILY EXERCISE-DIFFERENTIALS
o The pre-contest month comprises of final preparation for the contest.
o This month of the period of progressive resistance training comprises of 25 training session, spread over the four weeks of the month, **Table 13.10**.
o There is significant cut in the number of monthly sessions. The month's total lifts of 1684 are the lowest in the four-month period.
o The first half of the month comprises of eight weekly sessions that are performed in consecutive daily sequence of 2-1-0-2-1-2-0. The second half of the month shows decrease in the number of weekly sessions and increase in intensity, with six
o sessions in the third week and three sessions in the last.

Table 13.10. Total daily exercise sets during the **Pre-contest Month**, of the four-month training cycle.

	Week 1					Week 2					Week 3				Week 4			Total Exercise sets
Sessions / Day	2	1	2	1	2	2	1	2	1	2	2	1	2	1	1	1	1	
Day Number	1	2	3	4	5	6	7	8	9	10	11	12	13	14	15	16	17	
Exercises								Exercise sets										
Classic Snatch	16		24			16		24			24		24			18		146
Power Snatch		24		16			24		24			24			12		15	139
Hang Snatch			15		24			12		24					16			91
Snatch Pull		15		15	12		12		12	12	4		15		9		9	115
Jump Squat																12		12
Classic Clean and Jerk		24		24			24		24		24		24			18		162
Power Clean and Jerk	24		16			24		24				24			12		15	139
Hang Clean				24					24				24					72
Clean Pull	15		12			12		12				12		8	9	9		89
Jerk from Rack	12			8		12			8		12		12					64
Front Squat	24		18			18		18			18		18		10			124
Back Squat		12		24			18		18			18	12	18		9		129
Shoulder Press	12		12		12	12		12		18		12		12				102
Isometric Clean Pull					40													40
Eccentric											36							36
Back Exercise		32	32		32		32	32			32		32					224
Total Daily sets	103	107	129	87	144	94	110	134	86	114	114	90	137	78	52	54	51	1684

13.4.18. THIRTEENTH- WEEK DAILY EXERCISE-DIFFERENTIALS

Table 13.10.1 shows the breakdown of load volume and intensity, during the first week of the pre-contest month, of the four-month period.
o From this week on, intensity or resistance will start to increase. After warm-ups, all lifts will start with 70% 1RM, instead of 60% in the previous weeks.
o The net total weekly lifts are 570.
o The daily number of exercises follows the formula 6-5-7-5-6.
o The net weekly load volume is **54.01 tons,** based on a 100 kg-1RM in all lifts.
o The increase of resistance occurs every two sets, in most cases.
o This is the most intense and voluminous week of the sixteen weeks, *Figure 13.1*.

Table 13.10.1. Daily exercise sequence, sets, repetition, and percentage of 1RM during the **First Week** of the pre-contest month.

WEIGHTLIFTING EXERCISES	Time of day	100 kg-1RM Daily Volume Differential, kg	Sequence	Sets x Percentage x Repetitions					100 kg-1RM Exercise Volume Differential, kg
Snatch, Classic	AM	Day 1 9770	1	2 x 70 x 30	2 x 80 x 2	2 x 90 x 1	2 x 95 x 1	2 x 95 x 1	4890
Power Clean and Jerk	AM		2	4 x 70 x 3	4 x 80 x 2				1480
Power Clean and Jerk			3	2 x 70 x 3	2 x 80 x 2				740
Clean Pull			4	1 x 80 x 3	2 x 90 x 2	2 x 100 x 2	1 x 110 x 2	1 x 110 x 2	1220
Shoulder Press	PM		5	4 x 70 x 3					840
Squat			6	1 x 70 x 4	1 x 80 x 4		2 x 100 x 3	2 x 100 x 3	600
Power Snatch	AM	Day 2 13560	1	4 x 70 x 30	4 x 80 x 2	2 x 90 x 1	2 x 95 x 1	2 x 95 x 1	9410
Classic Clean and Jerk			2	2 x 70 x 2	2 x 80 x 2	2 x 90 x 2			960
Snatch Pull			3	2 x 70 x 3	1 x 80 x 2	2 x 100 x 3	1 x 110 x 2	1 x 110 x 2	1400
Back Squat			4	1 x 80 x 4	1 x 90 x 3				590
Jump Goodmorning			5	4 x 100 x 3					1200
Hang Snatch	AM	Day 4 14050	1	3 x 70 x 30	2 x 80 x 2				6620
Snatch, Classic			2	2 x 80 x 3	2 x 80 x 3	3 x 90 x 2			1500
Shoulder Press			3	2 x 70 x 4	2 x 80 x 3				1040
Back Exercise			4	4 x 100 x 3					1200
Power Clean and Jerk	PM		5	2 x 70 x 2	2 x 80 x 2	2 x 90 x 2	2 x 95 x 1	2 x 95 x 1	1150
Clean Pull			6	1 x 70 x 3	2 x 80 x 3	1 x 90 x 3			960
Front Squat			7	2 x 70 x 4	2 x 80 x 3	2 x 90 x 3			1580
Power Snatch	AM	Day 5 5540	1	2 x 70 x 2	2 x 80 x 2	2 x 90 x 2	2 x 95 x 1	2 x 95 x 1	1150
Classic Clean and Jerk			2	4 x 70 x 2	4 x 80 x 2				1200
Jerk from Rack			3	1 x 80 x 2	1 x 90 x 2	1 x 100 x 2			540
Snatch Pull			4	1 x 80 x 3	1 x 90 x 3	2 x 100 x 2			910
Back Squat			5	2 x 70 x 4	2 x 80 x 4	2 x 90 x 3			1740
Hang Snatch	AM	Day 6 11090	1	3 x 70 x 2	2 x 80 x 2	3 x 80 x 2			1220
Hang Clean			2	3 x 70 x 2	3 x 80 x 2	2 x 90 x 2			1260
Back Exercise			3	3 x 100 x 8					2400
Shoulder Press			4	2 x 70 x 2	2 x 80 x 3	1 x 90 x 2			940
Snatch Pull	PM		5	1 x 70 x 3	3 x 80 x 3	1 x 90 x 2	1 x 100 x 2	1 x 100 x 2	1310
Isometric			6	6 x 110 x 6					3960
Total of 100 kg-1RM, kg =									**54010**

13.4.19. FOURTEENTH-WEEK DAILY EXERCISE-DIFFERENTIALS

Table 13.10.2 shows the breakdown of load volume and intensity, during the second week of the pre-contest month, of the four-month period.
o   This week constitutes the beginning in tapering down of intense training in preparation for the contest, *Figure 13.1*.
o   All lifts start at 70% 1RM, and some reach 100%.
o   The number of daily picked exercises follows the formula 6-5-7-5-5.
o   The number of weekly sessions is still maintained at eight, spread on five days.
o   The net weekly lifts are 538, of 60% 1RM or higher.
o   The net weekly load volume is **40.21 tons,** based on a 100 kg-1RM in all lifts. This is a week of buildup and maintenance, rather than stimulation.

Table 13.10.2. Daily exercise sequence, sets, repetition, and percentage of 1RM during the **Second Week** of the pre-contest month.

WEIGHTLIFTING EXERCISES	Time of day	100 kg-1RM Daily Volume Differential, kg	Sequence	Sets x Percentage x Repetitions				100 kg-1RM Exercise Volume Differential, kg
Snatch, Classic	AM	Day 1 7330	1	2 x 70 x 3	2 x 80 x 2	2 x 90 x 1	2 x 100 x 1	1120
Power Clean and Jerk			2	3 x 70 x 3	3 x 80 x 3	2 x 90 x 2		1710
Jerk from Rack			3	1 x 70 x 3	2 x 80 x 3	1 x 90 x 2		870
Clean Pull			4	2 x 80 x 3	1 x 90 x 3	1 x 100 x 3		1050
Shoulder Press	PM		5	2 x 70 x 4	2 x 80 x 3			1040
Front Squat			6	1 x 70 x 5	1 x 80 x 4	1 x 90 x 3	2 x 100 x 3	1540
Classic Clean and Jerk	AM	Day 2 8080	1	2 x 70 x 2	2 x 80 x 2	2 x 90 x 2	2 x 100 x 1	1160
Power Snatch			2	3 x 70 x 3	3 x 80 x 2	2 x 85 x 2		1450
Snatch Pull			3	1 x 70 x 3	1 x 80 x 2	1 x 90 x 3	1 x 100 x 2	840
Back Exercise			4	4 x 100 x 8				3200
Back Squat			5	1 x 70 x 4	2 x 80 x 3	1 x 90 x 3	2 x 100 x 2	1430
Snatch, Classic	AM	Day 3 10840	1	3 x 70 x 3	2 x 80 x 3	3 x 90 x 3		1920
Hang Snatch			2	2 x 70 x 3	2 x 80 x 3			900
Back Exercise			3	4 x 100 x 8				3200
Shoulder Press			4	1 x 70 x 3	2 x 80 x 3	1 x 90 x 2		870
Power Clean and Jerk	PM		5	2 x 70 x 2	2 x 80 x 2	2 x 90 x 2	2 x 95 x 2	1340
Clean Pull			6	1 x 70 x 3	2 x 80 x 3	1 x 90 x 2		870
Front Squat			7	2 x 70 x 4	2 x 80 x 4	2 x 90 x 3		1740
Power Snatch	AM	Day 4 5720	1	2 x 70 x 2	2 x 80 x 2	2 x 90 x 2	2 x 95 x 1	1150
Classic Clean and Jerk			2	3 x 70 x 2	2 x 80 x 2	3 x 90 x 2		1280
Jerk from Rack			3	1 x 80 x 2	2 x 90 x 2	3 x 100 x 1		820
Snatch Pull			4	2 x 80 x 3	1 x 90 x 3	2 x 100 x 2		1150
Back Squat			5	2 x 80 x 3	2 x 90 x 3	1 x 100 x 3		1320
Hang Snatch	AM	Day 5 8240	1	3 x 70 x 3	2 x 80 x 3	2 x 90 x 2		1310
Hang Clean			2	2 x 70 x 3	4 x 80 x 2	2 x 90 x 2		1420
Eccentric			3	6 x 100 x 6				3600
Snatch Pull	PM		4	1 x 70 x 3	2 x 80 x 3	1 x 90 x 2		870
Shoulder Press			5	2 x 70 x 4	2 x 80 x 3			1040
Total of 100 kg-1RM, kg =								40210

13.4.20. FIFTEENTH-WEEK DAILY EXERCISE-DIFFERENTIALS

Table 13.10.3 shows the breakdown of load volume and intensity, during the third week of the pre-contest month, of the four-month period. This week precedes the week of the contest. It is, therefore, has reduced number of days, four instead of five, and reduced number of sessions, six instead of eight.
o   It is one of the least voluminous, yet most intense, weeks in the fifteen weeks.
o   Resistance starts with 70% 1RM and hikes to 100%.
o   It is the last week for any controlled high-tension exercise, such as Back Squat, Shoulder Press, or Goodmorning.
o   The net weekly lifts are 419, of 70% 1RM or higher.
o   The daily number of exercises follows the formula 6-5-6-5.
o   The net weekly load volume is **30 tons**, based on a 100 kg-1RM in all lifts.

Table 13.10.3. Daily exercise sequence, sets, repetition, and percentage of 1RM during the **Third Week** of the pre-contest month.

WEIGHTLIFTING EXERCISES	Time of day	100 kg-1RM Daily Volume Differential, kg	Sequence	Sets x Percentage x Repetitions				100 kg-1RM Exercise Volume Differential, kg
Snatch, Classic	AM	Day 1 8730	1	3 x 70 x 3	3 x 80 x 2	2 x 90 x 2		1470
Snatch Pull			2	1 x 70 x 3	1 x 80 x 3	1 x 90 x 3	1 x 100 x 2	920
Goodmorning			3	4 x 100 x 8				3200
Classic Clean and Jerk			4	2 x 70 x 2	2 x 80 x 2	2 x 90 x 1	2 x 100 x 1	980
Jerk from Rack	PM		5	1 x 80 x 2	2 x 90 x 2	1 x 100 x 2		720
Front Squat			6	2 x 70 x 3	2 x 80 x 3	2 x 90 x 3		1440
Power Snatch	AM	Day 2 6490	1	3 x 70 x 2	2 x 80 x 2	3 x 90 x 2		1280
Power Clean and Jerk			2	3 x 70 x 2	3 x 80 x 2	2 x 90 x 2		1260
Clean Pull			3	1 x 80 x 3	2 x 90 x 3	1 x 100 x 2		980
Back Squat			4	3 x 80 x 4	2 x 90 x 3	2 x 100 x 3		2100
Shoulder Press			5	1 x 70 x 3	2 x 80 x 3	1 x 90 x 2		870
Snatch, Classic	AM	Day 4 9280	1	2 x 70 x 2	2 x 80 x 2	2 x 90 x 1	2 x 100 x 1	980
Snatch Pull			2	2 x 70 x 3	3 x 80 x 3			1140
Stiff-legged Deadlift			3	4 x 100 x 8				3200
Classic Clean and Jerk			4	3 x 70 x 3	3 x 80 x 3	2 x 90 x 2		1710
Jerk from Rack	PM		5	1 x 70 x 2	1 x 80 x 2	2 x 90 x 2		660
Front Squat			6	1 x 70 x 4	2 x 80 x 4	1 x 90 x 3	2 x 100 x 2	1590
Hang Snatch	AM	Day 6 5500	1	3 x 70 x 2	2 x 80 x 2			740
Hang Clean and Jerk			2	3 x 70 x 2	3 x 80 x 2	2 x 90 x 2		1260
Clean Pull			3	2 x 80 x 3	2 x 90 x 2			840
Back Squat			4	2 x 70 x 4	2 x 80 x 3	2 x 90 x 4		1760
Shoulder Press			5	2 x 70 x 3	2 x 80 x 3			900
				Total of 100 kg-1RM, kg =				30000

13 MANAGING LOAD VOLUME AND INTENSITY

13.4.21. SIXTEENTH- WEEK DAILY EXERCISE-DIFFERENTIALS

Table 13.10.4 shows the breakdown of load volume and intensity, during the fourth week of the pre-contest month, of the four-month period. This week precedes the contest date.

o   This week only comprises of three morning sessions.
o   Exercises are cut down to four or five per day.
o   Also, assisting exercises are reduced to Front Squat, Clean and Snatch Pulls.
o   No Back Squat, Spinal erector, Eccentric, or Isometric exercises are included in this last week. This allows maximum buildup of physical strength for contest.
o   Intensity of resistance is also reduced at this low weekly volume.
o   The net weekly lifts are 157, of 60% 1RM or higher.
o   The daily number of exercises follows the formula 5-4-4
o   The net weekly load volume is **10.40 tons**, based on a 100 kg-1RM in all lifts. This is the lowest load volume of the sixteen-week period.

Table 13.10.4. Daily exercise sequence, sets, repetition, and percentage of 1RM during the **Fourth Week** of the pre-contest month.

WEIGHTLIFTING EXERCISES	Time of day	100 kg-1RM Daily Volume Differential, kg	Sequence	Sets x Percentage x Repetitions				100 kg-1RM Exercise Volume Differential, kg
Power Snatch	AM	Day 1 4020	1	2 x 70 x 2	2 x 80 x 2	2 x 90 x 1		780
Hang Clean and Jerk			2	2 x 70 x 2	2 x 80 x 2	2 x 90 x 1		780
Snatch Pull			3	2 x 80 x 2	2 x 90 x 4			1040
Clean Pull			4	1 x 80 x 2	1 x 90 x 2		1 x 90 x 2	340
Front Squat			5	2 x 70 x 3	2 x 80 x 3	1 x 90 x 2		1080
Snatch, Classic	AM	Day 3 3640	1	2 x 60 x 3	2 x 70 x 2	2 x 80 x 2	2 x 85 x 2	1300
Classic Clean and Jerk			2	2 x 60 x 3	2 x 70 x 2	2 x 80 x 2	2 x 85 x 1	1130
Clean Pull			3	1 x 70 x 3	1 x 80 x 2	1 x 90 x 2		550
Back Squat			4	2 x 70 x 3	1 x 80 x 3			660
Power Snatch	AM PM	Day 5 2740	1	2 x 60 x 3	3 x 70 x 2			780
Power Clean and Jerk			2	2 x 60 x 3	3 x 70 x 2			780
Jump Squat			3	4 x 50 x 3				600
Snatch Pull			4	2 x 70 x 3	1 x 80 x 2			580
Total of 100 kg-1RM, kg =								10400

13.5. PERSONAL ACCOUNT WITH MANAGING VOLUME AND INTENSITY

The following photographs depict the tale of growing up with Weightlifting training, living the experiment of the predecessors, and witnessing the emergence of a new breed of luckier and more knowledgeable Weightlifters.

MANAGING LOAD VOLUME AND INTENSITY

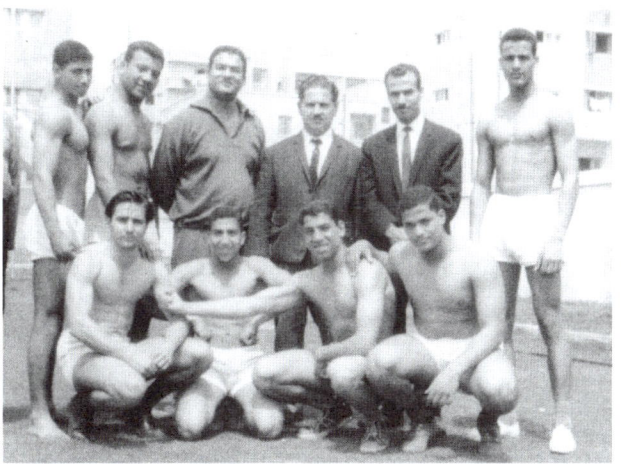

Figure 13.2. The factory of champions.

There was no shortage in Olympic or International Weightlifting champions in the city of Alexandria, Egypt. Mahmoud Fayad, the standing short man, is the Weightlifting Olympic gold medallist of 1948 Olympic games. He is considered an Egyptian icon in Weightlifting. Ahmed Mutawa, the slim man to his left, is the first coach that introduced the author to the sport of Weightlifting. He competed in Moscow in 1956 and died from rheumatic heart disease in his thirties. His talent and dream to reach the top Olympic games were lost a stenosed mitral valve that was not amenable to surgical treatment in 1960's. Al-Kassabany, the man in training suite, has coached the author in Weightlifting for seventeen years. **Year 1967.**

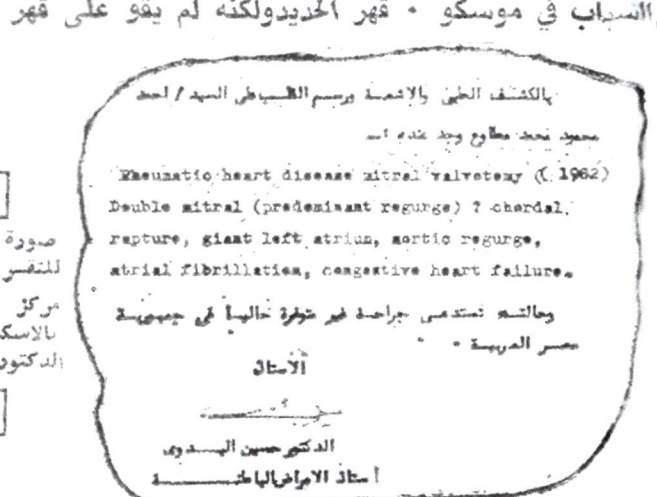

Figure 13.3. A diseased Champion.

Ahmed Mutawa, the first coach that introduced the author to Weightlifting, was diagnosed in 1962 to have both mitral and aortic regurge, chordal rupture, and congestive heart failure. He competed in Moscow 1956 in Weightlifting and died late 1969 from the complication of rheumatic fever. This photo was an excerpt form a national newspaper that aimed to seek his medical treatment abroad. Open heart surgery was unknown those days.

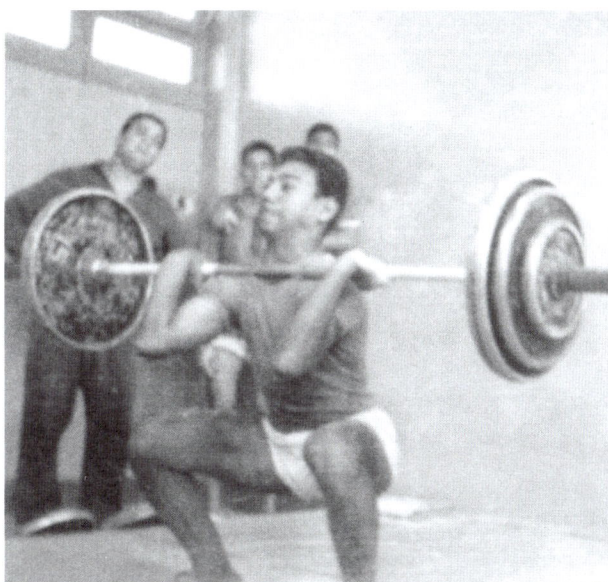

Figure 13.4. Introducing Full Squat lifting.

After finishing his research in Weightlifting in East Germany, Al-Kassabany (seen in the back) was the first coach to teach us the Full Squat Clean and Snatch. The author was in junior high school in this photo. It became apparent that the new lifting technique required consistent strengthening of the legs, back, and shoulders. The old and obsolete leg springing will not be practiced anymore. The new era of Weightlifting had to foster flexibility, coordination, strength, and speed. From mid 1960's, Weightlifting training required serious and consistent practice than earlier years did. The new technique of lifting proved very effective in building strength in few months. This 95 kg Clean was a great accomplishment in high school years. **Year 1967.**

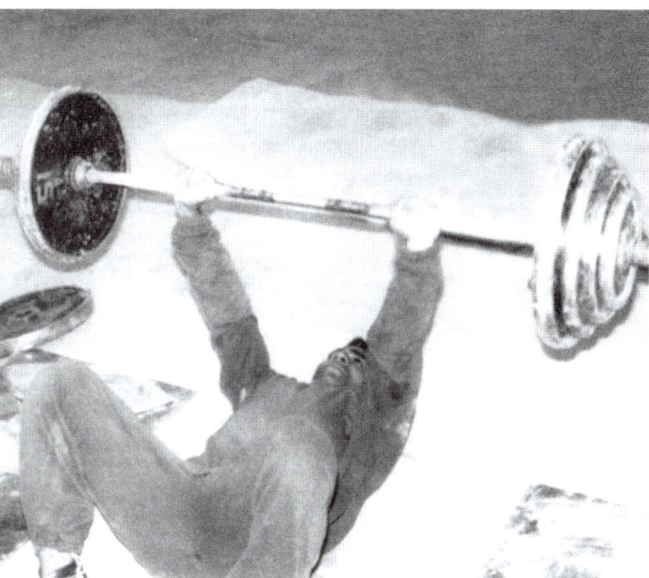

Figure 13.5. Down to earth exercises.

Platform Press was introduced by Al-Kassabany in order to encourage Weightlifters to use this assisting exercise before rushing to the locker room. Many Weightlifters skip this vital exercise when benches are remotely placed or unavailable. Platform Press utilizes the 20-centimeter radius of the plates as a stopping distance. In addition, getting to the floor, and lying on the back, enhances flexibility, in a sport that is geared to sole strengthening. **Year 1970.**

13 MANAGING LOAD VOLUME AND INTENSITY

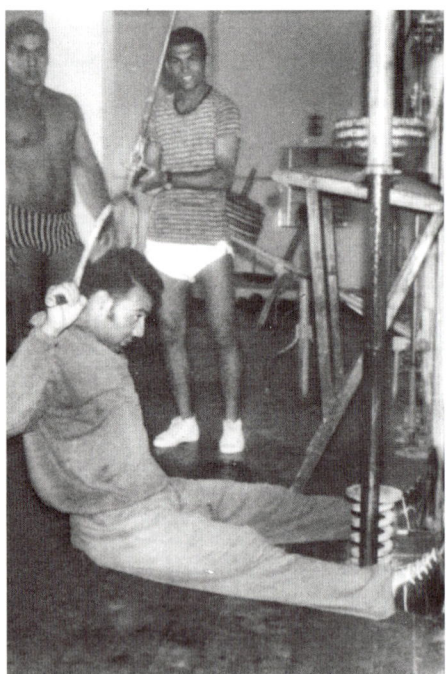

Figure 13.6. Down to earth exercises. Cable pulldown while sitting on the floor was superior to seated cable pulldown. Floor sitting stretches the Hamstrings, tones the Iliopsoas, and foster postural spinal erection for long duration. **Year 1970.**

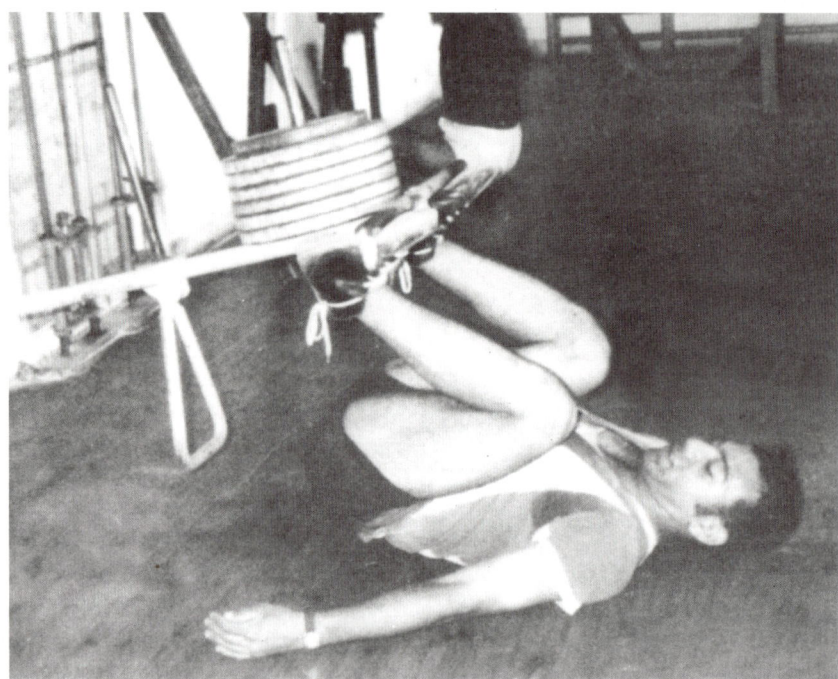

Figure 13.7. Down to earth exercises. Leg Press machines were as simple as few rods, welded to a joint. This inexpensive design achieves better results than today's fancy machines. Leg Pressing, lying on the floor, fosters natural flexibility. **Year 1970.**

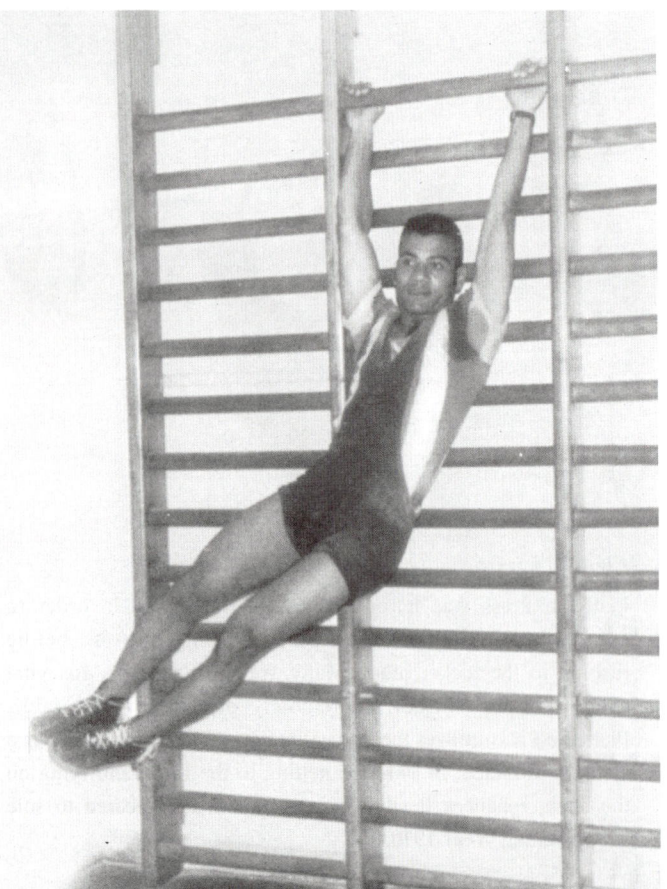

Figure 13.8. Wall ladders were essential part of training rooms. They were utilized in stretching and upper body exercises. **Year 1970.**

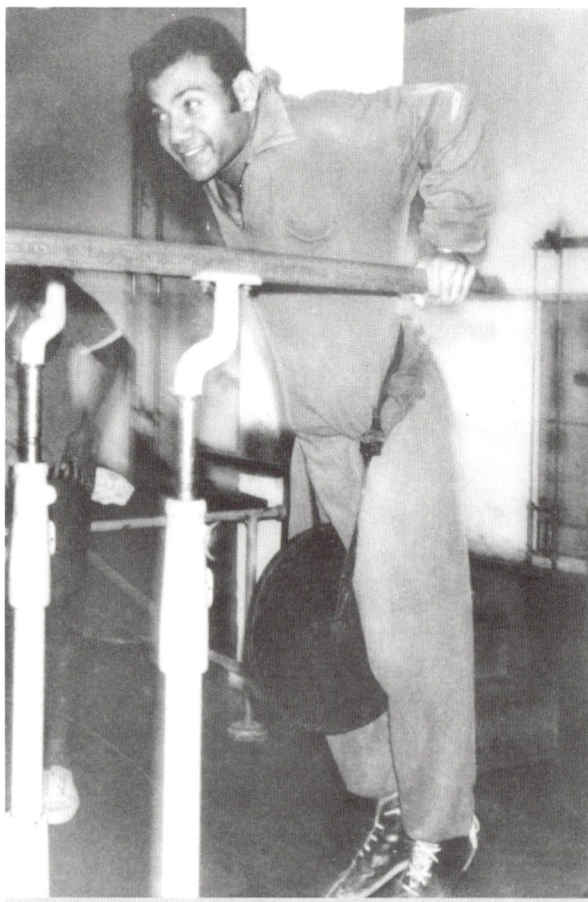

Figure 13.9. Basic upper body strengthening. Weighted parallel bar dips are basic upper body assisting exercise for Weightlifting. Suspending a 45 lb plate around the waist does not require special tools. **Year 1970.**

MANAGING LOAD VOLUME AND INTENSITY

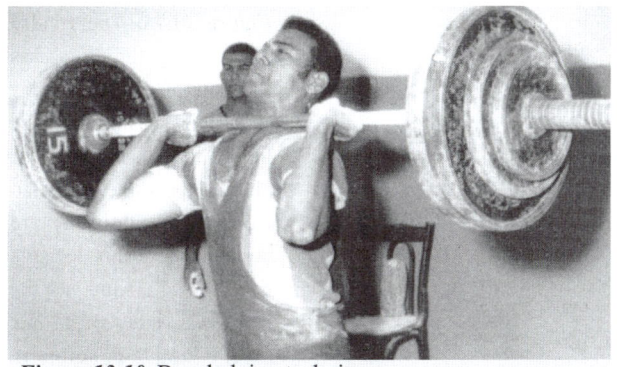

Figure 13.10. Bar shelving technique.

Shelving the bar on the top of the sternum and pushing the vital neck structures backwards, was a basic lesson for the beginners. This will enhance the elevation of the clavicles and strengthen the suspension of the chest cage from the vertebral axis. **Year 1970.**

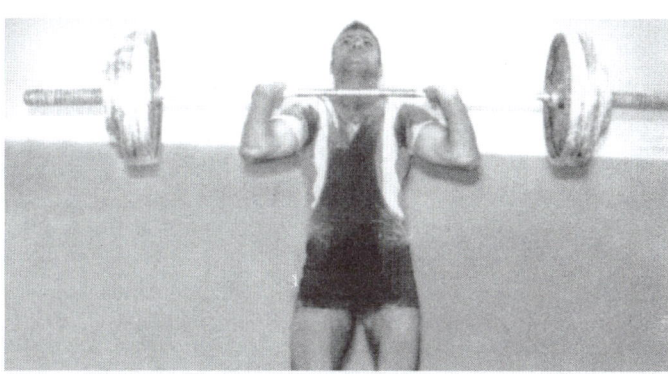

Figure 13.11. Bar shelving technique.

The coach has to find ways to explain the role of the scapulas and the Deltoids. If the lifter learns how to engage the Serratus in widening the sides under the arms pits, then he would be able to flex the shoulders high, under the bar, by the Deltoid action. Thus, the bar will rest in the groove between the Deltoids and the Trapezius, instead of sitting on the chest cage alone. **Year 1970.**

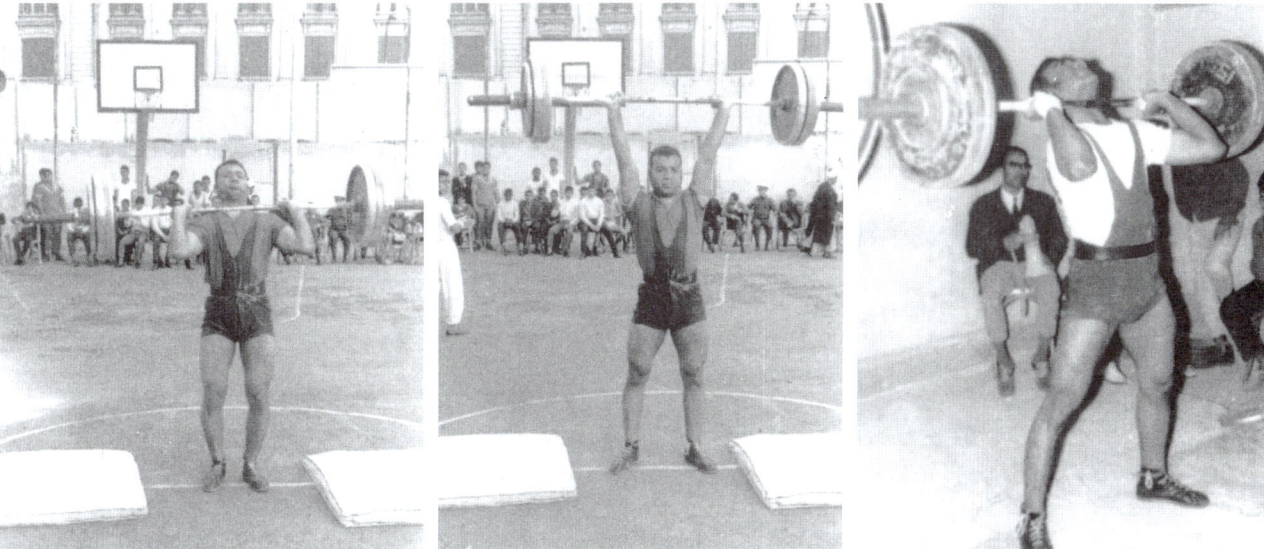

Figure 13.12. Promoting the sport of Weightlifting.

In an effort to publicize the sport of Weightlifting, Al-Kassabany worked hard to convince school officials that Weightlifting is not as complicated as many people perceived it. Lifting heavyweight on the grass was not a wise idea. However, no matter how compelling new ideas were, school officials were indifferent to any idea that does not bring immediate and substantial revenues. **Year 1970.**

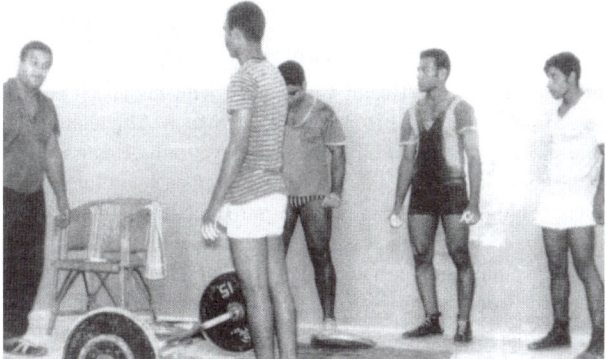

Figure 13.13. Coaching in training.

Three years later, Al-Kassabany managed to get a new training room in a larger Health Club. Our team started growing. The author was a senior member and a magnet to new comers. We also got new platform and new Russian barbell. That was a great gift from the government at that time. The Russian barbell came with lubricating kits that made lifting less traumatic and fun. The roughness of the bar surface was meticulously machined to suit heavy lifting. The serration of the plate cylinders was very ingenious in preventing the plates from sliding, without using a lock. **Year 1970.**

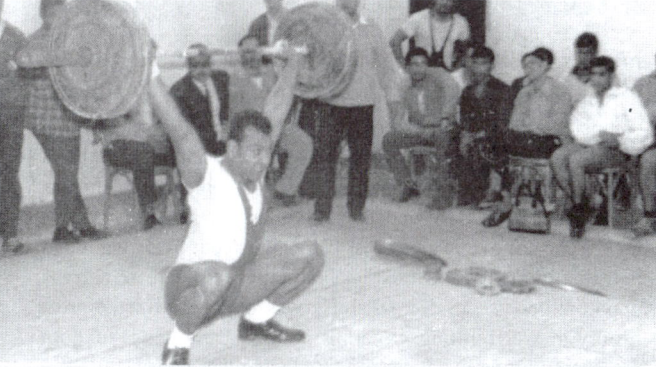

Figure 13.14. Coaching in contests.

After five years of training, Al-Kassabany started seeing the fruits of his efforts as a coach. In this college contest, the author lifted 110 kg in the Snatch and 135 kg in the Clean and Jerk, in the 82.5 kg. That was a great accomplishment in college Weightlifting. It also proved that Weightlifting is not a monopoly of the blue color workers. This was the first college contest that witnessed the new Full Squat lifting style and the first participation from the college of engineering. The opponent of the author was a Bodybuilder who bench-presses over 180 kg, yet failed to lift 105 kg in the Clean and Jerk. **Year 1973.**

13 MANAGING LOAD VOLUME AND INTENSITY

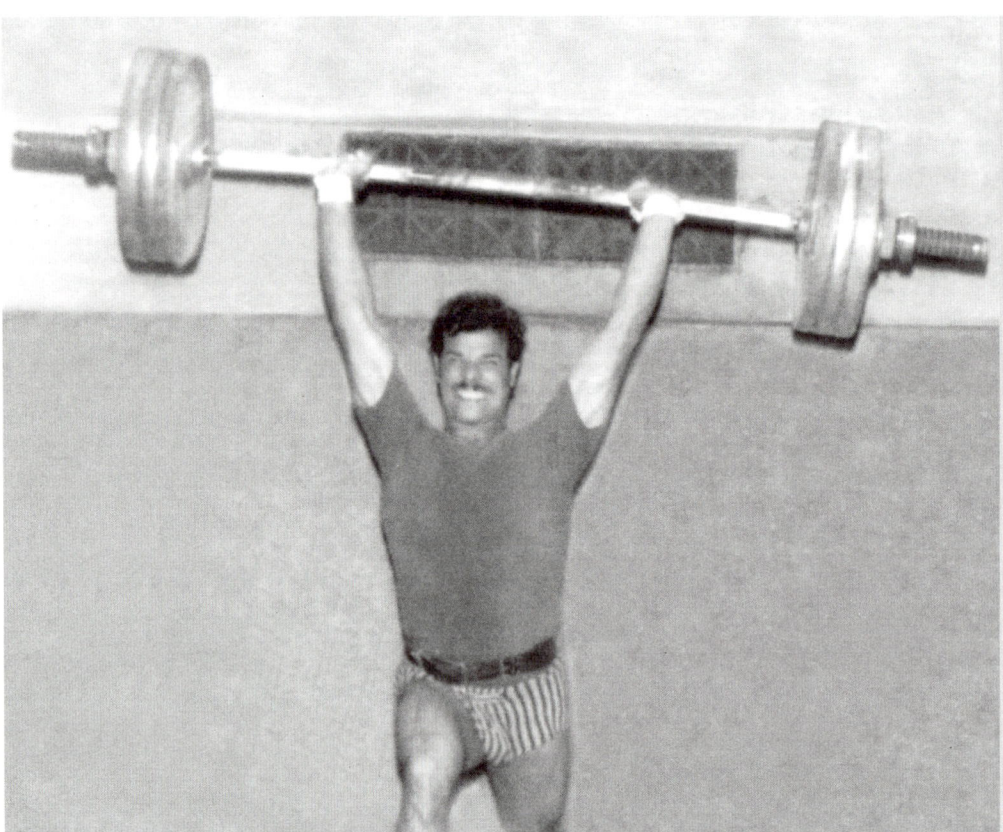

Figure 13.15. The rivalry of three Weightlifting coaches and icons. Competing on the state level was a challenge for college students. In these photos, the three Egyptian icons of Weightlifting are nervous about this decisive lift. Al-Kassabany, to the right, was the first to use paper and pencil in documenting Weightlifting events. He was ridiculed by others for being literate. The Olympic gold medallist Fayad, second from right, is more nervous because this lifter is his trainee and he has to prove his superiority over Al-Kassabany. The third Egyptian legend, Gaber Hafez, far to left, is also anxious to see his partner dominates his weight class. **Year 1973.**

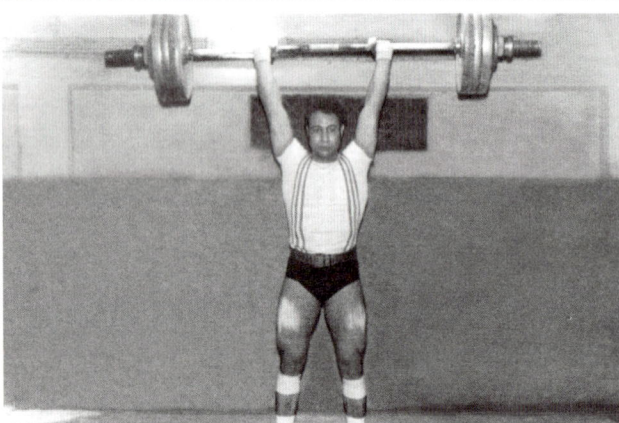

Figure 13.16. A rising star flunking the Olympic dream.

In our old Health Club, we invited outsiders to come and compete. This young man was a rising star. He trained at a private, outdoor, poor gym. He climbed to the national level and competed in few international contests. His biggest problem was lack of education. That undermined his financial security and, in the absence of public awareness campaign about overweight and nutrition in his days, caused his bodyweight to increase and his opportunities to win decreased. He was destined to make great history in Weightlifting, if not his poor education and stubborn mistrust in professional coaches. Realizing that he can lift more than those coaches did in their competitive years, he only relied on his sole method of training. **Year 1973.**

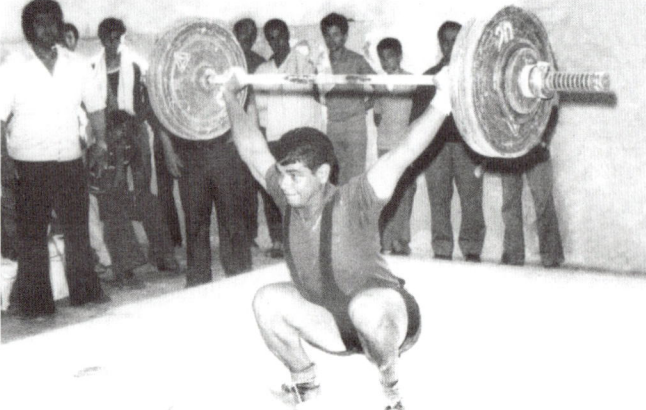

Figure 13.17. Competing and coaching.

Another visitor to our Health Club, came with his coach Gaber Hafez, to show his unique technique in the Snatch. Although many people started practicing Full Squat lifting, yet only Al-Kassabany was the most knowledgeable of the requirements for long term planning of this new technique. He introduced at least two leg exercises in each training sessions. His balanced emphasis on the shoulder, spinal, and pelvic proportions of strengthening was unmatched. Comparing a self-taught coach such as Gaber Hafez with a College graduate coach such as Al-Kassabany was like comparing the math skills of a layman to those of a mathematician. The latter, planned for years of remedial strategies to deal with each individual problem. **Year 1973.**

MANAGING LOAD VOLUME AND INTENSITY

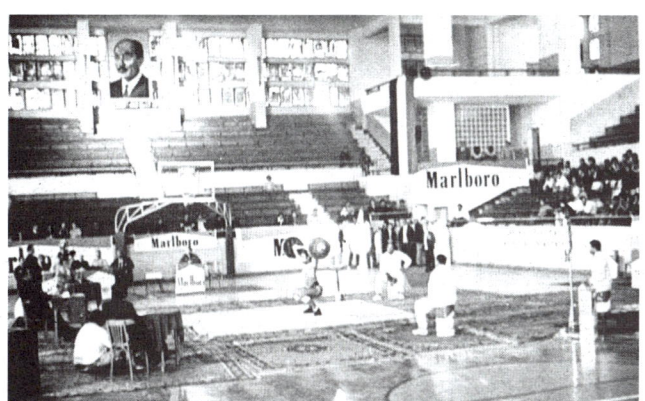

Figure 13.18. The theatre of International Weightlifting Championships.

The first international championship the author has witnessed was sponsored by Marlboro. The organizers also claimed that President Sadat (his photograph is seen on the wall) was supervising its arrangement. This was a great opportunity to watch diverse international methods of training, competing, and expressing emotion of success and failure. The sponsorship by cigarette manufacturer attests to lack of awareness of the public about the harm of smoking. Even until the present time, many third world countries do not view smoking as public health menace. Moreover, since smoking was not mentioned literally in the Holy Quran, while alcohol was, therefore, many muslim countries do not prohibit smoking. Yet, the Holy Quran encompasses many verses that prohibit destructive habits and wasteful conduct. **Year 1973.**

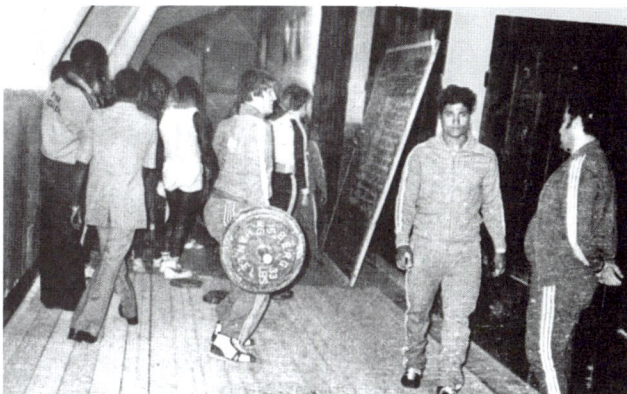

Figure 13.19. Warming up in International contests.

The warm-up room in that international championship in Weightlifting was a chaotic and messy place. On the wall, a blackboard shows the news of the competition and the turns of the lifters. Since each lifter has a set-time to show up on the platform when called on, therefore, warm-up was the worst part of the contest. This competitor has to warm up in the middle of all these irrelevant people. Many contest failures are attributed to hasty warm-up, rather than to poor training. The beginning of warm-up has to be timed with the first lift in the contest. If too much or too little time elapses between warm-up and commencing the contest, then chances of failure increase. **Year 1973.**

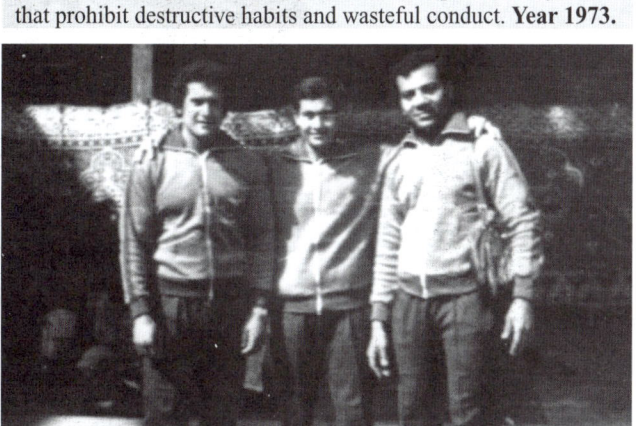

Figure 13.20. College Weightlifting.

Ibrahim Abu Kalila (left) had joined our Weightlifting team in 1973. He converted from Bodybuilding and excelled in Weightlifting beyond any expectation. In this photo, he became a student in the college of law and competed with the author (right) in the college championship, in Cairo. Advancing to the Olympic level was not a mere accident. The personality attributes of Abu Kalila led him to the top. His aggressive attitude made him view social relationships as short-lived and money-driven. His friendship with others was very short. He even fought the coach who had made him a champion, when suspected of foul play against him. His weight training was self-taught and unique, in hard and long hours of working out, and innovative and diverse exercises. His biggest asset was his farming background. That had helped him greatly in believing in natural food and simple life. Such aggressive personality, combined with hard training, and financial resources to avail himself to long hours of training, and demanding nutritional needs, put him on the top of all of us, in Weightlifting. **Year 1978.**

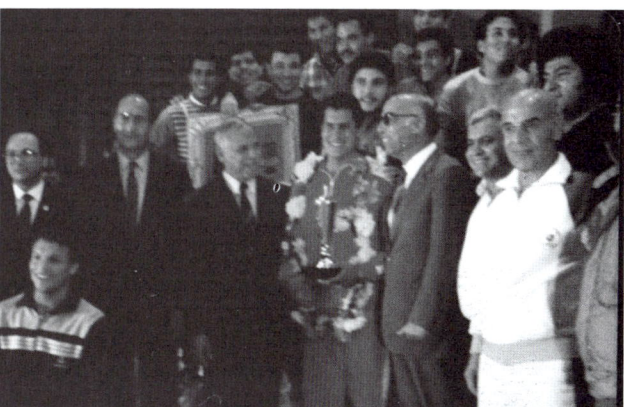

Figure 13.21. Winning in Olympic games.

Abu Kalila was celebrated as a national icon after his participation in the Los Angeles Olympic games in 1984. Gameel Hana, right to Abu Kalila, was the President of the Egyptian Federation of Weightlifting. He and his brother had competed, coached, and managed that organization for many years. Gaber Hafez (far right, back row) was now slipping away from his glorious days as a national champion. Yet, all these men had contributed to refining the method of managing load volume and intensity throughout the training cycles.

The most puzzling mystery to the author, is the great number of people who devoted their life, lobbying for the sport of Weightlifting, and promoting it in every occasion, despite the lack of adequate financial gain. In each contest, there would be at least one or few famous international champions, watching, managing, or judging. The fact that most of these people do not worry about owning cars, or homes, or making millions of dollars, may explain their genuine passion towards the real sport testing of human strength. **Year 1984.**

13 MANAGING LOAD VOLUME AND INTENSITY

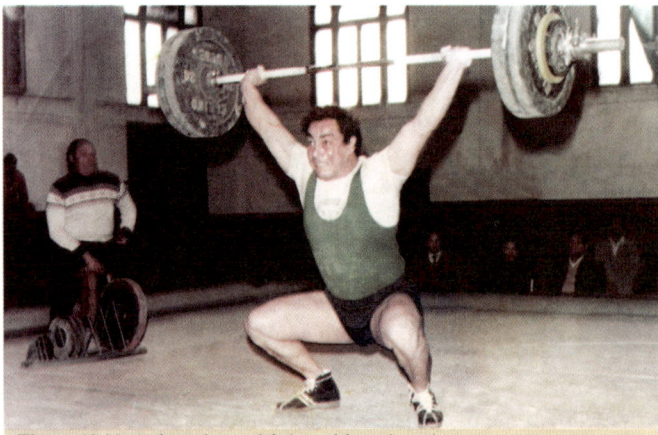

Figure 13.22. A champion and father of four champions.
Ramadan Abdel Mouety competed with the author, in Alexandria, Egypt, in 1971. He will never lose affection to the sport of Weightlifting, and the Club he trained in, and represented in championships. He will train all his four children on Weightlifting. Two of his daughters will reach international level and travel allover the world, training and competing. Although he never lifted heavier than 110 kg Snatch and 140 kg Clean and Jerk, yet, in 1971, we did not know about the daily double-session training, nor did we know about the simplification of exercise picking to four or six. His daughter, Nahla Ramadan, will surpass him by 116.5 kg Snatch and 147.5 kg Clean and Jerk, in year 2003, in Mexico, World Junior Championship. His daughter trained twice daily, full time, and with the state financial support and supervision. **Year 1971.**

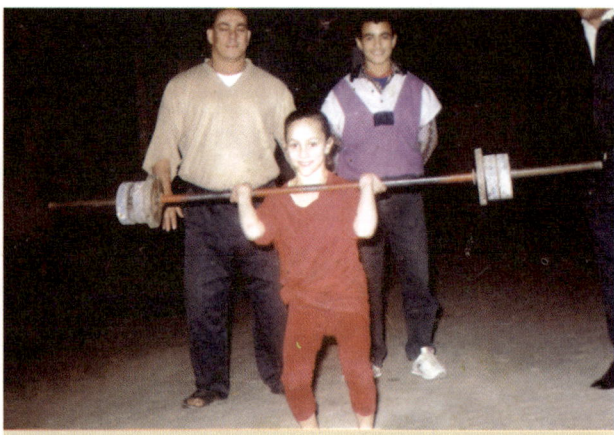

Figure 13.23 The young girl and future Weightlifting gold medallist.
Ramadan (left) started training his daughter Nahla at the age of seven. He built this homemade barbell and started a gym on the street, in front of his house. This young girl will lift 116.5 kg in the Snatch and 147.5 in the Clean and Jerk, in May 2003, in the weight class 75 kg. Nahla was born in 1985, the fourth child and the second daughter. The neighbors accused the street coach, and the father and trainer of his four children, of being insane. His elation of seeing his kids lift weights, Olympic style, was overwhelming. None of his children dared not to lift weights in order to win the smile of their weight-possessed father. Although he lived in a religious society that is very restrictive to women's rights, yet his poor education had spared him the inclination to and the obsession of the believes of the predecessors. He devised his own world, set his own rules, and turned deaf ears to the insanity accusation.

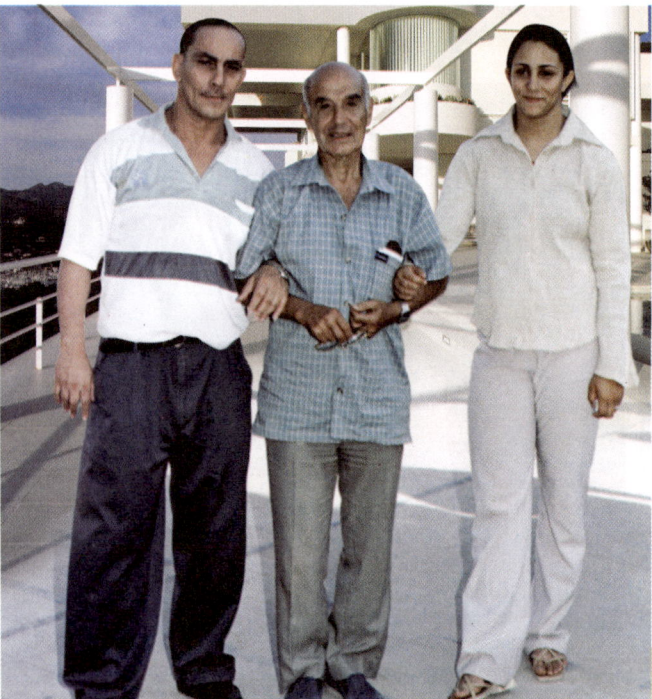

Figure 13.24. The new and old gold medallists.
Ramadan and his daughter Nahla (now international champion in Weightlifting) seen with Kamal Mahgoob, the 1951 Weightlifting champion. Kamal had given Olympic Weightlifting over fifty years of his life. He attended most of the contests and meetings, and talked to thousands of common people and politicians about the sport. His contribution to the popularity of this sport, in Egypt, is undeniably immense. The unique story of Nahla is that she is a muslim women, born and raised in Islamic culture, yet excelled to the top International Weightlifting and broke the records at the age of twenty-one. Despites her father's poverty, she took pride in his great effort to make her different and unique. The conservative Islamic tradition had contributed to her acceptance to her father's shortcomings, her belief is marriage as the only setup for sexual life, and her abstinence from alcohol and smoking. Without such cultural and traditional influence on her character, she might have never stuck with her father's extreme views until that age.

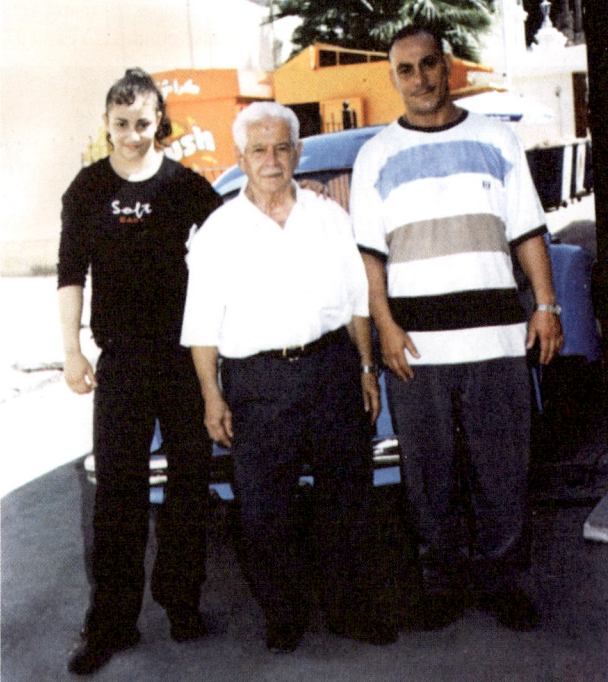

Figure 13.25. The new and old gold medallists Ramadan and his champion daughter Nahla seen with Mahoud Fayad, the 1948 Olympic gold medallist, see also Figure 13.2. Although, Fayad was not an active speaker, he never missed a Weightlifting contest until his death in December 2002. Almost every Weightlifter in Egypt must have taken a photograph with Fayad. This is the first photograph, where Fayad was seen without a suite and tie. He attended all public gathering in formal dress, owing to his days during King Farouk of Egypt, when formality meant respect, wealth, and power. That impressive social appeal had attracted many young people to the sport of Weightlifting. Many had aspired to the seriousness and the tough outlook of retired Weightlifters. **Year 2002.**

MANAGING LOAD VOLUME AND INTENSITY

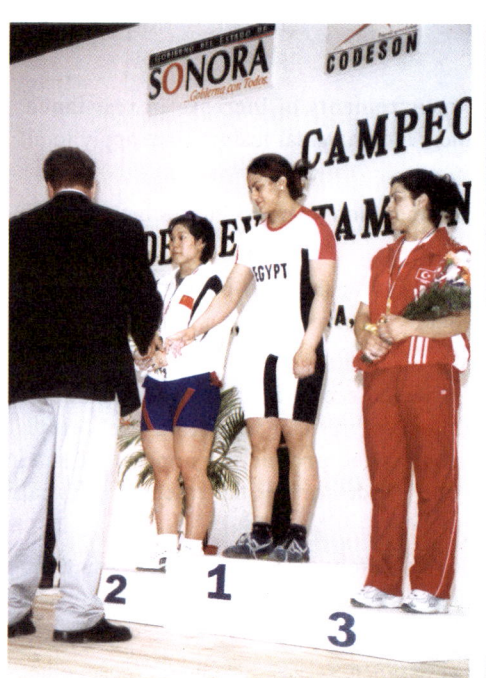

Figure 13.26. Gold medal at twenty-one.

Nahla Ramadan Mohamed became a gold medallist in the 75 kg weight class and made two international records for junior women. She was born in 1985. Despite the altra-conservative Egyptian society, on women's rights, Nahla has followed her passionate father and trainer. Her full time training with the Egyptian national team, in addition to her training by the Bulgarian method, helped her excel to the top. **Year 2003.**

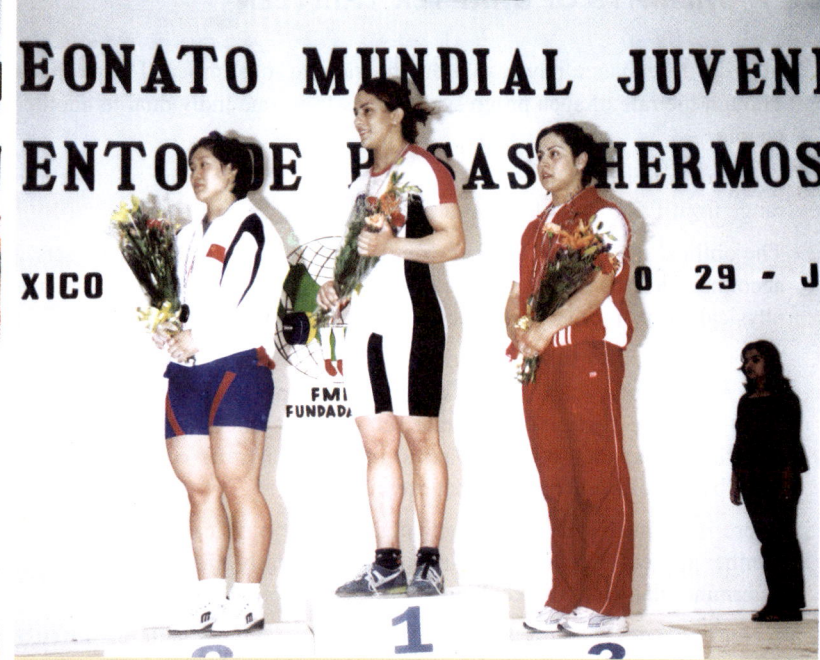

Figure 13.27. Earning flower with life sweat.

A great moment for a young girl, a passionate father, and a misperceived nation. Not every one appreciates these flowers as much as this twenty-one year young, muslim, poor woman. Her father and her three siblings struggled for fourteen years to see this dream become reality. No one ever thought that her father will win the gamble of training his daughter on Weightlifting and smashing international records. Although, her father was thought to be insane, by his neighbors, for training his kids on the street, yet these flowers vindicate her father's passionate intention. In this photo, Nahla is seen with other two winners:

1. Nahla Ramadan (born 1985), from Egypt, weighing 73.40 kg, lifted 116.5 kg Snatch, 147.5 Clean and Jerk, and totaled 262.5 kg.
2. Chunhong Liu (born 1985), from China, weighing 70.80 kg, lifted 112.5 kg Snatch, 147.5 Clean and Jerk, and totaled 260.0 kg.
3. Sibel Simsek (born 1984), from Turkey, weighing 71.30 kg, lifted 100 kg Snatch, 130 Clean and Jerk, and totaled 230 kg.

Year 2003.

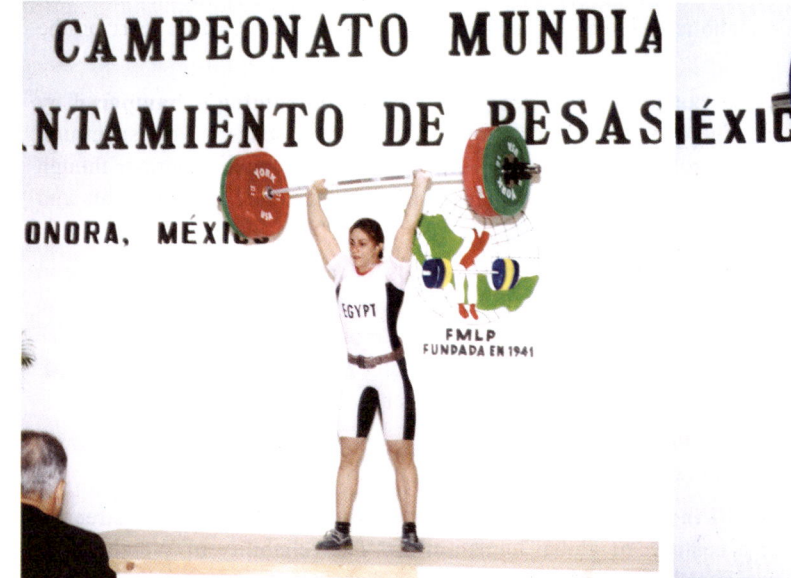

Figure 13.28. Clean and Jerk of double-bodyweight by 18-year old muslim girl.

2003 Junior World Championships, Hermosillo, Mexico. 147.5 kg Clean and Jerk, bodyweight 73.40 kg. **Year 2003.**

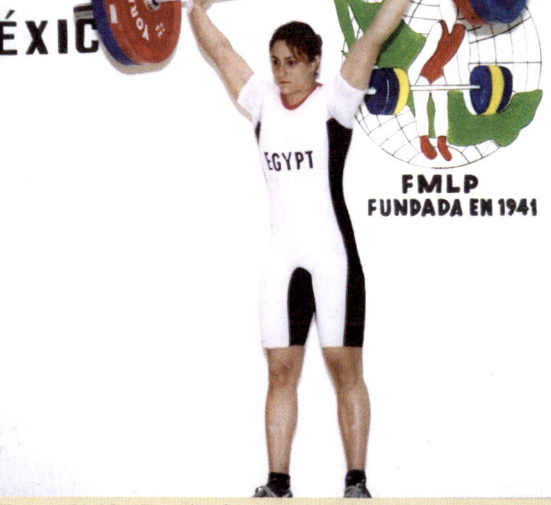

Figure 13.29. Snatch of one-and-half bodyweight by 18-year old muslim girl.

2003 Junior World Championships, Hermosillo, Mexico. 116.5 kg Snatch. **Year 2003.**

13 MANAGING LOAD VOLUME AND INTENSITY

13.6. HIGHLIGHTS OF CHAPTER THIRTEEN

1. In order to enhance physical strength, training must proceed in **progressive increments of increase in resistance**. Though the rate of such progression varies from one individual to another, there are universal features that apply to all people.

2. A **set** of exercise group is defined as the starting and ending of an exercise, without long pauses. Pauses between sets range from 1.5 minutes to 3 minutes.

3. The optimal number of sets, per exercise group, is between 2 and 5 sets. The reason for the **multiple-set routine** is to accommodate for neuromuscular, cardiopulmonary, and cardiovascular adaptation. These require a total net of high physical work, in order to produce significant changes in structures

4. A set of exercise may comprise of multiple repetition, of a cycle of concentric and eccentric muscular contractions. The number of cycles per set constitutes "**repetition**". Also, the magnitude of resistance, during each cycle, constitutes the "**intensity**" of that set. The net intensity of an exercise group is the **product of number of sets, repetition, and magnitude of resistance**. This is referred to as "load volume". It determines the extent of physical work by muscles and heart, in that exercise.

5. There is a limit on trying to manipulate the net physical work, per exercise, by merely increasing or decreasing the number of sets, repetition, or intensity. The daily and weekly sum, of all differential work of various exercises, determines daily and weekly **load volumes**, respectively.

6. Increasing weekly load-volume, or session load-volume, with **low intensity resistance**, serves different purpose, other than developing strength. That is enhancing aerobic oxidation by muscles, and depleting fuel depots.

7. Although intense resistance does not consume body fat, at least immediately and during exercise, it induces active, after-exercise, cycling of byproducts and replenishing consumed substrates. In fact, anaerobic activity utilizes only less than 5% of the energy available for fast **fuel supply**.

8. **Recuperative intervals** between intense training sessions are typically 12-24 hours. High performance athletes can train twice daily, every other day, and alternate with once daily, every other day, in the remaining days of the week.

9. Multiple sets enhance the **neuromuscular adaptation** and power output, required for freestyle lifting. Yet, the cost of these accomplishments is abbreviating the number of exercise groups and repetitions, per set, in daily sessions.

10. The final results of managing load volume and intensity are judged by reducing burning of contractile tissues and enhancing their strength and mass. In other words, maximizing a **good mix of endurance and strength** is the ultimate goal of wise management of strength training. Lack of understanding, of the relationship between resistance and physiologic adaptation, leads to poor mix, such as reaching plateau in endurance level because of decline in basic strength, or reaching plateau in power output because of sluggish recuperative endurance.

11. Overtraining can be defined as a shift in metabolism towards the catabolic side. Such shift is caused by exerting **physical work** in excess of the body's ability to regenerate consumed energy molecules and re-synthesize essential cellular components necessary for anabolism. Catabolic shift might occur in vital organs such as the heart or the nervous system.

12. Whatever the cause of overtraining may be, the final outcome is that **progress in strength training is hampered** by the lack of anabolic shift of cellular metabolism. The clinical manifestation of overtraining scans a wide spectrum, from mild fatigue, brief and extreme exhaustion, to protracted weariness. Trainees can still make progress, though overtrained, but not at the expected performance, as if they were not overtrained. The quick recognition and management of overtraining can prevent its chronic and grave consequences.

13. **Remedial approach to overtraining.** These comprise of taking mini break periods, occasional changes in routine in order to avoid boredom, long recovery period, or modifications to the intensity-volume plan of workout. Also modification of exercise picking can dramatically resolve overtraining. For example, cross training between endurance and strength can be counterproductive if the athlete fails to understand that the two are mutually exclusive, in maxima. Exercise picking should follow similar metabolic pathways and motor skills needed for that particular sport.

14. **Powerlifting training** has major flaws and complies with no known expert professional planning. It is a haphazard way of massing muscles, yet compromises flexibility and predisposes to injury.

15. Managing the load-volume and intensity in **Weightlifting** is more problematic. It must account for form and strength. It also has been enhanced and refined, for over a century, of global human effort. The reliability of Weightlifting periodization of volume and intensity is well manifested in Olympic game records that do not cease to climb, game after game.

Chapter 14
Health and Fitness

14.1. ROLE OF EXERCISE IN HEALTH

14.1.1. BODY SYSTEMS OF MOTION
o **Living in motion:** Humans are not created to idle in couches. Only plants exist in a state of motionlessness, because they do not have hearts, blood vessels or nervous systems. Nature did not equip humans with those three systems in vain. Without daily exercise, the blood vessels transform into hardened tubes that mimic those of the trees. Hardened blood vessels are silent killers. Even if you are good in avoiding unhealthy food, smoking, alcohol, and drugs and, above all, you enjoy optimum bodyweight, you still belong to the animal kingdom and exercise is your best bid to stay an agile creature. Relaxing, sitting, and drinking claim more lives than all wars and epidemics of the entire human history.

o **Atomic participation:** Indeed, physical activity is a lifelong prerequisite for health and longevity. That is because every atom in the living matter has a definite lifetime to participate in the process of life. Such participation might be in the form in enzymatic, hormonal, mineral, or chemical substrate that operate the biological processes. The main role for atomic participation might come down to the very basic task of utilizing energy. This is obvious in the role of the calcium and phosphate minerals in the physiology of bone. Physical activity increases the participation of the calcium and phosphate in building up stronger bones, while immobility causes thinning of bones and loss of calcium in urine. Thus, atoms and molecules seem to follow very precise laws in the biological process of life and exercise might be the main tool that makes these laws work in our favor.

o **Dynamic milieu:** Each atom enters the body composition only stays there for specific lifetime. Afterwards, it departs the body just to be replaced by another atom. This applies to all food ingredients and molecules of air that enter into the body composition. Thus, the animal body constitutes a very dynamic congregation of atoms, each has specific role to play in certain time span, of a matter of days, not years or decades. What makes the body so fluid and dynamic is the very nature of energy. Exercise activity fosters energy flow, be it physical or spiritual, in such manner as to allow constant growth and reproduction of body cells. Recall that cells do not choose their chemical processes based on emotion, intellect, or behavior, but rather on, more or less, rigorous physical laws. Thus, activity or inactivity is dealt with, by the cells, in the form of alteration of the level of activity of enzymes, concentrations of accessory cofactors, and genetic transcription[1] of major chemical catalysts. Such cellular adaptation to activity or inactivity determines the outcome of health or disease.

14.1.2. CELLULAR ADAPTATION TO EXERCISE
The human body demonstrates diverse specialized cellular functions. These functions serve the purpose of refining, storing, burning, and managing fuel resources.
o The liver refines synthesis and production of glucose from carbohydrates, proteins, and glycerol.
o Fat cells store highly condensed fuel sources in the form of neutral fat.
o Muscle cells burn glucose and fatty acids in greater rates than any other cells.
o The nervous system manages the mental and physical regulation of muscular activity.

Table 14.1 lists some differences in function between these four types of cells. It shows the purposeful designation of tasks of various organs, which make human life a fascinating design of energy management.

---
[1] Genetic transcription is a process that takes place within the cell nucleus, by which messenger ribonucleic acids mRNA is synthesized from a DNA template, resulting in the transfer of genetic information from the DNA molecule to the mRNA. These exit the nucleus and translate their genetic information into new protein synthesis, in the cytoplasm.

Table 14.1. Difference in function of various types of cells of the human body.

Functions	Liver Cells	Muscle Cells	Fat Cells	Brain cells
Glucose uptake	Highest rate of **glucose uptake**, without the need for insulin or calcium ions, due to possessing glucose transport protein GLUT-2. **Synthesize glycogen** and fatty acids. Possess specific **glucokinase** to trap glucose in the form G6P. This is a biologically active form of glucose.	Require insulin or calcium ions to stimulate transport, via transport protein GLUT-4. Only 1/10th of liver uptake. **Synthesize glycogen** and perform anaerobic oxidation.	Like muscle cells	Have non-specific **hexokinase** capable of trapping glucose in the form G6P within the cell.
Glucose breakdown	All cells can perform anaerobic glucose oxidation to pyruvate and lactates. The ATP molecules generated from this process are utilized as high-energy currency for various biological processes. Only muscle cells can utilize ATP in producing kinetic energy.			
Glycogen synthesis	The liver stores ~150-200 g glycogen. Possess only one **glycogen phosphorylase** enzyme for breakdown of glycogen into G1P. This enzyme does not inhibit liver Glycogen synthase.	Muscles store ~ **300 gm** glycogen. Possess **two phosphorylase** enzymes for the breakdown glycogen into G1P. One is induced by cAMP, calcium ions, and insulin and inhibits glycogen synthase, while the other is induced by G6P.		Very small glycogen formation.
Fat synthesis	Can operate hexose monophosphate pathway and produce glycerol and pentose sugars form glucose. Thus, synthesize fat, steroids, phospholipids, and lipoproteins. Synthesized steroids regulate activity. Synthesized lipoprotein regulates fat transport.	Cannot produce glycerol or pentose from glucose.	Like liver, can manufacture glycerol and pentose from glucose, and fatty acids from amino acids and carbohydrates via acetyl CoA.	Can synthesize fatty acids in the cytoplasm.
Fatty acid oxidation	Can operate fatty acid oxidation. Can phosphorylate[2] glycerol and convert it to dihydroacetone phosphate to be oxidized anaeobically.	Can operate fatty acid oxidation. Cannot metabolize glycerol.		Can operate fatty acid oxidation.
Cholesterol synthesis	Can synthesize 1-1.5 g/day. This is about 5 times dietary intake. Inhibited by dietary intake.	Cannot synthesize cholesterol.		Can synthesize cholesterol.
Amino acid breakdown	Liver cells possess arginase enzyme and can cleave urea from the amino acid arginine. This is the main process of clearing nitrogen from the body, since urea is excreted by the kidneys.			Glutamic acid is the only amino acid metabolized and accepts ammonia to form glutamine.
Gluconeo-genesis	Can synthesize glucose from glucogenic amino acids, lactic acid, glycerol, and other ketoacids. Possess G6P phosphatase and can **synthesis glucose and release** it to blood.	Deficient in G6P-phosphatase and **cannot release** glucose to blood.		
Tricarboxylic acid cycle	Cycling depends on the need for ATP for gluconeogenesis, lipogenesis, and amino acid synthesis.	Cycling depends on calcium ion release and ATP demand by **contracting muscles.**	Cycling depends on fat synthesis and fat breakdown.	
Ketogenesis	Can oxidize fatty acids into **ketone bodies** but cannot use them.	Can oxidize ketone bodies.		Can oxidize ketone bodies.
Creatine Phosphate-ATP		Possess creatine phosphate shuttle for immediate supply of ATP.		
Hormone receptors	Insulin induces fatty acid synthesis from glucose. Adrenalin and glucagon induce conversion of glycogen into glucose.	Insulin induces glycogen synthesis from glucose. Adrenalin induces conversion of glycogen into G6P. Glucagon has NO effect.	Cortisol induces fat breakdown.	

---

[2] Phosphorylation refers to the process of adding phosphate ions to a chemical substrate. This converts substrates to active form. It is catalyzed by **phosphorylase** enzymes. The reverse is removing phosphate ions from substrates to render it inactive. This is catalyzed by **phosphatase** enzymes.

14.1.3. PHYSICAL APPEARANCE

Exercise gives the sense of being stronger, more accomplished, and less afraid. It induces the protein machine within the cellular DNA to make anew muscle protein and convert the mushy look of tissues into firm and vibrant **appearance.** Without exercise, most of the excess energy in the food we consume is stored in the form of fat. Fat not only accumulates under the skin, but also deposits within the entire connective tissues, wherever they are found. Fat accumulates in the walls of the blood vessels, in the tissues that suspend the intestines, and in the heart. Thus, fat permeates throughout our internal organs as well as under our skin. The change in the outer appearance with exercise gives an assurance that parallel changes are taking place internally as well.

14.1.3.1. Managing Body Fat

o   At certain age, our body has the resilience to rebel the incursion of fat on vital blood capillaries and arterial system, even after calcification has been settled. Yet, if major deformations of the blood vessels are extensive, due to fat deposition, calcification, and sclerosis, then total recovery diminishes. The excess body fat is rich in cholesterol, which is a precursor for the hormones mineralocorticosteroids, glucocorticosteroids, and sex hormones. Thus, excess fat provides anomalous sources of adrenal and gonadal hormones. Excess in mineralocorticosteroids cause high blood pressure, glucocorticosteroids suppress the immune system and cause cancer, and sex hormones cause cancer of the breast, uterus, and prostate.

o   Managing excess fat deposition requires reduction in bodyweight and enhancement of muscular mass through balancing the calories you eat with your physical activity choices[3], as follows.

> **Tip # 1***
> **CHOOSE SENSIBLE PORTION SIZES**
>
> - If you're eating out, choose small portion sizes, share an entree with a friend, or take part of the food home (if you can chill it right away).
> - Check product labels to learn how much food is considered to be a serving, and how many calories, grams of fat, and so forth are in the food. Many items sold as single portions actually provide two servings or more. Examples include a 20-ounce container of soft drink, a 12-ounce steak, a 3-ounce bag of chips, and a large bagel.
> - Be especially careful to limit portion size of foods high in calories, such as cookies, cakes, other sweets, French fries, and fats, oils, and spreads.
>
> * NUTRITION AND YOUR HEALTH: DIETARY GUIDELINES FOR AMERICANS, published by the Department of Health and Human Services (HHS) and the Department of Agriculture (USDA).

   i. Choose a **healthful assortment of foods** that includes vegetables, fruits, grains (especially whole grains), skim milk, and fish, lean meat, poultry, or beans. This prevents deficiencies of various essential nutritional elements.
   ii. Choose foods that are **low in fat** in order to reduce major source of excess calories.
   iii. Choose foods **low in added sugars**, since extra sugars are added to low-fat muffins or desserts, for example, and they may be just as high in calories as fat containing foods.
   iv. Whatever the food, eat a **sensible portion size**, *Tip # 1.* Snacks and meals eaten away from home provide a large part of daily calories for many people. Choose them wisely. Try fruits, vegetables, whole grain foods, or a cup of low-fat milk or yogurt for a snack.
   v. Muscle mass can increase with activity. Try to **be more active throughout the day**, preferably all days of the week. Since older people tend to lose muscle mass, regular physical activity is a valuable part of a weight-loss plan. Building or maintaining muscle helps keep older adults active and reduces their risk of falls and fractures. Staying active throughout your adult years, helps maintain muscle mass and bone strength for your later years.
   vi. Adopt **consistent sleep and rest regimen.** Remember that promoting health depends on a regulated system of diet, rest, and activity in order to enhance biological harmony of growth and healing.
   vii. **Encourage healthy weight in children.** Children need enough food for proper growth, but too many calories and too little physical activity lead to overweight. The number of overweight U.S. children has risen dramatically in recent years. Encourage healthy weight by offering children grain products; vegetables and fruits; low-fat dairy products; and beans, lean meat, poultry, fish, or nuts—and let them see you enjoy eating the same foods. Let the child decide how much of these foods to eat. Encourage children to take part in vigorous activities (and join them whenever possible). Limit the time they spend in sedentary activities like watching television or playing computer or video games. Make small changes. For example, serve low-fat milk rather than whole milk and offer one cookie instead of two. Since children still need to grow, weight loss is not recommended unless guided by a health care provider.

14.1.3.2. Muscular Machinery

Human appearance thus signifies the type of energy machinery we labor to build. Inactivity causes the cells of the body to divert all excess sources of energy from food into stored fat, which are fat cells loaded with triglycerides. These consist of glycerol and fatty acids that carry plenty of carbon dioxide molecules fixed into long chains fatty acids. Fat cells are equipped with receptors that detect blood levels of glucose and low-density lipoproteins. Cell receptors regulate the

---

[3] NUTRITION AND YOUR HEALTH: DIETARY GUIDELINES FOR AMERICANS, published by the Department of Health and Human Services (HHS) and the Department of Agriculture (USDA).

returning of the stored fat to the circulation, if the body demands persistent fuel supply. The demand for fuel comes from activity of muscles. Physical activity increases glucagon, adrenalin, growth hormone, and testosterone, which all stimulate fat cells to hydrolyze triglycerides and pump fatty acids into circulation. Regular, long, and intense activity alters body appearance by diminishing fat depots and enhancing musculoskeletal outlook.

14.1.4. MOBILITY

This is most the important insurance we have for freedom. It is prudent to plan our lives, and the lives of those for whom we are responsible, for life-long ability to move free from disease. Starting exercise at early life has greatest potential for shaping the heart, bones, and joints for the challenging demands of active life. Athletes from both sexes enjoy wide range of activities and better chances of getting the right jobs than non-athletes get. People who admire mobility find themselves more knowledgeable of the world they live in and expand their repertoire of skills and potentials to improve society. The author recalls an art teacher's comment on how artists differ from common people in their ability to notice and cherish the variation in shades and colors in every step of their lives. People must take those steps in order to enrich their appreciation of nature. Besides, the mental gain of moving around, starting exercise at any age improves strength, flexibility, coordination, sense of worthiness, and problem solving ability. Lack of mobility is a real danger for the elderly. It causes renal failure due to the decrease in the cardiac output, infection that is life threatening to the elderly with low immune defense, hip fracture due to poor coordination and weakness, and stroke due to thickening of the sluggish blood flow in the brain.

According the Dietary Guidelines for Americans, published by the department of Health and Human Services, the proper way to enhance mobility is as follows.

o Be physically active each day. A moderate physical activity is any activity that requires about as much energy as walking 2 miles in 30 minutes. Aim to accumulate at least 30 minutes (adults) or 60 minutes (children) of moderate physical activity most days of the week, preferably daily. You can gain even more health benefits by increasing the amount of time that you are physically active or by taking part in more vigorous activities.

o Make physical activity a regular part of your routine. No one is too young or too old to enjoy the benefits of regular physical activity. Choose activities that you enjoy and that you can do regularly, *Tip # 2*. Some people prefer activities that fit into their daily routine, like gardening or taking extra trips up and down stairs. Others prefer a regular exercise program, such as a physical activity program at their worksite. Some do both. The important thing is to be physically active every day.

o Most adults do not need to see their health care provider before starting to become more physically active. However, if you are planning to start a vigorous activity plan and have one or more of the conditions below, consult your health care provider:
   i.   Chronic health problem such as heart disease, hypertension, diabetes, osteoporosis, or obesity.
   ii. High risk for heart disease.
   iii. Over age 40 for men or 50 for women.

o Two types of physical activity are especially beneficial:
   i.   Aerobic activities speed your heart rate and breathing. They help cardiovascular fitness.
   ii. Activities for strength and flexibility. Developing strength may help build and maintain your bones. Carrying groceries and lifting weights are two strength-building activities. Gentle stretching, dancing, or yoga can increase flexibility.

Tip # 2*
EXAMPLES OF PHYSICAL ACTIVITIES FOR ADULTS

For at least 30 minutes most days of the week, preferably daily, do any one of the activities listed below—or combine activities. Look for additional opportunities among other activities that you enjoy.

As part of your routine activities:
- Walk, wheel, or bike ride more, drive less.
- Walk up stairs instead of taking an elevator.
- Get off the bus a few stops early and walk or wheel the remaining distance.
- Mow the lawn with a push mower.
- Rake leaves.
- Garden.
- Push a stroller.
- Clean the house.
- Do exercises or pedal a stationary bike while watching television.
- Play actively with children.
- Take a brisk 10-minute walk or wheel in the morning, at lunch, and after dinner.

As part of your exercise or recreational routine:
- Walk, wheel, or jog.
- Bicycle or use an arm pedal bicycle.
- Swim or do water aerobics.
- Play racket or wheelchair sports.
- Golf (pull cart or carry clubs).
- Canoe.
- Cross-country ski.
- Play basketball.
- Dance.
- Take part in an exercise program at work, home, school, or gym.

* NUTRITION AND YOUR HEALTH: DIETARY GUIDELINES FOR AMERICANS, published by the Department of Health and Human Services (HHS) and the Department of Agriculture (USDA).

- o Help children be physically active. Children and adolescents benefit from physical activity in many ways. They need at least 60 minutes of physical activity daily, *Tip # 3*. Parents can help:
    - i. Set a good example. For example, arrange active family events in which everyone takes part. Join your children in physical activities.
    - ii. Encourage your children to be physically active at home, at school, and with friends by jumping rope, playing tag, riding a bike.
    - iii. Limit television watching, computer games, and other inactive forms of play by alternating with periods of physical activity.
- o Older people need to be physically active too. Engage in moderate physical activity for at least 30 minutes most days of the week, preferably daily and taking part in activities to strengthen muscles and to improve flexibility. Staying strong and flexible can reduce your risk of falling and breaking bones, preserve muscle, and improve your ability to live independently. Lifting small weights and carrying groceries are two ways to include strength building into your routine.

14.1.5. GASTROINTESTINAL HEALTH

- o **Food demands:** Mammals are created big in body and brain in order to perform many complex mental functions. Such big body size causes mammals to have voluminous storing capacity of toxic waste in the guts. Birds dispose of their excreta on the fly since they carry less weight and possess lesser cerebral faculties. The large size of mammals does not come without a price. Colon diseases are most probably the cost that we have to pay for such luxury of continent digestive system. Exercise stimulates the digestive juices to flow, the intestinal contents to mix and transit the intestine hastily, and the intestinal epithelium to regenerate normally.
- o **Elimination demands:** Without exercise, digestive juices stagnate and become viscid, bacterial growth increases in virulence and quantity, and the intestinal linings fight harder to

> **Tip # 3***
> **PHYSICAL ACTIVITIES FOR CHILDREN AND TEENS**
>
> *Aim for at least 60 minutes total per day:*
> - Be spontaneously active.
> - Play tag.
> - Jump rope.
> - Ride a bicycle or tricycle.
> - Walk, wheel, skip, or run.
> - Play actively during school recess.
> - Roller skate or in-line skate.
> - Take part in physical education activity classes during school.
> - Join after-school or community physical activity programs.
> - Dance.
>
> * NUTRITION AND YOUR HEALTH: DIETARY GUIDELINES FOR AMERICANS, published by the Department of Health and Human Services (HHS) and the Department of Agriculture (USDA).

contain such lethally toxic milieu from harming the host. Many people with chronic digestive troubles have insidiously succumbed to such maladies by losing insight into the difficulties they face. You might have wondered how some people got to the point of developing such humongous size of intestine without being alerted earlier. Unfortunately, the problem of developing such excessively huge belly, though sounds simple, is not easily amenable to reversal. Once our intestine enlarges for few months, a setup of internal reflexes works hard to keep perception in concert with the new state of body condition. People find it very difficult to alter their habits without taking new and aggressive measures to restore new healthy outlook.

14.2. FLAGS OF ALARM

14.2.1. HEADACHE

- o **Silent malady:** Many people go through years of their life performing daily activities without complaint of ill health despite the presence of alarming signs that should have urged them to exercise sooner. Many interpret headache, after a strenuous workday, as a natural consequence to fatigue. Yet, headache is a sign of a malady within the brain that is most probably arisen as a result of poor cellular respiration, after strenuous work. Since both physical and mental work requires energy, brain cells work harder during physical activity. In addition, the brain depends on the systemic circulation to supply glucose and oxygen that are affected by the body condition after long day of work.
- o **Privileged organ:** Headache, thus, arises because, either the brain cells do not have sufficient supply of nutrients to produce energy, or the energy production is inadequate to fuel brain activity, or the intermediate substrates of energy production are falling short. Such fuel shortage is caused by excessive utilization of fuel by processes other than energy production. There are few reasons that explain the common occurrence of headache symptoms. First, the brain is located at the highest elevation of the body, which renders the brain circulation susceptible to postural changes and sympathetic regulation of blood flow more than any other organ in the body. Second, the brain possesses blood-membrane barrier that facilitates selective diffusion of blood constituents, in and out of the brain, but that also requires energy to perform such selective transport. Third, the brain performs extensive and active regulation control of the entire body functions and thus requires more oxygen and glucose[4] than any other organ in the body.

---

[4] The average human brain weighs 1400 g, has blood flow rate of 770 ml/min, and consumes 46 ml Oxygen/min. This is about 20% of whole body oxygen requirement and amounts to 20 watts (12.20 Cal/hour) of energy utilization. The brain uses 110 g glucose/day. Source: Textbook of Physiology and Biochemistry, by Bell, Davidson, and Scarborough, Edinburgh, UK. 1970. Pages 361 and 980.

- **Cellular respiration**: Exercise alleviates headache by conditioning all body cells to develop active respiratory machinery that can efficiently cycle the ingredients of food intake into the cellular furnace of TCA cycle. The fundamental role of exercise on the body physiology is the extraction of energy from food ingredients and transporting the carbon atoms of these ingredients to combine oxygen. The formed carbon dioxide exits the cellular membrane to the external atmosphere. Without efficient cellular respiration, carbon dioxide accumulates in the body and faces different fates such as being fixed in fat depots. The enhanced cellular respiration facilitates the biological cellular functions of synthesis, breakdown, transport of elements, and response to body control.
- **Systemic fuelling**: The cells that are mostly affected by exercise are those of the muscles, heart, blood vessels, liver, and fat cells. The hearts of exercising folks could handle fatigue much better than those of inactive folks do. That is because of greater availability of substrates in the intermediate cycling of the food fuel and the enrichment with energy transport molecules. These sustain vital reaction of synthesis of cellular elements and prevent the prevalence of destruction over regeneration. The heart cells undergo extensive destruction and regeneration processes, every minute during contraction, relaxation, and conduction. Enhanced cellular respiration fosters generation of new circulation, removal of byproducts, and maintaining active heart tissue. Thus, the heart relieves the brain with efficient circulation during long and tiring work
- Exercise also expands **muscular storage** of glycogen, through enlarging muscle mass, thus reduces body dependence on the liver glycogen for glucose supply. Recall that muscles can store glycogen but cannot maintain blood glucose, while the liver can do both, *Table 14.1*. Thus, the outcome of inactivity is shrinking the muscular boost of excess reserve of immediate fuel supply and expanding the carbon dioxide load on the brain metabolism. Active muscles can do more with fatty acid oxidation than the liver alone can do. Therefore, exercise facilitates clearing the circulation of accumulated fat blockages and consequently facilitates brain circulation.

14.2.2. CONSTIPATION AND INDIGESTION

- **Healthy gut**: Constipation and indigestion, after strenuous work, are attributed to factors other than just poor eating habits. After physical work, all the cells of the body have to deal with the excess byproducts of metabolism, the diminished blood flow due to tired heart, and the depletion of the body enzymatic resources, used to generate energy for the daily work. Indigestion may result from poor circulation to the gastrointestinal tract, diminished digestive juices, incoordination of peristalsis, or accumulation of toxic fecal constituents. The worst scenario plays when the byproducts of catabolism trigger autoimmune disease that causes indigestion. In addition, lack of exercise contributes to the low tone of the abdominal muscles, the respiratory muscles, and the intestinal muscles.
- **Insults to intestine**: These are caused by the protracted putrefaction of undigested food remains within the colon. You would not go around sedentary people without noticing bulging of bellies due to lack of exercise. The relationship between food and cancer, particularly colon cancer, is centered on the changes that take place in animal protein. It is thought that certain amino acids in animal proteins could cause colon cancer. Yet, the effect of lack of exercise, in creating unhealthy sluggishness of the intestinal tone, could cause colon cancer in response to protracted putrefaction and bacterial overgrowth.
- **Managing elimination**: Exercise is more demanded for meat eaters in order to avoid the toxic effects of animal protein on the intestine, liver, and brain. These effects are due to the excessive production of ammonia from amino acid metabolism. Ammonia is transported on one of the intermediate substrates of the TCA cycle, oxaloacetic acid, and is used in the formation of urea by the liver. Urea is finally excreted by the kidneys. In addition, production of ammonia increases during the catabolism of nucleic acids in growth and reproduction, which signifies the role of exercise during these vital biological processes. In the brain, the active cycling of the TCA cycle enhances the production of the amino acid; glutamic acid, which helps the brain clear ammonia at greater rates with exercise. Thus, exercise enhances the body's ability to clear the highly toxic ammonia and thus sustain vital biological reactions.

14.2.3. MUSCLE PAIN AND STIFFNESS

- **Insults to muscle**: These are not necessarily attributed to old age or to excessive physical work. The fact that muscle cells perform great regeneration of tissue, oxidation of fatty acids, and production of kinetic energy, makes muscles the most active organ in the body. High activity does not come cheap! Muscles require more than basic food materials to maintain function. They require active enzyme complexes and blood supply to perform their robust respiratory function. Deficiency of thiamin, niacin, flavoprotein, or calcium may amount to severe muscular dysfunction. Such disease process as **polymyositis, polymyalgia rheumatica, and fibromyalgia**, mostly affect elderly and women, and all have no definite cause to treat. Autoimmune reaction is used to explain the inflammation around the blood capillaries of the muscles that causes pain, tenderness, of atrophy.

o **Managing byproducts of metabolism:** Exercise might have prevented the very instigator of autoimmune disease, the byproducts of catabolism that accumulate within the extracellular space, and unduly stay there for longer periods due to lack of circulation, Figure 14.1. Exercising muscles have higher capacity to eliminate insults and recover without triggering global inflammation of the blood capillaries. Thus, when getting up in the morning becomes troubling, lifting a limb causes pain or difficulty, or rising from a chair becomes more trying, the long term solution is most probably exercising, not painkillers or stimulants. However, short-term treatment of acute pain might entail chemical therapy in order to relieve acute inflammation before exercise can be tolerated.

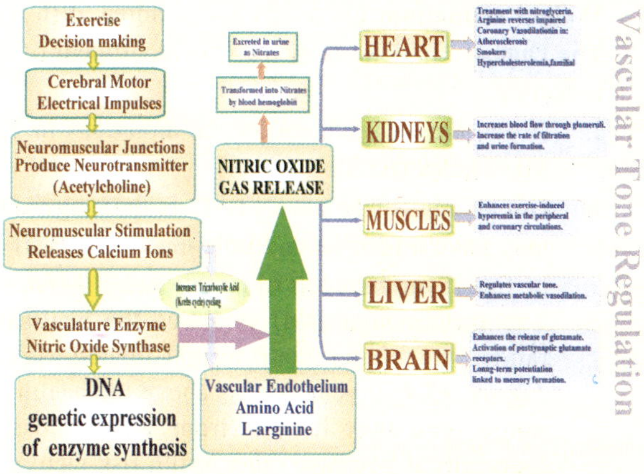

14.3. THE PEARLS OF FITNESS

14.3.1. WALKING EXERCISE

Figure 14.1. The L-Arginine-Nitric Oxide Pathway relates physical activity to new angiogenesis.[5]

o **Total harmony:** We take our ability to stand and walk for granted. Walking is the most graceful activity that all humans can do. A lot is involved in walking. The very coordinated neuromuscular system works hard to support the movement of the body. It seems that human genes have evolved over many millions of years before we were able to master the rules of mechanics. Walking is the simplest way of staying fit and healthy. It stimulates the muscles to expend energy, invigorates blood flow and cellular nutrition, not only in the working muscles, but also in every live cell in the body. The non-working muscles and organs also benefit from walking through the binding effect of the circulation. The vitalized muscles create an abundant blood pool around the joints, which encircles the joints in the front, back, above, and below the moving surface of joints. Even with chronic arthritis, the vitalized muscles of athletes make living with arthritis a whole lot easier than non-athletes do.

o **Muscular balance:** Walking has a particular advantage over many other exercises, in that it maintains the optimum balance of muscular strength without the grotesque appearance of preferentially enhanced weight-trained muscles. It also maintain balanced function of the body in real life, without the risks of flawed weight training that, most of the time, causes life long stiffness, muscular imbalance, and limited mobility. What walking can offer you, that weight training cannot, is the conditioning of the slow twitching muscles and the endurance devices of the cells that operate slowly, but for longer duration. Conditioning these elements of endurance promotes general health of the heart, liver, brain, kidneys, nervous system, and intestine. These vital organs need more than vigorous work to maintain basic life functions.

o Brisk walking combines **the vigor and endurance** in exercise. Thirty minutes of daily brisk walking induces the cellular respiration to mobilize fats from adipose tissues and then pump it into the cellular furnace, thus reducing bodyweight. The activity of walking induces the mind faculties and activates the brain cells to produce more energy and substrates to attend its basic needs. In addition, regular brisk walking expands the cellular metabolism of the precursors of cholesterol; the acetyl units, and thus can substantially lower blood pressure and raise levels of HDL[6]. HDL keeps LDL from building up in the coronary arteries that causes heart disease.

> **Tip # 4 ***
> **HOW TO EVALUATE YOUR WEIGHT (ADULTS)**
> Weigh yourself and have your height measured. Find your BMI category in *Figure 15.4*, Chapter 15. The higher your BMI category is, the greater is the risk for health problems.
> Measure around your waist, just above your hip bones, while standing. Health risks increase as waist measurement increases, particularly if waist is greater than 35 inches for women or 40 inches for men. Excess abdominal fat may place you at greater risk of health problems, even if your BMI is about right.
> Use *Tip # 5* to find out how many other risk factors you have. The higher your BMI and waist measurement, and the more risk factors you have from *Tip # 5*, the more you are likely to benefit from weight loss.
> NOTE: Weight loss is usually not advisable for pregnant women.
> * NUTRITION AND YOUR HEALTH: DIETARY GUIDELINES FOR AMERICANS, published by the Department of Health and Human Services (HHS) and the Department of Agriculture (USDA).

---

[5] Also, see these two articles: Salvador Moncada, and Annie Higgs, "The L-Arginine-Nitric Oxide Pathway", The New England Journal of Medicine,1993 Dec; 329(27): 2002-2012. And Shen W, Zhang X, Zhao G, Wolin MS, Sessa W, Hintze TH, "Nitric oxide production and NO synthase gene expression contribute to vascular regulation during exercise", Med Sci Sports Exerc 1995 Aug; 27(8): 1125-34.

[6] Lipoproteins are transport vehicles, synthesized by the liver in the form of very low-density lipoproteins (VLDL). They contain triglycerides and cholesterol ester core, covered with lipoprotein and phospholipid coat. Muscle and fat cells remove the triglycerides core for fat storage and burnout, respectively. The remaining of the VLDL's are the low density lipoproteins (LDL), which are rich in cholesterol and poor in triglycerides. The liver cells regulate the LDL level according to cholesterol balance. Efficient clearance of LDL, by the liver, leaves lipoproteins with lowest cholesterol and triglycerides content, termed high-density lipoprotein (HDL). Thus, high level of HDL signifies low blood cholesterol and triglycerides.

HEALTH AND FITNESS

14.3.2. OPTIMUM BODYWEIGHT

o **Weight reduction:** For adults and children, different methods are used to find out if weight is about right for height. The Dietary Guidelines, of the US Department of Health and Human Services, offer the following advices for weight reduction.

   i. If you are an adult, follow the directions in *Tip # 4* to evaluate your weight in relation to your height, or Body Mass Index (BMI).

   ii. Not all adults who have a BMI, in the range labeled "healthy", are at their most healthy weight. For example, some may have lots of fat and little muscle. A BMI above the healthy range is less healthy for most people; but it may be fine if you have lots of muscle and little fat.

   iii. The further your BMI is above the healthy range, the higher your weight-related risk, *Figure 15.4.* If your BMI is above the healthy range, you may benefit from weight loss, especially if you have other health risk factors, *Tip # 5.*

   iv. BMI's slightly below the healthy range may still be healthy unless they result from illness. If your BMI is below the healthy range, you may have increased risk of menstrual irregularity, infertility, and osteoporosis.

   v. If you lose weight suddenly or for unknown reasons, see a health care provider. Unexplained weight loss may be an early clue to a hea-lth problem. Keep track of your weight and your waist measurement, and take action if either of them increases.

   vi. If your BMI is greater than 25, or even if it is in the "healthy" range, at least try to avoid further weight gain. If your waist measurement increases, you are probably gaining fat. If so, take steps to eat fewer calories and become more active.

> **Tip # 5 ***
> **FIND OUT YOUR OTHER RISK FACTORS FOR CHRONIC DISEASE**
>
> The more of these risk factors you have, the more you are likely to benefit from weight loss if you are overweight or obese.
>
> - Do you have a personal or family history of heart disease?
> - Are you a male older than 45 years or a postmenopausal female?
> - Do you smoke cigarettes?
> - Do you have a sedentary lifestyle?
> - Has your doctor told you that you have
>   i. High blood pressure?
>   ii. Abnormal blood lipids (high LDL cholesterol, low HDL cholesterol, high triglycerides)?
>   iii. Diabetes?
>
> * NUTRITION AND YOUR HEALTH: DIETARY GUIDELINES FOR AMERICANS, published by the Department of Health and Human Services (HHS) and the Department of Agriculture (USDA).

   vii. **If you need to lose weight, do so gradually**. If you are overweight, loss of 5 to 15 percent of your body weight may improve your health, ability to function, and quality of life. Aim to lose about 10 percent of your weight over about 6 months. This would be 20 pounds of weight loss for someone who weighs 200 pounds. Loss of 1/2 to 2 pounds per week is usually safe. Even if you have regained weight in the past, it's worthwhile to try again.

14.3.3. AEROBICS

o **Relics of the past:** The author's first exposure to aerobics was in 1957, in an Egyptian city. There was a sort of an annual family arrangement in the neighborhood. That arrangement was made to treat a family member from possession by evil spirits, which we now call "depression". In that setting, a large crowd gathers in a circle around the possessed person and beat their drums, the whole night long. The possessed girl jumps and bends forwards and backwards until totally exhausted. That was the cure for depression prior to the invention of antidepressant medications. Now, aerobics has spread allover the globe as an awesome way to stay fit and healthy.

o **Modern aerobics:** Doing aerobic exercises, you could watch your weight drops in hours, not days or weeks. In addition, you are on a safe track to fitness, rather than being on weight-shedding medication that might cost you your life. The argument that "such fast weight loss is quickly reversed by drinking fluids" is misleading. Because if you continue aerobic exercises three to five times a week, you will see the fat melting away, faster than any other exercise program can do. Most weight reduction medications either directly increase the heart rate, via adrenergic stimulation (ephedrine), or stimulate the thyroid to speed metabolism. Both are risky. Weight reduction by blocking fat absorption would not work with carbohydrate calories. Supplements that claim enhancing the enzymatic complexes of the cells to pump pyruvate into the cellular furnace, the TCA cycle, must be kidding people to believe in illusive myth.

o **Burning efficiency:** Why aerobic exercises reserve such undisputable reputation of being the best in fitness? The answer is that they engage all systems in utilizing energy. In aerobic exercise, each cell in the body has to rise to the challenge of playing its assigned role in the survival of the organism. Aerobic energy production is an active process that has to take place only in the mitochondriated cells, via specialized system of membranes, enzymes, and catalysts. These concert extracting energy from the calories of food intake. Aerobic production of energy operates at about 40% efficiency of oxidation of glucose, compared to only 2% efficiency of anaerobic energy production (weight and resistance training). In addition, aerobic folks are not only rich in energy transport substances, but also in the availability of the precursors for synthesis of vital biological substances.

- o **Mental drive:** On the top of the body are the **brain cells.** This makes it possible to engage in playful activity that does not directly seem to serve purposeful gain. It might be the innate instincts, which drive the brain cells to endure the pain of aerobics. Definitely, the brain that engages in aerobic could not be either depressed or psychotic. It might be possible to prevent depression by creating proper environment to play and tide the mind over gloomy moments of life.
- o **Neural control:** The nerve cells are the first to suffer from any disturbance in health. Many people suffer from paralysis after common viral infections, from neurological disturbances due to malnutrition, diabetes, or chronic alcoholism. That is because the nerve cells require exquisitely complex nutritional needs in order to be able to perform their function. That consists of transferring ions and charges, for long distances, from the brain to all organs, without mixing different massages during the transmission process. Like hair follicles, skin cell, and gut lining cells, nerve cells are first to be struck when health deteriorates. That is because these organs are active in production and growth thus generate greater amounts of ammonia and require greater amounts of caloric substrates.
- o **Muscular stimulation:** You might believe that electrical stimulators, advertised on TV ads, might do the job of strengthening, without sweat. That is a fallacy. Exercise requires neuromuscular feedback, not just at the nerve level, but also at the brain level. Electrical stimulators stimulate the nerve or the muscle directly, without proper feedback control on the cerebral signal pattern. This is required to recruit definite muscle pools that are needed to perform purposeful motion. Direct muscular stimulation does not sense the depletion of the resources of muscles during extreme exhaustion. On the other hand, aerobic exercise helps regenerate new neural dendrites and synapses to make you better, day after day, as long as you persevere in exercising.
- o **Systemic harmony:** The reason that exercise is beneficial, to every system in the body, stems from the process of evolution of living cells. Before cells aggregate to form multi-cellular organisms that possess systems, which in turn consist of organs, cells are driven by an essential need to utilize energy. Even in the harshest conditions and in the absence of oxygen, cells adapt in astonishing manner to existing environment, for the sake of utilizing energy. Thus, no wonder why each cell in our body, not just the working organs and systems, benefits from exercise. Exercise is the language of living cells in mastering the economy of energy.
- o **Fueling energy:** Where does the fat go after exercise? That is analogous to asking, "where does gasoline go after driving your automobile, for a distance long enough to consume all the fuel in the gas tank?" The principle of "conservation of energy" governs all kinds of energy transactions. The conversion of the chemical energy of the gasoline into kinetic energy and heat is governed by the same principles that govern the burning of body fat by exercise. Performing office jobs, reading, or watching TV for hours, necessitate serious consideration of engaging in exercise in order to sustain body management of food intake and organ health.
- o **Buildup versus burnout**: Exercise does not only burn the fat under the skin, but also the internal fat, anywhere in the body, and in some order of priorities. Exercise diverts the precursors of fat, the **acetyl CoA**, from the process of fat synthesis into the energy production process. Fat synthesis entails either condensation of acetyl CoA with carbon dioxide, to form fatty acids, or condensation of acetyl CoA molecules, to form **cholesterol.** On the other hand, energy production entails cleaving carbon dioxide from acetyl CoA and producing energy.
- o **Cholesterol buildup**: Cholesterol hardens the blood vessels, renders them immobile, causing high blood pressure and vascular blockage. Some people misinterpret the **high blood pressure** as plenty of blood flowing to the organs. The truth is that because the blood could not flow fast enough, at adequate rate to the cells, therefore it suffers from high resistance to its molecules. Thus, the high vascular resistance that causes high blood pressure deprives the cells from adequate nutrition. On the long run, high blood pressure causes cellular death, which in turn causes organ death. This occurs in the form of infarctions, strokes, paralysis, gangrene, or weakness. Cardiac infarction is the fatal disease of modern times that could be easily prevented by regular exercise and balanced diet. Sexual dysfunction due to inadequate blood flow to the pelvic organs is another preventable condition. Narcolepsy is the sudden collapse into sleep state due to inadequate blood flow through the entire body. In short, exercise maintains open blood vessels, strong heart pump, and healthy cells that could take advantage of enhanced blood flow, in fulfilling their need.
- o **Adequate exercise**: The proper amount of exercise that is required by people in urban societies is surprisingly greater than many people can endure.[7] The premise made by some, that 30 minutes of daily exercise is adequate, has no scientific grounds. In order to alter body chemistry, longer and regular exercise is needed. Olympic athletes can perform way out of proportion of the average population. This proves that there is plenty of room for improvement, when exercise is taken seriously. Substantial change in body appearance and ability to perform daily duties can only occur with at least 60 minutes of vigorous daily exercise. With advanced training, people get better grasp on how to make use of such 60 minutes.

---

[7] "Every hour spent in vigorous exercise as an adult is repaid with two hours of additional life span" and "If you worked out twelve hours every day, statistically you'd never die." By Dr. Ralph Paffenbarger, Stanford University, from an article titled "Fighting Back, with Sweat", by Jerry Adler and Joan Raymond, Newsweek Special Issue, page 36, Fall and Winter, year 2001.

14.3.4. CARING FOR ACHING JOINTS

- **Improving circulation:** One of the greatest fallacies of modern times is that, many people, young and old, believe that once they suffer from joint pain they are doomed forever to inactive life. It takes more than just good reasoning to convince lay folks that exercise is beneficial for joints, both in health and in disease. Joint health relies greatly on the adequate blood flow, supplied through fleshy muscular coating around the joints. As soon as pain subsides, joint exercises dramatically advance joint health.
- **Avoiding faulty exercise:** Of course, faulty exercise does more harm than good. Exercise that could benefit joints should adhere to the anatomical and physiological needs of joints. Examples of harmful exercises are:
  i. Using excessive weight, for longer duration, and for partial range of motion. For example, heavy Deadlift that far exceeds the ability to lift in the Clean lift can cause more harm than good.
  ii. Improper balancing of opposing groups of muscles by exercise. For example, heavy Bench Press that far exceeds the ability to lift from the floor can also cause more harm than good. .
  iii. Improper balancing of different groups of muscles that assist in specific motions, such as having well trained Biceps without proportionately trained shoulder.
  iv. Performing exercises that violate the normal anatomical function of joints, such as leaning forwards or hunching the upper back while squatting.
- Faulty exercise can damage the cartilage within the joint, shorten or tear the ligaments or tendons. Injured cartilages do not heal on their own. Torn ligaments require many months to recover and endure strain. Therefore, the long recovery needed to undo the harm, of faulty exercise, causes deterioration in other systems. Long recovery wastes bone calcium and causes bone thinning and kidney problems. The heart does not fare well during long recovery from injury. In addition, the entire neuromuscular system is impacted by long recovery from injury.
- **Planning for exercise:** Exercise should not be blamed for pain in the knees and joint after training. Modifying rest breaks, intermission intervals, intensity of exercise, and range of motion, should take the blame off exercise and put it onto the planning of exercise. Even little exercise would induce substantial benefits. The greatest benefits of exercise or physical activity are vividly demonstrated in menial workers and in athletes who train daily and diversify between endurance and strength training. Of course, gradual progressive training is a necessity, in order to allow body systems to build up necessary infrastructures for high-energy production. Lack of exercise causes weak muscles, which leads to unstable joints. Unstable joints wiggle excessively causing internal injury to the joint. Internal joint injuries heal by scars. Scarred ligaments, cartilages, and bones, result in chondro-osteo-arthritis, which is a condition of inflammation of the cartilage and bone of the joint. Without daily exercise, these degenerative conditions progress relentlessly after the age of forty.

14.3.5. DAILY ACTIVITIES

When not exercising, all activities in the off-training interval determine your fitness condition, when you return to training. In order to maintain robust and invigorated strength, maintain constant state of activity whenever you feel you can do so (see *Tips # 2 and 3*), as follows.

- **Walking** to and from your car or work can account for extra expenditure of calories and eases your mind in the future when repeating these non-obligatory rituals. In addition, you would not have to worry about bitty conflicts with others about parking spaces that are fewer feet closer to your door or messy traffic in busy streets.
- **Take the stairs** instead of the elevator. Though little strength is gained that way, yet activity adds up on the long term and gradually maintains your health in better condition.
- Make up occasions for walking out of your room, office, home, or any place you are destined to be, even if you do not have specific tasks to attend. Since most of our workday entails these long and personal time, it is wise to make use of few **walks every hour or so** in order to avoid insidious development of sneaky problems such as lower back weakness, upper back hunching, belly distention, or loss of stamina.
- Remember that we can perform any long and demanding job if we are given sufficient time for that purpose. We thus can do the car repair, laundry, and household duties if we space these tasks into tiny pieces over few days, instead of simultaneously. **Thinking strategically** in this manner is the highest function of the human brain. That is superior to other mammals that put all attention to single moments of life without planning for protracted periods of time.
- Listen to music and change your exercise routine constantly in order to **avoid monotony** and falling into stages of mental stagnation and isolation from the world. Short and frequent talks with new others are also stimulating and can bring you precious feedback and encouragement.

o Tap into **diverse resources of information,** from magazines, videotapes, books, or real events that might change your perception of the world and further promote your enthusiasm for exercise.

14.3.6. HEALTHY DIET

Food intake is an integral aspect of health and fitness. The following dietary guidelines are recommended for enhancing health and fitness, *Figure 14.2* and *Tip # 6*.

o Carbohydrates from various sources of whole grains should constitute the basic healthy daily consumption of food.
o Fruits and vegetables should constitute another major portion of daily consumption of food. Variation of consumed food ensures availability of various nutrients. Fatty fish contains omega-3 fatty acids and should be consumed at least once every week.
o Reduce saturated fat intake from food such as full-fat milk products, fatty meats, tropical oils, partially hydrogenated vegetable oils and egg yolks. These can be replaced by skim milk, skinless, poultry and lean meats. Unsaturated fats supply the required fat intake and are found in vegetable oils, *Table 14.5*.
o Count your caloric intake. This is the total caloric content of all daily-consumed food and drinks. The body needs between 13 and 15 Calories per each pound (25 Cal/kg) of bodyweight in adults. Children require more calories, depending on their age.
o Reduce daily salt intake to less than one teaspoon of salt. Carbonated soft drinks contain sodium, which should also be watched in order to reduce daily sodium intake.

14.4. SOURCE OF INFORMATION

The promise of bettering health by activities or products invites many people to the field of health and fitness. This new field is proliferating rapidly, particularly in big cities around the world. You should apply few rules in order to distinguish between myth and truth, in what different parties can offer to promote health. The following are recommended tips.

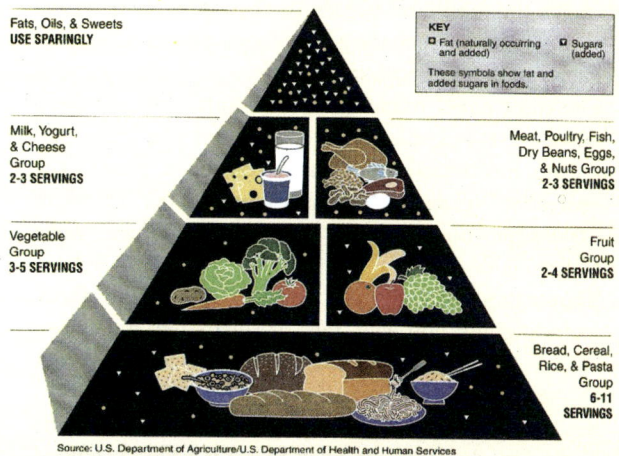

Figure 14.2. Recommended daily food servings from the "DIETARY GUIDELINES FOR AMERICANS", published by the Department of Health and Human Services (HHS) and the Department of Agriculture (USDA).

Tip # 6 *
WHAT COUNTS AS A SERVING?

Bread, Cereal, Rice, and Pasta Group (Grains Group)—whole grain and refined
- 1 slice of bread
- About 1 cup of ready-to-eat cereal
- 1/2 cup of cooked cereal, rice, or pasta

Vegetable Group
- 1 cup of raw leafy vegetables
- 1/2 cup of other vegetables cooked or raw
- 3/4 cup of vegetable juice

Fruit Group
- 1 medium apple, banana, orange, pear
- 1/2 cup of chopped, cooked, or canned fruit
- 3/4 cup of fruit juice

Milk, Yogurt, and Cheese Group (Milk Group) +
- 1 cup of milk** or yogurt**
- 1 1/2 ounces of natural cheese** (such as Cheddar)
- 2 ounces of processed cheese** (such as American)

Meat, Poultry, Fish, Dry Beans, Eggs, and Nuts Group (Meat and Beans Group)
- 2-3 ounces of cooked lean meat, poultry, or fish
- 1/2 cup of cooked dry beans# or 1/2 cup of tofu counts as 1 ounce of lean meat
- 2 1/2-ounce soy burger or 1 egg counts as 1 ounce of lean meat
- 2 tablespoons of peanut butter or 1/3 cup of nuts counts as 1 ounce of meat

NOTE: Many of the serving sizes given above are smaller than those on the Nutrition Facts Label. For example, 1 serving of cooked cereal, rice, or pasta is 1 cup for the label but only 1/2 cup for the Pyramid, *Figure 14.2.*
+ This includes lactose-free and lactose-reduced milk products. One cup of soy-based beverage with added calcium is an option for those who prefer a non-dairy source of calcium.
** Choose fat-free or reduced-fat dairy products most often.
\# Dry beans, peas, and lentils can be counted as servings in either the meat and beans group or the vegetable group. As a vegetable, 1/2 cup of cooked, dry beans counts as 1 serving. As a meat substitute, 1 cup of cooked, dry beans counts as 1 serving (2 ounces of meat).

* NUTRITION AND YOUR HEALTH: DIETARY GUIDELINES FOR AMERICANS, published by the Department of Health and Human Services (HHS) and the Department of Agriculture (USDA).

HEALTH AND FITNESS

- Food contents are displayed in food labels on most sold food products. These provide significant information about the nutritional value of food, as follows, *Figure 14.3*.
  i. Check the food label before you buy. Food labels have several parts, including the front panel, Nutrition Facts, and ingredient list.
  ii. The front panel often tells you if nutrients have been added—for example, "iodized salt" lets you know that iodine has been added, and "enriched pasta" (or "enriched" grain of any type) means that thiamin, riboflavin, niacin, iron, and folic acid have been added.
  iii. The ingredient list tells you what's in the food, including any nutrients, fats, or sugars that have been added. The ingredients are listed in descending order by weight.
  iv. See *Figure 14.3* to learn how to read the Nutrition Facts. Use the Nutrition Facts to see if a food is a good source of a nutrient or to compare similar foods—for example, to find which brand of frozen dinner is lower in saturated fat, or which kind of breakfast cereal contains more folic acid.
  v. Look at the Percentage Daily Value (%DV) column to see whether a food is high or low in nutrients. If you want to limit a nutrient (such as fat, saturated fat, cholesterol, sodium), try to choose foods with a lower %DV. If you want to consume more of a nutrient (such as calcium, other vitamins and minerals, fiber), try to choose foods with a higher %DV. As a guide, foods with 5%DV or less contribute a small amount of That nutrient to your eating pattern, while those with 20% or more contribute a large amount.
  vi. Remember, Nutrition Facts serving sizes may differ from those used in the Food Guide Pyramid, *Tip # 6*. For example, 2 ounces of dry macaroni yields about 1 cup cooked, or two (1/2 cup) Pyramid servings.

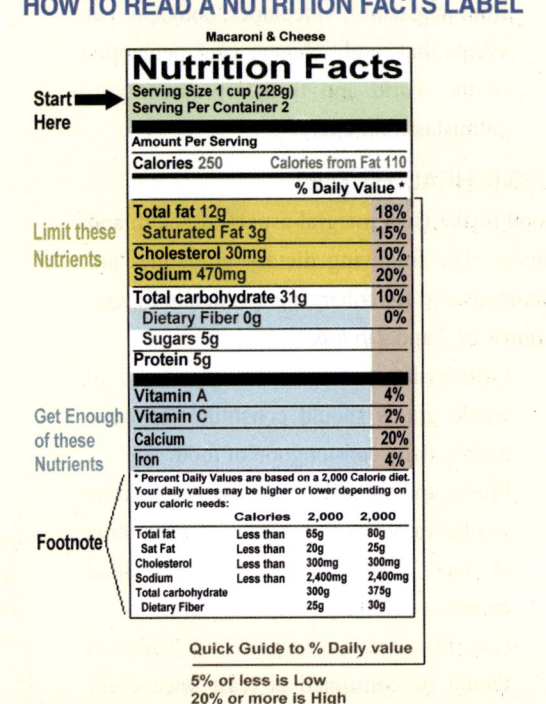

Figure 14.3. Reading Food labels. Most food products, that are produced in large volume, carry commercial brand names, have food labels. Food products that are prepared on site such as cakes, sandwiches, French fries, etc, do not have food labels. Yet, some food outlets might display their food contents on posters and brochures.

- The source of information conveys the level of scrutiny of its authenticity. For example, growth hormone administration, chelation therapy, antioxidant vitamins, and magnetic mattresses are heavily promoted commercially for enhancing health, while, in reality, they hold no value in the purpose they were promoted to serve. The commercial nature of the source should arouse your suspicion on the validity of their claim.
- **Statistical flaws** are common among commercial promotion of products, not necessarily for the purpose of deception, but might be due to enthusiasm towards certain approach or other. These flaws include overlooking significant factors, limited group size of population under study, lack of control groups, bias of observers or subjects, geographical fallacy, flawed randomization of trial subjects, or flawed arithmetic analysis. Statistical information is meant to glorify the mathematical power to people fascinated with the ingenuity of science and mathematics without understanding them.
- **Flawed application** such as trying to strengthen muscles by electrical stimulators. While this approach is useful in cases of rehabilitation or paralysis, it has no value in fitness training since it bypasses the central nervous system and applies peripheral stimulation. Also testing drugs on animals does not guarantee their equivalent effect on humans, due to the difference in size, biochemistry, and ability to express symptoms.
- **Track history** of success of the proposed method of promoting health. Anabolic steroids for example foster strength in few months' period but cause serious long-term effects that render them dangerous to health. In addition, creatine phosphate might help developing stronger muscles but its long effect on health is unknown.
- **Plausibility and validity** are important when judging new means of promoting health. You might question the plausibility of aerobic exercises since they entail excessive jolting and twisting that apparently seem to traumatize body structures. Yet, experience has shown the validity of such means of fitness when performed reasonably and regularly.

14.5. FOOD AND HEALTH

Food sustains life through two basic chemical groups of substances. The first group of substances is the **macronutrients** that provide fuel needed for energy and molecules needed for synthesis of cellular elements. The second group is the **micronutrients** needed for operating chemical reactions.

Table 14.2. List of percentage of weight of constituents of samples of major food ingredients.

Food description	C % of weight		O % of weight		H % of weight	
Glucose	40		53.28	↑	6.713	↓
Glycerol	39.12		52.11	↑	8.755	↓
Saturated fatty acids						
Butyric acid	54.52	↑	36.31	↓	9.151	↑
Caproic acid	62.04	↑	27.54	↓	10.41	↑
Palmitic acid	74.99	↑	12.47	↓	12.57	↑
Stearic acid	75.99	↑	11.24	↓	12.75	↑
Lignoceric acid	78.19	↑	8.680	↓	13.12	↑
Unsaturated Fatty acids						
Oleic acid	76.53		11.32		12.13	
Linolenic acid	76.81		11.36		11.81	
Amino acids					N % of weight	
Glycine	32	↓	42.62		6.713	18.65 ↑
Alanine	31.16	↓	41.51		9.152	17.17 ↑
Glutamic acid	54.93	↓	24.39		9.988	10.67 ↑

14.5.1. MACRONUTRIENTS

Food substances that constitute the **bulk of consumption** by mammals are carbohydrates, protein, and fat. These substances provide the body with building elements and energy supply, as follows.

o **Carbohydrates** are richest in oxygen content and poorest in hydrogen content, *Table 14.2*. Carbohydrates carry higher oxygen percentage per weight and are necessary for immediate energy production. **Fruits**, green plants, and whole grains provide adequate carbohydrate requirements. Refined flour and sugar should be reduced to a minimum. The most common among these refined carbohydrates are listed in *Table 14.3*. These have highest carbohydrate contents, over 88 g/ 100 g. These are mainly candies, sugar, desserts, and cereals.

o **Fat** contains fatty acids and glycerol; the former is richest in carbon and hydrogen content and poorest in oxygen content, *Table 14.2*. Fats provide greater amounts of carbon and protons (hydrogen) and thus are reserved for construction tasks. Unless carbohydrates are depleted, then fats will be oxidized to provide energy. Saturated fats are mostly obtained from animal source, *Table 14.4*. These include butter, beef, pork, and poultry. Saturated fats are known to cause many diseases in human. Unsaturated fat enhances cardiovascular health and are mostly obtained from plant source, *Table 14.5*. **Vegetables** contain simple carbohydrates, fibers, and plenty of vitamins and minerals, except vitamin B_{12} and cholesterol. The fiber roughage of vegetables, the low nitrogen contents, and the lack of saturated fatty acids maintains healthy digestive system and reduces the toxic load of ammonia and cholesterol on the body. **Nuts and whole grains** can provide most protein needs for human, in addition to unsaturated fatty acids, minerals, vitamins, and roughage that maintain short transit time in the guts and prevents overgrowth of bacteria. **Cholesterol** exists mainly in food from animal source. *Table 14.6* lists foodstuff that contain the highest contents of cholesterol. Animal brains (veal, pork, and lamb) and eggs are top contenders for cholesterol content. Omega-3 fatty acids, in **fish liver** oil, make arteries more flexible and in part by reducing inflammation, which plays a role in heart disease.

o **Amino acids** have higher oxygen content, lower hydrogen content, in addition to having nitrogen, *Table 14.2*. Proteins contain nitrogen, that enters in the nucleic acid and protein synthesis and thus are used for growth and reproduction functions. *Table 14.7* lists foodstuff with highest protein content. Although, animal products are richer in protein, yet, soy, sesame, and almond also compete in the top highest protein containing food. Healthy dietary guidelines require restricted red meat and saturated fats and substituting with grass fed beef, instead of traditional grain fed. This meat is leaner and contains higher levels of essential omega-3 fatty acids. **Fish** supplies most of the essential amino acids that are deficient in vegetarian food in addition to omega-3 essential fatty acids, which improve cardiovascular health.

14.5.2. MICRONUTRIENTS

o In addition to providing building elements, food also provides **catalysts** to the enzymatic reaction that direct the biochemical reactions within living cellular organisms. These catalysts are minerals and vitamins that occur in food from animal and plant sources. *Tables 14.8 thru 14.24* list foodstuff with highest content of traditional vitamins. **Fish liver oils are** rich source of the omega-3 long chain polyunsaturates, as well as vitamins A and D. Most of the long chain omega-3 polyunsaturates are formed in the microscopic algae, plankton and planktonic crustacea at the bottom of the marine food chain. These are then passed up the food chain into the higher fish, and, of course, ultimately to humans.

o **Vitamins** are essential to life as accessory factors to carbohydrates, protein, and fat, as follows.
   i. Though vitamins are required in minute amounts, yet life cannot be sustained without them. Deficiency of vitamins cause many diseases that range from severe psychosis, heart failure, bone deformities, blindness, to skin disorders.

ii. Athletes require extra amounts of vitamins if their diet is restricted or their load volume is excessive. Since exercise activity involves energy production, and synthesis and breakdown of substrates, it will undoubtedly require more vitamins than resting conditions in order to operate such extensive cellular activities.
iii. Some people need vitamin-mineral supplements to meet specific nutrient needs. For example, women who could become pregnant are advised to eat foods fortified with folic acid or to take a folic acid supplement in addition to consuming folate-rich foods to reduce the risk of some serious birth defects. Older adults and people with little exposure to sunlight may need a vitamin D supplement. People who seldom eat dairy products or other rich sources of calcium need a calcium supplement, and people who eat no animal foods need to take a vitamin B_{12} supplement.
iv. Sometimes vitamins or minerals are prescribed for meeting nutrient needs or for therapeutic purposes. For example, health care providers may advise pregnant women to take an iron supplement, and adults over age 50 to get their vitamin B_{12} from a supplement or from fortified foods.
v. Supplements of some nutrients, such as vitamin A and selenium, can be harmful if taken in large amounts.
vi. Because foods contain many substances that promote health, use the **Food Guide Pyramid** when choosing foods, *Figure 14.2 and Tip # 6.* Don't depend on supplements to meet your usual nutrient needs.
vii. Dietary supplements include, vitamins and minerals, amino acids, fiber, herbal products, and many other substances that are widely available. Herbal products usually provide a very small amount of vitamins and minerals. The value of herbal products for health is currently being studied. Standards for their purity, potency, and composition are being developed.

The following are the main vitamins that play significant role in human health.[8]

i. **Vitamin A (retinal)**, *Table 14.20*, occurs, in the form of fat-soluble calciferol, in food of animal origin such as milk, eggs, and liver, as well as in yellow and green vegetables such as carrots, tomatoes, and peaches. Vitamin A deficiency impairs the integrity of the skin and other epithelial tissue, causing dryness and excess keratin formation on the skin and cornea of the eye. Deficiency renders the body susceptible to microbial invasion. That is because vitamin A affects the formation of the cell membrane. Vitamin A also is crucial to the integrity of the retina and its deficiency impairs vision and causes Night Blindness. Since vitamin A is fat-soluble, it is deficient in low fat diet. In addition, excess vitamin A is toxic to the mitochondria of cells of active organs, such as liver, and it impairs oxidative phosphorylation, which is essential in pumping degraded food substrates (pyruvates, amino acids, and fatty acids) into the TCA cycle for cellular respiration and energy production.
ii. **Vitamin D** occurs mainly in fish livers, eggs, and butter as fat soluble sterols. It affects absorption of calcium and phosphate from the intestinal wall by increasing the biosynthesis of special transport proteins. In the body, vitamin D is activated by the liver and kidney into a form that controls the mobility of bone calcium in response to the hormonal regulation by the parathyroid gland. Thus, deficiency of vitamin D affects bone integrity, muscular contraction, cardiovascular function, and neuromuscular coordination through the calcium balance in the body. Vitamin D deficiency causes the diseases of Rickets and Osteoporosis. Since calcium is essential in most chemical reactions that deal with energy production, therefore, vitamin D deficiency may present in the form of generalized fatigue and lack of energy. Older adults need extra vitamin D in order to avert osteoporosis.
iii. **Iron.** Young children, teenage girls, and women of childbearing age need enough good sources of iron, such as lean meats and cereals with added nutrients, to keep up their iron stores, *Table 14.21* and *Tip # 7.*

> **Tip # 7 ***
> **SOME SOURCES OF IRON+**
>
> - Shellfish like shrimp, clams, mussels, and oysters
> - Lean meats (especially beef), liver** and other organ meats**
> - Ready-to-eat cereals with added iron
> - Turkey dark meat (remove skin to reduce fat)
> - Sardines†
> - Spinach
> - Cooked dry beans (such as kidney beans and pinto beans), peas (such as black-eyed peas), and lentils
> - Enriched and whole grain breads
>
> \+ Read food labels for brand-specific information.
> ** Very high in cholesterol.
> † High in salt.
>
> * NUTRITION AND YOUR HEALTH: DIETARY GUIDELINES FOR AMERICANS, published by the Department of Health and Human Services (HHS) and the Department of Agriculture (USDA).

iv. **Calcium.** If you usually avoid all foods from one or two of the food groups, be sure to get enough nutrients from other food groups. For example, if you choose not to eat milk products because of intolerance to lactose or for other reasons, choose other foods that are good sources of calcium, *Tip # 8*, and be sure to get enough vitamin D, *Table 14.8*. Meat, fish, and poultry are major contributors of iron, zinc, and B-vitamins in most American diets. If you choose to avoid all or most animal products, be sure to get enough iron, vitamin B_{12}, calcium, and zinc from other sources. Vegetarian diets can be consistent with the Dietary Guidelines for Americans, and meet Recommended Dietary Allowances for nutrients. GROWING children, teenagers, women, and older adults have higher needs for some nutrients. Adolescents and adults over age 50 have an especially high need for calcium, but most people need to eat plenty of good sources of calcium for healthy bones throughout life. When selecting dairy products to get enough calcium, choose those that are low in fat or fat-free to avoid getting too much saturated fat.

---

[8] "The Vitamins in Medicine" by Franklin Bicknell and Frederick Prescott, William Heinemann Medical Books, London (1948).

v. **Vitamin E** occurs in food of animal origin and plant oils as a fat-soluble tocopherol. Heating and freezing of food lowers the vitamin concentration. It acts as antioxidant that prevents the formation of peroxides from the oxidation of polyunsaturated fatty acids by molecular oxygen from ozone or nitrogen dioxide polluted air. Vitamin E deficiency causes rupture of the red blood cells due to accumulated peroxides thus causing hemolysis and anemia, which is treatable by administration of vitamin E. Deficiency is more apparent when intake of polyunsaturated fatty acids increases in normal people or when diet consists of artificial formulas such in infants commercial formulas.

vi. **Vitamin K** occurs in green vegetables such as spinach, cabbage, cauliflower, and peas in the form of fat-soluble quinone compound. The vitamin is also manufactured by intestinal microorganisms, in the human guts, and becomes deficient in cases of chronic malabsorption, diarrhea, antibiotic oral administration, or in newborn infants. Vitamin K is crucial for the regulation of synthesis of prothrombin and other plasma clotting factors by the liver, which is essential for blood clotting. Vitamin K also may play a role in the formation of Coenzyme-Q that is essential in oxidative phosphorylation in the electron transport chain of the mitochondria. Currently, vitamin K is used to treat hemorrhage due to low prothrombin formation by the liver.

Tip # 8 *
SOME SOURCES OF CALCIUM +

- Yogurt#
- Milk**#
- Natural cheeses such as Mozzarella, Cheddar, Swiss, and Parmesan#
- Soy-based beverage with added calcium
- Tofu, if made with calcium sulfate (read the ingredient list)
- Breakfast cereal with added calcium
- Canned fish with soft bones such as salmon, sardines†
- Fruit juice with added calcium
- Pudding made with milk#
- Soup made with milk#
- Dark-green leafy vegetables such as collards, turnip greens

+ Read food labels for brand-specific information.
** This includes lactose-free and lactose-reduced milk.
# Choose low-fat or fat-free milk products most often.
† High in salt.

* NUTRITION AND YOUR HEALTH: DIETARY GUIDELINES FOR AMERICANS, published by the Department of Health and Human Services (HHS) and the Department of Agriculture (USDA).

---

vii. **Vitamin C**, *Table 14.14,* (ascorbic acid) occurs in citric fruits and green vegetable as water-soluble monosaccharide, which is easily destroyed by cooking and storage of food. Human body cannot synthesize vitamin C, which has to be supplied in food. The vitamin has a half-life time of 16 days in man and its deficiency for few months causes Scurvy. This disease afflicts connective tissues by the lack of formation of supporting tissue such as cartilage, bone, dentine, and collagen. It is characterized by bleeding gums, loosening of teeth, impaired wound healing, and fragile bones. Vitamin C also plays important role in mitochondrial oxidation in maintaining the transport of proton along the electron transport chain. This serves the purpose of production of energy by oxidizing NADH into NAD and loading the proton onto the oxygen molecules.

viii. **Vitamin B_1 (Thiamin)**, *Table 14.18,* occurs in unrefined cereal grains and food of animal origin, in water-soluble form. The vitamin is destroyed by heat and alkaline solution and is lost if water solution is drained out of food. Thiamin is part of the PDH complex that converts pyruvates to acetyl CoA for energy production and plays a role in regulating Na-K pump across cellular membranes. Its deficiency causes the Beriberi disease that afflicts the nervous and cardiovascular system.

ix. **Vitamin B_2 (Riboflavin)**, *Table 14.19,* occurs in milk and other food from animal origin as well as in plants. It is not destroyed with heat but is destroyed by light since it is fluorescent pigment. It is part of the oxidative tissue enzymes cytochrome-c reductase, amino acid dehydrogenase, acetyl-CoA dehydrogenase, and cofactor FAD and thus affects utilization of caloric contents of all food by cells. Riboflavin deficiency causes symptoms limited to the face in the form of fissures mouth angles, dermatitis, inflammation of the tongue, and eye disorders.

x. **Niacin**, *Table 14.17,* occurs in green vegetables and food of animal origin. Niacin enters in the formation of the hydrogen transport coenzyme NAD and NADP. These are vital cofactors in transport of protons and electrons in oxidation and reduction reactions both, in the cytoplasm and mitochondria of cells. They perform both anaerobic and aerobic energy production for all sorts of cellular activities. Niacin deficiency causes the disease of Pellagra, which presents with inflammation of skin, tongue, and mouth, diarrhea and loss of metal capacity. The disease is treatable by niacin administration.

xi. **Vitamin B_6 (Pyridoxine)**, *Table 14.13,* occurs in green vegetables and food from animal origin. It is essential in the metabolism of amino acid such as tyrosine, arginine, serine, threonine, and tryptophan. The vitamin thus affects muscle, nerves, connective tissue, and brain functions. Its deficiency causes impaired growth, muscular weakness, convulsive seizures and irritability, anemia, and edema of the connective tissue due to low plasma protein level. Protein loss in urine due to vitamin B_6 deficiency can be treated with administration of the vitamin especially in pregnant women.

xii. **Pantothenic acid** is one of the vitamin-B complex family and occurs in food from animal sources, legumes, and whole grain cereals. It is a constituent of coenzyme-A that plays important role in transferring substrates onto active molecules. In the conversion of food energy into ATP energy, CoA is essentials in condensing acetic acid with oxaloacetic. This forms citrates in the TCA cycle that produces energy to supply cellular demands. In the hemoglobin synthesis, CoA plays crucial role in condensing succinate and glycine in the process of heme biosynthesis. In the liver, CoA makes possible the condensing of acetyl groups to produce cholesterol or ketone bodies. In addition, pantothonic acid enters into the acyl carrier protein that builds up longer chains of fatty acids.

HEALTH AND FITNESS

xiii. **Lipoic acid** is one of the vitamin-B complex that is involved in the pyruvate conversion into acetyl CoA with the rest of the PDH complex. It is not required in the diet of humans.

xiv. **Biotin** occurs widely in natural food. Biotin acts as coenzyme in transferring carbon dioxide into substrates such as acetyl CoA in fatty acid synthesis. Biotin fixation of carbon dioxide is an anabolic process of generation of fatty acids as well as other biological substances.

xv. **Folic acid**, *Table 14.15*, is water-soluble and heat labile vitamin that is commonly deficient in many people consuming cooked food. It occurs in green vegetables. It is vital in cell growth and reproduction through the synthesis of nucleic acids, which enter into the DNA formation. Fast reproducing organs such as the bone marrow are greatly affected by folic acid deficiency, which results in megaloblastic anemia. Since the half-life time of red blood cells is about 120 days, therefore, folic acid deficiency for 4 months would undoubtedly cause anemia. In addition, women who could become pregnant need extra folic acid in order to prevent birth defects.

xvi. **Vitamin B_{12} (Cyanocobalamin)**, *Table 14.16*, occurs mainly in food of animal origin and is deficient in vegetarian diets. Only microorganism can manufacture this vitamin in the intestine of animals and it, thereafter, is kept bound to protein in the tissue of animals. Most of the ingested vitamin is absorbed in the ileum part of the intestine by selective absorption through an intrinsic factor secreted by the stomach and calcium ions. This vitamin enters into many coenzymes that affect nucleic acid formation in bone marrow, epithelial cells, and nervous system. It is alone used in the treatment of megaloblastic anemia and neural abnormalities due to impaired nucleic acid formation.

14.6. FOOD CONTENTS

This section presents twenty-two tables that contain food representatives of the top 100 high-density of essential macro- and micronutrients, as follows.

Tables 14.3 thru 14.24 are compiled from the United States Department of Agriculture Internet web site: http://www.nal.usda.gov/fnic/foodcomp/Data.

Table 14.3. Foodstuff with high **Carbohydrate** contents.	*Table 14.14.* Foodstuff with high **Vitamin C** contents.
Table 14.4. Foodstuff with high **Polysaturated fatty acids** contents.	*Table 14.15.* Foodstuff with high **Folate** contents.
Table 14.5. Foodstuff with high **Polyunsaturated fatty acids** contents.	*Table 14.16.* Foodstuff with high **Vitamin B12** contents.
Table 14.6. Foodstuff with high **Cholesterol** contents.	*Table 14.17.* Foodstuff with high **Niacin** contents.
Table 14.7. Foodstuff with high **Protein** contents.	*Table 14.18.* Foodstuff with high **Thiamin** contents.
Table 14.8. Foodstuff with high **Calcium** contents.	*Table 14.19.* Foodstuff with high **Riboflavin** contents.
Table 14.9. Foodstuff with high **Fiber** contents.	*Table 14.20.* Foodstuff with high **Vitamin A** contents.
Table 14.10. Foodstuff with high **Phosphorus** contents.	*Table 14.21.* Foodstuff with high **Iron** contents.
Table 14.11. Foodstuff with high **Sodium** contents.	*Table 14.22.* Foodstuff with high **Zinc** contents.
Table 14.12. Foodstuff with high **Potassium** contents.	*Table 14.23.* Foodstuff with high **Copper** contents.
Table 14.13. Foodstuff with high **Vitamin B-6** contents.	*Table 14.24.* Foodstuff with high **Selenium** contents.

Abbreviation in *Tables 14.3 thru 14.24*.

BEV	Beverage	CRM	Cream	KRNLS	Kernels	PROC	Processed	USDA	US Department of Agriculture
BF	Beef	DEHYD	Dehydrated	LIQ	Liquid	PROD	Product	VAR	Variety
BKD	Baked	DI NA PO4	Di-sodium phosphates	LN	Lean	PROT	Protein		
BLD	Blend	DRK	Drink	LO	Low	REG	Regular	VEG	Vegetable
BNLESS	Boneless	DRND	Dried	LRG	Large	RND	Round	VIT	Vitamin
BNS	Beans	DRSNG	Dressing	mcg	Microgram	RSTD	Roasted	WHL	Whole
BRKFST	Breakfast	ENGL	England	mg	Milligram	SAU	Sauce	1 Cup	218 grams
BRLD	Broiled	ENR	Enriched	mgm	Milligram	SD	Seed	1 tbsp	13.6 grams
CA	Calcium	EX	Extra	MSHD	Mashed	SHLDR	Shoulder	1 tsp	4.5 grams
CD	Code	FLAV	Flavored	MT	Meeting	SKN	Skin		
CHOC	Chocolate	FLR	Flour	NA	Sodium	SML	Small		
CHOIC	Choice	FORT	Fortified	NAT	Natural				
CHS	Cheese	FRSH	Fresh	PDR	Powder	SOYBN	Soybeans		
CINN	Cinnamon	FRZ	Frozen	PK	Pack	SP	Species		
CKD	Cooked	gm	Gram	PLN	Plain	SWT	Sweet		
CND	Canned	GRN	Grain	PNUT	Peanut	SWTND	Sweetened		
COCNT	Coconut	HI	High	PRCD	Product Code	UNCKD	Uncooked		
COMM	Common	HVY	Heavy	PRECKD	Precooked	UNDIL	Undiluted		
COMP	Compressed	INST	Instantaneous	PREP	Prepared	UNENR	Unenriched		
CONC	Concentrated	IU	International Unit	PREP	Prepared	UNSWTND	Unsweetened		
CRL	Cereal	JUC	Juice	PRK	Pork				

HEALTH AND FITNESS

The top ten contenders for Carbohydrate density are: **SUGARS, STRAWBERRY BEVERAGE, DESSERTS VANILLA, CANDIES STARCH JELLY, LEMONADE POWDER, FRUIT PUNCH FLAVOR DRINK, EGGNOG FLAVOR MIX POWDER, ALCOHOLIC BEVERAGE WHISKEY SOUR, CHEWING GUM, AND FROSTINGS WHITE FLUFFY.**

Table 14.3. Foodstuff with high **Carbohydrate** contents.

Carbohydrate, gm/100 gm	Description	Carbohydrate, gm/100 gm	Description
100	SUGARS, GRANULATED	83	PEACHES, DEHYD (LOW-MOISTURE), SULFURED, UNCKD
99	STRAWBERRY-FLAVOR BEV MIX, PDR	83	POTATO FLOUR
99	DESSERTS, RENNIN, VANILLA, DRY MIX	83	APRICOTS, DEHYD (LOW-MOISTURE), SULFURED, UNCKD
99	CANDIES, GUMDROPS, STARCH JELLY PIECES	82	HONEY, STR OR EXTRACTED
99	LEMONADE, POWDER	82	CRACKERS, SALTINES, FAT-FREE, LOW-SODIUM
98	FRUIT PUNCH-FLAVOR DRK, PDR, W/ NA	82	CANDIES, FUDGE, VANILLA, PREPARED-FROM-RECIPE
98	TEA, INST, SWTND W/SUGAR, LEMON-FLAVORED, WO/ VIT C, PDR	82	BABYFOOD, PRETZELS
97	EGGNOG-FLAVOR MIX, POWDER	82	CEREALS RTE, WHEAT CHEX, (WHEAT)
97	ALCOHOLIC BEV, WHISKEY SOUR MIX, PDR	82	CRACKERS, CRISPBREAD, RYE
97	CHEWING GUM	82	RICE, WHITE, LONG-GRAIN, PARBLD, DRY, ENR
96	SAUCE, SWT & SOUR, DEHYD, DRY	81	CHESTNUTS, JAPANESE, DRIED
95	DESSERTS, PUDD, LEMON, DRY MIX, INST	81	COFFEE SUB, CRL GRAIN BEV, PDR
95	FROSTINGS, WHITE, FLUFFY, DRY MIX	81	CAKE, WHITE, DRY MIX, PUDDING-TYPE, ENR
94	DESSERTS, PUDD, TAPIOCA, DRY MIX	81	PRETZELS, HARD, WHOLE-WHEAT
94	FROSTINGS, VANILLA, CREAMY, DRY MIX	81	CHESTNUTS, JAPANESE, DRIED
94	APPLES, DEHYD (LO MOIST), SULFURED, UNCKD	81	SEAWEED, AGAR, DRIED
93	CAROB-FLAVOR BEV MIX, PDR	81	POPCORN, CARAMEL-COATED, W/PNUTS
93	CANDIES, JELLYBEANS	80	COOKIES, BROWNIES, DRY MIX, SPL DIETARY
92	CEREALS RTE, KELLOGG, KELLOGG'S CORN POPS	80	CRACKERS, RYE, WAFERS, PLAIN
91	CORNSTARCH	80	CEREALS RTE, KELLOGG, KELLOGG'S LOFAT GRANOLA WO/RAISINS
91	CEREALS RTE, KELLOGG, KELLOGG'S FRSTD FLAKES	80	RYE FLOUR, LIGHT
91	DESSERTS, PUDD, RICE, DRY MIX	81	SEAWEED, AGAR, DRIED
90	PECTIN, UNSWTND, DRY MIX	79	ICE CRM CONES, CAKE OR WAFER-TYPE
90	CHOCOLATE-FLAVOR BEV MIX, PDR	79	TOPPINGS, MARSHMLLW CRM
89	PRUNES, DEHYD (LOW-MOISTURE), UNCKD	79	CAKE, CHOC, DRY MIX, PUDDING-TYPE
88	BANANAS, DEHYD, OR BANANA PDR	79	FRUIT LEATHER, BARS
85	CAKE, ANGELFOOD, DRY MIX	78	RAISINS, SEEDED
85	CANDIES, M & M MARS, STARBURST FRUIT CHEWS	79	ICE CRM CONES, CAKE OR WAFER-TYPE
84	MALTED MILK-FLAVOR MIX, CHOC, ADDED NUTR, PDR	78	CORNMEAL, DEGERMED, UNENR, WHITE
84	FRUIT LEATHER, ROLLS	77	BAKING CHOC, MEXICAN, SQUARES
84	ICE CRM CONES, SUGAR, ROLLED-TYPE	75	SPAGHETTI, DRY, ENRICHED
84	CAKE, YELLOW, DRY MIX, LIGHT	75	MACARONI, DRY, UNENRICHED
84	CRACKERS, MATZO, PLAIN	75	TOMATO POWDER
84	CEREALS RTE, KELLOGG, KELLOGG'S NUT & HONEY CRUNCH	75	LEEKS, (BULB & LOWER-LEAF PORTION), FREEZE-DRIED
84	RICE, WHITE, LONG-GRAIN, PRECKD OR INST, ENR, DRY	75	SORGHUM
83	CORN CAKES	75	NOODLES, JAPANESE, SOBA, DRY
85	CAKE, ANGELFOOD, DRY MIX	75	CAKE, GINGERBREAD, DRY MIX
83	ONIONS, DEHYDRATED FLAKES	73	BARLEY
83	RICE NOODLES, DRY	73	WHEY, ACID, DRIED

HEALTH AND FITNESS

The top ten contenders for Polysaturated fatty acids density are: **FISH OIL MENHADEN FULLY HYDRATED, SHORTENING CONFECTIONERY COCCONUT, OIL VEGETABLE NUTMEG BUTTER, VEGETABLE OIL COCONUT, OIL VEGETABLE UCUHUBA BUTTER, VEGETABLE OIL PALM KERNEL, OIL VEGETABLE BABASSU, SHORTENING CONFECTIONERY FRACTIONATED PALM, BUTTER OIL ANHYDROUS, AND COCONUT MEAT DRIED (DESICCATED).**

Table 14.4. Foodstuff with high Polysaturated fatty acids contents.

Total saturated FA, gm/100 gm	Description	Total saturated FA, gm/100 gm	Description
96	FISH OIL, MENHADEN, FULLY HYDR	32	PORK, FRESH, BACKFAT, RAW
91	SHORTENING CONFECTIONERY, COCNT (HYDR) & OR PALM KERNEL (HYDR)	32	MARGARINE, REG, HARD, LARD (HYDR)
90	OIL, VEG, NUTMEG BUTTER	31	COCONUT MEAT, DRIED (DESICCATED), SWTND, SHREDDED
87	VEGETABLE OIL, COCONUT	31	PILINUTS-CANARYTREE, DRIED
85	OIL, VEG, UCUHUBA BUTTER	31	
82	VEGETABLE OIL, PALM KERNEL	30	FISH OIL, MENHADEN
81	OIL, VEGETABLE, BABASSU	30	SHORTENING, MULTIPURPOSE, SOYBN (HYDR) & PALM (HYDR)
66	SHORTENING, CONFECTIONERY, FRACTIONATED PALM	30	FISH OIL, SARDINE
62	BUTTER OIL, ANHYDROUS	30	FAT, CHICKEN
61	COCONUT MEAT, DRIED (DESICCATED), CRMD	30	COCONUT MEAT, RAW
60	OIL, VEG, COCOA BUTTER	29	BEEF, RTL CUTS, FAT, RAW
57	COCONUT MEAT, DRIED (DESICCATED), NOT SWTND	29	FAT, TURKEY
57	MARGARINE, REG, HARD, COCNT (HYDR & REG) & SAFFLOWER & PALM (HYDR)	29	PORK, CURED, SALT PORK, RAW
53	OIL, VEGETABLE, CUPU ASSU	29	CANDIES, CAROB
52	BEEF, VAR MEATS & BY-PRODUCTS, SUET, RAW	29	BANANA CHIPS
50	BUTTER	29	SHORTENING, SPL PURPOSE FOR BAKING, SOYBN (HYDR) PALM & CTTNSD
50	FAT, BEEF TALLOW	29	COCONUT MEAT, DRIED (DESICCATED), SWTND, FLAKED, PACKAGED
49	OIL, VEGETABLE, PALM	29	BEEF, RTL CUTS, FAT, CKD
48	SHORTENING FRYING (HVY DUTY), PALM (HYDR)	28	MARGARINE-BUTTER BLEND, 60% CORN OIL MARGARINE & 40% BUTTER
47	FAT, MUTTON TALLOW	28	COCONUT MEAT, DRIED (DESICCATED), SWTND, FLAKED, CND
47	OIL, VEGETABLE, SHEANUT	28	FAT, GOOSE
45	PORK, FRSH, VAR MEATS & BY-PRODUCTS, LEAF FAT, RAW	27	SHORTENING CAKE MIX, SOYBN (HYDR) & CTTNSD (HYDR)
45	SHORTENING FRYING (HVY DUTY), BF TALLOW & CTTNSD	27	SAUCE, HOLLANDAISE, W/BUTTER FAT, DEHYD, DRY
42	COCONUT MEAT, DRIED (DESICCATED), TSTD	27	LAMB, DOM, COMP OF RTL CUTS, FAT, 1/4"FAT, CHOIC, CKD
40	SHORTENING, HOUSEHOLD, LARD & VEG OIL	27	CORN-BASED, EXTRUDED, CONES, NACHO-FLAVOR
39	LARD	26	NUTMEG, GROUND
37	DESSERT TOPPING, POWDERED	26	OIL, VEG, CTTNSD, SALAD OR COOKING
36	SHORTENING INDUSTRIAL, LARD & VEG OIL	26	COFFEE, INST, W/SUGAR, FRENCH-FLAVOR, PDR
35	LAMB, NZ, IMP, FRZ, COMP OF RTL CUTS, FAT, RAW	26	SHORTENING INDUSTRIAL, SOYBN (HYDR) & CTTNSD
33	FAT, DUCK	25	BAKING CHOC, UNSWTND, LIQ
33	VEAL, COMP OF RTL CUTS, FAT, RAW	25	PORK, FRSH, VAR MEATS & BY-PRODUCTS, JOWL, RAW
33	BAKING CHOC, UNSWTND, SQUARES	25	SHORTENING HOUSEHOLD SOYBN (HYDR) & PALM
33	CREAM SUBSTITUTE, POWDERED	22	CHEESE, CREAM

The top ten contenders for Polyunsaturated fatty acids density are: **OIL VEG SAFFLOWER SALAD, OIL VEGETABLE GRAPESEED, OIL VEG, SUNFLOWER LINOLEIC, OIL VEGETABLE WALNUT, OIL VEGETABLE POPPYSEED, OIL VEG CORN SALAD, OIL SOYBN SALAD OR COOKING, SALAD DRESSING MAYO SOYBN & SAFFLOWER OIL, OIL VEGETABLE TOMATOSEED, OIL VEGETABLE COTTONSEED SALAD OR COOKING, MARGARINE SOFT SAFFLOWER & COTTONSEED (HYDR) & PEANUT (HYDR).**

Table 14.5. Foodstuff with high **Polyunsaturated fatty acids** contents.

Total Poly-unsaturated FA, gm/100 gm	Description	Total Poly-unsaturated FA, gm/100 gm	Description
75	OIL, VEG SAFFLOWER, SALAD OR COOKING, LINOLEIC, (OVER 70%)	36	OIL, VEG, SUNFLOWER, LINOLEIC, (HYDR)
70	OIL, VEGETABLE, GRAPESEED	36	MARGARINE, REG, LIQ, SOYBN (HYDR & REG) & CTTNSD
66	OIL, VEG, SUNFLOWER, LINOLEIC, (60% & OVER)	35	MARGARINE, SOFT, SOYBN (HYDR) & SAFFLOWER
63	OIL, VEGETABLE, WALNUT	35	OIL, VEGETABLE, RICE BRAN
62	OIL, VEGETABLE, POPPYSEED	34	FISH OIL, MENHADEN
59	OIL, VEG CORN, SALAD OR COOKING	34	SALAD DRSNG, FRENCH, HOME RECIPE
58	OIL, SOYBN, SALAD OR COOKING	34	SHORTENING FRYING HVY DUTY, SOYBN HYDR, LINOLEIC 30% W/SILICON
55	SALAD DRSNG, MAYO, SOYBN & SAFFLOWER OIL, W/SALT	33	SUNFLOWER SD KRNLS, DRY RSTD, WO/SALT
53	OIL, VEGETABLE, TOMATOSEED	32	OIL, PNUT, SALAD OR COOKING
52	OIL, VEG, CTTNSD, SALAD OR COOKING	32	FISH OIL, SARDINE
50	MARGARINE, SOFT, SAFFLOWER & CTTNSD (HYDR) & PNUT (HYDR)	32	SUNFLOWER SD BUTTER, WO/SALT
48	OIL, SOYBN, SALAD OR COOKING, (HYDR) & CTTNSD	31	POPPY SEED
45	VEGETABLE OIL, SOYBN LECITHIN	30	VEGETABLE OIL, CANOLA
45	MARGARINE, SOFT, SAFFLOWER (HYDR & REG)	29	SALAD DRSNG, RUSSIAN, W/SALT
43	BUTTERNUTS, DRIED	29	OIL, VEG, APRICOT KERNEL
42	OIL, SESAME, SALAD OR COOKING	29	MARGARINE, SOFT, SOYBN (HYDR) & CTTNSD
41	SALAD DRSNG, MAYO, SOYBN OIL, W/SALT	28	WATERMELON SD KRNLS, DRIED
41	VEGETABLE OIL, OAT	28	SALAD DRSNG, ITALIAN, COMM, REG, W/SALT
41	MARGARINE, REG, HARD, SAFFLOWER & SOYBN (HYDR) & CTTNSD (HYDR)	23	FAT, TURKEY
41	SHORTENING BREAD, SOYBN (HYDR) & CTTNSD	23	FORMULATED, WHEAT-BASED, UNFLAVORED, W/SALT
40	FISH OIL, SALMON	23	FISH OIL, COD LIVER
40	OIL, VEG, SUNFLOWER, LINOLEIC (LESS THAN 60%)	22	SESAME BUTTER, PASTE
39	WALNUTS, ENG OR PERSIAN, DRIED	22	PUFF PASTRY, FRZ, RTB, BKD
38	SHORTENING, SPL PURPOSE FOR CAKES & FROSTINGS, SOYBN (HYDR)	22	SHORTENING FRYING (REG), SOYBN (HYDR) & CTTNSD (HYDR)
38	SUNFLOWER SD KRNLS, OIL RSTD, WO/SALT	22	HICKORYNUTS, DRIED
38	OIL, SOYBN, SALAD OR COOKING, (HYDR)	22	FORMULATED, WHEAT-BASED, FLAV, MACADAMIA FLAV, WO/SALT
38	SUNFLOWER SD KRNLS, TSTD, WO/SALT	22	SESAME SEEDS, WHOLE, DRIED
38	SUNFLOWER SD KRNLS, TSTD, W/SALT	22	SALAD DRSNG, FRENCH, COMM, REG, W/SALT
37	WALNUTS, BLACK, DRIED	21	PINE NUTS, PIGNOLIA, DRIED
37	SHORTENING, SPL PURPOSE FOR BAKING, SOYBN (HYDR) PALM & CTTNSD	21	VEGETABLE OIL, MUSTARD
37	SALAD DRSNG, MAYO, SOYBN OIL, WO/SALT	21	SESAME SEEDS, WHL, RSTD & TSTD
37	MARGARINE, REG, HARD, SUNFLOWER & SOYBN (HYDR) & CTTNSD (HYDR)	19	PUMPKIN & SQUASH SD KRNLS, RSTD, WO/SALT

HEALTH AND FITNESS

The top ten contenders for Cholesterol density are: **VEAL VAR MEATS & BY-PRODUCTS BRAIN, PORK FRSH, VAR MEATS & BY-PRODUCTS BRAIN, AND LAMB VAR MEATS & BY-PRODUCTS BRAIN, PAN-FRIED EGG YOLK DRIED, BEEF VAR MEATS & BY-PRODUCTS BRAIN, EGG WHOLE DRIED, VEAL VAR MEATS & BY-PRODUCTS, KIDNEYS, FISH OIL HERRING, FISH OIL SARDINE, AND CHICKEN LIVER.**

Table 14.6. Foodstuff with high **Cholesterol** contents.

Cholesterol, mgm/100 gm	Description	Cholesterol, mgm/100 gm	Description
3100	VEAL, VAR MEATS & BY-PRODUCTS, BRAIN, CKD, BRSD	260	SQUID, MXD SP, CKD, FRIED
2552	PORK, FRSH, VAR MEATS & BY-PRODUCTS, BRAIN, CKD, BRSD	256	BUTTER OIL, ANHYDROUS
2504	LAMB, VAR MEATS & BY-PRODUCTS, BRAIN, CKD, PAN-FRIED	240	CHICKEN, STEWING, GIBLETS, RAW
2335	EGG, YOLK, DRIED	238	VEAL, VAR MEATS & BY-PRODUCTS, TONGUE, CKD, BRSD
2054	BEEF, VAR MEATS & BY-PRODUCTS, BRAIN, CKD, SIMMRD	236	CHICKEN, ROASTING, GIBLETS, RAW
2017	EGG, WHL, DRIED, STABILIZED, GLUCOSE RED	235	FAST FOODS, BISCUIT, W/EGG & BACON
1715	EGG, WHOLE, DRIED	233	SQUID, MIXED SPECIES, RAW
791	VEAL, VAR MEATS & BY-PRODUCTS, KIDNEYS, CKD, BRSD	232	TURKEY, GIZZARD, ALL CLASSES, CKD, SIMMRD
766	FISH OIL, HERRING	229	VEAL, VAR MEATS & BY-PRODUCTS, LUNGS, RAW
710	FISH OIL, SARDINE	226	TURKEY, HEART, ALL CLASSES, CKD, SIMMRD
631	CHICKEN, LIVER, ALL CLASSES, CKD, SIMMRD	224	CUTTLEFISH, MXD SP, CKD, MOIST HEAT
626	TURKEY, LIVER, ALL CLASSES, CKD, SIMMRD	223	BEEF, VAR MEATS & BY-PRODUCTS, THYMUS, RAW
588	CAVIAR, BLACK & RED, GRANULAR	221	PORK, FRSH, VAR MEATS & BY-PRODUCTS, HEART, CKD, BRSD
572	EGG SUBSTITUTE, POWDER	221	CAKE, POUND, COMMLY PREP, BUTTER
570	FISH OIL, COD LIVER	219	BUTTER, WITH SALT
565	LAMB, VAR MEATS & BY-PRODUCTS, KIDNEYS, CKD, BRSD	260	SQUID, MXD SP, CKD, FRIED
561	VEAL, VAR MEATS & BY-PRODUCTS, LIVER, CKD, BRSD	173	SHRIMP, MXD SP, CND
565	LAMB, VAR MEATS & BY-PRODUCTS, KIDNEYS, CKD, BRSD	172	FAST FOODS, HAM, EGG, & CHS SNDWCH
561	VEAL, VAR MEATS & BY-PRODUCTS, LIVER, CKD, BRSD	171	FAST FOODS, BISCUIT, W/EGG
521	FISH OIL, MENHADEN	139	VEAL, RIB, LN & FAT, CKD, BRSD
515	DUCK, DOMESTICATED, LIVER, RAW	137	CREAM, FLUID, HVY WHIPPING
515	GOOSE, LIVER, RAW	137	CRAYFISH, MXD SP, FARMED, CKD, MOIST HEAT
504	PORK, FRSH, VAR MEATS & BY-PRODUCTS, SPLEEN, CKD, BRSD	137	ENTREES, CRAB CAKE
501	LAMB, VAR MEATS & BY-PRODUCTS, LIVER, CKD, BRSD	136	CHICKEN, HEART, ALL CLASSES, RAW
500	FISH OIL, MENHADEN, FULLY HYDR	136	DUCK, YNG DUCKLING, DOM, WH PEKIN, BRST, MEAT & SKN, BNLESS, CKD, RSTD
493	LAMB, VAR MEATS & BY-PRODUCTS, LIVER, CKD, PAN-FRIED	136	SNACKS, M & M MARS, KUDOS WHL GRAIN BARS, CHOC CHIP
485	FISH OIL, SALMON	135	SPINACH SOUFFLE, HOME-PREPARED
482	BEEF, VAR MEATS & BY-PRODUCTS, LIVER, CKD, PAN-FRIED	139	VEAL, RIB, LN & FAT, CKD, BRSD

Table 14.7. Foodstuff with high **Protein** contents.

Protein, gm/100 gm	Description	Protein, gm/100 gm	Description
88	SOY PROT ISOLATE, K TYPE, CRUDE PROT BASIS	36	LAMB, DOM, SHLDR, ARM, LN, 1/4"FAT, CHOIC, CKD, BRSD
86	DESSERTS, GELATINS, DRY PDR, UNSWTND	36	MILK, DRY, NONFAT, CA RED
82	EGG, WHITE, DRIED, PDR, GLUCOSE RED	35	GELATIN, DRINKING, ORANGE-FLAVOR, PDR
81	SOY PROT ISOLATE, K TYPE	35	SOYBEANS, MATURE SEEDS, RSTD, SALTED
63	COD, ATLANTIC, DRIED & SALTED	23	WHITEFISH, MXD SP, SMOKED
61	PORK SKINS, PLAIN	23	TUNA, FRESH, YELLOWFIN, RAW
58	SOY PROT CONC, PRODUCED BY ALCOHOL EXTRACTION	23	CHEESE, CHESHIRE
58	PORK SKINS, BARBECUE-FLAVOR	23	BEANS, WHITE, MATURE SEEDS, RAW
57	SEAWEED, SPIRULINA, DRIED	23	CHICKEN, CORNISH GAME HENS, MEAT ONLY, CKD, RSTD
56	EGG SUBSTITUTE, POWDER	23	GAME MEAT, BEEFALO, COMP OF CUTS, RAW
52	PEANUT FLOUR, DEFATTED	23	WHITEFISH, MXD SP, SMOKED
51	SOY FLR, DEFATTED, CRUDE PROT BASIS (N X 6.25)	22	CHEESE, PAST PROCESS, AMERICAN, WO/DI NA PO4
51	SOY FLR, LOW-FAT, CRUDE PROT BASIS (N x 6.25)	22	TURKEY, FRYER-ROASTERS, MEAT & SKN & GIBLETS & NECK, RAW
50	SESAME FLOUR, LOW-FAT	22	BUTTERFISH, CKD, DRY HEAT
50	COTTONSEED FLR, LOFAT (GLANDLESS)	22	CHEESE, PAST PROCESS, PIMENTO
49	COTTONSEED MEAL, PART DEFATTED (GLANDLESS)	22	LAMB, DOM, RIB, LN & FAT, 1/4"FAT, CHOIC, CKD, BRLD
48	SUNFLOWER SD FLR, PART DEFATTED	22	SALMON, ATLANTIC, FARMED, CKD, DRY HEAT
48	TOFU, DRIED-FROZEN (KOYADOFU)	22	PORK, FRSH, VAR MEATS & BY-PRODUCTS, FEET, RAW
48	WHELK, UNSPEC, CKD, MOIST HEAT	22	BEEF, RND, TOP RND, LN & FAT, 1/4"FAT, PRIME, RAW
47	EGG, WHOLE, DRIED	22	RIB-B-Q, FL BR LOWER FAT BEEF RIB-BQ.
47	SOY FLOUR, DEFATTED	22	PORK, FRSH, LOIN, CNTR LOIN (CHOPS OR ROASTS), BONE-IN, LN, Ried AW
45	SOY MEAL, DEFATTED, RAW	20	PIERRE, FLAME BROILED BEEF TWO-FERS, PROD CD 9684
42	CHEESE, PARMESAN, GRATED	20	SOUP, MINESTRONE, DEHYD, DRY
41	COTTONSEED FLR, PART DEFATTED (GLANDLESS)	20	BEEF, VAR MEATS & BY-PRODUCTS, LIVER, RAW
40	SESAME FLR, PART DEFATTED	20	LAMB, DOM, SHLDR, ARM, LN, 1/4"FAT, CHOIC, RAW
40	SOYBEANS, MATURE SEEDS, DRY RSTD	20	LAMB, DOM, RIB, LN, 1/4"FAT, CHOIC, RAW
40	ALMOND MEAL, PART DEFATTED, W/SALT	20	VEAL, RIB, LN, RAW
38	LEAVENING AGENTS, YEAST, BAKER'S, ACTIVE DRY	20	RIB-B-Q, FL BR LEAN MAGIC PRK RIB-BQ WONDRBT DPR, PROD CD 3830
38	MEAT EXTENDER	20	DILL WEED, DRIED
38	CHEESE, PARMESAN, SHREDDED	20	ALMONDS, DRIED, UNBLANCHED
37	ALMOND PDR, PART DEFATTED	20	SALMON, PINK, RAW
37	VEAL, LEG (TOP RND), LN, CKD, BRSD	20	SPEARMINT, DRIED
36	SOYBEANS, MATURE SEEDS, RAW	20	TURKEY, YOUNG HEN, WING, MEAT & SKN, RAW
36	LUPINS, MATURE SEEDS, RAW	20	BEEF, RND, EYE OF RND, LN & FAT, 1/2"FAT, PRIME, RAW
36	MILK, DRY, NONFAT, REG, WO/ VIT A	20	PORK, FRSH, LOIN, CNTR RIB (CHOPS OR ROASTS), BNLESS, LN & FAT, RAW
36	VEAL, LEG (TOP RND), LN & FAT, CKD, BRSD	20	SALMON, ATLANTIC, FARMED, RAW
36	BEEF, RND, TOP RND, LN, 1/4"FAT, ALL GRDS, CKD, BRSD	20	TURKEY, FRYER-ROASTERS, BACK, MEAT & SKN, RAW
36	BABYFOOD, CRL, HI PROT, DRY	19	VEAL, SHLDR, ARM, LN & FAT, RAW
36	CHEESE, PARMESAN, HARD	19	SUNFLOWER SD KRNLS, DRY RSTD, WO/SALT
36	VEAL, SHLDR, ARM, LN, CKD, BRSD	19	SUNFLOWER SD KRNLS, DRY RSTD, W/SALT
36	SAFFLOWER SD MEAL, PART DEFATTED	19	BEEF, SHRT LOIN, TOP LOIN, LN & FAT, 1/8"FAT, CHOIC, RAW

HEALTH AND FITNESS

Table 14.8. Foodstuff with high **Calcium** contents.

Calcium, gm/100 gm	Description	Calcium, gm/100 gm	Description
7364	LEAVENING AGENTS, BAKING PDR, DOUBLE-ACTING, STRAIGHT PO4	931	CUMIN SEED
5876	LEAVENING AGENTS, BAKING PDR, DOUBLE-ACTING, NA AL SULFATE	912	MILK, DRY, WHOLE
4332	LEAVENING AGENTS, BAKING PDR, LOW-SODIUM	895	CHEESE, GOAT, HARD TYPE
3733	DESSERTS, RENNIN, TABLETS, UNSWTND	880	DAIRY DRK MIX, CHOC, RED CAL, W/ASPRT, PDR
3098	LEMONADE, LO CAL, W/ASPRT, PDR	861	CEREALS RTE, GENERAL MILLS, TOTAL
2134	TOFU, DRIED-FROZEN (KOYADOFU), PREP W/CA SULFATE	860	MOLASSES, BLACKSTRAP
2132	SAVORY, GROUND	850	BABYFOOD, CEREAL, RICE, DRY
2113	BASIL, GROUND	834	BAY LEAF, CRUMBLED
2054	WHEY, ACID, DRIED	823	COCOA MIX, NESTLE, CARNATION NO SUGAR HOT COCOA MIX
1990	MARJORAM, DRIED	813	CHIVES, FREEZE-DRIED
1890	THYME, GROUND	796	WHEY, SWEET, DRIED
1784	DILL WEED, DRIED	795	BABYFOOD, CRL, BARLEY, DRY
1767	CELERY SEED	795	SAUCE, CHS, DEHYD, DRY
1661	GRAVY, CUSTOM FOODS, RED LABEL AU JUS BASE, DRY	790	CEREALS RTE, GENERAL MILLS, TOTAL CORN FLAKES
1652	SAGE, GROUND	783	SNACKS, M & M MARS, KUDOS WHL GRAIN BARS, CHOC CHIP
1633	SISYMBRIUM SP. SEEDS, WHL, DRIED	772	CHEESE, PAST PROCESS, SWISS, W/DI NA PO4
1576	OREGANO, GROUND	772	CHEESE, PAST PROCESS, SWISS, WO/DI NA PO4
1516	DILL SEED	756	CHEESE, PROVOLONE
1488	SPEARMINT, DRIED	751	BABYFOOD, CRL, HI PROT, W/APPL & ORANGE, DRY
1468	PARSLEY, DRIED	746	CHEESE, MONTEREY
1448	POPPY SEED	733	BABYFOOD, CEREAL, MIXED, DRY
1440	COCOA MIX, W/ASPRT, PDR, W/ CA P, WO/NA OR VIT A	733	BABYFOOD, CRL, OATMEAL, DRY
1376	CHEESE, PARMESAN, GRATED	731	CHEESE, MOZZARELLA, PART SKIM MILK, LO MOIST
1346	CHERVIL, DRIED	731	CHEESE, EDAM
1280	ROSEMARY, DRIED	724	BABYFOOD, CRL, HI PROT, DRY
1257	MILK, DRY, NONFAT, REG, WO/ VIT A	723	CHEESE FD, PAST PROCESS, SWISS
1257	MILK, DRY, NONFAT, REG, W/ VIT A	721	CHEESE, CHEDDAR
1253	CHEESE, PARMESAN, SHREDDED	717	CHEESE, MUENSTER
1246	CORIANDER LEAF, DRIED	709	CORIANDER SEED
1231	MILK, DRY, NONFAT, INST, WO/ VIT A	703	CHEESE, LOW-SODIUM, CHEDDAR OR COLBY
1231	MILK, DRY, NONFAT, INST, W/ VIT A	700	CHEESE, TILSIT
1229	TOFU, SALTED & FERMENTED (FUYU), PREP W/CA SULFATE	700	CHEESE, GOUDA
1228	CINNAMON, GROUND	696	BABYFOOD, CRL, MXD, W/BANANAS, DRY
1196	FENNEL SEED	691	BABYFOOD, CRL, RICE, W/BANANAS, DRY
1184	MILK, BUTTERMILK, DRIED	689	CARAWAY SEED
1184	CHEESE, PARMESAN, HARD	685	CHEESE, COLBY
1154	BABYFOOD, CRL, OATMEAL, W/HONEY, DRY	683	TOFU, RAW, FIRM, PREP W/CA SULFATE
1139	TARRAGON, GROUND	682	PUMPKIN PIE SPICE
1064	CHEESE, ROMANO	680	CHEESE, MEXICAN, QUESO ANEJO
1011	CHEESE, GRUYERE	674	SAUCE, WHITE, DEHYD, DRY
996	POULTRY SEASONING	674	CHEESE, BRICK
989	SESAME SEEDS, WHL, RSTD & TSTD	673	CHEESE, CARAWAY
975	SESAME SEEDS, WHOLE, DRIED	667	SAUCE, STROGANOFF, DEHYD, DRY
961	TOFU, FRIED, PREP W/CA SULFATE	662	CHEESE, ROQUEFORT
961	CHEESE, SWISS	661	CHEESE, MEXICAN, QUESO ASADERO
960	SESAME BUTTER, PASTE	661	ALLSPICE, GROUND

Table 14.9. Foodstuff with high **Fiber** contents.

Fiber, total dietary, gm/100 gm	Description	Fiber, total dietary, gm/100 gm	Description
86	CORN BRAN, CRUDE	25	BROADBEANS (FAVA BNS), MATURE SEEDS, RAW
70	FUNGI, CLOUD EARS, DRIED	25	BEANS, BLACK TURTLE SOUP, MATURE SEEDS, RAW
54	CINNAMON, GROUND	24	BEANS, PINTO, MATURE SEEDS, RAW
51	CEREALS, RTE, KELLOGG, KELLOGG'S ALL-BRAN W/EX FIBER	23	CRACKERS, RYE, WAFERS, PLAIN
48	CEREALS RTE, GENERAL MILLS, FIBER ONE	22	ALLSPICE, GROUND
46	SAVORY, GROUND	22	PEPPER, ANCHO, DRIED
43	OREGANO, GROUND	21	PEPPERS, SWT, GRN, FREEZE-DRIED
43	WHEAT BRAN, CRUDE	21	PEPPERS, SWT, RED, FREEZE-DRIED
43	ROSEMARY, DRIED	21	DILL SEED
42	CORIANDER SEED	21	TURMERIC, GROUND
41	BASIL, GROUND	21	LEAVENING AGENTS, YEAST, BAKER'S, ACTIVE DRY
40	MARJORAM, DRIED	21	RICE BRAN, CRUDE
40	SAGE, GROUND	21	PAPRIKA
40	CEREALS RTE, KELLOGG, KELLOGG'S ALL-BRAN BRAN BUDS	21	CRACKERS, RYE, WAFERS, SEASONED
40	FENNEL SEED	21	NUTMEG, GROUND
40	CAROB FLOUR	21	LIMA BNS, THIN SEEDED (BABY), MATURE SEEDS, RAW
38	CARAWAY SEED	20	MACE, GROUND
37	THYME, GROUND	20	BEANS, GREAT NORTHERN, MATURE SEEDS, RAW
34	CHILI POWDER	19	LIMA BNS, LRG, MATURE SEEDS, RAW
34	CLOVES, GROUND	18	MUNGO BNS, MATURE SEEDS, RAW
33	CURRY POWDER	18	BULGUR, DRY
33	COCOA, DRY PDR, UNSWTND	18	BAKING CHOC, UNSWTND, LIQ
33	PARSLEY, FREEZE-DRIED	18	CEREALS, ROMAN MEAL, PLN, DRY, (WHEAT W/OTHER GRAINS)
32	CEREALS RTE, KELLOGG, KELLOGG'S ALL-BRAN	18	CEREALS RTE, QUAKER, QUAKER CRUNCHY BRAN
31	SOUP, BEAN W/BACON, DEHYD, DRY MIX	18	SOYBEANS, MATURE SEEDS, RSTD, SALTED
31	LENTILS, MATURE SEEDS, RAW	18	SOYBEANS, MATURE SEEDS, RSTED, NO SALT ADDED
30	PARSLEY, DRIED	18	MEAT EXTENDER
30	SPEARMINT, DRIED	18	SOY FLOUR, DEFATTED
30	COCOA, DRY PDR, UNSWTND, PROC W/ALKALI	18	SOY FLR, DEFATTED, CRUDE PROT BASIS (N X 6.25)
30	CEREALS RTE, 100% BRAN, (WHEAT BRAN, BARLEY)	17	CHICKPEAS (GARBANZO BNS, BENGAL GM), MATURE SEEDS, RAW
29	COCOA, DRY PDR, UNSWTND, HERSHEY, HERSHEY'S EUROPEAN STYLE COCOA	17	BARLEY
29	PEPPERS, HOT CHILE, SUN-DRIED	17	SESAME SD KRNLS, TSTD, WO/SALT (DECORT)
28	CARDAMON, GROUND	17	TOMATO POWDER
27	PEPPER, RED OR CAYENNE	17	CRACKERS, CRISPBREAD, RYE
27	PEPPERS, PASILLA, DRIED	16	COCONUT MEAT, DRIED (DESICCATED), NOT SWTND
27	PEPPER, BLACK	16	MUNG BNS, MATURE SEEDS, RAW
26	BAY LEAF, CRUMBLED	16	CEREALS RTE, BRAN CHEX, (WHEAT BRAN, CORN)
26	PEPPER, WHITE	16	PEANUT FLOUR, DEFATTED
26	CHIVES, FREEZE-DRIED	16	PEANUT FLOUR, LOW FAT
26	PEAS, SPLIT, MATURE SEEDS, RAW	16	BARLEY, PEARLED, RAW
25	BEANS, FRENCH, MATURE SEEDS, RAW	15	BAKING CHOC, UNSWTND, SQUARES
25	BEANS, YEL, MATURE SEEDS, RAW	15	OAT BRAN, RAW

HEALTH AND FITNESS

Table 14.10. Foodstuff with high **Phosphorus** contents.

Phosphorus, mgm/100 gm	Description	Phosphorus, mgm/100 gm	Description
9918	LEAVENING AGENTS, BAKING PDR, DOUBLE-ACTING, STRAIGHT PO4	875	CHEESE SPRD, PAST PROCESS, AMERICAN, W/DI NA PO4
6869	LEAVENING AGENTS, BAKING PDR, LOW-SODIUM	853	DAIRY DRK MIX, CHOC, RED CAL, W/ASPRT, PDR
2191	LEAVENING AGENTS, BAKING PDR, DOUBLE-ACTING, NA AL SULFATE	849	POPPY SEED
1684	COTTONSEED MEAL, PART DEFATTED (GLANDLESS)	842	WHEAT GERM, CRUDE
1677	RICE BRAN, CRUDE	841	MUSTARD SEED, YELLOW
1630	COCOA MIX, W/ASPRT, PDR, W/ CA P, WO/ NA OR VIT A	839	SOY PROT CONC, PRODUCED BY ALCOHOL EXTRACTION
1597	COTTONSEED FLR, PART DEFATTED (GLANDLESS)	831	EGG, WHOLE, DRIED
1587	COTTONSEED FLR, LOFAT (GLANDLESS)	815	CEREALS RTE, WAFFELOS, (WHEAT W/OTHER GRAINS)
1554	LEMONADE, LO CAL, W/ASPRT, PDR	810	SESAME FLR, PART DEFATTED
1349	WHEY, ACID, DRIED	807	CHEESE, PARMESAN, GRATED
1293	DESSERTS, GELATINS, DRY MIX, RED CAL, W/ASPRT	807	SESAME FLOUR, HIGH-FAT
1290	LEAVENING AGENTS, YEAST, BAKER'S, ACTIVE DRY	804	DESSERTS, PUDD, BANANA, DRY MIX, INST
1214	CEREALS RTE, 100% BRAN, (WHEAT BRAN, BARLEY)	800	COTTONSEED KRNLS, RSTD (GLANDLESS)
1174	PUMPKIN & SQUASH SD KRNLS, DRIED	790	SESAME BUTTER, TAHINI, FROM UNROASTED KRNLS
1172	PUMPKIN & SQUASH SD KRNLS, RSTD, WO/SALT	782	PANCAKES, WHOLE-WHEAT, DRY MIX, INCOMPLETE
1172	PUMPKIN & SQUASH SD KRNLS, RSTD, W/SALT	776	SESAME SD KRNLS, DRIED (DECORT)
1158	SUNFLOWER SD KRNLS, TSTD, WO/SALT	776	SOY PROTEIN ISOLATE
1146	CEREALS RTE, WHEAT GERM, TSTD, PLN, (WHEAT GERM)	776	MILK, DRY, WHOLE
1139	SUNFLOWER SD KRNLS, OIL RSTD, WO/SALT	774	SESAME SD KRNLS, TSTD, WO/SALT (DECORT)
1139	SUNFLOWER SD KRNLS, OIL RSTD, W/SALT	762	CHEESE, PAST PROCESS, SWISS, W/DI NA PO4
1013	WHEAT BRAN, CRUDE	760	CHEESE, ROMANO
1011	MILK, DRY, NONFAT, CA RED	760	PEANUT FLOUR, DEFATTED
1011	CEREALS RTE, QUAKER, KRETSCHMER HONEY CRUNCH WHEAT GERM	755	WATERMELON SD KRNLS, DRIED
985	MILK, DRY, NONFAT, INST, WO/ VIT A	754	CHEESE FD, PAST PROCESS, AMERICAN, W/DI NA PO4
985	MILK, DRY, NONFAT, INST, W/ VIT A	752	SESAME BUTTER, TAHINI, FROM RAW & STONE GROUND KRNLS
980	CEREALS RTE, KELLOGG, KELLOGG'S ALL-BRAN	752	DESSERTS, PUDD, LEMON, DRY MIX, INST
968	MILK, DRY, NONFAT, REG, WO/ VIT A	745	CHEESE, PAST PROCESS, AMERICAN, W/DI NA PO4
958	CEREALS, RTE, KELLOGG, KELLOGG'S ALL-BRAN W/EX FIBER	744	CHEESE, PAST PROCESS, PIMENTO
950	COD, ATLANTIC, DRIED & SALTED	736	SUNFLOWER SD BUTTER, WO/SALT
933	MILK, BUTTERMILK, DRIED	735	CHEESE, PARMESAN, SHREDDED
932	WHEY, SWEET, DRIED	734	COCOA, DRY PDR, UNSWTND
920	EGG, YOLK, DRIED	734	OAT BRAN, RAW
914	ALMOND MEAL, PART DEFATTED, WO/SALT	733	BABYFOOD, CRL, OATMEAL, W/HONEY, DRY
913	PANCAKES, BUCKWHEAT, DRY MIX, INCOMPLETE	728	COCOA, DRY PDR, UNSWTND, PROC W/ALKALI
900	COCOA MIX, NESTLE, CARNATION NO SUGAR HOT COCOA MIX	518	CHIVES, FREEZE-DRIED
893	COCOA MIX, W/ASPRT, PDR, WO/ CA OR P, W/ NA & VIT A	518	ALMOND BUTTER, HONEY & CINN, WO/SALT

Table 14.11. Foodstuff with high **Sodium** contents.

Sodium, mgm/100 gm	Description	Sodium, mgm/100 gm	Description
38758	SALT, TABLE	4980	SOUP, CRM OF ASPARAGUS, DEHYD, DRY MIX
27360	LEAVENING AGENTS, BAKING SODA	4843	GRAVY, BROWN, DRY
26200	SOUP, CONSOMME W/GELATIN, DEHYD, DRY	4825	SAUCE, CUSTOM FOODS, SUPERB INST CHEDDAR CHS SAU MIX, DRY
26050	DESSERTS, RENNIN, TABLETS, UNSWTND	4681	SOUP, MUSHROOM, DEHYD, DRY
24000	SOUP, BEEF BROTH, CUBED, DRY	4620	SOUP, MINESTRONE, DEHYD, DRY
18623	GRAVY, CUSTOM FOODS, RED LABEL AU JUS BASE, DRY	4605	GRAVY, CUSTOM FOODS, SUPERB INST CHICK GRAVY MIX, DRY
18586	SOUP, CHICK BROTH OR BOUILLON, DEHYD, DRY	4450	SOUP, CAULIFLOWER, DEHYD, DRY MIX
16982	SOUP, BF BROTH OR BOUILLON, PDR, DRY	4392	GRAVY, TURKEY, DRY
13300	GRAVY, NESTLE, TRIO AU JUS GRAVY MIX, DRY	4363	GRAVY, NESTLE, TRIO BROWN GRAVY MIX, DRY
11063	GRAVY, CUSTOM FOODS, SUPERB INST AU JUS MIX, DRY	4186	GRAVY, ONION, DEHYD, DRY
10600	LEAVENING AGENTS, BAKING PDR, DOUBLE-ACTING, NA AL SULFATE	4152	GRAVY, CHICKEN, DRY
10400	SAUCE, TERIYAKI, DEHYD, DRY	4110	SAUCE, CHS, DEHYD, DRY
9420	SAUCE, SPAGHETTI W/MUSHROOMS, DEHYD, DRY	4090	GRAVY, CUSTOM FOODS, SUPERB INST TURKEY GRAVY MIX, DRY
8957	SOUP, ONION MIX, DEHYD, DRY FORM	4080	SAUCE, CURRY, DEHYD, DRY
8480	SAUCE, SPAGHETTI, DEHYD, DRY	4050	SAUCE, STROGANOFF, DEHYD, DRY
8408	SOUP, BF NOODLE MIX, DEHYD, DRY FORM	3833	SAUCE, TERIYAKI, RTS
8391	SOUP, CHICK NOODLE MIX, DEHYD, DRY FORM	3780	EGG, YOLK, RAW, FRZ, SALTED
7893	LEAVENING AGENTS, BAKING PDR, DOUBLE-ACTING, STRAIGHT PO4	3668	ANCHOVY, EUROPEAN, CND IN OIL, DRND SOL
7720	SAUCE, FISH, READY-TO-SERVE	3650	SAUCE, HOLLANDAISE, W/BUTTER FAT, DEHYD, DRY
7070	SOUP, CLAM CHOWDER, MANHATTAN STYLE, DEHYD, DRY	3647	MISO
7027	COD, ATLANTIC, DRIED & SALTED	3566	GRAVY, NESTLE, TRIO SUPREME CHICK GRAVY MIX, DRY
6722	SOUP, TOMATO VEG MIX, DEHYD, DRY FORM	3471	BEEF, CURED, DRIED BEEF
6580	GRAVY, MUSHROOM, DEHYD, DRY	3410	SAUCE, WHITE, DEHYD, DRY
6460	SOUP, OXTAIL, DEHYD, DRY	3390	SAUCE, BEARNAISE, DEHYD, DRY
6460	SOUP, VEG BF, DEHYD, DRY	3387	GRAVY, NESTLE, TRIO TURKEY GRAVY MIX, DRY
6416	SAUCE, CUSTOM FOODS, RED LABEL ALLPURP ITALIAN SAU MIX, DRY	3333	SOY SAU MADE FROM SOY & WHEAT (SHOYU), LO NA
6230	SAUCE, MUSHROOM, DEHYD, DRY	3319	SOUP, TOMATO, DEHYD, DRY
6048	SOUP, CHICK RICE MIX, DEHYD, DRY FORM	3283	SOUP, CLAM CHOWDER, NEW ENGLAND, DEHYD, DRY
5730	GRAVY, UNSPEC TYPE, DRY	3275	SOUP, BEAN W/BACON, DEHYD, DRY MIX
5715	SOY SAU MADE FROM SOY & WHEAT (SHOYU)	3263	SOUP, PEA, GRN, MIX, DEHYD, DRY FORM
5698	SOUP, CHICK VEG, DEHYD, DRY	2873	TOFU, SALTED & FERMENTED (FUYU)
5689	SOY SAU MADE FROM HYDROLYZED VEG PROT	2873	TOFU, SALTED & FERMENTED (FUYU), PREP W/CA SULFATE
5586	SOY SAU MADE FROM SOY (TAMARI)	2853	GRAPE LEAVES, CND
5356	GRAVY, PORK, DRY	2820	SAUCE, NESTLE, TRIO NACHO CHS SAU MIX, DRY
5053	GRAVY, CUSTOM FOODS, SUPERB INST BROWN GRAVY MIX, DRY	2751	DESSERTS, GELATINS, DRY MIX, RED CAL, W/ASPRT, P, K, NA, VIT C
5000	GRAVY, NESTLE, TRIO SUPREME BROWN GRAVY MIX, DRY	2733	SAUCE, OYSTER, RTS

Table 14.12. Foodstuff with high **Potassium** contents.

Potassium, mgm/100 gm	Description	Potassium, mgm/100 gm	Description
16500	LEAVENING AGENTS, CRM OF TARTAR	1921	COCOA MIX, NESTLE, CARNATION NO SUGAR HOT COCOA MIX
10100	LEAVENING AGENTS, BAKING PDR, LOW-SODIUM	1916	CHILI POWDER
6596	TEA, INST, UNSWTND, PDR	1902	MEAT EXTENDER
6300	PARSLEY, FREEZE-DRIED	1870	PEPPERS, HOT CHILE, SUN-DRIED
5075	COCOA, DRY PDR, UNSWTND, HERSHEY, HERSHEY'S EUROPEAN STYLE COCOA	1869	COTTONSEED MEAL, PART DEFATTED (GLANDLESS)
4740	CHERVIL, DRIED	1850	APRICOTS, DEHYD (LOW-MOISTURE), SULFURED, UNCKD
4466	CORIANDER LEAF, DRIED	1848	POTATOES, MSHD, DEHYD, GRANULES W/MILK, DRY FORM
3805	PARSLEY, DRIED	1840	COFFEE SUB, CRL GRAIN BEV, PDR
3535	COFFEE, INST, REG, PDR	1797	SOYBEANS, MATURE SEEDS, RAW
3494	RADISHES, ORIENTAL, DRIED	1795	BEANS, WHITE, MATURE SEEDS, RAW
3453	TEA, INST, UNSWTND, LEMON-FLAVORED, PDR	1794	MILK, DRY, NONFAT, REG, WO/ VIT A
3433	BASIL, GROUND	1788	CUMIN SEED
3427	TOMATOES, SUN-DRIED	1772	COTTONSEED FLR, PART DEFATTED (GLANDLESS)
3308	DILL WEED, DRIED	1761	COTTONSEED FLR, LOFAT (GLANDLESS)
3170	PEPPERS, SWT, GRN, FREEZE-DRIED	1744	POTATO CHIPS, LIGHT
3020	TARRAGON, GROUND	1724	SAFFRON
2960	CHIVES, FREEZE-DRIED	1724	LIMA BNS, LRG, MATURE SEEDS, RAW
2702	COCOA MIX, W/ASPRT, PDR, WO/CA OR P, W/NA & VIT A	1694	FENNEL SEED
2570	SOY FLOUR, LOW-FAT	1669	OREGANO, GROUND
2550	TEA, INST, SWTND W/NA SACCHARIN, LEMON-FLAVORED, PDR	1650	SHALLOTS, FREEZE-DRIED
2525	TURMERIC, GROUND	1622	ONIONS, DEHYDRATED FLAKES
2515	SOY FLOUR, FULL-FAT, RAW	1582	KANPYO, (DRIED GOURD STRIPS)
2492	MOLASSES, BLACKSTRAP	1565	TOMATOES, SUN-DRIED, PACKED IN OIL, DRND
2490	SOY MEAL, DEFATTED, RAW	1543	CURRY POWDER
2411	PEPPER, ANCHO, DRIED	1542	BEANS, SML WHITE, MATURE SEEDS, RAW
2400	LEEKS, (BULB & LOWER-LEAF PORTION), FREEZE-DRIED	1534	MUSHROOMS, SHIITAKE, DRIED
2384	SOY FLOUR, DEFATTED	1530	SOUP, MINESTRONE, DEHYD, DRY
2222	PEPPERS, PASILLA, DRIED	1528	POTATO CHIPS, CHEESE-FLAVOR
2130	SISYMBRIUM SP. SEEDS, WHL, DRIED	1524	COCOA, DRY PDR, UNSWTND
2080	WHEY, SWEET, DRIED	1522	MARJORAM, DRIED
2014	PEPPER, RED OR CAYENNE	1464	BEANS, PINK, MATURE SEEDS, RAW
2011	BREADNUTTREE SEEDS, DRIED	1464	MOLASSES
2000	LEAVENING AGENTS, YEAST, BAKER'S, ACTIVE DRY	1458	COD, ATLANTIC, DRIED & SALTED
1985	DESSERTS, GELATINS, DRY MIX, RED CAL, W/ASPRT, P, K, NA, VIT C	1441	ANISE SEED
1927	TOMATO POWDER	1409	CHEESE, GJETOST
1924	SPEARMINT, DRIED	1406	BEANS, KIDNEY, ALL TYPES, MATURE SEEDS, RAW

Table 14.13. Foodstuff with high **Vitamin B-6** contents.

Potassium, mgm/100 gm	Description	Potassium, mgm/100 gm	Description
7	CEREALS RTE, KELLOGG, KELLOGG'S PRODUCT 19	2	CEREALS RTE, FRSTD RICE KRINKLES, (RICE)
7	CEREALS RTE, GENERAL MILLS, TOTAL	2	CEREALS RTE, HONEYBRAN, (WHEAT)
		2	CEREALS RTE, RICE CHEX, (RICE)
6	BABYFOOD, COOKIES	2	CEREALS RTE, SUGAR SPARKLED FLAKES, (CORN)
4	MALTED MILK-FLAVOR MIX, CHOC, ADDED NUTR, PDR	2	CEREALS RTE, WAFFELOS, (WHEAT W/OTHER GRAINS)
4	PEPPERS, PASILLA, DRIED	2	CEREALS RTE, WHEAT CHEX, (WHEAT)
4	RICE BRAN, CRUDE	2	CEREALS RTE, KELLOGG, KELLOGG'S COMPLETE WHEAT BRAN FLAKES
4	CEREALS RTE, GENERAL MILLS, TOTAL RAISIN BRAN	2	CEREALS RTE, KELLOGG, KELLOGG'S FROOT LOOPS
4	MALTED MILK-FLAVOR MIX, NAT, ADDED NUTR, PDR	2	CEREALS RTE, KELLOGG, KELLOGG'S RICE KRISPIES
4	PEPPER, ANCHO, DRIED	2	CEREALS RTE, KELLOGG, KELLOGG'S CORN POPS
3	CEREALS RTE, 100% BRAN, (WHEAT BRAN, BARLEY)	2	CEREALS RTE, KELLOGG, KELLOGG'S APPLE-CINNAMON RICE KRISPIES
3	GARLIC POWDER	2	CEREALS RTE, KELLOGG, TEMPTATIONS, HONEY RSTD PECAN
3	CEREALS, OATS, INST, FORT, PLN, DRY, (OATS)	2	CEREALS RTE, KELLOGG, KELLOGG'S CINN MINI BUNS
3	SPEARMINT, DRIED	2	CEREALS RTE, KELLOGG, KELLOGG'S COMMON SENSE OAT BRAN FLAKES
2	CEREALS RTE, CRISPY RICE, (RICE)	2	CEREALS RTE, KELLOGG, KELLOGG'S CRISPIX
2	CEREALS RTE, KELLOGG, KELLOGG'S SPL K	2	CEREALS RTE, KELLOGG, KELLOGG'S DOUBLE DIP CRUNCH
2	PEPPERS, SWT, GRN, FREEZE-DRIED	2	CEREALS RTE, KELLOGG, KELLOGG'S RICE KRISPIES TREATS CRL
2	CEREALS, MAYPO, DRY, (OATS W/OTHER GRAINS)	2	CEREALS RTE, KELLOGG, KELLOGG'S NUTRI-GRAIN WHEAT
2	CHIVES, FREEZE-DRIED	2	CEREALS RTE, KELLOGG, KELLOGG'S HONEY CRUNCH CORN FLAKES
2	CEREALS RTE, QUAKER, CAP'N CRUNCH'S CRUNCHBERRIES	2	CEREALS RTE, QUAKER, KING VITAMAN
2	CEREALS RTE, KELLOGG, KELLOGG'S FRSTD KRISPIES	2	SHALLOTS, FREEZE-DRIED
2	CEREALS RTE, KELLOGG, KELLOGG'S SMACKS	2	CEREALS RTE, GENERAL MILLS, KIX
2	CEREALS RTE, KELLOGG, TEMPTATIONS, FRENCH VANILLA ALMOND	2	CHEX MIX
2	CEREALS, RTE, KELLOGG, KELLOGG'S ALL-BRAN W/EX FIBER	2	LEAVENING AGENTS, YEAST, BAKER'S, ACTIVE DRY
2	CEREALS RTE, QUAKER, SWT CRUNCH/QUISP	2	CEREALS RTE, KELLOGG, POP-TARTS CRUNCH FRSTD STRAWBERRY
2	CHILI POWDER	2	CEREALS, QUAKER, OATMEAL, INST, LO NA, DRY
2	CEREALS RTE, QUAKER, CAP'N CRUNCH	1	CRACKERS, CHS, SANDWICH-TYPE W/PNUT BUTTER FILLING
2	CEREALS RTE, QUAKER, CAP'N CRUNCH'S PNUT BUTTER CRUNCH	1	DILL WEED, DRIED
2	CEREALS RTE, QUAKER, QUAKER CRUNCHY BRAN	1	CEREALS, QUAKER, OATMEAL, MICROWAVE, QUICK 'N HEARTY, REG FLAVOR
2	CEREALS RTE, QUAKER, HONEY GRAHAM	1	BEEF, VAR MEATS & BY-PRODUCTS, LIVER, CKD, PAN-FRIED
2	TURMERIC, GROUND	1	CEREALS, CRM OF WHEAT, MIX'N EAT, APPL, BANANA & MAPLE FLAV, DRY
2	CEREALS RTE, BRAN CHEX, (WHEAT BRAN, CORN)	1	SNACKS, KELLOGG, KELLOGG'S NUTRI-GRAIN CRL BARS, FRUIT

Table 14.14. Foodstuff with high **Vitamin C** contents.

Vitamin C mgm/100 gm	Description	Vitamin C mgm/100 gm	Description
1900	PEPPERS, SWT, GRN, FREEZE-DRIED	122	PARSLEY, DRIED
1900	PEPPERS, SWT, RED, FREEZE-DRIED	122	FRUIT PUNCH-FLAVOR DRK, PDR, W/ NA
1678	ACEROLA, (WEST INDIAN CHERRY), RAW	122	FRUIT PUNCH-FLAVOR DRK, PDR, WO/ NA
1600	ACEROLA JUICE, RAW	120	KALE, RAW
660	CHIVES, FREEZE-DRIED	120	GRAPEFRUIT JUC, FRZ CONC, UNSWTND, UNDIL
567	CORIANDER LEAF, DRIED	118	LEEKS, (BULB & LOWER-LEAF PORTION), FREEZE-DRIED
490	DESSERTS, GELATINS, DRY MIX, RED CAL, W/ASPRT, P, K, NA, VIT C	117	TOMATO POWDER
394	LEMONADE, LO CAL, W/ASPRT, PDR	117	LEMONADE-FLAVOR DRK, PDR
289	GELATIN, DRINKING, ORANGE-FLAVOR, PDR	113	BABYFOOD, FRUIT, PAPAYA & APPLSAUC W/TAPIOCA, STR
243	ORANGE-FLAVOR DRK, BRKFST TYPE, W/PULP, FRZ CONC	102	VINESPINACH, (BASELLA), RAW
243	PEPPERS, HOT CHILI, GRN, RAW	102	TOMATOES, SUN-DRIED, PACKED IN OIL, DRND
243	PEPPERS, HOT CHILI, RED, RAW	100	TEA, INST, SWTND W/SUGAR, LEMON-FLAVORED, W/ VIT C, PDR
240	ORANGE-FLAVOR DRK, BRKFST TYPE, PDR	98	KIWI FRUIT, (CHINESE GOOSEBERRIES), FRSH, RAW
200	CEREALS RTE, KELLOGG, KELLOGG'S PRODUCT 19	97	HORSERADISH-TREE, PODS, CKD, BLD, DRND, WO/SALT
200	CEREALS RTE, GENERAL MILLS, TOTAL	97	HORSERADISH-TREE, PODS, CKD, BLD, DRND, W/SALT
200	CEREALS RTE, GENERAL MILLS, TOTAL CORN FLAKES	96	TARO, TAHITIAN, RAW
190	PEPPERS, SWEET, RED, RAW	95	CITRUS FRUIT JUC DRK, FRZ CONC
190	ORANGE DRK, BRKFST TYPE, W/JUC & PULP, FRZ CONC	95	CEREALS RTE, 100% BRAN, (WHEAT BRAN, BARLEY)
184	GUAVAS, COMMON, RAW	94	PEACHES, FRZ, SLICED, SWTND
184	PEPPERS, SWEET, YELLOW, RAW	93	BROCCOLI, RAW
183	LITCHIS, DRIED	93	BROCCOLI, LEAVES, RAW
181	CURRANTS, EUROPEAN BLACK, RAW	93	BROCCOLI, FLOWER CLUSTERS, RAW
171	PEPPERS, SWT, RED, CKD, BLD, engl, WO/SALT	93	BROCCOLI, STALKS, RAW
171	PEPPERS, SWT, RED, CKD, BLD, DRND, W/SALT	93	PEPPERS, HUNGARIAN, RAW
160	THYME, FRESH	89	PEPPERS, SWEET, GREEN, RAW
156	FRUIT PUNCH DRK, FRZ CONC	89	APPLE JUC, FRZ CONC, UNSWTND, UNDIL, W/ VIT C
150	MALTED MILK-FLAVOR MIX, CHOC, ADDED NUTR, PDR	88	CAULIFLOWER, GREEN, RAW
149	PARSLEY, FREEZE-DRIED	88	BALSAM-PEAR (BITTER GOURD), LEAFY TIPS, RAW
146	GUAVA SAUCE, COOKED	86	BABYFOOD, JUC, ORANGE & APRICOT
141	HORSERADISH-TREE, PODS, RAW	85	TANGERINE JUC, FRZ CONC, SWTND, UNDIL
138	ORANGE JUC, FRZ CONC, UNSWTND, UNDIL	85	DILL WEED, FRESH
136	ORANGE PEEL, RAW	85	BRUSSELS SPROUTS, RAW

Table 14.15. Foodstuff with high **Folate** contents.

Folate, mcg/100 gm	Description	Folate, mcg/100 gm	Description
2340	LEAVENING AGENTS, YEAST, BAKER'S, ACTIVE DRY	400	LIMA BNS, THIN SEEDED (BABY), MATURE SEEDS, RAW
1535	PARSLEY, FREEZE-DRIED	400	CEREALS RTE, KELLOGG, KELLOGG'S FRSTD KRISPIES
1333	CEREALS RTE, GENERAL MILLS, TOTAL	400	LAMB, VAR MEATS & BY-PRODUCTS, LIVER, CKD, PAN-FRIED
1333	CEREALS RTE, GENERAL MILLS, TOTAL CORN FLAKES	399	BEANS, FRENCH, MATURE SEEDS, RAW
1300	CEREALS RTE, KELLOGG, KELLOGG'S PRODUCT 19	395	LIMA BNS, LRG, MATURE SEEDS, RAW
785	LEAVENING AGENTS, YEAST, BAKER'S, COMPRESSED	394	BEANS, KIDNEY, ALL TYPES, MATURE SEEDS, RAW
770	CHICKEN, LIVER, ALL CLASSES, CKD, SIMMRD	394	CHICKEN, CAPONS, GIBLETS, RAW
759	VEAL, VAR MEATS & BY-PRODUCTS, LIVER, CKD, BRSD	393	BEANS, KIDNEY, ROYAL RED, MATURE SEEDS, RAW
738	CHICKEN, LIVER, ALL CLASSES, RAW	385	CEREALS RTE, QUAKER, CAP'N CRUNCH'S CRUNCHBERRIES
738	DUCK, DOMESTICATED, LIVER, RAW	379	CHICKEN, BROILERS OR FRYERS, GIBLETS, CKD, FRIED
738	GOOSE, LIVER, RAW	377	CEREALS RTE, QUAKER, SWT CRUNCH/QUISP
738	TURKEY, LIVER, ALL CLASSES, RAW	376	CHICKEN, BROILERS OR FRYERS, GIBLETS, CKD, SIMMRD
727	CEREALS RTE, GENERAL MILLS, TOTAL RAISIN BRAN	375	SOYBEANS, MATURE SEEDS, RAW
666	TURKEY, LIVER, ALL CLASSES, CKD, SIMMRD	372	CEREALS RTE, QUAKER, HONEY GRAHAM
658	YARDLONG BNS, MATURE SEEDS, RAW	371	CEREALS RTE, QUAKER, CAP'N CRUNCH
649	MOTHBEANS, MATURE SEEDS, RAW	367	CHICKEN, STEWING, GIBLETS, CKD, SIMMRD
642	VEAL, VAR MEATS & BY-PRODUCTS, LIVER, RAW	366	LEEKS, (BULB & LOWER-LEAF PORTION), FREEZE-DRIED
639	COWPEAS, CATJANG, MATURE SEEDS, RAW	365	CEREALS, OATS, INST, FORT, W/BRAN & RAISINS, DRY, (OATS, WHEAT BRAN)
633	COWPEAS, COMMON (BLACKEYES, CROWDER, SOUTHERN), MTRE SEEDS, RAW	357	CEREALS, CRM OF WHEAT, INST, DRY, (WHEAT)
625	MUNG BNS, MATURE SEEDS, RAW	355	LUPINS, MATURE SEEDS, RAW
622	BEANS, ADZUKI, MATURE SEEDS, RAW	345	TURKEY, ALL CLASSES, GIBLETS, CKD, SIMMRD, SOME GIBLET FAT
604	BEANS, CRANBERRY (ROMAN), MATURE SEEDS, RAW	345	SOY FLOUR, FULL-FAT, RAW
580	SEAWEED, AGAR, DRIED	345	SOY FLR, FULL-FAT, RAW, CRUDE PROT BASIS (N X 6.25)
557	CHICKPEAS (GARBANZO BNS, BENGAL GM), MATURE SEEDS, RAW	342	TURKEY, ALL CLASSES, GIBLETS, RAW
531	CEREALS, OATS, INST, FORT, PLN, DRY, (OATS)	340	SOY PROT CONC, PRODUCED BY ALCOHOL EXTRACTION
530	SPEARMINT, DRIED	340	SOY PROT CONC, PRODUCED BY ACID WASH
506	BEANS, PINTO, MATURE SEEDS, RAW	340	SOY PROT CONC, CRUDE PROT BASIS (N X 6.25), ACID WASH
494	CEREALS RTE, CRISPY RICE, (RICE)	338	ARROWROOT, RAW
482	BEANS, GREAT NORTHERN, MATURE SEEDS, RAW	321	PATE, CHICKEN LIVER, CANNED
463	BEANS, PINK, MATURE SEEDS, RAW	320	VEAL, VAR MEATS & BY-PRODUCTS, LIVER, CKD, PAN-FRIED
456	PIGEON PEAS (RED GM), MATURE SEEDS, RAW	305	SOY FLOUR, DEFATTED
444	BEANS, BLACK, MATURE SEEDS, RAW	305	SOY FLR, DEFATTED, CRUDE PROT BASIS (N X 6.25)

HEALTH AND FITNESS

Table 14.16. Foodstuff with high **Vitamin B$_{12}$** contents.

Vitamin B12, mcg/100 gm	Description	Vitamin B12, mcg/100 gm	Description
112	BEEF, VAR MEATS & BY-PRODUCTS, LIVER, CKD, PAN-FRIED	23	SOUP, CLAM CHOWDER, MANHATTAN STYLE, DEHYD, DRY
99	CLAM, MXD SP, CKD, MOIST HEAT	23	CHICKEN, LIVER, ALL CLASSES, RAW
99	CLAM, MXD SP, CND, DRND SOL	21	VEAL, VAR MEATS & BY-PRODUCTS, BRAIN, CKD, PAN-FRIED
90	LAMB, VAR MEATS & BY-PRODUCTS, LIVER, RAW	20	BRAUNSCHWEIGER (A LIVER SAUSAGE), PORK
86	LAMB, VAR MEATS & BY-PRODUCTS, LIVER, CKD, PAN-FRIED	20	CEREALS RTE, KELLOGG, KELLOGG'S PRODUCT 19
79	LAMB, VAR MEATS & BY-PRODUCTS, KIDNEYS, CKD, BRSD	20	CAVIAR, BLACK & RED, GRANULAR
77	LAMB, VAR MEATS & BY-PRODUCTS, LIVER, CKD, BRSD	20	OCTOPUS, COMMON, RAW
71	BEEF, VAR MEATS & BY-PRODUCTS, LIVER, CKD, BRSD	19	OYSTER, EASTERN, WILD, RAW
69	BEEF, VAR MEATS & BY-PRODUCTS, LIVER, RAW	19	CHICKEN, LIVER, ALL CLASSES, CKD, SIMMRD
64	VEAL, VAR MEATS & BY-PRODUCTS, LIVER, CKD, PAN-FRIED	19	OYSTER, EASTERN, CANNED
63	TURKEY, LIVER, ALL CLASSES, RAW	19	MACKEREL, ATLANTIC, CKD, DRY HEAT
54	DUCK, DOMESTICATED, LIVER, RAW	19	OSCAR MAYER, BRAUNSCHWEIGER LIVER SAUSAGE (SLICED)
54	GOOSE, LIVER, RAW	19	HERRING, ATLANTIC, KIPPERED
52	LAMB, VAR MEATS & BY-PRODUCTS, KIDNEYS, RAW	19	PORK, FRSH, VAR MEATS & BY-PRODUCTS, LIVER, CKD, BRSD
51	BEEF, VAR MEATS & BY-PRODUCTS, KIDNEYS, CKD, SIMMRD	19	OSCAR MAYER, BRAUNSCHWEIGER LIVER SAUSAGE (SAREN TUBE)
49	CLAM, MIXED SPECIES, RAW	18	WHELK, UNSPEC, CKD, MOIST HEAT
48	TURKEY, LIVER, ALL CLASSES, CKD, SIMMRD	18	MACKEREL, KING, CKD, DRY HEAT
47	VEAL, VAR MEATS & BY-PRODUCTS, LIVER, RAW	17	VEAL, VAR MEATS & BY-PRODUCTS, PANCREAS, CKD, BRSD
40	CLAM, MXD SP, CKD, BREADED & FRIED	17	PORK, FRSH, VAR MEATS & BY-PRODUCTS, PANCREAS, CKD, BRSD
39	SOUP, CLAM CHOWDER, NEW ENGLAND, DEHYD, DRY	17	BEEF, VAR MEATS & BY-PRODUCTS, PANCREAS, CKD, BRSD
37	VEAL, VAR MEATS & BY-PRODUCTS, KIDNEYS, CKD, BRSD	16	PORK, FRSH, VAR MEATS & BY-PRODUCTS, PANCREAS, RAW
37	VEAL, VAR MEATS & BY-PRODUCTS, LIVER, CKD, BRSD	16	OYSTER, EASTERN, FARMED, RAW
36	OCTOPUS, COMMON, CKD, MOIST HEAT	16	OYSTER, PACIFIC, RAW
35	OYSTER, EASTERN, WILD, CKD, MOIST HEAT	16	OYSTER, EASTERN, CKD, BREADED & FRIED
31	CLAM & TOMATO JUC, CND	16	MACKEREL, KING, RAW
29	OYSTER, PACIFIC, CKD, MOIST HEAT	15	BEEF, VAR MEATS & BY-PRODUCTS, BRAIN, CKD, PAN-FRIED
28	TURKEY, ALL CLASSES, GIBLETS, RAW	14	VEAL, VAR MEATS & BY-PRODUCTS, HEART, CKD, BRSD
28	VEAL, VAR MEATS & BY-PRODUCTS, KIDNEYS, RAW	14	BEEF, VAR MEATS & BY-PRODUCTS, HEART, CKD, SIMMRD
28	OYSTER, EASTERN, WILD, CKD, DRY HEAT	14	BEEF, VAR MEATS & BY-PRODUCTS, PANCREAS, RAW
27	CEREALS RTE, GENERAL MILLS, TOTAL CORN FLAKES	14	VEAL, VAR MEATS & BY-PRODUCTS, HEART, RAW
27	BEEF, VAR MEATS & BY-PRODUCTS, KIDNEYS, RAW	14	HERRING, ATLANTIC, RAW
26	PORK, FRSH, VAR MEATS & BY-PRODUCTS, LIVER, RAW	14	BEEF, VAR MEATS & BY-PRODUCTS, HEART, RAW

Table 14.17. Foodstuff with high **Niacin** contents.

Niacin, mgm/100 gm	Description	Niacin, mgm/100 gm	Description
67	CEREALS RTE, GENERAL MILLS, TOTAL	14	SNACKS, KELLOGG, KELLOGG'S NUTRI-GRAIN CRL BARS, FRUIT
51	MALTED MILK-FLAVOR MIX, CHOC, ADDED NUTR, PDR	13	PEANUT BUTTER, SMOOTH STYLE, W/SALT
49	MALTED MILK-FLAVOR MIX, NAT, ADDED NUTR, PDR	13	SESAME FLOUR, HIGH-FAT
40	LEAVENING AGENTS, YEAST, BAKER'S, ACTIVE DRY	13	CHICKEN, BROILERS OR FRYERS, LT MEAT, MEAT ONLY, CKD, FRIED
36	CEREALS RTE, GENERAL MILLS, TOTAL RAISIN BRAN	13	TUNA, LT, CND IN H2O, DRND SOL
36	BABYFOOD, CRL, OATMEAL, W/HONEY, DRY	13	CEREALS RTE, RAISIN BRAN, RALSTON PURINA, (WHEAT)
34	BABYFOOD, CRL, HI PROT, DRY	13	CEREALS RTE, HEALTHY CHOIC, KELLOGG'S TSTD BROWN SUGAR SQUARES
34	RICE BRAN, CRUDE	13	PEANUTS, VALENCIA, RAW
34	CHOCOLATE SYRUP, W/ADDED NUTR	13	SEAWEED, SPIRULINA, DRIED
32	CEREALS RTE, 100% BRAN, (WHEAT BRAN, BARLEY)	13	SESAME MEAL, PART DEFATTED
31	BABYFOOD, CEREAL, RICE, DRY	13	BEEF, VAR MEATS & BY-PRODUCTS, LIVER, RAW
22	MEAT EXTENDER	13	CHICKEN, BROILERS OR FRYERS, BREAST, MEAT & SKN, CKD, RSTD
20	ANCHOVY, EUROPEAN, CND IN OIL, DRND SOL	13	VEAL, LEG (TOP RND), LN, CKD, PAN-FRIED, NOT BREADED
19	TUNA, SKIPJACK, FRSH, CKD, DRY HEAT	13	TEA, INST, UNSWTND, PDR
19	CEREALS RTE, QUAKER, HONEY GRAHAM	13	SESAME FLOUR, LOW-FAT
19	CEREALS RTE, QUAKER, CAP'N CRUNCH	12	CHICKEN, BROILERS OR FRYERS, LT MEAT, MEAT ONLY, CKD, RSTD
17	VEAL, VAR MEATS & BY-PRODUCTS, LIVER, CKD, PAN-FRIED	12	TUNA, LT, CND IN OIL, DRND SOL
16	PEANUTS, SPANISH, RAW	12	LEAVENING AGENTS, YEAST, BAKER'S, COMPRESSED
15	TUNA, FRESH, SKIPJACK, RAW	12	LAMB, VAR MEATS & BY-PRODUCTS, LIVER, CKD, BRSD
15	PAPRIKA	12	CEREALS RTE, HEALTHY CHOIC, KELLOGG'S ALMOND CRUNCH W/RAISINS
15	PORK, FRSH, VAR MEATS & BY-PRODUCTS, LIVER, RAW	12	TUNA, WHITE, CND IN OIL, WO/SALT, DRND SOL
15	CEREALS RTE, KELLOGG, POP-TARTS CRUNCH FRSTD STRAWBERRY	11	PEANUT FLOUR, LOW FAT
15	CEREALS, QUAKER, OATMEAL, INST, LO NA, DRY	11	CEREALS, QUAKER, OATMEAL, INST, RAISINS, DATES & WALNUTS, DRY
14	ANCHOVY, EUROPEAN, RAW	11	SAUSAGE, MEATLESS
14	CHICKEN, BROILERS OR FRYERS, BREAST, MEAT & SKN, CKD, FRIED, FLR	11	CHICKEN, BROILERS OR FRYERS, BREAST, MEAT ONLY, RAW
14	CHICKEN, BROILERS OR FRYERS, BREAST, MEAT ONLY, CKD, RSTD	11	CHICKEN, BROILERS OR FRYERS, LT MEAT, MEAT & SKN, CKD, RSTD
14	PEANUT BUTTER, CHUNK STYLE, W/SALT	11	STURGEON, MXD SP, SMOKED
14	PEANUT BUTTER, CHUNK STYLE, WO/SALT	11	SOUP, CRM OF CHICK, DEHYD, DRY
14	WHEAT BRAN, CRUDE	11	CHICKEN, BROILERS OR FRYERS, GIBLETS, CKD, FRIED
14	ANCHOVY, EUROPEAN, RAW	11	VEAL, LEG (TOP RND), LN, CKD, PAN-FRIED, BREADED
14	CHICKEN, BROILERS OR FRYERS, BREAST, MEAT & SKN, CKD, FRIED, FLR	11	SHAD, AMERICAN, CKD, DRY HEAT
14	PEANUTS, ALL TYPES, DRY-ROASTED, WO/SALT	11	BEEF, VAR MEATS & BY-PRODUCTS, LIVER, CKD, BRSD

HEALTH AND FITNESS

Table 14.18. Foodstuff with high **Thiamin** contents.

Thiamin, mg/100 gm	Description	Thiamin, mg/100 gm	Description
14	WORTHINGTON FOODS, MORNINGSTAR FARMS BRKFST PATTIES	2	LEAVENING AGENTS, YEAST, BAKER'S, COMPRESSED
10	WORTHINGTON FOODS, MORNINGSTAR FARMS, SPICY BLACK BEAN BURGER	2	CEREALS, OATS, INST, FORT, PLN, DRY, (OATS)
10	WORTHINGTON FOODS, MORNINGSTAR FARMS GARDEN VEGE PATTIES, FRZ	2	CEREALS RTE, CRISPY RICE, (RICE)
9	WORTHINGTON FOODS, MORNINGSTAR FARMS "BURGER"CRUMBLES	2	SAUCE, STROGANOFF, DEHYD, DRY
5	SOUP, CRM OF VEG, DEHYD, DRY	2	CEREALS RTE, HEALTHY CHOIC FROM KELLOGG'S MULTI-GRAIN FLAKES
5	CEREALS RTE, KELLOGG, KELLOGG'S PRODUCT 19	2	CEREALS RTE, KELLOGG, KELLOGG'S SPL K
5	CEREALS RTE, GENERAL MILLS, TOTAL	2	CEREALS RTE, WHEAT GERM, TSTD, PLN, (WHEAT GERM)
5	CEREALS RTE, GENERAL MILLS, TOTAL CORN FLAKES	2	CEREALS, MAYPO, DRY, (OATS W/OTHER GRAINS)
4	BACON, MEATLESS	2	SESAME BUTTER, TAHINI, FROM UNROASTED KRNLS
4	BABYFOOD, CRL, RICE, W/BANANAS, DRY	2	CHEX MIX
4	BABYFOOD, CRL, HI PROT, W/APPL & ORANGE, DRY	1	BABYFOOD, COOKIES
4	BABYFOOD, CRL, MXD, W/BANANAS, DRY	1	CEREALS RTE, QUAKER, CAP'N CRUNCH'S CRUNCHBERRIES
4	BABYFOOD, CRL, OATMEAL, W/BANANAS, DRY	1	CORN FLOUR, MASA, ENRICHED
3	SUNFLOWER SD FLR, PART DEFATTED	1	CORN FLR, MASA, ENR, YEL
3	MALTED MILK-FLAVOR MIX, CHOC, ADDED NUTR, PDR	1	CEREALS RTE, QUAKER, SWT CRUNCH/QUISP
3	MALTED MILK-FLAVOR MIX, NAT, ADDED NUTR, PDR	1	CEREALS RTE, KELLOGG, KELLOGG'S FRSTD KRISPIES
3	BABYFOOD, CRL, OATMEAL, DRY	1	CEREALS RTE, KELLOGG, KELLOGG'S SMACKS
3	BABYFOOD, CRL, OATMEAL, W/HONEY, DRY	1	CEREALS RTE, KELLOGG, TEMPTATIONS, FRENCH VANILLA ALMOND
3	RICE BRAN, CRUDE	1	CEREALS, RTE, KELLOGG, KELLOGG'S ALL-BRAN W/EX FIBER
3	BABYFOOD, CRL, BARLEY, DRY	1	CEREALS RTE, QUAKER, CAP'N CRUNCH
3	CEREALS RTE, GENERAL MILLS, TOTAL RAISIN BRAN	1	CEREALS RTE, QUAKER, CAP'N CRUNCH'S PNUT BUTTER CRUNCH
3	SESAME FLOUR, HIGH-FAT	1	CEREALS RTE, QUAKER, HONEY GRAHAM
3	BABYFOOD, CRL, HI PROT, DRY	1	CEREALS RTE, QUAKER, KRETSCHMER HONEY CRUNCH WHEAT GERM
3	BABYFOOD, CEREAL, RICE, DRY	1	CEREALS, OATS, INST, FORT, W/BRAN & RAISINS, DRY, (OATS, WHEAT BRAN)
3	CEREALS RTE, RICE, PUFFED, FORT, (RICE)	1	CEREALS RTE, KELLOGG, KELLOGG'S ALL-BRAN
3	CEREALS RTE, WHEAT, PUFFED, FORT	1	CEREALS RTE, KELLOGG, KELLOGG'S APPL JACKS
3	SESAME MEAL, PART DEFATTED	1	CEREALS RTE, KELLOGG, KELLOGG'S ALL-BRAN BRAN BUDS
3	SESAME FLR, PART DEFATTED	1	CEREALS RTE, BRAN CHEX, (WHEAT BRAN, CORN)
3	SESAME FLOUR, LOW-FAT	1	CEREALS RTE, COOKIE-CRISP, CHOC CHIP & VANILLA
2	BABYFOOD, CEREAL, MIXED, DRY	1	CEREALS RTE, CORN CHEX, (CORN)
2	CEREALS RTE, 100% BRAN, (WHEAT BRAN, BARLEY)	1	CEREALS RTE, KELLOGG, KELLOGG'S CORN FLAKES
2	SEAWEED, SPIRULINA, DRIED	1	CEREALS RTE, KELLOGG, KELLOGG'S COMPLETE WHEAT BRAN FLAKES

Table 14.19. Foodstuff with high **Riboflavin** contents.

Riboflavin, mg/100 gm	Description	Riboflavin, mg/100 gm	Description
6	CEREALS RTE, KELLOGG, KELLOGG'S PRODUCT 19	2	OSCAR MAYER, LIVER CHS (PORK FAT WRAPPED)
6	CEREALS RTE, GENERAL MILLS, TOTAL	2	PORK, FRSH, VAR MEATS & BY-PRODUCTS, LIVER, CKD, BRSD
6	CEREALS RTE, GENERAL MILLS, TOTAL CORN FLAKES	2	TURKEY, LIVER, ALL CLASSES, RAW
5	LEAVENING AGENTS, YEAST, BAKER'S, ACTIVE DRY	2	EGG, WHITE, DRIED, FLAKES, GLUCOSE RED
5	LAMB, VAR MEATS & BY-PRODUCTS, LIVER, CKD, PAN-FRIED	2	CEREALS RTE, CRISPY RICE, (RICE)
4	BABYFOOD, CRL, HI PROT, W/APPL & ORANGE, DRY	2	LAMB, VAR MEATS & BY-PRODUCTS, KIDNEYS, CKD, BRSD
4	BEEF, VAR MEATS & BY-PRODUCTS, LIVER, CKD, PAN-FRIED	2	WHEY, ACID, DRIED
4	MALTED MILK-FLAVOR MIX, CHOC, ADDED NUTR, PDR	2	CEREALS RTE, HEALTHY CHOIC FROM KELLOGG'S MULTI-GRAIN FLAKES
4	BEEF, VAR MEATS & BY-PRODUCTS, LIVER, CKD, BRSD	2	VEAL, VAR MEATS & BY-PRODUCTS, KIDNEYS, CKD, BRSD
4	BEEF, VAR MEATS & BY-PRODUCTS, KIDNEYS, CKD, SIMMRD	2	CHICKEN, LIVER, ALL CLASSES, RAW
4	LAMB, VAR MEATS & BY-PRODUCTS, LIVER, CKD, BRSD	2	VEAL, VAR MEATS & BY-PRODUCTS, LIVER, CKD, BRSD
4	BABYFOOD, CRL, RICE, W/BANANAS, DRY	2	DAIRY DRK MIX, CHOC, RED CAL, W/ASPRT, PDR
4	BABYFOOD, CRL, OATMEAL, W/BANANAS, DRY	2	CEREALS RTE, KELLOGG, KELLOGG'S SPL K
4	SEAWEED, SPIRULINA, DRIED	2	VEAL, VAR MEATS & BY-PRODUCTS, KIDNEYS, RAW
4	LAMB, VAR MEATS & BY-PRODUCTS, LIVER, RAW	2	EGG, YOLK, DRIED
4	ORANGE DRK, BRKFST TYPE, W/JUC & PULP, FRZ CONC	2	CEREALS, MAYPO, DRY, (OATS W/OTHER GRAINS)
4	MALTED MILK-FLAVOR MIX, NAT, ADDED NUTR, PDR	2	CEREALS RTE, RICE, PUFFED, FORT, (RICE)
4	BABYFOOD, CRL, MXD, W/BANANAS, DRY	2	CEREALS RTE, WHEAT, PUFFED, FORT
3	VEAL, VAR MEATS & BY-PRODUCTS, LIVER, CKD, PAN-FRIED	2	EGG SUBSTITUTE, POWDER
3	BABYFOOD, COOKIES	2	VEAL, VAR MEATS & BY-PRODUCTS, LIVER, RAW
3	PEPPERS, PASILLA, DRIED	2	CHICKEN, LIVER, ALL CLASSES, CKD, SIMMRD
3	CEREALS RTE, GENERAL MILLS, TOTAL RAISIN BRAN	2	MILK, DRY, NONFAT, INST, W/ VIT A
3	PORK, FRSH, VAR MEATS & BY-PRODUCTS, LIVER, RAW	2	MILK, DRY, NONFAT, INST, WO/ VIT A
3	BABYFOOD, CRL, OATMEAL, W/HONEY, DRY	2	PAPRIKA
3	BEEF, VAR MEATS & BY-PRODUCTS, LIVER, RAW	2	CUTTLEFISH, MXD SP, CKD, MOIST HEAT
3	BABYFOOD, CEREAL, MIXED, DRY	2	PORK, FRSH, VAR MEATS & BY-PRODUCTS, HEART, CKD, BRSD
3	BABYFOOD, CRL, HI PROT, DRY	2	PORK, FRSH, VAR MEATS & BY-PRODUCTS, KIDNEYS, RAW
3	CEREALS RTE, 100% BRAN, (WHEAT BRAN, BARLEY)	2	ALMOND MEAL, PART DEFATTED, WO/SALT
3	BABYFOOD, CRL, BARLEY, DRY	2	ALMOND MEAL, PART DEFATTED, W/SALT
3	BABYFOOD, CRL, OATMEAL, DRY	2	MILK, DRY, NONFAT, CA RED
3	BEEF, VAR MEATS & BY-PRODUCTS, KIDNEYS, RAW	2	CEREALS RTE, QUAKER, CAP'N CRUNCH'S CRUNCHBERRIES
3	EGG, WHITE, DRIED	2	OSCAR MAYER, BRAUNSCHWEIGER LIVER SAUSAGE (SLICED)

HEALTH AND FITNESS

Table 14.20. Foodstuff with high **Vitamin A** contents.

Vitamin A, IU/100 gm	Description	Vitamin A, IU/100 gm	Description
100000	FISH OIL, COD LIVER	17702	CARROTS, FRZ, CKD, BLD, DRND, WO/SALT
77261	PEPPERS, SWT, RED, FREEZE-DRIED	17702	CARROTS, FRZ, CKD, BLD, DRND, W/SALT
68300	CHIVES, FREEZE-DRIED	17490	LIVER CHEESE, PORK
63240	PARSLEY, FREEZE-DRIED	17247	TOMATO POWDER
60604	PAPRIKA	17054	SWEETPOTATO, CKD, BLD, WO/SKN, WO/SALT
56099	SHALLOTS, FREEZE-DRIED	17054	SWEETPOTATO, CKD, BLD, WO/SKN, W/SALT
41610	PEPPER, RED OR CAYENNE	16670	OSCAR MAYER, BRAUNSCHWEIGER LIVER SAUSAGE (SAREN TUBE)
39907	DUCK, DOMESTICATED, LIVER, RAW	16410	SWEETPOTATO, FRZ, CKD, BKD, WO/SALT
36105	BEEF, VAR MEATS & BY-PRODUCTS, LIVER, CKD, PAN-FRIED	16410	SWEETPOTATO, FRZ, CKD, BKD, W/SALT
35760	PEPPERS, PASILLA, DRIED	16375	CHICKEN, LIVER, ALL CLASSES, CKD, SIMMRD
35679	BEEF, VAR MEATS & BY-PRODUCTS, LIVER, CKD, BRSD	16000	BROCCOLI, LEAVES, RAW
35346	BEEF, VAR MEATS & BY-PRODUCTS, LIVER, RAW	15728	OSCAR MAYER, BRAUNSCHWEIGER LIVER SAUSAGE (SLICED)
34927	CHILI POWDER	15126	SWEETPOTATO, CANNED, MASHED
30998	GOOSE, LIVER, RAW	15010	CARROTS, BABY, RAW
28129	CARROTS, RAW	14744	VEAL, VAR MEATS & BY-PRODUCTS, LIVER, RAW
27667	LIVER SAUSAGE, LIVERWURST, PORK	14675	CHRYSANTHEMUM, GARLAND, RAW
26993	GRAPE LEAVES, RAW	14566	CHICKEN, CAPONS, GIBLETS, RAW
26883	VEAL, VAR MEATS & BY-PRODUCTS, LIVER, CKD, BRSD	14452	BABYFOOD, CARROTS & BF, STR
26488	PEPPERS, HOT CHILE, SUN-DRIED	14051	BRAUNSCHWEIGER (A LIVER SAUSAGE), PORK
25998	LAMB, VAR MEATS & BY-PRODUCTS, LIVER, CKD, PAN-FRIED	14000	DANDELION GREENS, RAW
24945	LAMB, VAR MEATS & BY-PRODUCTS, LIVER, CKD, BRSD	13774	CARROTS, CND, REG PK, DRND SOL
24612	LAMB, VAR MEATS & BY-PRODUCTS, LIVER, RAW	13774	CARROTS, CND, NO SALT, DRND SOL
24554	CARROTS, CKD, BLD, DRND, WO/SALT	13266	CHICKEN, CAPONS, GIBLETS, CKD, SIMMRD
24554	CARROTS, CKD, BLD, DRND, W/SALT	13098	MALTED MILK-FLAVOR MIX, CHOC, ADDED NUTR, PDR
23340	PARSLEY, DRIED	12669	APRICOTS, DEHYD (LOW-MOISTURE), SULFURED, UNCKD
22604	OSCAR MAYER, LIVER CHS (PORK FAT WRAPPED)	12581	TURKEY, LIVER, ALL CLASSES, CKD, SIMMRD
22056	PUMPKIN, CND, WO/SALT	11929	CHICKEN, BROILERS OR FRYERS, GIBLETS, CKD, FRIED
22056	PUMPKIN, CANNED, WITH SALT	11892	PEPPERS, HOT CHILI, RED, CND, EXCLUDING SEEDS, SOL & LIQUIDS
21822	SWEETPOTATO, CKD, BKD IN SKN, WO/SALT	11810	BABYFOOD, VEG, CARROTS, JR
21822	SWEETPOTATO, CKD, BKD IN SKN, W/SALT	11700	DANDELION GRNS, CKD, BLD, DRND, WO/SALT
21650	PORK, FRSH, VAR MEATS & BY-PRODUCTS, LIVER, RAW	11700	DANDELION GRNS, CKD, BLD, DRND, W/SALT
21282	CARROTS, FROZEN, UNPREPARED	11647	VEGETABLES, MXD, CND, DRND SOL

Table 14.21. Foodstuff with high **Iron** contents.

Iron, Fe, mg/100 gm	Description	Iron, Fe, mg/100 gm	Description
124	THYME, GROUND	29	CEREALS, QUAKER, CORN GRITS, INST, CHEDDAR CHS FLAVOR, DRY
98	PARSLEY, DRIED	29	PEPPER, BLACK
87	SPEARMINT, DRIED	29	GRAVY, CUSTOM FOODS, SUPERB INST AU JUS MIX, DRY
83	MARJORAM, DRIED	29	SEAWEED, SPIRULINA, DRIED
67	BABYFOOD, CRL, OATMEAL, W/HONEY, DRY	28	SAGE, GROUND
66	CUMIN SEED	28	CLAM, MXD SP, CKD, MOIST HEAT
60	CEREALS RTE, KELLOGG, KELLOGG'S	20	PUMPKIN PIE SPICE
54	PARSLEY, FREEZE-DRIED	20	SAUCE, CUSTOM FOODS, RED LABEL ALLPURP ITALIAN SAU MIX, DRY
49	CEREALS RTE, RAISIN BRAN, RALSTON PURINA, (WHEAT)	19	SESAME BUTTER, PASTE
49	DILL WEED, DRIED	19	CEREALS, MAYPO, DRY, (OATS W/OTHER GRAINS)
48	BABYFOOD, CRL, BARLEY, DRY	19	PORK, FRSH, VAR MEATS & BY-PRODUCTS, LUNGS, RAW
48	BABYFOOD, CRL, HI PROT, DRY	19	RICE BRAN, CRUDE
45	CELERY SEED	19	FENNEL SEED
45	BEEF, VAR MEATS & BY-PRODUCTS, SPLEEN, RAW	18	MOLASSES, BLACKSTRAP
44	OREGANO, GROUND	17	THYME, FRESH
43	BAY LEAF, CRUMBLED	17	MALTED MILK-FLAVOR MIX, CHOC, ADDED NUTR, PDR
42	CORIANDER LEAF, DRIED	17	MALTED MILK-FLAVOR MIX, NAT, ADDED NUTR, PDR
42	BASIL, GROUND	17	LEAVENING AGENTS, YEAST, BAKER'S, ACTIVE DRY
42	COCOA, DRY PDR, UNSWTND, HERSHEY, HERSHEY'S EUROPEAN STYLE COCOA	16	PORK, FRSH, VAR MEATS & BY-PRODUCTS, LUNGS, CKD, BRSD
42	LAMB, VAR MEATS & BY-PRODUCTS, SPLEEN, RAW	16	DILL SEED
41	TURMERIC, GROUND	15	SOY PROTEIN ISOLATE
39	BEEF, VAR MEATS & BY-PRODUCTS, SPLEEN, CKD, BRSD	15	SOY PROT ISOLATE, K TYPE, CRUDE PROT BASIS
39	LAMB, VAR MEATS & BY-PRODUCTS, SPLEEN, CKD, BRSD	14	BABYFOOD, CRL, HI PROT, W/APPL & ORANGE, PREP W/WHL MILK
32	TARRAGON, GROUND	14	BABYFOOD, OATMEAL CRL W/FRUIT, DRY, INST, TODD
32	CHERVIL, DRIED	14	SESAME FLR, PART DEFATTED
32	CEREALS RTE, RICE, PUFFED, FORT, (RICE)	14	CHILI POWDER
32	CEREALS RTE, WHEAT, PUFFED, FORT	14	SESAME FLOUR, LOW-FAT
31	CEREALS RTE, KELLOGG, KELLOGG'S CORN FLAKES	14	CEREALS RTE, KELLOGG, KELLOGG'S FROOT LOOPS
31	CEREALS RTE, KELLOGG, KELLOGG'S RAISIN SQUARES MINI-WHEATS	14	CLAM, MIXED SPECIES, RAW
31	DUCK, DOMESTICATED, LIVER, RAW	14	CARDAMON, GROUND
31	GOOSE, LIVER, RAW	14	CHOCOLATE SYRUP, W/ADDED NUTR
30	CEREALS, QUAKER, CORN GRITS, INST, PLN, DRY	13	WINGED BNS, MATURE SEEDS, RAW

HEALTH AND FITNESS

Table 14.22. Foodstuff with high **Zinc** contents.

Zinc, Zn, mg/100 gm	Description	Zinc, Zn, mg/100 gm	Description
182	OYSTER, EASTERN, WILD, CKD, MOIST HEAT	9	CHERVIL, DRIED
91	OYSTER, EASTERN, CANNED	9	BEEF, CHUCK, BLADE RST, LN & FAT, 0"FAT, SEL, CKD, BRSD
91	OYSTER, EASTERN, WILD, RAW	9	CEREALS RTE, 100% BRAN, (WHEAT BRAN, BARLEY)
87	OYSTER, EASTERN, CKD, BREADED & FRIED	9	LAMB, DOM, FORESHANK, LN, 1/4"FAT, CHOIC, CKD, BRSD
74	OYSTER, EASTERN, WILD, CKD, DRY HEAT	9	BEEF, CHUCK, BLADE RST, LN & FAT, 1/8"FAT, SEL, CKD, BRSD
50	CEREALS RTE, KELLOGG, KELLOGG'S PRODUCT 19	7	BEEF, RIB, LRG END (RIBS 6-9), LN, 1/2"FAT, PRIME, CKD, RSTD
50	CEREALS RTE, GENERAL MILLS, TOTAL	7	PUMPKIN & SQUASH SD KRNLS, RSTD, WO/SALT
50	CEREALS RTE, GENERAL MILLS, TOTAL CORN FLAKES	7	PUMPKIN & SQUASH SD KRNLS, RSTD, W/SALT
45	OYSTER, EASTERN, FARMED, CKD, DRY HEAT	7	BEEF, BRISKET, POINT HALF, LN, 1/4"FAT, ALL GRDS, CKD, BRSD
38	OYSTER, EASTERN, FARMED, RAW	7	BEEF, BRISKET, POINT HALF, LN, 0"FAT, ALL GRDS, CKD, BRSD
33	OYSTER, PACIFIC, CKD, MOIST HEAT	7	VEAL, SHLDR, BLADE, LN, CKD, BRSD
27	CEREALS RTE, GENERAL MILLS, TOTAL RAISIN BRAN	7	BEEF, CHUCK, ARM POT RST, LN & FAT, 1/8"FAT, SEL, CKD, BRSD
22	CEREALS RTE, KELLOGG, KELLOGG'S ALL-BRAN BRAN BUDS	7	CHICKEN, HEART, ALL CLASSES, CKD, SIMMRD
17	CEREALS RTE, WHEAT GERM, TSTD, PLN, (WHEAT GERM)	7	LAMB, DOM, SHLDR, ARM, LN, 1/4"FAT, CHOIC, CKD, BRSD
17	OYSTER, PACIFIC, RAW	7	SESAME BUTTER, PASTE
15	CEREALS RTE, QUAKER, CAP'N CRUNCH'S CRUNCHBERRIES	7	SPINY LOBSTER, MXD SP, CKD, MOIST HEAT
12	WHEAT GERM, CRUDE	7	WHEAT BRAN, CRUDE
12	CEREALS RTE, KELLOGG, KELLOGG'S SPL K	7	PIERRE, FLAME BROILED MESQUITE BEEF PATTY, PROD CD 3870
12	COTTONSEED FLR, PART DEFATTED (GLANDLESS)	7	PIERRE, FLAME BROILED MESQUITE BEEF PATTY, PROD CD 3880
11	CEREALS RTE, KELLOGG, POP-TARTS CRUNCH FRSTD STRAWBERRY	7	BEEF, RND, TIP RND, LN & FAT, 1/4"FAT, ALL GRDS, CKD, RSTD
11	FAST FOODS, OYSTERS, BATTERED OR BREADED, & FRIED	6	LAMB, DOM, SHLDR, BLADE, LN, 1/4"FAT, CHOIC, CKD, BRLD
11	SESAME FLR, PART DEFATTED	6	LAMB, DOM, SHLDR, BLADE, LN, 1/4"FAT, CHOIC, CKD, RSTD
11	CEREALS RTE, COOKIE-CRISP, CHOC CHIP & VANILLA	6	PIERRE, FLAME BROILED BEEF & ONION PATTY, PROD CD 3879
10	BEEF, SHANK CROSSCUTS, LN, 1/4"FAT, CHOIC, CKD, SIMMRD	6	BEEF, GROUND, EX LN, CKD, BRLD, WELL DONE
10	SESAME BUTTER, TAHINI, FROM UNROASTED KRNLS	6	BEEF, CHUCK, ARM POT RST, LN & FAT, 1/2"FAT, PRIME, CKD, BRSD
10	PUMPKIN & SQUASH SEEDS, WHL, RSTD, WO/SALT	6	WONDERBITES DIPPERS, FL BR BF FAJITA WONDRBTS DIPR, PR CD 9971
10	PUMPKIN & SQUASH SEEDS, WHL, RSTD, W/SALT	6	BEEF, SHANK CROSSCUTS, LN & FAT, 1/4"FAT, CHOIC, RAW
10	BEEF, CHUCK, BLADE RST, LN, 1/4"FAT, ALL GRDS, CKD, BRSD	6	BEEF, TOP SIRLOIN, LN, 1/4"FAT, CHOIC, CKD, PAN-FRIED
10	LEAVENING AGENTS, YEAST, BAKER'S, COMPRESSED	6	GAME MEAT, BEEFALO, COMP OF CUTS, CKD, RSTD
10	VEAL, VAR MEATS & BY-PRODUCTS, LIVER, CKD, BRSD	6	LEAVENING AGENTS, YEAST, BAKER'S, ACTIVE DRY
9	BEEF, SHANK CROSSCUTS, LN & FAT, 1/4"FAT, CHOIC, CKD, SIMMRD	6	BEEF, RND, TIP RND, LN & FAT, 1/4"FAT, CHOIC, CKD, RSTD
9	HYACINTH BNS, MATURE SEEDS, RAW	6	BEEF, CURED, BRKFST STRIPS, CKD

Table 14.23. Foodstuff with high **Copper** contents.

Copper, Cu, mg/100 gm	Description	Copper, Cu, mg/100 gm	Description
9.88	VEAL, VAR MEATS & BY-PRODUCTS, LIVER, CKD, PAN-FRIED	2.17	CASHEW NUTS, OIL RSTD, W/SALT
9.83	LAMB, VAR MEATS & BY-PRODUCTS, LIVER, CKD, PAN-FRIED	2.17	BAKING CHOC, UNSWTND, SQUARES
7.95	VEAL, VAR MEATS & BY-PRODUCTS, LIVER, CKD, BRSD	2.16	DESSERTS, GELATINS, DRY PDR, UNSWTND
7.57	OYSTER, EASTERN, WILD, CKD, MOIST HEAT	2.11	SQUID, MXD SP, CKD, FRIED
7.52	GOOSE, LIVER, RAW	2.06	WHELK, UNSPEC, CKD, MOIST HEAT
7.07	LAMB, VAR MEATS & BY-PRODUCTS, LIVER, CKD, BRSD	2.04	MOLASSES, BLACKSTRAP
6.98	LAMB, VAR MEATS & BY-PRODUCTS, LIVER, RAW	2.04	PEANUT FLOUR, LOW FAT
6.10	SEAWEED, SPIRULINA, DRIED	2.00	SOY MEAL, DEFATTED, RAW
5.96	DUCK, DOMESTICATED, LIVER, RAW	2.00	SOY MEAL, DEFATTED, RAW, CRUDE PROT BASIS (N X 6.25)
5.83	VEAL, VAR MEATS & BY-PRODUCTS, LIVER, RAW	1.94	LOBSTER, NORTHERN, CKD, MOIST HEAT
5.17	MUSHROOMS, SHIITAKE, DRIED	1.91	BAKING CHOC, UNSWTND, LIQ
5.08	SOY FLOUR, LOW-FAT	1.89	SQUID, MIXED SPECIES, RAW
5.07	JEW'S EAR, (PEPEAO), DRIED	1.84	GRAPE LEAVES, CND
4.51	BEEF, VAR MEATS & BY-PRODUCTS, LIVER, CKD, BRSD	1.83	SUNFLOWER SD KRNLS, TSTD, WO/SALT
4.47	BEEF, VAR MEATS & BY-PRODUCTS, LIVER, CKD, PAN-FRIED	1.83	SUNFLOWER SD KRNLS, TSTD, W/SALT
4.46	OYSTER, EASTERN, CANNED	1.80	PEANUT FLOUR, DEFATTED
4.45	OYSTER, EASTERN, WILD, RAW	1.80	MIXED NUTS, OIL RSTD, WO/PNUTS, WO/SALT
4.29	OYSTER, EASTERN, CKD, BREADED & FRIED	1.79	CORIANDER LEAF, DRIED
4.21	SESAME BUTTER, PASTE	1.77	BRAZILNUTS, DRIED, UNBLANCHED
4.08	SESAME SEEDS, WHOLE, DRIED	1.63	POPPY SEED
4.07	SOY FLOUR, DEFATTED	1.63	RADISHES, ORIENTAL, DRIED
4.07	SOY FLR, DEFATTED, CRUDE PROT BASIS (N X 6.25)	1.62	SESAME BUTTER, TAHINI, FROM RAW & STONE GROUND KRNLS
3.79	COCOA, DRY PDR, UNSWTND	1.61	SESAME BUTTER, TAHINI, FROM RSTD & TSTD KRNLS (MOST COMMON TYPE)
3.61	COCOA, DRY PDR, UNSWTND, PROC W/ALKALI	1.60	SOY PROTEIN ISOLATE
3.46	OYSTER, EASTERN, WILD, CKD, DRY HEAT	1.58	CEREALS RTE, 100% BRAN, (WHEAT BRAN, BARLEY)
3.34	BEEF, VAR MEATS & BY-PRODUCTS, LIVER, RAW	1.58	FILBERTS OR HAZELNUTS, OIL RSTD, UNBLANCHED, WO/SALT
2.92	SOY FLOUR, FULL-FAT, RAW	1.58	OYSTER, PACIFIC, RAW
2.92	SOY FLR, FULL-FAT, RAW, CRUDE PROT BASIS (N X 6.25)	1.51	FILBERTS OR HAZELNUTS, DRIED, UNBLANCHED
2.88	WINGED BNS, MATURE SEEDS, RAW	1.49	SESAME BUTTER, TAHINI, FROM UNROASTED KRNLS
2.68	OYSTER, PACIFIC, CKD, MOIST HEAT	1.42	TOMATOES, SUN-DRIED
2.47	SESAME SEEDS, WHL, RSTD & TSTD	1.39	PEPPERS, SWT, GRN, FREEZE-DRIED
2.19	CASHEW BUTTER, PLN, WO/SALT	1.37	CELERY SEED

HEALTH AND FITNESS

Table 14.24. Foodstuff with high **Selenium** contents.

Selenium, Se, mcg/100 gm	Description	Selenium, Se, mcg/100 gm	Description
2960	BRAZILNUTS, DRIED, UNBLANCHED	71	WHEAT, HARD RED SPRING
422	MIXED NUTS, WO/PNUTS, OIL RSTD, W/SALT	68	ANCHOVY, EUROPEAN, CND IN OIL, DRND SOL
421	MIXED NUTS, OIL RSTD, W/PNUTS, W/SALT	68	PORK, FRSH, VAR MEATS & BY-PRODUCTS, LIVER, CKD, BRSD
312	PORK, FRSH, VAR MEATS & BY-PRODUCTS, KIDNEYS, CKD, BRSD	67	OYSTER, EASTERN, CKD, BREADED & FRIED
190	PORK, FRSH, VAR MEATS & BY-PRODUCTS, KIDNEYS, RAW	66	FAST FOODS, OYSTERS, BATTERED OR BREADED, & FRIED
154	OYSTER, PACIFIC, CKD, MOIST HEAT	66	TUNA, WHITE, CND IN H2O, DRND SOL
149	BEEF, VAR MEATS & BY-PRODUCTS, KIDNEYS, RAW		
148	COD, ATLANTIC, DRIED & SALTED	66	CAVIAR, BLACK & RED, GRANULAR
136	MUSHROOMS, SHIITAKE, DRIED	65	CEREALS RTE, WHEAT GERM, TSTD, PLN, (WHEAT GERM)
134	MUSTARD SEED, YELLOW	64	CHICKEN, LIVER, ALL CLASSES, RAW
133	JEW'S EAR, (PEPEAO), DRIED	64	CLAM, MXD SP, CKD, MOIST HEAT
128	FUNGI, CLOUD EARS, DRIED	62	SUNFLOWER SD KRNLS, TSTD, W/SALT
128	EGG SUBSTITUTE, POWDER	62	MACARONI, DRY, ENRICHED
127	LAMB, VAR MEATS & BY-PRODUCTS, KIDNEYS, RAW	59	NOODLES, EGG, DRY, ENRICHED
125	EGG, WHITE, DRIED, PDR, GLUCOSE RED	59	NOODLES, EGG, DRY, UNENR
123	CEREALS RTE, QUAKER, QUAKER PUFFED WHEAT	59	CEREALS, ROMAN MEAL W/OATS, DRY, (WHEAT W/OTHER GRAINS)
90	MUSSEL, BLUE, CKD, MOIST HEAT	59	HERRING, ATLANTIC, PICKLED
90	WHELK, UNSPEC, CKD, MOIST HEAT	58	SUNFLOWER SD FLR, PART DEFATTED
90	CUTTLEFISH, MXD SP, CKD, MOIST HEAT	58	FLATFISH (FLOUNDER & SOLE SP), CKD, DRY HEAT
90	OCTOPUS, COMMON, CKD, MOIST HEAT	58	BRAUNSCHWEIGER (A LIVER SAUSAGE), PORK
89	WHEAT, DURUM	58	LIVER SAUSAGE, LIVERWURST, PORK
87	EGG, YOLK, DRIED	58	CEREALS RTE, QUAKER, KRETSCHMER HONEY CRUNCH WHEAT GERM
82	LAMB, VAR MEATS & BY-PRODUCTS, LIVER, RAW	57	SALMON, PINK, CKD, DRY HEAT
80	TUNA, LT, CND IN H2O, DRND SOL	57	BEEF, VAR MEATS & BY-PRODUCTS, LIVER, CKD, PAN-FRIED
79	SUNFLOWER SD KRNLS, DRY RSTD, WO/SALT	56	OCEAN PERCH, ATLANTIC, CKD, DRY HEAT
76	TUNA, LT, CND IN OIL, DRND SOL	55	CRACKERS, MELBA TOAST, WHEAT
76	TUNA, LT, CND IN OIL, WO/SALT, DRND SOL	55	CEREALS RTE, KELLOGG, KELLOGG'S SPL K
75	CRACKERS, MATZO, WHOLE-WHEAT	54	TOFU, DRIED-FROZEN (KOYADOFU)
73	SPAGHETTI, WHOLE-WHEAT, DRY	54	TOFU, DRIED-FROZEN (KOYADOFU), PREP W/CA SULFATE
73	PORK, FRSH, VAR MEATS & BY-PRODUCTS, PANCREAS, CKD, BRSD	53	PORK, FRSH, VAR MEATS & BY-PRODUCTS, LIVER, RAW
72	OYSTER, EASTERN, WILD, CKD, DRY HEAT	53	SARDINE, ATLANTIC, CND IN OIL, DRND SOL W/BONE
72	OYSTER, EASTERN, WILD, CKD, MOIST HEAT	53	HERRING, ATLANTIC, KIPPERED
71	CEREALS, MALTEX, DRY, (WHEAT)	52	ABALONE, MXD SP, CKD, FRIED

Chapter 15: Exercise and Preventable Diseases

15.1. PREVETABLE CAUSES OF DEATH IN THE USA

15.1.1. NEW CHALLENGES OF URBANIZATION

The relationship between exercise, nutrition, and the heart are better understood today than just few decades ago. Half a century ago, the main emphasis of medical sciences was to halt epidemic infectious diseases and urgent saving of lives. With triumphant victories over infectious diseases, many people live longer and healthier than in the past. The emergence of new challenges such as heart disease, diabetes, cancer, and AIDS had farther emphasized the crucial role of behavior on acquiring chronic diseases. Exercise tops the list of behavioral habits that prevent the diseases of the era of urbanization. Nutrition becomes a pressing national issue due to the influence of industrialization of packaged food products and the rise of fast food industries.

15.1.2. HEALTH TRENDS OF MODERN AMERICAN SOCIETY

o The effect of a common culture shapes the lifestyle of an individual according to the norms of that milieu. Statistical analysis of the **health habits**, of most Americans, point to the following trends:
  i. Smoking is involved in one of each five deaths due to cardiovascular diseases.
  ii. Regular physical activity is practiced daily by only one in five adults
  iii. Fat consumption constitutes about one-third of the diets of most Americans.
  iv. Overweight affects over one-third of all Americans.
  v. Blood cholesterol level is above normal in one-half of the population.
  vi. Medical prescriptions are used by one-half of the population.
  vii. Recreational drugs are prevalent in more than two-thirds of the population.

o The major preventable causes of death of over 1.2 million Americans annually, between 1994 and 1999, are heart diseases, smoking, and alcohol, *Table 15.1*.

o **Recreational drugs** are other detrimental health factors, *Table 15.2*. Recreational drugs afflict the nervous system most. Illicit drugs are not manufactured according controlled quality standards and might have lethal toxins and concentration, as follows.
  i. Stimulants such as **amphetamines and cocaine** can cause fatal irregularities of the heartbeats or sudden death in people with coronary heart disease. In addition, many people with coronary heart disease do not know they have it.
  ii. Narcotics such as **heroin and opiates** may cause fatal respiratory failure, particularly in smokers with chronic lung diseases.
  iii. Intravenous injection of **septic matter**[1] causes infection in the heart inner lining, the liver, lungs, and brain, in the form of abscess or general septicemia. These serious medical conditions require hospitalization and parenteral antibiotics but may lead to death.
  iv. Some of these potentially fatal complications can occur in a first-time user. Older people with abnormal coronary arteries and diseased blood vessels in the brain vessels are at greater risk.
  v. Recreational drugs cause birth defects when consumed during pregnancy or even prior to conception.

Table 15.1. Major causes of **preventable deaths** in USA, 1994-1999.

Causes of Death	No. of Deaths	Rates per 100,000
Coronary heart disease	529,659	202.63
Tobacco	395,000	151.11
Alcohol	150,000	57.39
Hypertension	44,435	17.00
Diabetes mellitus, women	37,249	15.25
Diabetes mellitus, men	31,150	11.92
Drug overdose	20,500	7.84
Caffeine	5,500	2.10
Cardiovascular defects	4,657	1.78
Illicit drugs overdose	4500	1.72
Aspirin	500	0.19

Compiled from data published by The federal government's Bureau of Mortality Statistics and Centers for Disease Control and Prevention.

Table 15.2. Annual prevalence of substance use in USA, in 1993. From the National Household Survey on Drug Abuse.

Alcohol	66.50%
Smoking	29.40%
Illicit drugs	11.80%
Cannabis	9.00%
Cocaine	2.20%

---
[1] In this context, septic matter is any substance that is not sterilized and authorized for injection by health experts

15 EXERCISE AND PREVENTABLE DISEASES

15.2. PREVALENCE OF CARDIOVASCULAR DISEASES

o The diseases of the heart and blood vessels are the major causes of death worldwide. These include the following disorders:

   i. Hypertension (high blood pressure).
   ii. Coronary heart disease (heart attack and angina).
   iii. Cerebrovascular disease (stroke).
   iv. Peripheral vascular disease (reduced blood flow).
   v. Heart failure (failure to pump blood).
   vi. Rheumatic heart disease (inflammatory disease).
   vii. Congenital heart disease (birth defects).
   viii. Cardiomyopathies (other heart diseases).

o In the USA, **the morbidity rates of cardiovascular diseases** are staggering. According to the data published by the federal government's Bureau of Mortality Statistics and Centers for Disease Control and Prevention, *Table 15.3*, the following are the national trends of cardiovascular diseases in USA.

Table 15.3. 1988 annual prevalence of cardiovascular diseases in USA Centers for Disease Control and Prevention.

Causes of Morbidity	Total No.
Heart Disease	58,800,000
High blood Pressure	50,000,000
Coronary artery disease	12,000,000
Heart attacks	7,000,000
Angina pectoris	6,200,000
Congestive heart failure	4,600,000
Stroke	4,400,000
Rheumatic heart disease	1,800,000
Congenital cardiovascular defects	1,000,000

   i. Heart disease has no geographic, gender or socio-economic boundaries.
   ii. Heart diseases afflict one fourth of the population of the USA.
   iii. Heart diseases cause 47% of all deaths in the USA, but 33% of all deaths worldwide.
   iv. Cardiovascular diseases kill fifteen million a year, worldwide.
   v. Heart diseases alone kill seven million in the world, each year.
   vi. Heart diseases cause 53% of all female deaths in America.
   vii. Heart attacks kill one person every minute in the USA.
   viii. Stroke kills one person every four minute in the USA.
   ix. At least 250,000 people die of heart attacks each year before they reach a hospital.
   x. Heart attacks will kill 38% of women compared with 25% of men, within one year after onset.
   xi. Sudden deaths, without previous symptoms from coronary heart disease, are reported in 57% of men and 64% of women.

o The **major risk factors** for cardiovascular diseases are preventable and controllable. However, millions are dying in middle age every day from these preventable risks:

   i. Tobacco use increases the risk of dying from cardiovascular disease by 2 to 3 folds.
   ii. Unhealthy diet promotes obesity, overweight, diabetes mellitus, and high blood pressure.
   iii. Physical inactivity leads to cardiovascular compromise, overweight, and psychological disorders.
   iv. Hereditable diseases, some of which can be modified with behavior change, by exercise, avoiding smoking and alcohol, in addition to medical prescription of drugs and genetic counseling.

15.3. HEART DISEASES

The heart is a sacred organ. Heart disease impacts all aspects of the life of the individual. It presents in one of these forms: **heart attack, heart failure, cardiac arrest, cardiac arrhythmia, and myocardial infarction.** General understanding of what these terms mean helps understand how they happen and how to deal with them. Not all heart diseases afflict old people or people with previous symptoms of diseases.

15.3.1. CURRENT STATE OF KNOWLEDGE

o Great progress has been made in **understanding and treating heart disease** of modern day living. We now know, for fact, that diet, activity, and inherited conditions affect the heart, in many ways. The course of development of many heart diseases is well researched and understood than in the past. This allows us to interfere with developing disease conditions and modify their outcome to our favor. Even in genetically inherited condition, such as familial hypercholesterolemia, there are various options to help the patient manage their condition and live regular life. Cholesterol lowering drugs are examples of reducing the internal production of cholesterol by the liver cells and hence saving many lives from coronary occlusive vascular diseases. When coronary occlusion progresses to serious levels, there still options for invasive procedures to dilate the occlusion by stents or angioplasty. More advanced occlusion can be further treated by complete reconstruction with vascular transplants obtained from the leg veins.

o **Advent in modern imaging** by magnetic resonance, ultrasound, and radioactive labeling enabled physicians to even visualize cerebral stroke and coronary occlusions while they actually happen, not after organic damage has already occurred. In the past, physicians relied on EKG [2] and blood chemistry of cardiac enzymes in order to diagnose heart diseases after they already afflicted the patient. Today, both live-visualization of internal organs and live-analysis of their functions are available to physicians and offer emergency treatment to save life. In addition, the advent in biochemical science offers new means to analyze cellular functions, in time to correct many disease conditions. The analysis of blood gases, ions, cellular elements, and complex proteins has made modern medicine very effective in treating and preventing many diseases. Thus, physicians can now foster their clinical skill with advanced laboratory workup and offer patients helpful counseling. Physicians today can injects clot-busting drugs in time to avoid brain, lung, or heart damage by clot occlusion, with the help of nuclear imaging, blood chemistry, and clinical skill. Follow-up with magnetic resonance imaging can actually show the effect of treatment in improving blood flow and the degree of reversal of the heart or brain damage. Thus, patients and doctors can have better idea of the prognosis of disease conditions

o However, such advent is research is creating a real crisis in the health industry of increasing cost of health care and **lack of access** to the majority of the population. It is impossible to rely entirely on health care in treating most preventable diseases. Therefore, the advent in medical technology does not benefit everybody, particularly those indulged in sedentary lifestyle and other destructive habits. Above all, the advent in medical science has revolutionized our understanding of the role of exercise in preventing diseases. Today, we see many doctors becoming involved in fitness training and nutrition counseling. In the near past, doctors were secluded in study rooms, laboratories, and clinics.

o With advent in biochemical sciences, we now understand the role of diet on health better than few decades ago. **Diets rich in fruits and vegetables,** olive oil, nuts and fish protect the heart and blood vessels. Fruits and vegetables have traditional vitamins, minerals, and fiber, in addition flavonoids and organosulfur compounds. Flavonoids improve the elasticity of blood vessels and thin the blood that enhances blood flow. Organosulfur compounds increase levels of HDL cholesterol. Of course, one of the classic ways of reducing heart disease risk is to eliminate saturated fat, which is found in meat, full-fat dairy products and tropical oils, and to replace it with monounsaturates (in olive oil and avocados) and polyunsaturated omega-3 oils (found in fish, walnuts, flaxseed, and canola oil). Saturated fat raises levels of 'bad' cholesterol. Even worse are the so-called trans fats, the hydrogenated vegetable oils, which both raise bad cholesterol and lower the good cholesterol [3].

15.3.2. HEART ATTACK

This is an episodic mishap to the vitality of the heart. During the attack, the heart fails to pump blood to body organs as well as to its own arteries, the coronary arteries. If not caught and treated immediately, heart attacks are fatal.

o **Causes:**
  i. **Reduced blood volume:** This happens in situations such as acute burn, extreme fright, and shock due to blood loss, severe dehydration, or sudden excessive physical exhaustion. In these conditions, either the blood is lost to the outside of the body or the blood is trapped inside the body, without access to flow freely with the circulation. Burn victims, for example, experience enormous stress such that, any fluid or food supplied by mouth would lead to obstruction of the intestine. Intestinal obstruction causes severe trapping of blood inside abdominal organs. In addition, a frightened person might lose most of his or her blood trapped inside the terminal blood vessels, due to the failure of the nervous system to regulate the flow of circulation.
  ii. **Narrowed coronary arteries:** This is common in coronary artery diseases, the major killer in almost all cultures. In this disease, the coronary arteries lose their smooth and malleable nature by aging, high blood cholesterol, and other insults such as infections and inflammation. Diseased coronary arteries act like rigid tubes that do not comply with turbulent blood flow or excessive needs of circulation. This disease is heavily targeted by all fitness and nutrition experts, due to the high potential of prevention and saving lives.
  iii. **Hyperviscous blood:** This is encountered in severe dehydration, heat stroke, and other hyperviscosity disorders. Severe loss of flood or the over production of blood elements leads to sluggish blood flow and deprivation of the heart cells from nutrients.

o **Clinical manifestation:**
  i. Heart attack might present as **angina pectoris**, which varies from mild unnoticeable discomfort on exertion, to severe pain in the chest, arms, neck, chin, or back. Minor functional angina pectoris lasts up to 20 minutes and

---

[2] EKG or ECG refers to "electrocardiography". This is a method of recording the propagation of electric stimulation of the heart by means of surface electrodes. This method documents heart rate irregularities, pumping forces, defects in conduction, orientation of the heart, and many other physiological parameters.

[3] High-density lipoproteins (HDL) contain about equal proportions of protein and fat, by weight. Ideal blood concentration of HDL falls in the range 350 to 650 mg/L. About 15% of their fat is made of cholesterol and 3% of triglycerides. Low- density lipoproteins (LDL) contain about 25% protein and 75% fat (that is the reason for having low density). Ideal blood concentration of LDL falls in the range 600 to 1600 mg/L About 50% of their fat is made of cholesterol and 10% of triglycerides. Thus, LDL's are major cholesterol carriers. Source: "The Merck Manual of Medical Information", ISBN: 0-671-02726-3, 1997, and "Biochemistry" by Ian D. K. Halkerston, ISBN: 0-471-85554-5, 1988.

recurs on exertion.
ii. Full-blown heart attack is the severest crushing chest pain, caused by physical damage to the heart muscle- **infarction**. The patient with severe heart attack presents in a **state of shock**. He or she looks pale, diaphoretic (soaked in sweat), has clammy skin, and appears dyspneic (breathless).
iii. Heart attacks may happen in **any age**, even in the fittest athletes. These should be highly suspected whenever a questionable or vague sudden inconvenience is encountered, such as fatigue, weakness or anxiety.
iv. The sooner emergency medical care is sought, the better are the chances of saving life. Cardiopulmonary resuscitation and immediate oxygen administration, prior to arrival to the intensive care unit, are crucial to survival

15.3.3. HEART FAILURE
The heart may fail to pump blood and to maintain adequate circulation for many reasons. Such pumping inadequacy might not be severe enough to cause complete heart attack. Thus, patients with heart failure can live for many years with troubled heart.

o **Causes:**
  i. The **heart muscle** is diseased. This could happen due to medications, toxins, smoking, or diseases that disturb metabolism. Fatigue and overtraining produce sufficient metabolites and deplete vital resources to the extent of failure.
  ii. The **heart mechanics** are impaired. Disease that damages the heart valves and causes prolapse, hardening, or narrowing, disrupts the work of the heart. Rheumatic fever was a major cause of valvular heart diseases before the discovery of antibiotics, *Figure 13.3*. Intravenous drug use is the major preventable cause among drug users.
  iii. The **heart electricity** is malfunctioning. Disease that impairs the generation and conduction of electricity through the heart causes failure. Thyroid disease, alcoholism, smoking, and vitamin deficiency (thiamin) affect the integrity of neurocardiac regulation.
  iv. **Fluid imbalance,** due to excessive intake and reduced excretion by the kidneys, leads to pump failure. Kidney diseases and over consumption of salted food (sodium) cause fluid imbalance and induce heart failure.

o **Clinical manifestation:**
It is very important to know when the heart is the source of a problem. All athletes and every individual engaged in physical activity are subjected to heart challenge. Heart failure could be concealed in many ways. Children in particular have to be considered subjects, until proven otherwise. Heart failure may reverse itself with adequate rest, sleep, reduction of resistance, or absolute rest for days. Heart failure due to recognized structural causes require medical interference to correct the problem. The following are common presentation of a failing heart.
  i. **Breathlessness:** Even with slightly failing heart, the lungs become jammed with slow circulation. In overweight people, this problem is compounded with excess burden of larger fluid volume.
  ii. **Weakness:** All forms of activities become tiring. Even flipping a page in a book, keeping the head upright, or moving the eyes around, all give the feeling of weariness. Resorting to full rest is wiser than seeking a stimulating drink or drug.
  iii. **Heart racing:** The weakened heart could not fulfill the needs of mobility and, thus, responds with faster beating on any effort.
  iv. **Pain:** Pushing beyond your limits, when your heart is sick, causes other organs to fails as well. Headache indicates that the brain is troubled with poor circulation. Severe injuries to joints, muscles, or major life threatening accidents occur, when the heart's calls for rest are unheeded.
  v. **Worry:** Mental awareness of vague or eminent changes in the body due to troubled heart could be interpreted as stress or anxiety. Alcohol and other recreational drugs camouflage these symptoms and cause the individual to breach his or her limits.
  vi. **Swelling:** Accumulation of fluids in the limbs is a sign of circulatory failure, due to heart failure.

15.3.4. CARDIAC ARREST
Cardiac arrest is an immediate cessation of heart beating. It leads to the loss of the vital signs of life such as responsiveness, breathing, heart beating, movement, and coughing.

o **Causes:**
  i. Severe reduction in the **blood supply** to the heart muscle. Massive blood clotting could entirely block the blood flow to the heart causing arrest, such as in case of severe burn. Working your heart to barely deal with minimal daily activities, denies the heart the potential to build higher threshold for the unexpected, such as snow shoveling, lifting of a child, or stepping outdoors in a hostile weather.
  ii. Disruption of the **electric circuits** or the electric generators of the heart; conducting bundles and nodes. Electrocution overrides the electric harmony of the heart and induces the quickest arrest. The most dreaded

cardiac arrests are those that afflict young and healthy people. Tackling demanding tasks, with less sleep, under the effect of caffeine, alcohol, of other drugs, or after heavy meals, is a recipe for heart trouble.
   iii. Severe loss of **vitality of the heart muscle**. Carbon monoxides and toxins render the heart muscle irresponsive to electrical stimulation and cause the heart to stop beating. Fire fighters are at higher risk of carbon monoxide induced cardiac arrest.

15.3.5. CARDIAC ARRHYTHMIA

o Arrhythmia is a condition of irregular heart beating. Irregular heart beating demands serious medical attention since it could lead to cardiac arrest, heart attack, or myocardial infarction. Arrhythmia might be transient or permanent, due to functional causes or structural ones, and with various degrees of seriousness. Irregular heart beating interferes with the timing of opening and closing the heart valves and the strength of the heart pump.

o **Experienced planning of exercise** differs from improvised training in preventing such tragic loss of lives due to episodic arrhythmias. The individual adhering to experienced planning learns the following phases of training.
   i. **Drug-free** body is essential to getting organs to function normally and predictably, without surprising failure.
   ii. **Total load:** The sum of all loads involved in resistance exercises that exceed ordinary limits (>50% of maximum) are monitored daily. Gradual increase of the total load, over months of regular training, guarantees increase of heart reserve. The increased heart reserve is attributed to the increase of mitochondria in the cardiac muscle. High mitochondrial density generates energy at higher rates. Increased cardiac reserve is also attributed to the enriched circulation of the heart muscle. This helps the heart to contract vigorously and recover faster. High cardiac reserve enables the heart to respond timely to rhythmic stimulation, without falling out-of-rhythm. Accelerated training and poor preparation leave the heart reserve lagging behind its demands and predispose to arrhythmias.
   iii. **Intensity:** Gradual and calculated increase in intensity of exercise of major muscle groups is another crucial factor in preparing the shock organs to deal with transient changes. Intense training of one preferred group of muscles, such as the chest or the arms, is ineffective in inducing cardiac adaptation. Intense training must focus on function that deals with the host's mobility and agility.
   iv. **Regular exercise:** Interruption of exercise routine for more than two days sets things back to the starting point. A person without documented long record of regular training should not be put in challenging situations for fear of sudden arrhythmia. This is particularly true in old age and in people with ill heart.

15.3.6. MYOCARDIAL INFARCTION

o This is a damage of the heart wall due to blocked circulation. The main cause of blockage is coronary artery disease. In this disease, the coronary arteries are damaged by deposits of fat, calcium, and fibers (hardened or atherosclerotic coronary arteries). Part of the heart muscle suffers sudden blockage of circulation that results in death of the muscle. The dead portion of the heart wall loses its ability to contract, to conduct electricity, or to allow blood flow to adjacent tissue. It might rupture, causing sudden internal bleeding. It also might bulge outside of the heart wall, forming aneurysm, which might rupture, sooner or latter, causing sudden death. Atherosclerosis is overwhelmingly the first killer in developed countries.

o **Prevalence trends:**
   i. The principal victims are men in the prime of their productive lives.
   ii. It is a preventable cause of death since it varies from culture to culture. In Japan death rate among men is one-fifth that in the USA.
   iii. The main lesion is a blockage of the muscular arteries (of medium and large size) by a defect consisting of cholesterol and calcium (atheroma).
   iv. Atheroma of the arteries takes 20 to 40 years or longer to manifest clinically.
   v. Main risk factors are high level of blood lipids, hypertension, cigarette smoking, and diabetes. Serum cholesterol level 265 mg/dl, or over, associates with a five times higher risk of coronary artery disease, than at levels below 220.
   vi. Surgical repair of myocardial infarction has saved many lives. Many infarction patients were able to walk the streets within two weeks of the heart repair and many others return to the gym within few months and enjoyed life to the fullest.

15.3.7. RHEUMATIC HEART DISEASE

o Rheumatic heart disease is initiated by throat infection with streptococcus bacteria of specific type. The infection triggers autoimmune disease of the heart valves and muscle. It is a plague of the pre-antibiotics era, before WWII. Today it afflicts the poor and uneducated social class.

o The author arose amongst such class and witnessed the tragic loss of lives of friends, relatives, neighbors, and daily encounters to that crippling disease. The first Weightlifting coach, who introduced the author to this sport, died in his early thirties from rheumatic mitral valve stenosis, **Figure 13.3**. Another childhood's friend lost his two daughters to rheumatic heart diseases, before they reached their twenties.

15 EXERCISE AND PREVENTABLE DISEASES

o   In USA, rheumatic fever and rheumatic heart disease killed 3,676 Americans in 1999 (28.4 % males and 71.6% females). In 1950, about 15,000 Americans died of these diseases. From 1989 to 1999, the death rate from rheumatic heart disease fell 34.6 %.[4]

o   Since rheumatic fever afflicts children most, it is very important to treat any kind of fever or joint pain in children with utmost medical care. Antibiotics, steroids, and aspirin saved many inflamed hearts from the damage of rheumatic fever, yet absolute rest during treatment enhances recovery in children. All children planning to engage in physical activities should be screened for rheumatic heart disease and treated if found affected. Low socioeconomic status and unstable family environment should alert the teacher, coach, or health care provider to screen a child for valve murmurs or thrills on the chest area. A child found to have rheumatic heart disease should never be allowed to engage in physical activities without rigorous treatment of his or her heart condition. Physical activities with inflamed heart cause damage to the heart valves, which leads to rupture, scar, narrowing, or prolapse.

15.4. HEART DISEASE AND CULTURAL DIFFERENCES

Prevention of heart diseases is a realistic mean to minimize human suffering. Cultural norms seem to play major role in increasing or decreasing the risk for contracting diseases. *Figure 15.1* shows the very high relative risk form dying from circulatory diseases and AIDS in USA over Japan. In addition, there is quite high relative risk from dying from arteriosclerosis, ischemic heart, hypertension, accidents, diabetes, and digestive disease, of Americans compared to Japanese. Japanese only outpace Americans, in annual risk of death from liver disease, suicide, kidney disease, cerebrovascular disease, chronic lung disease, and pneumonia. Therefore, there must be something wrong in the American culture that causes the high risk of death from certain disease. The same can be said about the Japanese culture and its elected high-risk diseases. *Table 15.4* lists statistics on causes of death for both sexes in USA and Japan.

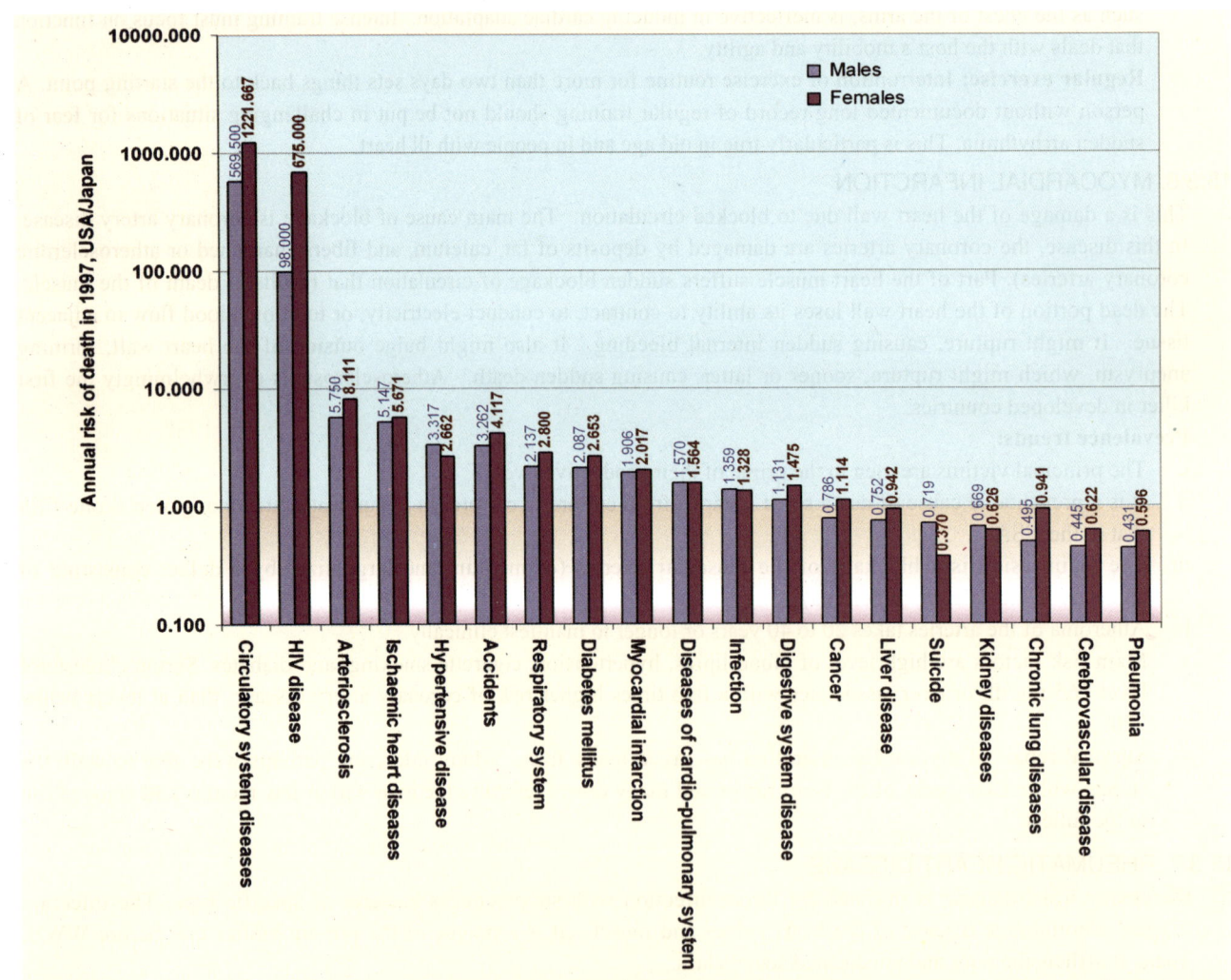

Figure 15.1. Relative annual risk of death from disease in USA and Japan, 1997. Annual rate of death is the number of deaths per 100,000 populations per year. Data compiled from publication of the World Health Organization, *Table 15.4,* below. Note the logarithmic scale.

---

[4] National Center for Health Statistics, http://www.cdc.gov/nchs/fastats/rheumat.htm

Table 15.4. Annual Rate of Death per 100,000 population and Number of Annual Death, in USA and Japan, in 1997, from the various causes. Published by permission of World Health Organization, Information Management and Dissemination WHO, Geneva, Switzerland.

Causes of Death	Japan				USA			
	Females Number of annual death	Females Annual rate of death per 100,000	Males Number of annual death	Males Annual rate of death per 100,000	Females Number of annual death	Females Annual rate of death per 100,000	Males Number of annual death	Males Annual rate of death per 100,000
All causes	415606	651.90	497796	813.3	1160206	849.2	1154039	880.8
Arteriosclerosis	593	0.90	492	0.8	10038	7.3	6019	4.6
Cancer	108337	169.90	167076	273	258465	189.2	281110	215.6
Diseases of cardio-pulmonary system	36296	56.90	31317	51.2	121552	89	105276	80.4
Cerebrovascular disease	72907	115.40	65790	107.5	97227	71.2	62564	47.8
Chronic lung diseases	6515	10.20	12231	20	13064	9.6	12943	9.9
Circulatory system diseases	181	0.30	357	0.6	500725	366.5	447687	341.7
Diabetes mellitus	6075	9.50	6295	10.3	34449	25.2	28187	21.5
Digestive system disease	7553	11.80	7466	12.2	23827	17.4	18059	13.8
HIV disease	3	0.00	72	0.1	3624	2.7	12892	9.8
Hypertensive disease	4347	6.80	2537	4.1	24709	18.1	17856	13.6
Infection	7988	12.50	10238	16.7	22642	16.6	29729	22.7
Ischemic heart diseases	10853	17.00	11633	19	131728	96.4	128161	97.8
Kidney diseases	9899	15.50	8525	13.9	13191	9.7	12140	9.3
Liver disease	4380	6.90	10113	16.5	8915	6.5	16260	12.4
Myocardial infarction	22459	35.20	26772	43.7	97041	71	109171	83.3
Pneumonia	36590	57.40	42314	69.1	46716	34.2	39013	29.8
Respiratory system	9230	15.50	12972	21.2	55422	40.6	59403	45.3
Suicide	7593	11.90	15901	26	6043	4.4	24492	18.7
Accidents	3847	6.00	8847	15.5	33681	24.7	61963	47.3
Mental disorders					28886	21.1	18595	15.2
Other accidents					5853	4.3	8944	6.8
Septicemia					12741	9.3	9655	7.4
Traffic accidents					14427	10.6	27913	21.3
Accidental falls					7742	5.7	7705	5.9
Ill-defined conditions					10704	7.8	12331	9.4
Homicide					4384	3.2	15107	11.5
Vascular diseases					12683	9.3	15109	11.5
Nervous system diseases					28820	21.1		
Infection					22642	16.6		

15.5. RISK FACTORS FOR HEART DISEASES

Heart diseases can be prevented when risk factors are known and manageable, such as cigarette smoking, high blood pressure, high blood cholesterol, and overweight. In other cases, heart disease can be brought under control by medical treatment with aspirin, beta-blockers, ACE-inhibitors (angiotensin converting enzyme inhibitors), thrombolytics (clot-busters), and coronary artery surgery, which are bringing hope to heart disease patients. The following are the major culprits in predisposing to heart disease.

15.5.1. AGE

o   Aging brings about many maladies. The heavy burden of cultural taboos and inhered customs and habits contribute to the repeated mistakes all people make, and in many instances, fail to recognize or rectify. The best example, is the great progress made in medicine in the last three hundred years that helped millions of people to live longer. Yet, many more millions overlook the greatest scientific discoveries, and easily succumb to preventable diseases. Aging presents the culmination of life-long mistakes of poor dieting and inactivity.

15 EXERCISE AND PREVENTABLE DISEASES

o The wisest approach to better the life as we grow older is constant and calculated mobility. With balanced diet, and awareness of the essential need for hydration, mobility invigorates the circulation of the heart muscle, which positively affects all organs. An effort to determine the deficits in diet and physical activity and correct them could greatly improve the quality of life of the aged. As we age, we could experiment many things that can advance our health, as follows.

   i. **Diets** that cause you to sleep less comfortably, to hardly move your bowels, or hikes your bodyweight, might need be modified or substituted.
   ii. Pain that arises after exercise, but improves within days, and doesn't disturb night sleep, might give a clue to a point of weakness. Such discovery of weakness needs more persistence and continuation of the **exercise** that caused the pain, but with modified load volume and **intensity**.
   iii. Movements that seem tiring to perform should be assisted with **relevant exercise**, with lighter resistance and more repetitions, or with aiding machines that help ease the high repetitive nature.
   iv. Heart rate that hikes for days, **after exercise**, signals heart stress. Either the load of exercise has to be reduced or ceased, until the heart beating levels to normal and stays there for few weeks, or other causes of the increased heart rate have to be sought.

15.5.2. GENDER

o Women are more likely to die from **heart disease** than from cancer, chronic lung disease, pneumonia, diabetes, accidents and AIDS combined, *Table 15.4* and *Figure 15.2*. The prevalence rate of circulatory disease in women is 366.5 per 100,000 populations, compared to 341.7 for men in 1997 (USA). However, men have a greater prevalence of myocardial infarction, with prevalence rate of 83.3 per 100,000 populations, compared to 71 for women.

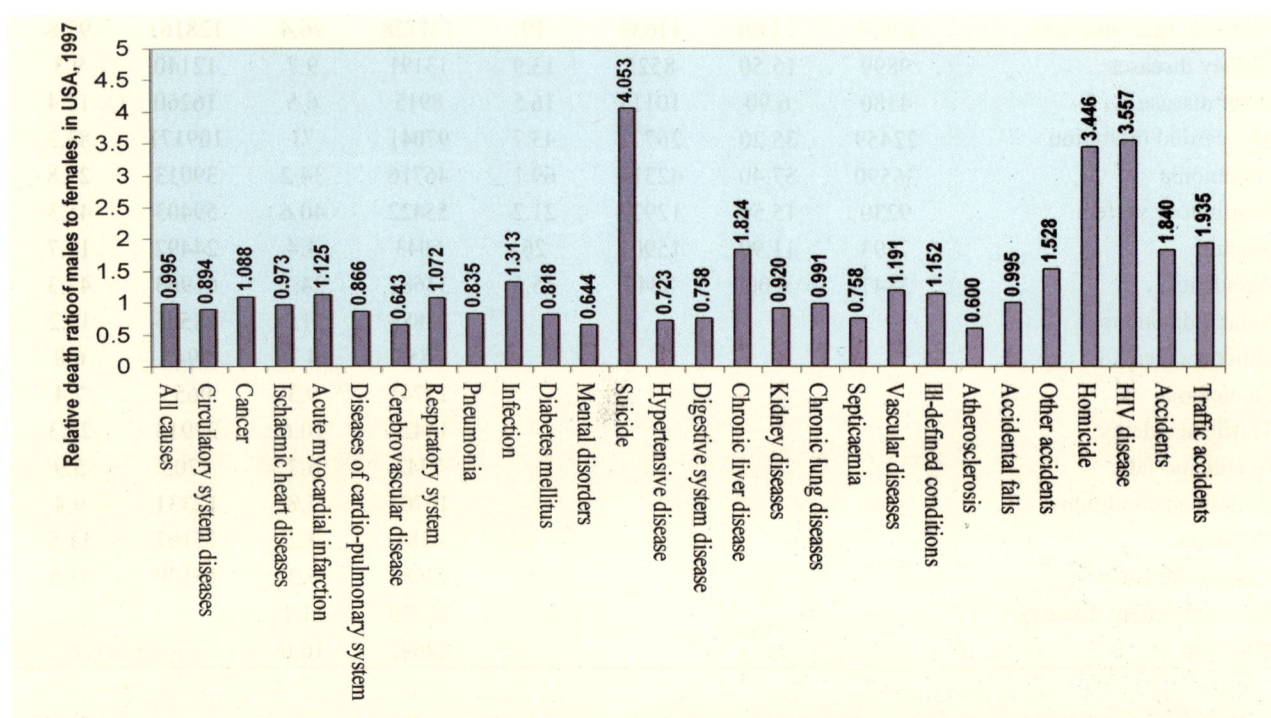

Figure 15.2. Gender breakdown of annual relative death ratio from various diseases in USA, 1997. Compiled from *Table 15.4*.

o Women need exercise as much as men do, because **exercise** is the major stimulant to **cellular viability**. Gender plays important part at the primitive instinct level. This is clear form the difference in the prevalence rates of diseases. Men are curiously interested in gaining strength, since it is the pass for many opportunities in the men's world, with much less interest in the quality of diet. Women are better in exploring delicious food and less interested in strength exercise. Bridging the two worlds complements healthy living. Getting strong, at any cost, might cut short the longevity of an athlete. Since our systems live in harmony, forcing one system to work harder, out of rhythm, could impair other systems. Women are less risky in using force and in experimenting with unfamiliar activities. This reduces the women risk from episodic disease such as heart attacks.

o **Sex hormones** seem to play a role in heart disease. It is well known that men have more heart attacks than pre-menopausal women do. The loss of natural estrogen, as women age, may contribute to a higher risk of heart disease after menopause. Hormones also affect blood cholesterol. Female hormones tend to raise HDL ("good") cholesterol and lower total blood cholesterol. Male hormones do the opposite. If you've had a natural or surgical menopause, you may be considering estrogen replacement therapy (ERT) or hormone replacement therapy (HRT). ERT and HRT may increase your risk of some diseases and health conditions. The early forms of birth control pills, with higher doses of estrogen and progestin, increased a woman's risk of heart disease and stroke. That's especially true for older women who smoked for many years. Newer, lower-dose oral contraceptives carry a much lower risk of cardiovascular disease, except for women who smoke or have high blood pressure. If a woman taking oral contraceptives has other risk factors (and especially if she smokes), her risk of developing blood clots and having a heart attack goes up. If you take birth control pills, get your blood pressure, triglycerides and glucose levels checked yearly.

15.5.3. ALCOHOL

About two thirds of Americans consume alcohol, *Table 15.2*. The health care authorities seem to suffer from the same malady they are set to prevent. Instead of alerting the public that no minimal amount of alcohol is good for health, medical authorities publish data about how moderate drinking is beneficial for the heart. The basic fact about alcohol consumption is that it has never been good to health in any way, as follows.

o Health and fitness require **clear mind, planning, and daily dedication** to avoid falling in the traps of chronic and lasting troubles. Alcohol interferes with many hours worth of planning and delays workout for days. This delay is sufficient to undermine regular serious training.
o The reduction in LDL cholesterol in people who drink moderately, for years, is judge based on **comparison with excessive drinker and nondrinker** and not in comparison with physically active people who do not drink.
o People who drink do not do so to lower their bad cholesterol, but rather, to relieve stress. Asking stressed people to moderate in drinking might only lead to subjective response.
o The benefit of lowering cholesterol or protecting against myocardial infarction, by moderate alcohol consumption, is counteracted with much harm of **inactivity, depression, addiction, and lowered autoimmune defenses**.
o The irresponsible publishing of misleading data about the benefits of alcohol neglects seeking data about the number of people who could adhere to moderate drinking and remain actively fit and healthy. Such course of events requires many years of follow up and expensively detailed research.
o Alcoholic beverages supply calories but few nutrients. Alcoholic beverages are harmful when consumed in excess, and some people should not drink at all. Excess alcohol alters judgment and can lead to dependency and a great many other serious health problems.
o Taking more than one drink per day for women or two drinks per day for men (see *Tip # 1*, below, Section 15.11) can raise the risk for motor vehicle crashes, other injuries, high blood pressure, stroke, violence, suicide, and certain types of cancer.
o Even one drink per day can slightly raise the risk of breast cancer. Alcohol consumption during pregnancy increases risk of birth defects.
o Too much alcohol may cause social and psychological problems, cirrhosis of the liver, inflammation of the pancreas, and damage to the brain and heart. Heavy drinkers also are at risk of malnutrition because alcohol contains calories that may substitute for those in nutritious foods. If adults choose to drink alcoholic beverages, they should consume them only in moderation and with meals to slow alcohol absorption.
o Drinking in moderation may lower risk for coronary heart disease, mainly among men over age 45 and women over age 55. However, there are other factors that reduce the risk of heart disease, including a healthy diet, physical activity, avoidance of smoking, and maintenance of a healthy bodyweight.
o Moderate consumption provides little, if any, health benefit for younger people. Risk of alcohol abuse increases when drinking starts at an early age. Some studies suggest that older people may become more sensitive to the effects of alcohol as they age.
o Some people should **NOT** drink alcoholic beverages at all. These include:
  i. Children and adolescents.
  ii. Individuals of any age who cannot restrict their drinking to moderate levels. This is a special concern for recovering alcoholics, problem drinkers, and people whose family members have alcohol problems.
  iii. Women who may become pregnant or who are pregnant. A safe level of alcohol intake has not been established for women at any time during pregnancy, including the first few weeks. Major birth defects, including fetal alcohol syndrome, can be caused by heavy drinking by the pregnant mother. Other fetal alcohol effects may occur at lower levels.
  iv. Individuals who plan to drive, operate machinery, or take part in other activities that require attention, skill, or coordination. Most people retain some alcohol in the blood up to 2 to 3 hours after a single drink.
  v. Individuals taking prescription or over-the-counter medications that can interact with alcohol. Alcohol alters the effectiveness or toxicity of many medications, and some medications may increase blood alcohol levels. If you take medications, ask your health care provider for advice about alcohol intake, especially if you are an older adult.
  vi. Of course, Weightlifting and strength training necessitates abstinence from alcohol as well as from drugs and smoking. Abstinence is a humble choice that attests to our recognition of the complexity of human physiology.

15.5.4. HEREDITY
o Heredity plays **an important role** in health issues. Advances in genomic knowledge made it possible for determined people to do better than their parents did. Yet, there are many instances when the parents surpassed their offspring!

15 EXERCISE AND PREVENTABLE DISEASES

When physical labor was the only option for making living, less air pollution, and less prevalent fast-food industry, many modern diseases were delayed to advanced age.
- **Genetic predisposition**, however, does not always amount to life sentence of doom and gloom. Many variables play in acquiring skills and modifying gene expressions. For example, the common belief that physical strength is mainly hereditary raises suspicion. If no specific pathological defect could be detected, one can assume that champions are not born stronger than others are. That is because children do not express the peak level of strength that is reached by adulthood. Another example is attributing fractures of osteoporotic people to genetic predisposition after engaging in exercise. This hypothesis omits the fact that exercise might have been improperly planned and performed. Genetic predisposition should not be overcharged as an excuse for succumbing to maladies that could otherwise be prevented.
- Acquired skills greatly improve the outcomes of our inhered limitations. Unhealthy habits do more harm, as follows.
    i. **Genetics is not responsible** for the damage incurred by *smoking cigarettes*.
    ii. Genetics is also not responsible for the harm incurred by *eating junk food* without knowing the ingredients of its contents.
    iii. Genetics also is not responsible for the irreversible harm incurred by *sitting immobile,* for long hours, everyday.

15.5.5. SMOKING
- Smoking affects cellular respiration by undermining oxygen delivery to cells, as follows.
    i. Firstly, smoking generates **carbon monoxide** that has greater affinity to blood hemoglobin than inhaled oxygen does. The compound carboxyhemoglobin reduces blood capacity to transport oxygen to the cells.
    ii. Secondly, smoking introduces **nicotine** into the circulation, which acts as constrictor to small blood vessels, thus further reduces blood flow to the tissue.
    iii. Thirdly, smoking introduces **inorganic particles** into the pulmonary and vascular tissue, which causes local destruction and inflammation, thus, further reduces pulmonary capacity.
- The three mechanisms of depriving tissue of oxygen lead to accumulation of protons in the body, diminish cellular production of life sustaining substrates, and subsequently affect all cells in the body, not only the lungs.
- The increase in **obesity and smoking** among women are major risk factors for ailing hearts. The rise in cost of living contributes to stress and lack of resources to exercise and learn about pressing health issues. Such lifestyle leads to high blood pressure, the main culprit in causing heart disease in women. In men, the decline in **smoking** seems to have contributed most to the reduction in the risk of heart disease, particularly in developed nations. Litigation against the tobacco industries has raised public awareness about the menace of smoking, or that might be just a wishful thought. Countries that lack active campaign of public awareness, such as the developing nations, are lagging behind in prevention.
- Smoking interferes with the basic functions that all living cells learned to master through evolution. That is converting the chemical energy stored in foodstuff into kinetic energy, water, and carbon dioxide. The most sensitive cells, first to suffer, are those that have high turnover rate, such as the **nerve cells** and **the endothelium,** which cover the inside of hollow organs and vessels. The endothelium of the blood capillaries is afflicted, allover the body, with slow and silent deprivation of life in all body organs. The damaged blood capillaries heal by scar tissue and fat deposits, leading to narrowing and obstruction. All sorts of disease could be attributed to smoking. On the top of the list are cardiovascular diseases.
- **Stopping smoking** significantly decreases the risk of myocardial infarction, stroke and peripheral vascular disease, over the first two years. Continuing to smoke after myocardial infarction or coronary revascularization can have serious clinical consequences. Even eight years after myocardial infarction, the mortality of post-myocardial infarction patients who continue to smoke is double that of quitters. Further, those who do not stop smoking after coronary revascularization also have a two-fold higher risk of re-infarction and death. Studies indicate that although doctors are knowledgeable about the risks of cardiovascular diseases (CVDs) associated with tobacco smoking, they are not sufficiently prepared to help their patients stop smoking.
- Even though physicians identify a substantial number of smokers during consultations, for example, many patients do not receive counseling to help them quit. Smoking cessation is the most cost-effective intervention for patients with documented CVDs. The challenge is to get doctors and nurses to encourage patients to stop smoking.

15.5.6. HIGH BLOOD PRESSURE
- **Cause:**
    i. High blood pressure is a symptom of many diseases, which affect the body's ability to balance and circulate fluids. The simple fact about how the body balances fluids is as follows.
        a. The intestines absorb fluid intake.
        b. The heart and muscles circulate the body fluids
        c. The kidney drains some and withholds some.
        d. The lungs provide gas exchange, to utilize the withheld portion of the intake, to replenish the body resources.
    ii. High blood pressure signifies a **jam in such balance of body fluids**, as follows.
        a. Either the body resources are not being properly replenished.
        b. The intake is too excessive.

EXERCISE AND PREVENTABLE DISEASES

            c. The outlet is too restricted.
            d. Alternatively, the circulation is too congested.
        iii. Such jamming of fluid balance is due to either **overactive autonomic nervous** system that squeezes the blood vessels, or **diseased organ** (kidneys withhold sodium, over intake of sodium, or weakening heart) that impairs fluid balance. When the exact cause is not found, it is called **essential hypertension**. It is treatable, and its treatment prevents fatal diseases.

- **Effect:** When left untreated, high blood pressure does more harm to the vital systems. Hypertension causes **strokes, heart disease, and kidney failure**. The fallacy that high blood pressure amounts to high blood flow is prevalent among lay folks and health professionals. Yet, hypertension is a silent killer, as follows.
    i. In High blood pressure, the arteries are narrower than normal, making it harder on the heart to pump blood. Thus, the heart might fail.
    ii. The high velocity, high-pressure blood flow might damage the arteries causing stroke, hemorrhage, or aneurysm.
    iii. It might damage the kidneys causing kidney failure.
    iv. In terminal tissues, the high blood pressure creates turbulence and negative pressure that deprives tissue from nutrition. The constant knocking of the walls of the arteries, by turbulent blood flow, causes injuries to the inner wall of the vessels. Such injuries attract cholesterol and calcium to form plaques and harden the arterial walls.

- **Prevalence:** The following are published statistics on the impact of hypertension on public health.
    i. High blood pressure (hypertension) was the primary cause of death for **42,555** Americans in 1997 (24709 women and 17856 men). It afflicts about 50 million Americans aged 6 and older, *Table 15.4*.
    ii. One in five Americans (and one in four adults) has high blood pressure. Blacks are afflicted 3.5 times as whites, in the annual rate of death, *Figure 15.3*.
    iii. The annual mortality rate per 100,000, in 1997, due to hypertensive diseases, was **18.1** for American women compared to **6.8** for Japanese women. It was **13.6** for American men compared to **4.1** for Japanese men.
    iv. Many people with the disease do not know they have it.

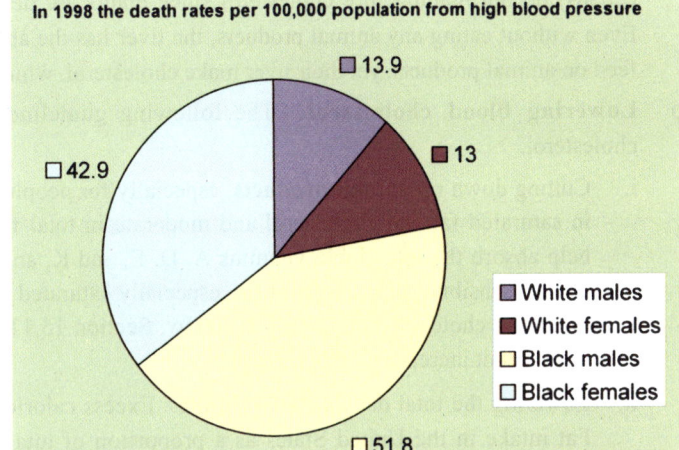

Figure 15.3. Racial and gender breakdown of annual death rate from hypertension in USA, 1998. Source: USA Centers for Disease Control and Prevention.

   v. It afflicts males more than females, the poor more than the rich, Americans more than Japanese.
   vi. Low-cholesterol, low-saturated-fat, polyunsaturated-rich diet lower plasma level of cholesterol by 10-20% and reduce the risk of coronary heart disease.
   vii. Blood pressure higher than 160/95 in men, 45 to 62 years age, is associated with more than five times incidence off coronary heart disease compared to men with blood pressure less than 140/90.
   viii. Diastolic hypertension is more important, 105 mm Hg associates with four times incidence of coronary heart disease than with individuals with 84 mm Hg or less.
   ix. After age 45, hypertension is a greater risk factor than hypercholesterolemia.

- **Role of diet:**
    i. Many people can reduce their chances of developing high blood pressure by consuming **less salt**. Several other steps can also help keep your blood pressure in the healthy range (see *Tip #2*, below, Section 15.11). In the body, sodium-which you get mainly from salt-plays an essential role in regulating fluids and blood pressure.
    ii. Many studies in diverse populations have shown that a high sodium intake is associated with higher blood pressure. There is no way to tell who might develop high blood pressure from eating **too much salt**. However, consuming less salt or sodium is not harmful and can be recommended for the healthy, normal person (see *Tip # 3*, below, Section 15.11).
    iii. At present, the firmest link between salt intake and health relates to blood pressure. High salt intake also increases the amount of calcium excreted in the urine. Eating less salt may decrease the **loss of calcium** from bone. Loss of too much calcium from bone increases the risk of osteoporosis and bone fractures.
    iv. Salt is found mainly in processed and prepared foods. Salt (sodium chloride) is the main source of sodium in foods (see *Tip # 4*, below, Section 15.11). Only small amounts of salt occur naturally in foods. Most of the salt

EXERCISE AND PREVENTABLE DISEASES

you eat comes from foods that have salt added during **food processing** or during preparation in a restaurant or at home. Some recipes include table salt or a salty broth or sauce, and some cooking styles call for adding a very salty seasoning such as soy sauce. Not all foods with added salt taste salty. Some people add salt or a salty seasoning to their food at the table. Your preference for salt may decrease if you gradually add smaller amounts of salt or salty seasonings to your food over a period of time.

    v. Aim for a moderate sodium intake. Most people consume too much salt; so moderate your salt intake. Healthy children and adults need to consume only small amounts of salt to meet their sodium needs—less than 1/4 teaspoon of salt daily. The Nutrition Facts Label lists a Daily Value of 2,400 mg of sodium per day. This is the amount of sodium in about 1 teaspoon of salt. See *Tip # 5*, below, Section 15.11, for helpful hints on how to keep your sodium intake moderate.

15.5.7. CHOLESTEROL

o **Role of cholesterol:** Although, Cholesterol has a bad rap as a culprit in many diseases that claim the lives of millions every year, it is also a vital substance in the existence of animal life. From cholesterol, many hormones are made that defines sexuality, control metabolism, and allow the nervous system to exist and function. It is only found in animal products such as meats, whole milk dairy foods, egg yolks, poultry and fish. Plants (vegetables, fruits, grains, and cereals) do not manufacture cholesterol since plants are devoid of hormones, nerves, or complex endocrine system. Even without eating any animal products, the liver has the ability to make cholesterol. Herbivores, for example, do not feed on animal products, yet their liver make cholesterol, which we consume.

o **Lowering blood cholesterol:** The following guidelines are universally accepted in dealing with high blood cholesterol:

    i. Cutting down on **animal products**, especially for people with hereditary hyperlipidemia. Choose a diet that is low in saturated fat and cholesterol and moderate in total fat. Fats supply energy and essential fatty acids, and they help absorb the fat-soluble vitamins A, D, E, and K, and carotenoids. You need some fat in the food you eat, but choose sensibly. Some kinds of fat, especially saturated fats, increase the risk for coronary heart disease by raising the blood cholesterol (see *Tip # 6*, below, Section 15.11). In contrast, unsaturated fats (found mainly in vegetable oils) do not increase blood cholesterol.

    ii. Lowering the total daily **caloric intake**. Excess calories are stored as fat depot that drives cholesterol synthesis. Fat intake in the United States as a proportion of total calories is lower than it was many years ago, but most people still eat too much saturated fat. Eating lots of fat of any type can provide excess calories. See *Tip # 7*, below, Section 15.11, for tips on limiting the amount of saturated fat and cholesterol you get from your food. Taking these steps can go a long way in helping to keep your blood cholesterol level low.

    iii. Following the tips in the *Tip # 7* will help you keep your intake of saturated fat at less than 10 percent of calories. They will also help you keep your cholesterol intake less than the **Daily Value of 300 mg/day** listed on the **Nutrition Facts Label**. If you want more flexibility, see *Tip # 8* below, to find out your saturated fat limit in grams. The maximum number of saturated fat grams depends on the amount of calories you get daily. Use Nutrition Facts Labels to find out how much saturated fat is in prepared foods. If you choose one food that is higher in saturated fat, make your other choices lower in saturated fat. This will help you stay under your saturated fat limit for the day.

    iv. **Different forms of the same food** may be very different in their content of saturated fat. *Tip # 9,* below, provides some examples. Try to choose the forms of food that are lower in saturated fat most often.

    v. Keep total fat intake moderate. Aim for a total **fat intake of no more than 30 percent of calories**. If you need to reduce your fat intake to achieve this level, do so primarily by cutting back on saturated and trans fats. Check *Tip # 8* to find out how many grams of fat you can have for the number of calories you need. For example, at 2,200 calories per day, your suggested upper limit on fat intake would be about 73 grams. If you are at a healthy weight and you eat little saturated fat, you'll have leeway to eat some plant foods that are high in unsaturated fats.

    vi. Beginning at age 2, **children** should get most of their calories from grain products; fruits; vegetables; low-fat dairy products; and beans, lean meat and poultry, fish, or nuts. Be careful, nuts may cause choking in 2 to 3 year olds.

    vii. Increasing the **energy expenditure** through physical activity and exercise. Daily activities around the home or at work are not always sufficient to burn calories.

    viii. Cholesterol lowering **medications** are prescribed when diet and exercise aren't enough. Medications have to be combined with exercise in order to be effective. Medications work on the liver synthesis of cholesterol, while exercise depletes the substrates of the process of synthesis of cholesterol.

EXERCISE AND PREVENTABLE DISEASES

15.5.8. OVERWEIGHT AND OBESITY

15.5.8.1. Obesity

o Obesity signifies inadequate **cellular respiration**. When caloric intakes exceeds caloric expenditure then cellular respiration falls short of pumping enough fuel into the cellular furnace of energy production, the TCA cycle. The excess byproducts of food are diverted to adipose tissue for storage. Thus, inefficient cellular respiration, during inactivity, activates building fatty acids and storing them as triglycerides. It also activates manufacturing more cholesterol and depositing it into the walls of blood vessels. Obesity thus deprives the body cells from energy rich molecules and biochemical substrates that are vital to life.

o Obesity is defined as too much body fat. A person might not be overweight yet obese due to lack of exercise and wasting of muscles. It is very important to stress that with lack of physical activity, all ingredients of food (carbohydrate, protein, and fat) will be converted to fat, if in excess of body needs. It is also very important to point out that, apparent fat deposition at the waist and buttocks is only part of the total fat deposition. Fat deposits inside the walls of the blood vessels and around the internal organs, as early as the age of 20. When planning to lose fat, one has to keep in mind that the liver is the pivotal organ in that process. Fast fat reduction could harm the liver, reverse the process, and ail the entire health.

o In order to assess body fat content, the following empirical methods of measuring body fat are used:

i. **Waistline measurement** indicates obesity in the following conditions:
   a. Women waistline over 35 inches.
   b. Men waistline over 40 inches.

ii. **Body mass index (BMI)** is defined as the "quotient of the bodyweight by the square of the height." It is widely used to determined fluid needs in states of medical emergency. The division of bodyweight by square of height estimates the amount of area needed per each unit of the bodyweight. Thus, it indicates the availability of surface area to dump heat and excess byproducts of the body metabolism. It is estimated as follows, *Table 15.5* and *Figure 15.4*.

Table 15.5. Body mass index for obesity and overweight (National Center for Health Statistics).

Body conditions	B.M.I
Healthy	18.5 – 24.9
Underweight	Less than 18.5
Overweight	25.0 – 29.9
Obesity	30 - up

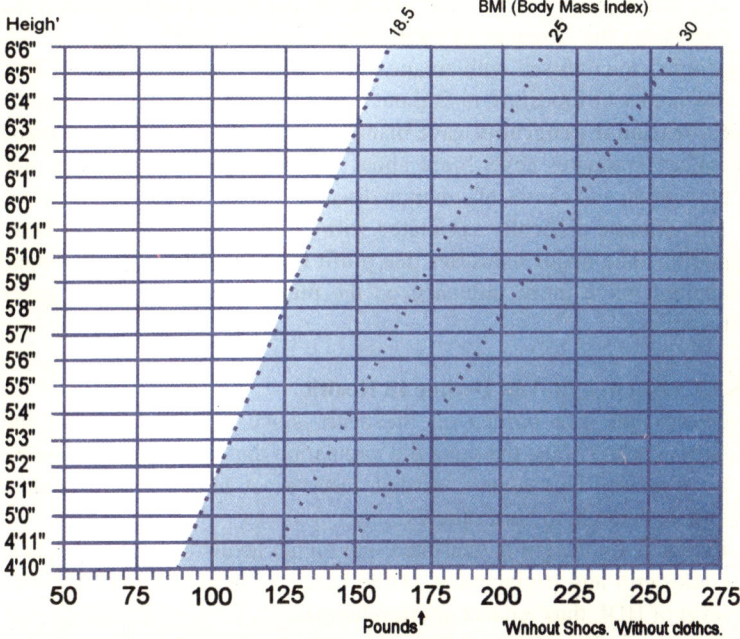

Figure 15.4. BMI measures weight in relation to height. The BMI ranges shown above are for adults. They are not exact ranges of healthy and unhealthy weights. However, they show that health risk increases at higher levels of overweight and obesity. Even within the healthy BMI range, weight gains can carry health risks for adults.

Directions: Find your weight on the bottom of the graph. Go straight up from that point until you come to the line that matches your height. Then look to find your weight group.

Healthy Weight BMI from 18.5 up to 25 refers to a healthy weight.

Overweight BMI from 25 up to 30 refers to overweight.

Obese BMI 30 or higher refers to obesity. Obese persons are also overweight.

Source: *Report of the Dietary Guidelines Advisory Committee on the Dietary Guidelines for American.*

BMI = Weight (kilogram) / Square of Height (meter)^2 = 703 x Weight (pounds) / Square of Height (inch)^2

EXERCISE AND PREVENTABLE DISEASES

15.5.8.2. Overweight
Overweight is defined as body weight that is in excess to the norms of the population of the same height as the individual. In addition, an overweight athlete might not be obese due to increase of muscle mass. Overweight and obesity is a national public health problem in many developed countries. Lack of dietary knowledge, combined with physical inactivity and the large-scale availability of junk food, are the main causes of the obesity and overweight epidemic, as follows.

o Many people consume excess amounts of food rich in **carbohydrates and fat**. The cheapest food products in the market are made of carbohydrates and fat.
o People believe that their body knows how to live, regardless of their behavior. **Fatalistic thinking** is predominant in all cultures and leads to dissociation of knowledge and habits.
o Exercise requires **resources** such as transportation, participation fees, dedication, and long learning of how to get results.
o Overweight **drains resources** such as money spent on food and special clothes, loss of job opportunities, cost of health expenses, and lack of energy to deal with the multifaceted problem of overweight.
o Some cultural traditions emphasize on eating as a **strengthening bond** between individuals.
o The method of **communicating knowledge** to the consumer is arcane. The majority of the public has hard time relating terms such as "energy imbalance", "Calories", "carbohydrates", "protein", or "fat", to issues of bulging bellies and excess bodyweight. The lay public is not well familiar with the structured world of chemistry and physics that dominates the language of publications, radio, and television. In America, as well as in the middle of Africa, many people are confused with arcane terms such as "carbohydrates". To hide their embarrassment, they might enumerate few names of foodstuff, to find out if "carbohydrates" refers to something they know.
o **Educational programs** leave many people in utter darkness, in many areas of life, such as health and fitness. Many college graduates never heard about "hypertension" or "diabetes mellitus" or they do not know the basic facts about prevention and causes of common diseases.
o The extreme difficulty associated with efforts to reduce excess bodyweight calls for radical measures to protect the public. The major industries that profit from the sale of predominantly carbohydrate- and fat- rich food, tobacco, and alcohol, have more influence on the public interest and the governments than all **public health advocacies** put together.

15.5.8.3. Overweight And Decline In Health
o Overweight is a burden on the heart, since the heart doesn't increase in size in proportion to the increase in bodyweight. Thus, the same old circulation that used to supply nutrients to the body, is now stretched to supply more body mass. This reduces cardiac reserve. A heavy person could not perform **physical activities** long enough, or intense enough, to burn calories.
o Excess body weight is translated into higher levels of **LDL**. This is a fraction of the blood lipoproteins that are rich in cholesterol and triglycerides. High LDL causes fat deposition inside the walls of the arteries. Exercise elevates the level of HDL thus reduces arteriosclerosis.
o Overweight is a *bitter challenge* to millions of people around the world. Most of the time, people lose the battle, to reduce their bodyweight, to **diseases** such as diabetes, high blood pressure, heart and kidney failure.

15.5.8.4. Failure To Reduce Bodyweight
o Body **hormones and endocrine** system overzealously work to maintain *existing body conditions,* even if they are harmful to health. Trials to lose weight cause craving, headache, and anxiety, which lead to failure to comply with a weight-reduction plan.
o Many people desire to reverse the weight, gained in months and years, in shorter period. By the time the weight reduction plan starts showing results, and the body hormones and endocrine start *resetting their threshold* to new bodily conditions, many people become frustrated or have sensed that they have already been punished enough.
o Reducing bodyweight by calculating calories and engaging in physical activities might not suffice, if other *factors are in work in favor of weight gain.* A **job** that requires long hours of immobility and mental stress would defeat any good that comes from short hours of exercise. A **favored kind** of food such as pizza or ice cream, even though total calories are in check, would require extended hours of calorie-burning exercise, in excess of one's normal ability.
o Obsession of health habits is ridiculed in some **cultures**. Life-long trends are more important than transient efforts. Aggravating factors such as alcohol and smoking make it harder to break the cycle of weight gain. If little alcohol protects your heart a bit, it impairs your ability to exercise afterwards, or in the next day, depriving you from any gain. If smoking is magical in suppressing pain and lifting your spirit for few hours, it snatches away your livelihood to endure lengthy physical activity.

15.5.8.5. Obesity And Overweight In Children
o Children develop their self-esteem from their ability to excel in entirely new activities. Overweight denies the young a chance to join his or her peers in the daunting task of play. It is much easier to control bodyweight in younger children than in older ones. The following guidelines are recommended in dealing with dietary issues in children.

i. Younger children should not be subjected to strict reduction in dietary fat since the **brain development** requires fat for growth.
ii. **Parents' behavior** is a crucial factor in picking and choosing food. Consumption of **excess** amounts of sweet, bread, pizza, rice, ice creams, or butter should be rigorously reduced, in order to see any drop in body fat and weight. If one sort of carbohydrate or fat is consumed in abundance, the other sources should be eliminated. Thus, the quantity of intake can be used as a reliable index of caloric intake.
iii. Strict rules on the times of meals become ingrained in the minds of the young with some consistent and stable home environment.
o Children older than 10 years could master complex sports and participate in lengthy training planning according to their age. There is no need to fear for children participation in sport, since their future success depends on their early childhood learning.

15.6. COST-EFFECTIVE AND REALISTIC PREVENTION OF HEART DISEASES

In order to prevent heart disease, one should adopt the most reliable method of combining healthy diet with exercise, on a daily basis. This helps control bodyweight and promotes fitness, as follows.

15.6.1. HEALTHY EATING
o **Variation:** different foods contain different nutrients and other healthful substances. No single food can supply all the nutrients in the amounts you need. For example, oranges provide vitamin-C and folate but no vitamin-B_{12}; cheese provides calcium and vitamin-B_{12}; but no vitamin-C. Choose the recommended number of daily servings from each of the five major food groups, *Tip # 10* below. If you avoid all foods from any of the five food groups, seek guidance to help ensure that you get all the nutrients you need. Choose a variety of foods for good nutrition. Since foods within most food groups differ in their content of nutrients and other beneficial substances, choosing a variety helps you get all the nutrients and fiber you need. It can also help keep your meals interesting from day to day.
o **The food pyramid:** use plant foods as the foundation of your meals. There are many ways to create a healthy eating pattern, but they all start with the three food groups at the base of the Pyramid: grains, fruits, and vegetables. Eating a variety of grains (especially whole grain foods), fruits, and vegetables is the basis of healthy eating. Enjoy meals that have rice, pasta, tortillas, or whole grain bread at the center of the plate, accompanied by plenty of fruits and vegetables and a moderate amount of low-fat foods from the milk group and the meat and beans group. Go easy on foods high in fat or sugars.
o **Serving size:** keep an eye on servings. Compare the recommended number of servings in *Tip # 10* with what you usually eat. If you don't need many calories (because you're inactive, for example), aim for the lower number of servings. Young children 2 to 3 years old need the same number of servings as others, but smaller serving sizes except for milk. In addition, notice that many of the meals and snacks you eat contain items from several food groups. For example, a sandwich may provide bread from the grains group, turkey from the meat and beans group, and cheese from the milk group.
o **Serving methods:** Try serving fruits and vegetables in new ways, such as follows:
i. Raw vegetables with a low- or reduced-fat dip.
ii. Vegetables stir-fried in a small amount of vegetable oil.
iii. Fruits or vegetables mixed with other foods in salads, soups, and sauces (for example, add shredded vegetables when making meatloaf).
iv. Find ways to include plenty of different fruits and vegetables in your meals and snacks
v. Buy wisely. Frozen or canned fruits and vegetables are sometimes best buys, and they are rich in nutrients. If fresh fruit is very ripe, buy only enough to use right away.
vi. Store properly to maintain quality. Refrigerate most fresh fruits (not bananas) and vegetables (not potatoes or tomatoes) for longer storage, and arrange them so you'll use up the ripest ones first. If you cut them up or open a can, cover and refrigerate afterward.
vii. Keep ready-to-eat raw vegetables handy in a clear container in the front of your refrigerator for snacks or meals-on-the-go.
viii. Keep a day's supply of fresh or dried fruit handy on the table or counter.
ix. Enjoy fruits as a naturally sweet end to a meal.
x. When eating out, choose a variety of vegetables at a salad bar.
o **Fruits and vegetables:** Choose a variety of fruits and vegetables daily.
i. Fruits and vegetables are key parts of your daily diet. Eating plenty of fruits and vegetables of different kinds may help protect you against many chronic diseases. It also promotes healthy bowel function. Fruits and vegetables provide essential vitamins and minerals, fiber, and other substances that are important for good health.
ii. Most people, including children, eat fewer servings of fruits and vegetables than are recommended. To promote your health, eat a variety of fruits and vegetables—at least 2 servings of fruits and 3 servings of vegetables—each day.

15 EXERCISE AND PREVENTABLE DISEASES

  iii. Different fruits and vegetables are rich in different nutrients (see *Tip # 11* below). Some fruits and vegetables are excellent sources of carotenoids, including those which form vitamin-A, while others may be rich in vitamin-C, folate, or potassium. Fruits and vegetables, especially dry beans and peas, also contain fiber and other substances that are associated with good health. Dark-green leafy vegetables, deeply colored fruits, and dry beans and peas are especially rich in many nutrients.
  iv. Most fruits and vegetables are naturally low in fat and calories and are filling. Some are high in fiber, and many are quick to prepare and easy to eat. Choose whole or cut-up fruits and vegetables rather than juices most often. Juices contain little or no fiber.
- **Whole grains** are the best source of carbohydrates and vitamins such as niacin.
  i. This should be consumed on daily basis. High sugar containing food undermines the body metabolism. Thus, sweet food and drinks should be kept minimum or eliminated from daily intake.
  ii. Foods made from grains (wheat, rice, and oats) help form the foundation of a nutritious diet. They provide vitamins, minerals, carbohydrates (starch and dietary fiber), and other substances that are important for good health.
  iii. Grain products are low in fat, unless fat is added in processing, in preparation, or at the table.
  iv. Whole grains differ from refined grains in the amount of fiber and nutrients they provide, and different whole grain foods differ in nutrient content, so choose a variety of whole and enriched grains. Eating plenty of whole grains, such as whole wheat bread or oatmeal (see *Tip # 12* below), as part of the healthful eating patterns may help protect you against many chronic diseases.
  v. Aim for at least six servings of grain products per day—more if you are an older child or teenager, an adult man, or an active woman (see *Tip # 10*)—and include several servings of whole grain foods.
  vi. Vitamins, minerals, fiber, and other protective substances in whole grain foods contribute to the health benefits of whole grains. Refined grains are low in fiber and in the protective substances that accompany fiber. Eating plenty of fiber-containing foods, such as whole grains (and also many fruits and vegetables) promotes proper bowel function.
  vii. The high fiber content of many whole grains may also help you to feel full with fewer calories. Fiber is best obtained from foods like whole grains, fruits, and vegetables rather than from fiber supplements for several reasons. There are many types of fiber, the composition of fiber is poorly understood, and other protective substances accompany fiber in foods. Use the Nutrition Facts Label to help choose grains that are rich in fiber and low in saturated fat and sodium.
  viii. Enriched grains are a new source of folic acid. Folic acid, a form of folate, is now added to all enriched grain products (thiamin, riboflavin, niacin, and iron have been added to enriched grains for many years). Folate is a B-vitamin that reduces the risk of some serious types of birth defects when consumed before and during early pregnancy. Studies are underway to clarify whether it decreases risk for coronary heart disease, stroke, and certain types of cancer. Whole grain foods naturally contain some folate, but only a few (mainly ready-to-eat breakfast cereals) contain added folic acid as well. Read the ingredient label to find out if folic acid and other nutrients have been added, and check the Nutrition Facts Label to compare the nutrient content of foods like breakfast cereals.
- **Food borne illness:** Keep food safe to eat. Foods that are safe from harmful bacteria, viruses, parasites, and chemical contaminants are vital for healthful eating. Safe means that the food poses little risk of food borne illness (see *Tip # 13* below). Farmers, food producers, markets, food service establishments, and other food preparers have a role to keep food as safe as possible. However, we also need to keep and prepare foods safely in the home, and be alert when eating out. Follow the steps below to keep your food safe. Be very careful with perishable foods such as eggs, meats, poultry, fish, shellfish, milk products, and fresh fruits and vegetables. If you are at high risk of foodborne illness, be extra careful (see *Tip # 14* below).
  i. **Clean:** Wash hands and surfaces often. Wash your hands with warm soapy water for 20 seconds (count to 30) before you handle food or food utensils. Wash your hands after handling or preparing food, especially after handling raw meat, poultry, fish, shellfish, or eggs. Right after you prepare these raw foods, clean the utensils and surfaces you used with hot soapy water. Replace cutting boards once they have become worn or develop hard-to-clean grooves. Wash raw fruit and vegetables under running water before eating. Use a vegetable brush to remove surface dirt if necessary. Always wash your hands after using the bathroom, changing diapers, or playing with pets. When eating out, if the tables, dinnerware, and restrooms look dirty, the kitchen may be, too—so you may want to eat somewhere else.
  ii. **Separate:** Separate raw, cooked, and ready-to-eat foods while shopping, preparing, or storing. Keep raw meat, poultry, eggs, fish, and shellfish away from other foods, surfaces, utensils, or serving plates. This prevents cross-contamination from one food to another. Store raw meat, poultry, fish, and shellfish in containers in the refrigerator so that the juices don't drip onto other foods.
  iii. **Cook:** Cook foods to a safe temperature. Uncooked and undercooked animal foods are potentially unsafe. Proper cooking makes most uncooked foods safe. The best way to tell if meat, poultry, or egg dishes are cooked to a safe temperature is to use a food thermometer, *Figure 15.5*. Several kinds of inexpensive food thermometers are available in many stores. Reheat sauces, soups, marinades, and gravies to a boil. Reheat leftovers thoroughly to at

least 165° F. If using a microwave oven, cover the container and turn or stir the food to make sure it is heated evenly throughout. Cook eggs until whites and yolks are firm. Don't eat raw or partially cooked eggs, or foods containing raw eggs, raw (unpasteurized) milk, or cheeses made with raw milk. Choose pasteurized juices. The risk of contamination is high from undercooked hamburger, and from raw fish (including sushi), clams, and oysters. Cook fish and shellfish until it is opaque; fish should flake easily with a fork. When eating out, order foods thoroughly cooked and make sure they are served piping hot.

iv. **Chill** : Refrigerate perishable foods promptly. When shopping, buy perishable foods last, and take them straight home. At home, refrigerate or freeze meat, poultry, eggs, fish, shellfish, ready-to-eat foods, and leftovers promptly. Refrigerate within 2 hours of purchasing or preparation—and within 1 hour if the air temperature is above 90° F. Refrigerate at or below 40° F, or freeze at or below 0° F. Use refrigerated leftovers within 3 to 4 days. Freeze fresh meat, poultry, fish, and shellfish that cannot be used in a few days. Thaw frozen meat, poultry, fish, and shellfish in the refrigerator, microwave, or cold water changed every 30 minutes. (This keeps the surface chilled.) Cook foods immediately after thawing. Never thaw meat, poultry, fish, or shellfish at room temperature. When eating out, make sure that any foods you order that should be refrigerated are served chilled.

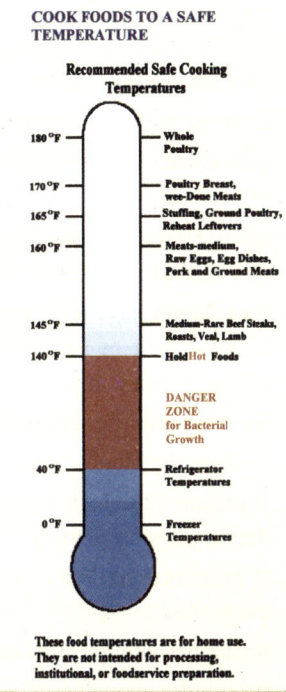

Figure 15.5. Safe cooking and chilling temperatures for food.

v. **Follow the label:** Read the label and follow safety instructions on the package such as "KEEP REFRIGERATED" and the "SAFE HANDLING INSTRUCTIONS."

vi. **Serve safely** : Keep hot foods hot (140° F or above) and cold foods cold (40° F or below). Harmful bacteria can grow rapidly in the "danger zone" between these temperatures. Whether raw or cooked, never leave meat, poultry, eggs, fish, or shellfish out at room temperature for more than 2 hours (1 hour in hot weather 90° F or above). Be sure to chill leftovers as soon as you are finished eating. These guidelines also apply to carryout meals, restaurant leftovers, and home-packed meals-to-go.

vii. **When in doubt, throw it out** : If you aren't sure that food has been prepared, served, or stored safely, throw it out. You may not be able to make food safe if it has been handled in an unsafe manner. For example, a food that has been left at room temperature too long may contain a toxin produced by bacteria—one that can't be destroyed by cooking. So, if meat, poultry, fish, shellfish, or eggs have been left out for more than 2 hours, or if the food has been kept in the refrigerator too long, don't taste it. Just throw it out. Even if it looks and smells fine, it may not be safe to eat. If you have doubt when you're shopping or eating out, choose something else.

15.6.2. EXERCISE

o Do not think of exercise as something that only other folks can do. **Exercise is for everybody**. The ability to move, kicks, and scream is vital to the survival of a newborn, and is still vital to grown adults, to sustain mobility. It becomes more vital as we get older. Humans spend their first 10 years working harder on physical skills than in development of intellectual maturity. Afterwards, in the next10 to 20 years, physical activity declines while intellectual maturity peaks. What happen after 30 years of life are complacence, boredom, and distraction with vanities.

o **Exercise now. Exercise anywhere**. Be patient. It will pay back in weeks, not months. The longer you exercise the livelier you get. Even if you have done poorly, for so long, exercise and patience could pull you out of the deep. Weighing the danger of destructive behavior in social interactions and the desire to "fit in" social groups, against personal health, is greatly overlooked amongst all social classes.

o **What should you do to exercise, now?**
  i. Go for a walk.
  ii. Kick away chairs and sofa out of your way and do things while standing or moving.
  iii. Then read more about how to proceed slowly along the tracks, others have followed.
  iv. Start with very simple routines, of three exercises, for an hour, three to four times a week.
  v. Never shy from dreaming to be in the same shoes of the best, even if you keep that ambition secretive.

15 EXERCISE AND PREVENTABLE DISEASES

vi. The most complicated exercises start with simple movements, lightest resistance, and visual training, prior to stepping into tougher routines.

- **Why is exercise important?**
    i. Exercise adds fuel to the fire. Every cell in our body perfects the science of mastering the fire of life.
    ii. Live creatures have warm body, breathe and exhale warm air, and secrete warm byproducts of that biological fire of life within us.
    iii. Intense exercise could increase the amount of blood, the heart pumps every minute, **from 5 liters to 25 liters**. It also could increase the volume of airflow to the lungs every minute, **from 7 liter to 100 liters**.
    iv. You do not have to be a scientist to understand that when the body needs that much air during exercise there must be some sort of fuel burning within the body. There also have to be some sort of mechanism to facilitate the energy burning in fit people, better than in the unfit.
    v. Exercise modifies each cell in the body to work in harmony, to deal with the fire of life.
    vi. It clears the blood vessel highways from the junk of cholesterol plaques that clogs the traffic of blood flow
    vii. It prepares the highway controllers of pressure and gas sensors to react promptly and efficiently as the fire flares during physical activity.
    viii. It prepares the body inlets (intestine) and the body outlets (kidneys, skin, lungs) of the highways to avoid congestion.
    ix. It supplies enough provision of coronary blood flow to the heart, to maintain the circulation of the blood.
    x. It provides enough provision to the brain, to maintain the central control commanding of all vital operations.
    xi. It provides enough provision to the bone, muscles, tendons, and joints to stand the forces of gravity.

Look at the faces of children who do not exercise. They lack the joy of active living. Regular physical activity increases your capacity for exercise. It also plays a role in both primary and secondary prevention of cardiovascular disease

- **Prerequisites to exercise:** Though exercise is always praised for goodness to health, it nevertheless requires certain minimal health conditions to avoid harm. The following are some conditions that need attention by physicians prior to and along with exercise
    i. Heart conditions that have past long record, or those that arise as a result of physical activity, should seek medical advice prior to exercise.
    ii. Pain on exertion, shortness of breath, and general sense of imbalance or dizziness are signs that require immediate cessation of physical activity and subsequent medical attention.
    iii. Cerebrovascular conditions (stroke) that interfere with motor or sensory activities require expert health care.
    iv. Long history of unexplained fatigue or loss of energy might indicate hidden medical problems that should be corrected prior to engagement in strenuous activities.
    v. Use of medication for existing medical problems such as high blood pressure, heart condition or a stroke should exercise only under the supervision of professional medical care. Many medications can induce sudden arrhythmias, suppress the sympathetic nervous system, and thus lead to unpredictable outcome during exercise.
    vi. Medical conditions that might worsen by the proposed physical activity need individualized expert planning.
    vii. Extremes of bodyweight, age, and fitness status should be advised and supervised by health experts.

15.7. CANCER

- **Aging:** The prevalence of cancer among the elderly population accounts for about 80% of annually diagnosed cases of all types of cancer. The common denominator, among most cases of cancer, is the compromised immune system. Whatever causes the immune system to crumble is most probably responsible for triggering the new growth of pathological cells.
- **Autoimmune decline:** Age plays multiple roles in impairing the autoimmune system. The long duration of individual habits, add up to insidious and chronic development of pathological processes. Physical inactivity for few decades is sufficient to cause multiple systemic problems, including the cardiovascular, musculoskeletal, and the digestive system. The slow and constant decline in health over the years takes its serious toll over the age of 50. The fact that the body can cope with so many insults and poor health habits for so many years, before it start to protest, attests to the marvelous design of the biological system.

EXERCISE AND PREVENTABLE DISEASES

- o **Obesity:** Inactivity affects the molecules of the body cells in very direct manner. This occurs through the biochemical signals that regulate maturation, proliferation and death, among neighboring cells. Disturbed biochemical communication alters that social network between cells, organs, and systems, resulting in the evasion of the immune defense system by cancer cells. Examples of the high prevalence of cancer due to immune suppression are seen in cases of organ transplant and AIDS patients. Inactivity induces active synthesis of fat, from all sorts of foodstuff, but with minimal creation of new blood capillaries. Such process of mass production of fat, with limited blood supply, might induce the body to activate a parasitic form of angiogenesis. This serves as circulatory access to the fat cells. Parasitic angiogenesis is peculiar to cancerous cells and might have stemmed from processes similar to fat deposition. That may explain the well-known trend of high cancer prevalence among obese people. Modern and future chemotherapy for cancer focuses on the disturbed molecular conditions that led to cancer. Thus, chemical drugs are designed to inhibit the malfunctioning molecules of cancer cells. In addition, vaccines can induce the body to produce anti-cancer antibodies.
- o **Winning the battle:** Early detection of some kinds of cancers can help in lasting treatments. Colon cancer for example can be detected early with simple stool test, or colonoscopy, with great accuracy. Mammography and genetic analysis may detect early breast cancer and guide management plans. In addition, urine test for specific cell division proteins can detect bladder cancer before imaging techniques. The new approach for searching for abnormal molecules of cancerous tumors in the body fluids might be promising in earlier detection or correction of carcinogenesis. The role of exercise is more emphasized after the rectification of pathological causes and during chemotherapy. The famous story of the basketball layer Magic Johnson is a testimony for the crucial role of exercise in augmenting chemotherapy for AIDS treatment and preventing cancer related problems. In 1991, Johnson stunned the world with the announcement that he had tested positive for the HIV virus and was retiring from the NBA. He began a campaign to promote AIDS awareness. Johnson went on to play for the 1992 U.S. Olympic Dream Team. In addition to his genuine understanding of the need for compliance with rigorous medical treatment, he also adhered to very active training plan to enhance his muscular strength.
- o **Role of diet:** Vegetables help reduce cancer risk. At least five servings of fruits and vegetables a day are recommended to reduce cancer incidence. Animal food products and greater alcohol consumption induce abnormal cells to develop into tumors. Eating less meat helps fight cancers in part because saturated fats are thought to promote certain cancers, and also because high temperature cooking generates carcinogenic amines in meat.

15.8. CEREBROVASCULAR DISEASE
- o Stroke is a brain accident. It results from either blockage of the blood flow or hemorrhage. The following are the trends in stroke affliction in the USA, *Table 15.4.*
    - i. Stroke is the third largest cause of death, ranking behind diseases of the heart and cancer.
    - ii. About 4,500,000 stroke survivors are alive today.
    - iii. About 600,000 people suffer a new or recurrent stroke.
    - iv. Female's account for over 60% of stroke deaths.
    - v. All functions controlled by the affected site of the brain could be impaired. Therefore, a person with stroke might complain of:
        - a. Loss of sensation or numbness of one side of the body (face, arm, or leg, or the entire side).
        - b. Paralysis or weakness of limbs, eye, or tongue.
        - c. Mental disorders (confusion, loss of vision, speech, hearing, smelling, headache, imbalance, or dizziness).

- o Physical activity is crucial to the survival of the individual after recovering from the acute phase of stroke. Exercise can reverse loss of function, both in the periphery and in the brain. Since activity enhances circulation and respiration, it fosters recovery of afflicted organs.

15.9. AUTOIMMUNE SYSTEM
- o **Internal policing:** As with any large community, law and order are essential for the community to work and produce, without wasting resources in trivial internal conflicts. The autoimmune system of humans performs the task of internal policing of the body molecules, as follows.
    - i. The immune system of mammals is so sophisticated as to distinguish foreign from self-elements, be they cells or molecules.

EXERCISE AND PREVENTABLE DISEASES

-
  - ii. It has the means to disable foreign cells and neutralize foreign molecules in order to maintain secure and balanced biological milieu.
  - iii. Our immune system can even be educated to recognize foreign bodies and manufacture antibodies to prevent their disruption to the internal milieu of the body. This defense system operates by both fluid and cellular components that can present their actions, either in vivo or in vitro.
  - iv. Like any other cells, the cells of the immune system perform energy production, synthesize protein, and communicate with the network of body cells through circulation. Yet, immune cells are always on alert, surveying the internal environment for order. Thus, immune cells perform very active synthesis and energy production.

- **Autoimmune intolerance:** Disturbance in communication between immune cells and the network of body cells results in mistaken identification of law-breakers. The immune system might err in identifying self-cells as foreign, attack them causing a wide spectrum of autoimmune diseases, as follows.
  - i. Immune-system cells attack the connective tissues of joints causing rheumatoid arthritis.
  - ii. They attack multiple organs, in Lupus erythromatosus. This disease afflicts many organs and target women more than men. If untreated, it causes major organ failures
  - iii. They attack the coating of nerves, in multiple sclerosis. This disease afflicts the nervous system and impacts the entire health of the individual.
  - iv. They attack specific liver cells, in sclerosing cholangitis. This disease diminishes the liver's ability to excrete bile. Thus, it causes serious malabsorption and accumulation of bilirubin in the blood. It necessitates liver transplant.
  - v. They attack stomach cells, in pernicious anemia. This prevents the intestinal absorption of vitamin-B_{12} due to the lack of a stomach protein, the intrinsic factor. Pernicious anemia diminishes the delivery of nutrients to all organs, particularly, the nervous system.
  - vi. They attack transplant organs with different antigenic makeup. This causes organ transplant failure and may necessitate aggressive immune suppressive therapy or re-transplantation.
  - vii. They attack the pancreatic cells that produce insulin or the insulin receptors on target cells causing diabetes, and so on.

- **Causes of intolerance:** Such disturbance in autoimmune identification can come about by various conditions.
  - i. Viruses and microorganism can induce the immune system to attack self-cells such as in rheumatic fever and post-viral fevers.
  - ii. Inactivity can also trigger the immune system by undermining the availability of energy molecules and biological substrates of synthesis and reproduction by the immune cells.
  - iii. Genetic defects in genes can cause deficiency in the cellular or antibody elements of the defense system.
  - iv. Long before our current understanding of immunology, old medicine relied on herbs and rituals to treat autoimmune diseases. In many remote communities, people believed in certain food or plant ingredient that may cure such mysterious diseases.
  - v. Modern treatments, though guided with immense chemical knowledge, fall short of curing autoimmune diseases. They suppress the autoimmune system when inflammation or rejection flares up, and induce the system to produce antibodies when foreign insults are expected to afflict the body.

15.10. DIABETES MELLITUS

15.10.1. IMPACT ON PUBLIC HEALTH
- Diabetes mellitus killed 28,187 men and 34,449 women in USA in 1997. This amounts to annual mortality rates of 21.5 per 100,000 for men and 25.2 per 100,000 for women.
- In contrast, the annual mortality rate due to diabetes mellitus in Japan in 1997 was 10.3 for men and 9.5 for women.
- It is a disturbing fact that risk of American women of dying from diabetes mellitus is 2.65 times that for Japanese women. The risk of American men of dying from diabetes is 2.09 times that for Japanese men.
- Most diabetics are overweight or obese, have high blood pressure, and aren't physically active.
- In USA, 10,600,000 Americans have physician-diagnosed diabetes.
- In USA, 798,000 new cases of adult-onset diabetes are diagnosed every year.
- Two-thirds of people with diabetes mellitus die of some form of cardiovascular disease.

15.10.2. GLUCOSE FUEL

o Diabetes mellitus is thought of as the man-made disease that was born with the discovery of refined sugars. Extracting sugars from fruits created an abundant food supply of **fast absorbable carbohydrate**. Within 30 minutes after ingestion, the consumed refined sugar appears in the blood as a hike in the blood glucose level. This creates irresistible desire to consume sweets without discretion. In response to the rise in glucose, the pancreas secretes insulin. The secreted hormone circulates in the blood and reaches all cells in few seconds. Insulin helps uptake of blood glucose by the cells of many organs. Cells either store glucose in the form of glycogen or burn it for energy.

o Diabetes mellitus is a disease that affects the ability of the cells of the body to **uptake glucose** from the blood, which fuels cellular energy demands. Glucose is a byproduct of breakdown of ingested carbohydrates. It is the basic fuel for anaerobic energy production in the cytoplasm of all cells. Without glucose, cells cannot meet their energy needs for synthesis and metabolism of the biological ingredients of life. Diabetes mellitus develops when the insulin hormone secreted by the pancreas is, either insufficient for adequate glucose transport, or the target cells become insensitive to insulin. Insulin regulates the storage of glucose in the liver and the muscles and the uptake of glucose by the cells.

o Whatever the cause may be, diabetes means **fuel deprivation** of cells of vital organs. The brain and the nervous system, the kidneys, the eyes, and the blood vessels suffer most in diabetes. Exercise, if tolerated, induces all body cells to operate the TCA cycle at higher rates and thus increases the production of ATP molecules, as well as the vital intermediate substrates of the cycle that enter in all biological processes. Exercise thus synchronizes most of the biological functions of the body and enhances the different systems to deal with energy expenditure. It is both preventive and beneficial for those who already developed the disease.

15.10.3. INSULIN ROLE

o Insulin is secreted by the b-cells of the pancreas[5]. These constitute a tiny portion of the pancreas, weighing about one gram. In normal people, the b-cells secrete 2 mg of insulin per day. The **β-cells** have exquisite features, as follows.
  i. They snuggle close to the blood capillaries of the pancreas, to detect any changes in the blood glucose level.
  ii. They store insulin in the form of crystals of protein, prior to release into the circulation. The stored crystals are coated granules.
  iii. Insulin is manufactured on ribosomes, on the granular endoplasmic reticulum of the cytoplasm, by translating the mRNA codes made in the nucleus of these specialized cells. The genetic codes of the nucleus transcribe the mRNA templates for the synthesis of the protein of insulin molecules.

o Consuming excessive amounts of carbohydrates, for longer times, exceeds the ability of the pancreas to secrete adequate amount of insulin. The **excess glucose**, left in the blood, destroys the blood vessels and/or the b-cells, causing the complications of diabetes mellitus. Excessive intake of carbohydrates, combined with inactivity, cause over production of insulin and diminished burning of carbohydrates. This causes overweight. The excess gain in bodyweight stretches the duties of the pancreas and heart, impairing their functions.

o Diabetes, that is not genetically inherited (adult-onset or **type II diabetes**), is caused by obesity, inactivity, stress, and smoking. Lack of exercise affects the ability of all cells to produce energy through the cellular respiration process. The diminished cellular respiration amounts to the deficiency of energy molecules and intermediate byproducts of respiration that is crucial for cellular life. Thus, physical inactivity hinders the ability of cells to sustain life, to respond to insulin signal, or for the pancreas to secrete insulin.

o Cells respond to insulin signals by membrane receptors and cytoplasm transport-protein. The transport protein moves to the periphery of the cell in response to the insulin signal. Both, the synthesis of glucose transport protein and its response to insulin, require efficient cellular respiration by exercise. In addition, the synthesis of insulin in the _-islet cells of the pancreas requires energy and substrates from cellular respiration that is also enhanced by exercise.

15.10.4. PREVENTIVE DIET

o Choose beverages and foods that are low in sugar content in order to moderate your intake of sugars. **Sugars are** carbohydrates and a source of energy (calories). Dietary carbohydrates also include the complex carbohydrates starch and dietary fiber. During digestion, all carbohydrates, except fiber, break down into sugars. Sugars and starches occur naturally in many foods that also supply other nutrients. Examples of these foods include milk, fruits, some vegetables, breads, cereals, and grains.

o Foods containing sugars and starches can promote **tooth decay**. The amount of bacteria in your mouth and lack of exposure to fluorides also promote tooth decay. These bacteria use sugars and starches to produce the acid that causes tooth decay. The more often you eat foods that contain sugars and starches, and the longer these foods remain in your mouth before you brush your teeth, the greater your risk for tooth decay. Frequent eating or drinking sweet or starch

---

[5] "Basic Histology" Junqueira, et al. (1975), pages 390-1. ISBN 0-87041-200-0

EXERCISE AND PREVENTABLE DISEASES

- foods between meals is more likely to harm teeth than eating the same foods at meals and then brushing. Daily dental hygiene, including brushing with fluoride toothpaste and flossing, and adequate intake of fluorides will help prevent tooth decay. Follow the tips in *Tip # 15* below, for healthy teeth.
o **Added sugars** are sugars and syrups added to foods in processing or preparation, not the naturally occurring sugars in foods like fruit or milk. The body cannot tell the difference between naturally occurring and added sugars because they are identical chemically. Foods containing added sugars provide calories, but may have few vitamins and minerals. In the United States, the number one source of added sugars is nondiet soft drinks (soda or pop). Sweets and candies, cakes and cookies, and fruit drinks and fruitades are also major sources of added sugars.
o Intake of a lot of foods high in added sugars, like soft drinks, is of concern. Consuming **excess calories** from these foods may contribute to weight gain or lower consumption of more nutritious foods. Use *Tip # 16* below, to identify the most commonly eaten foods that are high in added sugars (unless they are labeled "sugar free" or "diet"). Limit your use of these beverages and foods. Drink water to quench your thirst, and offer it to children. Some foods with added sugars, like chocolate milk, presweetened cereals, and sweetened canned fruits are high in vitamins and minerals. These foods may provide extra calories along with the nutrients and are fine if you need the extra calories.
o The **Nutrition Facts Label** gives the content of sugars from all sources (naturally occurring sugars plus added sugars, if any). You can use the Nutrition Facts Label to compare the amount of total sugars among similar products. To find out if sugars have been added, you also need to look at the food label ingredient list. Use *Tip # 17* below; to identify names of some added sugars.
o **Sugar substitutes** such as saccharin, aspartame, acesulfame potassium, and sucralose are extremely low in calories. Some people find them useful if they want a sweet taste without the calories. Some foods that contain sugar substitutes, however, still have calories. Unless you reduce the total calories you eat or increase your physical activity, using sugar substitutes will not cause you to lose weight.
o Intake of sugars does not appear to affect **children's behavior** patterns or their ability to learn. Many scientific studies conclude that sugars do not cause hyperactivity in children.
o Foods that are high in sugars but low in essential nutrients primarily contribute calories to the diet. When you take in extra calories and don't offset them by increasing your **physical activity**, you will gain weight. As you aim for a healthy weight and fitness, keep an eye on portion size for all foods and beverages, not only those high in sugars.

15.10.5. CLINICAL MANIFESTATION

o Diabetes mellitus is a progressive disease that affect metabolism. It is clinically defined as fasting blood glucose of 126 mg/dl, or more, measured on two occasions. **Adult-onset diabetes (type II)** is the most common form of acquired diabetes and appears in middle-aged adults. **Insulin-dependent diabetes (type I, juvenile diabetes)** is inherited from parents and appears at younger ages. Because diabetes affects the metabolism of all cells, no organ escapes its harm. Uncontrolled diabetes mellitus can manifest as:
  i. Hunger: Frequent and lasts as long as the diabetes remained untreated.
  ii. Extreme thirst: This is due to the loss of fluids from the cells to the blood because of high blood glucose. The kidneys filter excessive fluids.
  iii. Frequent urination: Blood glucose exceeds kidney threshold of excreting glucose (usually 180 mg/dl).
  iv. Weight loss: Cells could not utilize glucose energy. Thus, synthesis of fat, protein, and carbohydrates is diminished.
  v. Fatigue: Cells lack energy. Muscles loss mass and strength.
  vi. Blurry vision: Nerves are deprived from nutrients, mainly glucose.
  vii. The damage to nerves causes numbness, accidents, and blindness.
  viii. The damage of the blood vessels results in limb amputations, blindness, and kidney diseases.
  ix. The wasting of muscles causes debility and inactivity.
  x. The poor quality of life leads to psychiatric illnesses.

15.11. HIGHLIGHTS OF CHAPTER FIFTEEN

The following seventeen tips are published by the Department of Health and Human Services (HHS) and the Department of Agriculture (USDA), in "NUTRITION AND YOUR HEALTH: DIETARY GUIDELINES FOR AMERICANS."

Tip # 1: On moderation in alcohol drinking.

WHAT IS DRINKING IN MODERATION ?

Moderation is defined as no more than one drink per day for women and no more than two drinks per day for men. This limit is based on differences between the sexes in both weight and metabolism.

Count as a drink—
- 12 ounces of regular beer (150 calories).
- 5 ounces of wine (100 calori).
- 1.5 ounces of 80-proof distilled spirits (100 calories).

NOTE: Even moderate drinking provides extra calories

Tip # 2 : On preventing hypertension.

STEPS THAT MAY HELP KEEP BLOOD PRESSURE IN A HEALTHY RANGE

- Choose and prepare foods with less salt.
- Aim for a healthy weight: blood pressure increases with increases in body weight and decreases when excess weight is reduced.
- Increase physical activity: it helps lower blood pressure, reduce risk of other chronic diseases, and manage weight.
- Eat fruits and vegetables. They are naturally low in salt and calories. They are also rich in potassium (see **Tip # 11**), which may help decrease blood pressure.
- If you drink alcoholic beverages, do so in moderation. Excessive alcohol consumption has been associated with high blood pressure.

Tip # 3 : On the role of dietary salt intake.

IS LOWERING SALT INTAKE SAFE?

- Eating too little salt is not generally a concern for healthy people. If you are being treated for a chronic health problem, ask your doctor about whether it is safe for you to reduce your salt intake.
- Some table salt is fortified with iodine. If you use table salt to meet your need for iodine, a small amount—about 1/4 teaspoon of iodized salt—provides more than half the daily iodine allowance.
- Your body can adjust to prevent too much sodium loss when you exercise heavily or when it is very hot. However,
- if you plan to reduce your salt intake and you exercise vigorously, it is sensible to decrease gradually the amount of salt you consume.

Tip # 4 : On lowering sodium intake.

SALT VERSUS SODIUM

- Salt contains sodium. Sodium is a substance that affects blood pressure.
- The best way to cut back on sodium is to cut back on salt and salty foods and seasonings.
- When reading a Nutrition Facts Label, look for the sodium content. Foods that are low in sodium (less than 5% of the Daily Value or DV) are low in salt.

EXERCISE AND PREVENTABLE DISEASES

Tip # 5: On lowering salt intake.

WAYS TO DECREASE YOUR SALT INTAKE

At the Store
- Choose fresh, plain frozen, or canned vegetables without added salt most often—they're low in salt.
- Choose fresh or frozen fish, shellfish, poultry, and meat most often. They are lower in salt than most canned and processed forms.
- Read the Nutrition Facts Label to compare the amount of sodium in processed foods— such as frozen dinners, packaged mixes, cereals, cheese, breads, soups, salad dressings, and sauces. The amount in different types and brands often varies widely.
- Look for labels that say "low-sodium." They contain 140 mg (about 5% of the Daily Value) or less of sodium per serving.
- Ask your grocer or supermarket to offer more low sodium foods.

Cooking and Eating at Home
- If you salt foods in cooking or at the table, add small amounts. Learn to use spices and herbs, rather than salt, to enhance the flavor of food.
- Go easy on condiments such as soy sauce, ketchup, mustard, pickles, and olives—they can add a lot of salt to your food.
- Leave the salt shaker in a cupboard.

Eating Out
- Choose plain foods like grilled or roasted entrees, baked potatoes, and salad with oil and vinegar. Butter-fried foods tend to be high in salt, as do combination dishes like stews or pasta with sauce.
- Ask to have no salt added when the food is prepared.

Any Time
- Choose fruits and vegetables often.
- Drink water freely. It is usually very low in sodium.
- Check the label on bottled water for sodium content.

Tip # 6 : On the variety of dietary fat.

KNOW THE DIFFERENT TYPES OF FATS

Saturated Fats

Foods high in saturated fats tend to raise blood cholesterol. These foods include high-fat dairy products (like cheese, whole milk, cream, butter, and regular ice cream), fatty fresh and processed meats, the skin and fat of poultry, lard, palm oil, and coconut oil. Keep your intake of these foods low.

Dietary Cholesterol

Foods that are high in cholesterol also tend to raise blood cholesterol. These foods include liver and other organ meats, egg yolks, and dairy fats.

Trans Fatty Acids

Foods high in trans fatty acids tend to raise blood cholesterol. These foods include those high in partially hydrogenated vegetable oils, such as many hard margarines and shortenings. Foods with a high amount of these ingredients include some commercially fried foods and some bakery goods.

Unsaturated Fats

Unsaturated fats (oils) do not raise blood cholesterol. Unsaturated fats occur in vegetable oils, most nuts, olives, avocados, and fatty fish like salmon. Unsaturated oils include both monounsaturated fats and polyunsaturated fats. Olive, canola, sunflower, and peanut oils are some of the oils high in monounsaturated fats. Vegetable oils such as soybean oil, corn oil, and cottonseed oil and many kinds of nuts are good sources of polyunsaturated fats. Some fish, such as salmon, tuna, and mackerel, contain omega-3 fatty acids that are being studied to determine if they offer protection against heart disease. Use moderate amounts of food high in unsaturated fats, taking care to avoid excess calories.

Tip # 7 : On lowering dietary saturated fat and cholesterol.

FOOD CHOICES LOW IN SATURATED FAT AND CHOLESTEROL AND MODERATE IN TOTAL FAT
Get most of your calories from plant foods (grains, fruits, vegetables). If you eat foods high in saturated fat for a special occasion, return to foods that are low in saturated fat the next day.
Fats and Oils <ul><li>Choose vegetable oils rather than solid fats (meat and dairy fats, shortening).</li><li>If you need fewer calories, decrease the amount of fat you use in cooking and at the table.</li></ul> *Meat, Poultry, Fish, Shellfish, Eggs, Beans, and Nuts* <ul><li>Choose 2 to 3 servings of fish, shellfish, lean poultry, other lean meats, beans, or nuts daily. Trim fat from meat and take skin off poultry. Choose dry beans, peas, or lentils often.</li><li>Limit your intake of high-fat processed meats such as bacon, sausages, salami, bologna, and other cold cuts. Try the lower fat varieties (check the Nutrition Facts Label).</li><li>Limit your intake of liver and other organ meats. Use egg yolks and whole eggs in moderation. Use egg whites and egg substitutes freely when cooking since they contain no cholesterol and little or no fat.</li></ul> *Dairy Products* <ul><li>Choose fat-free or low-fat milk, fat-free or low-fat yogurt, and low-fat cheese most often. Try switching from whole to fat-free or low-fat milk. This decreases the saturated fat and calories but keeps all other nutrients the same.</li></ul> *Prepared Foods* <ul><li>Check the Nutrition Facts Label to see how much saturated fat and cholesterol are in a serving of prepared food.</li><li>Choose foods lower in saturated fat and cholesterol.</li></ul> *Foods at Restaurants or Other Eating Establishments* <ul><li>Choose fish or lean meats as suggested above. Limit ground meat and fatty processed meats, marbled steaks, and cheese.</li><li>Limit your intake of foods with creamy sauces, and add little or no butter to your food.</li><li>Choose fruits as desserts most often.</li></ul>

Tip # 8 : On daily limit of fat Calories intake.

WHAT IS YOUR UPPER LIMIT ON FAT FOR THE CALORIES YOU CONSUME?		
Total Calories per Day	*Saturated Fat in Grams*	*Total Fat in Grams*
1,600	18 or less	53
2,000*	20 or less	65
2,200	24 or less	73
2,500*	25 or less	80
2,800	31 or less	93
* Percent Daily Values on Nutrition Facts Labels are based on a 2,000 Calorie diet. Values for 2,000 and 2,500 Calories are rounded to the nearest 5 grams to be consistent with the Nutrition Facts Label.		

EXERCISE AND PREVENTABLE DISEASES

Tip # 9 : On saturated fat content of different foods.

A COMPARISON OF SATURATED FAT IN SOME FOODS		
Food Category	Portion	Saturated Fat Content in Grams
Cheese		
Regular Cheddar cheese	1 oz	6.0
Low-fat Cheddar cheese*	1 oz.	1.2
Ground Beef		
Regular ground beef	3 oz. cooked	7.2
Extra lean ground beef*	3 oz. cooked	5.3
Milk		
Whole milk	1 cup	5.1
Low-fat (1%) milk*	1 cup	1.6
Breads		
Croissant	1 medium	6.6
Bagel*	1 medium	0.1
Frozen Desserts		
Regular ice cream	1/2 cup	4.5
Frozen yogurt*	1/2 cup	2.5
Table Spreads		
Butter	1 tsp.	2.4
Soft margarine*	1 tsp.	0.7
NOTE: The food categories listed are among the major food sources of saturated fat for U.S. adults and children. * Choice that is lower in saturated fat.		

Tip # 10 : On saturated fat content of different foods.

HOW MANY SERVINGS DO YOU NEED EACH DAY?			
Food group	Daily Caloric Intake		
	1,600 §	2,200 §§	2,800 §§§
Bread, Cereal, Rice, and Pasta Group (Grains Group)—especially whole grain	6	9	11
Vegetable Group	3	4	5
Fruit Group	2	3	4
Milk, Yogurt, and Cheese Group (Milk Group)—preferably fat free or low fat	2 or 3*	2 or 3*	2 or 3*
Meat, Poultry, Fish, Dry Beans, Eggs, and Nuts Group (Meat and Beans Group)—preferably lean or low fat	2, for a total of 5 ounces	2, for a total of 6 ounces	3, for a total of 7 ounces
Adapted from U.S. Department of Agriculture, Center for Nutrition Policy and Promotion. The Food Guide Pyramid, Home and Garden Bulletin Number 252, 1996. § Children ages 2 to 6 years, women, some older adults §§ Older children, teen girls, active women, most men §§§ Teen boys, active men * The number of servings depends on your age. Older children and teenagers (ages 9 to 18 years) and adults over the age of 50 need 3 servings daily. Others need 2 servings daily. During pregnancy and lactation, the recommended number of milk group servings is the same as for nonpregnant women.			

EXERCISE AND PREVENTABLE DISEASES

Tip # 11 : On nutritional value of fruits and vegetables.

WHICH FRUITS AND VEGETABLES PROVIDE THE MOST NUTRIENTS?

The lists below show which fruits and vegetables are the best sources of vitamin-A (carotenoids), vitamin-C, folate, and potassium. Eat at least 2 servings of fruits and at least 3 servings of vegetables each day:

Sources of vitamin-A (carotenoids)
- Orange vegetables like carrots, sweet potatoes, pumpkin.
- Dark-green leafy vegetables such as spinach, collards, turnip greens.
- Orange fruits like mango, cantaloupe, apricots.
- Tomatoes.

Sources of vitamin-C
- Citrus fruits and juices, kiwi fruit, strawberries, cantaloupe.
- Broccoli, peppers, tomatoes, cabbage, potatoes.
- Leafy greens such as romaine lettuce, turnip greens, spinach.

Sources of folate
- Cooked dry beans and peas, peanuts.
- Oranges, orange juice.
- Dark-green leafy vegetables like spinach and mustard greens, romaine lettuce.
- Green peas.

Sources of potassium
- Baked white or sweet potato, cooked greens (such as spinach), winter (orange) squash.
- Bananas, plantains, dried fruits such as apricots and prunes, orange juice.
- Cooked dry beans (such as baked beans) and lentils.

NOTE: Read Nutrition Facts Labels for product-specific information, especially for processed fruits and vegetables.

Tip # 12 : On intake of whole grain food.

HOW TO INCREASE YOUR INTAKE OF WHOLE GRAIN FOODS

Choose foods that name one of the following ingredients first on the label's ingredient list.
- Brown rice.
- Oatmeal.
- Whole oats.
- Bulgur (cracked wheat).
- Popcorn.
- Whole rye.
- Graham flour.
- Pearl barley.
- Whole wheat.
- Whole grain corn.

Try some of these whole grain foods: whole wheat bread, whole grain ready-to-eat cereal, low-fat whole wheat crackers, oatmeal, whole wheat pasta, whole barley in soup, tabouli salad.

NOTE: "Wheat flour," "enriched flour," and "degerminated corn meal" are not whole grains.

Tip # 13 : On food borne illness.

WHAT IS FOOD BORNE ILLNESS?

Food borne illness is caused by eating food that contains harmful bacteria, toxins, parasites, viruses, or chemical contaminants. Bacteria and viruses, especially Campylobacter, Salmonella, and Norwalk-like viruses, are among the most common causes of food borne illness we know about today. Eating even a small portion of an unsafe food may make you sick. Signs and symptoms may appear within half an hour of eating a contaminated food or may not develop for up to 3 weeks. Most food borne illness lasts a few hours or days. Some food borne illnesses have effects that go on for weeks, months, or even years. If you think you have become ill from eating a food, consult your health care provider.

EXERCISE AND PREVENTABLE DISEASES

Tip # 14 : On preventing food borne illness.

TIPS FOR THOSE AT HIGH RISK OF FOOD BORNE ILLNESS
Who is at high risk of food borne illness? <ul><li>Pregnant women.</li><li>Young children.</li><li>Older persons.</li><li>People with weakened immune systems or certain chronic illnesses.</li></ul> *Besides following the guidance in this guideline, some of the extra precautions those at high risk should take are :* <ul><li>Do not eat or drink unpasteurized juices, raw sprouts, raw (unpasteurized) milk and products made from unpasteurized milk.</li><li>Do not eat raw or undercooked meat, poultry, eggs, fish, and shellfish (clams, oysters, scallops, and mussels).</li></ul>

Tip # 15 : On dental health.

FOR HEALTHY TEETH AND GUMS
<ul><li>Between meals, eat few foods or beverages containing sugars or starches. If you do eat them, brush your teeth afterward to reduce risk of tooth decay.</li><li>Brush at least twice a day and floss daily. Use fluoride toothpaste.</li><li>Ask your dentist or health care provider about the need for supplemental fluoride, or dental sealants, especially for children and if your drinking water is not fluoridated.</li></ul>

Tip # 16 : On sources of added sugars.

MAJOR SOURCES* OF ADDED SUGARS IN THE UNITED STATES
<ul><li>Soft drinks.</li><li>Cakes, cookies, pies.</li><li>Fruitades and drinks such as fruit punch and lemonade.</li><li>Dairy desserts such as ice cream.</li><li>Candy.</li></ul> * All kinds, except diet or sugar-free.

Tip # 17: On names of added sugars.

NAMES FOR ADDED SUGARS THAT APPEAR ON FOOD LABELS			
A food is likely to be high in sugars if one of these names appears first or second in the ingredient list, or if several names are listed.			
Brown sugar	Fruit juice concentrate	Lactose	
Corn sweetener	Glucose	Malt syrup	Sucrose
Corn syrup	High-fructose corn syrup	Maltose	Syrup
Dextrose	Honey	Molasses	Table sugar
Fructose	Invert sugar	Raw sugar	

Chapter 16 Exercise & Injuries

16.1. WEAKNESSES AND INJURY

16.1.1. HIGHER NEURAL CAUSES OF MUSCULAR WEAKNESS

o   Muscles are controlled by the lower neural regulation that originates from the spinal cord neurons. These in turn are controlled by higher regulation from the brain neurons. Physical weakness can be attributed to many causes within the **motor units** that comprise of muscles, peripheral nerves, and spinal neurons. Alternatively, higher causes of weakness can reside in the **central nervous system** that comprises of the brain, brain stem, and descending and ascending nerve tracts that control the lower motor units. Weakness due to higher neural causes is caused by either failure of the brain to initiate effective control, or failure of the conducting neural tract to convey signals to and from the remote spinal neurons, as follows.

   i.   Examples of **organic brain failure** are headache, stroke, tumor, hemorrhage, or other mass lesions such as abscesses. These cause disruption of the cerebral neurons by physical destruction or compression.
   ii. Examples of **psychological brain failure** of causing weakness are conversion disorder (hysteria), depression, anxiety, and inattention. These are caused by either chemical imbalance, or diversion of mental activities to issues other than muscular regulation.
   iii. Examples of **failed conduction** are multiple sclerosis, fever, spinal cord lesion, isolated neural pinching conditions, pernicious anemia, and thiamin deficiency. These may result in loss of insulation of the conducting neural tracts, interruption of the neural tracts, or reduced neurotransmitters along the synaptic bridges.

o   **Higher neural causes** of physical weakness can be distinguished from other causes by the following:
   i.   Symptoms and signs of **brain affliction** are apparent and point to higher causes of weakness. In the case of neural tract causes, weakness is widespread along the anatomical distribution of the affected spinal tract. That might be motor, sensory, or both. Lack of training and unacquaintance with lifting styles simulate organic brain failure. Since the brain of the untrained person lacks any memory of performing the new action, therefore weakness appears vividly along the chain of lifting.
   ii. Muscular **spasticity** is associated with physical weakness. That is because of the diminished inhibition on the spinal motoneurons by descending tracts. Without regular axial training, all people, young and old, incur some degree of spasticity of unused muscles. That is because, lack of training leads to brain neglect of unused muscles.
   iii. Impaired **voluntary control** of limbs, sensation, or posture. Muscles that are not used in compound exercises lead to inability to initiate such compound motion, when need calls for it. For example, if you try a new postural movement or a movement that you have not performed for longtime, you feel the tremors and instability of the performing muscles.

16.1.2. LOWER NEURAL CAUSES OF MUSCULAR WEAKNESS

o   Weakness due to lower neural control originates from the spinal motor neurons, the peripheral nerves, or the terminal muscles, as follows.

   i.   Examples of **failed spinal motor control** are amyotrophic lateral sclerosis (ALS), poliomyelitis, and localized spinal cord injuries. These affect the spinal neurons that innervate peripheral organs, communicate with adjacent neurons, and receive higher signals.
   ii. Examples of **peripheral neural weakness** are various peripheral nerve injuries and peripheral neuritis after viral infection such as Guillain-Barré syndrome, or metabolic disorder such as diabetic neuropathy. These affect the peripheral nerves that originate from the spinal cord neurons and innervate muscles.
   iii. Examples of **neuromuscular junction failure** are Myasthenia gravis and Botulism. These affect groups of muscles, at the terminal joints of the nerve endings, on the muscle surface.
   iv. Examples of **muscular failure** are low blood calcium, failed sodium-potassium pump due to water intoxication or excess carbohydrate intake in some people, fever, inadequate muscle mass, starvation, fasting, or muscle damage due to viral, autoimmune, or genetic disorders. Peripheral muscular failure occurs at the level of muscle cells.

o   **Lower neural causes** of physical weakness can be distinguished from other causes by the following:

i. Symptoms and signs of motor unit affliction point to peripheral causes, **without relevant mental or psychiatric** causes. Thus, anatomical explanation of physical weakness points to LMNL (lower motor neuron lesion). Lack of strength training of peripheral muscles simulates LMNL. The untrained weak muscle fails to perform strongly or effectively, when need calls for it.
ii. Muscular **flaccidity** dominates physical weakness due to interrupted muscular innervation. Lack of training leads to diminished muscle size, as well as spinal neurons that regulate such reduced muscle mass. Thus, flaccidity signifies inadequacy of toned muscle fibers.
iii. Depending on the site of impairment, **motor control** is impaired in the afflicted muscles. Weak muscles can enter a stage of total irresponsiveness after minimal exhaustion. That is attributed to lack of adequate circulation, lack of sufficient CP and ATP reserve, low mitochondrial density, and poor innervation.

16.1.3. CAUSES OF PERIPHERAL MUSCULAR WEAKNESS
In this context, "**peripheral**" refers to the location within the nervous system, as compared to the previous usage in relation to the musculoskeletal system (see Chapter 11). The following are the main causes of physical weakness:

o The most common cause of weakness is **inactivity**. Inactivity diminishes protein synthesis in active muscles, undermines the integrity of heart, blood vessels, central control of circulation, and entire body control of metabolism. Thus, general weakness results from reduced metabolism that fits reduced activity.
o **Nutritional** causes of weakness are mainly either overeating or disinterest in healthy feeding habits. Specific deficiencies of vitamins, minerals, and proteins are common in women, children, elderly, and people with low socioeconomic and educational background. Overeating, in particular, crams the energy expenditure system and jeopardizes the harmonious control of general metabolism.
o Weakness of **specific body regions** is another imperative cause of injury. Weak thigh, pelvis, lower back, and shoulder muscles are prevalent in modern society because of the availability of all sorts of machines that replace human labor.
o Weakness due to lack of **coordination** is common in activities that do not enhance neuromuscular control. Exercising of isolated muscles without incorporating group coordination causes injuries. Walking or running prior to weight training strengthens group coordination of diverse muscles.
o **Diseases** cause weakness in many different ways. Fevers impair cellular respiration and denature essential proteins of active muscles. Viral infections undermine protein synthesis, at the transcription level within the nucleus, and impair both muscle and nerve functions. Genetic disorders that affect the metabolism of ATP, CK, and other essential enzymes of the muscle metabolism cause weakness, wasting, or paralysis.

16.2. GROUP MUSCLE WEAKNESSES

The following are common issues regarding weakness of the main groups of muscles.

16.2.1. ABDOMINAL WEAKNESS
o Abdominal muscles act as a voluntary diaphragm and blood pump during vigorous activities such as:
    i. Bearing down during labor, defecation, or vomiting.
    ii. Sneezing, coughing, screaming, or shouting.
    iii. Deadlifting, pulling for the Clean or Snatch.
    iv. Sprinting, jumping, diving, or aggressive swimming.

o The abdomen performs its dynamic reservoir action as follows.
    i. Contracting the abdominal muscles pushes the abdominal contents upwards and augments the diaphragm ascent, during expiration. The high abdominal tension squeezes major abdominal veins thus maintains adequate blood return.
    ii. Relaxing abdomen, after vigorous activity, causes the abdominal contents to descend precipitously and induce suction effect on the abdominal veins and diaphragm. Thus, both blood return from the legs and air entry into the lungs are enhanced by abdominal suction.
    iii. From the point of view of dynamic performance, the abdomen acts as a **soft pumping sac.** The soft sac produces waves of suction and compression in the fluid medium of the abdomen, utilizing the inertia of fluid density. When the intestines are full of gases, as in indigestion, the effect of abdominal pump is greatly diminished.
    iv. The chest acts as a **hard pumping cage.** The hard cage produces waves of compression and rarefaction in the gas medium of the lungs, utilizing the surface tension of the pleural space as well as the alveolar space. When the surface tension in the lungs is diminished, as in pneumonia, drowning, or pneumothorax, the effect of the chest pump is greatly impaired.

o Abdominal weakness interferes with the mechanisms of respiration, stabilization of the vertebral column, and circulation of blood, as follows.

EXERCISE & INJURIES

i. During deep inspiration, weak abdominal muscles do not exert **sufficient tension** to contain and prevent herniation of abdominal contents (escape of contents through weak points). This leads to constant buildup of gases and distension of the abdominal hollow organs, as well as insufficient pressure on major abdominal veins that augment venous return. On the long run, weak abdomen amounts to heart failure.

ii. Bulging abdomen weakens back and leg muscles due to venous congestion in the lower body. Because abdominal and Iliopsoas muscles (muscles that bend the thighs on the torso) oppose the back extensors (muscles in the back of the body), therefore, weak abdomen undermines the **support of the vertebral spines** during hip and back flexion and extension. Unsupported spinal discs slip very frequently in people with lax abdomen.

iii. Both, weak opposition (antagonism) of back muscles, and weak support to abdominal contents, interfere with all **vigorous and heavy strength training** exercises, such as the Clean and Jerk, the Snatch, Squat, and Deadlifts. Strengthening the four abdominal muscles (the two oblique muscles, transversus, and rectus) prevents abdominal weakness. Crunches work the abdominal rectus. Exercises that involve torso twisting strengthen the other three muscles.

o The most practical and efficient way to reduce abdominal bulging is through **healthy diet and exercise** (see Chapter 15 and Section 7.8 on "Strengthening the Abdominal Muscles").

i. Brisk walking offers the advantage of extending the duration of exercise. Long walking is superior to strength training in reducing bodyweight, since it burns aerobic fuels that is less taxing on the body and mind. Brisk walking for an hour or longer, daily, is the trick for trimming the waist girth. The swinging arms and shoulder oppose the briskly advancing legs and generate significant torque on the waist to mobilize intestine, mid-torso fat, abdominal belt of muscles, and lower body venous blood.

ii. Diet that is high in fibers, low in calories and fat will help hasten intestinal contents. This reduces colon toxicity and deflates abdomen. Such healthy diet will make the most benefit out of any exercise program, be it walking, running, or strength training.

16.2.2. HAMSTRINGS WEAKNESS

o This results from modern day lifestyle. Wasting of the Hamstring, Glutei, and back erectors results from lack of exercises that involve strength training, in bending positions. The Hamstrings and Quadriceps act on two joints (knee and hip, *Figure 7.63*) and their weakness increase the risk of injury of the back and knees. Weak and inflexible Hamstrings make torso bending risky, due to the weak anchoring of the pelvis during bending.

o The best Hamstrings strengthening exercises are the Goodmornings (even without weights, in sets of 20 to 50 repetitions and with varying speeds), the Clean, the Snatch, and the Deadlifts (see Section 7.5.1 on "Hip Extension"). Legs curls should only be performed during fatigue, injuries, or boredom, since they lack the effects of standing up. Sprinting is another highly effective exercise in strengthening the Hamstrings. Isometric exercising of the Hamstrings is heavily practiced in yoga training. This is as simple as folding the torso on the thighs, while standing, and staying in that folding position for long duration.

o Strengthening the Hamstrings and Quadriceps is of paramount importance in rehabilitating arthritis and recovery from knee injuries. After isolated specific exercises are performed to tide the person over advanced weakness of the knee muscle, general exercises of muscle groups should be gradually introduced. The long-term gains of persistent strengthening of the knee muscles are very gratifying, as follows.

i. The knee bones strengthen and thicken. This is slow, yet long and attainable outcome of regular strengthening. It requires many months to manifest real results.

ii. The muscles, tendons, and ligaments are strengthened and increase in bulk. This is quite faster process that requires only few months to show improvement.

iii. The capillary network around the knee is greatly enriched. The nervous control is also dramatically enhanced.

iv. The sensory nerve endings that trigger pain become less irritated and less annoying, after stress.

16.2.3. SUPRASPINATUS WEAKNESS

o Rotator cuff muscles anchor the shoulder balls in their socket, while the bigger muscles (such as Deltoid, Pectoralis, Latissimus dorsi) perform forceful resistance. All cuff rotators waste quickly with inactivity and require very careful and balanced shoulder training to regain strength. Training the cuff rotators is very tricky since they are not apparent from the outside surface of the shoulders. Omitting balanced shoulder training is very common practice.

o The Supraspinatus, the upper rotator cuff muscle, is located above and behind the shoulder ball (head of humerus), *Figure 7.22*. It is an extremely important muscle in lifting from the floor. Whether you lift a light object, a child, or you lift Olympic style or Deadlift; weak Supraspinatus increases the risk of injury during shoulder flexion and abduction. Thus, lifting anything, from below the chest level to a level above the eyebrows, is particularly impaired with weak rotator cuff.

o The best preventive exercises to Supraspinatus weakness are (see Section 7.4 on "Strengthening the Shoulders"):

i. **Lifting objects from floor** instead of lifting from racks or relying on machines. Freestyle lifting forces recruitment of muscles groups that are relevant to natural motion. Thus, proper recruitment of Supraspinatus adds

EXERCISE & INJURIES

more safety to preventing rupture or inflammation of this important muscle.

ii. **Olympic lifts** such as the Clean and the Snatch, with light weights, or performing similar exercises with medicine balls or other objects offer dynamic strength.

iii. Deadlift offers static strength, since the cuff rotators act isometrically in the limited range of motion of the Deadlift.

16.2.4. INFRASPINATUS WEAKNESS

o This rotator cuff muscle is located behind and below the shoulder ball, *Figure 7.24*. Its weakness affects exercises that involve pulling towards the body as in chin-ups, stabilizing the shoulder in pushing, pressing, and jerking.

o The Infraspinatus is a huge and fleshy muscle that covers the shoulder plate, below the spine of the scapula. Strengthening this muscle forces its opponent, the Serratus, to work hard to stabilize the shoulder plate while exercising. Thus, strong Infraspinatus strengthens both the chest cage (due to the pull of the Serratus) and the vertebral column (due to the pull of the Rhomboid muscles). This is best done by lifting from the floor, rather than performing sitting exercises. Floor lifting stimulates the vertebral, pelvic, and leg to endure the pull of the Infraspinatus.

o The best exercises to strengthen Infraspinatus are the Deadlift, the Olympic lifting, aided chin-ups; bend over-and-row, and cable rowing.

16.2.5. WEAKNESS OF SPINAL ERECTORS

This results from modern lifestyle of less bending and squatting activities. The following are facts about the strength training of the back erectors.

o Many people never figure out that without regular **bending and squatting** exercises, back erectors waste permanently, with little hope for regaining the same strength, had these muscles worked out daily and effectively.

o The muscles of the back are predominantly **tendinous in structure** and require persistent and regular training, just to maintain current strength, *Figure 7.80*. This is different from fleshy muscles such as the Quadriceps, which could be strengthened, in relatively short time, with many exercise options.

o Weak back manifests in many forms of ailments, from sciatica (disc material bugles and compresses sciatic nerve), muscle strain, inability to walk, lift, or stand up.

o If exercise is not commenced in young age, the weak spinal erectors cause **loss of lower back curvature.** This is noticed from the body contour and in the difficulty to keep waist-belt stay, without slipping downwards. Loss of depression in the center of the back, between the two bundles of spinal erectors on both sides, is a clear sign of weak erectors. This is most noticeable in children, women, obese people, and untrained individuals.

o The best strengthening exercises of the lower back are the Clean, Snatch, Goodmorning, Deadlift, sprinting, and brisk walking. The worst exercise of all is the stiff-legged Deadlift, which forces the Hamstrings to contract isometrically for longer time, inducing congestion of the lower legs, in addition to the dangerous horizontal position of the back during bending in stiff-legged Deadlift.

16.2.6. QUADRICEPS WEAKNESS

o The thigh muscles (Quadriceps femoris) have four fleshy and multi-pinnate heads, all of which are of utmost importance in controlling the knee motion, *Figure 7.62*. No other animal species has such complexity of motion as the knees of humans. Knees do not only bend and extend, but also lock and unlock, and stabilize in the most extremes of motions such as starting of motion and stabilizing vigorous dynamic motion.

o The four heads of the thigh muscle perform leverage actions in very narrow space such as to keep the knee size in such concise shape to accommodate graceful motions. The lateral head of the Quadriceps balances the action of the medial head. The intermediate head adds more stability to the Quadriceps tendon during protracted activities. The Quadratus femoris extends the knee, while stabilizing the hip. The four heads of the Quadriceps allow different directions of resisting forces to travel from the hip to the feet. Thus, pointing the knees in different directions, while squatting or running, affects different Quadriceps muscle and different side of the knee surface.

o In spite of such complex structure, leg exercises are as simple as squatting, running, lifting from the floor, Olympic styles. The most fundamental fact about Quadriceps strengthening is that it requires **strengthening in every training session**, in one way or another, either squatting, floor lifting, running, leg presses, leg extensions, or just brisk walking.

o Imbalance in the four heads of the Quadriceps leads to:

i. Wiggling of the three surfaces within the knee (tibia, femur, and patella) increases **wear and tear** of articulating cartilages.

ii. **Tearing menisci** due to excessive and pointed forces, acting in directions that shear the fixed menisci.

iii. Traumatizing ligaments and bones. Weak Quadriceps are poor on blood circulation and nervous control and easily expose the knee ligaments and bone to extreme forces that exceed their ability to remain intact.

iv. When one meniscus is torn, the Quadriceps can be trained to shift bodyweight onto the healthy meniscus side such that the athlete could still compete, with focusing on throwing his bodyweight on the healthy side of the knee.

16.3. SOFT TISSUE INJURIES

16.3.1. CAUSES OF INJURIES DUE TO PHYSICAL ACTIVITY

o The main soft tissue elements of the musculoskeletal system are muscles, tendons, and ligaments. They differ in function and structure as follows.
  i. **Muscles** are contractile elements that respond to electrical stimulation and neural discharge. They move bones and produce motion. The contractile protein fibrils transmit their forces through muscular connective tissue. This is a network of interlacing tissue between the bundles of muscle fibers. The muscular connective tissues converge onto terminal tendons thus transmit all forces of muscular fibrils onto tendons, which are anchored onto bones.
  ii. **Tendons** do not contract. They act as links between muscles and bones. They are tough and compact structures that can transmit large mechanical forces per relatively small cross sectional area. A tendon is wrapped with a closed sac of fluids that allow the tendon to slide on smooth curved surfaces thus transmitting muscular forces into different directions.
  iii. **Ligaments** share the same properties of toughness with tendons. They bridge bones, prevent disassembly, allow limited degree of motion, and stabilize joints. They are only connected to bones, on both ends. Shrunk and tight ligaments result from limited range of mobility. This impedes joint usage and, if not treated soon, will lead to loss of joint function.

o Structural soft tissues elements are injured when stretched beyond their maximal limits or traumatized by compression against solid objects such as in joint dislocation or impact accidents. The reaction of soft tissue to injury ranges from **inflammation** to total structural disruption. Injuries to these structures due to physical activity are caused by the following:
  i. **Excessive forces** that exceed the body's ability to resist cause imbalance, regardless of the direction of action. Lack of warm-up leads to inability of the neuromuscular system to coordinate muscles to resist forces that could otherwise be resisted had the warm-up been done.
  ii. Forces that act in **directions** that could not be opposed, by the natural course of action of muscles and joints, cause imbalance. Lifting from the floor without bending the knees put forces perpendicular on the vertebral spines and may cause disc slipping, ligament sprain, and muscle or tendon strain.
  iii. **Unfit body** fails to coordinate muscular efforts to maintain balance. Lack of regular physical activity undermines the integrity of the autonomous nervous system, which control respiration, circulation, and arousal. Inactivity also undermines the integrity of the voluntary nervous system, which control muscular balance, and muscular and skeletal strength that support the body under stress.
  iv. Lack of **acquaintance** with proper lifting techniques. The leverage actions of the joints account for amplification of forces of moving bodies. Moving the head, for example, amounts for an equivalent force plus a torque at the lower back or feet, depending on the distance between the head and lower back and feet, respectively. The generated torque eludes many people and can cause injuries and fall. Watch a young toddler sustain sudden fall due to unexpected movement of the head.

16.3.2. ALLEVIATING PHYSICAL INJURIES OF SOFT TISSUES

Alleviation of inflammation by rest, cooling, compression, stretching, and, or analgesic medication, reduce tissue destruction and nerve irritation and may allow healing to progress, as follows.

o **Rest** should be limited to the injured body part and should not restrict daily activity, unless it worsens pain and swelling. Whole body rest is counterproductive to local injuries. Activity improves oxygen delivery, lactate clearance, and cellular metabolism thus enhances recovery of locally rested limbs.
o **Stretching** of muscle groups can be very effective tool of rehabilitation if conducted properly. Stretching might hold the secret for longevity in sport. Long duration of isometric and balanced stretching, in yoga, enables old and slim people to perform extraordinary movements. The role of mental will, in yoga, has its anatomical explanation in the role of the extrapyramidal neural system in motor control. Thus, yoga stretching modifies brain control over muscles, through modulating the spindle-reflex of muscles in response to voluntary control.
o **Cooling** is effective when there is hotness or redness at the site of injury. The purpose of cooling by ice is to reduce inflammation of the acute phase. After few days from the onset on injury, cooling may interfere with healing and reduce blood supply.
o **Compression** is applicable after the acute phase is managed. It should not cause discomfort. Compressing knees that swell quickly with exercise is a good idea, since it supports the synovial knee capsule to stand inner pressure and keep injured surfaces separated. In the past, compression was reported to cause amputation if compromised vital signs are omitted. Only light compression, that does not impair sensation or circulation, is safe. No compression is needed, at all, if there is no progressive swelling.

EXERCISE & INJURIES

- o **Analgesics** are helpful if pain is intolerable and may be given right after injury. They permit pursuing daily activities and continuing exercises that strengthen muscles and lead to weaning from analgesics. Most people with little medical background do not understand the effect of proper dose and proper blood level of analgesic that can alleviate pain. Aspirin may have the same effect of any expensive analgesic if given in proper dose and frequency. One or two tablets of 350 mg of aspirin, once or twice a day, would not do any good for tendonitis or strain. Up to 10 tablets of aspirin of 350 mg per day (3.5 gram/day), for few days, may relieve the most annoying pain. Of course, allergy to aspirin precludes some people from its usage.
- o **Immobilization** might be needed until severe pain subsides. Complete tears may require surgical repair.
- o **Elevation** of injured and swollen limb is entertained by many therapists to reduce swelling. This is particularly important in elderly, in people with unfit heart, and with extensive swelling.

16.3.3. LIGAMENT SPRAIN

- o Sprain affects the joint ligaments and presents with pain, tenderness, and swelling. Sprain results in inability to move that joint. It is caused by traumatic insult to the joint, as follows.
    i. Forces that tend to **vigorously disassemble** joints injure ligaments. Ligament injuries are incurred in extreme and aggressive physical activities, away beyond those that cause strain. Depending on the magnitude and direction of force and the distance of stretching, ligaments could be completely or partially torn or contused.
    ii. Blows to ligaments also cause contusion or tear. Accidents, falls, **excessive physical activities**, improper lifting or improper use of joints, generate traumatizing forces. Common joints that incur sprain are ankle, knee, hip, wrist, elbow, shoulder, and joints of the back and neck.
    iii. A characteristic feature of sprain is its **deep location**, closer to bone, gives the feeling of tight gripping and deep discomfort that prevents joint movement.
- o **Ankle sprains** are the commonest injury due to accidents that occur as results of walking, running, or falling. Sprains to the ankle are common while descending on a slope or landing in a jump, when the ankles are most unstable. The ankle ligaments are located on both sides of each ankle. They anchor the foot bones to the lower leg bones as they slide in anterior-posterior plane of motion. Sudden ankle inversion tears the outside ligament and produce swelling, pain, and sometimes internal bleeding at the ankle. The main causes of ankle sprains are:
    i. Wearing improper shoes.
    ii. Walking on uneven surface.
    iii. Poor neuromuscular balance.
    iv. Overweight.
    v. Muscular weakness.
    vi. Debilitating diseases.
    vii. Repeated and heavy physical activities.
- o **Knee ligaments** are located both on the sides of the knee and inside the knee cavity. Twisting the knees during falls (as in skiing accidents) traumatizes the outside ligaments. Forces that tend to translate the knee in forward and backward directions traumatize the internal cruciate ligaments. Immediate application of ice helps reduce swelling and pain. X-ray exclude fracture of bones, joint sublaxation, or presence of bone destruction or overgrowth due to tumors. MRI diagnoses internal knee disorganization.

16.3.4. MUSCLE AND TENDON STRAIN

- o Strain presents with pain, tenderness, swelling, or weakness due to injured muscles or tendons. It differs from ligament sprain in that strain is **related to the course of the muscle** and is not localized to the joint.
- o Strain is caused by traumatizing insults such as:
    i. Pulling, twisting, or impact forces
    ii. Forces that overstretch, tear, or contuse muscles or tendons.
    iii. Long-term repetitive injuries occur in people working in menial jobs or leading sedentary life
    iv. Without full-range exercising, strains heal by sclerosis, stiffness, and shortening of muscles.
    v. Injuries occur in the most vulnerable regions of the body, particularly the back, and the most used limbs.
    vi. Predisposing factors are muscle weakness, imbalanced exercise training, poor warm-up prior to physical activity, poor understanding of the proper lifting, pulling, or pushing techniques.
- o Muscle and tendon strains are the most commonly encountered symptoms in all populations. Muscle injury heals within days. It could be prevented from happening again by regular exercise and strengthening. Tendon injuries are notorious in their demands for local rest for long time, progressive exercises without aggravating pain, analgesics, and heat application.

16.3.5. BURSITIS

- o Bursas are flattened sacs of fluid (cysts), located between prominent parts of bones and tendons. They allow sliding of structures with minimal friction or heat production.

o   Excessive overuse of joints causes the lining of bursas to become inflamed. Normally, regular and continuous exercise affects the pace of secretion of fluids within bursas in a manner that permit normal movements.
o   **Sudden changes in exercise** activity, general illness (such as common cold), external trauma, or nutritional deficiency may impair the cellular function of the wall of bursa leading to poor absorption of fluids, swelling, and pain (bursitis).
o   Painful bursa can be very distressing (such as pinching inflamed bursa with fully extended elbow, between the two bones of elbow joint). Heat or cold application with local rest of the affected joint is the proper treatment. Elastic wrapping helps reduce pain and permits exercise. It must be remembered that most distressing pain due to bursitis subsides with rest alone.

16.3.6. COMPARTMENT SYNDROME

Muscle compartments are sacs of fibrous tissue that enclose a group of muscles of similar anatomical function. Compartments contain, in addition to muscles, blood vessels, nerves, and lymph vessels. Excessive training, trauma, or immune diseases may cause obstruction of lymph drainage and increase the internal pressure within muscle compartments. For example, excessive training of the Biceps or the calf muscles leads to solid rock feeling of these muscles. The increased internal pressure squeezes blood vessels and nerves. Since the veins are squeezed easier than the arteries, more blood flows into the muscle compartment than out of it. This leads to congestion, numbness, and tension. Compartment syndrome is differentiated from **nerve injury** by the increased pressure of fluids within the muscle compartments and by the defined anatomical boundaries of the tense compartment. Internal compartmental pressure is measured by introducing tiny catheter connected into manometer through a small incision into the muscle compartment. It is differentiated from **blood vessel injury** by presence of peripheral pulse, anatomical boundaries, and lack of color change of the skin. Compartment syndrome worsens by exercise as long as the cause is not eliminated.

16.3.7. SORENESS

o   Soreness is the feeling of dull ache in soft tissues (mainly muscles, ligaments, and tendons) in response to physical activity. Soreness differs from pain due to strain in that the latter is caused by pathological changes, ranging from simple inflammation to complete rupture. Soreness is attributed to the adaptation of muscles to physical work, as follows.
  i.   During any exercise activity, there is some degree of anaerobic oxidation of glucose (immediate supply of ATP energy to initiate contraction), which produces pyruvic acid and lactic acid. Acidity causes fatigue by blocking calcium release, hindering muscular contraction, and causes discomforting soreness. This **mid-exercise soreness** is relieved with rest, which allows time for lactates to diffuse outside the cells. In the blood, lactates are eliminated by liver and other organs that perform gluconeogenesis. Depending on your level of fitness, rest required for recovery may be short (few minutes), long (more than 3 minutes), or protracted (requires termination of training session). If you have plenty of mitochondria in your muscle cells and your decarboxylation enzymes are more active than untrained people, you might continue exercising without need for rest. The ability to endure beyond what untrained peoples cannot endure is attributed to your increased ability to shift fuel supply towards aerobic oxidation of fatty acids.
  ii. After exercise is over, other biochemical processes take place to replenish depleted reserves. Such processes are affected by changes of the body hormones. These **post-exercise** changes cause "delayed-onset muscle soreness" or DOMS (residual soreness, or after-exercise soreness). The stimulus for post-exercise changes is the exercise-induced hormonal increase in growth hormone, thyrotropin, prolactin, endorphins, vasopressin, cortisol, aldosterone, epinephrine, glucagons, parathormone, estrogen, progesterone, testosterone, and rennin. Hormonal changes affect protein synthesis, generation of mitochondria, and metabolism of fat and carbohydrates. Depending on prior physical fitness, post-exercise changes range from minor soreness, stiffness, or weakness, to extreme or even fatal cardiac arrest. For people without history of serious health problems and under age of 65, the majority of such changes are normal adaptation to changes in intensity or duration of physical activity. Post-exercise changes generally commence 12 hours after exercise and peak in 2 days before remitting.
  iii. Post-exercise soreness is substantial with exercises that involve resisting forces during muscular elongation of **eccentric contraction, or negative contraction**. Examples of such exercises are descending in Squat, descending in chin-ups, lowering weights, and descending downhill. Eccentric exercises involve heavy neuromuscular feedback and recruitment control. To resist weight while elongating, a muscle must relax a group of muscle fibers (to lower weight) then contract another group to catch the weight at a lower distance. The cycle of relaxing and contracting proceeds in stepwise, yet smooth fashion, to voluntarily control the rate of descent. Such demanding neuromuscular control taxes the reserves of the nervous elements and causes significant soreness. As the muscle elongates and resists force, the sliding filaments, within the sarcomere (thin Actin and thick Myosin myofilaments), progressively separate apart and lose pulling force. Thus, the effect of resistance on the elongating muscle, in eccentric contraction, is greatly enhanced as the muscle length increases. Muscles unaccustomed to new activities do not have sufficient connective tissue strength to prevent elongating muscles from exceeding traumatic thinness. As the muscle develops strength, both the supporting connective tissue and nervous control progress to protect elongating muscles from crushing their own weaker fibers.

EXERCISE & INJURIES

    iv. The **damaged muscle fibers** due to unaccustomed activity are thought as a cause of soreness. This microscopic muscle damage may be detected by measuring the enzyme **creatine kinase (CK),** in the blood serum, and the **myoglobin** content (chemical compound found in muscle), in the urine of the person suffering of soreness. The concentration of myoglobin and CK depend on the severity of muscle damage and intensity and duration of activity. Supposedly, damaged microfilaments are the most vulnerable ones and are replaced by stronger filaments that can tolerate the new stress. Thus, soreness signifies transition to stronger, firmer, and larger muscles than prior to the application of the stimulus of soreness.

    v. Another possible cause of muscle soreness is the buildup of **metabolites** including lactic acid, in excessive rates, to cause swelling and irritation of nerve fibers. Irritated nerve fibers cause the discomfort of soreness (sensory) and muscle **spasm** (motor). Both muscle swelling and spasm cause stiffness of sore muscles.

    vi. If the **connective tissue** other than the myofibrils is damaged, an increase in the urinary concentration of **hydroxproline** (a constituent of connective tissue) may be detected in biochemical urine analysis.

o Soreness is managed as follows.
    i. As soon as acute discomfort subsides, **stretching** a sore muscle helps reducing internal swelling, relieve discomfort, and expedite recovery.
    ii. **Cold** applications (ice or cold water) are useful if the sore muscle is generating too much local heat and discomfort. Cold reduces inflammatory reaction and oozing of fluids from dilated capillaries to extra cellular space.
    iii. **Hot applications** (sauna, Jacuzzi, deep heater creams) are useful with deeper discomfort, without surface hotness. Heat dilates skin circulation and increases local circulation. Both cold and hot stimuli act on the sympathetic nervous system to achieve their effect. Heat may also stimulate the hypothalamus to secrete hormones that facilitates relaxation and sleep.
    iv. Of course, the realistic management of soreness is continuous **regular exercise.** Exercise fosters the ability of tissue to repair damage and withstand higher stress. Gradual and progressive increase in intensity and duration of exercise, over several weeks, builds up the protein synthesis and cellular oxidation microstructures of muscles.
    v. Both protein synthesis and cellular respiration require adequate intervals of **rest** between sessions of exercise to restructure affected muscles and recuperate.

o The ability to differentiate between serious **damage** to the body and reversible reactive soreness, due to unaccustomed activities, is sometimes lacking, even in advanced athletes, as follows.
    i. Prior **experience** with soreness of various muscles allows the person to predict the fate of his or her condition. New unfamiliar injuries may not raise the trainee's suspicion of injury for quite some time.
    ii. Severe knee or hip trauma could be confused for normal soreness. Crushed knee **cartilages** during heavy half-Squat, Leg Press, or Deadlift, produce acute and tense feeling in the hip and knee and might be confused for soreness due to their shared symptoms of stiffness, swelling, discomfort, and limitation of motion. These injuries are very well limited to the joints, though they radiate pain and tenderness in the neighborhood of the injury.
    iii. Abnormal discomfort lasts longer than **few days** and evolves to local injury that lingers for certain course.

16.3.8. CRAMPS

Cramps are intense involuntary contractions of large number of muscle bundles. They are common on the lower legs. Cramps are caused by acute changes in the concentration of ions due to exercise, dehydration, or exhaustion. Ionic changes trigger an avalanche of calcium release or instability of discharge from nerves. Thus, groups of muscles simultaneously contract causing acute intolerable pain and general state of distress. Prior to cramps, many athletes feel tension and discomfort in the vulnerable muscles. Well-rested, hydrated, and relaxed individuals seldom have cramps. Cramps are best managed by gradual stretch of the affected muscle. On the long run, one should search for causative factors such as imbalanced diet, improper sleep cycle, overtraining, or poorly planned load volume and intensity program.

16.3.9. ROLE OF EXERCISE IN INJURY MANAGEMENT

Exercise is a natural approach in the management of injured soft tissue. It offers the benefits of immediate relieve of symptoms as well as in preventing future injuries, as follows.

o Soft tissue injuries are facts of everyday life. Minor injuries go unnoticed. Yet the **cumulative effects** of injuries, over the years, impact our posture, range of motion of joints, flexibility to perform our physical duties, and predisposition to further injuries. Exercise for life is intended to prevent cumulative effects of injury and inactivity.

o The outcome of any injury depends on the **degree of damage** to the structures, the wisdom of planning relief of inflammatory reactions, and commencing exercise without aggravating the incurred injury. Exercise builds up new tissues. This could fully reverse the side effects of many injuries. Yet, exercise has to commence as soon as possible before serious wasting of muscles and shortening of tendons ensue. Immediate exercise incorporation might catch defaulting organs, before progressing into states of chronic irreversible dysfunction.

EXERCISE & INJURIES

- o **Rehabilitating physical therapy** should deal with both local cause of injury as well as general body balance, strength, and endurance. Gradual stretching of muscles and general light aerobic activity, such as walking, jogging, or biking prepare and test the body systems for predictable outcome. The transition from inactive to active lifestyle is a tremendous challenge that needs strong will. It could be accomplished by persistent planning of regular activities on daily basis. Rehabilitative measures are constant aspect of regular exercise. You just have to keep maintaining your body performance as you advance or maintain your level of fitness.
- o Thorough **warm-up** before physical activity allows the person to exceed their preset goals since warm-up relieves annoying stiffness, tenderness, and pain and elevate spirit. Also, gradual increase of intensity and duration of physical activities should take into consideration various rates of growth of tissues. Inactive people should be taught about the basic concepts of body responses to activities. Muscles require few weeks to grow. Tendons and ligaments require few months. Bones require longer time to catch up with other tissues.
- o Weight training starts with lightweight that can be lifted repeatedly for up to 10 times per set, for up to 6 sets. **Gradual increase in weights** on weekly basis, or whenever condition allows, is fundamental to stimulate muscle, tendon, and bone growth. Activities that were not performed on regular basis, for up to 3 days prior to present training session, could cause injuries if intensity of exercise is increased abruptly.

16.4. KNEE INJURIES

16.4.1. MENISCUS INJURIES

The knee menisci are crescent cartilaginous structures attached to the lower knee bone (tibia) in the form of a pair per each knee. They are positioned on the sides of the surface of the tibia. They are anchored by ligaments, in front and back, to the underlying tibia. Thus, most of the meniscus surfaces are freely sliding, allowing some degree of mobility, in addition to the elasticity recoil of the cartilages. Menisci perform as cushioning elements and help distribute bodyweight on tibial upper surface. Menisci are injured as follows.

- o Forcible **knee twisting** tears the meniscus because it forces motion in the fixed direction, along the fixed front and back ends. Menisci are good in tolerating compression, but not twisting, due to their fixed configuration. Small tears do not disrupt attachments of the meniscus, while larger tears leave loose or hanging cartilages in the knee cavity.
- o The cardinal picture of meniscus injury is **pain and swelling**. These differ from soreness and tension of muscles due to excessive intense training in that pain due meniscus injury is maximal at the joint, not on the muscle. Swelling surrounds the joint and becomes tenser, with bending the joint. Excruciating pain, or pain that disturbs night sleep for long without response to painkillers, heat or cold application, or massage, indicates larger tear. Small meniscal tears and wearing may go unnoticed. The knee swelling results from inflammation of the synovial membrane of the knee and serves to reduce friction and possibly mediate healing.
- o Knowing which meniscus is the site of injury helps you alter your loading of the knee, by using the other side, of the same knee. This is done by concentrated slight eversion or inversion of the feet, while walking, lifting, or running. Quitting exercise altogether due to meniscus injury is unwise. **Exercise** enhances circulation and strengthens muscles thus prevents further damage and improves existing injury. Athletes with bad knees live better lives than non-athletes with weak knees do, as far as mobility is concerned. The pain of torn meniscus could impair the nervous control of the knee muscles and causes weakness or falls. With exercises and surgical trimming (if needed), stronger muscles eliminate further instability of the knee. When you bulk massive Quadriceps, you will be better in avoiding motions that provoke pain.
- o Injury to menisci is suspected from **the history** of the current condition. That includes the nature of activities, age, nature of pain, and past history. Inspection of recent active tears reveals swelling and limb on walking. Palpation reveals tense joint. Manipulation reveals limited range of motion and pain on twisting a bent knee. Radiography excludes fractures, aging conditions such artherosclerosis, and destructive tumors, but does not diagnose meniscus disorders. MRI is the best diagnostic tool for both cartilaginous and soft tissue injuries. Many **orthopedic surgeons** rely on strong history and clinical picture to perform arthroscopic trimming surgery for larger tears, *Figures 16.1 and 16.2*.
- o Minor tears that respond to analgesics (pain killers) are helped by leg **strengthening exercises**. Extensive tears and injuries to the articular cartilage progress faster to osteoarthritis, in the absence of exercise or in overweight people. Postoperative recovery takes about two months to regain full strength and walk without limb, provided that strengthening exercises are performed gradually during that period. Many return to competitive sport after recovery. Heavier weight in Deadlifts or Squats after surgery could be tolerated if extreme balance during the exercises is observed, without favoring one side of the knee. From time to time, swelling waxes and wanes depending on other factors such as excessive load volume, lack of sleep, improper shoes, long walking on uneven surface, or lack of rest. At least 24 hour of rest, after recurrence of swelling, helps abort a cycle of trauma and swelling from reaching intolerable level. Inactivity causes stiff knees, undermines balance control, and leads to disabling condition.

EXERCISE & INJURIES

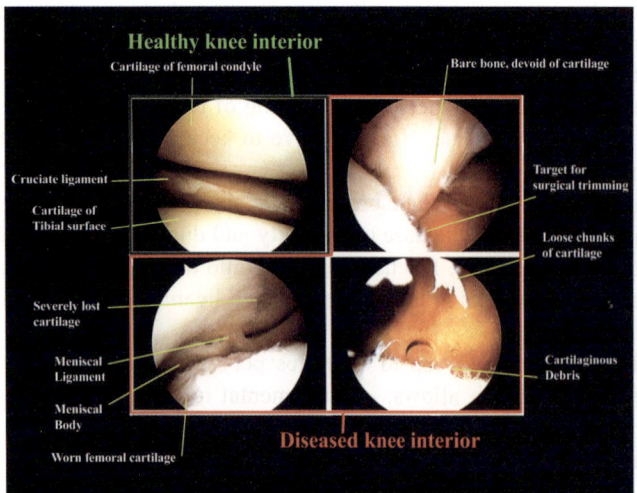
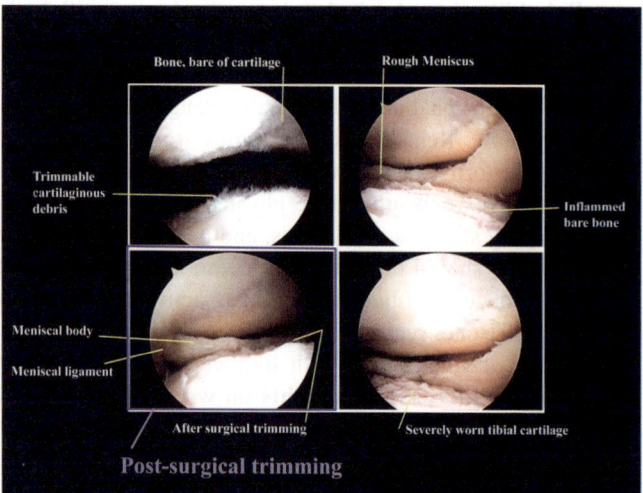

Figure 16.1. Arthroscopic photographs of the interior of the normal and diseased knee joints.
i. Upper left photo shows normal cartilaginous surfaces and healthy cruciate ligament, in between.
ii. Upper right photo shows worn cartilage.
iii. Lower left photo shows intact meniscus ligament and worn cartilage and meniscus.
iv. Lower right photo shows loose cartilaginous fragments.

Figure 16.2. Arthroscopic photographs of the interior of the knee joint, before and after surgical trimming.
i. Upper left photo shows rugged and worn cartilaginous surfaces.
ii. Upper right photo shows worn cartilage and inflamed red bone.
iii. Lower left photo shows surgically trimmed cartilage.
iv. Lower right photo shows badly worn cartilaginous surface and exposed bone.

16.4.2. CRUCIATE LIGAMENTS

o   The cruciate ligaments are two separate ligaments situated inside the knee cavity, in an anterior posterior vertical plane. They are not accessible from outside, *Figure 16.1*. Each ligament prevents the translation of the bones of the knees in one direction, the front or the back (anteriorly and posteriorly). Each ligament has an origin and an insertion in femoral and tibial surfaces of the knee. Thus, the two ligaments crisscross in the middle groove between the femoral epicondyles.

o   Since they are ligaments, they do not require stimulation to maintain tension. Thus, whether you are paying attention or not, the cruciate ligaments prevent knee-bones translation and spare the knees the serious dislocation, during bending and straight knee configurations. The knee muscles prevent translation only if they are voluntarily contracted.

o   The anterior cruciate prevents anterior sliding of the tibia on the femur. The posterior cruciate prevents posterior sliding of the lower legs on the femur. In either case, the direction of translation of knee bones is **perpendicular to the lines** of action of muscles, in front as well as behind the knee. Thus, the cruciates enhance involuntary knee stabilization. Excessive forces in the anterior-posterior plane disrupt the cruciate ligaments. Roller-skating is an example of sports where cruciate ligaments could be torn by either sudden cessation of the feet on an obstacle, while the body is speeding, or a turn that ends in halting the feet, while the body is turning. Other sports such as sprinting and skiing cause similar injuries.

o   Unless the muscles of the knees are strong enough, torn ligaments cause the knee to cave in to bodyweight on initiating standing. Clinical manipulation shows lack of anchorage of the knees, when pulled or pushed, while bent and relaxed. MRI detects large tears. Nowadays, Complete tears could be repaired. Partial tears are managed by supportive aids during walking and gradual exercise to strengthen tissues. Recovery might take up to 6 months.

16.4.3. COLLATERAL LIGAMENTS

Collateral ligaments are situated on both sides of each knee and are easily accessible from outside, since they have no much muscular covering. These ligaments are injured when overstretched. The medial collateral ligament of the knee is protected from some trauma by the other limb that prevents blows to the medial side of the limb. Blows to the side of the body, in sports or falls, avulse or overstretch the medial ligament and contuse the lateral ligament. Acute trauma invokes severe local pain, swelling, color changes, and/or apparent separation of the knee bones on the medial side. Partial tears recover with alleviation of inflammation, in the acute and chronic phases, and gradual strengthening exercises. Ice application may be required for few days or even weeks. Stiffness and tightness improve with movements.

16.4.4. ARTHRITIS

o   Arthritis is the condition of **inflammation** of joints. Inflammation produces symptoms such as pain, swelling, hotness, or discoloration, separate or combined, in different degrees, acute or chronic. Large swelling limits the range of motion of the inflamed joint. Inflammation can be caused by insulting agents such as infection, degeneration due to aging, overweight, physical abuse of sport or job, autoimmune reaction, or tumors. Some people confuse inflammation for

infection. Inflammation is a reaction to insult, while infection is a cause or insult to biological tissue.
- o If inflammation is not reduced quickly and the joint is not kept moving, then damage progresses at fast rate, as the inflammatory cells deposit fibrous proteins and cause adhesions within the joint interior.
- o The types of arthritis are named according to the cause of inflammation. Thus, arthritis can take the forms of infectious arthritis, osteoarthritis, or rheumatoid arthritis. These are characterized as follows.
    i. **Infectious arthritis.** Infections such as syphilis, gonorrhea, or tuberculosis have specific causative microbial agents. These are treated with antibiotics. Infection always yields the causative agent through laboratory tests. Tapping knee fluids for culture and microscopic analysis may diagnose infection. No vigorous exercise is recommended during antibiotic therapy, since vigorous exercise causes oxygen debt in tissues and hence hinders recovery.
    ii. **Osteoarthritis.** Aging, heavy lifting for many years, or overweight cause degeneration of cartilages. This is the most common type of arthritis in vigorous sports. Athletes incur injuries to cartilages and menisci due to heavy lifting and risky techniques that endanger the integrity of the knee. Damaged cartilages and menisci undermine the smoothness of sliding of the inner surfaces of the joint (articular surfaces) and create friction wear and tear and inflammation. Inflammation eats up the elastic slippery surface and adjacent bone. Inflamed bone is extremely painful and precludes joint use. Despite the high prevalence of osteoarthritis in athletes, the quality of life is much better with exercise than non-athletes. With stronger knee muscles, the knees are more stable, with less wiggling or wearing and tearing. Stronger muscles enhance circulation around the joint that promote alleviation of pain, reduce accumulation of fluids, and permit active movements. With activity, vital organs such as the heart, kidneys, and nervous system stay healthy. Osteoarthritis used to be the disease of old or overweight household wives, in the first half of last century. Today, with prevalence of less active lifestyle, osteoarthritis affects larger segments of society due to overweight. X-ray only shows advanced changes in bony surfaces or joint space. MRI is superior in visualizing changes in cartilage and menisci. Arthroscopy is now used to diagnose and repair many knee conditions. Knee inflammation is treated with painkillers (analgesics such as acetaminophen, ibuprofen, and indomethacin), exercise, physical therapy, and sometimes cortisone injection. The advantage of exercise, over other modalities, is that exercise improves function for many years by enhancing general health, in addition to alleviating arthritis. Analgesics have side effects and only relieve inflammation without enhancing circulation and balance. Analgesics are invaluable during acute pain.
    iii. **Rheumatoid arthritis** is thought to be autoimmune disease. The connective tissue structures of joints are attacked with antibodies. Thus, inflammation is self-induced. Unabated soft tissue inflammation destroys the articulating surface of the joint and causes disability. As soon the acute phase of inflammation is managed by corticosteroids or non-steroidal anti-inflammatory drugs (NSAID), regular exercise offer great hope in recovery.

16.4.5. TENDON INJURIES
- o The most common tendon injuries are inflammation due to overuse (tendonitis). People who **do not exercise** have thin and weak tendons with low threshold for overstretching. Overstretching squeezes the matrix of the tendon and damages its structure. Damaged tissue provokes inflammation. Inflamed tendons are predisposed to tear.
- o **Excessive explosive forces** avulse tendons from muscle or bone. Old age, overweight, lack of exercise, and poor nutrition also increase risk of tendon injury.
- o **Tears** of tendons may be partial or complete. Complete tear may present with apparent defect under skin and inability to move the affected part of the body. Completely torn large tendons require surgical repair. Partial tears are painful when the affected part starts moving.
- o **Inflamed tendons** require many months to heal. Inflammation of the flexor tendons of the fingers (on the front of the hand) is common in menial laborers and Weightlifters. **Cystic swelling** of the flexor tendons causes locking of fingers as the swollen tendon is trapped in the fibrous tunnel. At least six months might elapse before locked fingers recover, with massage and regular movements.
- o Wrist straps are common cause of inflammation of the extensor tendons on the back of the hand. They cause cystic swellings (ganglion) that move with the tendon. These may require few months to disappear.
- o Most exercise induced tendon injuries occur with interruption of training or with sudden changes in **exercise intensity** or performing new exercises with heavy weights. If you are not familiar with tendon injuries and their course of recovery, you may expose yourself to unnecessary surgery, because tendonitis presents with dramatic pain or loss of function for many weeks. If there is no structural damage, long course of physical therapy (up to 6 months) may completely restore function.
- o **Life long exercising** is crucial to prevent injuries to tendons. Lack of exercise cause thinning, weakness, shortening, and calcification of tendons and predispose to injuries, which might be life threatening. Tendonitis causes discomfort and pain at the beginning of warm-up. It improves as warm-up proceeds and returns to lesser degree after cessation of exercise. Inflammation diminishes with repeated, progressive, and incremental exercising, resulting in complete cure in most cases.

EXERCISE & INJURIES

16.5. INJURIES TO THE SHOULDER

16.5.1. ROTATOR CUFF TEAR

o   The rotator cuff consists of tendons of the four scapular muscles: Subscapularis, Infraspinatus, Supraspinatus, and Teres minor. The four tendons wrap around the shoulder ball and anchor the ball to its socket, while the bigger muscles perform the leverage movements. Seven external muscles perform shoulder motion, in addition to the internal cuff rotators. The seven muscles are: Deltoid, Coracobrachialis, Triceps, Biceps brachii, Pectoralis major, Teres major, and Latissimus dorsi. The four tendons of the cuff rotators are allowed to move freely on padding of fluids (synovial bursa).

o   Since shoulders are mainly mobility joints, wear and tear afflict the rotator cuff tendons due to excessive usage, repetitive heavy lifting, lack of strength training, degenerative changes of aging, falling on extended arm, and collision. Injuries of cuff rotators will remain real danger in exercise activity as long as education on exercise planning and execution is lacking. The main issues in educating people on preventing such injuries are: incremental training over many weeks, balanced shoulder exercising, and planning long term strategies in dealing with individual shortcomings.

o   Torn cuff presents with **pain** on the shoulder top on abducting or raising the arms. Totally torn cuff causes **popping** of the shoulder ball, when trying to move the shoulder or during sleep when the arms fall off the bed. This forces the patient to wake up and replace the shoulder back into its socket, using the other hand. Weakness is another symptom of torn cuff rotator.

o   X-ray imaging excludes bone fracture and MRI detects bursitis and larger tears. **Arthroscopy** might be needed to confirm diagnosis and repair tear. Initially, partial small tears are treated with anti-inflammatory medication, heat application, cortisone injection, and strength training.

o   In Weightlifting, full range of motion Shoulder Press prevents weakness of rotator cuff. Partial Shoulder Press, without lowering the bar to touch the shoulders, contributes to the stiffness and weakness of the rotator cuff. Extremely heavy one-hand Shoulder Press, with the aid of a partner, could tear the cuff, if the weight is lowered suddenly.

16.5.2. DISLOCATION

o   The high mobility of shoulder joint and the complexity of its structure render the shoulder vulnerable to disassembly under the influence of strong forces. These may operate in the direction of joint weakness or during inattentive state.

o   Dislocation amounts for separation of the ball and socket (of the shoulder joint) apart, completely, partially (sublaxation), or frequently (instability). The dislocated shoulder ball compress vessels, nerves, bursas, and ligaments around the joint. Thus, it causes pain, swelling, numbness, and apparent deformation of the contour of the shoulder.

o   X-ray is diagnostic. Immediate manual restitution of the joint prevents loss of limb due to obstruction of circulation and paralysis due to nerve interruption. Subsequent immobilization permits healing of inflammation.

o   Strength exercise should commence as soon as pain and inflammation subside, and should be gradually increased in intensity to build strong muscular support. Even with advanced arthritis, exercise is crucial to maintain shoulder mobility.

o   Badly disorganized joint requires arthroscopic or open surgery to restore mobility and prevent progressive development of artherosclerosis.

16.5.3. INFLAMMATION

o   Insults to the soft tissues of the shoulder cause irritation of the delicate structures of this highly mobile joint. As a result of irritation, inflammation ensues producing pain, swelling, and hotness. The inflamed deformed structures interfere with the smooth and frictionless mobility of the joint.

o   Cold trauma is the most common cause of shoulder inflammation leading to stiffness of the muscles, weakness, instability, and further internal inflammation.

o   Connective tissue disease such as rheumatoid arthritis is caused by autoimmune disorder.

o   Inactivity is another cause of shoulder inflammation. Inactive lifestyle causes muscular weakness and thinning of the tendons. Slightly excessive force causes pinching of the thinned and weak tendons causing inflammation (tendonitis). Bursas adjacent to inflamed tendons become inflamed too. Inactivity leads to adhesions within the inflamed structures and further increases vulnerability to future inflammation and stiffness.

o   Strength training builds circulation-rich muscular surrounding and enhances fast recovery of inflammation. In addition, strong tendons and muscles are less vulnerable to irritation. Although inflammatory pain of the shoulder is sometimes severe, mobility and gradual exercise improves the outcome of recovery better than complete shoulder rest.

o   Tendonitis requires up to six months, or more, for pain to fully subside. Bursitis and myositis requires few weeks to recover. The exclusion of fracture, dislocation, and tumor are important prior to embarking of the diagnosis of inflammation. If the swelling is very severe and does not respond to medication, heat, or ice application, fluid withdrawal from the joint becomes necessary to decompress structures and permit movement. Before resorting to steroid injection, alternating electric stimulation of the Deltoid might help alleviate inflammation and allow comfortable night sleep.

o   Rest of the inflamed joint may be the ultimate solution for alleviating pain, when there is no identifiable organic cause and when other treatment modalities fail to suppress pain. Recovery from shoulder tendonitis should not be hastened by aggressive intervention. This may do more harm than good.

16.5.4. FRACTURE
The shoulder joint is formed by three bones, the humerus (upper arm), clavicle (collar bone), and scapula (shoulder plate). Fractures of any of these bones result from accidents, falls, or a blow to the shoulder. These may be minor cracks, comminuted, closed, or open fractures. Severe localized pain, swelling, redness, and hotness are common in fractures. Immobilization is very crucial on suspicion of fracture. This prevents further soft tissue damage or interference between fractured segments. X-ray is diagnostic. Fractures are treated with restoration of alignments, either conservatively or surgically, then immobilization in a sling or cast until bone union is complete.

16.5.5. ADHESION
Immobility of the shoulders leads to sticking of internal soft tissues, due to inflammatory adhesions. Immobility may be caused by painful inflammation, paralysis of muscles, or connective tissue disease. The shoulder bursas, capsule, and tendon are prevented from sliding due to dryness of synovial fluid, adhesion, and pain. Partial or complete shoulder fixation due to adhesive capsule is common in alcoholics and smokers with inactive lifestyle. Active inflammation and total fixation of the joint causes pain on movement. In younger patients and short history of adhesions, stretching exercises may help improve the range of motion.

16.6. BACK INJURIES

16.6.1. CAUSES OF BACK INJURIES
Back injuries vary from minor strains to disabling paralysis. Not all injuries to the back afflict the intervertebral discs. The wide range of back injuries lead many people to attribute all back injuries to disc bulging.
o   Farmers working in hot climates sometimes confuse **kidney pain** for back pain and vice versa.
o   Back pain due to **improper alignment,** during sleeping, or cold trauma due to sleeping under **cold air** current, are mainly inflammation of soft tissues. Despite the feeling of stabbing pain, this kind of injury recovers completely within days. Heat application, exercise, and analgesics may hasten recovery.
o   Sharp pain, during physical activities without proper warm-up, usually leads to acute muscle or ligament pain. That also recovers completely and shortly.
o   Improper lifting, sitting, or bearing down cause intervertebral discs to push through their sheathes and bulge (herniated) causing nerve pinching, with local and remote changes in sensation or motor condition.

16.6.2. LOWER BACK PAIN
o   This is the most common problem in all cultures and, most probably, since man learned to walk on two limbs. The lower back endures both predictable static forces and sudden dynamic forces. Many people opt for less activity for the back for fear of incurring injury. Unfortunately, that is exactly the wrong approach to prevent back weakness. The back has to be conditioned to deal with extremes of forces that link the extreme parts of the body, head to toes, passing by the lower back.
o   The **soft tissues** of the lower back (muscles and ligaments) are pulled beyond their maximal tolerance by improper alignment, during forceful resisting or sudden yanking activities. Unconditioned muscles do not have the strength, neural control, or flexibility to stand unexpected extremes of forces. In addition to absence of strength training, smoking, alcohol, drugs (particularly cortisone), and diseases (such as osteoporosis) predispose lower back to strain.
o   The **bones and cartilages** of the body are also affected by the degenerative changes of aging, inflammatory diseases, and wear and tear of heavy long-term physical activities. Loss of cartilage due to degeneration exposes the bone for inflammation and scarring, creating spurs and sinusitis and loss of full range of motion with aging. Exercise is the best strategy to prevent disability and slow progress of degeneration.
o   Women in particular benefit more from exercise since women start losing bone minerals starting from their twenties before full-blown **osteoporosis** sets in, late in post-menopausal women. Even prior to menopause, **female hormones** relax muscles and ligaments and dispose to lower back pain. When active inflammation causes pain and discomfort analgesic, hot sauna, massage, and light activity alleviate symptoms. Strengthening exercises reduce ischemic pain (poor circulation) and promote neuromuscular balance. Abstinence from smoking eliminates the vasoconstrictive action of nicotine and the debilitating effects of carbon monoxide. Alcohol might improve spasm temporarily, but weaken muscles and depletes neuromuscular reserves, for many days after intake.

EXERCISE & INJURIES

16.6.3. HERNIATED DISC
o Intervertebral discs (spinal discs) consist of gelatinous material (nucleus pulposus) contained within sheaths of fibrous tissue (annulus fibrosus) and are sandwiched between the vertebras of the back. Intervertebral discs provide cushioning during movement, *Figure 2.21*.
o Discs act like shock absorbers in front of spinal cord and do not offer articulation between bones. Joints articulation is located behind the spinal cord and is surrounded by the back muscles. Thus, discs are kept contained within their annulus, as long as the covering fibrous tissue stands the pressure of the upper weight of the body.
o **Weakening of the disc sheath** leads to leaking of the gelatinous material, as bulging protrusion (herniated disc or slipped disc). The bulged material may compress nerve roots, the spinal cord, or adjacent blood vessels. Disc sheath are weakened or disrupted in the following situations.
   i. Improper straining postures such as bending on sink, or driving for long distances without breaks.
   ii. Improper lifting postures. See Chapter 2, *Table 2.1* on "Comparison between lordotic versus kyphotic postures, during lifting".
   iii. Degeneration of tissues due to inactivity, aging, drug use, malnutrition, or disease.
o Herniated discs present with localized pain on the site of injury, and along the central line of the back. The time of onset of the pain coincides with the time of herniation. Depending on the amount and direction of thrust of the leaked disc material, symptoms vary from aching pain, tingling, numbness, and weakness, to complete paralysis. These symptoms are related to the path of the compressed nerve root and the degree of compression, *Table 2.2*. Compression of the spinal cord, by backward **bulging of herniated disc,** disrupts neural function below level of compression, such as urination, defecation, sensation, walking, and voluntary control. If the bulged material penetrates through blood vessels, emboli of cartilaginous material could travel to remote location and cause granulomatous inflammation around the emboli.
o MRI is a perfect tool to visualize structural changes due to disc bulging. Monitoring the integrity of electrical conduction from nerves to muscles, and the responsiveness of muscles, help exclude disorders of the nerves and muscles other than the mechanical pinching due to disc protrusion. Most injuries to discs are **treated conservatively** with rest, until pain and inflammation subside and the person can tolerate exercise to strengthen back muscles. Anti-inflammatory medication and heat application speed up recovery within days. Wearing supportive waist wrapping help keep the back warm and enhance circulation, if wrapping is kept loose and soft. Sometimes disc injury requires surgery to remove blood clot, trim bulged disc, or decompress structures.
o Exercise is the golden rule of preventing disc herniation and improving weakness. Back muscles and structures do not fare well with inactivity. They stiffen, weaken, and waste, without strength training. Full recovery from herniated disc is usually the case, with appropriate rest and gradual increase in exercise activity. It is possible to regain full range of motion, strength, and freedom of pain and return to prior activities. Tall and thin people are at highest risk of repeated back injuries and lengthy recovery. These should be introduced to daily exercises to improve quality of life.
o Maintaining optimum bodyweight, regular and continuous exercise, and implementing healthy postural habits, during daily activities, prevents disc herniation. Exercises that undermine back performance are:
   i. Deadlifting heavy weights, in far excess of full range of motion lifting, such as the Clean or Snatch.
   ii. Weekly exercises that are devoid of proper portions of back strengthening.
   iii. Poor warm-up and lifting heavy weights without proper graduation from lighter weights.
   iv. Omitting flexibility and full range of motion training.
   v. Relying heavily on machines, benches, and waist belts stiffen the back.

16.6.4. WHIPLASH
o Whiplash is a soft tissue injury caused by forceful jerking of the head. This impulsive motion strains the spinal muscles and ligaments causing tension headache and neck stiffness, few days after the incident. In infants, such head jerking could cause brain stem injury and sudden death (shaken baby syndrome). In adults, car accidents, head traumas, or diving could cause whiplash, spinal cord injury, brain concussion or contusion.
o If no loss of function of the limbs, no changes in sensation, spinal x-ray shows no fractures or dislocation, and no loss of consciousness then local soft tissue inflammation is the most probable diagnosis.
o Like any acute soft tissue inflammation, cold application relives inflammation and analgesic might offer relief of pain.
o Slow and progressive neck exercises relieve the soft tissue inflammation, prevent stiffness, and strengthen neck muscles. Strained tendons and ligaments take months to recover full strength and flexibility. These withhold muscular recovery for the same duration, particularly for women and untrained people with weak neck structures. The combination of analgesics and exercise is the basic treatment of strained neck structures.
o Inactivity leads to chronic symptoms such as lower back pain, stiffness, nerve problems (numbness, dizziness, loss of memory, or insomnia), fatigue, weakness, and headache. These are probably caused by the inflamed and weakened neck structures.

16.6.5. PINCHED NECK NERVES
o The brachial plexus is the bundles of nerves that emerge from the spinal cord at the seven vertebras of the neck and run to the arm, shoulder plates, and chest. Injury to these nerves produce motor and sensory changes in the skin and muscles of the arms, upper back, and chest.
o Stretching the brachial plexus occurs during stretching the distance between the origin of the nerves and their fixed

peripheral side. Lifting exceedingly heavy weights such as dumbbells, twisting the neck such as in comatose states, or sleeping without pillows, or forced push on the head away from the shoulder (lateral) as in wrestling, pinch the nerve bundles and produce temporary sensory or motor changes in adults. In newborns, life long paralysis results from birth trauma to these nerve bundles.

- o Common nerve concussion is the transient sensation of acute shocking pain due to nerve stretch, with complete recovery within minutes. Organic changes such as disc herniation, fracture vertebra, tumor at the neck, or severed nerve, cause changes that lasts as long as the causative lesion exists. Motor changes such as paralysis and weakness, and sensory changes such as numbness, burning sensation, pain, or complete loss of sensation, are cues to organic nerve damage or substantial pinching of the nerve that require medical attention.
- o Preventive methods of neck injury include dynamic training, and warm-up of local and general body regions prior to physical activities, and paying attention to proper neck movements in daily activities. Lifting heavy dumbbells without proper warm-up might inflect injury to the long thoracic nerve at the neck, within the middle scalene muscle, leading to Serratus anterior paralysis and winging of the scapula. This injury requires over three months of therapy for the regrowth of the nerve. Weightlifters seldom incur such injury because of the regular and constant training of the Trapezius by the Deadlifts, Clean, and Snatch. These create roomy structures that protect the passages of long and delicate structures such as the long thoracic nerve.

16.7. CORTISONE INJECTIONS

- o **Cortisone** is synthesized, internally, from cholesterol in the cortex of the adrenal gland. It shares the steroid nucleus (that is formed by 17 carbon atoms in aromatic rings) with cholesterol and other steroids such as vitamin-D, bile salts, sex hormones, and other adrenal cortical hormones. Synthetic cortisone and other members of the glucocorticoids family are manufactured and distributed under many brand names that do not frankly or clearly mention their content of cortisone.
- o In the body, cortisone is modified by adding two hydrogen atoms to its 11th-carbon atom to produce **cortisol**, the active form of glucocorticoids. Cortisol has high biological value as a regulator of metabolism of fat, protein, carbohydrates, and minerals. Cortisol level in the blood increases and decreases over the 24-hour day, in a cycle that regulates metabolism, sleep, arousal, mood, and cognition.
- o Synthetic cortisones are used as an anti-inflammatory medication, only as the last resort, and only for acute short-term conditions, under the supervision of a medical doctor. Even medical doctors have hard time embarking on cortisone therapy because of its serious side effects and complex interaction with other drugs.
- o External administration of corticosteroids, for long time, suppresses the internal synthesis by blocking the feedback control of the hypothalamus-pituitary-adrenal through the blood level of cortisol and ACTH. A person using corticosteroids for long duration to treat arthritis, asthma, or autoimmune diseases, might die during surgical operations or stressful situation if not given corticosteroids by injection, on emergency basis. Indeed, corticosteroids are two-edged weapons. They alleviate many devastating immune conditions such as ulcerative colitis, sarcoidosis, temporal arteritis, lupus, to name a few. Yet, their long term side effects outweigh their benefits in many conditions that are manageable by other means.
- o Cortisone is the antidote for vitamin-D overdose since both of them descends from the steroid nucleus. Thus, corticosteroids undo the effects of vitamin-D by demineralizing the bones (reduce calcium and phosphate entry to build up bone structure), weakening muscles and tendons. Thinning of bone, in long-term cortisone usage, leads to fracture, joint replacements, morbidity due to rehabilitation and poor life quality after injury, and death due to complication of injuries. The wasting of tissues due to long term use of cortisone diminishes the blood supply to highly active joints causing "avascular necrosis" that results in destruction of bone.
- o Local cortisone injections are in common use in alleviating pain and swelling of inflamed joints and tendons. When inflammation does not respond to non-steroidal anti-inflammatory drugs (such aspirin, acetaminophen, or indomethacin), digestive difficulties preclude intake of such oral medications, pain is chronic and troubling, when fast recovery is desired, or no improvement is gained by physical therapy, then cortisone injections offer plausible alternative. Oily preparation of glucocorticoids injection allow for slow and protracted action of cortisone. This might last about a month long, at concentration higher than orally distributed cortisone. Conditions that are commonly alleviated by cortisone injection are **inflamed joints** (osteoarthritis, bursitis, epicondylitis) such as knee, hip, elbow, shoulder and **inflamed tendons** such as carpel tunnel syndrome (inflammation of wrist due to overuse). Alleviating inflammation might completely cure the condition if no long-term physical damage was done and no disruption of the joint or tendon structure was incurred. At least, remitting inflammation allows time for healing and minimizes chronic damage.
- o Some of the locally injected steroid leaks into the circulation and could cause systemic effects if they reach higher concentration for longer duration. Long term use of steroids reduce the immune defense and predispose to infection, interferes with calcium metabolism causing osteoporosis and muscular weakness particularly of the back erectors, interferes with fluid balance leading to edema, weight gain, and high blood pressure, introduce infection to the injection site and cause traumatic injury. Steroids induced cataract is of concern in the elderly with long-term use. The side effects of long term use of cortisone outweighs the benefits of alleviating inflammation, particularly the effects on bone and muscles that might render the individual inactive for many months.

EXERCISE & INJURIES

16.8. HIGHLIGHTS OF CHAPTER SIXTEEN

1. The most common cause of weakness is **inactivity**. Inactivity diminishes protein synthesis in active muscles, undermines the integrity of heart, blood vessels, central control of circulation, and entire body control of metabolism. Thus, general weakness results from reduced metabolism that fits reduced activity.

2. **Diseases cause weakness** in many different ways. Fevers impair cellular respiration and denature essential proteins of active muscles. Viral infections undermine protein synthesis, at the transcription level within the nucleus, and impair both muscle and nerve functions. Genetic disorders that affect the metabolism of ATP, CK, and other essential enzymes of the muscle metabolism cause weakness, wasting, or paralysis.

3. **Wasting of the Hamstring, Glutei, and back erectors** results from lack of exercises that involve strength training, in bending positions. The Hamstrings and Quadriceps act on two joints (knee and hip) and their weakness increase the risk of injury of the back and knees. Weak and inflexible Hamstrings make bending forwards risky, due to the weak anchoring of the pelvis during bending.

4. Many people never figure out that without **regular bending and squatting** exercises, back erectors waste permanently, with little hope for regaining strength.

5. Unfit body fails to coordinate muscular efforts to maintain balance. Lack of regular physical activity undermines the **integrity of the autonomous nervous system**, which controls respiration, circulation, and arousal. Inactivity also undermines the integrity of the voluntary nervous system, which controls muscular balance, and muscular and skeletal strength that support the body under stress.

6. When exercise is over, other processes take place to replenish depleted reserves. These are affected by changes of the body hormones. These post-exercise changes cause **"delayed-onset muscle soreness" or DOMS** (residual soreness, or after-exercise soreness). The stimulus for post-exercise changes is the exercise-induced hormonal increase in growth hormone, thyrotropin, prolactin, endorphins, vasopressin, cortisol, aldosterone, epinephrine, glucagons, parathormone, estrogen, progesterone, testosterone, and rennin.

7. The damaged muscle fibers due to unaccustomed activity are thought as a **cause of soreness**. This microscopic muscle damage may be detected by measuring the enzyme creatine kinase (CK), in the blood serum, and the myoglobin content (chemical compound found in muscle), in urine of the person suffering of soreness. The concentration of myoglobin and CK depend on the severity of muscle damage and intensity and duration of activity.

8. Soft tissue injuries are facts of everyday life. Minor injuries go unnoticed. Yet the **cumulative effects of injuries**, over the years, impact our posture, range of motion of joints, flexibility to perform our physical duties, and predisposition to further injuries. The widespread side effects of mismanaging these injuries are stiffness, limited range of motion, weakness, and predisposition to injuries of many people, whether they are exercising or not. Exercise for life is intended to prevent cumulative effects of injury and inactivity.

9. Exercise enhances circulation and strengthens muscles thus prevents further damage and improves existing injury. **Athletes with bad knees live better lives than non-athletes** with weak knees, as far as mobility is concerned. The pain of torn meniscus could impair the nervous control of the knee muscles and causes weakness or falls. With exercises and surgical trimming (if needed), stronger muscles eliminate further instability of the knee. When you bulk massive Quadriceps, you will be able to control how to avoid motions that provoke pain.

10. **Arthritis** is the condition of inflammation of joints. Inflammation amounts to symptoms such as pain, swelling, hotness, or discoloration, separate or combined, in different degrees, acute or chronic. The larger the swelling the more limited is the range of motion. Insulting agents such as infection, degeneration due to aging, overweight, physical abuse of sport or job, autoimmune reaction, or tumors, cause the inflammation of arthritis.

11. **Immobility of the shoulder** leads to sticking of internal soft tissues, due to inflammatory adhesions. Immobility may be caused by painful inflammation, paralysis of muscles, or connective tissue disease. The shoulder bursas, capsule, and tendon are prevented from sliding due to dryness of synovial fluid, adhesion, and pain.

12. **Back injuries** vary from minor strains to disabling paralysis. Not all injuries to the back afflict the intervertebral disc. The wide range of back injuries lead many people to attribute all back injuries to spinal disc bulging. Farmers working in hot climates sometimes confuse kidney pain for back pain and vise versa.

13. **Herniated discs** present with localized pain on the site of injury, and along the central line of the back. The time of occurrence of the pain coincides with the onset of herniation. Depending on the amount and direction of thrust of the leaked disc material, symptoms vary from aching pain, tingling, numbness, and weakness to complete paralysis.

14. **Lifting heavy dumbbells** without proper warm-up might inflict injury to the long thoracic nerve at the neck, within the middle scalene muscle, leading to Serratus anterior paralysis and winging of the scapula. This injury requires over three months of therapy for the re-growth of the nerve. Weightlifters seldom incur such injury because of the regular and constant training of the Trapezius by the Deadlifts, Clean, and Snatch.

Chapter 17
Exercise and Science

17.1. THE ENTITY OF ENERGY

17.1.1 DISTURBANCE VERSUS LIFE
We exercise to boost our energy. Understanding the nature of energy is crucial in managing many things in life, from exercise planning, dieting, home work, transportation, etc. For a layman, energy is life. For a scientist, energy is disturbance in space. No matter which definition we choose to describe energy, we can interpret many physical concepts with either definition. The genius of the human mind has gotten good grasp on such elusive being of energy. Our senses may never directly identify the subject of energy in the same way we can sense solid objects, fluids, and gases. Yet, our intellect is capable of extrapolating senses to include the mysterious quality of **fire, light, and heat** to the list of material subjects. Not only we were able to use energy the old fashion way of cooking, burning, or illuminating the dark, but also to figure out how energy disguises its existence in many intriguing ways. Energy is packaged and stored in foodstuff, in fuels, in electromagnetic field, in storms and winds. In fact, every being seems to be made of energy. Concepts such as **mass, inertia, force, gravitation, and momentum** are all fingerprints of energy, *Figure 17.1*.

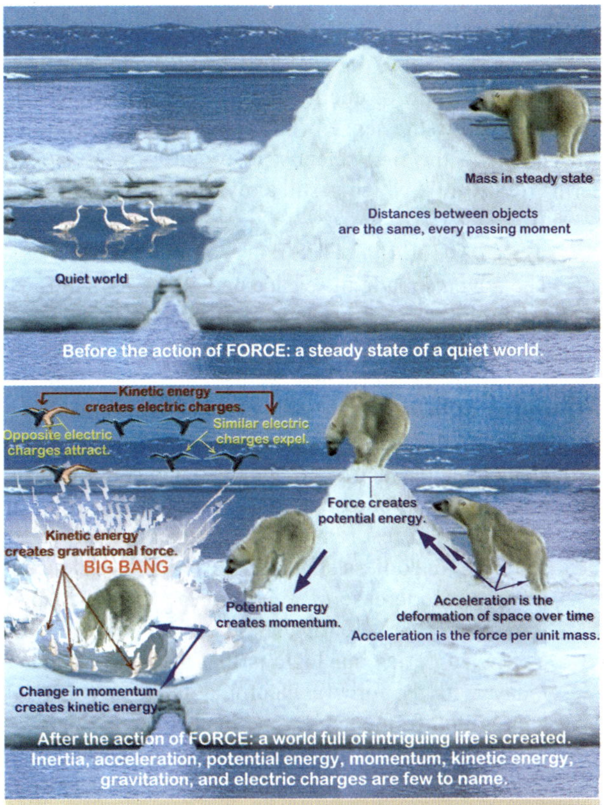

Man has struggled with the concepts of mass and weight for thousands of years until modern science has laid out a logical delineation for many physical phenomena. The bitter fact is that logical reasoning, in its own right, would have never led man to truly master the jinni of energy. Luck played substantial role in tweaking our logic to comprehend nature. Prior to the accidental discovery of radioactive material in late 1800's, the basic elements of the atom were entirely out of the scope of human imagination. In a very brief time on the scale of human history, scientists were able to guess the existence of a whole new world of subatomic structures, namely, the electron, proton, and neutron. With this evolution in knowledge, the 1900's started the new era of nuclear age, which was nothing more than finding out where and how energy disguises its entity. From now on, **mass** was no longer simplified as an aggregation of particles, as was the case with Newtonian classical mechanics. Consequently, **weight** is also no longer conceived as the mere effect of Earth on mass. A new definition of mass has to be undertaken. Since particles have mass and some have charges, therefore, the mass of particles has to be made of something other than particles. This we shall settle in the next few paragraphs.

Figure 17.1. Energy is a disturbance in the state of quiet. Mass, weight, acceleration, momentum, and force are all fingerprints of energy.

17.1.2. SPACE
If energy is disturbance in space, we do not know what is space made of, to assume that it could be disturbed. The old concept of ether, as a basic medium of space, was neither refuted nor substantiated. The assumption that space is an empty, endless, dark, and cold place does not render a medium for disturbance to take place. For, if space is empty, there is nothing to disturb. Here, we have to make a radical assumption to overcome our primitive perception of reality. If a single illogical assumption leads to the explanation of many natural phenomena, then we have reduced many unknowns into the single question: **what is energy?** To answer this question, we might also have to stretch our logic to accommodate the new reality of nature. We will assume that such **emptiness of all and every thing is an almighty state of reality**. Any disturbance to that state is energy or life.

17.1.3. DISTANCE
If disturbance were "squeezed" tightly in space, would it make mass? The answer is that there is no meaning for "tight space" without a mass reference. Thus, the initial existence of mass is a prerequisite for defining the sense of "tight"

space. That is distance. Since without the creation of mass there is no meaning for measuring distance. Therefore, distance is born when mass is created. Thus, we can claim that if energy shows in the form of mass, then, and only then, the sense of distance follows. That is, mass is energy that will create our sense of distance. Since distance defines sizes, lengths, and areas, all have to refer to a mass object. We know of no means to measure distance without mass reference.

17.1.4. TIME

If disturbance "spreads" in a wide space, would it make radiation? The answer is contingent on the existence of a defined space. Thus, if mass is initially defined then, and only then, we can speak of "wide" space, in relation to a concise mass. Thus, the initial existence of mass is a prerequisite for defining radiation. For, we know of no radiation that originates without mass. Radiation defines our sense of time, since it spreads over space. We measure time by observing the light emitting from the sun, while the Earth spins. All other means of measuring time have to refer to radiation and mass. The old water clock, uses the rate of waterfall to estimate time, has to be referred to the day and night cycle. The mechanical spring clock utilizes the recoil property of metals, which depends on the heat, a sort of radiation. At very high or very low temperatures, such clocks would not exist. The nuclear disintegration counters must be calibrated in reference to radiation and mass. Thus, distance and time are merely the **fingerprints of mass and radiation**, respectively. Both, the latter, are two different representations of energy, be it disturbance or life. The hypothesis that energy is a prerequisite for defining distance, time, mass, and radiation does not only explain many complex physical phenomena, but also led to the dramatic advances in nuclear technology. We now know how to unleash the enormous energy stored in the mass of nuclei, through well-engineered nuclear reactions.

17.1.5. LIGHT

By the end of the nineteenth century, man has come to grasp that radiation exhibits a unique property that correlates distance and time to radiation and mass. In accordance of what we have hypothesized previously, that radiation is the spread of energy in space, the speed of light was found to be a universal constant. Thus, energy spreads at speed independent of the speed of the Earth or the speed of the source that emits the light. Moreover, material particles were proven to **store energy** that is constantly in proportion to their mass. The square of the speed of light defines that constant proportion. Thereby, the speed of light, which describes the expansion of radiation on certain distance and time, is directly related to the ratio of energy and mass of a particle. Experiments support our postulation that the sense of distance and time are merely the sense of the two forms of energy: mass and radiation. Now, we talk about light in terms of "quanta". Max Planck[1], the first scientist to propose quantization of energy, was ridiculed for many years for daring to invent the term "**quantum**", which is still a mysterious but well accepted concept in modern science.

17.1.6. MOTION AND REST

o The advents made in science had all started with man's curiosity to understand the rules of common daily events. The principle of **permanency of objects** provides assurance that whatever man owns, and works hard to earn, won't disappear without cause. We take for granted the fact that, when we leave our homes and return by the end of the day, those must be still where we have left them. Otherwise, we seek explanation for any change in the state of events. The causes of motion were such primitive concepts that occupied scientists since the beginning of existence. Man observed that when objects move at constant speed, in straight line, they remain moving at the same speed, unless external elements alter their state. This is obvious in the difference of motion of a heavy object, such as an apple falling from a tree, or a light object, such as leaves falling from the same tree in the same time as the apple. Similarly, objects that are at state of rest remain at rest, unless disturbed by external force. Thus, both the apple and the leaves would not fall from the tree unless something external had induced them to do so. That might be blowing wind, an animal that shakes the tree, or increase of weight of the apple on ripeness. It is logical, according to our reasoning, to find the external force that causes the **disturbance of the state** of being.

o Yet, what defies our logic is that the state of constant speed, in straight line, is equivalent to the state of rest. Even today, with the forceful claim that the theory of relativity had settled that defiance, many scientists are skeptical of any gain gotten from such arcane mathematical theory. The theory still failed to vise the duality of energy and matter in a concrete approach. The discovery of the constancy of the speed of light led to the conclusion that **constant speed** only alters the energy to mass ratio of particles very negligibly. Let us imagine that an object consists of an aggregation of particles, not necessarily elementary masses, but units of disturbance that form the entire mass. These particles are the constituents of the proposed disturbance. On moving at a "constant speed" in straight line, each particle in the object moves at that constant speed. Therefore, the distances between all these particles, at any "point in time", will be constant and identical to the state of rest. The moving object retains its initial mass, energy, or disturbance, even though it is moving. Thus, if the "space to time" ratio, of all particles in an object, is constant, then the object is at state of relative rest.

17.1.7. ACCELERATION

o An object moving under constant acceleration does not remain accelerated, unless an external force maintains its state of acceleration. **Then why the effect of constant speed differs from that of constant acceleration?** Why does

---

[1] Max Planck, "The theory of heat radiation", Dover Publications, 1991. Pages 151-4. ISBN 0-486-66811-8.

maintaining a state of acceleration require energy? In order to answer this question we will dwell on the concept of disturbance. Thus, thinking along the previous lines, acceleration cannot occur unless there is mass. Particles that have no mass, such as photons, cannot be accelerated. Such particles travel at the speed of light. Since mass is a prerequisite for defining distance, therefore, each particle, or unit of disturbance, in the mass is at an initial distance from the rest of particles that constitute the mass. Such initial state of disturbance in space is changed, from time to time, only if an **external disturbance is superimposed** on it. Therefore, acceleration could be interpreted as a distortion in the state of space-time or mass-radiation. Thus, an accelerated object is a distorted object in the distances between its initial units, over time. As soon as the object restores its initial undistorted state, it resumes a constant speed in straight line. For example, an accelerated rocket egresses at a final constant speed that is determined by the amount of energy required to restore all its particles to the initial state.

o Newton's laws of mechanics implement the previous interpretation of acceleration in defining force as the acceleration of a whole mass. Thus, force is a distortion in the space and the time arrangement of a mass of particles. The concept of relating acceleration to force raises the question regarding still objects. **Static objects do not express apparent acceleration even though they are subjected to forces.** Take the example of lifting an object from the floor. Even if we exert force on the object, it will not move before a certain amount of force is imparted on it. What have happened to the force that is below that certain required magnitude of force? We forget that objects move as whole if, and only if, they have the strength to remain **whole** and are **free** to move. A ball of fluffy snow, for example, might not have the strength to move as whole. Acceleration deforms the snowball and scatters it all over. Therefore, it is crucial to realize that acceleration occurs as a microscopic internal distortion, before visible external motion takes place.

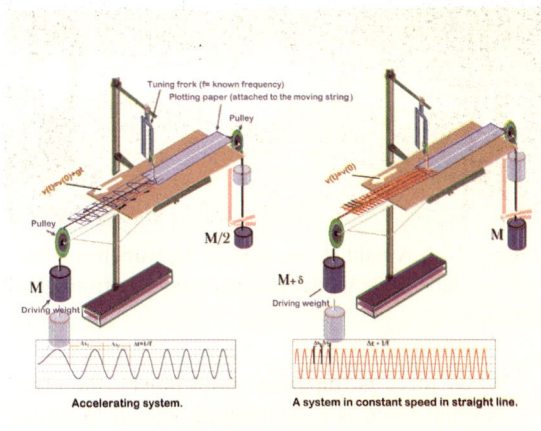

Figure 17.2. Laboratory measurements of acceleration and speed account for visible change in motion.

o If acceleration vanishes during lifting the object and before it starts moving, that violates the very basic definition of acceleration, *Figure 17.2*. For, while we are sitting still, we remain under the influence of gravitational acceleration. Why are we not moving while we are being accelerated? The better answer is to dwell on the **disturbance hypothesis** and recall that acceleration is a distortion of the state of distance-time. Each particle in our body is distorted as long as we remain within reach of the gravitational force "g". The ground we stand on has its particles distorted by our downward acceleration. That creates reaction.

o When lifting an object, the internal acceleration of the particles of the object, and the particles of our body, are accelerated in proportion to the force we are exerting on the object. This is true, whether the object is moving or not. Thus, an object yields to motion as a result of the total summation of acceleration of its entire particles. When forces are externally in balance, **acceleration does not vanish**. It just acts internally, until reaches a sensible level to express external motion. Weightlifting does not deal with free objects. Lifting a bar from the floor involves the recoil of the bar, the inertia of its mass, and the delayed articulation of our joints during conveying force to the lift.

17.1.8. FORCE

o We have used the subject of "force" without defining its meaning. We have postulated that force is acceleration of a mass and that mass is stored energy. We have interpreted acceleration as a distortion in the basic constituents of mass: distance and time. The distance constituents refer to those of the mass elements of the accelerated object. The time constituents are the periods during which distortion of those mass elements is taking place. We also stated that acceleration could not take place without mass. Thus, this question arises: **are force and energy the same thing?** To answer this question, we may proceed by assuming that, the subject of force instigates disturbance. We cannot exert force on something that has no mass. As time passes, an object under the effect of force has to change the distance of its constituents. If such change amounts to visible motion then the object is a "freely moving object". A bound object, however, changes its distance in relation to other objects, but in different directions that will not show as visible **translation**. For example, loading a heavy bar on the back of the shoulders during squatting, the force of the weight will deform all the cartilages of the weight-bearing joints. The changes in distance of these cartilages will not show noticeable visible shortening of the lifter.

o **What would happen if we exert force on an object that is not free to move?** The example of the "harmonic oscillator" is widely used by educators to explain the difference between visible work done by a free moving object and bound objects. Imagine that each element in a mass looks like a string in a piano. The string is fixed at both ends, like the elements in a mass that are fixed to other elements. A sensible mass is formed of almost infinite number of strings. Imposing force on the mass means altering the positions of these strings. Since force is a deformation, the strings will start moving back and forth. If, and only if, all the strings move in the same direction, and in the same time, then the entire mass will move in that direction. Then, we can say that the mass has performed work. This is

EXERCISE AND SCIENCE

similar to sliding a bar on the platform, *Figure 17.3*. If the object is hindered from moving by external force, such as gravity, then the strings of the harmonic oscillators will vibrate in directions that would not add up to a visible motion. Nevertheless, the work done by these strings is **converted into collisions** between themselves. Such internal collision generates heat without producing external motion. So, energy never vanishes in vain, it must be conserved in one form (motion) or another (heat). In *Figure 17.4*, whatever force the toddler exerts on this relatively enormous weight, deformation of the harmonic oscillators will take place, but not enough deformation to displace the barbell. The bar gets hot, not enough to move the mercury of a thermometer, but sufficient to make the toddler's palm turn red.

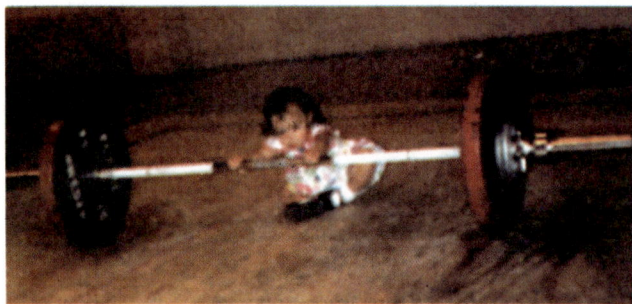 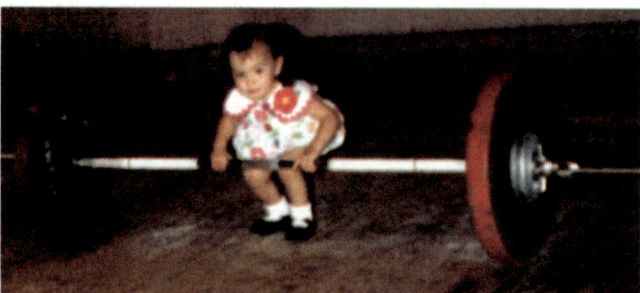

Figure 17.3. A toddler can push 75 kg barbell few inches. The bar has done some work because it was free from gravitational forces.

Figure 17.4. The energy spent by a toddler in trying to lift a 75 kg is never wasted in vain. It is just converted into heat.

o When force is imparted on an object, the object counteracts by **reaction.** The truth is that, the mass perceives the external force as a disturbance, adds it to its own initial disturbance. The mass is now at a higher level of disturbance by accommodating that new guest, the external force. Such accommodation depends on the mass's initial constituents. The opposite and equal reaction hypothesis is a trick to remedy our simple mathematical representation of balancing forces. It accounts for the missing energies, but disguises the real interpretation of nature. Consequently, we do not lose energy by trying to lift a weight that does move. That energy is converted to other forms of energy that might be insensible to us. This concept is used in **isometric** exercises, where effort is made to resist something that does not move. Isometric exercises are the essence of building impressively defined muscles.

17.1.9. INERTIA

o After exerting an amount of force, sufficient enough to equalize the weight of an object, would the object start moving upwards? The answer is: No. In order to move an object upwards, after eliminating the gravitational force of weight, an extra amount of force is needed to initiate moving. If the object has no mass, no such extra force would be required. Moving a massive object requires disturbing every particle in that mass. That is acceleration. The **bigger is the mass, the bigger the force** that is required to induce acceleration. Inertia is this property of massive objects of resisting change in state. Therefore, setting massive objects into motion, amounts to initiating acceleration. This means deforming, disturbing, or energizing a mass. The longer the time the change of state takes, the lesser the force that is required to move such mass. Vigorous yanking reduces the **time of change** and increases the force required to do so. That increase in force might exceed the ability of our tendons, ligaments, muscles, and bones to withstand, and might cause serious injury. Injuries due to sudden force range from acute disc herniation to permanent crippling back injury or paralysis.

o Many inexperienced trainees think that yanking weights from the floor would expedite the lifting. Such common misbelief stems from associating lifting with vigor (see Chapter 2). A well-trained Weightlifter, however, had long learned not to err on the side of yanking during lifting weights. Even without knowing what inertia is, Weightlifters are told, repeatedly, about the necessity of slow and strong initiation of motion during lifting. If you yank the bar vigorously, it would feel like a mountain of steel. Where did the increased force come from, when the object was yanked? The answer is that the inertia of mass resists **"change"** in the state of motion, but does not resist motion, once it remains steadily ongoing. Thus, **inertia** signifies the need to add disturbance to a mass to change its state. As soon as the motion of mass reaches steady state, the energy used in its disturbance is now "stored" in its motion as a projectile. The stored energy is called **"potential energy"**.

o A great part of the advance in Weightlifting is attributed to understanding and utilizing the concept of inertia. Training for Weightlifting deals with optimizing the delivery of energy to achieve maximum translation of the weight. Systemic training results in conditioning the body's proprioceptors that synchronize the recruitment of the needed motor units (neurons, nerves, nerve endings, and muscles) to achieve that goal. The most complex aspect of physical conditioning is developing adaptive flexion-extension reflexes that characterize highly skillful and technical lifting.

17.1.10. MOMENTUM

Momentum is the **amount of motion of objects**. It accounts for the mass content and the velocity state of the object, including the directions of the velocity. Thus, momentum is a vector. It has a direction and a magnitude. We define it by the product (mv), where (m) is the mass and (**v**) is the speed of the object. The direction of momentum is the direction of the speed (**v**). Thus, momentum is the energy that is stored in the mass of the moving object, carried with it in a specific direction, and is delivered if, and only if, the state of the object is altered. Man knew, for centuries, that there would be no momentum without the combined effect of mass and energy. Radiation carries momentum too, though it does not have mass. Although the momentum of radiation is negligible, yet it shook our way of relating mass to energy. We now perceive matter as having dual nature, wave and mass.

17.1.11. GRAVITY

We know that all massive objects fall toward the center of the Earth, with acceleration "g" equals to 32 ft/sec^2 or 981 cm/sec^2. Yet, in the early formation of the Earth, the Earth was a cloud of hot gases. There was no heavy center inside the Earth to attract things towards it. So, how did gravity originate in the center of a cloud of gases? If we use the concept of disturbance, we can present a better answer to this question. Assume that the cloud of gases is a mass or disturbance, which the almighty space tries to contain. Thus, the space presses the disturbance in order to quiet it. This is much better way to explain gravity than to assume that a magical origin is located at the center of the planet Earth, which did not exist in its early formation. Thus, being in the neighborhood of a massive object is equivalent to being close to a massive disturbance. Again, mass and energy explain well the concept of gravity. Another observation is that, if gravitational forces can penetrate the entire thickness of Earth to reach the moon, the question that arises is that: how can such force spread efficiently in two different media: Earth's solids and space? The same can be said on the gravitational pull of the sun to the remote planets. How would such force spread on such widespread universe? A plausible answer is that a space pressing on disturbances would do much better. Therefore, one can define gravity as the effect of the disturbance of a huge mass on the space, which leads to space's pressure to quell the disturbance.

17.1.12. CHARGE

o Electric charges are best described as "**the mediators of energy**". Everything that surrounds us owes its existence to electric charges. The reason why objects permanently exist, the way we know them, is because electric charges are "at work". Electric charges are thought to carry energy in strictly specific amounts; each corresponds to a state of existence. This concept was borrowed from astronomy by observing the constancy of planetary orbits over many years. Thus, water remains in a state of flowing, as long as the electronic charges of its molecules are at specific level of energy. The buildings we inhabit remain in the same state, as long as the electric charges of each particle in them are in constant states of energy. Fire alters the energy state and causes loss of property.

o Electric charges were discovered only few centuries ago. They have very **distinctive duality, positive and negative**. Positive charges deviate in magnetic fields in opposite direction compared to that of negative charge. Similar charges repel each other, while different charges attract each other. Charges exist only on matter, not on radiation. Furthermore, matter cannot emit radiation without a disturbance in its charges. In addition, radiation cannot affect matter without disturbing its charges. Thus, charges mediate the interaction between radiation and matter. We know of no electric charge that originates without mass. Mass is a prerequisite for the creation of the electric charge. Electrons and protons have masses and charges. Photons have neither masses nor charges. Neutrons can disintegrate to produce protons and electrons. Therefore, the electric charge is another expression of disturbance. The attraction of opposite charges and the repulsion of similar charges are not hard to explain in terms of disturbance in space but, furthermore, they give the space **orientation.** You are able to distinguish between right and left, up and down, far and close, only because electric charges possess the property of duality. The eye muscles elongate and shorten to deviate the eyes or adjust the depth of focus by muscular contraction and relaxation, which is basically, governed by the work of electric charges. These act on the protein fibrils inside the extrinsic muscles of the eyeballs. The muscle cells evolved to learn how to increase or decrease the work of electric charges. Thus, muscles perform physical activity according to your "will", which is also (the will of the mind) a result of electronic work.

o The very fundamental occupation of all living cells is how to manage electric charges. Everything we eat, inhale, or come in contact with, goes through a process of rearrangement of its electric charges by our cells. These cellular processes extract energy and pick and choose the atoms needed to build up the body. Consider, for example, that you need to make a choice between buying creatine supplement, amino acid pills, or fried chicken. The cells know one way or arranging the electric charges, to grab what they need, and to dispose of the remainder.

17.1.13. HEAT

Heat is the oldest form of energy known to man. Our efforts to understand why hot objects aren't different in weight from cold objects had extended over millions of years. We stumbled upon myriad of ideas in our endeavor to uncover the secret of heat. We thought of the sun as the heavenly God of warmth, whereas darkness as the God of cold. We toped the millions of years of endeavor by the bizarre idea of "disturbance", as the ultimate explanation for energy. Yet, we benefited greatly from our efforts to understand the entity of heat. Today, we perfected various industries that process energy, from the silicon industry that deals with channeling electrons through controlled circuits, to the jet propulsion industry that mastered flight. We observed that whenever there is heat there is also motion. Any time we exercise, we feel warm. Automobiles generate heat to run. Even subways, which are operated with electricity, utilize a remote source of heat to generate electricity. **Why then heat accompanies motion?** The answer is that: heat is produced when the electronic charges of an object are disturbed. Radiation cannot produce heat unless it strikes objects, since only material objects possess electric charges. The disturbed charges move to different vicinities, seeking quiet and tranquility at new energy levels. Such movements of electronic charges generate pressure that drives winds, pushes pistons in fuel combustion engines or steam engines, propels rockets, moves particles across media inside our cells and all media surrounding us, and gives life the sense of motion.

17.1.14. ENERGY DISGUISES

o The most intriguing myth about energy is that, despite its various disguises, it strictly follows the **conservation principle**. We can trace all forms of energy, in precise quantitative manner, to solar origin. When conservation is breached, scientists detect new mysteries, as follows.
   i. The chase for the neutrinos exemplifies such scientific chase to account for imbalance in conservation.
   ii. The oldest known disguise is the solar light. This strikes the Earth surface, heating its matter and creating vapor, clouds, fog, air, and water. Without the solar energy, the Earth would be cold, solid rock.
   iii. The solar light ionizes the clouds, creating lightening. Lightening emits from electric discharge in atmospheric plasma corona. The energy of lightening activates atmospheric nitrogen and oxygen to interact and produce nitric oxide. The fall of nitrates on the Earth sustains organic life. This source of nitrates must have preceded the existence of nitrate-fixing bacteria.
   iv. Plants photosynthesize the solar energy and store it on chemical compounds, by generating carbohydrates from atmospheric oxygen and carbon dioxide.
   v. Bacteria and animals feed on plants, creating more complex amino acids and nucleic acids.
   vi. These acids miraculously conspire to build the matter of life, the DNA. The DNA stores all our features and secrets in billions of "top-secret files" called genes.
   vii. Demised plants and animals biodegrade creating petroleum and rich cultivable soil.
   viii. Petroleum is extracted from underground and refined to produce fuel for automotive and complex petrochemical industries.

o In each form of energy disguise, there seem to be strict **"rules of conduct" of energy**, as follows.
   i. All forms of storage of transferred energy happen at the electronic level of atoms, leaving the nuclei untouched.
   ii. Energy is stored in physical states as in water, ice, fog, clouds, and air. Loss or gain of energy amounts to alteration in physical state from freezing, vaporization, and turbulence, to liquefaction.
   iii. Energy is stored in chemical state as in carbohydrates, fat, protein, and all organic matter. These trade energy within complex organic systems in living animals and microorganisms.
   iv. Energy is stored in kinetic form as in winds, waves, and running water. These forms of energy are converted into electricity in electromagnetic generators, which are driven by turbines. Turbines operate by the kinetic energy of moving media.
   v. Energy is stored in potential form, in masses restrained from moving by balancing forces. Waterfalls exemplify a practical way of converting potential energy into kinetic energy, then into electricity.
   vi. Energy is stored in electromagnetic form in highly oscillating atomic particles. X-ray, MRI, and radio-transmission exemplify this sort of energy.

o The conversion of energy from one form to another is the ultimate goal of life of any form, as follows.
   i. The tiniest virus particles, though lifeless, are capable of utilizing cells to manufacture new viruses through energy conversion processes.
   ii. Bigger cells such as bacteria have specialized structures that independently convert energy, multiply, and furthermore alter the environment.
   iii. Plants develop global factories of capturing the solar energy and rendering planet Earth livable by other creatures.
   iv. Animals consume energy-rich plants and develop highly sophisticated systems that are capable of mobility and intellectualization.

o The rationale behind the hypothesis of energy as a sole link among all these processes of transformation from light, to chemical energy, to living plants and animals, to nuclear energy, is the conservation principle. The only available approach that interprets how energy performs its disguises is the "electron wave theory". The "wave theory" postulates that the electrons of an atom represent waves. The waves have specific energy levels that depend on the mix of different atoms in a mass. The energy levels of the electron waves are supposed to account for all physical and chemical properties of atoms. Though successful in simulating simple atoms and molecules, the wave theory offers no clue on how atoms proceed in making proteins and DNA and initiate life. The practical observation of living cells offers more facts than current theoretical methods could grasp.

EXERCISE AND SCIENCE 17

17.2. THE HUMAN ORGANISM

17.2.1 PURPOSEFUL CREATURE

o We know from our long observation that life starts in tiny microscopic cells. Both animal and plant life originates in the cell. Here, in the cell, lie all intriguing and fascinating processes of manufacturing the elements of biological life. Our complex body is a constellation of trillions of member cells. Biological cells have specialized to form organs that make up our complex body. In each of these cells lie our genetic database and control codes in the form of genes, enzymes, and complex factory of biological reactions. The health of the human organism is determined by how we maintain and nurture this very complex harmony of biochemical and physical processes within our body. This entire organism is meant to perform one and only one function that **is energy utilization.**

o All biological functions are precursors of that single function. Even our cognitive functions are geared to aid in utilizing energy to the best of our ability. Animals that fail to compete for energy utilization are denied the benefits of life. It seems that energy utilization is not just securing food, consuming it, and roaming around the globe. The exquisite structure of biological nature indicates that there is more purpose to energy utilization than just balancing the daily inventory of energy. The exquisite nature of the universe points out to greater causes of existence than just enhancing health and fitness on the physical scale. People do not live happily, just because of strong bodies, otherwise, chimpanzees would surpass human in happiness. The role of the human mind seems to aim for **greater mission** than physical health. Exercise and balanced diet are simple tools to motivate the mind to trace the right straights to logical reasoning that is conducive to the greater missions of human life. No other animal species were able to uncover the secrets of atoms and the outer space and utilize them in fostering its existence than humans.

17.2.2. WHOLESOME NATURE

o Somehow, the trillions of cells that make up our body have long been dedicated to specializing in various tasks that benefit the constellation, as well as the individual cells. Congregated cells form defense system in which the cells divided into outer, intermediate, and inner cells called, respectively, ectoderm, mesoderm, and endoderm. The three layers of cells thus distinguish themselves from the outside as an individual creature. The three cell layers then specialized further into systems and organs. These possess independent identity, almost to the extent that organs could not be transplanted from one individual to another without long and complex immunosuppressive medication. Wholesome existence thrives in the dedication of each system in the body to fulfill its obligation towards the entire constellation of cells. The major test for organism dedication to survival is **activity**. Physical activity demands every cell, organ, and system to prove its ability to function when energy demands change. Here comes the role of exercise.

o Exercise is a nurturing process of our entire systems to live in harmony. If you believe that exercise will keep your heart healthy and your blood vessels free from cholesterol plaques, what good are these if other organs are being neglected? For example, you can have perfectly healthy heart that might keep beating for another hundred years, however, bad knees due to overweight or imbalanced exercise can spoil your whole well being. A global approach to health is not only a wise choice; it is the only choice to make exercise do any good. No matter what approach you choose to enhance your health, the basic approach is balancing **diet, exercise, and rest**. This is simple, cheap, and efficacious, but is always overlooked.

o The best approach for planning your own health strategy is skepticism of any habit that violates these instinctual rules, as follows.
   i. Superficial knowledge of what we consume exposes us to preventable causes of harm. Consuming **alcohol** as a stimulant overlooks the long-term consequences of depressing the immune system and the cognition process. Consuming **delicious foods** clouds our judgment regarding balanced hormonal regulation of biological needs.
   ii. Superficial knowledge of disorders that relentlessly afflict humans, due to well recognize risky habits, make us repeat the same foolish mistakes other have made. People with cystic fibrosis, for example, hardly live past the age of twenty due a defect in the cellular mechanism of regulating sodium and potassium. Cystic fibrosis patients die from lung failure, liver failure, pancreatic failure, severe malnutrition, and fracture, just because their cells default in one function. Smokers on the other hand do not appreciate the great privilege of having healthy lungs, which cystic fibrosis patients are deprived from, that make them live past the thirties and the forties, before they realize the irreversible harm of **smoking.**
   iii. Superficial knowledge of fitness exposes us to preventable causes of harm as well. Physical activities that lack balance between endurance and strength are problematic. Running for example is beneficial for heart, nervous system, and digestion, yet it wastes muscles and bone, if not supplemented with strength training. **Strength straining** without some understanding of flexibility, balanced proportion, and full range of motion of joints, causes stiffness and injuries.

17.2.3. BASIC STRUCTURE

In our study of biology, we describe a biological organism in its simplest form by three constituents: **cells, matrix, and connective tissue.** The cells are the privileged constituents that master life. Without cells, there is no organism to speak of. Cells run the show of life of the organism. The matrix is the medium where the cells inhabit and function. Cells take and give products to the medium. The medium might be liquid, solid, or gas, such as those of blood, bone, and lung, respectively. The medium is the highway that the cells use to communicate with their world. The connective tissue is the constituent of the medium that specializes in transmitting information between the cells and the medium. Nerves are connective tissue that transmits electric messages (electric energy). Muscles are connective tissue that transmits dynamical messages (kinetic energy). Bones are connective tissue that transmits support signals (potential energy). Blood is a connective tissue that transmits chemical signals (chemical energy), and so on.

17.2.4. MUSCLES

Without muscles, an organism would have to depend on external forces to move it around. Muscles are specialized tissue that utilizes energy and convert it to force. Muscles that pull on bones are called skeletal muscle and are voluntary. They can be controlled by the will of the individual. Skeletal muscles are specialized in exerting larger forces that move larger masses. Muscles that pull on soft tissue are called visceral muscles. Visceral muscles exert smaller, yet frequent, forces that control internal organs. Both groups of muscles are meant to do one thing that is **moving products between cells,** as follows.

- o In animals, motion is exclusively produced by muscles. Muscles have proteins (actin and myosin) specialized in converting chemical energy into kinetic energy. Muscular motion results from sliding of microscopic strands of muscle protein. These dynamic elements exist in the skeletal muscles, heart muscles, in the walls of arteries allover the body, and in the wall of patents tubes, such as bronchioles, intestines, pile ducts, ducts of glands, urethra, ureter, and so on. Thus, muscles exist in every macroscopic part of animal flesh.
- o Motion results from proteins and, in the same time, motion stimulates synthesis of proteins. Without exercise, proteins are destined to demise. When we do not exercise our muscles waste away (atrophy). These include all sorts of muscles, skeletal, cardiac, arterial wall muscles, and ductal muscles. Thus, activity affects every macroscopic piece of animal flesh.
- o Protein holds the secret for life. Though protein is formed from amino acids, we do not know how the aggregation of atoms in amino acids, in certain configuration, starts life. We know few ways that explain why exercise is beneficial, but there might be other unknown reasons for our instinctive drive to play.
- o When exercise stimulates the protein molecules to regenerate, we should be grateful to have the privilege of managing our health by such willful behavior. Many disabled people lack such livelihood gift of benefiting from activity. In muscular dystrophy, for example, patients that used to enjoy mobility, during earlier years of their life, lose such privilege, when the disease progresses and muscles disintegrate.
- o Therefore, exercise does not only affect the exercising muscles, but also all muscles, allover the body. Through blood circulation and nervous system, exercise affects all arterial wall muscles in the brain, heart, liver, kidneys, endocrine glands, and lungs. Exercise affects all ductal wall muscles such as those of lungs, intestine, endocrine and exocrine ducts. Thus, **exercise mobilizes fluids in the high-pressure fluid system of animal tissues**. Fruits and vegetables have low-pressure fluid system, and hence possess mushy texture, simply because they are devoid of the high mobility systems of animals. These possess dense tissue texture and rely heavily on exercise to maintain fluid flow to their internal cells.

17.2.5. REGENERATION

- o This is a vital function to live organisms. Constant **repair and overhaul** of expired elements in the organism is the essence life. Muscle cells do not increase in numbers after birth, yet they efficiently regenerate and adapt to activity. Thus, a newborn baby is thought to have the same number of muscle cells as an advanced Bodybuilder. Muscular hypertrophy is attributed to the increase in the myoactin fibrils in the cytoplasm of muscle cells. Muscular hyperplasia is not new growth, but rather a stimulation of the stem cells of muscles that would decline without exercise.
- o Slow exercise activities stimulate slow twitching muscle fibers, whereas ballistic activities stimulate fast twitching fibers. If a muscle cell loses its nucleus, it ceases to live. Activity thus stimulates muscle protein by signaling the cell DNA to manufacture new off springs of its own protein. The DNA expresses it genetic wonders through the synthesis of **adaptive protein enzymes**. Thus, exercise activity invigorates the DNA machine shop to reproduce and grow new muscles.
- o Thus, exercise touches life in its atomic affairs. It directs life into a certain direction, be it health, if exercise is mastered intelligently, or ill health, if exercise is performed with poor knowledge. Having built up a protein-living machine shop, all other operations related to **energy management** are then conducted expeditiously. Fat is burned out, if it exceeds optimum needs of making cushioning tissue and hormones. Carbohydrates are refined and processed according to demands. Even protein itself is managed wisely. Minerals also fuel the energy currency system with little delinquency.
- o Muscles cannot be exercised without depending on other tissues such as the nervous system, bones, cartilages, tendons, heart, liver, kidneys and endocrine glands. **Too much muscle mass** has the following drawbacks:
  i. Add extra weight on cartilages and shorten their already-limited life span.
  ii. Limit mobility and deprive the animal from long life of exercising.
  iii. Require excessive effort to stay on the edge, otherwise, muscles turn into fat and worsen the situation.

EXERCISE AND SCIENCE 17

- o Too **small muscle mass** increase the propensity of bone fractures and organs injury due to lack of support. If muscles fail to perform efficiently, the following would be the outcome.
    i. Cells ail because of lack of necessary substrates, or over accumulation of byproducts.
    ii. Muscles ail because the cells, the masters of life, are ailing.
    iii. Cellular products accumulate in improper sites, blocking the conducting channels: blood vessels and lymphatics.
    iv. Bones ail because, both their cells and the muscles acting on them, are ailing.
    v. Blood vessels lose their vigor of contractions to mobilize blood, lose their channel space to accommodate flow of blood, and lose their vitality to deliver and uptake products, to and from cells.
    vi. The heart loses its vital cells, as well as its ability to deal with ailing, clogged, rigid blood vessels to deliver blood flow.
    vii. The nervous system is the most sensitive system to ailing musculature. Accumulation of unnecessary cellular byproducts, because of inefficient muscular function, impairs the ravenous needs of energy by the nervous system.
    viii. Intestinal walls fail to mobilize nutrients and slow our entire utilization of nutrition. Loss of intestinal muscular contraction leads to fatal accumulation of toxins in the abdomen.
    ix. Lungs fail to deliver the needed oxygen and rid of the carbon dioxide we produce. Loss of muscular contractions of the blood vessels and lung tissues hinders any exchange process and threatens life.
- o Thus, cellular synthesis depends fully on the health environment within the body that is kept by activity. Synthesis of various biological ingredients occurs allover the body in **response to exercise activity**.

17.2.6. FAT METABOLISM

- o Fat synthesis is vital to animal cells. Fats constitute a structural component of all cell membranes. Fats also play important role in the metabolism of hormones. Fatty acid biosynthesis occurs in the cytoplasm of all cells, but predominantly in the liver and to a lesser extent in adipose tissue. It starts with the citrate of CoA, an intermediate substrate of the TCA cycle in the Mitochondria. In the cytoplasm of cells, the enzyme ATP-citrate lyase cleaves the citrate CoA into oxaloacetate and acetyl CoA. The latter begins fatty acid biosynthesis by **carboxylation** (adding carbon dioxide) into malonyl CoA. Carboxylation is catalyzed by the enzyme acetyl CoA carboxylase and the stimulation of both insulin and citrate. Thus, fat synthesis is merely a **trap for carbon dioxide** into long chains of fatty acids. The carbon originates from food intake, whereas oxygen originates from inhaled air.
- o The specific features of fat synthesis are reduction by capturing hydrogen ions and carboxylation by capturing carbon dioxide. **Physical inactivity** stimulates fat synthesis mainly through accumulation of hydrogen and carbon dioxide in the body. Activity clears both, hydrogen and carbon dioxide, by oxidation and power production. Therefore, fatty acid synthesis occurs when the TCA cycle is slow, i.e., during inactivity. The acetyl CoA is decarboxylated by the TCA during activity and energy demand, while it is carboxylated into fatty acids during inactivity and low energy demands.
- o In addition, physical inactivity produces excess acetyl CoA that condenses to synthesize **Cholesterol** in the cytoplasm of liver cells. Acetyl CoA first forms acetoacetyl CoA, by thiolase enzyme. The latter product is then condenses with another acetyl CoA to form HMG-CoA, by the enzyme HMG-CoA synthase.[2] The third step comprises of reduction of HMG-CoA to form mevalonic acid (MVA), using two NADPH molecules. This is the rate-limiting step in cholesterol biosynthesis and is regulated by phosphorylation, gene expression, and dietary intake of cholesterol.
- o Cholesterol is only synthesized by animal cells and used as a precursor for all **corticosteroid hormones**: androgens, estrogens, progesterone, and the corticosteroids. It is also secreted into the intestine in the form of bile salts, where it emulsifies dietary fats. The gallbladder stores bile salts for future heavy digestion of fatty meals.
- o The liver codes Cholesterol and triglycerides and delivers them to cells on tiny particles called "very low-density lipoproteins", or **VLDL**. These have phospholipids and protein code molecules on their coat. The coded lipoproteins are recognizable by **receptors on cellular membranes**. The number of cellular receptors to LDL, the concentration of blood cholesterol, and dietary intake determine the uptake of the blood cholesterol by cells. Cellular uptake of cholesterol lowers blood level and consumes cholesterol in hormone synthesis processes.
- o If dietary supply of cholesterol is high, then the synthesis (nuclear transcription) of the enzyme HMG-CoA reductase is decreased and less endogenous cholesterol is manufactured. In addition, the high uptake of cholesterol by cells decreases the LDL receptors on the cell membranes and thus slows farther cellular uptake of cholesterol. In meat eaters, the enzyme HMG-CoA reductase is inhibited to lesser extent by **Cholesterol lowering drugs**, than in vegetarians. The former ingests more dietary cholesterol and synthesizes less endogenous cholesterol than the latter. Meat eaters thus have less effect of drugs on endogenous cholesterol biosynthesis. Thus, treatment with Cholesterol lowering drugs alters the serum cholesterol levels of vegetarians more effectively than in meat eaters, despites the need of the latter group for more cholesterol reduction. This is best treated by combination of a cholesterol free diet, Cholesterol lowering drugs, and exercise.
- o In genetic disorders, such as familial hyperlipidemia, defects in the LDL receptors on the cell membrane block the removal of cholesterol from plasma and increases LDL concentration in serum to high level.

---

[2] HMG-CoA refers to the chemical compound: Hydroxy Methyl Glutaryl Coenzyme A.

- **Ketone body** formation (ketogenesis) occurs in liver mitochondria, in a process similar to the synthesis of cholesterol, but with the cleavage of the HMG-CoA to form acetoacetate. This is followed by reduction to form β-hydroxybutyrate or cleavage to form acetone. Whereas cholesterol and fat biosynthesis occur by fixation of carbon dioxide and addition of protons (Hydrogen ions) to acetyl CoA, in the cytoplasm of fat and liver cells, during inactivity, ketone synthesis (**ketosis**) operates only in the mitochondria of liver cells by cleavage and reduction of fatty acids products (acetoacetyl CoA, acetyl CoA, and HMG-CoA) during fasting and activity.

17.2.7. CARBON SCAVENGING

Herbivores can make animal protein by just eating carbohydrates. Alternatively, high protein intake by animals can supply caloric needs in place of carbohydrates. Thus, animals have the biological machinery to conserve carbon atoms and reconstruct skeletons of many chemical ingredients. Such biochemical reactions add hydrogen, oxygen, and so many other groups to the carbon-skeleton to sythesize fat, carbohydrates, or proteins. Gluconeogenesis is the process that utilizes various kinds of substrates (from amino acids, glycerol, lactate, to pyruvate) in order to remanufacture glucose anew. It is activated when glucose needs to be replenished, particularly when liver glycogen supplies are low. If dietary intake of carbohydrates is low, the body utilizes other ingredients such as the amino acids of proteins in order to manufacture glycogen. Excess amino acids are deaminated (cleared from their amine group) and their amine groups enter urea formation. Urea is then excreted in urine. The remaining carbon atoms are converted to acetyl CoA and used in gluconeogenesis, fat synthesis, or ketone body synthesis. The complete pathway of Gluconeogenesis operates in the liver, and to a lesser extent in the kidney. This pathway uses more phosphate bonds (4 ATP and 2 GTP) to make glucose than from its breakdown by glycolysis, which produces 2 ATP moles per each glucose mole.

17.2.8. NITROGEN METABOLISM

- Biological life depends on the chemical element Nitrogen in the synthesis of amino acids and nucleic acids. Nitrogen exists in abundance in the Earth's atmosphere as a partial constituent of the air. As a gaseous element, Nitrogen has to be converted into water-soluble compounds that can be absorbed by plants. One physical way of converting Nitrogen into nitrates is through lightening. Another organic way of fixing Nitrogen requires the nitrogenase enzyme. This is found in **nitrogen fixing organisms** that are capable for converting nitrogen into ammonium. A molecule of nitrogen requires about 16 ATP to be converted into two molecules of ammonium (NH_3), as follows.

$$N_2 + 8H + 16\,ATP \rightarrow 2NH_3 + H_2 + 16\,ADP + 16P_i$$

- **Ammonium** is then taken up by plants and utilized in amino acid synthesis. Plants are consumed by animals. Ammonium is used for the synthesis of amino acid glutamate by the enzyme Glutamate dehydrogenase. The amino acid glutamate transfers its amino group to ketoacids and thus forms the **non-essential amino acids**. Essential amino acids cannot be synthesized by humans and must be included in the diet.
- In the mitochondria of animal cells, the enzyme "Carbamoyl phosphate synthase" phosphorylates bicarbonates (adds phosphate to bicarbonates to make them active), which converts ammonium to **urea**. This reaction consumes 2 ATP and requires N-acetylglutamate for activation. Urea is excreted by the kidneys. Thus, urea eliminates spent Nitrogen compounds from the animal system.
- Glutamine also mediates the synthesis of pyrimidine, a **nucleic acid**, by donating an amide group, obtained from ammonium, by the help of the enzyme Glutamine synthase in the cell cytosol.
- Thus, both, the atmosphere of Earth and bacteria, concert the generation of amino acids and nucleic acids that make up life molecules. Of course, there must be **protein enzymes** at the very beginning of creation to initiate nitrogen fixation.
- Ingested amino acids enter in protein synthesis in the cytosol of nucleated cells. The nucleus of the cell sends mRNA (messenger ribonucleic acid) signals to be translated in the cytoplasm to form specific chains of amino acids called polypeptides. These are chunks of protein molecules. The cytosol of cells has protein-manufacturing elements called ribosomes, embedded within the ER (endoplasmic retinaculum). The synthesis of polypeptides from amino acids by the cytoplasmic ribosomes and mRNA is guided by signal recognition protein issued by the nuclear DNA coding. Thus, muscles, enzymes, and all protein dependent ingredients of life drive their origin from the **atmosphere and the solar energy**.

17.2.9. BIOLOGICAL ENERGY

- Today, scientists deal with energy in very sound quantitative manner. The concept of disturbance or life is practically quantified as "high-energy phosphate bonds". These chemical bonds occur in certain substances such as the **adenosine tri-phosphate (ATP)** and **adenosine di-phosphate (ADP)**. An ATP mole carries free energy of hydrolysis equivalent to 7300 calories. The consumption or production of ATP molecules, during biological reactions, designates consumption or production of energy, respectively. The reason that some substances have high energy bonds, while other do not, is attributed to the electronic arrangements in the atomic shells of the molecules of these substances. Since various substances have different atomic configuration, therefore, such **electronic configuration** determines the nature of "disturbance" or bonding energy that hold the atoms together. Such explanation of chemical energy was untenable by the classical theory of Newtonian mechanics, until the dual nature of matter was recognized in the late

EXERCISE AND SCIENCE

1900's. Modern Physics perceived chemical energy as quantized states of disturbance, which the electrons assume during their steady state wave propagation around the nuclei of atoms. When molecules of various substances are created by chemical reactions, such states of disturbances will assume specific values of quanta, which characterizes specific substances.

- Why certain substances carry high **energy bonds** different from the rest of substances? This question arises from the fact that certain substances are required, in very specific amounts, in order for specific chemical reactions to take place. For this reason, physicists strived to delineate the laws of nature that govern such process of energy transport. The explanation that physics offer, for reasons of possessing high-energy bond, is founded on the following three rules of modern physics.
    i. First, electrons are proposed as the main vehicles of transporting energy between chemical atoms. Likening electrons and nuclei with planets and stars, respectively, electrons are thought to revolve is specific orbits around the nuclei of atoms. Such **electronic orbits** depend on the amount of energy they possess. Electrons with higher energies can spin faster closer to the nucleus, while electrons with lower energies spin slowly, farther way from the nucleus.
    i. Second, electrons are proposed to behave as **waves**. Thus, they have to revolve in orbits with integers of wavelengths. That means that electrons cannot revolve at random, at any distance from the nucleus, but rather in specific levels of orbits. Thus, orbits with shorter or longer circumferences than whole integers of wavelength would be eliminated.
    i. Third, electronic orbits at specific energy levels have **limited occupancy**, in order to avoid colliding of electrons with each other. The allowed orbital occupancy was determined by mathematical probability. This gives each atomic configuration very distinguished identity. Thus, energy level imposes characteristic electronic configuration on atoms and molecules.
- These three rules result in practical conclusion, as follows.
    i. In **stable chemical substances**, electrons can only stay stable in specific energy levels. They cannot remain stable in between these levels. Electrons "in-between" energy levels have to radiate or absorb energy to relocate to nearest **allowable level**.
    i. Energy lost by electrons of one atom is gained by electrons of another atom, through **electronic collisions**.
    i. If a group of atoms possesses stable electron levels, in a specific configuration, they will form a molecule of a **new substance**.
    i. Hence, energy transport is determined mainly by the probability of finding the configuration of atoms that can stay stable by simple electronic collisions and arrangement of atoms, in compliance with the laws of modern physics of **dual nature of matter**.
- Hopefully, the previous explanation of how substances hold up energy in chemical form suffices the purpose for proceeding in the simple arithmetic's of energy balance. In this arithmetic, ATP will be used as the "**currency of biological energy**". *Table 17.1* lists energy demands of major biological pathways, where ATP net balance accounts for consumption or production of energy. The total production of ATP from aerobic oxidation of glucose accounts for 40% efficiency of the energy of hydrolysis of glucose (686,000 calories / mole of glucose or 3.8 Calories /gram). This is calculated by multiplying 7300 by the number of ATP molecules of 38, and dividing by the energy of hydrolysis. Anaerobic energy production accounts for 2.1% efficiency, since only 2 ATP molecules are produced for each glucose molecule (2 x 7300 / 686000).

Table 17.1. Energy transport in major metabolic pathways.

Pathway	Substrates	Products	Location	Net Energy
Glycolysis	1 glucose + 2 ADP + 2Pi	2 Pyruvate + 2 ATP Produces energy.	Cytoplasm of all cells	2 ATP moles /1 mole Glucose (Anaerobic)
Gluconeogenesis (From lactate, glucogenic amino acids, and glycerol.)	2 Pyruvate + 4 ATP + 2 GTP	1 glucose + 4 ADP + 2GDP + 6Pi Consumes energy.	Mitochondria of cells of Liver and Kidney	- 3 ATP/ 1 mole Pyruvic acid
Hexose Monophosphate Shunt	G6P *	F6P, glyceraldehydes-3-P, CO_2, NADPH, H^+	Cytoplasm of cells of active organs: Liver, lactating mammary gland, fat cells, adrenal glands, testis, and leucocytes. Not in muscles	2 $NADPH_2$ / 1mole G6P
β - oxidation fatty acid	Fatty acid	Acetyl CoA	Mitochondria of all cells	$FADH_2$ + $NADH_2$ per 2 carbon atoms
Tricarboxylic Acid Cycle (Of pyruvate, fatty acids, and amino acids)	Acetyl CoA	2 CO_2 , 3 NADH, FAD, GTP Produces great amount energy.	Mitochondria of all cells	30 ATP moles/ 1 mole glucose, starting from glycolysis

---

* G6P and G1P refer to the biological active compounds glucose-6-phosphate and glucose-1-phosphate, respectively. These phosphorylated forms of glucose are capable of engaging in glycolytic reactions.

17 EXERCISE AND SCIENCE

- o In the absence of oxygen, cells extract energy from glucose breakdown through the pathway of **Glycolysis**. This takes place in the cytosol of all cells. It converts glucose into two pyruvate molecules with concomitant production of ATP (source of chemical energy). Strength training comprises of such condition when the TCA cycle cannot generate $NADH$ [3] in sufficient quantities to keep glycolysis going. Thus, the pyruvates produced from glycolysis convert into lactate, in a reaction that consumes $NADH^{2+}$ and produces NAD^+. Even though the buildup of lactate can lead to muscle aches and cramps, it is nevertheless another way of regenerating NAD^+ for glycolysis to continue, and so to continue to supply energy to the cell, at rather low efficiency. When oxygen is abundant, during rest or aerobic activities, the byproducts of glycolysis enter the TCA for complete oxidation to CO_2 and H_2O.
- o Strength training decreases the **concentration of ATP**, which also stimulates the rate of the enzyme phosphofructokinase (PFK). This enzyme keeps glycolysis going by irreversibly converting F6P to F-1,6-Diphosphate. PFK is not activated by insulin, glucagon, phosphorylation, or the intake of carbohydrate. Therefore, exercise directly enhances **trapping of glucose** byproducts within working cells, through PFK enzyme. The fuel for glycolysis is the G6P. That is sequestered by cells that have hexokinase or glucokinase enzymes. G6P is isomerized[4] by an isomerase enzyme into F6P. In a muscle cell, if the concentration of F6P is high, then glucose is unlikely to be converted into G6P. In addition, if the concentration of G6P is high, then the G6P will inhibit hexokinase, preventing any more glucose conversion.
- o The fate of pyruvate, the byproduct of glycolysis, is determined by the **activity of PDH** complex.
    i. If PDH is inactive (during anaerobic condition and lack of oxygen) then the Pyruvate is reduced anaerobically to lactate (by lactate-dehydrogenase, LDH) in order to oxidize $NADH^{2+}$ into NAD^+. Pyruvate is then sent back to the liver for gluconeogenesis, whereas NAD^+ enters the respiratory chain of the mitochondria to produce ATP molecules from ADP. This occurs during fasting and strength training when muscle cells convert most pyruvate into lactate. The heart can use lactate as a fuel for the Krebs cycle since it contains large amounts of LDH.
    ii. If PDH is active then cells convert pyruvate into acetyl CoA and run it through the TCA, after transporting Pyruvate from the cytoplasm to the mitochondrial matrix by a specific transporter. This full aerobic oxidation of glucose (during endurance training) yields about 30 ATP moles per each glucose mole consumed.

17.2.10. MUSCULAR ENERGY

- o We have attributed every purpose in life to energy utilization. All live cells have the machinery of transporting energy, from the ingredients of food intake onto the high-energy molecules of ATP.
- o Muscle cells are capable of utilizing ATP molecules in the production of kinetic energy. In the muscle cells, the ATP molecules bind the Actin protein of the muscle fibrils. These are the protein fibrils that constitute the I-band of the muscle that slides into the A-band during contraction. The **Actin** fibrils are about 6 nm is diameter, sandwiched at both ends within the A-band. This is formed by the protein filaments of **Myosin**, about 16 nm diameter. Calcium release, by neuromuscular excitation, triggers the hydrolysis of ATP to ADP and Pi. This releases energy for contraction of Actomyosin complex. This complex performs acceleration, which is deforming of space and time.
- o During inactivity, excess energy accumulates as fat in many parts of our bodies. Excess fat deposits limit our ability to move, breath, digest, or even earn our living. On the other hand, when there is energy deficit during activity, the organism taps into available alternative stocks of stored fuel. Muscles manage energy expenditure differently from other tissues. The blood glucose and the widespread body fat are drafted for burning by active muscles, at different levels of physical activities, as follows.
    i. **Sudden physical activities** are dealt with direct energy transport from the energy-rich molecules of **ATP**. These are capable of immediate delivery of energy, at much higher rates than glucose, in the absence of Oxygen (anaerobic). The available amount of ATP in the muscle determines the length of possible anaerobic contractions.
    ii. **Immediate replenishment** of spent ATP occurs through another muscle-specific, energy-rich mediator, **creatine phosphate (CP)**. The amount of CP available in the muscle determines the duration of maximal work, in the absence of oxygen. The CP-ATP shuttle cuts down the time needed to deliver energy by glucose and works in the absence of oxygen.
    iii. **Prolonged replenishment**: The regeneration of CP occurs either through glycolysis, during anaerobic oxidation at efficiency of 2.1%, or the TCA cycle during aerobic oxidation at efficiency of 40%.
    iv. **Blood glucose fuelling** of physical work operates through oxidation of glucose by anaerobic glycolysis. This produces 2 ATP and 2 pyruvates molecules for each molecule of glucose. Since blood glucose is crucial to brain

---

[3] NADP refers to nicotinamide adenine dinucleotide phosphate. NAD and NADP are major hydrogen carriers. Their production requires energy. Such energy is used in carrying the oxygen ion, of water hydrolysis, along the respiratory chain and adding it to carbon atoms to produce carbon dioxide.

[4] Isomers of chemical compounds are similar to their original compounds, except in the configuration of one atom or group of atoms. Thus, G6F is an isomer of F6P, and vice versa. The different configurations of atoms alter their chemical properties. This may enhance solubility, diffusion, or ability to bind with other reactants. Thus, isomeration helps alter the outcome of chemical reactions.

metabolism, it cannot be totally consumed by muscles, unless for brief and sudden work. The liver cells can maintain blood glucose level, but within the limited storage of their glycogen. Glycogen fuel comes from the liver, which stores about 108 g, and muscles, which stores about 235 g, in a 70 kg adult. Such amount of fuel can produce about 1400 Calories.

v. **Fatty acid oxidation** fuels prolonged exercise. This pathway of fuelling is not as robust as CP-ATP shuttle or anaerobic glycolysis. It requires inactivation of the PDH complex, activation of lipase enzymes, and Carnitine shuttling of fatty acids from the cytoplasm into the mitochondria, for repeated oxidative decarboxylation. You cannot perform vigorous physical work on fatty acid oxidation.

vi. **Limiting forces**: Lack of adequate oxygen, for the level of exercise intensity, fosters anaerobic glycolysis with the formation of lactic acid as a byproduct of glucose oxidation. Lactic acid alters the pH of the blood and the inside of the muscle thus limits muscle contraction. Lactate accumulation causes fatigue and exhaustion that forces the individual to cease activity in order to replenish the glycogen and creatine phosphate reserves.

vii. **Continuous long-term energy supply**: Prolonged muscular activity taps into other sources of fuel. The influx of glucose from the blood into the muscle is accompanied by the liver activity to make up for the extra needs for glucose by gluconeogenesis. Yet, this process, in itself, requires ATP and GTP in order to synthesize glucose from pyruvate, *Table 17.1*.

17.3. THE CELLULAR FURNACE OF CHEMICAL FUEL

17.3.1. THE TRICARBOXYLIC ACID CYCLE (TCA OR THE KREBS' CYCLE)

o Most of the **energy** contained in foodstuff is **extracted** in the TCA cycle and transported on specialized chemical compounds. The cycle operates in the mitochondrial matrix of cells (not the red blood cells). Carbohydrates, fats, and proteins enter the cycle after converting into acetyl CoA, through the pathways of glycolysis, fatty acid oxidation, and gluconeogenesis, respectively.

o The cycle's main function is to **oxidize the 2-carbon atoms** that originated from pyruvates into carbon dioxide. To accomplish this goal, the cycle splits water by hydrolysis, combines the carbon with the water oxygen, and loads the water hydrogen on the hydrogen acceptors NAD and FAD. The energy of hydrolysis is extracted on GTP molecules and the oxidization of the NADH and FADH, in the electron transport process in the mitochondria. The net energy product is the ATP. The TCA cycle starts with the citric acid (6C), which has three carboxylic groups (COOH) formed by the condensation of acetyl CoA (2C) and Oxaloacetic acid (4C).

o TCA cycle operates maximally during exercise when the **demand for ATP** is highest. The cycling rate is determined by relative proportion of reduction and oxidation reactions within the mitochondria. This is determined by the ratio of concentration of [NADH]/[NAD$^+$]. For every NADH mole, the cycle produces about 2.5 moles of ATP. The pace of the TCA cycle is determined by the activity of the oxidization of citrates by the enzyme Isocitrate dehydrogenase. That cleaves 2 protons from the acid and loads them on NAD, with the help of magnesium ions and ADP. The concentration of oxaloacetate carrier and acetyl CoA dictates the number of TCA cycling.

o The Krebs **cycle yields** three molecules of NADH, one molecule of FADH$_2$, two molecules of carbon dioxide, and one molecule of GTP (guanidine tri-phosphate) for each consumed molecule of acetyl CoA. At the end of the cycle, another oxaloacetate molecule is generated and is ready to combine with another molecule of acetyl CoA. NADH and FADH$_2$ are recycled through the electron transport chain. ATP that is produced from the recycling in the electron transport chain in the mitochondrial matrix crosses to the cytoplasm by a specific translocase enzyme. CO_2 is removed via the blood stream.

o The **CO_2** produced by the TCA cycle ultimately comes from the glucose or fatty acids, but it takes a few cycles before the carbons from a particular glucose or fatty acid are found in the CO_2. The production of CO_2 by decarboxylation is the rate limiting of the TCA cycle. Both ADP and Ca_2^{++} ions, produced by muscle contraction through the regulation of dehydrogenase enzymes, activate decarboxylation.

o It is very evident that the TCA cycle mainly **joggles protons and electrons** between water, on one side, and NAD and carbon atoms on the other side. The electron joggling that takes place within the mitochondria induces the molecules on the cytoplasmic side of the membrane to joggle their electrons and protons too. The reduction of NAD$^+$ to NADH is carried out by three dehydrogenase enzymes (isocitrate, 2-oxoglutarate, and malate) on the matrix of the mitochondria. This reduction process induces oxidization of the NADH on the cytoplasmic side of the mitochondrial membrane, through the aspartate-malate shuttle. Reduction can also induce glycerol-3-phosphate oxidization to dihydroxyacetone phosphate with the reduction of FADH$_2$.

17.3.2. ELECTRONIC JOGGLING

o The basic chemical reactions that sustain biological life comprise of managing the interplay of four main elements: Hydrogen, Oxygen, Carbon, and Nitrogen, which are derived from the **atmosphere of Earth**. Such reactions take place between the outer electrons of these elements, when one ion is brought closer to the other and with sufficient energy to allow binding of ions into molecules.

EXERCISE AND SCIENCE

- o Chemical oxidation constitutes donating electrons [e⁻] by the interacting ions, whereas chemical reduction constitutes accepting electrons by the other ions. The hypothesis of electronic joggling, as a mean to interpret energy transport between chemical elements, was introduced by mathematicians as a solution of the **wave equation** of elementary particles. That mandates specified quantization of levels, based on electron occupancy, and radius of orbits around the nucleus.
- o The hypothesis of electronic joggling offered chemists a tool of quantifying **energy balance** of chemical reactions. The biological significance of this hypothesis is the understanding of the processes of activation, stimulation, and catalysis of reactions by mere electronic joggling. That alters rates of reaction or changes their direction. In every chemical process, the terms "activation", "stimulation", and catalysis" will carry such sinister process of electronic joggling to achieve specific end products.
- o Such processes offer some explanation on the underlying causes of **physical strength**, on why some people are stronger than others, and on how exercise fosters the mysterious intricacies of chemical strength. Definitely, the size of muscles, nutrition, the volume or intensity of exercises is not what make physical strength so variable among different people. These mentioned factors only play on the activity of the cellular enzymes, substrates, and end products, through the electronic joggling process. Thus, one can comfortably claim that athletes with exceptional strength may have developed exceptional functional chemical ingredients that can joggle electrons in the most efficient manner, which others cannot perform.
- o Hydrogen and Oxygen are the major players in such biological interplay. Cells get their oxygen and hydrogen supply loaded on skeletons of carbon atoms that comprise all foodstuffs consumed by animals. The carbon atoms may combine with oxygen and exit to the atmosphere as carbon dioxide. Alternatively, carbon atoms may dissolve in water and form carbonic acid that plays important role at the stomach and kidney, in the generation hydrochloric acid and acidic urine, respectively. Carbon atoms also enter in the synthesis of the main skeleton of fat, protein, and carbohydrate. The hydrogen atoms will be carried to interact with oxygen on special hydrogen carrier factors. The fourth element, nitrogen enters in the synthesis of the basic life molecules of amino acids and nucleic acids and thus plays major role in structural elements of cellular reaction. Such interplay of ions requires **physical design** that separates ions in distinct compartments and transport molecules that move these ions according to logical regime of chemical production. The cell provides such physical design in the form of cellular membrane, cytoplasm, mitochondria, nucleus, endoplasmic reticulum, and so on. These structures have sets of rules of transporting ions and their carriers in such manner as to allow the execution of the chemical algorithm of the living organism. Without such cellular design, chemical reaction would proceed in chaotic purposeless fashion.
- o **Mitochondria:** These are unique structures that possess enzymes, cofactors, and structures that foster proton and electron transfer exchange between molecules The electron transport chain in the matrix of mitochondria of cells carries out oxidation of NADH and reduction of molecular oxygen to water. It does that by shuffling electrons and protons between molecules, with the assistance of enzymes (dehydrogenase enzymes) and cofactors ($NADP^+$ and FAD), along a chain of exchange reactions. Thus, NADH is oxidized to NAD while giving away H^+ and e^-. The produced electrons are transferred upstream in a chain of reactions between various transport carriers (coenzyme Q, flavoprotein, and non-heme iron) until they reach molecular oxygen. The mitochondrial double membrane plays an active role in maintaining proton gradient, with higher concentration of protons downstream of the chain. Thus, molecular Oxygen ($\_O_2^+$) is reduced to H_2O by acquiring $2H^+ + 2e^-$.
- o The following processes characterize mitochondrial design.
  i. Cofactor complexes act as electron acceptors that maintain proton gradient across the membrane. People with partial defects in these complexes suffer from lactic acidosis, i.e. high serum lactate level. A partial defect in any of these complexes prevents the formation of the proton gradient and impedes ATP formation and oxidation of NADH. Pyruvate builds up and converts to lactate, with the accumulation of NADH. High blood lactate decreases muscular power during work.
  ii. The enzyme F_1/F_0-ATP synthase mobilizes protons (H^+) and maintains O_2 consumption. Mutation in the gene of the enzyme ATP synthase may prevent ATP release, though it is being catalyzed. Acidic environment creates proton gradient across the mitochondrial membrane that fuels ATP formation, even if electron transport is blocked. Poisons such as Cyanide poisoning binds to the ferric form of cytochrome a_3 and blocks oxygen consumption.
  iii. The enzyme ATP/ADP translocase transports ATP out and ADP in, across the membrane, thus mobilizes protons across the membrane.
- o **Cytoplasm:** Outside the mitochondria of mammalian cells, there exist enzymes (dehydrogenase enzymes) that are capable of performing oxidation, in the absence of oxygen, by activating the transport of protons from NADH to Pyruvate. This reduces Pyruvate to lactates by the enzyme lactate dehydrogenase (LDH) in order to produce NAD^+ from $NADH^{2+}$. Ultimately, NAD^+ produces ATP in the TCA cycle.. The bacterial electron transport complexes are located in the plasma cell membrane. This cytoplasmic phosphorylation produces ATP in the course of a reaction by the phosphorylation of ADP. The energy for this phosphorylation comes from inorganic phosphates. This is different from mitochondrial Oxidative phosphorylation, which produces ATP from energy, derived from the transfer of electrons and the formation of a proton gradient across the mitochondrial membrane. Many enzymes and cofactors, in addition to selective filtering membranes, heavily regulate the mitochondrial processes.

17.3.3. THE ENZYMATIC FUEL GUARDIAN

o One of the enzymatic complexes, in the cellular mitochondria, that guard fuel consumption by biological organisms is the pyruvate dehydrogenase complex (**PDH**). It is comprised of a sequence of enzymes and cofactors that cleaves CO_2 off pyruvate (CH_3COOH) (oxidative decarboxylation) and converts the reminder into active acetate, in the form of acetyl CoA (CH_3CO-$SCoA$). This complex comprises of Thiamine Pyrophosphate (TPP), Lipoic acid, Coenzyme-A, riboflavin-containing coenzyme (FAD), a niacin-containing coenzyme (NAD), and Pyruvic acid dehydrogenase enzyme. These constituents of PDH serve the following roles.
  i. **TPP** catalyses the transfer of pyruvate and its decarboxylation by Pyruvate Dehydrogenase enzyme, with the release of CO_2, as follows.
      a. TPP also activates the **sodium-potassium** ion pump across the membrane of muscle and nerve cells during the transfer of action potential. These activations are crucial for energy production and neuromuscular action. A varied diet should provide most individuals with adequate thiamin to prevent deficiency.
      b. Without thiamine, pyruvate would not be decarboxylated to lactic acid. It will build up causing the disease of **Beriberi**, which affects the cardiovascular, nervous, muscular, and gastrointestinal systems.
      c. Thiamin deficiency can also result in a form of dementia (**Wernicke-Korsakoff** syndrome), impaired cardiac function and ultimately congestive heart failure.
      d. Thiamin deficiency is caused by inadequate thiamin intake particularly in the underdeveloped countries where diets are high in carbohydrate. In developed countries, thiamine deficiency afflicts **alcoholics** due to the low intake of thiamine among other nutrients. See *Table 14.18* on "Foodstuff with high **Thiamin** contents".
      e. **Deficiency** can also result from increased requirement for thiamine due to strenuous exertion, diseases, fever, pregnancy, breastfeeding, and growth or excessive loss of thiamine in kidney failure and high fluid intake and urine flow rate.
  ii. **FAD** catalyzes the oxidation of lipoic acid $L(SH)_2$ into LS_2 and the reduction of NAD^+ to NADH. The oxidized lipoic acid transfers the acetyl group to CoA and produces Acetyl CoA.
  iii. **Lipoic** acid helps transfer the acyl group that resulted from decarboxylation of pyruvate to lactate to CoA by reacting with TPP. Without lipoic acid, the acyl group converts to acetaldehyde or aldehyde and NAD^+ ions could not be reduced to NADH. A deficiency in lipoic acid prevents the production of acetyl CoA and thus directly inhibits the PDH complex. This affects one's ability to produce energy.

o The rate of production of the PDH complex varies according to **rest, eating, activity, and fasting**, but the net reaction is as follows.

$$CH_3COOH + HSCoA + NAD^+ \rightarrow CH_3CO\text{-}SCoA + CO_2 + NADH + H^+$$

o **Rest versus activity:** The normal activity of PDH complex at rest is balanced by the activities of its phosphatase and kinase enzymes. PDH kinase signals starvation and fat breakdown and thus inhibits the PDH complex, whereas PDH phosphatase signals muscle activity and thus stimulates the PDH complex, as follows.
  i. At **rest**, the PDH complex is about 80% phosphorylated, with plenty of room for activation by phosphatase enzyme, once exercise starts.
  ii. During **starvation or long activity**, muscle oxidizes ketone bodies and release acetyl CoA. This activates the PDH kinase and inhibits PDH complex thus preventing further glycolysis.
  iii. Optimal glycolysis is maintained by PDH phosphatase. That remains active during muscle contraction. It activates the PDH complex enough to maintain steady blood glucose level, for the sake of maintaining **brain fuel**. The activity of the PDH complex in the brain depends on the NADH/NAD+ ratio and not the acetyl CoA. The brain does not have access to fatty acids, by virtue of its membrane barrier. Thus, long activities do not increase acetyl CoA in the brain. The brain only gets its energy from glucose.

o **Switching signals:** Short term sustained activity, less than 15 minutes, activates the PDH complex to meet urgent fuel demands. Activation declines soon as fatty acids start oxidization. This transition is signaled by Ca^{++} ions of muscle contraction on the PDH phosphatase enzyme. The PDH complex does not work actively under anaerobic conditions. Cessation of exercise raises blood glucose level and slows down the TCA cycle, as the demand for ATP diminishes. This inactivates PFK enzyme and reduces pumping of glucose into the pyruvate production. In other words, the decrease of glucose oxidation and fatty acid oxidation causes glycolysis to decrease. This normalizes the PDH complex.

17.3.4. GLUCOSE TRANSPORT

In addition to the well regulated mitochondrial processes of fuel conversion and oxidation, live cells possess another mechanism of selectively grabbing glucose from the external matrix. That is supplied by blood glucose. Brain, muscle, and liver cells, for example, differ in their ability to uptake glucose. This selective transport of glucose is undertaken by specialized membrane proteins, known as **glucose transporters** (GLUTs). Different isoforms of GLUTs are expressed in different tissues. Their molecular weight varies from 40 to 60 kDa. The discovery of GLUT's enables us to understand how the cells of different organs react differently in response to food intake, hormonal regulation, disease, and stress, as follows.

- o **GLUT-1** has a high affinity to glucose, with reactivity constant, Km^5, ranges from 1 to 5 mM. It mediates passive transport of glucose into most cells, such as embryo tissues, kidney, muscles, liver, tumor cells, red cells, and throughout the blood brain barrier. Red blood cells have GLUT-1 transporters only and must use glucose as fuel, since they do not carry out the Krebs cycle. GLUT-1 transporters also take up Fructose, either from sucrose or ingested as free fructose, at a faster rate than glucose, in both, muscle and fat cells. It doesn't need insulin for high levels of uptake. Therefore, fructose is converted to fat more directly than glucose. Inside the cells, Fructose can be converted to F6P by hexokinase and pumped into the glycolysis pathway for anaerobic energy production.
- o **GLUT-2** transporters occur in the cells of the liver and the pancreas. The liver cells do not require insulin to stimulate glucose transport. They contain pathways for glycogen synthesis, lipogenesis, and gluconeogenesis. These transporters allow high rates of glucose influx from blood, into and out of liver cells (high Km for glucose ~60 mM). This translates to high G6P concentration in the liver, because of the presence of liver glucokinase enzyme.
- o **GLUT-3** has a high affinity to glucose (Km ~1 -5 mM). It is the main transporter in brain (neurons).
- o **GLUT-4** transporters are brought to the cell surface, in response to insulin, in fat cells or muscle after a meal, but not in liver. Ca_2^{++} also bring the GLUT-4 to the cellular surface of muscles during exercise. Once insulin is withdrawn, these transporters are slowly sequestered back to the Golgi apparatus. These are micro-organelles within the cytoplasm of cells. If muscle cells were deficient in GLUT-4 transporters then it would not be able to increase glucose uptake in response to insulin. Fat cells have GLUT-4 transporters, have the enzymes Acetyl CoA Carboxylase and G6P dehydrogenase, and have receptors for glucagon and insulin. Muscle has the GLUT-4's but no receptors for glucagon.
- o **GLUT-5** transports Fructose in intestine and testis.

17.4. POWER PRODUCTION BY HUMAN BODY

17.4.1. INSTINCT

- o Movement and strength are vital to animal life. **Plants** adapt to still existence that does not require heart and blood vessels, lungs and kidneys, or central and peripheral nervous systems. Animals differ from plants in possessing specialized systems that adapt to movement. Such adaptation accounts for sudden variation in demand for energy and accumulation of byproducts.
- o A newborn **jackass** stands and walks away from his mother, within few hours, *Figure 17.5*. Even before his amniotic fluid dries, he possesses both motor and the sensory abilities far superior to those of a human newborn. His rear limbs get stronger by the minutes. His exquisite hearing ability enables him to track the breathing sound of his mother. His visual awareness in viewing his mother, as well as exploring the new world, will prove vital to his role in this rural Egyptian desert. By the time the villagers return from shopping at this Monday's market, a fully independent new guest would be ready to join the crowd. A year later, this jackass would become an invaluable mean of transportation, at moonless nights and on muddy dirt road, when pickup trucks are stranded at the nearest towns.

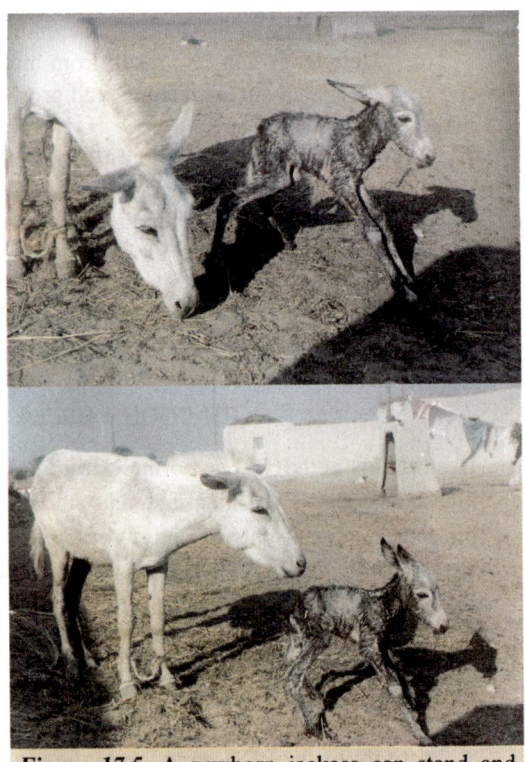

Figure 17.5. A newborn jackass can stand and walk in few hours after birth.

- o A **human newborn** devotes the first month of life preparing for lifting his, or her, own head. This entails frequent feeding, extended sleeping periods, and frequent kicking exercises. These concert all biological functions for the sake of developing strength. The three instincts, of feeding, resting, and exercise, constitute the fundamental rules of developing strength. In the first year of human life, many inherited reflexes operate and help sustain life of the newborn. The newborn can start suckling breast milk immediately after birth and can direct his head and mouth towards any nearby objects. As soon as the infant gains weight, he will develop other reflexes that helps him push up his body, when left face down, and twist, turn, kick, and scream in order to reach objects. These and other innate drives demonstrate the role of instinct in governing our unconscious mind in search for exercise.
- o How did we inhere such drive to initiate an act that will benefit our future needs, rather than our immediately pressing gratification? From my own observation, I witnessed fellows who have spent many years of their prime life practicing sport and were determined to pass that passion to their offspring, as well as to other kids. The following figures depict such driving passion to spread sport among younger generations.

---

[5] Km refers to reactivity constant. It is the ratio of the arithmetic products of concentrations of byproducts to those of substrates. Thus, for a reaction such as A+B→C+D, Km =[C][D]/[A][B]. Where [ ] refers to the concentration of the reactants A, B, C, and D.

- o In *Figure 17.6*, the 9-year old girl is the daughter of a colleague and companion in Weightlifting. She is one of four siblings who excelled in gymnastics and Weightlifting. She spends 8 hours every weekday, after school, in training. Her father is government clerk, making about 300 Egyptian pounds a month. That is barely enough to buy groceries to feed his kids. Her coach is an ex-champion in gymnastic and a high school teacher with three daughters of her own. The youngest is the 6-month old baby, in her hand. The gym they train in is a poorly equipped warehouse that is provided by the government. Explaining the technique to the 9-year old is a daunting task that

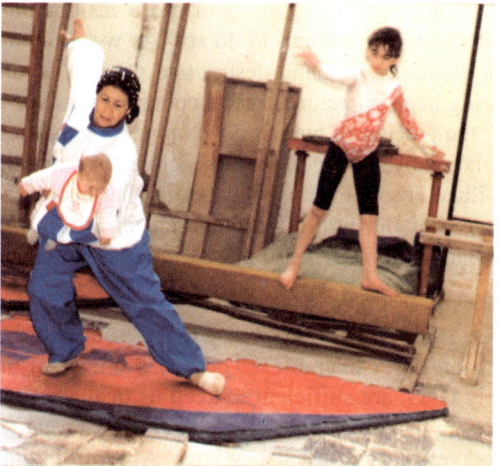

Figure 17.6. Explaining the technique of execution among three generations of two different families ensures better and wider spread of human ingenuity.

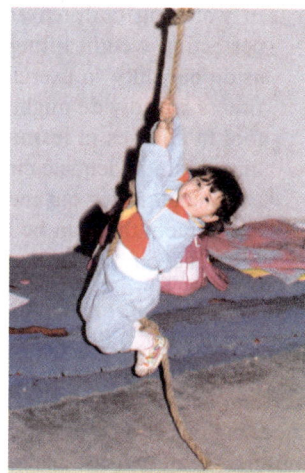

Figure 17.7. A champion in the making, borne, and grown up among people dedicated to sport.

consumes many hours on daily basis and for many years, before performance peaks. In *Figure 17.7*, the 4-year old girl, the other daughter of the coach, is enjoying the playful atmosphere, where her mother spends most of the time. She has no fear doing any thing older others champions can do.

- o In *Figure 17.8*, an 8-year-old boy is competing with his other two older brothers, by lifting a 30 kg barbell by the Olympic Snatch style. This is the earliest development of awesome strong back, pelvis, and shoulders. Within few years, this boy will be completely distinguished from others with strength, coordination, and spontaneity of performance.
- o There are many similar stories of family dedication despite dire financial needs and against all odds, *Figures 19.1* thru *19.10*, Chapter 19. What drives such a concerted group of people to leave their homes, devote such tremendous portions of their lives to make other children carry a unique mission of performing better than they had done? None of these people earns substantial incentive.

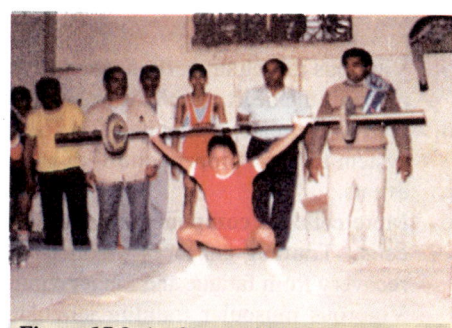

Figure 17.8. An 8-year-old boy snatching 30 kg barbell with perfect technique.

17.4.2. HUMAN DEVELOPMENT

- o The goal of lifting one's own head is celebrated by the very first smile in life an infant exhibits. Not before two more months, when an infant could lift his or her own body and turn from side to side. This landmark in muscular development prevents the growing infant, if laid face down, from suffocating of its own soft abdominal organs. It takes at least eight months for an infant to be able to lift its own bodyweight and start walking. Three years later, a child develops stronger bony skeleton. This accommodates his guts from bulging and shelters them in roomier pelvic cavity. Further **developmental changes** enable the growing child to perform new functions, as follows.
  - i. Shock organs such as the heart, lungs, nervous system, and endocrine systems deal with immediate events
  - ii. Relief organs such as the kidneys, liver, intestine, and blood adjust the milieu within our body in order to sustain cellular demands for the length of their life.
  - iii. Adaptation systems such as the cellular devices of respiration and metabolic enzymes that evolve with environmental challenges in order to catch up with changes in muscles, bones, and tendons.
- o If children are trained properly, by **regular and continuous activities**, the following benefits are gained.
  - i. The most apparent and significant improvement of a physically active child, over others, is the dipping of the lower part of vertebral column, between bulky erector muscles, on both sides. Untrained children do not develop **strong extensors** of the back and do not suffer back injuries due to lifting, until adolescence. Childhood back injuries have to be looked with suspicion of pathological underlying causes, such as cancer and genetic deformities.
  - ii. The bulking of the **shoulder muscles** and hiding of the borders of the shoulder plates (the scapulae) under thick muscular covering.
  - iii. The developing of the **leg muscles** is faster in trained children and speeds in growth after puberty. The back, shoulders, and thighs are the most resilient regions for gaining strength and mass if training is delayed to advanced ages.
  - iv. Strong, yet flexible, **joints** could only be developed by early training, prior to permanent shortening of tendons and ligaments.

17 EXERCISE AND SCIENCE

o   In watching children and animals growing, we gain more insight into our way of thinking. As life begins with perfecting weight lifting, it ends when we fail to do so. As we grow up, we take our strength for granted. We push aside our duty to exercise, enjoy life in many destructive ways. Yet, the last few decades of promoting exercise and fitness worldwide might bring hope in restoring good common sense of healthy living. Exercise is a great educational tool to all ages in learning the process of human development. It teaches us how to prevent many maladies by simply maintaining adequate circulation by staying physically active. We mature with exercise and learn how much activity is good enough for our individual needs. Exercise teaches us that maladies are not our natural fate, but are rather causes and effects that can be altered by our willful participation in life. It might not even be true that we have to face the same fate our predecessors had faced, if we learn more about our potential to stay active.

17.4.3. STRENGTH TRAINING

No matter what walk of life you come from, your ability to lift your own head and shoulders and walk on strong healthy legs is what makes your living on Earth tolerable. There is a universal misbelief that daily activities such as walking, moving, and executing our daily tasks, are sufficient to keep us healthy. However, industrialization and urbanization have squeezed our stretch of activities to dangerously low levels. We all forget that healthy walking requires healthy breathing muscles, healthy heart and blood vessels, not just strong legs. Apart from other sorts of physical activities, strength training offers the following benefits.

o   Strength training is performed by alternately contracting and relaxing muscle during lifting. This workout expends **kinetic energy** by balanced proportions of muscles, and their antagonists, utilizing the organs of immediate fuel supply.
o   Postural training is performed by balancing the body during the support of heavy weights. This workout expends **thermal energy,** causes greater internal heat generation, and increases vascularity. The increase of local chemical byproducts causes local vasodilatation and expedites repair and regeneration processes.
o   Vigorous muscular work increases oxygen supply to the muscles, with up to 500 times resting levels. It proportionately increases larger quantities of the metabolic breakdown products. The removal of such excess metabolites and the replenishment of excessively depleted reserves stimulate the body to function at **higher metabolic rates**.
o   Vigorous muscular work increases **cardiac output,** from 5 L/min at rest up to 30 L/min during peak resistance. This prepares the heart muscle to withstand extremes of stress.
o   During exercise, **pulmonary ventilation** peaks to 100 L/min, from 7 L/min at rest. This prepares the respiratory system to exert proper control of humidification, expectoration, and spontaneous opening of closed alveoli at stressful events.
o   More **cellular components** are generated to deal with excessive oxidation of glucose and protein synthesis in muscle cells. Training enhances the metabolism of lactate removal and glucose and fatty acid oxidation, permitting faster recovery from fatigue and longer duration of feeling of strength.
o   Vigorous muscular training stimulates the generation of **neuro-transmitting chemicals and neural synapses** networks that control muscular balance at higher resistance

17.4.4. MODERN HISTORY OF WEIGHTLIFTING

o   In this book, the author has studied how man has refined the playful activities of strength training, from mere improvised play to well-structured, long term, and purposeful endeavor. More than a hundred years of **experimentation with Weightlifting** methods have uncovered the ultimate capacity of human strength. Many people thought that there must be a limit to man's ability to lift weights. Yet, new lifting records are being made every year. In few centuries, human civilization has advanced tremendously in understanding the laws of the universe. It might be said that harnessing the physical resources of energy, such as steam, electricity, fossil, and nuclear, are more difficult than experimenting with human biology. Yet, every progress made in one field has impacted other fields. From the Olympic games of the year 1920 through 2000, accomplishments in the sport of Weightlifting were a bona fide witness to the progresses made in all physical and social sciences.
o   Although unpopular, Weightlifting represents our genuine awareness of our instincts to become strong. Like many new concepts that had their seeds planted many centuries before becoming popular, Weightlifting is in its infancy as a convincing way of **healthy life in the age of urbanization,** as follows.
   i.   The twentieth century's history of Weightlifting has paralleled **the international conflicts** of the century. When many nations were preparing for World War I, those unaffected nations had enjoyed monopoly of Weightlifting. America, Egypt, and Sweden had dominated Weightlifting by virtue of their tranquil social lives. Yet, that generation of Weightlifters was poorly equipped with scientific methods, were amateur athletes who happen to inhabit urban cities and be exposed to entertaining and gambling activities of urban life.
   ii. By the end of World War II, new players entered the race. The communist countries had learned the lesson form the aggressors and were set to prove strong militarily and physically. As a **military asset**, Weightlifting was thrust by intense Russian experimentation, national zealousness, and desire to turn every unturned stone to avert the bitter experience of defeat by aggressors.
   iii. Then came the widespread use of **radio and automotive means** that increased the pool of Weightlifters to include rural and remote villages. Coincided with a revolution in health sciences, invention of antibiotics, that curtailed the stampede of epidemic diseases such as cholera, tuberculosis, and typhoid fever, many young people start living disease-free and able to participate in sport.

iv. In the postwar era, communist athletes dominated individual sports. Excelling is sport, in communist regimes, was the only available avenue to escape hard labor and enjoy **privileged life**.
v. After the cold war era, new players are emerging. Yet, the sport in general has to pass another tough test. The **commercialization of the health-and-fitness industry** is driven by overzealous profiteers. Heavy emphasis on **drug use** to better health is poisoning the minds of the youth. Too many **attractive exercise machines** are introduced that promise false gains. Very tempting electronic gadgets are introduced that occupy the time and attention of youth and keep them away from basic training. Although, better and wide communication might advance new ideas to the front, yet there are too many ideas to choose from, and more confusion than facts.
vi. The twentieth century had witnessed both increased life expectancy and physical strength, *Table 17.2*. Why are we lifting more today than in 1920? The answer is that we have refined better technique of lifting, better understanding of how much to lift and how frequent, how to plan for long term buildup of strength, new well educated and diverse athletes, and specialized and caring organizations have joined the sport.

Table 17.2. Data compiled from records of the Olympic games of Weightlifting since 1920 and other sources of health statistics.

Year	1920	1990
Life expectancy in years	54	72
Lifting strength per bodyweight in the Clean and Jerk style	1.5	2.5
Lifting strength per bodyweight in the Snatch style	1.2	3.0

17.5. ENERGY FLOW IN HUMAN BODY

17.5.1. PHYSIOLOGICAL CHANGES DUE TO EXERCISE

Exercise is not about just strengthening this muscle group and that other group. Exercise serves the need of the very peculiar nature of animal physiology that mandates constant mobility. Animal tissues differ from plant tissues in the need for highly pressurized fluid flow. That requires both, efficient pumping power, and efficient clearance of passages of fluid flow, as follows

o Exercise is a **surveillance process** of what goes in and out of our body. We consume food and inhale air, but we do not know how good they are, until we test and tune up our body by exercise. Even good food could do harm if we do not consume it wisely. Regular exercise is our best litmus test to survey internal changes before maladies set in. Inadequate food intake can also be monitored by our level of performance of exercise and can be remedied before long-term effects occur.

o Exercise builds **healthy muscles,** not only on bones, ligaments, and tendons, but also everywhere muscles exist, such as heart, arteries, and intestines. Arterial wall muscles waste and calcify by arteriosclerosis when inactivity and excess intake of calories dominate our life. Muscles are the stockpiles of protein in the body, which the body renews by degradation and synthesis, at a rate of 4 to 6 days half-life cycle. They store carbohydrates, creatinine phosphate, and ATP and utilize them as an immediate response system. This arrangement helps the body cope with extremes of emotion and environment, such as laughter, anger, fright, fight, chills, cold, etc.

o Healthy muscles **burn excess calories** and prevent them from depositing as fat plaques in our arteries. Managing energy fuel stocks and mobilizing them to meet the body needs, immediate and latent, requires active muscle machinery that is capable of making decisions of which fuel source to use, and when to use, and how much to use. Only muscles could operate the TCA cycle harder and longer to consume the final byproducts of breakdown of fatty acids oxidation and glycolysis. Only fat cells can store fat when the TCA cycle is sluggish during inactivity.

o **Ridding of excess calories** guarantees access of circulation, by unblocked arteries, to vital organs such as bones, brain, lungs, kidney, liver, and endocrine system. If you try to burn fat, without long and systemic building of healthy muscles, you might confront the following problems:
  i. Your **coronary arteries** remain narrow and rigid to tolerate any excess cardiac work.
  ii. The vascular **baroreceptors** are sluggish because of the rigid arteries that put blood pressure out of control, in response to any physical activity.
  iii. Your heart force and rate will not correlate with your voluntary work. You might have heard about many accidents where people collapse after sudden exertion such as the heart attacks that afflict fire fighters and people who shuffle snow in extreme weather. Thus, fitness is mastered through your **circulatory sensors**, which are conditioned by regular and systemic exercise.
  iv. When the **chemoreceptors** are blocked by fat deposits on the arterial walls, they fail to regulate the force and rate of your breathing during activity. Thus, heart rate will not cooperate with your working and breathing demands. Your blood will pour into the muscular bed and severe drop in the blood pressure will force you to collapse or quit. Your best choice is exercise for life to keep building the protein machinery and wrecking the fat army, in order to keep the elasticity and vitality to your sensors, for as long as you need them to work.

o Exercise **strengthens bones**. Healthy, strong bones are very reliable mineral depot, *Figure 17.9*. Healthy muscles have to be anchored to strong bones that require adequate, unhindered circulation. Our bones are dynamic store of minerals. Bone delivers and receives minerals every moment in our life. Mammals are different from microorganism in that they have relatively very huge body mass. Thus, for mammals to provide adequate and prompt energy supply to their gigantic groups of cells, they have to store abundant fuel stock to sustain both immediate and protracted needs. Bones store abundant stock of calcium and phosphate, which are essential in all cellular chemical reactions. Without immediate supply of calcium, the heart will stop beating and all cell reactions will come to halt. Phosphate is the basic currency of energy transport between reactions. Bones keep constant exchange of these minerals with the blood, in every second of our life.

o   Strong bones fulfill the needs of cells in extremes of **stressful life conditions**. Cells utilize and dispose of minerals in every step of their metabolic activities. Each cell requires the flow of certain amounts of nutrients to metabolize its own constituents, and a way to discharge its waste products. Having accomplished its vital functions, these basic units rely on the lungs and the kidneys to filter the entire bodily byproducts. The lungs function as fast body filter of gas exchange, while the kidneys function as slow body filter of ionic exchange. Both, fast and slow, filters rely heavily on exercise to enhance circulation, which drives filtering of bodily gases and fluids.

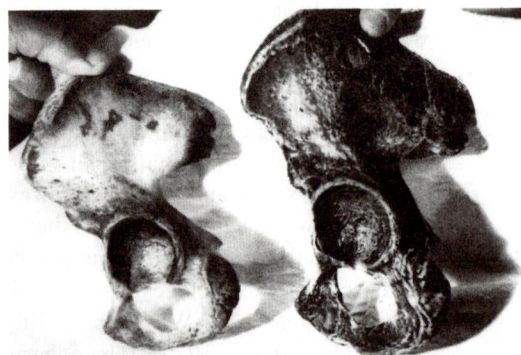

Figure 17.9. Effect of exercise on the pelvic bones. The right bone comes from male athlete. The left comes from female. Faculty of medicine, Alexandria University, Egypt.

o   Exercise helps cells **obtain their basic demands** of nutrients and discharging byproducts by building strong dynamic muscular mass, which enhances breathing and overall circulation. The dynamic nature of active musculature and healthy bone accomplishes the task of mobilization of fluids, which ensures constant processing of nutrients.

o   Walking alone does not work out the massive groups of muscle of the shoulder, back, or abdomen. Executing our daily activities prejudices all groups of muscle that are not used in that sort of activities. Strength training is a prescription for health for our generation. **Strength training** catches the body before falling apart into debility, wasting, and disease. It stimulates the forgotten functions of regeneration and readiness for the unexpected of everyday life.

17.5.2. CLINICAL CHANGES DUE TO EXERCISE

No such single activity has such immense impact on our health as exercising our muscles, as follows.

o   Physicians can draw many conclusions, about one's health, by just inspecting the individual's muscular condition. Even before the patient tells his or her side of the story, a physician can glance swiftly on the general outlook of his patient to guide his suspicion of what might be ailing. Wasted muscles and thinned bones are cues of a debilitating process.

o   A long history of psychiatric problems would be consistent with lack of well-structured history of exercise and imbalanced muscular appearance. Preoccupation with drugs, sex, or food is a sign of anxious minds that thwart planning an exercise program.

o   General systemic diseases such as hypertension, diabetes, chronic fatigue, and depression, all are caused by no single identifiable culprit other than poor management of energy, as follows.
   i.   The poor circulatory passages that cause hypertension result from excessive energy accumulation in the body.
   ii. The excessive energy accumulation that cause acquired diabetes results from excessive eating and inactivity.
   iii. The wasting of muscles that causes chronic fatigue results from inactivity and diminished metabolism.
   iv. The imbalanced brain stimulation in depressed people is, in part, due to imbalanced physical activity.

o   Nowadays, physicians advise their patients to start exercise as soon as they can tolerate its effect. Since exercise modifies the basic essence of existence, energy, it impacts all aspects of health. You do not have to understand all this metaphor to believe that exercise is your ultimate solution. No matter what problem is occupying your mind, exercise helps find different approaches to long-standing conflicts.

17.5.3. MANAGING THE FLOW OF ENERGY

Now, you have a clear idea about the fate of the food we consume and the air we breathe. We have attributed all actions to the messengers of energy, the electronic charges, and we concluded that our "mental will" is but a form of electric charges put to work. Therefore, our mind is thought to evolve to perfect the flow of energy in our body. The mind and the body orchestrate the flow of energy, as follows.

o   Life depends on **heart beating** to keep energy flowing. The following biological data give you an idea about the marvelous design of the biological system of the human organism.
   i.   The heart pump has the size of clenched fist, weighing 300 g, in a 70 kg adult, compared to the brain that weighs about 1400 g.
   ii. In 70 years of human life span, the two heart ventricles pump 400 million liters of blood (2 ventricles x 5.5 liter x 60 min x 24 hr x 365 day x 70 year).
   iii. Each liter of blood contains 5.5 trillion red blood cells. Each cell has average half-life of 120 days. The red blood cells exit the heart at a rate of 5.4 liters/min, through the aortic valve, with a cross section of 4 cm^2, at average speed of 22.5 cm/sec.

iv. Each blood cell travels an average of 2333 km during its half-life time of 120 days (22.5 cm/sec x 3600 x 24 hr x 120 day x 10^{-5} km). Each second, the red blood cells have to cover as distance of 6.19 billion kilometers, during rest (5L x 10^6 x 5.5 x 10^6 x 22.5 cm/sec x 10^{-5} km). This distance is equivalent to 153851 times the circumference of Earth.

v. From such marvelous mechanical design, it is evident that energy flow is paramount to life. Without regular, frequent, and intelligently planned physical activities, excess energy would be stored in redundant locations. This falls along the circulatory system that clogs the flow of energy and squeezes life out of functioning cells. Clogged arteries occur in arteriosclerosis that causes high blood pressure, heart disease, and stroke. Blocked energy flow also leads to other myriad of maladies ranging from wasting of organs to developing cancer. In addition, balanced diet with watchful eyes on caloric needs ensures that energy assets do not interfere with energy flow.

o Other habits also affect flow of energy in our body. Smoking blocks energy flow, via the effect of its carbon monoxide on **blood hemoglobin and cellular enzymes**, the effect of nicotine on narrowing the blood vessels, and the toxic inorganic ashes that destroy cells on contact.

o Although we have dwelled on the concept of "disturbance" to characterize energy, it seems that our health and fitness are enhanced by controlling such disturbance, in the form of "righteous flow of energy". Our mind works that way too, by gating energy into channels of logical reasoning. We learned that in modern industries of high technological performance by merely channeling electrons and photons to flow according to smart logic. Mental and psychological maladies are mostly attributed to either, **acquired disturbances** to our process of thinking, perception, and behavior, or to inherited abnormalities, in the chemical processes of the central nervous system. Humans are still in the process of understanding how the mind works. We invented religions, rituals, art activities, and playful sports, in an effort to unravel the mysteries of the mind. Exercise falls under these ventures to heal the body and mind.

o A balanced muscular system is a system that permits mobility, stability, efficient circulation, which allows efficient management of fuel stocks. Exercise is the willful activity that perfects energy management, since nature had enabled us to impose voluntary control on our muscles but much less control on our internal organs. The latter are regulated by the autonomic nervous system. You cannot control how your stomach digests, how your intestine absorbs, how your lungs exchange gases, or how your brain memorizes. Yet, you have **the privilege to control your muscles** by exercise. At rest, your entire blood vessels might contain 5 liters of blood, of those 0.8 liter goes through the muscles. When you exercise, the muscles can handle as much as 80% of the entire blood volume and can use such power to make your heart healthier, muscular, and efficient.

o We have utilized motion to develop our brain, in millions of years of evolution. We have tested the laws of nature by movement and learned how to use these laws better and better in miniscule steps. Thus, the benefits of play, movement, and exercise do not vanish when we die, but rather pass through our genes to our off springs. Not necessarily through direct birth, but probably even through communication of ideas, as when we share our experience by language or other means. Above all, lifeless object do not move on their own, since willful movement is the essence of life. The most intriguing nature of play is that it does not sound to have a direct immediate purpose, while it prepare the animal for future tasks that cannot be accomplished without prior preparation and polishing of skills.

17.6. EFFECTS OF EXERCISE ON THE BODY

17.6.1. DIGESTION

The common reason people cite for joining a gym is to slim their waist size. Without activity, the movement of the food we intake becomes sluggish. Because our digestive tract is made to retain the remains of the final products of digestion, the elimination process depends on strong abdominal muscles and efficient respiratory and cardiac functions. Many people suffer from digestive problems and abdominal distension when they do not move adequately. As digestive function slows down, during inactivity, the toxic effects, of sluggish elimination and hyperpopulation of bacterial flora in our intestine, negatively affects every aspect of our life. Birds lack the ability to retain digestive remains and evacuate as soon as absorption and digestion is complete. Thus, they can fly light. Yet, humans can carry massive amounts of feces in their large intestine, for days, with many adverse effects on health. Exercise tests your health during performance and alerts you to potential problems that need your immediate attention. If abdominal muscles are lax, you will find out that your intestine would not propel their contents where you want them to go, but rather will swell in front of you. Then you have to increase your waist strength and mobility. If fluid intake is low, you will find out that the large colon is too solid and dry to let you exercise comfortably. Then you have to increase your fluid intake to maintain some fluidity within the abdominal content. If your caloric intake is excessive, then you will find out the progressive increase in your waist size, and so on.

17.6.2. RESPIRATION

When our abdominal muscles waste, due to inactivity, our lungs are hampered with the extra weight in the abdominal cavity that results from slowed elimination. Loaded guts prevent adequate breathing, by limiting the upward and downward excursions of the diaphragm. Many people would describe it as a heavy dragging load in the abdomen that bothers their breathing and that worsens at night. This is attributed both, to the natural decrease in the sympathetic activity on sleeping, and to the positional situation of the heavy abdominal contents on the major blood vessels, during lying down. Deficient oxygenation of the entire body tissues, due to lack of exercise, causes headache, mal-absorption, general weakness, depression, and endless cycles of impaired biological functions. Exercise does more to respiration than just lifting the abdominal contents. It strengthens the cardiac pump and conditions the pulmonary vasculature, vascular baroreceptors, and chemoreceptors, to adapt to active lifestyle.

EXERCISE AND SCIENCE

17.6.3. CARDIOVASCULAR

Lack of exercise is the major cause of high blood pressure, heart attacks, stroke, and cancer. When our ability to secure enough oxygen for our tissue on all times, and particularly in times of stress, the first tissues that are heavily afflicted are the minute blood vessels that supply the bigger blood vessels. The blood vessels are organs in themselves. They have tiny blood vessels, vasa vasora, that run along their walls to supply nutrients to their cells. The vasa vasora, because of their very delicate structure, are the first victims to poor oxygenation of the body. They succumb to lack of oxygen, die (atrophies), and degenerate into fat tissue (plaque streaks), along the walls of the bigger blood vessels. This is the main cause of the common disease of atherosclerosis, the deposition of atheromas into the wall of the blood vessel. Having impaired blood vessels is like having flawed highway system in a big city. Eventually, the city will fail to exist as the traffic of essentials necessities of life is halted. That mimics the stroke and heart attacks in humans. Exercise in any age can stimulate the stem cells of these tiny blood vessels and foster the new growth of abundant circulatory networks, allover the body.

17.6.4. IMMUNE DEFENSE

o   When tissues lack oxygen, the immune defense system is impaired too, and malignancies flourish. It is a vicious circuit. When something goes wrong, a chain reaction of many subsequent mishaps ensues. Thus, not only the lack of oxygen due to poor lung function that disturbs the tissue, but also the extra nutrients, which are not being utilized by physical exercise, deposit as fat. Cholesterol plaques in the damaged vessels, and in fat storage areas of the body, compound the dilemma of atherosclerosis. In such compromised cellular environment, pathogens and malignancies flourish.

o   Pathogens such as microorganisms, viruses, and foreign antigens attack cellular structures, since immune defense is crippled. Lack of oxygen diminishes both cellular and humoral immune mechanisms and allows attackers to roam free, inflicting damage on cells and organs.

o   Malignancies rise in compromised cellular environments. Thus, even normal cells might resort to malignant tactics in order to obtain necessities of survival. Such tactics may involve developing malignant blood vessels, blocking circulation to other tissues, fast multiplication, and metastasizing to remote locations.

17.6.5. KIDNEYS

o   The kidneys do not possess pumping power to excel the urine downstream through the ureters, without the aid of gravity. When we do not exercise, the flow of urine, down the ureters, is sluggish, particularly, during inactivity. Stagnation of urine causes infection, stone, and inflammation of the genitourinary tract.

o   When the blood vessels are affected by atherosclerosis, the kidneys sense the drop in the systemic blood pressure. They use their own devices, the juxtaglomerular sensor, to restore the blood pressure back to normal. This is achieved by excreting the hormone renin. This compounds the problem and worsens the high blood pressure furthermore, since the physical deposits of atheromas permanently damage the vascular system. Yet, this kidney's mechanism prevents immediate shock due to low blood pressure. It gives us plenty of time to interfere and save our life by doing something positive. That may entail medical interference and dietary and exercise planning.

o   High blood pressure causes more damage to the kidney's vessels and its overall function. Diseased kidneys fail to regulate the body minerals resulting in osteoporosis and anemias. Calcium and phosphates are mainly regulated by the kidney filtering and their disturbances affect the metabolism of every cell in the body.

17.6.6. BONES

o   The bone is not just a solid frame that supports our muscles, but, in addition, is the powerhouse of the body. All cells in the body, without exception, need calcium ions for their biological reactions. **Calcium** is the major stored element in bone. Muscular contraction of the voluntary muscles, the cardiac muscles, and the visceral muscles, all, are conducted through calcium mediation. All energy carrying molecules (CP, ATP, GTP, and UTP) release **phosphate** when releasing energy and recapture phosphate when storing energy. Phosphate is another major stored mineral in bone.

o   We can endure many hours and days without sufficient dietary supply of calcium and phosphate. Our bones sustain us during those periods, until external supply becomes available. The stronger and healthier our bone is, the more tolerant we become to extremes of temperature, stress, and disease.

o   Exercise is the main stimulant for bone growth and maintenance. When we exercise, we need extra energy molecules of ATP. These drive the sliding protein strands against each other, in muscle cells, to create displacement. We also need extra calcium ions to flow through the muscles cells to trigger the ATP molecules to release their energy and initiate the displacement. Exercise enhances bone health through storing plenty of phosphate and calcium in viable bone matrix.

17.6.7. MIND

Exercise builds up the bricks of logic and structures our ability to judge things the way they are made, rather than the way our modest imagination perceives them to be. Our perception of reality stems from acquired lessons from constant play and exploration of our surroundings. There were times in our history when we thought that the stars are shinning pearls

EXERCISE AND SCIENCE

ornamenting the back roof of the heaven. As soon as we extrapolated the laws of nature, we soon realized that the stars obey the same laws that make an apple falls from a tree. We figured out why a rock keeps moving after falling from a mountain, does not stop by hitting another object, unless certain laws of mechanics are fulfilled.

17.7. MANAGING CHEMICAL ENERGY BY LIVE ORGANISMS

17.7.1. ENERGY IN FOOD INTAKE

o   The food we consume carries the **solar energy** in the form of chemical bonds between various atoms. In the beginning of the 20th century, scientists acknowledged the existence of specified energy levels, for all atoms, at which electrons with specific physical quantities reside. These energy levels account for the excitation of atoms by the solar radiation and hence the capture of the solar energy by moving electrons. These jump into higher energy levels and react with other atoms. The chemical energy stored in food can then be retrieved within the body, when needed for biological energy demands. Biological energy production is accomplished by devised systems of enzymes, catalysts, and selective membranes. The process of capturing solar energy starts by the green leaves that manufacture **carbohydrates** from solar energy, water, and carbon dioxide. Photosynthesis utilizes solar energy to add water molecules to carbon atoms that form the carbohydrate compound $C_x(H_2O)_y$. This process releases oxygen in the atmosphere and thus sustains breathing life. The essence of utilizing energy by live organisms is extracting energy from the breakdown of carbohydrates and releasing water and carbon dioxide to the surroundings. Carbohydrates, therefore, mediate the transfer of energy between the sun and living organisms. Thus, while plants utilize carbon dioxide and solar energy to produce carbohydrates and oxygen, animals consume carbohydrates and oxygen and produce carbon dioxide and energy. Such relation of mutual dependence of plants and animals is called "symbiosis".

o   **Proteins** are distinguished from carbohydrates by the presence of nitrogen atoms in their molecules. All amino acids that make up protein molecules have, in their structure, nitrogen atoms that are derived from the Earth atmosphere. Since proteins make up the enzymes that catalyze most biochemical reactions, therefore, proteins must had long existed before carbohydrates. Plants could not convert carbon dioxide, water, and solar energy into carbohydrates, without first possessing protein enzymes to operate such biological reaction. We do not know exactly how the first protein molecule been created. The presence of nitrogen in protein structure, and the essential role of protein in biological synthesis of other substances, raises many questions on the unique role on nitrogen in biological life. Thus, when we talk about **nitrogen balance** we mean protein-balance. Positive nitrogen balance signifies adding protein to the body, or building up, or anabolism. Negative nitrogen balance means wasting of protein or catabolism.

o   **Fats** are different from carbohydrates and proteins in containing hydroxyl groups in their molecules, $(C_5H_8)_y$. Fat synthesis also requires protein enzymes. Plants cannot synthesize complex fat compounds such as cholesterol. The apparent reason for synthesizing fat and carbohydrates, by protein enzymes, seems to be solely for energy storage purposes. Fats differ from carbohydrates in their energy storage density and the method of unleashing such energy into active form. Such distinguishing criteria between the basic organic matter, involved in food and body structure, facilitates the job of health and fitness professionals in managing nutrition. The three basic organic food stuff (carbohydrates, protein, and fat) when allowed to burn in controlled environment, with equal weights from each type, each yields an amount of heat estimated as 4 Calories (4000 calories) per gram of carbohydrates or protein, and 9 Calories (9000 calories) per gram of fat. For a layperson, such simplification of sorting foodstuff into three basic types, and assigning each type certain amount of energy content, reveals the "tricks of the trade" of the health profession. For example, it does no matter which part of the chicken flesh or cow beef you eat to accounts for protein. Nor does it matter if you pick rice over potato, or bread, to account for carbohydrates. Many people mistake the different appearance of foodstuff for different nutritional values. For example, combining rice, banana, and ice cream, in the same meal, undermines its nutritional balance, since the three foodstuffs are mainly carbohydrate-rich.

17.7.2. ENERGY FLOW WITHIN THE BODY

o   In the body, there exists an intricate system of chemical regulation that responds to states of basic metabolism, activity, growth, and regeneration. Again, **protein enzymes** master such biological response through activation and deactivation of reactants. The body extracts energy from food intake according to the demands of growth, activity, and regular maintenance requirements. In all these processes, chemical enzymes, vitamins, and enzyme helpers (cofactors) operate by chemical and physical signals. These comprise of chemical changes, modifying the level of their activity, and activating substrates to react in specific manners, to produce specific end-products, at specific rates.

o   The chemical orchestration of reactions of substrates is very similar to **electric switching systems** of digital circuitry. The parallel differences between the two are that the electronic elements of resistance, capacitors, inductors, transistors, sources, or motors are represented by chemical elements of hormones, enzymes, cofactors, vitamins, minerals, substrates, and end products. *Table 17.3* lists the major chemical elements involved in the flow of energy in the human body.

EXERCISE AND SCIENCE

Table 17.3. Major metabolic enzymes and their regulatory mechanisms.

Enzyme	Activated by	Inactivated by	Regulation and Products
PFK (Phosphofructokinase)	Increased AMP, decreased ATP) Uses ATP as substrates	ATP increases during inactivity. Reduces F6P concentration.	Regulated by the ratio of ATP/AMP. Muscle PFK is not stimulated by creatine phosphate. G6P → F6P. F6P prevents reversal of reaction.
cAMP dependent protein kinase (protein kinase A)	Starvation, cAMP binding.		
PEP Carboxykinase (PhosphoEnolPyruvate Carboxykinase)	Starvation. Requires GTP activation. Glucagon.	Glucose. Food intake. Insulin.	Reverses a step in the glycolysis pathway by converting oxaloacetate to phosphoenol pyruvate (PEP) and releases CO_2. PEP can be converted to glucose.
Adenylate Cyclase	Starvation, Hormones binding to the outside of the cell e.g. adrenalin and glucagon.		
Phosphodiesterase	Insulin binding to the outside of cells.	Starvation	Converts cAMP into 5'-AMP. Thus, it deactivates cAMP during fed state and inhibits glycogenolysis.
Hexokinase (all cells) : phosphorylates glucose	Mg^{++} and ATP	G6P G6P does not inhibit liver glucokinase.	Km = 0.1 mM hexokinase can trap glucose faster at low concentration. G → G6P, F → F6P
Glucokinase (Liver) : phosphorylates glucose	Mg^{++} and ATP	Phosphorylation, PDH-kinase	Km = 10 mM, Insulin regulation. Enables liver cells to remove glucose from the blood when blood [glucose] is high. G → G6P
PDH (Pyruvate Dehydrogenase Complex)	PDH-phosphatase: Cleaves phosphates from PDH, activity	PDH-kinase: phosphorylates PDH, starvation, fatty acid oxidation, Acetyl CoA	TPP, Lipoic acid, CoA, FAD, NAD, Pyruvic acid dehydrogenase
PDH-kinase	Allosteric activator Acetyl CoA, NADH, starvation,	Physical activity.	Inhibits the decarboxylation of pyruvate
PDH-phosphatase	Physical activity. Allosteric activator e.g. Ca_2^{++}	Decrease of Ca_2^{++} influx, starvation	Fosters the decarboxylation of pyruvate to Acetyl CoA
Phosphorylase (liver)	Starvation, phosphorylation		
FBPase (Fructose Diphosphate kinase)	Starvation	Glucose. Food intake. Insulin.	Reverses one step of glycolysis by converting $F1,6P_2$ into F6P, which can convert to glucose.
Glycogen phosphorylase (muscles)	Intracellular Ca_2^{++}, phosphorylation, [Pi] from hydrolysis of creatine phosphate, elevated [AMP]), adrenalin, or epinephrine	Eating Phosphatase G6P Insulin	Convert Glycogen to G1P, which enters glycolysis and supplies muscle energy.
GS (glycogen synthase) (muscle)	Insulin (via effect on Protein phosphatase 1). G6P	Starvation. Ca_2^{++} (muscular contraction)	Regulated by phosphorylation of glycogen into G1P. Glycogen synthesis in muscle.
Glycogen Synthase (liver)	Dephosphorylation Insulin	Starvation	Glycogen synthesis in liver.
G6P dehydrogenase	Eating (Insulin)		Regulated by the availability of NADP
Glycogen Synthase kinase (liver)	Starvation, phosphorylation		Glycogen breakdown in liver.
ACC (acetyl-CoA carboxylase)	Insulin via polymerization and phosphorylation	Starvation	Regulated by phosphorylation and citrate.
CK (Creatine kinase)	Low ATP/ADP ratio. Physical activity.	Physical inactivity.	
Pyruvate carboxylase	Starvation, Acetyl CoA activates.	Glucose. Food intake. Insulin.	Adds CO_2 into pyruvate converting it into oxaloacetate, which enters TCA cycle.

o Food intake and exercise induce the body to activate various biochemical pathways that deal with food and energy requirements. These pathways are chains of processes that operate in selective locations in the body. They are mostly regulated by hormones, enzymes, and the substrates upon which they act, *Table 17.3*, as follows.
  i. **During exercise**, the body fuels physical work through three biochemical pathways. Exercise manages these three pathways to the best ability of the body to fuel its energy demands, as follows.
     a. **Glycolysis** which produces 2 ATP moles, from the conversion of a mole of glucose to Pyruvate. This pathway operates when blood glucose level is adequate to fuel brain metabolism and physical activity of muscles.
     b. **Fatty acid oxidation** which produces acetyl CoA, for the TCA. This pathway operates when physical activity is extended such that it lowers blood glucose level and induces glucagon increase.
     c. The **TCA** cycle extracts energy molecules from acetyl CoA and releases carbon dioxide and water. This pathway operates when physical activity shifts to aerobic energy oxidation.
     d. The **CP-ATP** shuttle operates when muscular contraction demands immediate energy source. Neither glycolysis nor aerobic oxidation can supply energy to muscular contraction on urgent call.
  ii. **After food intake**, the body replenishes muscle and liver resources and fat depots by three biochemical pathways as follows.
     a. **Glycogenesis** restores depleted glycogen depots in liver and muscle cells.
     b. **Protein synthesis** builds up structural elements. Utilizes the byproducts of the TCA cycle in amino acid synthesis.
     c. **Fat synthesis** is at highest speed after meals due to the actions of insulin, thyroxin, growth hormone, and corticosteroids. The cell uses NADPH for fatty acid biosynthesis, at a rate limited by the enzyme ACC (acetyl-CoA carboxylase).
  iii. **During cellular growth,** the body manufactures nucleic acids through the Pentose Phosphate pathway. This pathway reduces NADP and synthesizes ribose-5-P, at a rate limited by the enzyme G6P dehydrogenase.

17.7.3. REST
Rest implies lower demands for glycolysis. This is slowed down by the low concentrations of G6P. Rest affects the liver and muscles in different ways, as follows.
o **In muscle**, the unused G6P, during rest, inhibits hexokinase enzyme thus reduces further production of G6P.
  i. Muscle content of **G6P** self-regulates glucose uptake from blood or glucose synthesis from glycogen breakdown.
  ii. **Insulin** activates GS (glycogen synthase) through the increase of phosphodiesterase activity and decrease of GS kinase activity.
  iii. Amplification of the effect of insulin on GS takes place through **Protein phosphatase-1 (PP1)**. Both, activation of GS, and the inhibition of its inactivation, are controlled by insulin, in muscle. Muscle glycogen stores are depleted in the absence of insulin, in uncontrolled diabetes.
o **In the liver**, G6P does not inhibit glucokinase enzyme, which enables the liver to constantly generate glucose to maintain blood level. This is vital to brain metabolism that is mostly glucose-dependent.
  i. The **liver glucokinase** has greater chemical reactivity constant of 100 times that of muscles' hexokinase, which enables the liver to consume too much substrates than the muscles. However, both muscle and liver convert G6P into glycogen, which is a compact form of storage of carbohydrates. This process is regulated by the effect of Insulin on the enzymes hexokinase and glucokinase
  ii. The high blood glucose is also more easily transported into liver cells than into muscle cells because of the specific **glucose transporter proteins** in the liver cells.
  iii. Glucose binds the **phosphorylated phosphorylase enzyme** complex, releasing the PP1. PP1 activates GS and inactivates phosphorylase thus stimulates glycogenesis and blocks glycogenolysis. Thus, activation of liver GS is induced by high glucose levels not insulin.
  iv. **Insulin** inhibits inactivation of liver GS. The low insulin level in diabetes allows GS kinase to inactivate GS and depletes liver glycogen stores.
  v. Mutation in **insulin receptor gene** mimics diabetic effects in diminishing glucose transport to cells after meal. Thus, cells would rely on fatty acid oxidation instead of glycolysis. This sort of muscle energy does not allow robust or vigorous physical activities, since it requires longer time to supply the needed ATP molecules.

17.7.4. EATING
o Dietary carbohydrates increase **blood glucose level**.
  i. This affects glucose transporters on both fat and muscle cells, increases the secretion of insulin, decreases the activity of liver glycogen phosphorylase, and increases G6P dehydrogenase activity.
  ii. **Insulin** activates the anabolic pathways of glycogen synthesis and fatty acid synthesis, while inhibits glycogen breakdown and gluconeogenesis. The activated anabolic processes depose the administered foodstuff, mostly glucose. This is transported from the blood into cells, by various cellular protein transporters.
  iii. **Glucose** is stored as glycogen in muscle and liver cells, converted to acetyl CoA by fat cells, processed through the pentose phosphate pathway to reduce NADP by fat and liver cells, or consumed in glycolysis by most cells. The excess dietary carbohydrates are first converted onto glycogen, until those stores are replenished, before they are taken up by fat cells.

EXERCISE AND SCIENCE

iv. **Glycogen** storage is limited to muscle, liver, and few other cells, while fat storage is unlimited. Active organs manufacture nucleic acids components from carbohydrates, through the pentose phosphate pathway. The main purpose of the pentose phosphate pathway is to regenerate NADPH from NADP+ through an oxidation/ reduction reaction and the formation of ribose 5-phosphate from glucose 6-phosphate. NADPH is used for reductive reactions in anabolism, especially in fatty acid synthesis.

o Dietary proteins are digested into **amino acids**, absorbed, and sent to the liver. Many of the amino acids are released into the bloodstream and taken up by the muscle for repair and synthesis. Muscles are the major protein depots in the body. Those amino acids, not required by the muscle cells, are converted into ketoacids[▼] and their carbon atoms are used in the TCA cycle. The amino groups, of the spent amino acids, are transaminated[♦] onto the pyruvate, in muscle cells, producing the amino acid Alanine. This is released into the bloodstream during activity. Nitrogen, over and above normal requirements, cannot be stored and is excreted by the kidneys as urea.

o Most dietary fat is ingested as **triglycerides**.
   i. After intake, triglycerides are emulsified by bile salts and then cleaved by pancreatic lipase enzyme, to **fatty acids** and **glycerol**.
   ii. Fatty acids pass into the intestinal epithelial cells, where they are esterified again to glycerol. In the intestinal wall, these are assembled with lipoproteins, produced by the liver, to form **chylomicrons**. These contain small amount of dietary cholesterol.
   iii. Chylomicrons are then taken up by the intestinal walls capillaries and transported into the lymphatic system. The latter empties into the systemic bloodstream and reaches peripheral tissues, before first being filtered in the liver. Chylomicrons are stripped of their lipids by extracellular lipoprotein lipase (LPL) enzyme, at the capillary surface of fat cells and converted into fatty acids and glycerol. Fatty acids are then hydrolyzed and taken up by fat cells for storage. The glycerol remainder of chylomicrons returns to the liver, where it can be converted to glucose, triglycerides, or acetyl CoA. Thus, the glycerol, in the dietary triglycerides, does not end directly to fat cells, but is rather processed by the liver. The remains of chylomicrons are taken up by the liver.
   iv. The **free fatty acids** are transported to the liver on plasma albumin, in the portal circulation.
   v. The transport molecules "**lipoproteins**" are made up of a core of triglycerides and cholesterol esters surrounded by a layer of phospholipids, with protein molecules inserted into it. The protein codes act as recognition sites for low-density lipoproteins (LDL) receptors, located on cell plasma membranes throughout the body. The circulating lipoproteins bind to specific receptors on the capillaries of muscle and adipose tissue. On the capillaries, a lipoprotein lipase enzyme hydrolyses the triglycerides and thus removes them from the circulation. These are stored mainly in fat cells. Inherited defects in the number or structure of LDL receptor cause elevated serum LDL levels.

o The slow conversion of dietary fat to triglycerides and chylomicrons, and the long detour through the lymphatic system prior to reaching the liver, explains the **steady effect of fats** on the body metabolism. That differs from the acute effect of carbohydrate intake. As the chylomicrons are distributed through the systemic circulation, the liver filters them and their triglycerides are resent into the circulation. Very Light Density Lipoproteins (VLDL) transport lipids from the liver to the circulation. These are stripped of their triglycerides by the action of lipoprotein lipases, at various tissues. Cholesterol returns back to the liver on High Density Lipoproteins (HDL). High serum HDL levels correlate with low risk of cardiovascular disease, since they contain low level of triglycerides and cholesterol, in comparison to LDL.

17.7.5. ACTIVITY

o The muscle and liver stored glycogen is utilized in the production of glucose when the body **demands ATP** molecules for energy supply. Such demand is signaled, biochemically, by increase in AMP (adenosine mono-phosphate), which activates the PFK enzyme, *Table 17.3*.

o The **PFK enzyme** prevents the buildup of G6P. It maintains the continuous breakdown of glycogen by blocking the inhibition of the hexokinase enzyme. Thus, activity increases glycogen degradation as well as clears G6P, the product of degradation, at a rate higher than that at rest. G6P sustains physical activity as the fuel of first choice through the activated pathways of glycolysis and Krebs cycle. This oxidizes blood glucose, produces CO_2, and generates ATP (hence named oxidative decarboxylation). Blood glucose level remains fairly steady, though it dips slightly, after about 15 minutes of exercise, and remains low, until after the demand for ATP has ceased.

o Thus, activity is associated by oxidation of the NADH molecules and increase electron transport during the mitochondrial oxidative phosphorylation. The net result of energy consumption is increase in ADP and NAD^+ concentration. Adrenalin stimulates activity by enhancing glycogen breakdown through the activation of adenylate cyclase enzyme, which increases cyclic **AMP production**. The increased cAMP activates glycogen breakdown and stimulates performance. Cyclic AMP is cleared by the enzyme phosphodiesterase. Inhibitors to the phosphodiesterase allow buildup of cAMP thus stimulate short-term performance, but prevent long-term glycogen replenishment after exercise.

[▼] **Amino acids** contain an amine group (NH_2) and mostly have the formula $RC(NH_2)COOH$. In **ketoacids**, the amine group is replaced by oxygen in the formula $RCOCOOH$. **Imino acids** are unsaturated form of amino acids and mostly have the formula $RC(NH)COOH$.

[♦] Transamination refers to transferring the amine group (NH_2) from an amino acid to a ketoacids in order to synthesize a required form of amino acid that is different from the existing one.

EXERCISE AND SCIENCE

o If intense physical activity is sustained beyond about 15 minutes, then changes occur in both muscle and liver. These changes comprise of glucose transporters on the surface of muscle cells (but not on fat cells), the activation of triglyceride lipase (TGL), the phosphorylation of PDH, and elevated glucagon levels in blood. These changes **switch fuel usage** from glycolysis to fatty acid oxidation.

17.7.6. FASTING

o Early, during the first 12-hour or so of fasting, liver **glycogen** suffices to maintain blood glucose.
o After liver glycogen is depleted, the body uses **fatty acids** for energy for most tissues, except the brain cells. These can rely on the ketone bodies produced by the liver. The drop in blood glucose due to reduced food intake induces the switch between glucose fuel and fatty acids. The low glucose level raises the level of glucagon hormone in the blood.
o **Glucagon** binds to receptors on fat cells and increases cAMP, which leads to the activation of protein kinase-A, which in turn phosphorylates and activates TGL enzyme.
o The **enzyme TGL** breaks down fat into fatty acids and glycerol. Muscle cells do not have glucagon receptors.
o Fatty acids reach muscle cells by blood flow. Inside muscle cells, fatty acids are transported to the mitochondria by the Carnitine shuttle and oxidized to acetyl CoA. That partially inactivates PDH and preserves the blood glucose from oxidation in the Krebs cycle. The limiting factor in the **oxidation of fatty acids** varies with the individuals, depending on the amount of Carnitine or the activity of oxidation enzymes. Carnitine shuttles fatty acids across the mitochondrial membrane and leaves the CoA in the cytoplasm. Prolonged fatty acid oxidation results in ketosis, i.e. formation of ketone bodies: acetoacetate and β-hydroxybutyrate, due to high levels of acetyl CoA.
o People with disorders of **gene mutation** of glucagon receptor experience difficulties tapping into fat depot for energy supply. This is attributed to lack of binding of glucagon to the adipose tissue receptors and their subsequent stimulation to release of fatty acids, when blood glucose falls during activity or fasting. The lack of acetyl CoA, due to blocked lipolysis, keeps PDH inactivated thus allowing glycolysis to continue unchecked to further lower blood glucose down to hypoglycemic level.
o Energy from fat lasts the longest since fat comprises the **largest store supply**. Each fatty acid, when oxidized, provides the most ATP. Protracted fasting, beyond 48 hours, farther activates TGL enzyme, inactivates PDH, elevates glucagon levels in blood, and activates gluconeogenesis pathway in the liver. These conserve carbohydrate carbon and form glucose from lactate, amino acids, and glycerol.

17.7.7. WARM-UP

The warm-up interval, between initiating physical activity and assuming a steady rate of ATP demand, is managed by the change in activity of the enzyme PDH phosphatase, *Table 17.3*. This increases at the beginning of activity and then falls at about 15 minutes, when the demands for steady ATP are met. The rise in PDH phosphatase activity is attributed to the increased intracellular Ca^{++} concentration. This enzyme activates the PDH complex and stimulates TCA cycle for production of NADH and ATP molecules. Thus, warm-up mainly signals the PDH-complex to run the wheels of the TCA cycles faster, while pumping pyruvates into it, from the glycolysis pathway. Warm-up begins with calcium release from muscles, signaling the PDH to begin its work. It ends up when glucagon hormone kicks in, as a result of glucose level drop.

17.7.8. VIGOROUS ACTIVITIES

o Vigorous exercise cannot rely on the slow breakdown of glucose to pyruvic acid, or the slow transport of glucose out of the liver into the blood stream, in order to supply the **urgently needed ATP** molecules.
o Furthermore, **high twitching muscles** used in such activities are poor in blood supply and have few mitochondria to operate sufficient Krebs cycles. Thus, glucose cannot fulfill the immediade demands of vigorous muscular work.
o Muscles are equipped with viable endogenous sources of intracellular ATP that is ready to deliver immediate energy and is replenished by a relatively slower shuttle of **creatine phosphate**. That leaves the NADH in the reduced state during anaerobic vigorous activity. The enzyme that regulates the concentration of these metabolites during vigorous activities is the creatine kinase, which hydrolyzes creatine phosphate and produces ATP molecules for muscular contraction. Low ATP/ADP levels further stimulate creatine kinase activity.
o **After vigorous work ceases**, blood glucose will replenish the glycogen stores of the muscles and replace the consumed ATP molecules This recuperative phase is fostered by the release of Adrenalin, Ca^{++}, inorganic phosphate P_i from the hydrolysis of creatine phosphate, and elevated AMP, which all activate muscle glycogen phosphorylase.
o Drugs that act as **analogue of cAMP** may inactivate protein kinase-A and hence affect phosphorylase kinase, GS enzyme, and access to glycogen fuel source. This may undermine fuel supply and sluggish performance during sustained vigorous activity that relies on muscle glycogen for energy, such as increased acceleration during climbing hills or increasing speed.

17.7.9. WARM-DOWN

o As demand for energy diminishes, Krebs cycle slows down and both ATP and NADH concentration increase.
o The rise in ATP concentration inhibits PFK enzyme and slows down glycolysis.
o Also, the decrease of Ca^{++} influx and decrease in acetyl CoA inactivate PDH phosphatase enzyme.
o Rise in blood glucose also causes glucagon hormone to fall, inhibits TGL enzyme, and slows the release of fatty acids, some time after exercise has stopped.

17 EXERCISE AND SCIENCE

17.8. HIGHLIGHTS OF CHAPTER SEVENTEEN

1. Emptiness of all and every thing is an almighty state of reality. Any disturbance to that state is **energy** or **life**.

2. **Mass** is a form of energy that creates our sense of distance. Since distance defines sizes, lengths, and areas, all have to refer to masses. We know of no means to measure distances without mass reference.

3. **Distance and time** are merely the fingerprints of mass and radiation, respectively. Both, the latter, are two different representations of energy, be it disturbance or life.

4. **Energy transport** is determined mainly by the probability of finding the configuration of atoms that can stay stable by simple electronic collisions and arrangement of atoms in compliance with the laws of modern physics of dual nature of matter.

5. The **principle of permanency of objects** provides assurance that whatever man owns and works hard to earn won't disappear without cause. We take for granted the fact that when we leave our homes and return by the end of the day those must be still where we left them, otherwise we seek explanation for any change in the state of events.

6. **Acceleration** could be interpreted as a distortion in the space-time state or mass-radiation state. An accelerated object is a distorted object in the distances between its initial units, over time. As soon as the object restores its initial undistorted state, it resumes a constant speed in straight line.

7. **Why are we not moving while we are being accelerated?** The better answer is to dwell on the disturbance hypothesis and recall that acceleration is a distortion of distance-time state. Each particle in our body is distorted, as long as it falls within the gravitational field.

8. When lifting an object, the **internal acceleration** of the particles of the object and the particles of our body are accelerated in proportion to the force we are exerting on the object, whether is it moving or not. Thus, an object yields to motion as a result of the total summation of acceleration of its entire particles. When forces are externally in balance, acceleration does not vanish. It just acts internally until reaches a sensible level to express external motion.

9. Weightlifting does not deal with free objects. Lifting a bar from the floor involves the recoil of the bar, the **inertia** of its mass, and the delayed articulation of our joints to convey force to the lift.

10. We cannot exert **force** on something that has no mass. As time passes, an object under the effect of force has to change the distance of its constituents. If such change amounts to visible motion then the object is a "freely moving object". A bound object, however, changes its distance in relation to other objects, but in different directions that will not show as visible translation.

11. If an object is hindered from moving by external force, such as gravity, its particles will vibrate in directions that would not add up to a visible motion. Nevertheless, the work done by these particles is converted into **collisions** between them and heat is generated. So, energy never vanishes in vain, it must be conserved into different forms,

12. A well-trained Weightlifter had long learned not to err on the side of **yanking weights**. Even without knowing what inertia is, Weightlifters are told, repeatedly, about the slow and strong initiation of motion of weights. If you yank the bar vigorously, it would feel like a mountain of steel.

13. As soon as the motion of a massive object reaches steady state, the energy used in its disturbance is now "stored" in its motion as a projectile. The stored energy is called "**potential energy**".

14. Everything that surrounds us owes its existence to **electric charges**. The reason why objects permanently exist the way we know them is because electric charges are "at work". Electric charges are thought to carry energy in strictly specific amounts; each corresponds to a state of existence.

15. The **conversion of energy** from one form to another is the ultimate goal of life of any form. Although we have dwelled on the concept of "disturbance" to characterize energy, it seems that our health and fitness are enhanced by controlling such disturbance in the form of "righteous flow of energy".

16. The tiniest virus particles, though lifeless, are capable of utilizing cells to manufacture new viruses through energy conversion processes. The health of human organism is determined by how we maintain and nurture this very complex harmony of all bodily organs. This entire organism is meant to perform one and only one function that is energy utilization. All biological functions are precursors of that single function. Even our cognitive functions are geared to aid in utilizing energy to the best of our ability. Animals that fail to compete for energy utilization are denied the benefits of life.

Chapter 18
Frequently Asked Questions

The samples of frequently asked questions, included in this chapter, are intended to represent a wide spectrum of concerns to strength trainees and are not, by any means, inclusive to all prominent issues.

18.1. DRUG USE

18.1.1. USE OF MONOAMINE OXIDASE INHIBITORS
Question: Can I take a combination of MAO inhibitors simultaneously? Would somebody taking one of these supplements want to stay away from any of the others? Do some of these supplements not interact well with others?

Comment:
o   MAO-Inhibitors (Monoamine oxidase inhibitors)[1] are drugs that interfere with monoamine oxidase, an important enzyme in the brain and nervous system. The targeted enzyme, monoamine oxidase, regulates the balance between generation and clearance of the monoamine substances in the brain. Monoamines are so called because they carry a single amine group in their chemical formula. Some of the brain neurotransmitters are monoamines such as **serotonin** and **norepinephrine**. Thus, MAO inhibitors cause accumulation of these neurotransmitters and promote the activity of the brain. For this reason they are used to treat depression and restore normal mood state.
o   The most common MAO-Inhibitors used are isocarboxazid (Marplan), tranylcypromine sulfate (Parnate) and phenelzine sulfate (Nardil). However, other drugs such as **fluoxetine** (Prozac) can cause selective accumulation of serotonin, but not of norepinephrine, by blocking uptake of serotonin by blood platelets.
o   MAO inhibitors interact with food and drugs that contain the amino acid **tyramine** and cause accumulation of tyramine in the blood, after intake of certain food or drugs such as alcohol, legumes such as fava and soy beans, cheese, fish, ginseng, meat, shrimp paste, and yeast extracts. Tyramine accumulation **causes elevation of blood pressure.** High blood pressure affects cerebral function in many ways, ranging from stroke to dizziness, fainting, headache, tremors, muscle twitching, confusion, memory impairment, anxiety, agitation, insomnia, drowsiness, chills, and blurred vision. It also affects the circulatory function and can cause heart attack, weakness, and heart palpitations.
o   Intake of food or drugs that contain tyramine, within 12 hours before or after taking MAO-inhibitors, leads to dangerous or even life-threatening side effects. The following substances can cause very dangerous side effects when taken with MAO inhibitors: **Sleeping pills, cocaine, amphetamines (speed), narcotics, alcohol, and ephedrine**.
o   The following substances can cause headaches or sickness also if taken 12 hours before or after taking a MAO-inhibitor: **Old cheese, ripe bananas, wine, liver, caffeine, figs, raisins, yogurt, pine-apple, meats, avocados, chocolate, nuts, and nutmeg.**
o   The interaction of MAO inhibitors with body enzymes makes it very difficult to predict the outcome of taking multiple drugs simultaneously. In addition, mood disorders that require drug prescription cannot be diagnosed or treated by the patient himself, since subjective thoughts may cause unjustified over-medication. Thus, the prescription of MAO inhibitors should be delegated to physicians with experience in the usage of such medication, as well as in psychiatric disorders.

18.1.2. ANABOLIC STEROIDS
Question: If someone was stacking 50 mgs D-Bol a day and wanted to switch over to Anadrol, what dosage would be a good replacement dose? I'm assuming that replacing it with 50 mgs Anadrol wouldn't be enough since Anadrol has a lower receptor affinity than D-Bol. My personal opinion is that Dianabol is a little more potent than Anadrol.
Comment:
o   D-Bol is Methandrostenol. It is the active ingredient in the anabolic steroid Dianabol. It is administered orally in tablet form. D-Bol is claimed to increase muscle strength and size by converting, in the body, into **testosterone** ester after its oral administration. Because of the unknown outcome of tampering with body hormones, D-Bol is not approved for recreational purposes.
o   Anadrol is the anabolic steroid Oxymetholone, used to treat aplastic anemia, and is administered by subdermal injection.
o   The two drugs are only prescribed by physicians for patients with aplastic anemia. During muscle bulking cycles, Bodybuilders use anabolic steroids surreptitiously, alone or stacked with other anabolic steroids.

---
[1] "The Merck Manual of Diagnosis and Therapy", 15th edition, 1987. Pages 1524-25. ISBN 0911910-06-9.

FREQUENTLY ASKED QUESTIONS

- o If these drugs are taken in high concentration, in daily single doses, they start producing acne and other side effect. Since the half-life of some of these drugs is short, thus spreading doses over multiple intervals achieves more steady blood level and probably less side effects, particularly liver injury. Spreading doses on the 24hr affects the 2 to 4 hourly burst rhythmic secretion of pituitary gonadotrophic hormones.[2]
- o Stacking drugs with oral and subdermal injection makes it difficult to control blood level and thus leads to unpredictable outcome. The interaction of multiple drugs (androgens, for example, up-regulate liver enzymes) alters the half-life of removal of the drug from the body.
- o Long cycles of surreptitious use of anabolic steroids of high concentration (few months for drugs with long half-life) increase the risk of developing side effects.

18.2. BODYBUILDING AND SELF-IMAGE

Question: I don't think I've ever seen a Bodybuilder that I'd call well endowed. Judging from what I can see of them in their posing trunks, they are all, at best, of average size. I wondered is Bodybuilding a way to compensate for other perceived shortcomings, or does heavy steroid use shrink men's genitalia?

Comment:
- o Integrating both personal talents and physical fitness in one's lifestyle requires hard work on both fields. Exercise alone cannot nourish the physical well being, without serious effort of gaining knowledge.
- o As far as sexual appearance of Bodybuilders is concerned, many factors affect the appearance of men's genitalia. Physical performance, anxiety, cold, stress excitement, and heavy steroid usage shrink the size of the testicles by increasing sympathetic activity. Shrinking occurs as a result of both reduced blood flow and muscular pull of the testicles due to sympathetic stimulation.
- o Erection does not occur during activities that distract the mind away from sexual thoughts, and thus the penis size cannot be judged during athletic competition. This augments sympathetic activity and thus adversely affects the sexual organs, which rely entirely on blood to "fill" them out.
- o In some individuals, however, extreme excitement, during combat for instance, may trigger the instinctive reaction of erection. Whether such erection is caused by brain control impulses, or due to stressful excitation of peripheral parasympathetic nerves, is debatable. Alcohol for example causes sexual arousal prior to the onset of numbness and so do other hypnotics and narcotics.

18.3. FAT BURNING WITH DIET AND EXERCISE

18.3.1. DAILY CALORIC INTAKE

Question: I'm female who is pretty new to regular exercise, having just begun this summer. I have quite a bit of body fat to lose, though I don't need to lose weight. A trainer once suggested to me to stick with 75 gm of protein a day and no more than 75 gm carbohydrates a day, and 20-25 gm of fat. However, I find if I get to the 75 gm protein, I've gone way over on carbohydrates (usually 100-150 gm), or the fat is way off (in either direction). My question is this: If I reach the recommended protein/day, does it matter if the carbohydrates are high if I'm still not eating an excessive number of calories? What's the key to getting all three areas to balance? I'm having a lot of trouble believing that healthy carbohydrates like fruits and vegetables should be limited to 75 gm carbohydrates. I realize some recommend much lower than 75 gm/day. I'm hearing so much conflicting advice. Some recommend lots of carbohydrates, while others recommend limiting carbohydrates.

Comment:
- o Intake of calories has to be gauged based on bodyweight and physical activity, not on absolute values. There are no absolute values of caloric intake for all people. An adult requires 25 Calories per kilogram bodyweight per day (11.6 C/pound/day) in order to fulfill the basic metabolic needs.
- o Since the caloric contents of carbohydrates, proteins, and fats are known from experiments (4 Calorie/gm, 4 Calorie/gm, and 9 Calorie/gm, respectively), thus 2 gm carbohydrate, 2 gm protein, and 1 gm fat would provide adequate calories to each kilogram of bodyweight, when equal calories are obtained from the three different food stuff. For example, a 70 kg adult would thus need 140 gm carbohydrates, 140 gm protein, and 70 gm fat, to provide 1750 Calories/day. However, lesser proportion of fat is recommended for modern healthy living. See Section 15.11, *Tip # 8* on "Daily limit of fat calories intake".
- o Above-basic activities require more calories to maintain bodyweight. This is empirically estimated by multiplying bodyweight, in pounds, by 13, for females, and by 15, for males, in order to obtain total daily caloric needs.
- o The proper proportion of carbohydrates, protein, and fat is very empirical. Carbohydrates promote weight gain by constantly enhancing anabolic processes in tissues. Fats reduce appetite when taken with little carbohydrates. Proteins

---
[2] "Color Atlas of Physiology", Agamemnon Despopoulos and Stefan Silbernagl, 1991. Page 270. ISBN 0-86577-382-3.

are crucial to muscular growth. Thus, the balance between tissue growth, appetite, and body strength determines the proper combination of these basic food ingredients.

18.3.2. EXERCISING FOR FAT BURNING

Question: I'm currently doing 4 days a week of 30-40 minutes of cardio, in addition to about 20-30 minutes of weight training. For faster fat loss, should I adjust this to 5 or 6 days a week and/or longer time, doing either the weights or cardio?

Comment:
o   Fat loss is better done on longer periods of regular exercise and diet, since fat regulating hormones and enzymes require long time to reach stable level of activity. Chaotic lifestyle might cause transient variation in body fat. Thus, permanent and lasting effects require lifelong pattern of balanced energy expenditure and food intake.
o   In order for weight training to be effective in building strong muscles, sessions should exceed the 45 minutes mark, for a minimum of three workouts every week.
o   Since fat burning is essentially aerobic, while weight training is essentially anaerobic, one has to adjust the intensity of weight training. Thus, when aerobic exercises exceed 30 minutes, then weight training should be kept low in intensity. Conversely, when aerobic exercises are brief, then the lifting intensity is increased. In simple words, keep your weight lifts under 75% of your maximal lifts on aerobic days and increase them on your strengthening days.

18.3.3. DIET AND MUSCLE MASS

Question: I'm a female who was an endurance runner and has currently been dieting approximately 3 weeks. I wonder if it is possible to avoid muscle loss with dieting and in the same time maintain lower bodyweight and body fat, for long time after dieting. I started out at 200 lbs bodyweight, on around 2500-3000 calories a day. I eat continuously (like 4 to 7 separate gorging), but not very much per serving and get my nutrients from the sources shown in *Table 18.1*.

Table 18.1. Food source related to Section 18.3.3.

Fat	Flax and olive oils, roast beef, eggs, fish (salmon specifically), and occasionally skim milk.
Protein	Roast beef, eggs, turkey, chicken, cottage cheese, milk, soy, peanut butter, whey, and tuna.
Carbohydrates	Cereal (raisin bran), Gatorade, fruit (plums, pears, bananas), bagels (not every day), fibrous vegetables (red peppers, broccoli, etc.).

I work out from 3 to 5 days a week, as shown in *Table 18.2* My body weight and body fat percentage have gone down, obviously. My pants are looser, my abs are much more visible. It appears that my weight has gone down faster than many people think it should for retention of muscle. I have set several personal bests in Deadlift, Shoulder Press, and Squat. My poundage's and repetitions are going up, too. So, I don't believe that I am losing much if any muscle. I think my years of experience as an endurance athlete has something to do with this. My body seems to shed the fat relatively easily. May be it remembers when I was a skinny runner. My endurance for a particular workout may be less. I seem to have less capacity for multiple sets. Since I am working out more days per week (even multiple times per day as I showed on a few occasions), I am very aware of the risk of overtraining, and I have been making sure to keep the volume of sets in control. I have been getting lots of sleep, from 7-12 hours a night. That how diet and workout routine has worked for me. I plan to stay dieting for several more weeks, and get down to somewhere between 180-185 lb bodyweight.

Table 18.2. Weekly exercise routine, related to Section 18.3.3.

Monday (Legs workout)	Warm-up for three sets, 1 set with just the bar and 2 sets with about 40% 1RM. Three sets back Squats (pyramid up from 12 to 6 repetitions), three sets front Squats and one set leg press. Sprinting-intervals on other days. Deadlifts on back day.
Tuesday (Chest workout)	Warm-up for two sets. Four sets flat bench (50% 1RM), two sets decline low chest press, and one set incline chest press.
Wednesday (Back workout)	Deadlift for two sets of low repetitions (1-3 repetitions) and two sets of 1RM. One set unweighted pull-up for max repetitions, two sets weighted pull-ups, and one set lateral pull-down, followed by two sets of strength row.
Friday (Shoulder and Biceps workout)	Warm-up for two sets of Shoulder Press with just the bar. Four sets standing Shoulder Press, two sets lateral dumbbell raises, two sets weighted close grip chin-up, one set straight bar curl, two set EZ curl bar, 3-6 sets of close grip Bench Press followed by either Triceps cable extensions, or hammer strength dip, or rope extensions.
Saturday (Cardio and abs workout)	Cardio in the morning, Triceps and abdominals in the evening. Five sets using weighted Swiss ball crunches; leg raises, and weighted incline crunches.

FREQUENTLY ASKED QUESTIONS

Comment:
o   Obviously, 3 weeks of dieting on 2500 Calories/day is not considered strenuous routine. Your increased strength is attributed to regular strength training, good nutrition, and adequate sleep.
o   In order to reduce bodyweight, daily caloric intake must be reduced below 2400 Calories. This is estimated by **multiplying your bodyweight of 185 pounds by 13**. The fact is that for a female, with bodyweight of 200 lb, to be healthy she should have BMI (body mass index) of 25 or less. Using the formula **BMI = 703 x Weight (pounds)/ Height ^{2} (inch) ^{2}**, one can estimate your height as 75 (6 feet 3, inches) inches, at least. See Section 15.5.8 on "Overweight and obesity"
o   Of course, such empirical estimation, of bodyweight to mass ratio, does not apply to athletic people with greater muscle mass and lower body fat, yet it serves as a rough guideline to optimum bodyweight requirement. Also, see Section 14.3.2, on "Optimum Bodyweight".

18.4. DEADLIFT

18.4.1. PROPER TECHNIQUE FOR DEADLIFT
Question: What is the proper technique for deadlifting?

Comment:
o   The Deadlift exercise is as simple as walking to the barbell, grabbing the bar with both hands, pulling it off the floor, and then lowering it down. The Deadlift has evolved to various styles of execution. Each style serves specific anatomical and functional purpose, as follows (see also Section 5.2.9.1 on "Description of the Deadlift" and Section 7.5.1.6 on "Deadlift").
   i.   Military lift to the midthigh level, with Sumo stance, classic Clean stance, or Snatch stance.
   ii. Above-the-knees Deadlift (the shrugs).
   iii. Stiff-legged Deadlift.
   iv. Pulls, from the level of the kneecaps to shoulder level, or slightly higher.

o   Since the Deadlift is performed with heavy weight, it requires a standardized technique of proper execution that is described as follows (see also Chapter 2 on "Proper Lifting Techniques").
   i.   A classical Deadlift is executed by **standing** with feet shoulder-width apart, or a little wider, toes turned out slightly (external leg rotation). See Section 2.2.3 on "Standing very close to the object".
   ii. Squat down to grab the bar with **overhand grip**. The bar is kept close against shins and bodyweight is balanced back on heels. Hips are typically a little higher than knees. This means that torso is slanted on the vertical plane.
   iii. **Lower back** should retain a slight lordotic (concave) curvature. Rounded back is prohibited. The slight concave curve provides a margin of safety, since it will be flattened by the forward pull of the heavy weight. See *Table 2.1* on "Comparison between lordotic versus kyphotic postures, during lifting".
   iv. **Shoulders** should be kept elevated and pushed behind the chest, by retracting the shoulder plates backwards.
   v.   When you **commence lifting**, you should be tight, from your head to your toes. This means that you should harden the Trapezius, midback, Latissimus dorsi, back erectors, Glutei, Hamstrings, and Quadriceps. See Section 2.10.2 on "Sequential hardening of muscles".
   vi. From this position, you **pull** with the hardened shoulders and torso and **push** from the backs of your feet, away from the floor, to break the bar off the floor. Be careful not to start this movement too fast or you will shoot your butt up and round your back. This overloads your spinal joints with excessive shear stresses. Your shoulders and hips should move upwards at the same speed initially. See Section 2.11.4 on "Synchronizing the Pull".
   vii. As the bar passes your knee, your torso should start to straighten up. You should end up with your body completely straightened, shoulders pulled back. The bar should stay as close to your legs as possible during the entire movement. In practice, this means **dragging it up** your shins and upper leg. A skilled lifter can keep the bar a hair's length from his shins through the entire movement. See Section 2.11.3 on "Torques and forces".
   viii. On the descent, begin by starting to bend the knees, which will force the bar to slide back down your legs. As the bar passes your knees on the way down, your torso should be more or less back to the same level of inclination it was to begin with. Then you squat the bar back down.

o   The Deadlift was originally introduced in strength training of Olympic lifting. This is described in Section 4.3, "Standard Weightlifting Training Sessions" and in *Table 13.5* on "Monthly Weightlifting **Exercise-Differentials** of load volume and number of lifts". It strengthens the early stage of the pull. This is slow, yet powerful pull of the bar, from the mid-chin level to the kneecap level. It was never meant to be a lift that is separated from complete range of lifting, from the floor to overheads. The main goal of Deadlift is strengthening of the body extensors. Emphasizing on the Deadlift, per se, and overlooking its intended purpose, runs the risk of stiffening the back and shoulder and limiting the flexibility of the entire body.

FREQUENTLY ASKED QUESTIONS 18

18.4.2. VARIANTS OF DEADLIFT STYLE

Question: When doing Deadlifts with a weight you can handle for 8-10 repetitions, or any rep range for that matter, do you lower the weight so that it touches the floor or do you lower it to an inch from the floor, before coming back up? It seems that there would be different benefits to each method.

Comment:
- o Don't slam the weights down on the floor. Touch and come straight up with a stretch. Lowering the weight to touch the floor increases the range of motion of the spinal muscle, Glutei, and thigh extensor muscles.
- o Complete drop to the floor, in-between repetitions, requires loosening and retightening the leg muscles. This process causes joint wiggling and requires extreme attention during repetitive lifting.
- o Repetitive lifting, without touching the floor, enhances eccentric contraction, yet hastens overtraining and aftereffects of exercise.
- o Younger, well rested, and well nourished lifters can develop exquisite strength, in short time, with repetitive no-touch lifting. Older lifters may develop spasticity and inflexibility with overloading muscles, because aerobic oxidation diminished with inadequate training in old age.

18.4.3. DEFINITION OF STRENGTH TRAINING

Question: The Deadlift has been a tested lift for thousands of years. It sure didn't start with Olympic lifting. The Deadlift is primitive, it is raw, and it is the best overall indicator of pure strength there is. Do you honestly believe that the sport of strength only started with Olympic lifting? There is a huge block of volcanic rock in what is now Italy, which bears the 6th century BC inscription, emulates the son of Critobulus lifting the rock from the ground. These historic figures might have never heard of Olympic lifting. Wherever strong men and women have gathered and tested themselves against each other, they challenged each other in Deadlifting.

Comment:
The sport of strength is as old as the history of the human race. Olympic lifting is not a sport of strength alone but an integration of strength, speed, coordination, and flexibility. Powerlifting, on the other hand, is a sport of strength, a mute form of Weightlifting, and does not participate in the Olympic games, though it is an international sport. If the Deadlift is not integrated into whole body training, it results in stiffness of muscles, tendons, and ligaments, which lead to joint freezing. Whole body training must serve the purpose of maintaining flexibility and normal range of motion of joints, with simultaneous strengthening and balancing. See *Table 13.5* on "Monthly weightlifting exercise-differentials of load volume and number of lifts".

18.4.4. ESSENCE OF DEADLIFTING

Question: I do not deadlift but I squat regularly. What do I need Deadlift for?

Comment:
- o If you squat more than you deadlift, you may lack wise supervision. You should strengthen the back by deadlifting to avoid spinal injury during squatting. Secure a strong back with deadlifting, along with targeting the Quadriceps and the Deltoids.
- o Olympic lifters are very well aware of the mechanics of lifting. This enables them to fully squat, during the Clean, and then ascend to jerk overheads, with heavy weight.
- o If you do not deadlift, you should stay away from heavy lifting. Deadlift is the mainstay of strengthening the paraspinal muscles, from the neck down to lumbar region, as follows.
    - i. Not all Deadlifts are the same. You can change the angles at the knees, hips, shoulders, and make the exercise very versatile. This strengthens various directions of the complex anatomical structures of the knees, hips, and spines.
    - ii. Deadlift increases bone density, because it is the heaviest lift you would ever lift. Deadlifts comprise of at least, lifting a weight equals your bodyweight. Less than that is a warm-up to the real Deadlift.
    - iii. Deadlift induces maximal pelvic blood supply. The increased blood flow to the genitalia enhances testosterone secretion, which enhances bones strength and sex life.
    - iv. Deadlift must precede the Squat and follow the upper body workout. Deadlift requires great upper body tone and warm-up in order to avoid spinal or shoulder injury. It has to precede the Squat since it requires greater Quadriceps, Gluteal, and Spinal reserve. The Deadlift before Squat will make squatting feels like a breeze.
- o You should never Deadlift on a cold back or legs. You must be will warmed up to deadlift.

18.4.5. SEQUENCE AND PERCENTAGE OF DEADLIFT

Question: What if you are not very strong? Many Powerlifters squat more than they deadlift. Why do I have to make more than 10% of my workout deadlifting? If Deadlift precedes the Squat and follows the upper body workout, I would cripple myself!

Comment:

You are afraid of fatiguing your back if you deadlift before squatting. You are using a logic that is completely alien to athletes. Weightlifters perform the Deadlift without a belt and squat heavily, in the same day. This includes an average of 35 sets, of three repetitions each, in daily sessions. Time, patience and guidance are keys to developing strength with progressive incremental resistance training. See Section 13.3.3 on "Weightlifting Periodization". On the other hand, Powerlifting records are not the best role models in strength training. Many Powerlifters have long and chronic form of inflexibility and limited range of motion.

18.4.6. DEADLIFT AND INTENSITY OF RESISTANCE

Question: Can other exercises achieve the same effects of the Deadlifts? You can develop every muscle to the max without Deadlift. Lots of other exercises hit the "paraspinals", one way or the other. Even isolation, one-joint exercises will increase bone density. Running a mile also increases bone density, without lifting. Although the Glutes are used heavily during Deadlifting and that increases blood flow to that area, however, heavy Deadlifts are not necessary for that. Reversed hyperextensions, for 15-20 repetitions, will also increase the blood flow to that area, without any weights. In addition, performing the Deadlift, in the order you described, hurts the feelings of a lot of lifters. How can you explain to them, they trained wrong all those years?

Comment:
o   Weight is resistance. The heavier the weight is the richer is the circulation in the working muscles.
o   Running and repetitive exercises will thin you out. Runners are not muscular unless they run aggressively fast.
o   Squatting is the last in the daily sequence of exercises in any Weightlifting workout, in all schools of strength training. You should not burden the knees with Squats then Deadlift.
o   The Squat tightens the upper body with intense isometric contraction, while it exhausts the lower body with intense eccentric and concentric contractions. This combination of tightness and exhaustion demands length rest.

18.4.7. ABOUT PELVIC CIRCULATION IN DEADLIFT

Question: How does an increased pelvic blood supply increase testosterone levels in males? Does doing Deadlifts increase testosterone levels by increasing blood supply to the pelvic region? This would be only true if the blood supply is somehow impaired there. The above can be true even if one was not deadlifting. You implied that Deadlift would increase testosterone levels.

Comment:

Regular serious exercise enhances testosterone secretion as a part of enhanced anabolic cellular metabolism. On the other hand, inactivity causes muscular weakness and sexual dysfunction. Intense muscular overload increases serum Testosterone, LH, and FH hormones. In addition, the clearance rate of these hormones increases in well-trained athlete (over 2 years serious training). The increased vascular perfusion to the pelvic region in heavy strength training, such as in the Deadlift, is a result of both local and systemic factors, since the hypothalamus and pituitary hormones control the gonads, thyroid, and adrenal glands. All these factors contribute to the production, clearance, and effect of the testosterone. In endurance training, testosterone levels are decreased due to decreased production and increased clearance.

18.4.8. DEADLIFT AND OLYMPIC WEIGHTLIFTING

Question: Olympic lifters only do each lift once at a time and with submaximal weights in training. They are known to do light singles for technique, taking long breaks between sets to ensure full recovery. Training for either Powerlifting or general strength has a totally different set of parameters than Olympic Weightlifting. You can't discuss the one by using the other. Weightlifting standards got nothing to do with the fact that you should be able to deadlift more than you can squat. Weightlifters rely on speed and technique above all. Strength is built specifically for the motions required. They would not do heavy Deadlifts for repetition, and then go and do heavy Squats for repetition. They might do a few pulls and then do some lightweight Squats for a stretch, but not for a training effect.

Comment:
o   There is a common denominator in all strength-training activities. That is improving strength and fitness. Powerlifting and weight training should not differ in this goal.
o   Weightlifters do not do single lifts, unless the weight exceeds 90% of maximum, or prior to contest (see Chapters 4 and 13). Again, Weightlifters do not take breaks longer than 3 minutes between sets, since they are bound by both, the duration of intense training, and certain load volume, per session.
o   The reason that the maximum of Squat should be lower than that of the Deadlift, in all weight training disciplines, is that, in the Squat, the load is already fully loaded on the back of the shoulders when you start. You can get buried at

FREQUENTLY ASKED QUESTIONS

the bottom with exceedingly heavy weight. However, in the Deadlift, the bar just won't move off the floor if your back is too tired. Thus strengthening the Deadlift, beyond the Squat level, guarantees exceedingly stronger and controllable back muscles that can assist in squatting.
- o There are individual variations, but the undisputable fact is the following. When an Olympic lifter pulls the Clean or the Snatch lifts, he has to start with Deadlifting, until the bar reaches the kneecaps. Then he has to squat to catch the bar at the shoulders, in the Clean, and overheads, in the Snatch. Then he has to ascend to jerk, in the Clean. The sequence of Deadlift, Squat, and Press is the foundation of Weightlifting. You do not talk to an Olympic lifter about fatiguing back. That what sound training achieves: extraordinary back performance.
- o The so-called pocket Hercules, Naim Suleymanoglu, Clean jerked 190 kg, while weighing 64 kg (three times body weight), for three gold Olympic medals. That is over 12 years of maximal strength performance.

18.4.9. DEADLIFT AS AN ASSISTING EXERCISE TO WEIGHTLIFTING

Question: Since there is no Squat or Deadlift scoring in Olympic Weightlifting, why do Weightlifters perform these exercises?.

Comment:
- o Weightlifters do not train on classical Olympic lifts all the time. They go through cycles of strength training, technique enhancements, and progressive intensity increase. They incorporate the Squat and Deadlift in calculable manner that does not undermine flexibility, while increases strength. See Section 4.3 on "Standard Weightlifting Training Sessions".
- o Strength training for Squat assists the Clean lifts during the ascending and descending phases.
- o Deadlift training is paramount to Weightlifting since it maintains robust body extensors.
- o In order to balance strength versus speed, most Olympic lifters follow an empirical ratio of maxima in the Squat and the Deadlift, in relation to the Clean poundage. For example, take the Turkish gold medallist Naim Suleymanoglu, who cleaned 190 kg, one can predict his training back Squat as 110% to 120% of the Clean maximum, and his Deadlift 120% to 140% the Clean maximum.
- o The most important fact is not the maximum of strength training lifts, but the organization of the training volume and intensity in a manner that promotes strength and health, without overtraining or inducing muscular imbalance.

18.4.10. LOAD VOLUME OF DEADLIFT

Question: In calculating the training load volume, we add the weight of the barbell, multiplied by the number of repetitions per set, and add all sets to get the tonnage per session. This does not factor "time under load" into this equation. I imagine training with an explosive concentric and a 2 second eccentric, for example, would vary a lot from super slow cadence, even if provided that set, weight, and repetition numbers were equal. This way, one can predict overtraining, progress, and plateauing from the tonnage-time curve. In addition, where does nutrition enter this equation? This is a biggie in determining what type of volume will result in a training response versus overtraining versus optimal results.

Comment:
- o Enhancing strength performance requires proper planning of load volume, nutrition, and the mode of muscular contraction. For the general purpose of designing a basic program, it makes sense to concentrate on the average energy consumption without indulging in distracting details.
- o Realistically, the load volume is calculated by multiplying the number of sets by repetitions by weight of full-range exercises. The load volume translates into energy through the range of moving weight, which represents mechanical work. For example, the work-done by a mass (m), moving a distance (f), with acceleration (g), equals the product (mfg). If the distance (f) is replaced by the product of the speed (v) by the time (t), that is (f = vt), then the Work-Done is given by the product (mvtg). Therefore, the energy consideration takes care of the rate issue (time under load). This can be explained as follows. Suppose that you want to climb a mountain for a certain distance, (f). You can do that in a short time or in a long time. Yet, the distance, your body weight, and the gravity are the only factors that determine how much energy you put into it.
- o Nutrition is paramount to enhancing performance. However, individual circumstances of personal knowledge and discretion influence the role of nutrition on athletic performance. Therefore, one has to content with the technical planning of training load volume and account for nutritional factors on separate settings.

18.4.11. STIFF-LEGGED DEADLIFTS AND LOCKED KNEES

Question: I would like to know the correct way to do stiff-legged Deadlifts (SLDL's). There seems to be a discrepancy because I have been told to never lock my knees. Yet, for this exercise, you are supposed to keep them locked. Which is right? I am concentrating on Hamstrings and Glutes. So, do I keep my legs straight with my knees locked, or do I have a slight bend to my knees. I am confused.

FREQUENTLY ASKED QUESTIONS

Comment:
- Locked knees stretch the Iliotibial tract, between the pelvis (iliac crest) and knees (lateral tibial condyle). This fascial tract supports the hip and knees on the sides of the body. The Hamstrings are also stretched in locked knee position, between the ischial tuberosity and the upper parts of tibia and fibula. Such stretch can be tolerated in advanced trainees and in thorough warm-up conditions.
- In beginners and in those who do not exercise regularly and seriously, locked knees can cause strains and sprains in addition to dizziness. Dizziness results from overstretching thin muscles over major blood vessels and nerves. This acts like knife-cutting squeeze of vital structures.
- Locked knees are insecure and imbalanced, which may predispose to chronic injury.
- The proper way of performing SLDL is by slightly bending the knees, arching the back (concave or inward depression not rounded), thrusting the chest (in order to support the weight, ease breathing, and ease heart beating). Keeping the weight light helps performing high repetitions. Keeping the motion slow, benefits eccentric and concentric contraction.

18.5. EXERCISE AND BLOOD DONATION

Question: Does exercise preclude women from donating blood? I went to give blood and was told that my hematocrit level is too low. I like to donate blood, I like to work out, and it appears that the two are not compatible. I didn't realize that I needed to pass the same hemoglobin test to be allowed to donate platelets that you do to donate whole blood. The minimum level to donate is 12.5 and I only had a hematocrit of 12.4. So, I'm perfectly healthy, just training too hard to donate. In addition to the usual food list, the nurse made the suggestion of a multi-vitamin and vitamin C at bedtime, claiming that this was the most effective time of day to take vitamins to help build my hematocrit level.

Comment:
- Low hematocrit in a female, in the childbearing age, is most probably due to iron deficiency. That is because iron loss in menstruation might exceed iron intake in diet. Laboratory tests (e.g., complete blood picture) may help diagnose iron-deficiency. This can be treated by iron (Ferrous Sulfate) supplements, and not vitamin C or other vitamins, assuming that there is no other source of iron losses. The physician must exclude that possibility before prescribing iron supplement. See *Table 14.21* on Foodstuff with high **Iron** contents.
- Hematocrit is defined as the ratio of the volume of red blood cells to the volume of plasma. In females, normal hematocrit is 35-45%, compared to 39-49% in males. Thus, hematocrit is a percentage and it tells you how red or how pale the blood is.
- There are other conditions that present with low Hematocrit. These are classified as anemia and are treated differently. Hemoglobin is an iron (heme) bound to protein (globin). It is measured in grams per deciliter (100 ml). In female, hemoglobin is 12.0-15.5 g/dl, compared to 13.5-17.5 g/dl for males.

18.6. RESISTANCE TRAINING VERSUS OTHER TYPES OF WORKOUTS

Question: I saw some sports guy on TV saying that resistance training is better than other types of workouts to get more muscles and burn more fat. I don't know which types he was referring to. Why do certain workouts categorize as "resistance training" and others not?

Comment:
- Resistance training is as simple as picking up something heavy and then putting it down. It is the physical effort, or force, exerted against some kind of resistance. Resistance can be some kind of weight, your own bodyweight, or barbells, dumbbells, or gym machines. Thus, all forms of weight training fall into the resistance-training category. If you're moving a weight then you are performing weight resistance training. For example, Bench Press with a barbell is resistance training because the bar and the weights provide resistance. In squatting without weight, pushups, chin-ups, and calisthenics, your bodyweight is providing resistance.
- Resistance training increases muscular power and size, if the resistance is sufficiently large that you can fatigue yourself in a relatively small number of repetitions. For example, if you perform Squats by standing up and sitting down in a chair and this fatigues you in 10-20 repetitions, then this would be an appropriate load for you. If you can do this easily for greater than about 25 repetitions, then it's time to increase the resistance by adding dumbbells or a barbell or do the exercise on a machine, for example.
- Muscles do not grow with sole good nutrition and rest. Therefore, resistance training is necessary to enhance muscular development. Enhancing skeletal muscles also leads to enhancing smooth muscles allover the body. This takes place through the linking circulatory blood flow through visceral tissues. Thus, strengthening skeletal muscles affects the arterial wall muscles in the lungs, brain, kidneys, liver, intestines, and so on.
- Since muscles are the main protein depots in the body, therefore, strength training expands total body's protein content.

18.7. STRUCTURING WORKOUT SESSIONS

18.7.1. TWO-DAY SPLIT WORKOUT

Question: When I bench, I do three sets of 8 to 12 repetitions of the following four exercises: flat barbell Bench Press, flat dumbbell Bench Press, incline dumbbell Bench Press, and dumbbell flys. Should I include some declines to my workout and what part of the chest do they work?

Comment:
o The classical **Bench Press** targets the chest adductors (Pectoralis major and Subscapularis), in addition to the scapula anchoring muscles (Serratus anterior).
o The **dumbbell Bench Press** offers greater control over muscles and eliminates the compensatory effect of the bar. It is paramount to excelling in Bench Press.
o The **incline Bench Press** targets the anterior Deltoid and the clavicular head of the Pectoralis major.
o **Dumbbell flys** differ from dumbbell Bench Press in their intense effect on the cuff rotators (Subscapularis) than the primary rotator (the Deltoid). The flys are used to increase the range of motion more than the strength of the shoulder. They also benefit muscular definition greatly.
o It is very important to remember that one-hand shoulder exercises require few days of relative rest, before shoulder strength peaks again. That is because one-hand shoulder exercises strain the delicate rotator cuff tendons and induce considerable shoulder congestion.
o The **decline Bench Press** differs from the flat Bench Press in that it involves the shoulder adductors that originate from the back (Latissimus dorsi, long head of Triceps, Subscapularis, and Teres), in addition to those that originate from the chest (Pectoralis major and Serratus anterior). Yet, the decline position distinguishes the decline Bench Press from the parallel bar dips (which involves muscles in similar fashion) in the excessive venous return, when the heart lies lower than the pelvis. This diminishes congestion of the lower body and stretches the cardiac muscles considerably, in comparison to the parallel bar dips.
o Basing workout plans on rigid list of exercises is counterproductive. It is wiser to add and skip exercises based on the need for specific goals. Thus, one can add dumbbell Bench Press one day if the barbell Bench Press is done at heavier volume and intensity. In addition, one can substitute the flys with decline bench on another day in order to work out different angle of the shoulder, and so on. Again, one can completely skip the dumbbell exercises of the Bench Press on other days in order to balance intensity and volume.

Question: I do two split workouts of ten exercises. Each exercise is performed in three sets of 8 to 12 repetitions per set. I can get my workouts done in about an hour and twenty minutes. I do cardio in-between days. *Table 18.3* shows the list of exercises and their sequence of execution. What changes can I make to enhance my progress?

Table 18.3. Daily exercise routine of Section 18.7.1.

	Chest, shoulder, Triceps days	Legs, Back, Biceps days
1.	Flat barbell bench.	Full Squats.
2.	Flat dumbbell bench.	Leg extensions.
3.	Incline dumbbell bench.	Flat bench leg curls.
4.	Dumbbell flys.	One legged dumbbell calf raises.
5.	Seated dumbbell presses.	Dumbbell rows.
6.	Dumbbell shrugs.	Wide grip cable pull-downs.
7.	Lying dumbbell Triceps ext.	Seated incline dumbbell curls.
8.	Triceps cable pull-downs.	Standing dumbbell hammer curls.
9.	Crunches.	Crunches.
10.	Cable pull-down crunches.	Goodmornings (light weight on bar).

Comment:
o It is clear that performing weight-training exercises, based on working out **isolated muscles**, is meant for strengthening alone with no regard to total fitness and whole body conditioning. There are other ways of training for bulking muscle mass, explosive power, and sport-specific conditioning. These do not adhere to the method of laundry–list of exercises, but rather to achieve specific goals.
o **Split sessions** (splitting workout for different parts of the body on different sessions) are ineffective if done every other day, since the worked part will be hit every four days (on 2-day split routine) or every six days (on 3-day split routine). That is too long intermission for muscles to develop strength, mass, or tone control. That is particularly true when the exercises are of local isolation nature. Inserting global exercises, such as the Power Clean, Power Snatch, and Deadlift, helps keep many major muscles strong and toned.
o Splitting strength workout on 3-day routine can be very effective if **global exercises** are included in order to link major muscle groups. This will also help reduce the number of exercises to six or less, which helps in increasing intensity and volume. With less number of exercises per session, you can increase the number of sets to five or more. You can also widen the range of resistance, between the first and last sets of an exercise group. The best options for strengthening splits are: back, legs, and shoulders days, with few global exercises included in each session.

18 FREQUENTLY ASKED QUESTIONS

- o The major muscle groups of legs, trunk, and shoulders vary in strength, from one person to other. These should be worked out on **individual basis**. A person with weak legs might think about including leg exercises in every session even if it is chest-shoulder day. Vice versa, a person with weak spinal erectors may do likewise.
- o Exercises that redundantly repeat the work of others such as the leg extension, leg curls, and dumbbell rows, can replace the **classical exercises** (Squat, Goodmorning, and barbell row, respectively) on days of low intensity.
- o Some muscles such as the Glutes, Quads, Hams, and back erectors are better hit repeatedly every split sessions, since they are crucial to lifting. Thus, do not over emphasize **equality between muscles**. In the beginning, you might feel that some exercises, such as the Deadlift, may interfere with the recovery from other exercises, such as the Squats. Yet, after a while, you will develop axial strength that enhances your recovery, as long as you train regularly.

18.7.2. ENDURANCE VERSUS WEIGHT TRAINING

Question: I lift weight three days a week, do cardio on other three days, and rest on Sunday. I would like to know if I am on the right track or not. Here is my workout routine. On Tuesday, Thursday, and Saturday I ride the mountain bike of an hour making 10 miles. The weight training is as follows. I do each exercise in three sets each from 10 to 14 repetitions, as shown in *Table 18.4*.

Table 18.4. Daily exercise routine of Section 18.7.2.

Monday (Arm day)	Wednesday (Chest day)	Friday (Legs, Shoulders, and Back)
1. Dumbbell Curls	1. Bench Press	1. Leg Extensions
2. Dumbbell Preacher Curls	2. Incline Dumbbell Bench	2. Leg Curls
3. Triceps Extensions	3. Dumbbell Flys	3. Squats
4. Seated Dumbbell Extensions	4. Dumbbell Pullovers	4. One Leg Dumbbell Calf Raises
5. Cable Triceps Pull-downs	5. Front Cable Pull-downs	5. Seated Dumbbell Press
6. Bent over Dumbbell Extensions		6. Wide Grip Cable Pull-downs
7. Biceps Barbell Curls		7. Bent over dumbbell Rows
8. Alternating Dumbbell Curls Seated 45 deg.		

Comment:
- o Such extensive mountain biking might drain you of strength, if you keep lifting hard. You might want to "cycle" your emphasis between the two. Hard endurance training and heavy weight lifting are incompatible, particularly when major muscles like legs, shoulders, and back are worked out in a single day.
- o You forgot the entire spinal regions. Goodmornings, Deadlifts, and shrugs. You focus on the details and overlook the fundamentals. You need to include compound exercises that link major muscle groups such as the legs, shoulders, and back. These should work out more than one day each week.
- o Deltoid, Quadriceps, spinals must get at least 20%, each, of your time. The Deltoid, Quadriceps, and spinal erectors are the foundation and central groups of a fit physique. The Biceps, Triceps, calves are peripheral muscles and do not deserve a full workout day, unless they are particularly targeted for extra strengthening.
- o Do not overload the knees by two similar exercises in the same setting. Target another area of the body to avoid long-term cartilage wear and tear.

18.7.3. WORKOUT AT HOME

Question: I am 17 years old, and I am quite tall and a little bit skinny too. The gyms around my area are all private membership, and I can't afford that, so I was wondering if I could build myself up at home. The thing is, I am going on holiday in 6 months, and my friends are all quite muscular, but I am quite skinny. So, I basically have 6 months worth of hard work to do, to get myself toned up. I mainly need to concentrate on my arms, shoulders, and pectorals, although I would also like to work on my calves and thighs. Tough call, huh? Well, if you can give me any tips of programs to follow, products to buy, drugs to take, then I would be grateful. I am not too bothered about being really fit, but I will work on that too if it is necessary to broaden myself up.

Comment:
- o You do not need a lot of money or a gym to be fit. Fancy equipments and prestigious gyms do not make great athletes.
- o Setting a deadline is not practical. At the age of 17, you have a good chance to do the best out of your life, not just impress few friends. Friends change many times throughout life, what endures is sound personal goals.
- o Fitness is an investment in your health. Working out for getting fit may help prevent many problems in the future. That is wiser than sitting and waiting for problems to happen and then seeking solutions that might be tough to find.
- o Here is practical training program that you can execute at home.
    i.   **Warm-up** whole body for 10 minutes. You can warm up by running a mile, or marching in place while raising your arms, from your sides to overhead. Five sets, of 5 to 10 reps of arm raising, are enough.
    ii. With both hands placed behind your head, **squat** 10 times. Take a short break then repeat the Squat, for total of 50. This works out the Quadriceps and may take 10 min to execute. When you get stronger, you can hold a heavy object (sand bag, medicine ball or a barbell) behind your back, while squatting.
    iii. Bend over, as if you say **Goodmorning** in Japanese style, for 10 repetitions. Take a short break then repeat the Goodmorning, for total of 50. This works out the spinal muscles.

FREQUENTLY ASKED QUESTIONS

- iv. Do floor **push-ups** for 5 to 10 reps. Take a short break then repeat the floor push-ups, for a total of 50. This works out the chest muscles.
- v. Do **Chin-ups**, if you can, by holding to a high support such as a steel bar or a tree branch. Pull up your bodyweight for 3 to 10 times if you can. Take a short break then repeat the chin-ups, for a total of 20. This works out arms and back muscles.
- vi. Hold a heavy object (such as a sand bag, a medicine ball, or a dumbbell) in front of your chest and raise it up then lower it down for 5 to 10 times. Take a short break then repeat this **Shoulder Press,** for total of 50. This works out the shoulder muscles.

o With this simple training plan, we have hit every muscle, Quads, shoulder, back, and chest, in addition to the cardio. You can increase the total number or repetitions, from 50 up, depending on your progress. You can increase the weight of the medicine ball or replace it with a barbell. As you progress, you may think about buying an adjustable dumbbell set at the local sporting goods store. As you get stronger, you can buy more plates. Alternatively, you can buy an Olympic barbell set for about $150. A good whole-body routine with Olympic barbell might be as follows: Squats or Split Squats or Lunges, Stiff-Legged Deadlifts, Bench Press (if you get a bench or see *Figure 13.5*) or Push-Ups, One-Arm Row or Bent-Over Row, Overhead Press or Hang Clean & Press, Chin-Ups (if you have a bar fixed to a wall), abdominal Crunches, Single-Calf Raises, and Wrist Curls.

18.7.4. SPLIT DAY WORKOUT

Question: I train 4 days per week with 4 to 5 exercises per session. Two of the four days are for leg and lower back exercises and are comprised of Squats, Deadlifts, and abdominal exercises. The other two days are for chest and shoulders and are comprised of Bench Press, Shoulder Press, and dips. I do variations of Deadlifts of different stance (normal, sumo, very wide sumo); different start point (by going off the rack or standing on platforms), and different acceleration (slow and pull-thrust). Heavy days consist of pyramiding up to doubles and singles of high percentage of 1RM. The following is usual week routine, which I like some critique on its soundness, shown in *Table 18.5*.

Table 18.5. Daily exercise routine of Section 18.7.4.

Monday (Legs)	Tuesday (Chest and Shoulders)	Thursday (Legs)	Saturday
1. Squats 8x3, 58-62%	1. Regular Bench 8x3, 58-62%	1. Front Squats	1. Wide Grip Bench
2. SLDL's 8x3, 58-62%	2. Close Grip Bench 8x3, 58-62%	2. Weighted Pull Ups	2. Close Grip Bench
3. Calf Raises	3. Dips 5x5	3. Deadlift	3. Lateral Raises
4. Unweighted crunches.	4. Standing Military Press 5x4, 60%.	4. Weighted Crunches	4. Skull Crunches.

Comment:
o The legs days that completely devoid of any upper bodywork, other than the Deadlift, will stiffen the upper body joints. If a military or power Clean or Snatch are introduced on the leg days as a preparation for the Deadlifts then better flexibility, balance, and coordination are achieved.
o The chest and shoulders days are devoid of any torso or leg training. Doing upper body lifting on cold lower back and legs will cause strain and sprain. Any lifting has to commence after progressive toning of the torso and legs. Also inserting the Clean or Snatch in the chest and shoulders days prepare the back and legs for upper body loading.
o The compound exercises such, as the Clean and Snatch do not have to exceed five or six sets, with 60% to 80% 1RM. These have to precede the aided exercises (Squat, Bench Press, Deadlift, Press, and Crunches).

18.8. SQUAT

18.8.1. FRONT SQUATS AND KNEE PAIN

Question: I've been squatting religiously for a couple of years, and I haven't had knee pains in ages. About four weeks ago I decided to ditch normal Squats for a while and, for the first time, do front Squats instead. Now, my knees or rather, the left knee, which has always been the wonky one, is acting up again. The pain isn't nearly as bad as it was back when I didn't squat deep, but it definitely is there for the first time in over two years, and it seems to be getting worse little by little. Is there something about front Squats that makes them more hazardous to your knees? Am I doing something wrong, or should I just give up and switch back to normal Squats? Is there some reason why front Squats don't seem to make my things anywhere near as sore as regular back Squats?

Comment:
o Front Squats shift the center of mass of the body and the barbell, so you are developing a muscular imbalance between the Quads and Hamstrings that could be affecting the mechanics of your knee. Try stopping the front Squats until the pain subsides. Then slowly reintroduce them into a balanced workout.
o It is important to identify the precise source of the pain. The distribution of the area where the pain is referred to gives an idea on whether the pain originates from the soft tissues or from the cartilages. Injuries to soft-tissues refer pain to

wide area around the knee and the pain lasts for short time (less than two week). Injuries to cartilages refer pain very close to the injured cartilage and last for longer times. Thus, a two-year-old bad knee hints to chronic injury. Measures of reducing the acute inflammation may help on the short term in continuing exercise and thus building supportive tissues. However, if substantial knee injury persists despite medical treatment then surgery may be the best alternative in preventing complication. See *Figures 16.1* and *16.2*, Chapter 16.

o A very useful and effective method of restoring knee function and eliminating pain is stretching. For stretching to produce sensible results, it must be executed for at least twenty minutes and must cover all directions of movement of the knee, hip, and ankle joints. Yoga stretching is magical in relieving knee pain and restoring mobility.

o Changing the way the knees are pointed and wearing more comfortable shoes, with soft and flat soles, may help reduce the inflammation. This would even the stresses on the knee-articulating surface. By pointing the knees more forward than lateral, the load would be evenly distributed on the knee-inner-surface and the pain may diminish (if there in no significant physical injury). If the pain persists or worsens then other measures should be perused such as rest or examination by a specialist.

18.8.2. BALANCING KNEE EXTENSORS AND FLEXORS
Question: What exercises can balance the knee joint?

Comment: Squats strengthen the Quadriceps. Stiff-legged Deadlift or Goodmorning strengthen the Hamstrings. Squatting can be done without weight, but with fast explosive downwards and or upwards force such that the Quadriceps would resist virtual forces due to higher acceleration, instead of due to heavier weights. This is the essence of Calisthenics. Squatting with weights enhances the slow control of recruitment of muscle fibers that is lacking in the fast process of **Calisthenics**. However, Squats are poor in Hamstring developing despite their use of hip extension. The Hamstrings act on two joints. They extend the hips and flex the knees. For complete development, movements that encompass both joints are necessary. Thus, even though Goodmornings and stiff-legged Deadlifts also involve the Glutes and spinal erectors, they are an integral component of Hamstrings regimen. Although leg curls achieve good Hamstrings development as well, they lack spinal strengthening of the latter two exercises. These exercises are as direct as you can get for hip extension and knee stabilizing movements.

18.8.3. ISOLATION VERSUS COMPOUND EXERCISES
Question: Why do some people think that doing **sit-ups** destroys your lower back by stretching the ligaments that support the spinal discs leading to weakening and destabilizing the lumbar area? Are doing crunches OK? I've seen statements like this for years, but it seems to contradict the normal philosophy of training in this group, i.e. doing compound movements rather than isolation moves. Everybody says do Squats rather than Leg Extensions, dips rather than bench presses, etc. So, why all of a sudden crunches are better than sit-ups? So sit-ups hit your hip flexors - what's wrong with getting strong hip flexors? Sit-ups are a natural movement, cavemen had to do them every time they woke up, so why would the body be engineered to be injured from them?

Comment:
o The "general" idea is that compound exercises should form the core of your workouts since they effectively integrate neuromuscular and cardiopulmonary functions. Isolation exercises on the other hand are added to remedy individual deficits. Thus, Squats will activate a lot more than Quads and Dips activate a lot more than Triceps. This doesn't mean leg extensions or bench presses have no value. They're different.

o Sit-ups cause some people back-trouble when the spines are over flexed particularly those with big bellies. Sit-ups are not bad in themselves, except they do not work abdominals that much. The hip flexors draws the body forwards, which puts extra strain on the lower back. As long as the body is balanced that won't happen. If you are comfortable doing sit-ups, and you feel your abdominal muscles and hip flexors benefit from doing them, then continue doing them. You should remember that if you exercise the hip flexors more frequently and intensely than the abdominals then you might limit your abdominal exercise to the crunches in order to increase the load volume on the abdominals and reduce it on the hip flexors.

o On the issue of nature, people plan their exercise based on reality not on historic or evolutionary facts. It is not so much if the movement is natural or unnatural. Meaning for instance, if someone did not work out regularly since childhood, you cannot require him or her to overdo exercises that exceed their limits. Many times gradual and progressive training reverses long acquired limitations but, sometimes, certain limitations are permanent or can be slightly modified. For example, many overweight people have back problems and have to pick exercises that help them solve either or both problems without causing a setback.

o It is not the sit-up's movement itself that causes damage, it's the repetition. Lower back pain in elderly people is a result of a longer life span than the body was really built for, and so parts start to wear out. With sit-ups, and without balanced strengthening of back erectors, you speed up the wear to the lower back, which can eventually cause irreversible damage.

o The spinal extensors are active until approximately two thirds of maximal spinal flexion has been attained, at which point they become electrically silent. Thus, control of flexion becomes the responsibility of the passive elastic response of the thoracolumbar fascia and posterior ligamentous system. The posterior ligaments (supraspinous and interspinous ligaments) have longer movement arms than the extensor muscles and thus have a mechanical advantage over the extensors. Both, back erectors and back ligaments, require strengthening exercises in order to balance hip flexors during sit-ups. This can be accomplished effectively by lifting from the floor such as in the Clean, Snatch, and Deadlift. The balance between the back erectors and hip flexors refutes the argument on the bad effects of sit-ups.

18.8.4. LEG EXTENSIONS AND SHEAR STRESSES

Question: My physiotherapist thinks that Leg Extension is dangerous when performed below the top third of the movement. There was a period of time where that is all I could do. Is there any proof that Leg Extensions hurt or help people? How do I know that a force is too high or too low to get a training effect? Wouldn't a rational person choose a weight level that let's them do the weakest part of the lift safely? Or, do the lift in two pieces, heavy weight for the first 2/3rds and lighter weight for the last third in another set?
Comment:
o Individual variation causes some people to have imbalanced knee structures at certain angles. Those have to be very careful with Leg Extensions or other exercises when imbalance is suspected, be that at the top 1/3rd of the movement or below that. However, near full Knee Extension, there are extreme forces on one of the key knee ligaments (**ACL**) due to the maximum forward translation of the top of the tibia. This might cause worrisome pain with heavy loads near full extension in some people.
o As the Quads contract at the top of the movement, the **kneecap** is pulled upwards, which could be problematic for people with certain kinds of internal knee injuries. There is a risk of lateral movement of the patella if supporting tissue is not strong and balanced.
o The top of the Leg Extension movement puts the most **shearing forces** on the knee ligaments. Shearing forces are perpendicular to both femur and tibia at that position. At the top of the movement, the Quads are unopposed by the Hamstrings. Thus, the ACL is the main opponent to the Quads in preventing the knee from getting split open. In Knee Extension, there are two players.
  i. Contractile element, **Quadriceps**. There is no other muscle, which aids the Quadriceps in its pull during seated full Knee Extension. The Hamstrings are dragged under the thigh, yet they are not participating in pulling. They are eliminated from knee extension by fixed ischial tuberosity and lack of resistance to the Hamstrings in seated leg extension.
  ii. Non-contractile element, **ACL**. This will only anchor the tibia to the femur to prevent forward translation. How does shearing vary with knee flexion? The answer is that the projected area of contact between the tibia and femur that faces the Quadriceps ligament is diminished with extension. Suppose that you are looking horizontally at the knee joint of a standing person. At full extension, the projected area is zero. At 90-degree flexion, the projected area is maximal (the entire surface of the tibial upper end). Therefore, shear tension is minimum at full flexion and maximum at full extension. It is a "cosine" shaped relation (shear increases as projected area decreases). What concerns you, as an athlete, is that shear maxima would not hurt you if you train regularly with progressive incremental resistance.
o The bottom part of the leg extension stretches the tendon of the muscle and thus it challenges your **tendon strength**. Some may have to go lighter in order to stretch the tendon safely. The bottom problem has to do more with modern day use of legs in limited range of motion thus leaving the bottom range weaker. In addition, people with chronic patellofemoral instability suffer most at the bottom position of the movement, regardless of shear forces, since the knee would be most vulnerable while the joint is widely open.
o Leg Extensions are invaluable during rehabilitation from injuries since they strengthen the knees **in isolation** from the hips and ankles. Even Leg Extension without weight can cause untrained legs to sore after few sets. If you are injured at the foot or ankle, and cannot do Squats for example, you can do leg press instead. At least with Leg Extensions you might prevent some atrophy. Few sets of Leg Extension, on regular basis, can undoubtedly alleviate recurrent patellar tendonitis in people with this condition, particularly when done on separate legs, with fairly lightweights. If you're able to squat, then you should use Leg Extensions, leg curls, or leg press, for conditioning purposes. Full Squats are good substitute for these exercises in heavy resistance. Squats recruit the hips, knees, and ankles in unison and thus synchronize the antagonistic actions of the extensors and flexors across the hips, knees, and ankles.
o The disadvantage of training with sole isolation exercises, such as the Leg Extension, is the lack of **biarticulate coordination** of the extensors and flexors (across two major joints). This applies to the Quadriceps that extend the knees and flex the hips, Hamstrings that extend the hips and flex the knees, and Gastrocnemius that flex the knees and extend the ankles. Such disadvantage is overcome by incorporating compound exercises such as Squats. The advantage of leg presses though is the specific strengthening of the knee muscles and internal ligaments (ACL), which can receive targeted high volume of strength training, along with whole limb conditioning. This specific strengthening improves dynamic control of tibial translation after ACL injury.
o Leg Extension is not equivalent to squatting because of the following:
  i. Leg Extension is a **Quadriceps-specific** exercise. All other muscles are mostly eliminated. No Hamstring counter-action, no Glutei contraction, and no adductors. So, what keeps the knees supported against the Quadriceps pull?

The answer is: the cruciate ligaments, ACL. Squatting does not target the cruciate ligaments as long as the Quads and the Hamstrings are in full opposition. ACL strain is reduced during squatting by virtue of the muscular antagonism.
  ii. Leg Extensions require **full control** over the Quadriceps. While in the Squats the Quadriceps and Hamstrings participate in the control of movement starting from minimal recruitment, on standing, to maximum on squatting. In leg extensions, the Quads are fully recruited from start to end. This is a unique advantage for bulking the Quadriceps. Squats would not accomplish neuromuscular control with such efficiency.
  iii. Leg Extension induces minimal **inner knee stress**. Squatting raises the stress inside the knees way above normal, which limits the longevity of the knee joint. Leg Extension causes minimal stress and extends the knee longevity. In short, Knee Extension is not a redundant type of leg exercise neither is equivalent to Squat. It has specific indication that is to secure agile knees.
o Squatting deep and heavy will secure slow moving knees. If you **jerked** your **knees by accident** then the ACL or PCL (Posterior Cruciate Ligament) will give away at low-tension threshold. Suppose you are a strong Weightlifter and someone pushed you from front or behind, unexpectedly, what prevents your knees from getting displaced is the ACL and the PCL not just the Quads and the Hamstrings. In spite of your strong muscles, you might incur a serious knee injury if you overlooked ACL and PCL.

18.8.5. LEANING OVER DURING SQUAT

Question: How can I avoid leaning over during Squat?

Comment:
o Leaning over may be a necessity for balance as well as a sign of muscular imbalance, as follows.
  i. If leaning over starts when you begin bending the knees then that may be attributed to spinal **balance**. Leaning in this early phase brings the center of gravity to the line of descent.
  ii. If leaning starts half way down then it may be due to **weak** upper back **musculature**.
  iii. If it starts in your way to ascend from deep then that may be explained by **unconditioned entire body**.
o The **threshold of resistance,** when leaning over starts to show, may hint to the cause of leaning over. If lighter weights do not cause leaning, then you have to be patient in gaining strength over time in order to raise the threshold for leaning, bit by bit. You should not squat with weights before first mastering the Squat technique without weight. An empty sole bar on a rack can do the magic in exercising healthy legs, without adding heavy plates. Squatting with weight should follow proper squatting without weight. This way you become aware of the limits of your own performance.
o There are very skilled athletes who could not overcome the leaning habit and who did very well in other fields. It is a **mind-set habit**, too.
o Because many people injure their lower back and herniate the lumber discs, many erroneously believe that weakness of the lower back is always the source of all troubles. The fact is that the lower back has very limited **range of motion**, compared to other joints. Thus, the lower back incurs injuries by throwing it in awkward positions, even if it was very strong. You can hurt your lower back by sitting on a soft couch or by leaning on the sink when you forget to keep your back straight.
o Leaning over can thus be attributed to the following causes.
  i. The **proportion of the distances** between the joints (ankle, knee, hip, shoulders) necessitates the forward leaning to balance the motion, e.g., long thighs and short trunk. The proportion of the upper bodyweight to the lower body weight necessitates the forward leaning, for the same reason, e.g., a person with heavy built thighs and narrow shoulders, as in females.
  ii. Habitual forward leaning: Some people used to lean forward to **tighten the back muscles** before beginning the Squat, as a sort of self-assurance.
  iii. **Imbalance** muscular support of the vertebral column in the upper region.
  iv. **Cardiopulmonary** reason (lack of conditioning, or lack of endurance). When we lean forwards, the chest cage drops forwards and allows more air to flow to the lungs. If you watch a dog or a cat, you notice that they cannot stand upright for too long because, in upright position, the ribs of their chest would drop down by gravity, the chest cage becomes smaller, and impairs breathing.

18.8.6. USING WAIST BELTS DURING SQUATS

Question: I've been doing Squats for about six months now. I usually work my legs about twice every eleven days or so. I also do stiff-legged Deadlifts and classic Deadlifts among other exercises. I always start with Squats and I wear a belt cinched very tight. I've been constantly reading about Squats and how to do them in an effort to continually improve my form and technique. I have a spotter who spots me for forced repetitions and safety and also critiques my form. I also stand in front of a mirror and feel that my form is pretty good. I keep my back as straight as humanly possible, feet just slightly wider than shoulder width apart and carry the bar high on my Traps. I'm working more towards size and leg development. However, I also want to increase strength. I usually develop a real tight pump in my lower back after about two sets and start to get a lactic acid burn in my lower back. It's not that I'm in any unusual pain, but my lower back fatigues and it becomes a lot harder during the rest of my sets. I cannot continue to keep good form and grind out as many repetitions without my back becoming the issue of the weak link. Is there a better way regarding tweaking my form or technique in order to prevent this from being a continuing problem? Or, is there anything else that I may be missing?

Comment:
- **Regarding Belts:** Many lifters have never used a weight belt in their entire life, particularly those who are obsessed with natural workout, believing that belts make back weak. The following issues concern belt users.
    i. Wearing a belt is **restrictive** and more traumatic to live tissues since belts do not comply with breathing motion of expansion and contraction. This means less mobility, which leads to stiffness, which leads to weakness, which leads to injury. If you have to use the belt, don't cinch the belt tight. Just loosen it since it doesn't protect your back by structurally supporting your vertebrae anyway, but rather supports your abdominal muscles.
    ii. Belts are not for training; they are for competition and **competition only**. The rationale that wearing a belt helps in using more weight, which then helps your legs grow stronger, is flawed. Since more weight does not always cause fast growth. If joints were not balanced, by well-trained opposing groups of muscles, then more weight may cause injury. If you do Deadlifts, Squats, and sit-ups on regular basis, I doubt that you would need additional lower back support. Belts should only be used for working with maximal weights, for example just before or during contests.
    iii. Plain old everyday squatting with a belt allows your body to rely exclusively on the belt for support, instead of its natural girdle of muscle. In addition, many folks using a belt to squat use them incorrectly. For example, if you are not warmed up adequately and try to depend on the waist belt to protect your back during heavy lifting then you are making a serious mistake. You must not forget that your warmed up muscles are your prime lifters, while the belt only warns you when misalignment ensues.
    iv. However, belts have reduced back injuries in many **industries** that demand physical labor.
    v. Belts also enhance **self-esteem** and make young people feel like real strong adults or real athletes.
    vi. For those who strive for perfection, belts can be substituted by little **training** on keeping the vertebrae aligned during the lifting. Without the belt, one has to contract the abdominal muscles during lifting in order to push the guts inward and upward. This relieves the diaphragm from the downward dragging weight of the guts and enhances efficient breathing, which enhances performance.
- **Back and Quad balance:** The lower back will almost always fatigue before the Quads. The following methods may enhance back endurance.
    i. If you are looking for development of the Quadriceps in particular, you could try **superset pre-exhaustion technique** such as combining Leg Extensions (this isolates the Quadriceps muscles) and Squats in alternating supersets. Your Quads will be tired, but your Glutes and Hamstrings will help you push it. You will need to squat a lighter weight than usual. Pre-exhaustion elevates lactates threshold by enhancing circulation.
    ii. In my opinion, you are taking to many days off between workouts. One to three days off is plenty of rest. To grow stronger, try shortening the time between workouts. **Daily and long physical activity** is the essence of building up strength.
    iii. **Warm-up** gradually. Use perfect form. Add direct lower back and abdominals assistance work, and try stretching between sets. Direct lower back assistance work (i.e. reverse hyperextension and side bends) prepares the back for heavy lifting.
    iv. **Stretch** suppresses the high tone of the frantic muscles spindles and alleviates spasm. If you start with Squats, you must warm up for at least 20 minutes without weight. Then increase the weight gradually, from 45 lb bar up.
- **Backache remedies:** There are empirical methods in dealing with backache and back weakness in common weight training.
    i. Some people use heavy-duty power **belts** or turn the belt around so the wide part is facing the front. This is meant to assist abdominal tone. Others keep chest out, breath deeply, and push the stomach against the belt as hard as possible. The last one is dangerous, since pushing the stomach requires diaphragmatic contraction and can predispose to hernia. Contracting the diaphragm for long time, in order to push the stomach against the belt, means staying too long in the inspiration phase of the breathing cycle. This drastically drops gas exchange, cuts oxygen supply to vital tissues, and hampers muscular activity.
    ii. Many people lock the lower back and keep it locked throughout. This ensures support to **spinal alignment**. Others check body forms to make sure that the bar stays over the heels through the movement and not let it come forwards or go backwards significantly. This requires lightweight that is easily controllable.
    iii. Some add reverse hyperextensions in upper body days. This stretches the Hamstrings, Glutei, and spinal erectors. **Spinal stretching** in various directions is superior in preventing and treating backache. Stretch eliminates edema and conditions the proprioceptors for balanced muscular activity.
    iv. Few practice icing the lower back following the workout. This is a bad habit since the back muscles fare better on **heat** not on cold.
- **Lower back balance:** Lower backache is caused by muscular imbalanced. To avoid this problem you may do the following:
    i. You may have to take it easy on the Squat for a while. Don't stop squatting, but just **go light** and get that back into shape.

ii. Do some light work to increase your lower back strength. You should add exercises that strengthen both the front and back vertebral muscles. **Sit-ups** strengthen the hip flexors and the anterior vertebral muscles that oppose the posterior spinal and vertebral ones. **Abdominal muscles** support the vertebral column in position when flexion is required such as overhead press and incline bench. Abdominals also support the abdominal contents and prevent herniation of the gut to the outside of the abdominal sac.

iii. Pending back injuries can be predicted by measuring the amount of **torque** generated by the back extensors and flexors, either in comparison to control groups or to standardizes values of torques (see Section 2.12.8 on "Spinoscopic Examination"). High torque signifies the ability of the back to resist shearing forces and thus prevent injury, while low torques signify the need to strengthen the weak side to avoid future back strain.

o **Squat frequency and volume:** Squatting three times per week may result in overtraining of the legs, unless you vary the intensity and weight load. Vary intensity, weight, and type of squatting (front, back, half-seated, full Squat, etc). The Quadriceps and Glutei waste very fast if you neglect them for two days. If you have no access to a gym, you should exercise on squatting without weights for a much as you can to exhaust the Quads. There is no magic in using a barbell or a rack if your form is incorrect or your muscles are sore.

o **The role of abdominal muscles:** The contraction of the inner abdominal muscles (transversus abdominis and internal oblique muscles), in the presence of a closed glottis, raises the intra-abdominal pressure. This puts venous return under complete control of the nervous system. With adequate venous return from the guts and lower body, the sympathetic system can function relatively smoothly during vigorous exercise. During the long hours of no lifting, the intra-abdominal pressure can generate substantial extension moments by passive tension in the posterior ligamentous system. The imbalance between abdominal muscles and back erectors is more crucial during no lifting hours than during brief lifting moments. Such imbalance exert **chronic congestion** on the spinal structures and weaken them causing back pain and injuries. Lifting on regular basis revitalizes the spinal structures even if without intense abdominal exercises. Yet, the stronger the abdominal musculature is, the easier is the chance for balancing the back and the abdomen.

18.8.7. PLATEAUING IN SQUAT

Question: I would like to say I suck at Squats. I don't know why though. I just can't seem to get any stronger on my Squats. I am about 5'9" 122 lbs and only 15 years of age. I have long legs and a short upper body. I don't think I'm really made for Squats. On Tuesday and Friday, I do a set of 10 then a set of 8 and I am just not gaining like I am on bench. I have gained about 20 lbs on my bench and can Bench Press 145 lb, but my Squat plateaus. I do have some knee problems at times. After I do Squats, my knees kill me going up steps. My knees always have bothered me at times though since about three years ago. Should I change my sets and repetitions or what?

Comment:
o You need to lower your Squat repetitions, increase the **numbers of sets**, and not do long exhaustive warm-up sets. Remember, the big weight is what does the work. Doing sets of ten with low weight are only counter-productive. You could always try giving the good Olympic lifting fashioned, five sets of five repetitions, a run for starters.
o Squatting for two sets twice a week is a joke. Strengthening the legs require more frequent sessions, more sets, more weight, and less repetitions. In addition, you need **assisting exercises** such as the Deadlift, Clean, Snatch, Goodmorning, and Bent-Over Rows. The strength of the legs depends on the whole body strength.
o At age of 15, your recovery from Squat should be fast if your **nutrition, rest, sleep, and working intensity** are in good order. The acute soreness may be attributed to the high repetitions and the fewer sets of acute exertion.
o There are no hard and fast rules on how many sets, days, or repetitions, and the level of intensity of **proper workout**. If your knees are sore, they have to rest at least a full day without lifting. The famous method of Powerlifting axial training that involves Squat, Deadlift, and Bench Press, three times weekly, is so famous because it optimizes the number of exercises to three, the number of weekly sessions to three, and the numbers of sets and repetitions per exercises to 5 x 5, or so. It is thus a great method for whole body strengthening.
o The **intensity** of your Squat workout should depend entirely on your individual circumstances. You are the one who have to do the lifting and bear the consequences. You cannot force yourself to lift in a tiring day. Yet, the rule of thumb is to progressively increase the weight, even if you have to drop the repetitions in order to gain strength.
o As far as the bothering knee, an **accurate assessment** is due in order to avoid flawed training. The knees can be problematic if their musculature is weak, overtrained, or improperly trained, or due to other anatomical flaws. Three years of knee troubles requires some attention to planning workout and medical evaluation. Most probably long term strengthening will require many months of slow and steady progress.

18.8.8. SQUATS AND SHOULDER PAIN

Question: I just started doing Squats and lunges and am experiencing a really annoying pain in my shoulders. The pain doesn't seem to be from the bar resting on my shoulders. The pain occurs about 1/2 way through a set and feels like an acute soreness in and surrounding the shoulder joint. I suspect it's from balancing the bar. Sometimes I have to stop a set before really challenging my lower body because of the pain in my shoulders. I'm a small woman with narrow shoulders and have been using a fairly wide grip to keep the bar balanced. I'm trying for higher repetitions with deeper movement (bar only for lunges, bar + 10 or 20 pounds for Squats, 8-12 repetitions per set), at least until I get accustomed to the movement. I also use one of those cylindrical pads around the bar. I do not experience DOMS in the shoulders from doing Squats and lunges, just soreness during and for a few minutes after the exercise. I have no history of joint distress. I do not experience this particular kind of pain in my shoulders when doing upper bodywork. Usually, I'm pretty good at figuring out what hurts, but, this time, I'm having a hard time identifying the source of the pain, whether it is in the actual joint, in the muscle, in the connective tissues, etc. Is this pain normal? Is it just a matter of strengthening the muscles used to balance the bar, or does it indicate faulty form on my part? Could the pad have something to do with it?

Comment:
o Because of modern day life, many people do not exercise the shoulders properly and therefore have troubles with a certain grip during Squat. This is a typical presentation of muscular imbalance. The imbalance presents with pain in certain shoulder position and after certain number of repetitions.
o Putting the bar lower down the Traps, below the Deltoids, with wider hand grips may relax the Supraspinatus and take the pain out of the shoulders. Many have trouble with the high bar Squat and narrow grips because our shoulders are weak, stiff, and insecure. Because of the weak musculature, the shoulder joint has a lot of play. If you voluntarily elevate your shoulders (tense your shoulders upwards), as if you are about to begin a military press, this might took some pressure off your shoulders and thus eliminate the pain during Squats.
o There is no guarantee that lowering the bar below the Trapezius or widening the grip would resolve the problem. The sharp pain that forces her to stop the squatting requires a search for the anatomical structures that cause such vulnerability and consequently strengthening them slowly and gradually.
o A combination of dumbbell Shoulder Press, dumbbell Inclined Press, dumbbell Bent-Over Rows, and front dumbbell arm-raises should balance the rotator cuff muscles. This should proceed from light weight and progress incrementally over a period of few weeks, before noticeable progress is felt.

18.8.9. SQUAT AND DEADLIFT ROTATION IN WORKOUT

Question: Currently I do Deadlifts on Tuesdays (Back & Biceps) and I do Squats on Thursdays (Legs & Shoulders). The problem I have is that my legs are still a little sore on Thursdays from doing Deadlifts on Tuesday. Do you think one should do Deadlifts on leg days with the Squat?

Comment:
Deadlifts and Squats work essentially the same muscle groups: Hamstrings, Glutes, spinal erectors, and shoulder girdle. There should be more rest between the two for sure. If you are a fan of split session, I suggest that you train four days per week, two days for the Bench Press and two for the Squat and Deadlift. For beginners, one day of rest between Squats and Deadlifts might not be enough rest. Usually, on a three day split, it's best to work bench in between. Thus, for example on Tuesday, you train the Back with Biceps, on Thursday the Chest and Triceps, and on Saturday the Legs and Shoulders. You also could swap Back and Biceps for legs and shoulders. Alternatively, you could move shoulders into the day of Chest and Triceps since many of those exercises hit a lot of the same muscles.

Weightlifters do train Squats and Deadlifts on the same day and get good results. They might alternate the Deadlifts with Goodmorning or pulls and the Squat with jump Squat, overhead Squat, front Squat, or lunges. Modern Weightlifters can Squat and Deadlift every day, as long as the load volume and intensity curve are being monitored. Thus, it seems that your soreness is attributed to excessive volume due to either high repetitions or excessive weight. In addition, the low frequency of training prevents progressive increase of tolerated load volume.

18.8.10. SQUATS AND BENCH PRESS SYNERGY

Question: I read an article that claims that squatting before the Bench Press is synergetic. It's got to do with the expansion of the ribcage or something...never heard of it. The article claims that when you are squatting by placing a heavy barbell on your neck, you stop the blood flow in a couple of veins in your neck. The body will react by asking more oxygen to compensate. Also, when you are squatting, you are using the biggest muscle group in the body, which asks a lot of extra oxygen. This extra demand of oxygen puts more stress on the lungs. You will try to breathe in more than the volume the lungs can take. The lungs will be stretched outwards and the tendon plate (above the sternum) will be pushed outwards. This will make the ribcage expand and stretch the pectoral muscles to the full. When the pectoral muscle is fully stretched, you will get optimal results out of the Bench Press or other pectoral exercise (this goes for all muscles).

Comment:
o We do not place a barbell on major veins during back Squat. We place it on the spine of shoulder plates. The tiny veins that were crushed by the barbell are of minor significance and their debris would trigger the development of a new cushioning layer of fat and fibrous tissue to support the barbell. That same process occurs in different parts of the body that deals with external pressure. Examples are the soles, palms, and buttocks. However, during front Squat, the bar might fall on the major vessels on the front of the neck and this has to be counter balanced by strong Deltoids. When

the Deltoids are weak, the bar in the front Squat stops the blood flow to the arms and head and causes failure or termination of lifting.
- The high demand for Oxygen does not come from over-inflated lungs. We breathe maximally when we perform instantaneously vigorous acts. Squatting is a prolonged act. Therefore, the extra demand for Oxygen comes from opening new vascular beds in the pulmonary parenchyma and by pumping more blood to the pulmonary circulation. Watch a person while squatting. He or she does not hyperventilate. Yet, their pulmonary circulation is enhanced. Like all resistance exercises, contracted muscles trigger the sympathetic system to increase heart rate and stoke volume. Thus, the fully stretched pectoral muscle during squatting is farfetched. I do think that alternating squatting and Bench-Pressing, in the same workout, are synergistic but through sympathetic control mechanisms.
- The common belief that Squat is more tiring and undermines the Bench Press is true for unconditioned people, but not in regular trainees. If you squat every day even at low volume and intensity you will be able to tolerate the Squat like any other convenient exercise.

18.8.11. SQUATTING WITH RAISED TOES OR HEELS

Question: Some people suggest placing a 25-pound plate under each foot, under the arch of the toes or under the heels during squatting. I have trouble enough keeping my balance when I am doing the Squats, but putting weights under my legs for any exercise would seem like suicide. Have I been doing my Squats wrong? Is it true that elevating the toes (as opposed to doing it on a block or flat-footed) isolates Hams and Glutes, and is easier on the lower back (which should stay arched)?

Comment:
- Raising the heels or toes during Squatting are old and well-known ways of enhancing the range of motion of ankles, knees, hips, back, and neck. This shifts the center of gravity of the body forwards (when heels are raised) or backwards (when toes are raised) thus forces all body joints to function differently in order to maintain body balance.
- Raised heels forces the lower back to exaggerate its inward arch and thus increases the work of the Iliopsoas and spinal erectors in stabilizing the pelvis.
- Raised toes over-stretch the Achilles tendon and put more emphasis on the Iliopsoas to pull the torso forward when the center of gravity is shifted backwards.
- Both positions should be practiced occasionally, using lightweights in order to gradually tolerate stretch. The problem you have described indicates poor conditioning allover the spinal axis. This requires adequate warm-up, stretching, progressive weight training, and diversity of exercises.

18.8.12. ROUNDED BACK DURING SQUATTING

Question: Many people advised me never to round my back in Squat claiming that that places tremendous pressure on the lower lumbar region and can lead to serious injury. I think that is total crap. Many people do Squat with a rounded back just as many people do Squat with arched back. There is not only one correct way to do the exercise. No matter how you do well in Squat, you are going to put stress on your lower back.

Comment:
- If many people perform Squats with a rounded back this doesn't make it right. Many people also are injured during training. Many people also don't have a clue as to how to exercise properly. Just because "many" people do things doesn't mean that it is correct. While certain aspects of a movement can be subject to individual interpretation, others are endemic to the move. What you're basically saying is that there is no basis for proper form. I can't disagree with you more. If you keep slightly lordotic back, the erectors will act as stabilizers during the movement. Keeping the lower back tight will greatly reduce the stress to this area. This isn't a debatable point. Keeping the spines in their natural alignment, means that the spines are correctly supported. Rounding the back means that load is being applied in directions it shouldn't be, and eventually weak links are going to crumble. See *Table 2.1* on "Comparison of lordotic versus kyphotic postures during lifting."
- With a rounded back, three major events may take place.
    i. First, the erector **spinal muscles** may shut off. This means that all the stress is now thrown onto the posterior ligaments of the spine. In the case of an injury, a ligamentous sprain takes a lot longer to heal than a muscular strain. You're looking at a few days for the strain, 2-3 months for the sprain.
    ii. Second, there is a posterior force imposed on the nucleus pulposus of the **spinal discs**. This can eventually lead to tearing of the annular fibers and a posterior disc herniation. Thus, rounding your back while performing any forceful work can cause crippling injuries. Because the vertebral support will be unbalanced and might cause the

discs to herniated. This can cause injuries ranging from benched peripheral nerve to total lower body paralysis.

iii. Third, the spinal cord can also suffer from venous congestion, which can cause internal bleeding inside the spinal cord, at the lumber region, without any herniation. Lifting can also cause paralysis in rare cases of spinal cord abnormalities without disc herniation but with internal spinal cord bleeding. In this case, total lower body paralysis ensues while trying to lift from the floor. Thus, sudden shearing forces can invoke the internal bleeding and paralysis.

- You seem to think that stressing the lower back is like stressing any other part of the body. The lower back carries the vital spinal cord and should be kept as straight as can be to secure that vital neural highway. Rounding the back is therefore wrong, whether done in Deadlift, in Leg Press, in Squat, or in Goodmorning. Your lower back should maintain a slight lordotic curve and remain tight throughout the move.

18.9. LEARNING THE HANG CLEAN

Question: I tried the hang Clean for the first time after reading a description of the lift. The Clean part of the movement is causing me some difficulty. I bend the knees slightly, try to do an explosive upright row-type movement without using leg drive to assist and my heels come up off the ground, throwing me forwards and off-balance slightly. Doesn't feel right, somehow, what am I doing wrong?

Comment:
- The forward hip drive puts you up on your toes and slightly off balance, or at least it will feel that way if you are new to it. In fact, if you're coming up on your toes, you're likely doing a lot of things right. You should be using leg and hip drive. The hang Clean isn't just about upper body strength. It is about coordinating complex reflexes.
- One thing to watch out for is allowing the bar to get too far out in front of you. Ideally, it will be a microscopic distance away from your shirt, but it is not an ideal world. This reduces the forward torque of displaced center of mass of the barbell.
- Since you are only one day old into the Hang Clean, you are on the right track. It would take weeks and months of improvements to get your neuromuscular balance to tip top shape. The Hang Clean is not Biceps curls, it cannot be executed with the Biceps drive. The main drive in the Hang Clean comes from the Trapezius. The Biceps only stabilize the elbows until the Trapezius and posterior Deltoids pull the arms and scapulas maximally upwards.
- The basic leverage in the Hang Clean comes from the forward bouncing of the head and backward bouncing of the hips, during the prestretch position, then the reversing of the bouncing of the head and hips by the explosive action of the spinal erectors. This explosive torso extension facilitates the action of the Trapezius and Deltoids in pulling the bar upwards.
- Thus, what is wrong with your technique is your short experience. You will not pull from the hang by Biceps curls when you advance in the Clean. You will rather learn how to create the momentum by speeding the upper body rotation on the hips and toes and transferring such momentum to the bar with solid and straight arms synchronized with robust Trapezius shrugging and Deltoid abduction of the shoulders. See Section 5.2.6 on "Hang Clean".

18.10. OVERHEAD DUMBBELL PRESS

Question: Back when I was tiny and using the 30-pound dumbbells for overhead presses, I had no problems. Even a few months ago when I would top out with the 70 pounders. There really wasn't much of a problem. But now I'm using 90 pound dumbbells and I'm having problems getting them up to my shoulders, especially when I do them later in the workout and I'm fatigued. I change my workout regularly. I've tried kicking them up off of my knees, and doing a sort of "cheat curl" as well. Both work to some extent, but not all the time. Any help with ways to get heavier dumbbells up to one's shoulders when training alone?

Comment:
- If it makes you feel any better, the handful (more like 2 or 3) of guys at my gym who can overhead press 90 lb dumbbells all require assistance to get the dumbbells in position. Usually, one or two guys will lift the dumbbells into position for them. Swinging 90 lb bells into position for an overhead press looks like a high-risk activity, from an injury point of view.
- Unless you have spotters, using your knees to get them up is about the only way you can do it unless you train on the Clean and Snatch styles of Weightlifting. It is easier if you start the dumbbell on the very end of the thigh, at the knee,

FREQUENTLY ASKED QUESTIONS

lean slightly forward and then lean back and push up with your knees at the same time. If this cheat curl-knee catapult preposition doesn't work, you probably need someone to help. This technique can be murder on you back, shoulders, and just about any other part of your body as well. Just make sure the arc is slightly towards the inside of your shoulder. If you use a strong kick, and the dumbbell winds up outside of your shoulder, you're setting yourself up for injury of the rotator cuff muscles.

o There are some nifty clamps that work well when you can't get help with heavy weights. They are about $40 and work as hangers that hold the dumbbells in position attached to a racked Olympic bar, so you can get under them. All you need is something that has an Olympic bar at the desired height, could be a power rack, Bench Press stand, or whatever. Put the clamps on the dumbbells, hoist the dumbbell/clamp with both hands onto the bar, do the other dumbbell and then take them off the bar. This is safer and easier on the back than any alternative one-hand lifting.

o An alternative routine is to do barbell presses first then do the dumbbell press when you will be more tired and not need as heavy dumbbells. Alternatively, do one hand at a time. Take one 90-pound dumbbell, lift it up with two hands and then do one set with one arm, then stop and repeat procedure for other arm. In addition, you can try lowering the dumbbell to the lowest point on the shoulder thus you can use a lighter weight and still get a good workout.

o Another alternative is to try to do them standing, and cleaning (using the Clean lift) the dumbbells into position. Thus, you can learn the dumbbell Clean in the process of Shoulder Press. To do that, kneel in front of rack and maneuver the two dumbbells onto shoulders then stand and walk to seat and sit down with them. Once you learn decent technique, a single Clean won't wear you down at all. This would be a perfect opportunity to learn the dumbbell Clean. Since in most gyms the dumbbell area is always crowded and doing standing Shoulder Press after the Clean will obviate the need for a bench. This helps incorporating some variety in your workout without messing up your shoulder or at least not stressing them very effectively.

o Modern machines can do the same effect of dumbbell press. The "Hammer Strength" Shoulder Press plate-loaded machine is an example of such modern day gadgets.

o Arthritic changes in the shoulder could set a plateau and a cessation of progress in getting stronger. You have to strengthen the entire envelope of the shoulder to breakthrough a plateau, not just Overhead Press with dumbbells. Spotting by others, with inflamed shoulder, induces more injury. If you cannot lift it freely and nicely from the floor, you should not try to fiddle with it, since you may incur serious injury if you force it on your poor shoulders.

o There is more to weight training than just getting fixated on a single dumbbells press exercise. Try new techniques, new bodily regions, or new approaches. The golden rules of fitness encompass elements other than strength alone, such as flexibility, endurance, coordination, and speed. It is very dangerous to assume that physical strength progresses linearly without supervised training program. The main reason that you have plateaued at 90 lb dumbbell press is that you have ignored the other elements of fitness. This resulted in weak axial muscles that cannot lift the dumbbells from the floor to your shoulders. You should strengthen the Deadlift, Pulls, and Clean muscles in order to prevent spinal injuries during the dumbbell press.

o All athletes plateau in their lifetime, temporarily or permanently. Because of boredom, overtraining, lack of training, etc. Do not limit your thinking to muscular power alone. There are times when your cardiovascular system cannot catch up with your musculoskeletal vigor. Turn your attention to other exercises until you accumulate strength in other areas of your body, then you can try to breakthrough the plateau of dumbbell pressing.

18.11. PERSONAL TRAINERS

Question: I'm interested in getting a personal trainer but want to get some information. Is there a difference between personal trainers who work at the gym versus those who don't?

Comment:

o A personal trainer is a great asset to encouraging trainees to learn and work out. For new beginners, trainers can foster social acquaintance with gym environment and alleviate anxiety of new comers. For little profit, they share their invaluable knowledge and motivation with the people they train.

o Trainers as well as book authors are not flawless. Yet, a personal trainer offers the greatest sacrifice of personal interaction and dedicated time of guidance and motivation. The live presence is very effective in conveying overwhelming wealth of knowledge in short time and with personal touch. This might require formidable effort without the generosity and dedication of personal trainers.

o It is very demanding to train people. It would take at least three years of hard work to see substantial results. It is thus a good idea to begin with any available trainer and improve later, either by finding another trainer with advanced knowledge, or by advancing you knowledge with other means such as reading books, browsing web sites, or talking to experts in the field.

o Trainer's certifications are easy to get for many people after browsing a textbook for a few hours. Even such task, of obtaining certification and studying for it, signifies the seriousness and curiosity of the person that is interested in training others.

o Young trainers, however, do bizarre things, which have a higher risk of injury and a lower chance of making you stronger than what a sensible and rational person would recommend. In addition, just because someone is muscular does not make him an expert on training.

18.12. POWERLIFTING VERSUS BODYBUILDING

Question: Which one builds muscle fast? All the Powerlifters I see are really big but usually not cut. What are the best routines for Powerlifting? I am thinking about going the power route.

Comment:
o Since you sound to be new to the field of strength training, judging by your concern about muscular appearance and the aura of power, I suggest that you keep open mind and start gathering information about physical fitness and muscular balance. The boundaries between Bodybuilding, Powerlifting, Weightlifting, and weight training are but artificial ones. These boundaries do not amount to any sound or reasonable route to fitness and health. Thus, do not become mystified by such apparently authoritative brand names of fitness sports.

o Bodybuilding can be part of all sports when muscle size and strength require specific attention. Bodybuilding for the mere purpose of cutting and appearance is fun and simple since there is not complex technique involved. It is possible to remedy the flaws of Bodybuilding routines by adding few compound exercises to daily workouts that enhance coordination and flexibility. Power Clean, Power Snatch and Jump Squat are examples of these remedial exercises.

o Powerlifting differs from Bodybuilding in the training time and intensity requirements. Powerlifters perform fewer exercises at higher intensity and concentrate on axial muscles. The drawbacks of Powerlifting when it is limited to the Bench Press, Squat, and Deadlifts and their assisting exercises are the lack of flexibility, agility, and coordination. All these flaws can be easily avoided if brought to attention and tackled by remedial exercises. Running, swimming, aerobics, and Calisthenics are examples of such remedial exercises.

18.13. SHAKINESS DURING RESISTANCE TRAINING

Question: I've run into this problem lately. By the time I reach my third set of upper body exercises, I notice that my arms begin to quiver when I push or pull up. I don't think it is weight-related because I feel no stress in lifting. However, something tells me it's related to "nutrition". Any ideas what I might be doing wrong? I certainly don't exercise on an empty stomach.

Comment:
o One possibility is that you might be out of your **weight range**. When you increase the weight beyond your ability and in fewer sets, your system may not be ready to integrate cardiopulmonary and neuromuscular function to the fullest. For starters, slowly increase the weight, drop your maximum poundage, and do the movement by feel, not ego. Proper technique is a good indication that your poundage range is appropriate for specific date and time of training. It's impossible to know without more specific information on your training. However, a likely cause is activation of your tendon sensors, the Golgi tendon organs. These are proprioceptors located in your tendons. When your muscles are sufficiently fatigued by the weight that is exceeding previously known resistance, these sensors signal your motoneurons to relax your working muscles to prevent overload. Thus, at the end of your set, your muscles are being placed under stress yet your nervous system is trying to stop them from contracting. This causes them to quiver.

FREQUENTLY ASKED QUESTIONS

- o   Another possibility is that your muscles are easily depleted from **ATP supply**. This happen in low intake of calories, long hours of exhaustion in other activities (such as endurance exercises), and lack of sleep. ATP is replenished by the Creatine Phosphate pump, which in turn is replenished by the break down of glycogen into lactates in order to generate more ATP molecules. Regular and serious training promote the enzymatic activity of the Glycogen-Creatine Phosphate-ATP cycles such that shaking is delayed or concealed during regular training.

- o   Shaking also is a sign of **intense physical effort**. Many people don't recognize it as such because they have never achieved that level of effort. When muscles contract intensely they trap the blood and reduce the venous return to the heart, which has to compensate by rising the heart rate of beating and the force of pumping per stroke. When such compensation is outpaced by muscular intensity, circulatory deprivation ensues and shaking occurs. It is a normal reaction for high intensity workout.

- o   Exercising on full stomach can cause shaking as well by hampering respiration and diverting blood from active muscles to the guts.

- o   **Arrhythmias** or irregular heart beats in reaction to resistance can be cause by caffeine, smoking, lack of sleep, overtraining, or organic causes and can cause shaking due to oxygen deprivation. Irregular heartbeats can also result from thiamine deficiency due to accumulation of pyruvic acid and diminished ability of cellular energy production. Thiamine is essential in converting pyruvate to Acyl-Coenzyme-A, which ready to enter the Citric acid cycle in the mitochondria of cells.

- o   **Muscular imbalance** is very common in people who do not exercise consistently. If your weekly training frequency is less than three sessions per week, your session duration less than an hour, and your exercise picking is not balancing major muscle groups, then your muscles will not be conditioned to deal with resistance for long.

Chapter 19
Training Women

19.1. LONG-TERM STRUCTURED TRAINING FOR WOMEN

19.1.1. NEW TRENDS

The dramatic increase in participation of women in sport could be easily attributed to the advent in modern communication. This has eliminated barriers of ignorance, regarding health concerns of half of the population. As is the case with other minority participation, women have contributed significantly to the evolution of sport. They have excelled in the healthy aspect of sport such as aerobics, yoga, and Olympic sports. The following issues are of particular concern regarding the participation of women in strength training.

o   Most if not all women trainees do not subscribe to **long-term structured training.** Even in developed countries, barriers still exist that limit women's rights to equal employment, equal burden in sharing family responsibility, and equal safety of mobility in urban an rural cities during all times of the day. For example, a single parent mom, who is stuck with the financial burden of raising children, is still required to pay the same membership fees to health clubs and endure all other expenses of transportation and auxiliary support, as does a single man.
o   Most if not all women view strength training as a secondary **nonessential activity**. The misperception that strength training and feminine appearance are exclusive has deterred many women from participation in weight training. Many women believe that physical strength is a man's only nature.
o   Many **diseases** that are exclusive to women could be prevented with structured weight training. Without exercise, modern women succumb to many preventable diseases that are caused by the new lifestyle of industrialized society. For the difference between women and men, in prevalence, incidence, and death rates from preventable diseases, see Chapter 15.
o   In complete opposite to men's involvement in weight training, women's involvement is mainly attributed to higher level of **education and social and economic awareness** of the impact of exercise on health. In the not so far past, as well as in many current third world nations, women perform very demanding physical activities that keep them healthier than man, in particular, in the absence of smoking, alcohol, and caffeine usage in that groups

19.1.2. DEVELOPMENT

o   Long-term exercise is required to build healthy body. The growth of a **developing newborn**, from infancy to childhood to adulthood, is real evidence that human body develops through well-defined sequence of changes before reaching maturity. While a developing child goes through many organ development, grown up trainees experience similar, but different sequence of changes, in response to exercise.
o   Take the example of learning to ride a pike. After few days of trying, a beginner could master the skill of balancing his body on a pike. The skill is refined as training continues. Yet, at certain ages, **specific skills** could not be mastered as good as in younger age. Many years after learning certain physical skills, many folks find it easy to perform the past-learned skill in relatively shorter time, compared to those without past exposure.
o   Physical skills are mastered by very **complex brain system**. Long-term exercise might reserve a specific brain area to store past experience. Unlike memory storage of dreams and feeling, performance memory stores various aspects of force, speed, balance, muscular recruitments, and visual and sensory coordination. Modern research on learning languages at old age points to the fact that a second learned language by an individual is dealt with in different brain areas than one's mother language. Apart from the effect of long-term training on the brain development and memory, concrete developments take place at the cellular level of exercising organs.

19.1.3. BRAIN AND BODY MASTERY

To understand the changes that take place in the human body, as a result of adherence to long-term exercise, one needs to have a general idea about how the human body performs motor functions. The lengthy physiological events that take place, from the beginning of an IDEA, to commencing EXERCISE, to the final reaction of the body to such an adventure, are summarized as follows.

- Most probably, the very first event takes place in the form of an **"idea"** and **"will" to initiate events**. No such idea would spring without external events such as visual observation or discussions. The brain is the center of intelligence and information about one's own body. Strong will is the result of all concerns a person has. The younger the person is the stronger the will to channel own resources to master a new activity.
- The second event would logically deals with how to **prioritize such new discovery** of participation in new activity, with respect to other concerns.
    i. Just few decades ago, exercise was viewed as clownish activity or a sort of keeping the young busy. Remnants of that old generation still exist who believe that exercise is a sort of trivial play of marginal folks. Many well-educated and influential figures of the past suffered unduly from diseases that are completely preventable by exercise and habit modification. The old perception of sport passes to the new generation through **familial** and **cultural** interaction and affects one's ability to prioritize the significance of participating in exercise.
    ii. The influence of **modern society** on promoting health and fitness awareness is driven by the economic cost of caring for preventable diseases. Thus, promoting participation in exercise by women may be the most cost-effective task that society can undertake to reduce the cost of health care. **Women's health** differs significantly from men's health in many aspects. Women have highly active physiological processes that affect the bone, kidneys, digestion, heart, blood vessels, and mental status. The periodic blood loss and active endocrine systems put the women's health on constant motion, as follows.
        a. The **thyroid** function sustains the bone morrow periodic extra activity.
        b. The **parathyroid** function balances the bone and kidney regulation of calcium and potassium.
        c. The **adrenal** function sustains the cardiovascular dynamics of such active physiological changes.
        d. The **pancreatic** function sustains the extra digestive effort needed to maintain balanced nutritional status.
        e. The **pituitary** and the **hypothalamus** master the entire woman physiology during these periodical changes.
        f. Long-term exercise promotes that entire endocrine system and stability in reacting to the stress of training. When exposed to **stressful events**, people who do not engage in long-term exercise suffer from circulatory disturbance that could precipitate falls, heart arrhythmias that could cause sudden death, long recovery from pain that could impair many organs, and transient traumatic episodes that could cause severe long-term injuries.
- Having initiated the will to exercise and prioritized its significance in one's daily activities, the brain conveys such messages to the limbs, internal organs, and sensors via bundles of nerves called **"neural tracts"**. The **first neural tract** originates from the brain and ends in the brain stem, midbrain, or cerebellum (right under the brain hemispheres). It coveys the brain's decision to the lower systems. The purpose of the first station (ending of neural tract and start of another) is obtaining vital data from the brain stem, midbrain, and cerebellum, along with the higher brain signal, to carry them to the second neural tract. This data regards consciousness, visual (eye), auditory (ears), olfactory (nose), respiratory, circulatory, and balance issues (inner ears).
- The **second neural tract** descends, from where the first ends, and travels along the spinal cord or brain stem to reach the second station, inside the central nervous system. The second neural tract has, in addition to higher brain messages, signals from vital regulatory centers to convey to other organs. For example, lifting one's leg in the air, while laying on the back, forces the other leg to push down against the ground to support the body from spinning. A dull will not show such reflex. Thus, one leg has to relate to the other, with and without the brain interference, but with the control of the equilibrium reflex in the inner ears.
- The **third neural tract** leaves the central nervous system, from where the second ends, and travels to the final destination to the organ it is destined to affect. The third component carries messages from parts of the body around the local parts of the spinal cord or brain stem they correspond to. This specialized communication between the brain and body organs, and in-between body organs, is affected greatly with long-term exercise. A talented golfer, for example, would have very efficient brain-to-body communication to be able to master his external environment in such way as to excel in golf.
- Long-term exercise affects the genetic expression of the **relay neurons** that transmit and generate signals between nerves. Genetic expression of enzymes, their level activity and abundance, and the sensitivity of their receptors and destructors, greatly affect the performance of the body. Such genetic modification in response to exercise might also transmit to off springs thus fosters the evolution theory.
- The **peripheral nerves**, the third neural tracts (the peripheral nerves), reach their destinations at the muscles, joints, tendons, blood vessels, internal organs, and sensors. At the muscles, the nerve ends on the muscle membrane at a specialized nerve-to-muscle conversion structure (**neuromuscular junction**). The nerve signal releases a chemical substance (**Acetylcholine**), which stimulates receptors on the muscle membrane. The stimulated receptors trigger the spread of electrical stimulation of as many muscle fibers. Conveying signals from nerves to muscles depends on the availability of the Acetylcholine secreted, their receptors, their duration of action, and the ability of the muscle membrane to respond.
- Long term training guarantees well developed muscles, neuromuscular joints and active mechanism of nerve-to-muscle communication. The amount and rates of secretion of Acetylcholine, and its breakdown, are dependent of long-term exercise. The muscle membrane responds to the nerve signal by pumping out potassium from inside its cells (from the

inside of the cell to the outside) and pumping in sodium from outside the cells. With simple physics, such pumping process spread **electrical stimulation along the muscle membrane**. That is because the ions of potassium differ from the ions of sodium in the number of electrons on their outer surface, at similar ion concentration.
- o The **pumping activity** of the muscle membrane is a highly complex enzymatic process, regulated by the cell genes. Long-term training develops properly responsive muscle membrane. In specific disease process, high intake of carbohydrates causes failure of the muscle membrane pump. This pump failure traps the **potassium** ions inside the cells and prevents their release. Such disease causes total muscular paralysis after carbohydrate ingestion and total recovery with potassium administration. Long-term training educates the person of the causes of his or her troubles in performing physical activities.
- o Having responded to nervous stimulation, the muscle membrane conveys the signals to specific structures inside the muscle fibers that release calcium ions when stimulated. Calcium release triggers the smallest muscle **protein units** (Actomyosin), within the tiniest muscle fibers, to slide and produce muscular contraction.
- o Cellular enzymes control both muscular contraction and relaxation. The activity and synthesis of cellular enzymes are affected by long-term exercises through genetic modification by exercises. **Endurance training** differs from **strength training** in regulating the manner the way cells produce enzymes and the way cells oxygenate byproducts. Endurance exercise requires very efficient mitochondria oxygenation process to deal with lengthy aerobic process, while strength training is mainly anaerobic. Such microscopic cellular adaptation to exercise does not take place in short-term casual exercise.
- o Contracting muscles impose certain demands on the body. Sudden **drop in blood return** to the heart follows even the slightest muscular contraction. This serves the purpose of providing the muscle with a rich pool of blood nutrients. The priorly mentioned nervous communication triggers the blood pressure sensors in the carotid arteries and blood gases sensors in the major blood vessels to detect the drop in blood return to the heart and correct the deficit by increasing the **heart rate and force of contraction**.

19.1.4. ADAPTATION TO LONG-TERM EXERCISE

Although physiological adaptations to exercise have been discussed in Chapters 10, 11, 14-16, they are rehashed below for the purpose of augmenting the present topic.
- o **Cardiovascular adaptation:** Long-term training refines this adaptation mechanism and saves the trainee the trouble of sudden heart attacks, coma in poorly conditioned people, or failure while lifting heavy weight. Regular vigorous exercise prepares the coronary arteries of the heart for episodic disturbance in blood flow during exercise. The fact that some well-trained athletes die from coronary heart disease at the peak of their performance does not negate against the importance of regular exercise in reducing the prevalence of heart disease. Heavy athletes, in particular, are at risk of coronary heart problems, while light athletes are at risk of heart rhythm irregularities. Even partially clogged coronary arteries can benefit from exercise by generating new coronary capillaries, in response to long-term exercise.
- o **Neural adaptation:** The quickness of response of the autonomic nervous system to the drop of blood return to the heart, due to muscular contraction, determines the **strength of the person**. A delay in response means that the blood flow in coronary arteries would drastically diminish, forcing the heart to reduce its ability to pump blood or even stop beating. Delayed response also mean less blood flow through the lungs. This forces the entire body to suffer from lack of oxygen with reduction in muscular strength or even paralysis and loss of oxygenation to the brain, causing syncope or even coma. A poorly conditioned person shows clear facial alteration to lividity, in response to slightest muscular contraction. This is attributed to the response of the autonomic nervous system to stress. With long-term training, better response of the autonomic system prioritizes blood flow to vital organs, during exercise, and reduces flow to the skin and nonessential areas of the body.
- o **Respiratory adaptation:** Blood flow through the lungs during exercise is a determining factor in physical fitness. Long-term training regulates the response of the lungs during stressful exercises. Unconditioned persons suffer sudden lung congestion, coughing, or asthma during stress. Not only the adequacy of blood flow through the lung that improves with lengthy training, but also the response of the lungs to the speedy air ventilation. In untrained people, this causes dryness and irritation during exercise. Interrupting training for few months reflects clearly in the inability of the lungs to deal with hyperventilation, during exercise, in the form of acute coughing and dryness of throat on performing exercises that were mastered in the past. Few days may elapse before the person could tolerate prior level of stressful training.
- o **Bone adaptation:** Women are not in lesser need for long-term training as men. Developing healthy heart, lung, and nervous control are the least benefits gained from strength training. The most specific issue to women health is bone integrity. Without proper exercise and nutrition, women are at higher risk of osteoporosis than males of the same age. Bone serves as a depot of solid fuel, in addition to its mechanical supportive function. During the lengthy hours between meals, and the longer hours or even days between ingestion of specific rare nutritional elements, bone supplies blood circulation with vital ions (phosphate and calcium) to sustain the different biological reactions, allover

the body. Phosphate is the major energy carrier in biological reactions, while calcium is the major regulator of such reactions. Thus, the maintenance of female reproductive function relies greatly on healthy bone. Lengthy training thickens and strengthens bone, which supplies nutrition and support to muscles. Immobility induces bone loss. The calcium produced by bone thinning might deposit in the blood vessels causing their hardening, or in the kidneys causing kidney stones.

- o **Mobility adaptation:** The above description of nervous control of muscular interaction with the central nervous system was simplified in order to address the general concept. The nervous system has many communicating tracts that convey messages from the muscles, tendons, joints, skin, and sensors to the brain and other organs. The two-way communication, between the central nervous system and active organs, explains the complexity of physical performance. Long-term exercise protects women from falls, fractures, and strained joints and help women enjoy healthy living to the most of their ability. The response of a trained woman to stumbling on an object, while walking or running or even after incurring traumatic accidents, is greatly enhanced by long term training that reduces adverse effects. Exercise benefits range from fast healing, avoidance of fall, better balance and agility, greater reserves of healing, cardiovascular, and respiratory power.

19.2. WOMEN'S VIEW OF STRENGTH TRAINING

- o **Masculine look:** Tackling the fallacy that strength training is exclusive to men might be the first step to be taken in training women of adult age. Many women with advanced muscular weakness and overweight due to lack of mobility would argue that they are frightened of working out to avoid looking masculine. The fact is that even very progressive strength training would not cause women to look masculine. Abnormal female masculinity is either due to internal physiological disorder or to intake of masculinizing hormones. Exercise does not deform feminine contours as long as the woman keeps optimum bodyweight.
- o **Fear of injuries:** Structured long-term training is the best learning activity; a person can indulge in, to understand the day-to-day alteration in bodily physiology. Common mishaps are attributed to one's misunderstanding of exercise. Consider the commonly back injuries as an example. Most back injuries recover by immediate exercise, as soon as the acute pain subsides. Back injuries are preventable by exercise and are precipitated by the lack of it. The same could be said about knee injuries. Knee injuries fare better when the muscles around the knee are kept robust by strength training. Thus, the second issue to tackle in training women is stressing the gainful aspect of exercise, even in case of injury.
- o **Muscles and systems:** Third, is the scope of time required to see fruitful results. Embarking on a proper training plan could quickly (in a matter of few weeks) improve the breathing ability and cardiovascular response to stressful exercises. Women are not different from men in the rate of gaining strength and coordination. Many women adhere to certain exercise routines, when they discover the benefits of such regimen. It is crucial to explain that muscles do not develop in vain apart from bone, heart, lungs, and nervous system. Although exercise appears to deal with muscles, muscles do not properly work without oxygen that is supplied by the lungs, in proportion to the increased stress, blood nutrients supplied by heart beating, nervous balance and control that is provided by the nerves and the brain. All organs participate in proportion of the level of difficulty of exercise. The longer is the time spent in training, the more apparent the gain would be.
- o **Adequate exercise:** Less than one hour of strength training, for at least three days every week, would not do much good. Injuries increase in incidence with lesser training times. Apparently, unconnected symptoms, such as headache, constipation, shoulder pain, or leg cramps might be all attributed to lack or inadequacy of exercise. Many other physical complaints fall in line with few explanations such as poor cardiovascular reserve, diminished pulmonary reserve, poor digestion, or lack of passion to invigorating sport or hobby.

19.3. WOMEN'S EXERCISE AND PREVENTABLE DISEASES

The major preventable maladies that prevail in women population due to lack of exercise are osteoporosis, coronary heart disease, arthritis, falls and fracture due to lack of coordination, obesity, depression, urinary incontinence due to lax pelvic muscles, and postural deformities due to weak muscular tone. These are briefly discussed in the following paragraphs.

- o **Osteoporosis:** This is a condition of bone thinning due to loss of calcium. Most causes of osteoporosis are preventable. Muscular strengthening stimulates the bone cells to strengthen its structure by depositing more minerals. Exercise, also, could reduce the overgrowth of intestinal bacteria by avoiding stagnation of intestinal contents for unduly lengthy periods. Overgrowth of intestinal bacteria hinders the absorption of vitamin D and calcium and worsens osteoporosis. In addition to exercise, balanced nutrition should be examined for the specific needs of the individual (see Section 14.3.6 on "Healthy Diet"). Osteoporosis that is caused by parathyroid tumor or diseases of the kidney, liver, or intestine requires more than just exercise and nutrition. The causative abnormality has to be corrected.

- **Coronary heart disease:** Long-term exercise, beginning at earlier age, enhances the vascular flow to the heart muscles and prevents the obstruction of blood vessels. Regular exercise prepares the heart for extreme unpredictable circumstances such as the stresses of the state of fright, extreme cold, heat stroke, overeating, indigestion, or even the stress of conducting daily physical duties, such as shoveling snow without prior conditioning. Since exercise forces the bone to mineralize, this prevents the calcium ions from depositing within the walls of the blood vessels but rather in the bone matrix. Some believe that even calcified hardened blood vessels could be chelated (removing the deposited calcium from their walls) by long term exercise. Healthy arteries are devoid from calcium deposits and tolerate both normal and turbulent blood flow without developing thrombi.
- **Arthritis** due to weak muscle is explained by the fact that weak muscular support of a joint leads to extreme events within that joint, when minor mishaps occur. Such unstable joint incurs damage to its articulating surface. Without exercise, frequent damage takes place. In addition, due to the weakness of the muscles around the joints, blood circulation is diminished, causing ischemia (poor circulation) and aggravating pain. Chronic pain forces the person to abstain from moving. This causes more weakness of muscles and more instability to the joint. The vicious cycle continues. Arthritis due inflammation of the soft tissues of the joint such as rheumatoid arthritis, might have been preventable if exercise was commenced early in life. The fact that rheumatoid arthritis is caused by antibody immune mechanism could be interpreted, in part, by the accumulation of oxidants byproducts due to the lack of exercise. Even developed rheumatoid arthritis benefits from regular exercise by preventing deformities of joints due the constant destruction by inflammation, lack of use, stiffness, and weakness of the joints.
- **Falls and fractures** in women could be certainly prevented by improving muscle tone, coordination of visual and motor sensors, strengthening of bone, and enhancing the response of the cardiovascular, pulmonary, and nervous systems to accidental impulses. Falls induce new bone formation in the fractured limb. Incidents of developing bone cancer after falls are well documented. This signifies the importance of exercise to stabilize the equilibrium of the bone minerals with body needs.
- **Obesity** is another complex issue that afflicts modern society. Exercise and mobility are keys to preventing obesity. To overcome obesity we still should not eat every thing we wish, even if we exercise. Exercise should be used as a gauge to guide our eating habits to stay light, strong, and agile. Food that gets into the body and stays, as extra weight, impedes our ability to exercise and should be sought and avoided (see Chapters 14 and 15 for tips on eating, bodyweight, and exercise). Exercise is therefore not only an energy-burning mean, but also a monitoring tool to remind the person when limits have been breached.
- **Depression** is more diagnosed nowadays than few decades ago. Although the physiological mechanism of depression is better understood than before, yet the real causes of depression remain unknown. Depression that is not attributed to physical organic diseases, drug use, or precipitating emotional crises could be avoided by enhancing the sense of self-worthiness. Exercise is an invaluable activity that reverses the many centuries of oppression and demeaning of women. The complex physiology of women during and after the child bearing years is better understood today than in the near past. Exercise regulates the many hormonal processes that dominate women's health. Depression might result from the woman feeling of lack of energy and strength, shortage of resources to enjoy life and seek new opportunities as her man counterpart. In addition to its health benefits, exercise offers opportunities of reasoning and problem solving that maintains the mental process on the edge of improving living, rather than succumbing to the perils of emptiness and stagnation of sedentary living.
- **Urinary incontinence** is exclusively a women's malady that starts as early as the age of twenties. The main determinants of urinary incontinence are urinary infection, weak pelvic hammock (that support elevating the bladder, uterus, and rectum in the pelvic cavity), irritable bladder muscles, nervous disease, or bladder deformity due to mass or cyst or external process. Exercise benefits best in strengthening the lower abdominal muscles that support the bladder, uterus, and colon during walking, coughing, exercising, or bearing down. Exercise also enhances general health, which help resist infection and fasten the recovery of already existing infection. Long-term exercise prevents adult-onset diabetes and improves the symptoms of child-onset diabetes with positive effect on the bladder control.
- **Postural deformities:** Acquired postural deformities are mostly due to muscular weakness in the early years of life. Exercise educates children of the healthy habits of good posture while walking, sitting, or running. Back, shoulder, and pelvic deformities are very common in modern society. Many parents assume that children are destined to develop God-given body, posture, and personality. Exercise modifies many of such traits. Early life exercise is an impetus to growing children to value their immense potential and better their lives and the lives of others. Children who exercise get real life lessons on the nature of fostering the health of body and mind. With interaction with mature adult trainers, children evolve to improve the existing ideas to better ones, *Figures 19.1* thru *19.10*. Raising children to believe that food, exercise, and behavior affect their well being, in strictly logical manner, is the best exercise could do to nurturing the young. Many grown adults do not associate habits with problems that are cause by such habits. You might have known someone who seeks all sorts of weight reduction methods but the one, and only, that caused overweight, that is overeating. Postural deformities could be alleviated even if they are permanent. Strengthening the entire body as well as the muscles that counteract that deformity could drastically improve the quality of life of a person with persistent postural deformity.

19.4. WOMEN'S PARTICIPATION IN SPORT VERSUS MEN'S PARTICIPATION

o **Choice of activity:** In a class of aerobics, one might notice the presence of two or three guys in a room full of women. The opposite is true in a Weightlifting rooms. Few decades ago, women were hardly seen in public gyms. These discrepancies in the behavior of the two genders could be easily attributed to the lack of systemic training in childhood for both sexes. Strength training should not be exclusive to men. It only requires resources and long social support to get women to enjoy the luxury of playful fun activities. Most women cannot afford the cost of transportation, the time spent in activities that returns no immediate income, or the joy of being free from home responsibilities. Such resources are vital in building physical strength.

o **Strength and flexibility:** As men grow **heavier and stiffer,** with lack of exercise, they favor weight training that entails sitting and slow movements that do not challenge the heart and joints. Weight training of grown up adults, who do not have long history of training, requires hard planning to balance the shortening of tendons, stiffness of joints, and wasting of major muscles. Women on the other hand maintain better **flexibility and laxity** of many joints, even without exercise. Due to their lower bodyweight, women could endure stressful cardiovascular training better than men. Even heavy weight women could do better than their men counterparts can, in endurance, flexibility, and coordination exercises.

o **Endocrine burden:** Physical weakness forces women to rest or sleep for longer periods in order to recover from fatigue, produced by daily physical activities. Without strength training, the following compensatory endocrine changes take place:
  i. The **thyroid glands** work harder to compensate for the excessive metabolism of excessive daily activities.
  ii. The **adrenals** work harder to lend a kick to the adrenalin dependent activities.
  iii. The **pancreas** has to work harder to compensate for the constantly fluctuating blood sugar due to overeating and inactivity.

Exercise builds the active tissues-the muscles-that acts as a buffer for all body systems. With their higher metabolic nature, muscles provide a stable source of heat by burning fuel for energy. Muscles aid circulation and alleviate the hard work of the heart (the real solo pump). Men do not experience the chaotic endocrine fluctuation of women physiology. Thus, men struggle less with planning strength training than women. Designing load intensity-volume profile for women is very challenging. The most crucial aspect of such challenge is keeping watchful eyes on the blood and bone morrow conditions through out the menstrual cycle. Anemias should be corrected before advancing to chronic states.

o **Many psychosomatic disorders** that are prevalent in women population are thought to have unknown origin in modern medicine. With the obvious difference between women's and men's participation in sport and the obvious increase in women participation, as time passes on, one expects better understanding of the effect of exercise on women's health in the near future.

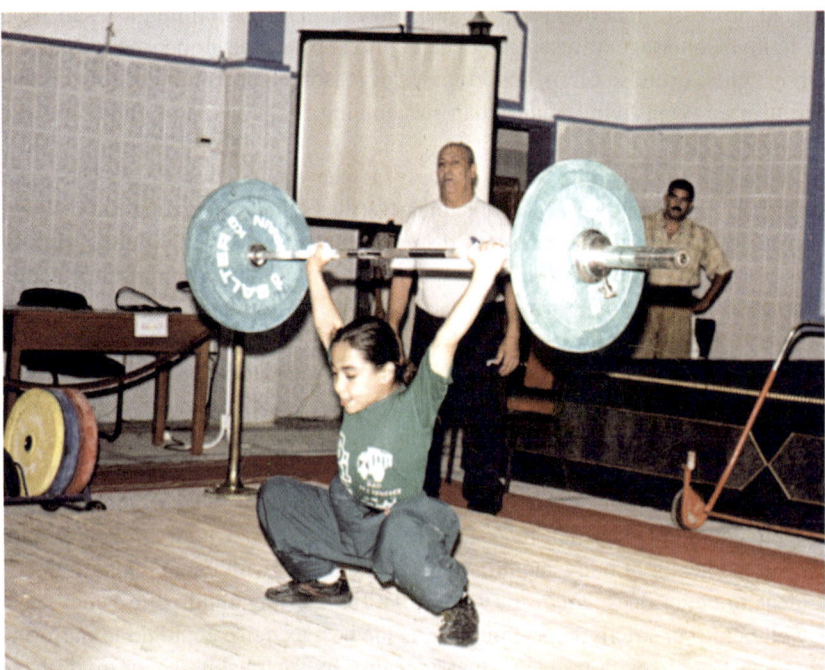

Figure 19.1. Young girls can learn and execute perfect Olympic style Snatch. This barbell weighs 45 kg. It is lifted with flawless technique, from the floor overheads, in full squatting position.

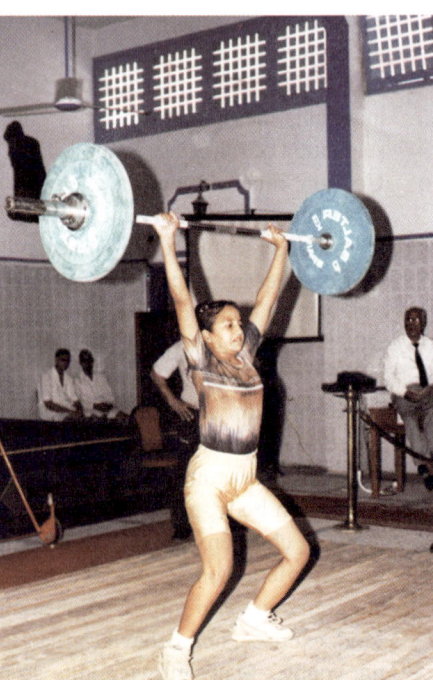

Figure 19.2. From the street gym to state gym and from the homemade barbell to the Olympic barbell. The eleven-year old can Clean and Jerk 45 kg with the new style of Jerk.

TRAINING WOMEN

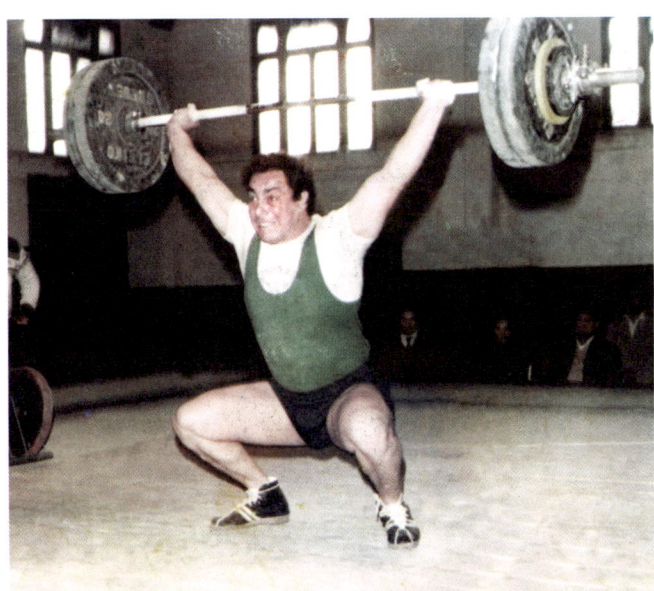

Figure 19.3. After competing in Weightlifting, Ramadan has coached his four children to lift weights, on the street, in front of his house. (See *Figure 13.22*). **Year 1971.**

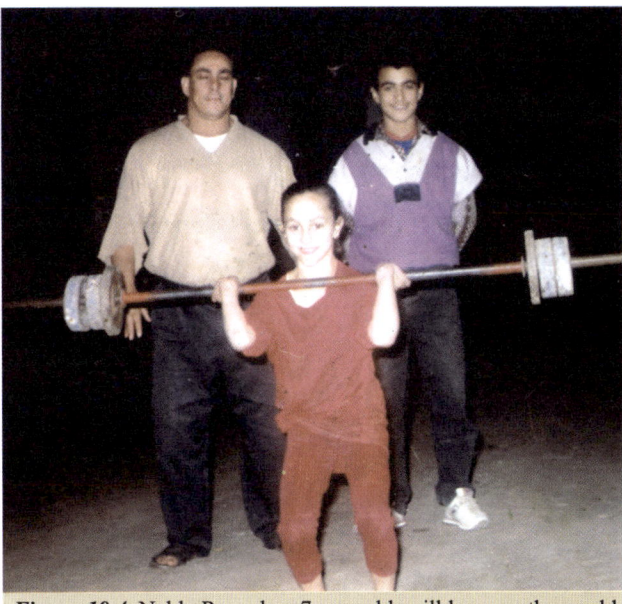

Figure 19.4. Nahla Ramadan, 7-year old, will become the world champion in 2003. (See *Figure 13.2*).

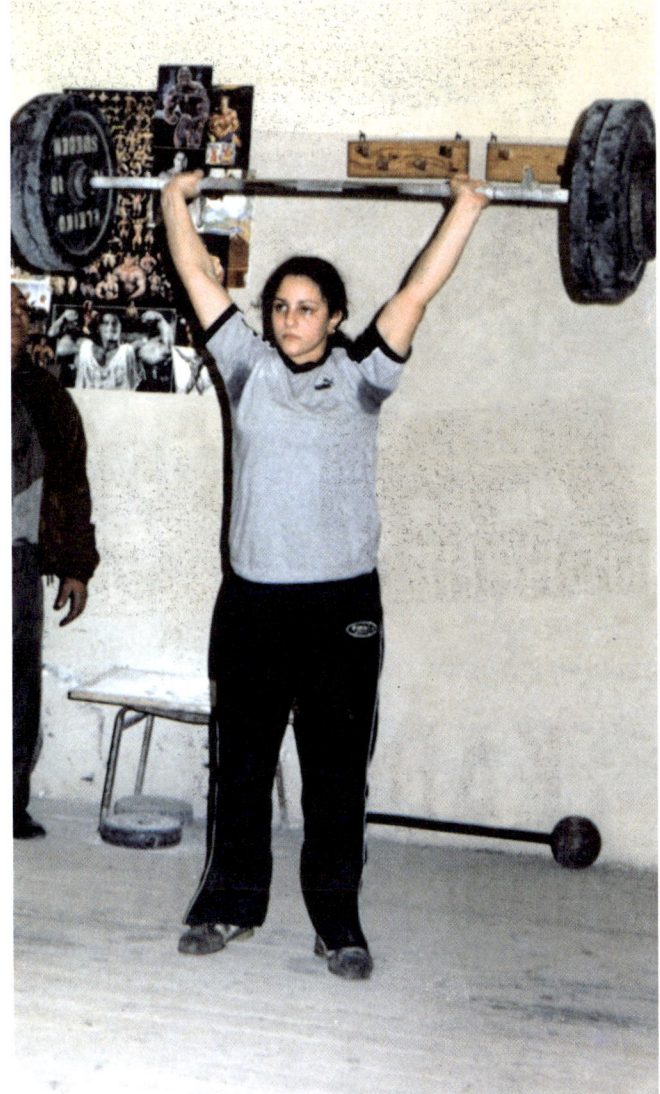

Figure 19.5. Nagham Ramadan, 15-year old. Training in front of their house on the Clean and Jerk of 110 kg. The father keeps close eyes on locking the elbows. **Year 2002.**

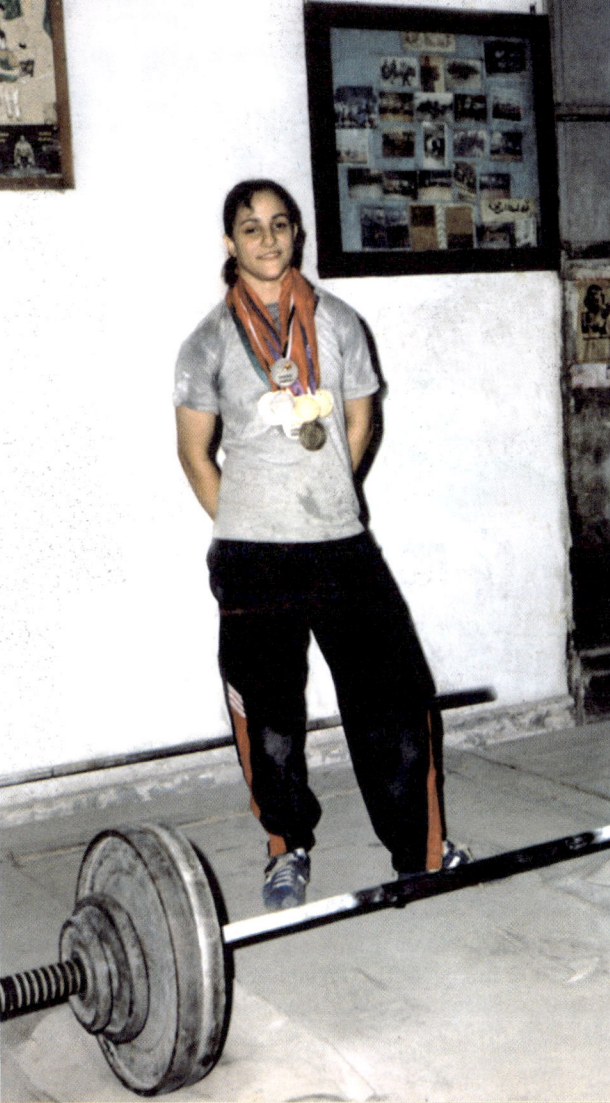

Figure 19.6. Wearing the medals on the street gym, in front of her house, Nahla shows her pride in everything her father has done for her and every sacrifice he had made to make her a champion.

TRAINING WOMEN

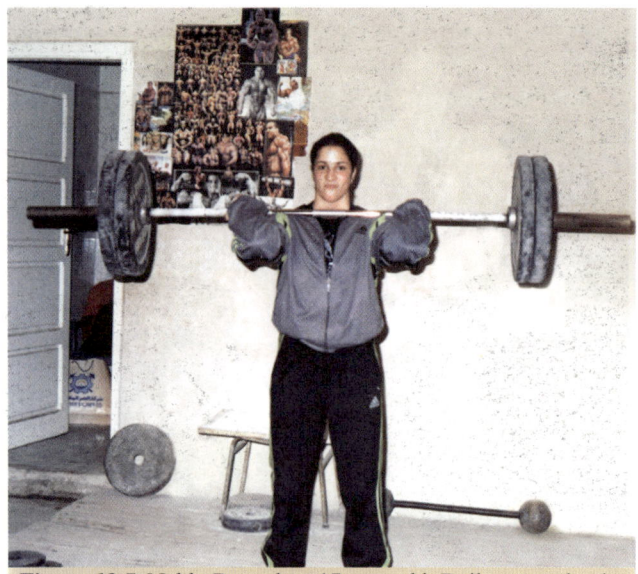

Figure 19.7. Nahla Ramadan, 17-year old. Daily strengthening with Power Clean exercise is done in front of her doorsteps. Nahla is two years older than Nagham.

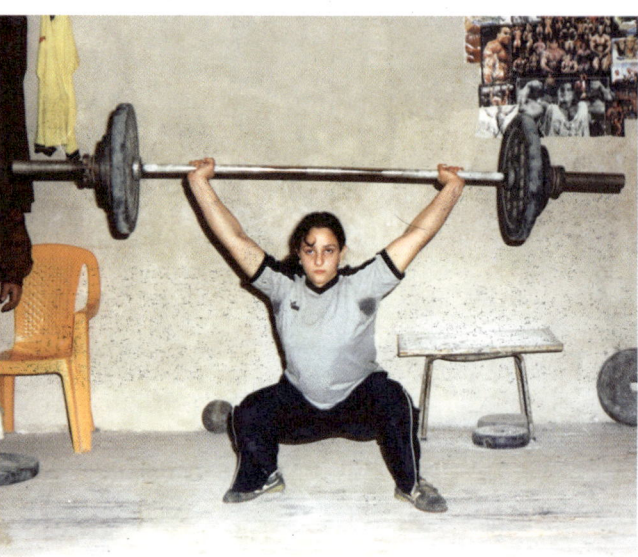

Figure 19.8. Nagham Ramadan, 15-year old. Squatting in this demanding lift, in front of her house, with 90 kg barbell has become a habit. This is a formidable lift even in well-equipped modern western gyms. She converted from track and field to Weightlifting and competed internationally in many countries.

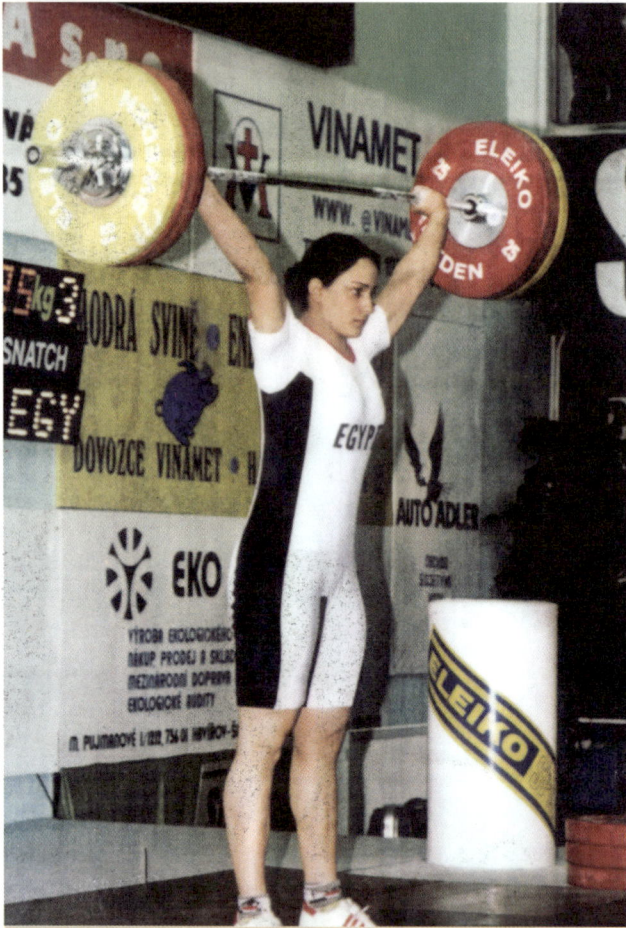

Figure 19.9. Nahla Ramadan, 17-year. Snatch of 102.5 kg. 2002 Junior World Championships, May 30 - June 5, Havarov, Czech Republic. She ranked third, as follows.

1) Chunhong Liu, CHN, bw: 68.52, Sn: 107.5, C & J: 147.5, Tot: 255.0.
2) Angela Medina, COL, bw: 68.72, Sn: 107.5, C & J: 125.0, Tot: 232.5.
3) Nahla Ramadan. Mohamed, EGY, bw: 68.81, Sn: 102.5, C & J: 127.5, Tot: 230.0.

(bw: bodyweight, Sn: Snatch, C&J: Clean and Jerk, Tot: Total weight.)

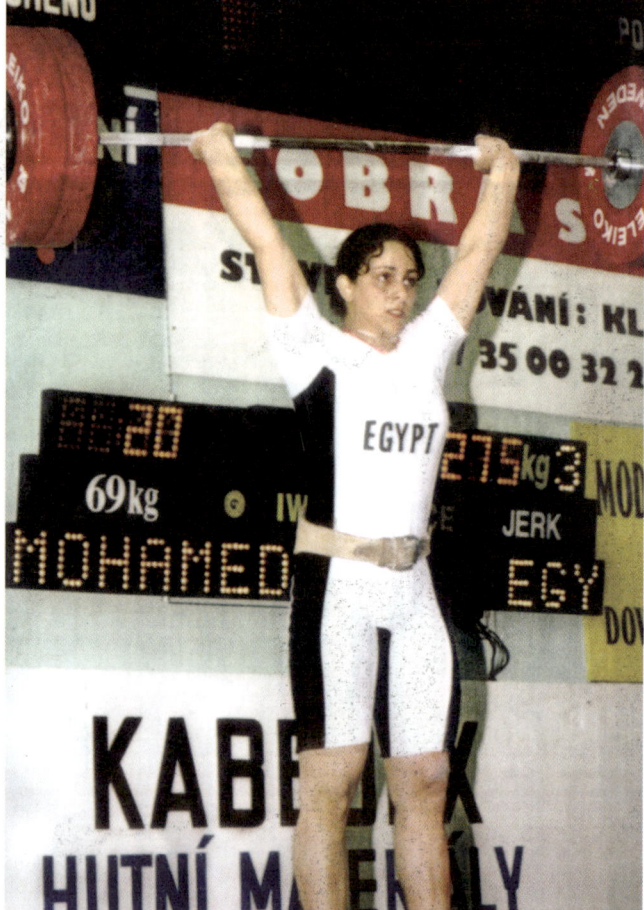

Figure 19.10. Nahla Ramadan. Clean and Jerk of 127.5 kg. 2002 Junior World Championships, May 30 - June 5, Havarov, Czech Republic.

19.5. TRAINING SCHEMES FOR WOMEN

Essential exercises for women are not greatly different from those for men. The common belief that women have inherently weaker upper body than men should not alter planning strength training. The fundamental rules of planning healthy training scheme is to give higher priority to the exercises that enhance general strength, in short time, and that lead to better athletic look on the long run. The following are main categories of exercises, in the descending order of priority.

1. Cardiovascular exercises.
2. Axial back exercises.
3. Pelvic girdle exercises.
4. Shoulder girdle exercises.
5. Peripheral Exercises.

19.5.1. CARDIOVASCULAR EXERCISES

o **Heart beating:** Proper exercise level, of heart beating rhythm, requires warm-up and preparation of the entire body, not just a particular region. What characterizes an exercise as "cardiovascular" is the potential of the exercise to increase the heart rate in a monotonously controlled fashion. For example, you could control the rate of increasing the heart rate by changing the pace of running.

o **Blood flow:** The main reason for putting your heart to test, prior to workout is to check your ability to endure stressful work, in that day and with your current condition. Initiating these exercises causes **"damming"** of the blood return within the exercising muscles. If the body were fit, then it would respond with appropriately increasing the heart rate in order to speed the circulation of the diminished blood return. If the increased heart beating is not too high, or too low, the rest of the vital organs would pass the test and you would not get warnings such as headache, dizziness, nausea, etc.

o **Lung perfusion and ventilation:** As the intensity of the exercise increases, the lungs have to pass the test of **exchanging** the carbon dioxide for oxygen at such increased heart beating. If the lungs are fit in structure and function and were conditioned before for stressful workout then new blood capillaries would open and begin gas exchange with alveolar air. If the arteries were not hardened, by arteriosclerosis, then the speeding blood flow, at higher heart beating, would not create serious turbulences within the vital organs. To recapitulate, cardiovascular exercises ensure that the vital organs are momentarily tuned up, for the excess demands of working out. During warm-up, one should be able to predict his or her own level of conditioning in that particular session.

o **Duration:** The duration of cardiovascular exercises depends on many factors.
   i. *Extra weight shedding:* If the trainee is overweight, the cardiovascular segment might be increased to a whole hour every training day. A minimal duration of 15 minutes of cardiovascular exercises, per training session, is reasonable.
   ii. *Ambient temperature:* In a hot sizzling summer, even with well-cooled gym, cardiovascular exercises have to be cut short to avoid exhaustion. When the room temperature is higher then the body temperature, cardiovascular workout could cause cellular damage, arrhythmias, and heart attack.
   iii. *Sleep condition:* On less than 7 hours of comfortable night sleep, cardiovascular intensity should be reduced. Caffeine would drastically speed the heart rate during cardiovascular warm-up and should be avoided long hours prior to workout.

o **Running:** The best and most complete cardiovascular exercise is running. Running with the upper back kept straight, the shoulder plates (scapulas) kept retracted (closer to each other), the head kept straight upright and swinging from side to side while running, provides general warm-up. Sloppy gait running does worse than good. Drooping arms, excessive forward leaning, uneven shoulder elevation, and back hunching all worsen postural deformities that require perseverance and constant awareness to rectify.

o **Aerobics:** An alternative to running is aerobic exercises without weights. You could easily use arm swinging sideways, forwards and upwards, to develop strong shoulders. You may start with swinging the arms for at least 20 repetitions. Increase the speed of swinging as tolerated and increase the total repetitions as much as you could tolerate. These exercises could be scattered between other exercises if shoulders fatigue quickly.

o **Torso warm-up:** The second region to warm up is the trunk (torso). You may perform the Goodmorning exercise (bending forwards, with slightly bent knees, to the horizontal level) for at least 20 repetitions and increase the speed and depth of bending as tolerated. This strengthens and warms up the entire back, from the back of the neck to the Glutei and Hamstrings.

o **Unweighted squatting:** The third region to warm up is the thigh. Squatting without weight, for at least 20 times, would prepare the heart, back, and legs to the extreme stress of strength training. Squatting could be flavored in many ways. Squatting with a jump, with feet brought close together, with widely kept apart feet, with knees pointed outwards, with descending on one leg while the other leg kept lax. All are ways to perform the most important exercise of all, squatting.

TRAINING WOMEN

- **Strengthening during warm-up:** Having warmed up the major body regions, you are now free to add extra warm-up exercise, and better even, focus on those parts of your body that demands special attention, such as the push-ups, the dips, and the chin-ups. In fact, with these cardiovascular exercises alone, you would have accomplished a full rounded session of strength training.
- **Muscular balance:** In those days when you would not like to approach weights or you find yourself away from training facilities, the warm-up described above suffices as a replacement of a whole training session. The smart way of assessing your routine of strength training is figuring out the proportion of exercises that entail **pushing** versus those that entail **pulling**. Balanced pushing and pulling ensures balanced extensors and flexors. As you might know, every joint in the body have flexors opposed by extensors. Alternatively, an acting group of muscles is always opposed by another group, since some joints perform abduction and adduction as well.

19.5.2. AXIAL BACK EXERCISES

- Before you think about your weak limbs, or the size of your waist, or the shape of your chest, you have to give serious consideration to your back condition. Strengthening the back muscles is a top priority for any strength training, particularly for women. The reasons for starting by back exercise are as follows.
    i. The arteries that supply the **spinal cord** are less than three millimeters in diameter, while those that supply the arm are at least three millimeter in diameter. The spinal cord arteries are long and torturous, while those of the **arms** are short and straight. The arms exercise every day and their arterial supply regenerates new capillaries with daily activities. The spinal cord does not enjoy such daily activity unless the person runs habitually, daily, for hours.
    ii. Axial back exercises increase the mass of the muscles in the proximity of the spinal cord, the **erectors**. With increased muscular vascularity, the spinal cord is enriched with plenty of circulation. As you might know, nerves that originate from the spinal cord supply all parts of the body, from the base of the skull all away down to the toes. Ensuring well perfused and well supported spinal cord, guarantees that the entire skeletal muscles of the limbs, truck, abdomen, and chest have healthy nervous control. In a layman words, strengthening the back guarantees sound and strong **center for the body** to depend on. Unprepared back muscles are your worst enemy, when it comes to physical performance.
    iii. Many if not all unsupervised trainees do not understand the real mechanism by which the condition of the vertebral column impacts our longevity in fitness. If the upper body is strong, while the back is not conditioned in proportion to the strength of the upper body, frequent **disabling injuries** are bound to occur. That is price we pay for being bipedal vertebrates. It is the vertebras that hold us together during moving our body mass.
    iv. The other very important fact about the back is that, without early life exercising of the back, it stays a weak link for rest of life. Neglecting the back muscles puts them in a state **atrophy and wasting** that is very difficult to change. Yet, it is rewarding to exercise the back muscles every day. That is because back injuries are the most frequent and most disabling injuries that result from unduly long inactivity, faulty lifting, or faulty planning of the order of execution of exercises.
- Axial back exercises should be performed from the floor, in standing position. Using machines to exercise the back should not be the rule, but rather the exception, or as augmenting to floor lifting. Lifting from the floor, conditions the nervous system to control the balance, and force of contraction, in normal daily activity. Lifting from the floor enhances the tone, coordination, and equilibrium of the whole body. Machine training deprives the nervous system from the ability to coordinate freestyle forceful motion, since machines restrict the trajectory of motion of the body. This eliminates whole groups of muscles from the dynamic process of lifting. Such selective workout with machines disturbs the equilibrium of mobility during physical performance. For the sake of recapitulation, the following standard axial back exercises are briefly discussed:
    1. The Clean lift.
    2. The Snatch lift.
    3. The Deadlift.
    4. The Bent-Over and Row.
    5. The Goodmorning.
    6. Shoulder Press and Jerk.
    7. Seated back pushing against resistance.
    8. Seated trunk twisting against resistance.
    9. Back extension.

19.5.2.1. The Clean Lift

- The Clean lift entails lifting a barbell from the floor to the shoulder level according to specific rules, as described in Section 5.2 on "Powerlifting Assisting Exercises". This **all-in-one** exercise enhances the entire body performance, including the cardiovascular, pulmonary, and neuromuscular functions. No other exercise accomplishes what the Clean lift from the floor does. It does not only strengthen the major axial muscles such as the Quadriceps, Glutei, back erectors, and Trapezius, but also coordinates these muscles' action and full range of motion. The axial muscles in the Clean lift do not default on balanced strengthening of opposing muscles, as is the case in isolated and aided exercises

TRAINING WOMEN

of individual muscles. Any lifting from the floor to the shoulder level, while standing freely on both feet, is considered a version of the Clean lift.
o   There are many ways to describe the various versions of the Clean, based on the body posture, grip width, and height of the pull prior to descent to retrieve the bar, as follows.

   i.   **Military Clean** entails lifting with stiffed knees, without descent under the barbell as it approaches the shoulder. The military Clean lift is intended to stretch the body extensors at higher resistance. This version of the Clean lift should not be habitually practiced as it induces stiffness and limited range of motion. The gained stretch is aimed at stimulating resiliently weak muscle to develop strength and grow massive.
   ii. **Power Clean** entails bending the knees at start position and squatting to some degree before the barbell approaches the shoulder level. The Power Clean is the mainstay of strength, flexibility, and endurance training. The trainee increases the weight of the barbell every other set or every two or three sets, depending on the intended load volume of exercise session.
   iii. **Classic Clean** encompasses four distinct phases, the Deadlift from the floor to slightly above the knees, followed by the pull up to the upper level of the thigh, followed by full Squat with shoulders and elbows flexion to retrieve the bar and shelve it on the shoulders, and finally ascending, with the barbell held in both hands on the shoulders. The Classic Clean tests the cumulative effects of basic classical training. It requires full preparedness and topnotch fitness to put all gained skills into full action.

o   The **basic rules** of the Clean lift are discussed in details in Section 9.1 on "Standard Technique of the Clean" and are summarized here as follows.
   i.   Stand at the bar with the front of the feet placed **under the bar**. The feet should be placed a foot apart.
   ii.   Bend the knees. Lower the thighs to horizontal that brings the hips to the level of the knees.
   iii. Keep the **elbows straight.** Grip the bar with both palms facing backwards.
   iv.   Bring the shoulder plates closer in the back. Move both shoulders behind the front of the chest cage, with the **chest cage thrust forwards**.
   v.   The **back is arched** to concave. If a flat board is placed on the back, it should touch the shoulder plates and the buttocks, but not the middle or the lower back.
   vi.   The lift **proceeds very slowly** with axial muscles hardened enough just to keep the posture stable, but not to the extent of total rigidity. The thighs drive the upward lifting, NOT the arms. The shoulders do not shrug but only sustain hardening to maintain the posture described in step (iv).
   vii. The slow upward lifting, to a level just above the kneecaps, is called **"Deadlift"** by virtue of its slowness. Having cleared the knees, **pulling with the shoulder,** NOT the Biceps, should start. The entire upper body bounces backwards pivoting on the feet balls. This is the fastest and strongest pulling phase.
   viii. Having reached the upper level of the thighs, four simultaneous joint movements take place.
       a. The shoulders shrug, abduct, adduct transversely, then flex, in a 'screw up" cadence, *Figures 9.17* thru *9.19*.
       b. The elbows bend and elevate, with the flexing shoulders, *Figure 9.21*.
       c. The hips descend and move backwards, while the knees bend and move forwards.
       d. The lower back is vigorously erected by the balanced actions of the spinal erectors and Iliopsoas muscles This thrusts the chest upwards, *Figure 9.25*.
   ix.   These four movements together bring the bar to its final destination on the shoulders. Ascending with the weight on the shoulders, and the elbows fully elevated up to the shoulder level to secure shelving on the outer parts of the collarbones, brings the Clean lift to finish. This constitutes a single **repetition** of the Clean lift. This may be repeated more than once to make up for a "**set**".

o   What have you accomplished by executing the Clean lift? The answer is not much that you would be able to notice in a mirror, in terms of new muscular development, particularly in the first few months of beginning this kind of training. The Clean works out the back extensors: the Hamstrings, Glutei, erectors, and Trapezius. After few months, other people would be able to notice your athletic look of slightly lordosed lower back, bulky Trapezius, and well-developed grove between the back erectors, which you could not notice yourself, in a front view mirror. Thus, you are building the frame of your body, not just the peripheral limbs.

19.5.2.2. The Snatch Lift
o   In the Snatch lift, the barbell travels from the floor straight overheads, without stationing at the shoulders, as described in details in Section 8.1 on "Standard Snatch technique". The added gains of performing the Snatch are strengthening the lifting muscles of the shoulder plates (the muscles that support the scapulas), the muscles that rotate shoulders, and enhancing of coordination of arms, back, and legs. The Snatch could be performed in many ways of different handgrips, height of pull prior to squatting, and stiffness of knees and hip during the lift.
o   What you accomplish by the Snatch lift, in excess of the Clean lift, is **stronger shoulder plates and rotators.** You would not gain such coordinated strength in performance by machine-aided or isolated exercises. With your feet on the floor and the barbell lifted high, an arm long above your shoulders, you are testing your cardiac performance to

eject blood to the highest possible **"head" of pressure**. The pressure head is the vertical distance of pumping to the highest body part. Remember that such human ability, to stand and lift high, demonstrates the genius of the neurovascular regulation of the brain and blood vessels. People with defective arterial regulation cannot even stand on their own feet without incapacitating hypotension.

o Why endure such troubles of challenge to your heart? The answer is that this exercise provides you with vital information on where your deficit lies. The Snatch lift uncovers weak links in the shoulder mobility, lower legs stability, and heart and lung reserve capacity, during this demanding exercise.

19.5.2.3. The Deadlift

Lifting barbell from the floor to any distance below the shoulder level is called Deadlift. See Section 5.2.9 on "Deadlift".
The lift is complete (dies) short of reaching the shoulders. The Deadlift is performed in many ways and serves different purposes, as follows.

o *Stiff-legged* Deadlift is similar to the early phases of the Clean, described above, but with straight knees. This is the most dangerous and flawed Deadlift that is practiced by uninformed trainees. Its danger lies in its potential to herniate spinal discs of the vertebral column. *Classic* Deadlift is performed in the same way as the early steps of the classical Clean lift. With bent knees and slanted and lordotic back, the lift proceeds slowly up to the level of midthighs.

o The Deadlift is the most stimulating resistance workout to the human musculoskeletal system. Weights lifted in Deadlift always exceed the trainee's bodyweight. After few weeks of performing Deadlift, your world would not be the same. You would get a sense of **mastering the forces** of gravity much better than before introducing this exercise into your routine. That is because deadlifting entails heavy resistance, with simple technique, that challenges the heart, lungs, nervous system, and musculoskeletal system. As your lifting exceeds your bodyweight, you will start feeling deep internal changes in your vascular system that signals your adaptation to heavy resistance. These constitute very high cardiac output and lung perfusion. If your heart and lungs are healthy, then such stressful transient changes last few minutes. Old or unhealthy heart and lungs might not tolerate such dose of acute stress. If you skip deadlifting for few weeks and then restart allover again, you will experience the same feeling over again. Too long omission of deadlifting could expose you to serious heart problem on restarting with heavy weight.

o The Deadlift increases the muscle mass of the major multi-pinnate muscles. These could not be worked out with any other isolated exercise. Yet, the very benefit of the Deadlift does not reside in its strengthening or bulking certain muscle groups, but in its **challenge to whole** body fitness. The Deadlift uncovers any hidden malady in the body. An unrecognized leaky heart valve, or irregular episodic heartbeat would seriously interfere with the Deadlift. Think about the Deadlift as the ultimate challenge to the heart's ability to eject blood in normal vessels without leaks, the lung's ability to increase its capacity to oxygenate excessive volumes of blood, the blood vessels' ability to tolerate extreme disturbance of blood flow, and the nervous system's ability to sustain acute harmonious physiological operation without failure.

o Therefore, the Deadlift could also lead to **serious heart problems** for people with prolapsed cardiac valves, or even worse, it could cause rupture corda tendinae (the tendons that pull open the mitral valves of the left heart). The Deadlift could cause many months of bed-ridden morbidity, if the trainee omits the importance of monitoring her or his heart rate and regularity of beating, during training and in the interval of days between the Deadlift sessions. Mandatory abstinence from all physical activities is essential for those who incur days of irregular, slow or fast heart beats after vigorous exercise.

19.5.2.4. Bend-Over-And Row (BOR)

o BOR targets the back muscles of the shoulder joint. Although these muscles could be trained with seated cable rowing, the BOR has the advantage of including two important regions for strengthening, the pelvic girdle and the lower back. Rowing, while bending with a barbell, offers the benefit of conditioning the autonomic nervous system to deal with resistance strength, while maintaining postural equilibrium.

o The observed results of few weeks of BOR is the enhanced ability of maintaining the shoulder plates closer to back of the chest cage even after lengthy hours of fatigue. This strengthened postural gain prevents the shoulders from caving forwards and hampering breathing. In other words, the breathing ability after lengthy standing or sitting improves with BOR.

19.5.2.5. Goodmorning Exercise

o Putting a barbell on the back of the shoulders and bending over, with it, is called **Goodmorning** exercise, from its resemblance to the Japanese way of saluting. See Section 7.5.1.2 on "Goodmorning Back Extension". If you are unfamiliar with Weightlifting, or never been exposed to strength training in your youth, this exercise might sound like total madness to you. Many people take for granted the fallacy that the back is destined to be a weak link in the human anatomy, and that there is nothing to do about it. The Goodmorning is the very proof that that fallacy is refutable. The human back could be trained to be a very secure and strong link.

o Whereas the Bent-Over-and Row, the Deadlift, and the Clean lift, all strengthen the back, the Goodmorning has a characteristic difference in that the center of the weight is placed right on the scapular spines (the back of the chest).

The other exercises place the weight in the hands, which transmit it to a wide range of spines, from the base of the skull down to top of the pelvic bones. Since the arms are not gripping the weight, in Goodmorning exercise, the shoulder plates are not pulled downwards. This permits maximal breathing while bending over.
- o For adults who never performed forward bending, with weights placed behind their shoulders, very gradual increase in the weight, over months, and regular execution of this exercise is very rewarding. In fact, the theme of this book is founded on the essential rule of "**progressive incremental strength training**". With little planning and patience, any person can overcome physical weakness by implementing such essential rule, as demonstrated in the following steps.
    i. Start any weight-exercise WITHOUT weight and execute the motion for at least TEN times.
    ii. Now, when you add weight, your ability to reach ten repetitions diminishes. A sensible low weight should make the 9th and 10th repetitions quite difficult, but should not cause the technique to default.
    iii. Determine the weight that can allow you to repeat the exercise up to six repetitions, but no more. Having identified your upper and lower maxima, you should perform two or more sets in each of the three splits between the maximum and the minimum. Thus, if your minimum and maximum in Goodmorning are 60 lb (10 reps) and 100 lb (6 reps), you should perform 2 sets in 60 lb, 2 sets in 80 lb, and 2 sets in 100 lb.
    iv. In order to progress incrementally, you will increase the reps in heavier weights, on the following sessions, such that the 100 lb will be performed 10 reps. That allows you to advance your maximum to 120 lb, in that example.
    v. In days when you feel tired, you should content yourself with lower than maximum. Yet, your curve will catch up soon after passing that tiring day.
    vi. Progress is visible in weeks, not months. This is particularly true in flexor strengthening such as the Biceps, abdominals, Deltoids, and Hamstrings.
- o The knees must bend slightly to avoid serious back injuries. Goodmorning with jumping, with and without weight, is an excellent exercise that prepares the spinal muscles to impulsive forces.
- o Goodmorning exercise should **NEVER** be attempted with any caving at the lower back. The slightest lower back hunching could cause serious injury, even after the workout session is over.

19.5.2.6. Shoulder Press and Jerk
- o Lifting weight from the shoulder level overheads is called either "Shoulder Press" or "Jerk", depending on which muscle groups initiates the lifting. The Press is performed without a drive from the lower legs. See Section 7.4.4.1 on "Barbell Shoulder Press". The Jerk is initiated with a dip at the knees and hips and an upward leg drive. See Section 9.2 on "Standard Technique of the Jerk".
- o The necessity of overhead lifting arises from the necessity to keep the **shoulder rotators balanced**. Lifting from the floor, without exceeding the shoulder level, causes serious imbalance at the shoulder joint and permanent freezing of the joint in a wide range of motion. The shoulder serves as a mobility joint and loss of mobility is dreadfully disadvantageous. Powerlifters omit overhead lifting and end up with stiffed shoulders for life, as do Bodybuilders. Stiffened shoulders are vulnerable to injuries.
- o Other than mobility, overhead lifting is an impetus both, to the heart and lungs that adapt to function at the increased **peripheral vascular resistance**. That arises from pumping blood all away up to the raised arms and though the entire body that is in state of total muscular hardening. Getting dizzy while pressing overheads is a common experience, when one's routine of sleep, nutrition, or emotion is upset, in one way or another.
- o Beginners of this exercise experience **upper middle-back muscular pain** when excess weight training is undertaken. That is because; overhead lifting engages two groups of shoulder rotators. The Deltoid lifts the humerus up to a horizontal level then the muscles attached to the inner border of the shoulder plates (the Serratus) rotates the shoulder plates to complete the shoulder rotation upwards. The upper middle-back muscles support the shoulder plates' upper inner corner, while they rotate.
- o The rhomboid area, behind the chest cage, is the main beneficiary of the overhead lifting. This is the area of the upper back, where hunching of osteoporosis occurs. Overhead lifting is therefore very taxing on people with **hunchback**. If performed regularly during the early years of adolescence, overhead lifting might prevent upper back hunching deformity. Once hunching occurs, the best hope is to keep improving the overhead press, both to halt further hunching and to ease the fatiguing effect of weak upper back.

19.5.2.7. Seated Back Pushing
- o Pushing backwards against resistance, while sitting at the back machine, is suitable in many circumstances as a substitute for other back exercises. Such circumstances are: injuries to the leg or arm, not feeling well enough to lift while standing, and desire to supplement freestyle training by focusing on particular region for strengthening.
- o Habitual seated training are not suitable for the youth, or people under fifty years of age, nor they are suitable for any age group for long times. Freestyle lifting, even with the slightest weight, or even mimicking lifting motion without weight, is crucial to developing and maintaining healthy equilibrium during mobility.

19.5.2.8. Seated Trunk Twisting
- o Resisting twisting, while sitting at an abdominal machine, is very innovative exercise for strengthening the abdominal oblique muscles. It parallels high impact aerobics is sliming the waist size. This is a precious exercise for folks with lax abdominal muscles. It helps mobilize the abdominal contents and improve the entire body's ability to breathe and

endures stress. Whereas crunches work out the abdominal rectus muscles that stretch from the chest cage down to the pelvic front bone (the symphysis pubis), few exercises work out the oblique muscles that sheath the sides of the waist (the flanks).
- o The abdominal girth correlates very well with health and fitness because strong abdominal muscles aid in the following:
    i. Move the bowels regularly. Highly tones abdominal muscles facilitate gas expulsion and mobilize intestinal contents. This enhances mixing, digestion, absorption, and elimination and reduces bacterial overgrowth.
    ii. Prevent congestion of the venous return in the abdomen due to lax muscles. Help maintain blood return to the heart that sustains the vital organs during activity.
    iii. Help in the extremes of breathing demands during vigorous activity.
    iv. Augment the blood flow to the spinal cord of the lower body. Lax abdomen steals blood from surroundings by trapping huge amount of fluids within the guts.
- o Many obese women and sedentary folks suffer from weak abdominal muscles and diminished ability to tolerate vigorous activity. A vicious cycle of weakness, intolerance to stress that causes further weakness, and decline in physical health is a common pattern of inactive life. In fact, soon after death, the abdomen distends significantly due to paralysis of visceral and skeletal muscles. Yet, many living people suffer from the extreme stress of distended bellies due to long inactivity.

19.5.2.9. Back Extension

Laying face down, with the lower body against a flat bench and the upper body freely projecting outside the bench, and the lower legs restrained to the bench, is another substitute to back exercises, specially in women who dread straining while standing. See Section 7.5.1.3 on "Horizontal Back Extension". When the head is lowered below the pelvis, the abdominal contents move away from the pelvic floor. Thus, this posture relieves pelvic congestion and enhances strengthening of the pelvic hammock. Urinary incontinence is exclusive to women particularly at advanced age and overweight. Incontinence that is due to weak pelvic hammock would greatly benefit from this and other exercises that strengthen the lower abdominal floor.

19.5.3. PELVIC GIRDLE EXERCISES

- o As with the case of axial exercises, many training programs in public health clubs never seriously consider planning workout based on skeletal integrity. Pelvic exercises work out the muscles that link the legs to the trunk. These muscles control our posture, while walking, standing, or sitting. With strong and sound pelvic muscles, we can carry our body gracefully with less strain on the heart and joints. Thus, the pelvic muscles deal with the body stability during motion. In folks with poor health such as alcoholics, smokers, and sedentary people, the first muscles that waste away are the Glutei, the thigh muscles, and the abdominal muscles. Such muscular wasting leads to thin legs, bulging abdomen, weak lower back, and unstable walking gait.
- o The basic exercises for the pelvic region, in addition to the above-mentioned axial exercises that overlap the truck and the pelvis, are:
    1. Squat.
    2. Abdominal Sit-ups.
    3. Leg Lunges.
    4. Leg Press.
    5. Leg Extension and Flexion.

19.5.3.1. Squat

- o Many new comers to the arena of strength training confuse Squat exercises for many other auxiliary exercises, in regards to the priority of execution. The Squat has to be executed **every training session**, whether in full load or in reduced load. The trend followed by Bodybuilders of splitting workout days, into upper and lower body sessions, is completely unscientific. Bodybuilders focus on the massive soft tissue bulging, while scientific training tackles the proper dynamics of motion fitness of the body. This comprises of enhancing reflex coordination and building sound spinal musculoskeletal frame. See Section 7.5.1.7 on "Back Squat".
- o The argument that squatting is very demanding and interferes with other exercises is a fallacy that has long propagated among late starters of strength training and uninformed trainees. Olympic Weightlifters work out the legs in **every training session**, for a minimum of 3 to 4 sets, each of 3 to 5 repetitions of squatting. The long-term perseverance, in training the thigh muscles, pays its rewards in reducing the demanding stress on other organs.
- o Traditional squatting comes in many styles.
    i. *Full* squat with the barbell placed behind the shoulders proceeds to full knees and hips flexion. This classical and common style works out the thighs, the Glutei, and the back.
    ii. Squatting with the barbell placed on the front of the shoulders, known as ***"front Squat"***, is an additional engagement of the shoulder muscles with the pelvic muscles. The front Squat does not work out different thigh muscles, but rather engages the shoulder muscles in lifting thus adds extra challenge on the chest cage, during

breathing. The front Squat forces the chest cage to elevate in order to support the barbell. This is an exquisite dual-purpose exercise of the chest and legs.

   iii. *Partial* Squat includes descending with the weight to a bench, placed behind the heels. This sort of squatting should not be the main routine of leg training since it does not strengthen the full range of motion of squatting. Partial squat could be very harmful when the trainee loads the barbell with very heavy load to prove his or her egoistic pride of strength. Partial squatting with extreme heavy load crush the knee cartilages and leads to life-long injury of osteochondritis. The rationale of practicing such dangerous style is to stretch and strengthen some of the short fibers of the Glutei and thighs that add extra stability under vigorous stress.

o Although squatting works out the thighs, as do the Deadlift and the Clean, Squat is unique in starting from minimal muscular recruitment, at full standing, and proceeding gradually for increased recruitment and with eccentric contraction, as descending proceeds. This gradual workout prepares the motor units of the lower body to develop, well beyond that could be achieved with other exercises alone.

19.5.3.2. Abdominal Sit-Ups

o The main purpose of the abdominal sit-ups is strengthening the muscles in front of the hip joints. See Section 7.5.2.4 on "Inclined Sit-ups". This counteracts those strengthened by squatting. The Iliopsoas, the muscles that brings the trunk closer to the thighs (the hip flexor) benefit most from abdominal sit-ups. The rectus abdominis is the muscle that brings the chest cage closer to the groin and endures stretch in this workout. If the chest bends on the truck, at the umbilicus level, the rectus abdominis (the front muscles that form 6 bags, 3 on each side of the midline of the abdomen) works out harder by elongation and contraction, rather than stretching alone.

o Working out the Iliopsoas and the abdominis rectus is crucially vital to healthy athletic living. The Iliopsoas is the bed upon which lie the major blood vessels to the lower limbs. The abdominis rectus is the ceiling under which lies these major vessels plus the abdominal contents.

o The sit-ups thus strengthen the muscles that **sandwich the major blood vessels** to the limbs and the abdominal contents. This improves the circulation to the limbs, the genitalia, and the pelvic and abdominal organs. Improvements are noticeable in the following functions:
   i. The back muscles develop strength faster.
   ii. The thighs gain mass and power faster.
   iii. The abdominal contents mobilize and evacuate the guts easier.
   iv. The sexual function sustains vitality for advanced age.
   v. The pelvic floor remains robust to sustain urinary continence, prevent uterus and rectum from congestion during bearing down (as in defecation, laughter, vigorous lifting, or coughing).

19.5.3.3. Leg lunges

o This an asymmetric exercises where the trainee puts the weight on the back or front of the shoulders and springs forwards with one leg. It serves the purpose of stretching the front ligaments of the leg that is lagging and lateral muscles of the hip that is leading. It does not strengthen the thighs as efficient as in squatting, since the weight is lighter and the range of motion is limited.

o Leg lunges are invaluable as stretching exercises, and enhancers of joint and muscle control. Their asymmetric posture prevents shortening of spinal, pelvic, and knee ligaments, particularly, when they are performed with fully flexed front knee and fully extended rear knee.

19.5.3.4. Leg Press

o This entails lying on the back and pushing upwards weights placed on the soles of the feet. See Section 7.5.1.5 on "Inclined Leg Press". Leg Press differs from the Squat in the following:
   i. No need for postural spinal balance. This is invaluable help in days of overtraining, fatigue, or sore joints.
   ii. Increased venous blood return to the heart in the elevated legs position. These make this exercise tolerable to many people and to those returning from long interruption of training routine.
   iii. High control on the leg flexion due to diminished need to spinal balance and enhanced upper body circulation. Thus, you can achieve very flexible knees and joints by dipping deeper with the weight. You can bring the knees to the chest, and the heels to the Hamstrings.

19.5.3.5. Leg Extension and Flexion

o Sitting on bench with weights attached to the upper surface of the feet, while extending the knees, is called **Leg Extension**. See Section 7.6.1.6 on "Seated Knee Extension". It works out not only the thigh muscles, but also the internal cruciate ligaments that resist forward translation of the lower legs at the knees. Here, the Hamstrings are almost eliminated from opposing the Quadriceps. Thus, the internal cruciate ligaments oppose the action of the Quadriceps to stabilize the knee.

o Laying face down on a bench or standing, with the weights attached to the back of the ankles, and bending the knees to pull the weight towards the back, is called **Leg Flexion**. See Section 7.6.2 on "Knee Flexion" and Section 7.6.2.1 on

"Leg Curls". It serves the opposing action of the leg extension by strengthening the Hamstrings and the other cruciate ligament that prevents backward translation of the lower legs on the thigh.

19.5.4. SHOULDER GIRDLE EXERCISES

o Looking at other people's shoulders tells a lot about their physical fitness. Full and round shoulders are signs of the athletic outlook of a person. Just by mere looking in a photograph of a person, one can judge his or her general level of activity by comparing the shoulder width to the chest and waist widths.

o The shoulders are the most complex joints in the body. They rotate in three planes and thus require at least two opposing exercises, in each plane, to guarantee mobile shoulder joint. Thus, shoulder exercises involve six basic movements. Flexion and extension are movements in a vertical plane that has forward and backward directions. Abduction and adduction are movements in a vertical plane that has lateral and medial directions. Elevation and depression are sliding movements in a vertical plane that has upward and downward directions.

o The basic shoulder exercises are:
1. Bench Press.
2. Seated Shoulder Press.
3. Cable Rowing.
4. Lateral Push and Pull.
5. Shoulder Shrugs.

19.5.4.1. Bench Press

o The fame of the Bench Press as a superior exercise for the development of strong chest muscles is well known worldwide. Anatomically speaking, the chest muscles are considered shoulder muscles, because the chest could not perform physical resistance without shoulders. The chest muscles also help voluntary respiration in stressful situation.

o The Bench Press could be performed in different forms by varying the inclination of the bench, from horizontal to inclined or declined, by varying the span of handgrips, or by using dumbbells in the place of barbells. See Section 7.4.4.12 on "Bench Press" and Section 7.4.4.13 on "Inclined Bench Press". Barbells eliminate the action of some muscles from the strengthening process, since the bar ties both arms together against the tension in the bar. Dumbbells add more active muscle to the motion, and strengthen the shoulders in a symmetrical manner. Dumbbells remedy the stiffness incurred by barbell limited range of motion, particularly in free arm rotation motions.

o Bench Press strengthens the front of the chest, using the shoulders in this respect. This could not be achieved unless the back of the chest is kept firmly hardened. Thus, the Bench Press induces the shoulder plates to adhere harder to the chest cage, as the weight is increased. Thus, the Bench Press forces the chest cage to resist both, from the front and the back. Resisting forces strengthen the chest cage and its attaching ligaments to the vertebral column.

o A strong chest cage provides roomy tunnels for the major blood vessels and air ducts that enter and exit the neck inlet. That guarantees adequate flow of air and blood both to the brain and the heart, during vigorous activity. It also provides roomy tunnels to the major vessels and nerve bundles passing under the clavicles (the collarbones) to reach the arms.

o Arms failure and collapse, during lifting heavy weight or after long hours of tiring workday, could easily be attributed to weak chest cage muscles. That fails to maintain adequate posture and permit adequate ventilation of the lungs or blood flow to the arms, brain, and heart.

19.5.4.2. Seated Shoulder Press

o Aside from its axial significance, the overhead Shoulder Press strengthens the vertical shoulder abductors. As with the Bench Press, the overhead press requires strong muscles that support the shoulder plates to the chest cage. Thus, pressing overhead also involves the scapular muscles (the Serratus anterior). Thrusting the chest forwards greatly enhances the benefits of the overhead Press. See Sections 7.4.4.1, 2, and 3 on "Shoulder Press".

o The three main groups of muscles that elevate the arms above the shoulders are the Deltoid, the Supraspinatus, and the Serratus anterior. The former two elevate the arms from its lowest position up to a horizontal upper arm. The Serratus rotate the scapulas from here on to the vertical position. Thus, performing overhead press from the level of the ears upwards neglects the crucial roles of the Supraspinatus; one of four shoulder's cuff rotators. It is essential to try to lift weight that are laying on the back or the front of the shoulders, in the overhead press, rather than dropping the weight from the rack to the level of the ears. This modification in Shoulder Press requires progressive incremental training in order to strengthen the internal shoulder structures.

o Incorporating overhead press in your daily workout sessions, with either one-handed dumbbells or barbell, could be the magical trick in enhancing your strength and fitness. As we have mentioned, shoulders and thighs must be worked out in **every training session** to guarantee advancing general strength. Strong thighs ensure your stability of gait, while strong shoulders ensure adequate blood flow to the brain and arms. Four to ten sets of overhead press, each set consists of 3 to 8 presses, three times weekly, might cause breakthrough in advancing your strength condition.

19.5.4.3. Cable Rowing
o   Pulling weight attached to cables, while sitting or standing, strengthens the muscles under the armpits. These muscles are attached to the shoulder plates. They adduct the arms. This exercise works out muscles that oppose those used in the Bench Press. See Section 7.4.3 on "Shoulder External Rotation".
o   As a rule, every exercise that entails pushing should be balanced by an exercise that entails pulling. This exercise also strengthens the chest cage and respiratory muscles. Since rowing strengthens the muscles that brings the arms closer to the body when pulling, rowing strengthen the lifting from the floor or pulling one's bodyweight upwards, as in climbing a rope and chin-ups. While performing cable rowing, a trainee could condition her or his entire arm by opening and closing the handgrip while pulling, and slowing the early arm bending to stimulate the Biceps.

19.5.4.4. Lateral Push and Pull
Pushing by the sides of the upper arms against resisting decks of a machine, which are attached to weights, strengthens the lateral fibers of the Deltoid and the Supraspinatus. Pulling a hand-gripped cable attached to weights towards the body sides strengthens the other shoulder rotators (the Infraspinatus, Subscapularis, and Teres minor), in addition to the Teres major and Latissimus dorsi. These exercises are introduced to supplement routine exercises, when a sense of lack on coverage, of some vital muscles by strength training, is suspected.

19.5.4.5. Shoulder Shrug
Shrugging the shoulders, with weight held in both hands, strengthens the shoulder elevators that lie at the upper back. Heavy weights are used for this purpose to strengthen and enlarge the Trapezius and shoulder plate elevators. Do not get addicted to shoulder shrugging. It should only be practiced occasionally to supplement the Clean lift. Lifting extremely heavy weights in this limited range of motion exercise, more than double one's bodyweight, is ridiculous, unless one could Clean lift at least more, something closer to one and half his own bodyweight. That is because shoulder shrugging causes stiffness allover the body and unnecessarily strains the knees in very localized spots.

19.5.5. PERIPHERAL EXERCISES
o   Though left to the end of this chapter, exercises that work out the peripheral parts of the body are over emphasized in most, if not all, public gyms. Due to their simplicity and the direct relationship between the exercise and the muscle it affect, many people indulge into these exercises as a sole workout routine. Exercises that target the Biceps, Triceps, forearms, and calves are the most famous exercise to folks who are not familiar with the long history of progress in strength training. Exercising the limbs, without a complete plan to shape the skeleton, results in many common body deformities. You might have noticed many trainees have well developed arm muscles that exceed the size of their thighs. Many others could bench press weight they could not use in squatting.
o   Yet exercising the limbs is as important as exercising the axial major muscles in the context of a complete and rounded exercise plan. The limbs feel the weight before the major axial muscles do. Thus, strong finger grip, Biceps pull, Triceps push, and calf drive are vital to lifting and mobility.
o   There is no shortage of machines and variety of gadgets that are used to exercise the limbs. The Biceps are worked out by pulling on a weight while bending the elbow joint as a pivot. See Section 7.2 on "Strengthening Elbow Flexors". The barbells used for **arm curls** have the advantage of symmetrical training. They strengthen the Biceps and the forearm flexors (muscles that bend wrist on the surface of the palm). Reversing the grip of the arm curls converts it to the reverse or **hammer curls.** This strengthens the Biceps, Brachialis, and the wrist extensors (the muscles that bend the wrist in the direction of the back of the hands).
o   The **Triceps** are worked out by pushing on a weight held in the hands while extending the elbows from a bent state. See Section 7.3 on "Strengthening Elbow Extensors". Thus, pushing and pulling a weight held in the hands and bending the elbows works out the upper arm muscles.
o   For many people, the limbs, particularly the **hand muscles,** are of concern since they suffer most of wasting with lengthy lack of exercise. This concern should be addressed in terms of overall look, by giving priority to axial training rather than getting distracted by a symptom that is resulted from lack of training. This approach would gain the confidence of the beginner when she or he feels the gain of well-planed overall training.

19.6. HIGHLIGHTS OF CHAPTER NINTEEN

1. People who do not engage in long-term exercise suffer from **circulatory disturbance** that could precipitate falls, heart arrhythmias that could cause sudden death, long recovery from pain that could impair many organs, and transient traumatic episodes that could cause severe long-term injuries. A poorly conditioned person shows clear alteration in the face circulation to lividity in response to slightest muscular contraction.

2. Long-term training refines this **adaptation mechanism** and saves the trainee the trouble of sudden heart attacks, coma in poorly conditioned people, or failure while lifting heavy weight. Regular vigorous exercise prepares the coronary arteries of the heart for episodic disturbance in blood flow during exercise. Long-term training regulates the response

TRAINING WOMEN

of the lungs during stressful exercises. Unconditioned persons suffer sudden lung congestion, coughing, or asthma during stress.

3. **Interrupting training** for few months reflects clearly on the inability of the lungs to deal with hyperventilation during exercise, in the form of acute coughing and dryness of throat

4. Long-term exercise protects women from **falls, fractures, strained joints** and help women enjoy healthy living to the most of their ability. The response of a trained woman to stumbling on an object, while walking or running or even after incurring traumatic accidents, is greatly enhanced by long term training. The enhanced level of health and fitness manifests in the form of fast healing, avoidance of fall, better balance and agility, greater reserves of healing, cardiovascular, and respiratory power.

5. **Immobility induces bone loss.** The calcium produced by bone thinning might deposit in the blood vessels causing their hardening or in the kidneys causing kidney stones. The major preventable maladies that prevail in women population due to lack of exercise are osteoporosis, coronary heart disease, arthritis, falls and fracture due to lack of coordination, obesity, depression, urinary incontinence due to lax pelvic muscles, and postural deformities due to weak muscular tone.

6. Even very progressive strength training would not cause women to **look masculine**. Masculinity on women is either due to internal physiological disorder or due to intake of masculinizing hormones.

7. Most **back injuries** recover by immediate exercise as soon as the acute pain subsides. Back injuries are preventable by exercise and are precipitated by the lack of it.

8. Many common exercises do not help advance physical performance. Embarking on a **proper training** plan could quickly (in a matter of few weeks) improve the breathing ability and cardiovascular response to stressful exercises. Less than one hour of strength training, for at least three days every week, will not do much good. Injuries increase in incidence with lesser training times.

9. In addition to its health benefits, exercise offers opportunities of reasoning and problem solving that maintains the mental process on the edge of **improving living** rather than succumbing to the perils of emptiness and stagnation of sedentary living.

10. To overcome **obesity,** we still should not eat every thing we wish, even if we exercise. Exercise should be used as a gauge to guide our eating habits to stay light, strong, and agile.

11. Since exercise forces the bone to mineralize, this prevents the calcium ions from depositing within the **walls of the blood vessels.** Thus, activity protects the blood vessels from hardening by depositing calcium in the bone matrix

12. Exercise benefits best in strengthening the lower **abdominal muscles** that support the bladder, uterus, and colon during walking, coughing, exercising, or bearing down.

13. The fundamental rules of planning healthy training scheme is to give higher priority to the exercises that enhance **general strength** in short time and that leave better athletic look for long term. Cardiovascular exercises ensure that the vital organs are momentarily tuned up for the excess demands of the workout. During warm-up exercises, one would be able to predict what kind of condition he or she is in that particular session. .

14. When the **room temperature** is higher then the body temperature cardiovascular workout could cause cellular damage, arrhythmias, and heart attack.

15. Drooping arms, excessive forward leaning, uneven shoulder elevation, and back hunching, all, worsen **postural deformities** that require perseverance and constant awareness to rectify.

16. **Unprepared back muscles** are your worst enemy when it comes to physical performance. Back injuries are the most frequent and most disabling injuries that result form unduly long inactivity, faulty lifting, or faulty planning of the order of execution of exercises.

17. After few weeks of performing the Deadlift, your world would not be the same. You would get a sense of mastering the forces of gravity much better than before introducing this exercise into your routine. However, the Deadlift could cause many months of bed-ridden morbidity if the trainee omit the importance of monitoring her or his heart rate and regularity of beating during training and in the interval of days between the Deadlift sessions. Mandatory abstinence from all physical activities is essential for those who incur days of irregular, slow or fast heart beats after vigorous exercise.

Chapter 20
Guidelines for Optimum Strength Training

20.1. NATURE OF PHYSICAL STRENGTH

20.1.1. WEIGHT TRAINING VERSUS ENDURANCE TRAINING

o **Regular weight training combined with aerobic exercise** decreases fat deposition and increases muscle mass. It does that by increasing the number of elements within the body cells that expend energy (muscle fibers) and those that metabolize foodstuff (mitochondria). During physical activity, the newly grown muscle fibers increase the conversion of chemical energy into kinetic energy and heat. However, during the recovery time between physical activities, the various sources of chemical energy (carbohydrates, fat, and aminoacids) provide the necessary fuel for reconstruction, within the mitochondria's citric acid cycle, thus replenish depleted resources. See Chapter 14, Section 14.1 on "Role of Exercise in Health".

o **Strength training** differs from endurance training in expanding the CP-ATP shuttle process within the muscle cells, whereas **endurance** training expands the mitochondrial processes. The former requires ample energy expenditure in brief duration, while the latter expends energy on protracted interval. Thus, strength training results in strong physiques with improved body appearance, curves, and shape. On the other hand, endurance training produces slim physiques; with least amounts of muscle mass that can efficiently moves the bodyweight. Light bodyweight slowly depletes ATP and CP and thus allows time for aerobic oxidation of fat. Aerobic exercise induces a state similar to fasting by depleting the reserves of carbohydrate and forcing the body to burn fat for energy. See Chapter 10, Section 10.1 on "Physical Endurance & Strength".

o **Axial weight training** exercises involve large muscle groups and induce greater changes in metabolism, in shorter duration compared to peripheral weight training. See Chapter 11, Table 11.1 on "Comparison between axial training and peripheral training". The effects of axial weight training last longer than those due to **peripheral training**. It is not true that weight training causes weight gain without excess caloric intake. Even weight training without aerobics does not drastically increase **bodyweight** unless the individual consumes greater amounts of calorie-rich foods. This induces Insulin and growth hormone, causing fast weight gain. Weightlifters learn how to develop lean bodies with minimal bodyweight as long as their diet is strictly controlled. Driven athletes cherish the principle of deprivation from tasty food that exceeds their basic needs of high performance. This does not mean that the author advocates deprivation as a mean to control bodyweight. The fact is that eating discipline induces a state of mind that is accustomed to avoid purposeless eating habits. Many researchers attribute such restrictive state of mind to the effect of controlled blood glucose level. They believe that excessive eating of carbohydrates causes frequent and common irregularities in blood glucose concentration, which stimulate many endocrine receptors to produce hormones that drive the person to consume unnecessarily large amounts of calories.

20.1.2. ESSENCE OF PHYSICAL OF STRENGTH

o **Synchrony of recruitment:** Consistent training increases the number of active nerve cells (motoneurons) in the spinal cord that control all aspects of muscle function below the brain level. Performing complex motor skills depends on the complexity of communication of nerve cells. Without training, muscular contraction occurs out of synchrony during purposeful tasks. In the untrained, agonist muscles oppose their antagonists, in random magnitudes and directions, leading to clumsy motion. During maximal strength, the greatest number of muscle fibers will synchronously experience the highest rate of tension and the maximum frequency of effective impulses. The duration of the up-to-the-limit tension is biggest in maximal strength, compared to that in submaximal activities. Thus, the greater synchronization of muscle fibers determines maximal strength through adaptive flexion and extension reflexes.

o **Compound exercises:** Multi-joint exercises modify harmonious recruitment and contraction of muscle fibers relevant to the intended activities. Thus, greater number of muscle units could simultaneously team up to perform high resistance movement. Daily inclusion of core compound exercises such as the Clean, Snatch, Deadlift, Bent-over row, Squat, Overhead Squat, Jerk, and Standing Shoulder Press fosters strength development of the whole body. The isolation approach of training Chest-Biceps, Shoulder-Triceps, Back-abdomen, and legs, on separate days, accomplished muscular hypertrophy but lacks whole proportional development or synchrony. Isolation and peripheral exercises should be reserved for off-session and recuperative periods.

- **Neural aspect:** Exercise modifies the continuous discharge of impulses from the higher neural centers of the brain as well as the lower neural centers of the spinal cord, in both magnitude of impulses and rate of discharge. Exercise also modifies the constitution of the cells that release the firing mediator, neurotransmitter (acetylcholine). These are located at the final destination of nerves, on the muscle surface (neuromuscular junctions). In trained people, neuromuscular junctions secrete sufficient amounts of mediators for strong contractions on timely manner. In addition, in the well-trained, neuromuscular junctions clear the spent mediators swiftly and efficiently. Exercise affects the response of the cellular membrane of muscle cells through the receptor molecules to hormones and blood nutrients. These receptors, in turn, modify the enzyme complexes that operate the Potassium-Sodium ion pump across the muscle membrane, in response to change of membrane potential. Here, reside most of the secrets of strength development, which may explain why some people have greater strength than others, or why some people can develop greater strength faster than others. Here, at the membrane of the muscle cells, all variation in human performance might be explicable within the response of the membrane enzymes, receptors, and glucose transport receptors to changes in ionic action potential and blood chemistry.

- **Cellular aspect:** Exercise increases the number of respiratory elements of the cells (the mitochondria) that burn foodstuff into energy by producing ATP, CO_2, water, and other byproducts. The mitochondrial ATP molecules are transported to the outer cytoplasm by specific enzyme transport system. In the cytoplasm, ATP is used in the contraction of the Actomyosin complex of the muscle fibers. Here, within the cell, also lie many secrets behind the variation of physical strength among humans. The cell has to make a chemical decision as to what source of food it will use to synthesize the high-energy molecules ATP, from ADP. The cell has the options of burning carbohydrates through glycolysis and pumping their pyruvate end products into the [TCA cycle-electron transport chain] in order to produce ATP. This decision is bound by the limited stock of glycogen in the liver and muscles that can only pump about 1400 Calories-worth of ATP and the high priority of the brain demands for glucose that have to supersede muscular needs. Alternatively, the cell has another option to burn fatty acids by β-oxidation and pump their end products, acetyl CoA, into the [TCA cycle-electron transport chain]. This decision is bound by the activity of the lipase enzymes at the vascular walls and the LDL-receptors on the fat cells that signal the need for fatty acid pumping into the circulation. If fat cells respond to such demands, they have to breakdown their stock of triglycerides into fatty acids and glycerol and pump them into circulation. Many tissues can then uptake the fatty acid into their cytoplasm and perform the oxidation of fatty acids, after first transporting them on the Carnitine shuttle into the mitochondria. Therefore, this decision is bound by many factors such as the ability of the liver to generate adequate lipoprotein carriers, the activity of the lipase enzymes, the response of the fat cell, and the transport of fatty acids on the Carnitine shuttle. Finally, the amount of ATP in muscles determines maximal contraction power of muscles and the duration of work.

- **Proprioception adaptation:** Stretching muscle fibers during weight training conditions the reflex mechanisms of muscular and tendinous proprioreceptors. These are reset to higher thresholds of firing for fiber recruitment and shut-off signals. Remember that we do not have any voluntary control on which portion of a muscle we may contract. For example, you can use your Biceps to pull your hand and forearm towards your body, but you cannot pick and choose which fibers of the Biceps can execute your motor signal. Although, such low level control of muscle fibers is trivial to our thinking, our inability to know what goes wrong within our muscles causes us to underestimate the value of strengthening. We might feel, from time to time, that we are weaker than we should and we should do something about it, but we do not know how much should we do to reach normalcy. We also do not have a wise voluntary mechanism to prevent tearing tendons with excessive weight. We must rely on the safety mechanism of tendon organs to shut off the motoneurons when newly heavier weight is excessively dangerous. Therefore, muscles have to take care of their welfare by spindle sensors that feedback the spinal nerve cells. These employ more or less units, only to execute the brain command that convey where, how, and when the weight will be lifted.

- **Cumulative effects:** Altering cells and their constituents and growing new nervous elements require time, continuity, and progressive increase in activity. The greater the weight of resistance, the greater is the need for cellular elements that produce energy, and the greater is the muscular strength. Working out with lighter weight enhances the aerobic trends of cells, which improves endurance, whereas heavier weights enhance anaerobic trends that improve strength. See Chapter 13, Section 13.3 on "Periodization of Load Intensity and Volume". How does strength grow with heavy lifting? It is easy to say that enzymes become more active, and energy cycles and transport shuttles become more dynamic, yet there must be a specific stimulus to strengthening other than mere chemical activation. It is thought that, heavier lifting rids of weaker muscle fibrils and stimulates their re-growth, in a process of hypertrophy. Or, the demised muscle fibers lead to stimulation of the stem cells of the muscles fibers to re-grow, in a process of hyperplasia of forming new muscle fibers. The newly hypertrophied or hyperplastic muscle fibers will carry the feature of the inducing activity, be they fast twitching or slow twitching. Repetitive weight training increases load volume at lower intensity and enhances growth of slow twitching muscle fibers. These are rich in blood supply and mitochondria, but can hinder ballistic activities of Olympic Weightlifting and other sports that require sudden and fast response. Thus, building huge muscles with high volume and low intensity causes hypertrophy of slow response muscle type. On the other side, high intensity ballistic exercises enhance the growth of the fast twitching muscles. These are poor in mitochondria and blood supply and rely heavily on anaerobic energy production. They can responds faster and produce high power by their efficient CP-ATP shuttle, which they have to replenish during longer rest breaks. Replenishment constitutes paying the oxygen debt aftereffect.

o **Dynamic gain and loss:** Muscular strength gained by training diminishes with inactivity. After six months intermission, more than 30% of the gained strength is reduced, and up 80% reduction by a year intermission. Reclaiming muscular loss does not happen over night, with quick and heavy exercise.[1] Training to reclaim loss of muscles alters the cellular strategies of managing energy. Long inactivity diverts excess food intake into fat. The amount of excess is determined based on the capacity of the muscle mass and liver to stock their glycogen depot by their specialized enzymes, Glycogen Synthase. Muscles can store more than twice as much glycogen as the liver. The liver converts excess amino acids into fuel form, after stripping them of their amine groups and converting them into acetyl CoA for fat synthesis. See Chapter 14, *Table 14.1* on "Difference in function of various types of cells of the human body". Thus, reclaiming muscular loss has to activate the fat breakdown in order to dig new routes of capillary circulation to active muscles. These new capillaries avail more acetyl CoA to the energy furnace of the [TCA cycle-electron transport chain]. Retraining has to proceed in slow and progressive manner in order to allow chemical changes to take place, according to the body's ability to tolerate changes.

o **Body and mind:** Of course, strength cannot be fostered without healthy biological milieu. This comprises of adequate rest, sufficient and balanced nutrients, and healthy neuromuscular and cardiopulmonary systems. You can account for all the training strategies of exercising and dieting, yet you have to integrate the body and mind into the equation of fitness. Some days you may feel very strong because all elements are accounted for, while other days strength might be reduced by imbalanced combination of training, rest, and nutrition. The part of the mind that we can enhance greatly lies in the cognitive and the memory departments. We can embark on interesting training plans that appeal to our cognitive faculties, as ways to enhance our understanding of the laws of nature, enhance health, and so on. Such self-convincing approach plays in committing ourselves to the venture of training. This opens new world of interactions with others and expands our memory in many dimensions that involve people, places, dates, and long accomplishments of successes and failures. I have met those who felt that training for six months is sufficient to equip them with all what they need to venture in the realm of fitness and health. Yet, I have spent over 40 years and still unconvinced that I have grasped all what I should have done. In fact, training is a growing up process. You will change your mind about many aspects of training, as you grow older.

o **Age:** is crucial to strength. Young age provides musculoskeletal system that can react to training, progressively and effectively. The young can better tolerate circulatory changes than adults do, by virtue of more elastic arterial system, more compliant heart, and more viable sympathetic reaction to vigorous exercise. At the peak of Weightlifting power, the slightest leak of the cardiac valves can cause sudden drop in strength. Also, the slightest delay of cardiac conduction of electricity, during peak performance, amounts to formidable plateau in strength. It is, therefore, not all muscle mass or nutrition that produce strength. Yet, we do not know for fact that aging is unavoidable fate. The common trend in aging is that people believe in counting the number of years elapsed and set themselves in accustomed lifestyle that is imposed by deceptive cultural norms. As far as science is concerned, the secret of aging is far from being known for sure.

o **Mode of muscular contraction:** Physical forces are produced by linear sliding of protein fibers by the action of forces of attraction produced by other protein fibers, within the muscle cells. The apparent movement of joints by muscular contraction is a net result of balance between external resistance and internal muscular attraction. The main regulator of internal affairs is the feedback mechanism of the nervous system. When the nervous system settles to overcome external work, by shortening of muscle fibers, then the result is dynamic concentric force. This sort of muscular contraction characterizes core-training exercises and is used for enhancing strength of major muscles, by increasing their ability to produce more power. When the nervous system settles to recede or yield to external resistance, by elongation of the muscle fibers, then the result is dynamic eccentric force. This sort of muscular contraction enhances hypertrophy of resilient muscles. Resisting external forces without altering muscle length is also a function of the nervous system that labors to exert isometric contraction with static force. Isometric training aims at enhancing motor control and fostering specific skill, such as strengthening weak links along chain of muscular contraction. In any case, the limitation to feedback is reached when muscular tension can no longer resist external forces. This is the point of

---

1 The false promise of altering physical condition in few weeks by serious exercise is unfounded, though propagated by some such as the book: "Body-for-life: 12 weeks to mental and physical strength" by Bill Phillips with Michael D'Orso, 1st edition. Harper Collins Publishers, New York, 1999.

maximal strength. The maximal strength of a muscle depends on the initial length of the fibers, the speed of contraction, and the time that is necessary to reach maximal tension. Simply said, this is proportional to the average acceleration of contraction given by Newton's law, $\mathbf{a} = (\mathbf{v}_i - \mathbf{v}_o)/\Delta t$. Thus, abrupt muscular contraction (short duration of Δt) requires greater forces than gradual contraction (large acceleration, $\mathbf{a}$). However, during eccentric dynamic force (as in lowering the weights), resistance forces are greater than in concentric dynamic forces, since both gravity and acceleration lie in one direction opposite to muscular resistance. This fact about eccentric contraction is utilized in developing maximal strength.

20.1.3. DEVELOPING STRENGTH

Muscular strength is promoted by mechanical work against resisting force. Since mechanical work is proportional to the magnitude of force and the distance traveled against that force, therefore, strength can be enhanced by either increasing the force or the distance of work, as follows.

o **Resisting maximal force**: Few repetitions of lifting heavy weights, or resisting greater forces, enhance the development of energy expenditure mechanism by anaerobic metabolism. The force of contraction of the muscle depends on the ATP concentration in the working muscle units. Maximal resistance enhances harmonious recruitment of large pool of muscle fibers and promotes neuromuscular coordination at higher stresses. This sort of strengthening is only recommended for advanced trainees, since maximal forces puts too much strain on the ligaments, tendons, and bone, which require many months of training to resist greater forces. Resisting greater forces with improper technique could lead to serious injuries to the joints. Forces over 60% of maximal lifts, in specific configuration, are considered "greater forces". Weights are lifted once to thrice per set, with rest intervals not longer than two minutes. If the weight could be lifted with ease, over three times, it is better to increase the weight rather than the repetitions. This approach is mainly anaerobic that is founded on the principle "deliver now, pay later".

o **Working longer distances:** Large number of repetitions of lifting sublimit weights increases the distance of work, in proportion to the number of repetitions and the range of motion. Fast repetitions also increase the virtual force (due to added acceleration). In fact, exercising without weight, at fast and jerky fashion, induces the same effect of weights but lacks the versatility of enhancing all possible directions of motion. For example, you can develop awesome thigh, abdominal, and shoulder muscles by just sprinting at top speed. The results of this alternative training are very gratifying. The total summation of work exhausts muscle reserves and generates sufficient lactates to induce local stimulation. This approach is mostly used for warm-up purposes, for learning new techniques by beginners, or for recuperation from long-term lack of training. Repeated lifting of lighter weights remedies the deficiencies in imbalance due to muscular instability. The protracted duration of high repetitive-work allows the accumulation of thermal energy, as the lactates interfere with local circulation. Locally generated heat alleviates spasm, strain, and enhances vascularity and muscular hypertrophy, afterwards. Light weights in the range from 40% to 60% of the maximum limits are repeated five to ten times, for three to six sets, depending on the desired extent of tension. Rest breaks between sets are less than three minutes. This approach is mainly aerobic that is founded on the principle "deliver as you pay". Thus, energy is produced as fat is being oxidized.

20.2. FUNDAMENTALS OF STRENGTH TRAINING

20.2.1. FREQUENCY

o **Weekly routine:** Exercise promotes health when it constitutes regular and continuous lifestyle activity. When performed regularly and for long time, it alters the structure and function of chemical agents, cellular elements, and organs, within the body. The apparent changes in the body and the feeling of wellness result from cumulative changes in all these biological entities. **Three days each week**, of at least an hour of vigorous exercise, should maintain your strength and health at a steady state. **Five days** of vigorous exercise per week will definitely breakthrough barriers of weaknesses and deficits of many systems of the body. **Random exercise** may cause injuries that might become lifelong problems. Of course, one should not attempt to make sudden changes in lifestyle by introducing strenuous activities all of a sudden. **Gradual increase** in intensity and frequency of strength training can only pull your health on the right path. Gradually, you can learn how to balance your fear from getting exhausted by heavy labor against your enthusiasm to promote your fitness and health. Go to the gym at least five days a week, even if you can grab few minutes of workout and more time in the saunas, whirlpool, or chatting with others. One of these days, that you might have thought being wasted in vain, may bring the greatest ideas to your life. Workout is, above all, just new ideas and new motivation that thrust your spirit and keep you going.

o For **late starters**, minimal number of exercise sessions is three sessions per week. Longer intervals between sessions lead to decline in strength and increase in injuries. The commonest injuries due to fewer weekly training sessions are strains of the wrist, ankle, back, and neck. These are the pivotal points of transfer of leverage forces from hands, to

GUIDELINES FOR OPTIMUM STRENGTH TRAINING

feet, to ground. In comparison to other professions that demand physical activities, farming produces natural strength that surpasses any strength gained from structured training, with the exception of lack of balanced strength in full range of motion. Prior to modern mechanization and in many third world countries, farmers perform heavy work from sunrise to sunset, with a brief mid-day nap.

o **Normal training** sessions are those that allow you to return to training within 24 hours, with normal heart rate and enough stamina to repeat the same workout and still feel comfortable. It is thought that vigorous training is controlled by bursts of testosterone excretion that starts, peaks, and drops within an hour period. It is a fact that you can have very effective workout within an hour, to an hour and half, and can repeat that more than once daily. Bear in mind that strength training is assisting to exercises that involve technique and speed and thus should follow such exercises, if these to be included in the same training session. A session is defined as a workout that is separated from a subsequent workout with at least few hours.

20.2.2. GYM

I am not an advocate for home exercise. If you enjoy hermitic life, you might have to weigh the consequences of repeating your own mistakes, over and over, without a clue of what goes wrong, versus the interaction with a world full of life that might teach you a better way of doing things, *Figures 20.1* and *20.2*. You never know whether your sources of information are up to date or entirely obsolete, until you see, talk, or listen to different opinions. Home exercise will limit you to books, television, radio, or Internet. Going to the gym, on the other side, is the greatest experience that you undertake. The gym is the biggest **live laboratory** of human achievements. Here, you can witness the constant effort made by people, from all walks of life, to overcome their difficulties. In the gym, you will be able to polish your theory about fitness and add or subtract methods and ways of doing things. Beside sharing information and learning the tricks of the trade from gym going, the essence of working out with and among others is that strength training is very complex and its consequences shape your lifestyle. You cannot grasp all the knowledge in functional anatomy, mechanical performance, physiological changes, and strategies of training by mere theoretical means. Take the example of learning the Power Clean. You can learn how to do that from a video or by reading books about it, but you will never be able to discover the accumulated knowledge of the hundred years of refining the technique on your own. You might guess that strong arms, back, and legs will do it. Yet, experience shows that it is not the strength of isolated body parts, but regular and constant neuromuscular coordination, that does it.

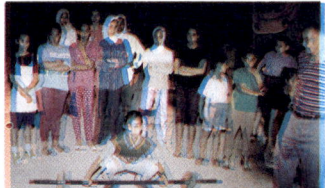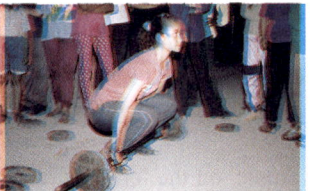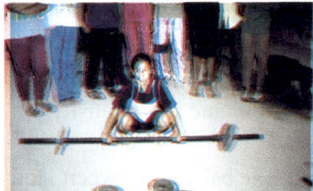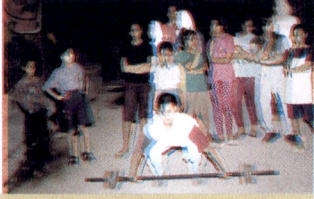

Figure 20.1. Weightlifting is an ancient folklore in some cultures. In these photos, kids gather and learn the start position of bending knees, thrusting chest, straightening back, and locking elbows. Spectators will make many comments when the technique deviates from ideal. Bear in mind the similarities of these photos with that story of a little old lady, Section 1.11. These kids are from Egypt, whereas lady's story from New York.

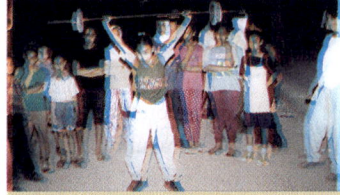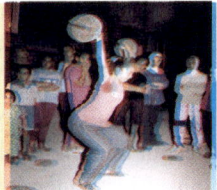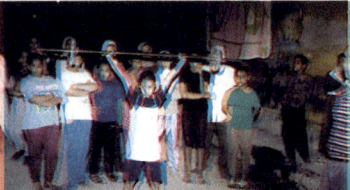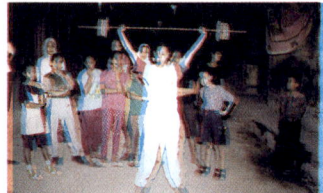

Figure 20.2. Lifting from the floor to overhead is all what these kids will do in this street gym. Note the perfect positioning of the head, back, legs, and arms. All the young lifters learn how to move the head and pelvis as the bar ascends from the floor to overhead. The final stance under the bar is also well mastered. That comprises of arched in lower back, straight and locked elbows, advanced head, thrust chest, and locked knees. (From Alexandria, Egypt. Courtesy of Dr. Salah F. El-Hewie.)

20.2.3. PROGRAM

o **Session details:** Exercise should be simplified in terms of the number of **exercise groups, sets per group, and repetitions** per set. To overcome boredom changes should be made frequently without undermining the basics of balanced exercise. The least number of exercise groups in a training session should be three. That is based on three body regions: pelvis, torso, and shoulders. The least number of sets per exercise is four, which enables you to gradually reach intense load. The maximum number of repetitions should not exceed ten (to avoid accumulation of lactic acid). Total sets per session should not exceed forty (to avoid boredom and exhaustion).

20 GUIDELINES FOR OPTIMUM STRENGTH TRAINING

- **Weekly details:** Weightlifting has come around almost a full circle, in the last century, in regard to the number of training exercises in weekly programs. In the 1920's and 1930's, Weightlifters practiced the three basic event lifts in their training. With the advances of the post-war sciences, weekly exercises were increased to assist in strengthening individual muscles on the premise that isolation exercises enhance whole body strength. Not so long until trainers discovered that strengthening individual muscles has very little to do with whole body performance. This discovery coincided with the elimination of the Clean and Press lift from the Olympic Weightlifting in 1972. Modern Weightlifting training is narrowed to less than **fifteen exercises per week**. These are, basically, the Clean and Jerk, Snatch, Pulls, Deadlift, Squat, and few variations of the same regarding the type of contraction and the phase of lifting process. Mainly, lifting the barbell from the floor is the fundamental principle in resistance training, *Figures 20.1* and *20.2*.

- **Anatomical details:** Factors that lead to incompliance and loss of interest are: complex session, lack of structured plan, unplanned total load strategy, too many repetition, sets, exercises, or inappropriate sequence of exercises. Although the most appropriate program varies from individual to individual, there still exist a basic rule of defining such program for all people. Such golden rule of embarking on an **effective strength-training program** is the inclusion of a substantial workout for each of the three body regions, each and every training session. For example, in the "chest- and arms-day", you can slightly touch on the torso and legs. In the "legs-day", you can slightly exercise the "shoulders and back". Also, in the "back-day", you can involve the legs and shoulders in light compound exercises. Such basic rule will prove effective after years of training, in the form of building sound musculoskeletal frame, balance proportions, and healthy cardiopulmonary and neuromuscular systems. The alternative of mere isolation days of training of body parts produce **disproportional deformities**, functional deficits such as incoordination and inflexibility, and reduced whole body strength.

20.2.4. INTENSITY OF RESISTANCE

- **Cumulative effects:** Strength and endurance do not happen overnight. Many changes in the body take place slowly and gradually to promote health. Many exercises require execution without weight, in order to master the technique, before increasing the resistance. Visual and mental efforts drive performance. Some regions of the body require slower gradient than others do. The forearms and the lower back regions take longer time to develop than the thighs and the shoulders. Yet, the most critical gradient is that of the **heart and lung development**. Patience and determination help advance performance. Whatever effort you undertake will produce cumulative effects as long as training continues. Such cumulative effects are quantified as **"the training volume"**, a term that become very familiar to all Weightlifters of modern times and signifies the whole body response to training on the long run. Modern Weightlifters average a daily volume of 30 to 40 tons of lifting in major exercises, with a maximum of 100 tons. The load volume is lowered two or three weeks before the contest in order to allow the athlete to build up strength. See Chapter 13 on "Managing Load Volume and Intensity".

- **Exertion versus stimulation:** The balance between load volume, on the long run, and load intensity, on the short run, determines the quality of strength training. Although the rule of thumb that "heavy weight does it" is a very precise mean of developing strength, yet the balance between lift tonnage and number of lift repetitions is critical. Efforts were made to find the proper balance between **lifting difficulty** due to heavier weight and lifting burnout due to higher repetitions. Some believe that if compound and competitive lifts (such as the Clean Jerk and Snatch) exceed two-thirds of all lifts, with average intensity (volume averaged over total number of lifts), then strength training becomes most effective. That is because compound lifts travel longer distances than isolated lifts and involves heavier weights.

- **Planning load intensity:** The pace at which you will increase the level of difficulty of resistance amounts to **"load intensity"** which signifies the short-term readiness to perform. Strength training implements the fundamental principle of progressive increase in load intensity in order to foster strength. This principle has undergone several phases of development before it culminates into modern day practice. Before the WWII, Weightlifters relied mainly on the buildup of psychological and physical energy prior to contest, in order to lift new records during contest. Famous stories I have personally heard from Ibrahim Shams (the Egyptian Olympic gold medallist in 1948, in the 67 kg class, Press 97.5, Snatch 115, Clean Jerk 147.5) that he used to limit his snatch maximum to 60 kg, in training. He focused on the speed and completely relied on his buildup of rest and mental concentration, during contest, when trying new records. Those who train with maximum lifts, every possible opportunity, had never succeeded in accomplishing new records. The rationale behind such old way of intense lifting, only during contest, stems from the old and long belief that **strength originates from the mind,** not the muscles. Modern Weightlifting has evolved to implementing attempts with maximum exertion during training as well. At present, the number of maximum exertion attempts during the Weightlifting training varies from training season to another. Few weeks prior to contest, the entire training session might be devoted to maximal exertion attempts in order to put the lifter in competitive mode.

GUIDELINES FOR OPTIMUM STRENGTH TRAINING

o **Tweaking maximal lifts:** Implementing intense training depends on the age and the current physical preparedness of the athletes. **Maximal intensity** can be breached with increase over, or decrease under, previous values. For example, an athlete who worked hard to foster shoulder strength might find that his maximal values of intensity can be easily surpassed in certain upper body exercises. Likewise, an athlete who omitted axial exercises for some time might have to lower his previous maximal intensity in freestyle lifting. Thus, the concept of defining maximal intensity should be versatile in accordance with current state of strength. The well-practiced method of working out with maximal loads is subtracting 10 or 20 kilograms of the maximum, as a guide for submaximal level

o **Periodization:** Efforts to balance breaching maximal strength (setting new record) and avoiding injury are made utilizing a **cycle of buildup** and exertion routines. The cycle starts with an introductory low intensity workout of less than 90% of maximal weigh, at less than 5 repetitions per set of exercises, for a week, or so. The second phase is basic average intensity training of up to 100% intensity, but at fewer total number of sets for a week, or so. The third phase of the cycle is a shock phase of great intensity, of greater number of sets, in the 100% or more of maximal intensity. The cycle ends with low intensity recovery week of less than 80% intensity. The cycle is then repeated with increased maximal strength level for another four weeks, and so on. See Chapter 13, Section 13.3 on "Periodization of Load Intensity and Volume".

o **Course of development:** The reason that many people get easily discouraged, when expected progress does not follow hard work, is the lack of understanding of the **time frame of physical development** and the significance of proper tweaking of efforts in order to foster development, *Figure 20.3* and *20.4*. Fast and hard work can cause overtraining and setback in your progress. Also, slow and minimal work may not suffice muscular stimulation and may not foster strengthening. Again, each day brings its own "music". You should not force yourself to engage in fatiguing workout if you do not feel good. There will come another day when you can perform at your best. You better save yourself from injuries to such moments. When it comes to training, a well-known fact is that some days may turn unexpectedly better than previously thought. When you do the right things, of proper sleep, nutrition, and regular training, your physical performance will outpace your psychological mood. Thus, when you feel down and bored, going to the gym and starting a regular routine of workout may demonstrate such superiority of physical dominance over mind.

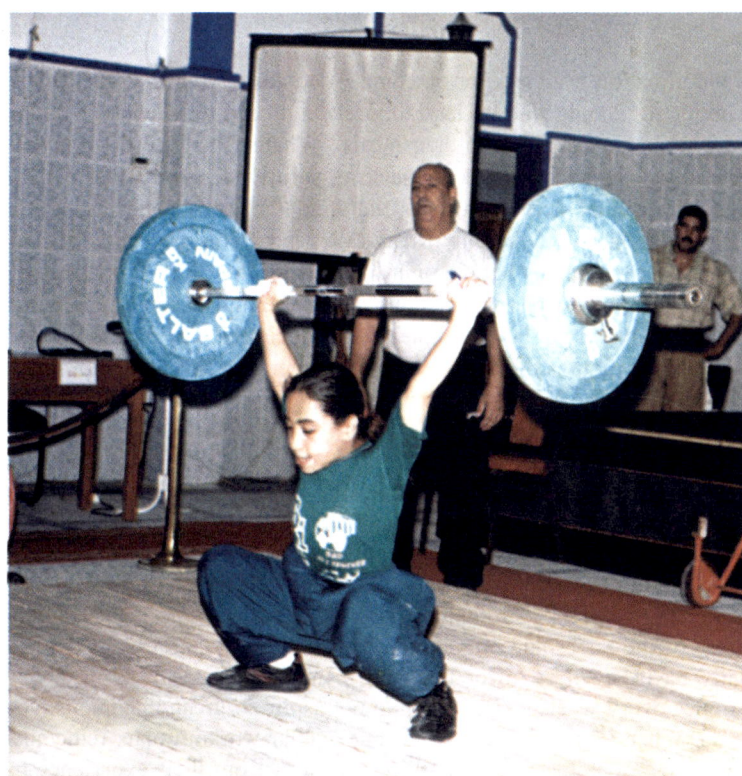

Figure 20.3. A twelve-year old girl lifting 45 kilograms in the Snatch, with outstanding Olympic technique. Whole body strength, coordination, and flexibility have little to do with muscular size. For this little girl, Weightlifting is very empowering. She can, not only perform perfect technique, but also dare to descend under such heavy steel barbell. (From Alexandria, Egypt. Courtesy of Dr. Salah F. El-Hewie.)

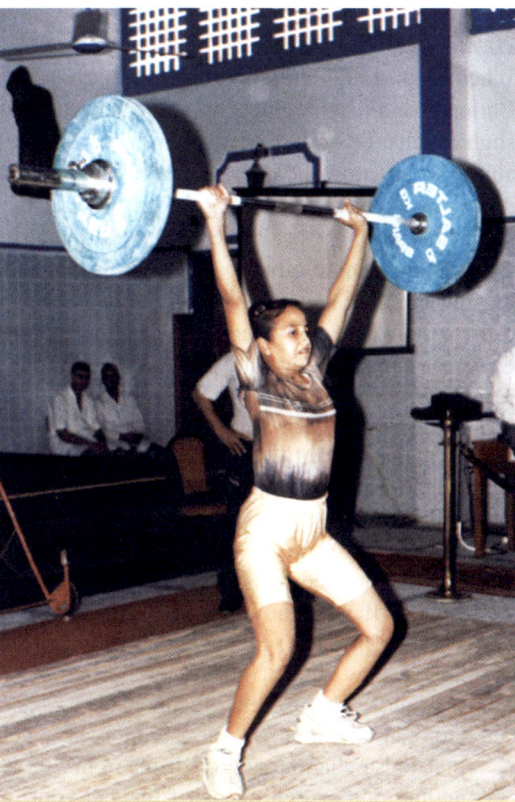

Figure 20.4. A twelve-year old girl lifting 45 kilograms in the Clean and Jerk. With little tweaking of the technique, this child lifter will remedy the weakness of the back and shoulders. (From Alexandria, Egypt. Courtesy of Dr. Salah F. El-Hewie.)

GUIDELINES FOR OPTIMUM STRENGTH TRAINING

20.2.5. GOALS
These evolve as training proceeds. The quality of the exercise plan, the adherence to, and compliance with the plan determine how far you can advance. Sometimes, you may discover a flaw in your program in time to correct without consequences. Other times, flaws are discovered too late. For example, young Bodybuilders may discover after few months that exercising at limited range of motion permanently limits the joint movement and denies the athlete opportunities to practice other sports. Early in training, many Bodybuilders enjoy the tight joints and stiff gait as a sign of toughness. Rectifying that flaw might require longer periods of stretching exercises, when the damage to the joints is still reversible. I recall my early days in Weightlifting when a coach excluded few new comers from training because they were over the age of sixteen, could not do ten pushups, ten Squats without weights, or three chin-ups. Simply, coaches are interested in those who can land on their feet and run for the medals. Yet, at young age, one can build up proper body proportion, in function and size, with considerable ease and certainty than at later years, *Figure 20.3*. Fortunately, with modern fitness technology and information every one can share the glory of promoting their health and fitness.

20.2.6. LIFESTYLE
Exercise alone does not promote health unless you adopt healthy habits in all aspects of your lifestyle. You do not have to know the caloric contents of each **foodstuff** in order to win the slimness contest. Yet, you need to know general ideas about healthy food. The role of thumb is that as little amounts of diverse food intake can maintain steady bodyweight and prevent excess calories and nutritional deficiencies. **Substance use** (including tobacco, alcohol, caffeine, and drug) may undermine any gain from exercise. Exercise relies on the liver, nervous system, and heart to expend muscular energy. Substance abuse afflicts these vital systems. Adherence to exercise program could greatly benefit from abstinence from those interfering factors. Also, regular and **adequate sleep** is crucial to benefiting from physical training. Sleeping in arbitrary hours, for irregular periods, at different times of the day, and in uncomfortable environments defeat the purpose of any physical training. The same can be said on **eating** in arbitrary hours, at different times of the days, and in unpleasant environments. Our inner and unconscious perception of the outer world affects how our body deals with health, growth, and fitness. Such hectic lifestyle afflicts our guts, circulation, and psyche. The large intestines are the first victim to chaotic lifestyle and can protest such chaos with complaints such as indigestion, constipation, and intestinal distention. The arterial system also is under the mercy of the sympathetic autonomic system that is afflicted with chaotic lifestyle. Also, the psyche of a person living in a fast pace urban community differs from that of country lifestyle. All such lifestyle habits play a major role in our ability to benefit from strength training.

20.2.7. ADJUSTMENT
When all plans do not work, there is still hope that a modification brings better outcome. You are not the first one to fail. Curiosity and listening to people might alert you to a problem. People who try hard to lose weight could be helped with the slightest change of avoiding sweet drinks or cutting down one source of fat in their meals. Whatever interferes with your ability to adapt to the demands of exercise could be easily remedied if you **keep seeking solutions**. Sometimes cutting down the volume of training altogether and focusing on areas of deficits such as the abdomen, chest, and legs could noticeably promote health better than an idealistic plan that is hard to adhere to. Many times, problems are caused by our unconscious denial, omission, or poor understanding. For example, many people omit lifting from the floor, exercising the legs every training session, or doing overhead exercises. Such omissions will undoubtedly undermine axial strength and afflicts the whole body performance. Confronting such problems might be as simple as introducing one or two compound exercises each sessions and monitoring the progress over many months of regular training. Sometimes, substantial progress requires few years of such modification of exercise plan in order to be noticeable.

20.2.8. INDIVIDUALIZATION
o   Past mistakes shape individual needs. Some people have hard time working their legs, some their shoulders, others their back. These major body regions suffer neglect and drastically impact health. Embark on an exercise plan that is tailored to remedy you **individual deficits**. Whether these deficits are in strength, flexibility, endurance, or coordination, correcting any aspect of deficit, on long-term plan, improves your entire health. Take the example of bad knees. If you know which aspect of the knee causes problem, you could modify your plan to target that deficit. Walking prior to running enhances postural balance of the knees and might make you run better than if start on cold knees. Few sets of quadriceps exercises on daily basis, even at lower intensities, tide your legs over prolonged weakness. This is better than exercising legs just once every week. Even if you do not aspire to great champions, you still can take them as reference to where you stand. When you have done with your regular workout plan, remember that those champions just differ from you in percentage of things and you still can benefit from their experience by adding one or two of their rituals to your routine. Do **Goodmorning, Squat, Bench Press, Deadlift, or Shoulder Press** for three to four light sets after the end of your routine, on regular cycle and depending on your needs. These great four exercises can easily be used to remedy most individual deficits, to the extent that they become the core exercises of Powerlifting and Weightlifting assistance training.

o   The principal rules of strength training that apply to all individuals are as follows. In building maximal strength, one should maintain the number of repetitions below five, with **maximal and sub-maximal weights** (above 60% of maximal) in each particular category of exercises. The total **duration of a session** is kept under an hour, in order to prevent severe exertion and protracted recovery. The fewer repetitions of strength training ensure slower heart rate (<120 bpm) and greater stroke volume per pulse.

20.2.9. DOCUMENTATION
Recording **daily exercises**, according to the body regions they act upon or the general action, gets you in the habit of swift planning and spotting deficits. Total sets and maximas of weights lifted or distances run on daily basis is a good habit to monitor progress or detect flaws. Dated **photographs** are the most invaluable documents you could have, especially in tracking the development of joint flexibility and technique refinement. In order to reach sound analysis of how deformities evolve, one may be helped by old photographs in answering questions regarding issues such as how deep could the person squat, how high can the person flex both shoulders in Front Squat, how straight can the back bend over in Goodmorning, and how oblique can the torso sustain in Deadlift. On the other hand, written records of daily workouts are invaluable in tracking imbalance training such as omissions of, and over-emphasis on certain muscles, movement, and load volume.

20.2.10. INSIGHT
Lack of insight is the worst enemy to exercisers. You might severely and unknowingly damage a joint, believing that pain precedes gain. Super heavy weight on half Squat or Deadlift is an example of many dangerous exercises that require insight. A coach, a training partner, reading, or other means of advancing your knowledge could enhance your insight into what you are up to. You might sense elation by shoulder pressing heavy weight so many times, while an outsider might notice your improper technique of incomplete range, imbalanced shoulder, or hunched back. Understanding how insight affects our life helps manage our affairs, as follows.

o   Insight is **totally or partially lost** in psychotic diseases such as schizophrenia and manic-depressive episodes. Also, insight could be temporarily lost in severe fever. An individual with fever might become unaware of hallucination and severe sickness because fever afflicts brain functions.
o   Insight is the **function of the cognitive sphere** of mind that constitutes one of three spheres, the other being mood and behavior. Cognition performs thinking, behavior manages our actions, and mood controls our feeling. The three spheres, or departments of the mind, are driven by instincts and censored by our ego that controls the psyche, in congruence with external reality. Instinctual forces aim at survival, reproduction, security of belonging, power of leading, and freedom from dangers, which all amount to mastering the environment of existence.
o   Common maladies, such as depression and anxiety, stem from the psyche mood and are alleviated by **fostering our insight** into the matters of affairs. This occurs in the playful activities of exercise, which are real interaction with methods and people. Sadly, despite our deep insight into many behavioral problems, we yet are unable to alter such behavior to alleviate suffering. Overeating and inactivity are examples of behavioral issues, with known causes but relentless progression.
o   Our **control over our mind**, to alter behavior that defies logic and learned knowledge, should be instilled in raising children prior to the development of long term unshakeable habits.
o   Understanding the nature of **conflict management** within the psyche aids us understand our complex and intriguing existence. Conflicts arise when our ego strives to reconcile our instinctual needs with realistic options. Wanting to become a gymnastic or a ballet dancer, while struggling with lack of training and opportunities, generates a conflict that might lead to anxiety. Insightful analysis helps assimilate various options to reach more plausible outcome, by seeking flexible and creative behaviors that may be more effective in our life.
o   Balancing the struggle of our ego, between our needs and realistic options, is greatly helped by expanding these options to new horizons. Exercise opens great spectrum of options for education that refines our motor skills and impacts our psyche in many ways. We think about how to **plan training**, act on complex and tricky strategies, and enjoy the success of getting that far. Even failure in sport leaves us with wealth of experience about miscalculating outcomes.

20.2.11. WEIGHT TRAINING GUIDELINES
o   On daily basis, perform a minimum of **three to six exercises** that work out the major muscle groups. Fewer exercises, with more sessions of workout per week, are superior to exhaustive exercises on three or four day's week. **Muscular hypertrophy** is promoted by higher training volume of average repetition, of six per set of 1RM. **Muscular power** is promoted by repetition under four per set, with many 1RM sets. Between sets, break should not exceed 3 minutes in order to sustain sympathetic stimulation and avoid drastic alteration in local muscular environment. **Endurance training** is promoted by higher repetitions. This drains immediate fuel supply and operates at fatty acid oxidation, with weaker power production
o   Programs longer than **one hour** are associated with higher drop out rates. In order to increase intensity of training, shorter sessions allow heavier training with faster recovery of systems.
o   Choose more compound, or **multi-joint exercises**, which involve more muscles with fewer exercises. Training groups of muscles leads to long-term improvement in systemic and local elements and foster proportionate growth and balanced functioning.
o   Exercises that comprise of **concentric muscle contraction** improve technique and muscular coordination and should constitute the bulk of your workout. Exercises that comprises of **eccentric muscle action** should be devoted for strengthening weaker links, since they work mostly on increasing strength, yet interfere with technique and relaxation.

GUIDELINES FOR OPTIMUM STRENGTH TRAINING

- o **Resilient muscles** such as the forearms, chest, shoulders may require higher repetition sets of 8 to 12 repetitions in order to induce volitional fatigue, which stimulate muscle growth.
- o **Major muscles** such as thighs, back erectors, shoulder plate muscles, and shoulders require 4 to 6 sets of progressive weight increase in order to maintain muscle strength.
- o Perform exercises at least 3 days per week. Training that is more frequent induces greater strength on the long term, if overtraining is carefully avoided. Recuperation between workouts may occur in few hours or longer. Some people train twice or thrice daily. The fact that menial workers develop outstanding strength attests to the effectiveness of **high frequency** and moderate intensity training.
- o **Proper performance** of exercise techniques guarantees strengthening of the muscles that exercises are intended to strengthen. Thus, deep squatting is superior to higher squatting, even if done at lower intensity, since it maintains stretchability of the Quadriceps and back erectors. Deviation from proper technique predisposes to ugly and distressing deformities that range from stiff and short ligaments and tendons, to deformed cartilages and bones.
- o The **range of motion** can be increased gradually and slowly over weeks or months, in almost all major joints, if regular and progressive training is maintained.
- o **Exercise sequence** should account for working major muscles, before small ones, through multiple-joint exercises and higher intensity, before lower intensity exercises. This guarantees utilization of major reserves of energy before the body switches to fat oxidation that is sluggish in producing muscular power.
- o **Warm-up** should not exceed fifteen minutes if one expects to reach high intensity during session. Full range of motion with progressive weights under 50% 1RM is ideal for warm-up. This prepares the neuromuscular system to stimulate the exact mechanics, which will be performed during the workout. It reduces muscle and joint injury and increases muscular recruitment through enhancing motor skill and breathing.

20.3. EFFECTS OF EXERCISE

20.3.1. MIND AND BODY

The instinctual drive to engage in physical activities serves the purpose of empowering the animal species with the capabilities to roam the universe in search for energy. Plants get their share of energy through symbiotic existence with animals. The mobility of animals sustains their participation in transmitting pollens, processing complex molecules for bacterial growth, and fertilization of the soil. In humans, it is feared that such instinctual drive to exercise might wane as urbanization proliferates through societies. Many animal species had ceased to exist, in part, due to failure to adapt to changes in environment. Such fear is fortified by the fact that the human brain is in constant process of evolution. The higher brain faculties of humans are far evolved beyond those of our closest relatives in the mammalian species. Our determination and thinking processes are believed to be localized in certain brain areas and governed by certain **chemical activities**. Thus, the instinctual drive to exercise is both originated in the brain and rejuvenated by its action to engage in physical work, through the activities of body cells, organs, and systems, as follows.

- o Exercise improves **mental health** by altering our emotion and mood, in a manner similar to what drugs do, yet more natural and safe. It fulfills the basic purpose of all animal life on earth, which is motion for search of specific energy resources. Exercise alleviates anxiety and depression through exposing the individual to **realistic activities** that proceed from cause to effect. It breaks the cycle of irrational fear of the unknown. It is self-empowering to engage in changing your fate from weakness and vulnerability to strength and assertiveness. After you get involved in gainful activity, your mind shifts its focus of passion towards the new challenge of more gainful activities.
- o Few weeks of training amounts to a transfer from the life of unfit survival to the **life of positive existence**. There are many new activities you can do with getting more fit. These range from mastering your immediate environment to improving your body image that you thought formidable. As long as you appreciate how the laws of nature govern its elements, you will be able to pace your endeavors in accordance to viable and reasonable goals.
- o To your surprise, changes in body image and feeling of wellness are surely accompanied with serious changes within you. Weightlifting in particular alters the body to perform forceful actions that make lifters more distinguished than others, in strength. Strength originates in the **ability of cells** to make new proteins and the ability of the nerve cells to manage those proteins within the muscles to generate forceful actions. The memory of strength resides in the molecules of life, the DNA, which custom-makes protein to fit exercise strategies. Thus, exercise affects the very essence of life codes, the DNA.
- o No such actions of strength are possible without a milieu conducive to **harmonious activities**. Exercise, and in particular strength training, advances such harmonious body activities to the highest efficacy. It prevents falls and dizziness due to sudden activities by conditioning the sympathetic system through the regulation of hormones (Norepinephrine, Epinephrine, ACTH, Cortisol, Dopamine, Serotonin, ß-Endorphin). Hormonal regulation controls the body metabolism and brain activity. The higher brain function that drives your will to engage in activities is over-stimulated by vigorous activities that require high arousal of lower brain centers (respiration, consciousness, cardiovascular activities, and reflexes). Less vigorous exercises induce boredom and mental fatigue.

20.3.2. ADAPTATION TO EXERCISE

- o Exercise is a willful activity that stems from mental drive, planning, motivation, and decision to act and follow up on the results. This impetus overcomes physical difficulties such as sweating, sunburns, friction injuries, strains of tendons, and even bone fractures. Incurring all such troubles, for the sake of **playful acts** that do not bring immediate material gains, cannot be explained without the innate drive to physical performance. In fact, playful activities seem to be more tempting to animals than mere search for food. Kids would rather play forever, if left on their own vices, than seek food.

o Persistent efforts to overcome difficulties lead to heightened endurance and strength, which reduce exhaustion over time. Without increasing stimulus, adaptation plateaus to steady state level. Planning exercise program with keen **integration of elements** of strength, endurance, flexibility, and coordination fosters adaptation of various systems of the body. For tough, young, and motivated people, the issues of integration of multi-systemic elements of fitness in exercise are hardly comprehensible unless imposed on them via institutional programs, with incentives to adherence, *Figure 20.3*. Amateur strength trainees do not foresee the consequences of deficient planning of exercise until irreversible changes take place.

o Today, the majority of strength trainees has difficulty balancing these elements and suffers stiff joints, limited mobility, vulnerable joints, reduced endurance, and lack of coordination. The basic advantage of integrated training is improving the harmony of recruitment of different muscle groups to perform different tasks. In layman words, this amounts to **graceful motion** in performance and in everyday activities. Bodybuilders incur common upper back deformities due to limited activities of free lifting from the floor. Powerlifters incur lifelong frozen joints, from damaged cartilages to calcified ligaments and tendons. Swimmers incur weak lower limbs due to limited squatting activities. Aerobic trainees incur weak upper limbs due to emphasis of light bodyweight. Gymnastics have weaker lower body due to focused upper body training. Weightlifters integrate most aspects of fitness to develop strength at full range of motion and flexibility, in major joints. They perform motions that emulate real life situations, yet lack impressive muscular appearance. If Weightlifters introduce adequate yoga-style stretching exercises, then they might be able to continue lifting effectively until old age.

20.3.3. IMMEDIATE EFFECTS OF STRENGTH EXERCISE

o **Tension:** Resistance exercise requires vigorous muscular contraction. That shuts off the blood flow exiting the active muscle, which leads to temporary trapping of blood in major muscles. Though most of the pooled blood returns to systemic circulation as soon as muscles relax, a substantial portion of the plasma fluid still accumulates within the extracellular space of the muscle. Heavy resistance exercise causes more accumulation of the byproducts in muscles, many hours after the exercise ends. That is because strength training relies on the ability of the muscle to amplify the energy obtained by burning glucose through the creatine phosphate and adenosine triphosphate replenishment. A molecule of glucose, when slowly metabolized in the cytoplasm of cells, yields two molecules of pyruvic acids and two molecules of ATP. Without oxygen, the pyruvic acid molecules snatch hydrogen from the hydrogen carrier molecules (NADH). This anaerobic reaction yields lactate and NAD molecules. Furthermore, those local byproducts increase fluid trapping in the muscle and lead to the sense of fullness and tension. As a muscle contracts, it squeezes any vein in its way thus pushes the venous blood towards the heart, but trap the arterial blood behind. Axial explosive exercises induce shocking, trapping, and pumping of massive amounts of blood within the major muscles. Thus, axial exercise reduces fluid trapping, and consequently the **swelling of the muscles with fluids**. Isometric exercise increases muscle size by protracted fluid trapping. This forces the tiny blood capillaries to find alternative routes to circulate fluids and, in the same time, induces angiogenesis, which makes muscles more vascular. Weightlifters resort to massage and steam sauna to reduce fluid trapping by warming the skin and inducing perspiration through superficial vasodilation. Many Weightlifters present with smooth muscle contours during rest, yet to show awesome definition during maximal lifting. The fluid clearance, by massage and sauna, aids muscles replenish reserves and reduce fluid congestion. In fact, without massaging and hot sauna many Weightlifters would not be able to lift such maximal weights or endure heavy lifting that many years. Both the Greek lifter **Pyrros Dimas** and the Turkish lifter **Naim Suleymanoglu** have hold the Olympic gold medals for 12 consecutive years, which is momentous task due to the fierce competition and performance on the global arena.

o **Soreness:** Strength related activities operate anaerobically and thus accumulate plenty of lactate in short duration. Lactates are produced from the reduction of pyruvate and oxidation of NADH into NAD. Lactates are acidic and cause sense of **exercise burning.** They block the calcium release within the muscle and cause decline in strength, until enough rest is taken to wash away lactate into circulation. The liver, kidney, intestine, and heart take up circulating lactates for gluconeogenesis, which converts lactates to glucose. The deceptive feeling of tightness of muscles after weight training leads people to believe that muscles grow instantaneously. In the past, we thought that the benefit of lactate burning and fatigue is the local stimulation of new vascularization and enhancement of circulation that lead to future growth. Recently, scientists discovered different mechanism for angiogenesis due to exercise. This takes place through the stimulation of the endothelium of blood vessels and the production of nitric oxide gas. The release of nitric oxide is governed by the presence of enzymes, amino acid substrates, genetic expression of enzymes, and exercise. This discovery bridges the gap between nature and nurture.

o **Injury:** Severe and lasting injuries may happen insidiously and may be confused for soreness. A tight joint after heavy partial range of motion could signal the early sign of **crushed cartilage or bone,** particularly if difficulty in moving the joint lasts for hours. Soreness is a muscular symptom that is limited to the topography of the workinga ctive muscle. However, joint tightness is due to swollen joint capsule. Knee injury due to heavy and high Squatr leg press is a typical example of common injuries that deceive many tough trainees and set an end to their career in competitive sports. Joint injury occurs once a heavy load exceeds the threshold of elasticity of the joint cartilage. Damaged cartilages are irreplaceable. These expose the bone underneath to direct trauma. Joint pain that resists medical treatment for weeks, or disturbs night sleep, is most probably due to cartilage injury.

20.3.4. FAT LOSS AND WEIGHT TRAINING
o   Fat is vital to all cellular functions since it enters in the formation of **cell membranes and hormone synthesis**. Without fat molecules, cell membranes would be porous to any water-soluble substance in their proximity, such as glucose and sodium. Thus, the presence of fat molecules and protein receptors on the cell membranes enables the cells to pick and choose, selectively, using the protein receptors as sensors and the fat layer as a barrier. Those guests that are welcome to enter the cells will be transported through the fat barrier by special transport protein. This portion of body fat is stable, even during dietary restriction.
o   There is another sort of fat storage in the body that accounts for excess caloric intake. Fat deposits at the midsection of the body, hips, and thighs because they are the least mobile areas of the body and contain large muscles that are rich in blood supply. Fat also deposits under the abdominal muscles, around the intestines, in the walls of the blood vessels, and other organs. This portion of body fat is the **labile fat storage.** It resides in the fat cells.
o   **Sustained and long exercise** that exceeds 15 minutes taps into fat depot. Here, the body spares glucose oxidation for the brain metabolism and turns to fat cells to pump fatty acids into the circulation. The limiting factors for this pathway of **fat oxidation** are as follows.
    i.   The ability of cellular mitochondria to uptake fatty acids and carry out oxidation. Long training enhances cellular mitochondrial density, which fosters fat burning.
    ii. The ability of muscles to wash away lactates before they interfere with the ion gradient across the mitochondrial membranes. Long training enhances new angiogenesis, which expedites recovery from lactate accumulation.
    iii. The response of fat cells to hormonal regulation. Fat cells possess a **lipase enzyme** that is inactivated by the actions of insulin and activated by the actions of glucagon, adrenalin, growth hormone, thyroxin, and cortisol. The lipase enzyme hydrolyses stored triglycerides into glycerol and fatty acids. The former is utilized by the liver and kidneys in gluconeogenesis, while the latter is utilized by most tissues, including muscles, in fatty acid oxidation for energy production.
    iv. Carbohydrate intake invokes insulin release and suppresses fat breakdowns. Prolonged activity reduces blood glucose level to minimal thus stimulates fat burning.
o   **Intense and short exercises** build big and strong muscles that possess greater number of mitochondrial elements capable of β- oxidation[2] of fatty acids and of producing greater amounts of ATP that are useful in many chemical reactions. Recall that fat deposit occurs during inactivity by combining carbon dioxide with acetyl CoA, whereas fat burning occurs during activity by cleaving carbon dioxide from fatty acids.
o   The **liver affects** fat utilization through its regulation of blood glucose level. Only the liver and kidney are efficient in constructing glucose molecules from non-carbohydrate sources such as glycerol, aminoacids, and fatty acids. Thus, the liver sustains the fuel supply of vital endocrine organs that secrete hormones and regulate fat breakdown. The liver is also capable of utilizing fatty acids to form ketone bodies through ketogenesis. Exercise affects the liver through the feedback of end products of glycolysis and the activated TCA cycle. As a strength trainee, you should know how the liver affects performance, as follows. See *Table 14.1* on "Difference in function of various types of cells of the human body".
    i.   Dizzy spells when attempting to exercise, after whole night sleep, and without breakfast, should alert you to the fact that your brain is protesting the shortage of glucose. You have to stop working out and ingest some carbohydrates in small amounts; otherwise, you might fall and incur injury. Although the liver produces glucose from non-carbohydrate sources, and was able to make you moving, its production may not be adequate for vigorous exercise unless you ingest some food.
    ii. Voluminous drinking of bland water, prior to exercise, dilutes the blood glucose concentration. This also produces dizzy spells, or worse, water intoxication. Although drinking sweetened fluids supplies immediate glucose to the blood, yet excessive drinking can also disrupt muscular function. Excess blood glucose prevents potassium ions from exiting the intracellular space, thus produces muscular relaxation, or worse, loss of muscular control.
    iii inInsults to the liver affect your mental state through the supply of liver glucose to the brain, when food intake is sparse. Examples of these insults are alcohol, drugs, smoking, excess saturated fat, parasitic and viral infection, and inactivity. Of course, cancer and benign tumors that afflict the liver also cause relentless signs of liver dysfunction.

20.3.5. ABDOMINAL GIRTH
o   The increase in the waist size of the average population is well acknowledged, particularly in developed countries. People are accustomed to eat more and move less than earlier generations. The abdominal girth correlates well with

---
[2] β-oxidation refers to the oxidation of the carbon atom that lies next to the first carbon atom in the formula of a fatty acid. The first carbon atom is referred to as α, the second as β, and the third as γ, and so on.

excess caloric intake. Yet the most significant factor in swelling of abdomen is the intake of **fat and protein** that produce toxic undigested products, which disrupt the digestive process. Proteins interfere with the putrefaction process of the large colon and cause lazy and enlarged guts. In addition, **animal fat** slows the digestive process and, on the long run, causes narrowing of the blood vessels and further slow absorption and motility of the guts, as well as the whole body. Vegetarians, on the other hand, have less putrefaction in the large intestine and shorter transit time.

o **External abdominal muscles** form a portion of the abdominal sac. The other portions of the sac are the diaphragm and the pelvic floor. The diaphragm is used for respiration, while the pelvic floor is used to support the pelvic organs. Weak abdominal sac leads to disturbance in digestion, absorption, and evacuation of the guts. The distended intestine, due to weak abdomen, presses against the vital organs such as the kidney, adrenal glands, and vena cava. Also, the large intestine can press against the spines, by virtue of its retroperitoneal location, particularly when it is loaded with feces.

o Exercise can take care of the muscular element of the abdominal girth, but the **internal environment,** within the guts, has to be controlled through balanced diet. The most practical force to use to strengthen the abdominal muscles is the **diaphragm excursion** during running, walking, twisting, or jumping. Isolated abdominal exercises strengthen the abdominal muscles, mostly by isotonic contraction, such as in Leg raises, Sit-ups, and Crunches. Activities that involve vigorous breathing work out the abdominal muscles, through the excursion of diaphragm and the tightening of the pelvic floor. Running and brisk walking efficiently work out the abdominal muscles for lasting results.

o Losing fat from the waist region is not the only factor in reducing waist size. The abdomen contains cavities within the hollow organs, fat within the mesenteries and around the solid organs, and fat and muscles within the abdominal wall. The body resists any changes in the present conditions by means of different reflexes. As soon as the intestine is evacuated, the cologastric reflex urges the person to eat or drink to refill the evacuated intestine. **Fat within the abdomen** is as important as fat within the walls of the abdomen. Thus, running or long walking depletes the whole fat content of the abdomen, in addition to desensitizing the person to the state of empty guts. Vigorous and lengthy activities increase the tone of the abdominal sac, in all directions, and maintain the guts compressed without annoying impulses of hunger and thirst. The suppression of hunger impulses has to be caused by inducing the hypothalamus to deal with other process than just satiety.

20.3.6. MUSCLE FUEL

Vigorous physical activity operates in the absence of oxygen. In such anaerobic process, muscles consume **ATP** molecules and produce ADP that requires **CP** to replenish spent ATP. Light physical activity allows diverse recruitment of various muscle bundles, by allowing some bundles to replenish while others contract. Longer physical activity operates in the presence of oxygen and leads to utilization of the **fat depot** for supplying energy. High repetitions of weight training fatigue the muscle fast and undermine fat utilization. Yet, the long-term effects of weight training is clearly the development of efficient oxidation machinery within the cell mitochondria that burns all fuel sources (fat, carbohydrates, and protein) more robust in trainees than others. This developed cellular oxidation presents as extended burning of calories even after exercise ceases. Fat people who do not exercise suffer from fast unrelenting weight gain than athletes. That is due to the deficient cellular oxidation without exercise. Aerobic exercise could be made both vigorous and light. Thus, it allows extension of duration of physical activity to develop both muscles and cellular oxidation machinery that burn fat. Very light brief exercise does little to grow muscles and slow the progress of burning fat. Thus, it seems that optimum combination of vigorous and protracted light exercises exists for individual conditions.

20.3.7. AEROBIC EXERCISE

o Aerobic activity amounts for production of energy with direct production of carbon dioxide and water. The carbon atoms of the carbon dioxide originate from the foodstuff consumed by humans. The oxygen of both water and carbon dioxide mostly originates from the air we inhale during respiration. Activity induces the body to transport the protons (hydrogen ions) from the carbon skeleton of the foodstuff to the inhaled oxygen, in order to produce water and transport energy into the ATP molecules. Thus, the **lungs** perform the respiration of the whole body by exchanging the byproducts of metabolism for ambient gases. The **mitochondria,** within the cytoplasm of the cells, perform the respiration of the cells by consuming chemical compounds and generating carbon dioxide, water, and energy.

o The **cellular respiration** utilizes different types of chemical compounds, carbohydrates, fat, and proteins. Aerobic activities refer to cellular respiration that consumes pyruvate to produce water, carbon dioxide, and energy production. The main difference between aerobic activities and strength training is that aerobic activities proceed at the pace of ATP-CP replenishment rate. This allows constant carbohydrate burning and depletion of carbohydrate reserve. Because of the abundance of oxygen in aerobic training, minimal accumulation of lactates occurs, which allows long training sessions and fat burning.

o Unfortunately, some conservative health-care professionals consider aerobic-training a **high-risk activity** that leads to orthopedic injuries for people with little preparation or medical knowledge. This disclaimer relieves health providers from legal litigation when injuries occur. The truth is that anybody, even with past surgical history of the knees, could advance his or her ability to benefit from aerobic training. Gradual and slow increase of duration and intensity of training are crucial to prevent injuries. As an example, weak or bad knees could be prepared to sprint with little trickery. Walking for half a mile, at brisk rate, increases the isotonic contractions around the knees, and generates enough heat and circulation to alleviate most pain. Thus, warm-up could help a person, who never ran before to feel strong with stable knees, to run again. If you are deterred by pain and stiffness of knees, you should start with progressive stretching, then try that trick of 15 minutes of walking. If running is still impossible, walking is still a

superb aerobic activity. You can utilize the arm swings with the shoulder, during walking, to twist the torso as vigorous as running could do for you. The twisting of torso is meant to involve the sides of the abdominal muscles.
- The whole concept of aerobic exercise is lightening slow fire within the cells. The more oxygen thrown to the fire, the longer the burning would last. The cardiovascular system delivers the oxygen gotten by the lungs to the body cells. Thus, aerobic fitness is equivalent to cardiovascular fitness. The harder the heart works to deliver oxygen and removes byproducts, the longer the fire lasts. Either the length of exercise or the intensity of exercise defines the **fitness of the cardiovascular system**.

20.3.8. OVERTRAINING

- Recreational physical activities encounter unique problems such as **overtraining, individualization, and conflicting strategies of planning long-term programs**. Beginner athletes are not born, nor raised, prepared for the sport they are about to dedicate their future for. Advanced athletes are also confronting the same issues due to the **"interval nature"** of recreational training. With such discrete intervals of intense physical activities, the body cells, organs, and systems do not have adequate time to adapt and evolve with training. The rate of increase of intensity (increase of resistance over time) could outpace the body's ability to replenish reserves and regenerate essential biological needs. This may lead to overtraining. Unlike lifelong physical careers, such as farming and factory work, recreational workout encounters problems with the pace of increasing load. Therefore, intensive and progressive strength training, that aims to elevate performance to unknown higher levels, produces unknown consequences. The most meticulous planning might still betray many talented beginners who might require different pace of preparation to remedy past acquired deficits.
- In any case, progressive increase in intensity of training is prescribed for improvement of strength. Simple biological needs such as supply of energy products or removal of byproducts (lactates and carbon dioxide) could be swiftly fulfilled within minutes or hours of rest. Yet, complex biological needs such as synthesis of proteins and neurotransmitters might lag behind the pace of recuperation. Such asynchrony between **recuperation and load** might presents as an isolated event such as sprain, strain, inflexibility, or weakness of a muscle, joint, or tendon. It might also present as transient deterioration in overall performance, insomnia, indigestion, anxiety, or fatigue. It is worthwhile to mention that in the complete absence of recreational training, similar states of chronic fatigue and exhaustion do occur, for the same exact causes of asynchrony between physical exertion and physiological recuperation. Yet, overtrained athletes develop more efficient recovery system than do chronically fatigued non-athletes who might have long depleted their biological resources, beyond reversal.
- Severe overtraining presents with incapacitating **feeling of weariness**. This is aggravated by other factors such as old age, poor sleeping or nutritional habits, common illnesses such as cold, alcohol consumption, or smoking. Severe overtraining could reach the point of irreversible injury to vital organs such as the heart valves, joint cartilage, or ligaments. The most noticeable signs of severe over training is the total loss of strength, even the strength to talk, listen to loud sounds, look to bright lights, or move the slightest objects. Heart racing is easily provoked by any effort. Even changing position in bed can cause heart racing in overtrained athletes. This syndrome is attributed to depletion of body reserves. Absolute rest and light meals are advised until normalcy is restituted and maintained, for at least a week of feeling of wellness, during performing normal duties. See Chapter 13, *Table 13.1* on "Signs of Overtraining".
- Factors that lead to overtraining are the peaking of the **rate of increase of load** by an individual with short history of engagement in fitness activities. This includes higher number of exercises that demand heavy resistances such as the Deadlift, Squat, and leg press, and leg extension, in the same training session, or ignoring states of **fever or lack of sleep** in heavy workout days. Also, **nutrition** cannot be overlooked in dealing with overtraining since a poorly nourished performer will undoubtedly succumb to overtraining at lower threshold than well-nourished performers. The length of duration that is required by an afflicted performer, to recover from overtraining state to normalcy, emphasizes that not only macronutrients intake is responsible for slower recuperation but also the deficient of more complex nutrients that causes lagging recuperation. Abundant calories require many enzymes, mineral catalysts, and mediators in order to complete their biochemical pathway of metabolism. Such nutritional factors have immense implication in developing strength that scan the spectrum from that of top Olympic performers to that of the average person.
- The question, whether overtraining is a **vague entity** caused by excessive exhaustion, or a specific deficiency of nutrients, could not be answered without further research. Thiamin (vitamin-B_1) deficiency, for example, can present with wide spread symptoms from neural difficulties, cardiovascular problems, and poor muscular performance that mimics overtraining. Also, niacin and lipoic acid deficiency cause similar problems due to accumulation of pyruvate in the cells and failure to produce energy through the TCA cycle. Niacin and flavoprotein deficiencies both impact the transfer of protons between reactants and thus interfere with energy production.

20.4. TRAINING PSYCHOLOGY

As a great nurturing milieu, training provides ample interaction between trainees and trainers. The years of training experience may be the most influential years in forming one's identity and self-rapport. Through training, athletes are introduced to the world through the vision of older predecessors, viable options of achieving substantial results, and means to deal with failure, recovery, and triumphant comeback. What else is greater than such milieu of nurturing?

20.4.1. DRIVE AND THE PSYCHE

I do not appreciate deterring ideas that attribute success to genetics, drugs, or mystical causes. You are not different from those at the top of any field. Circumstances play a role in many ventures, but if you keep your spirit high, plan, and learn from failure, you will pioneer a new experiment of success, as did our predecessors. High feelings of self-worth and your potential to play a valued role in society help your performance and drive to improve your skill level on a consistent basis. The drive to engage in physical activities does not die with life crisis and unresolved psychological conflicts. Many people find sport a haven for recuperation from major life crisis with newer reinstatement of goals. Our drive is a powerful force that can alter our behavior and mood.

20.4.2. PAST EXPERIENCE

Young and old trainees engage in training for various reasons. The young are driven by instincts and curiosity to untangle the governing laws of nature. Choosing the right sport for the young is crucial for their future success. Difficulties in excelling in a sport generate fear of failure. Young trainees could benefit greatly from parental, institutional, or peer support in overcoming difficulties in adjustment and progress. Adult trainees are captives of old habits that influence their set of priorities. Habits are amenable to change no matter how deeply ingrained in the mind of the individual. The drive to overcome difficulties and reach your goal stems from your unconscious sense of immortality, against the sense of fear of failure. Past experience and knowledge about the value of exercise influence our drive, as follows.

o The benefits of engaging in exercise are weighed against other interests and **responsibilities** of daily life such as caring for a family, attending school, or responsibilities of stressful job duties. Exercise outcomes depend on **reinforcing factors** such education, awareness of balanced lifestyle, or instinctual drive to lead healthy and clean life, removed from the temptation of modernity. These factors are well demonstrated in the choices made by the three lifters shown in *Figures 20.5 thru 20.7*.

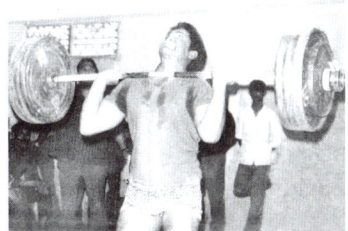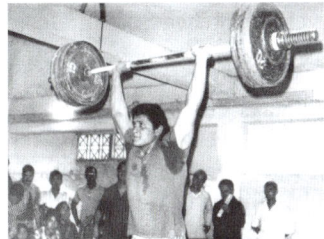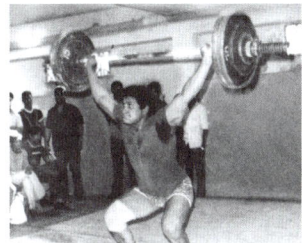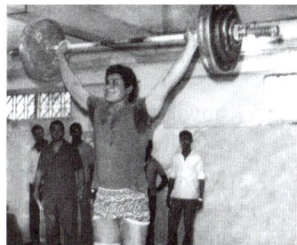

Figure 20.5. Abu Kalila, converted from Bodybuilding to Weightlifting at the age of eighteen. His Bodybuilding training of supersets of diverse exercises helped him surpass many others and excel to the top. His background in agriculture gave him advantage in maintaining the best nutritional regime for a Weightlifter. His family traded in diary products, which enhanced his understanding of role of healthy diet on building muscles. He started working in his father's shop since childhood, which imposed some discipline on his behavior. He worked nights, went to school in the morning, and trained afternoon, and often walked with blue rings under his eyes due to the hard work and lack of sleep. His conviction to advance his education got him to the law school and helped him work out with great confidence and ambition to climb to the highest ranks in society. In 1984, he competed in Los Angeles Olympic games, and ranked fifth in the 82.5 kg class. In 1988, he competed in Barcelona Olympic games at heavies weight class. His Olympic career ended as soon as he abandoned academics and started private business in wholesale. He became a national icon as an Olympic Weightlifter and a lawyer, a combination that seldom existed in this sport. Although he did not win even the Olympic bronze medal, his fifth ranking is a great achievement with regard to his balanced priorities and success in academics and business.

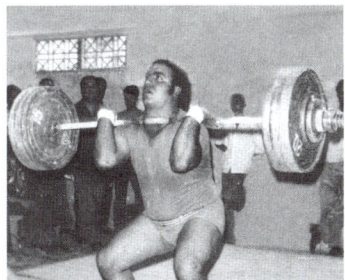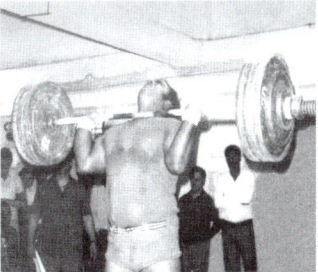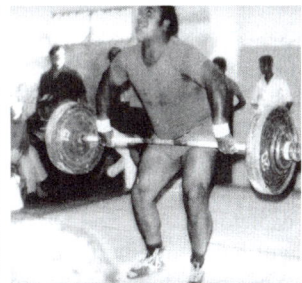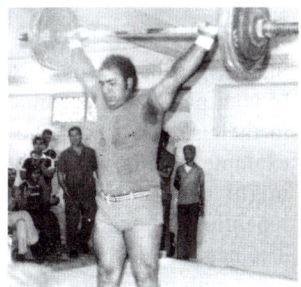

Figure 20.6. Ibrahim Safa grown up with well built musculature. His coach dreamed of him becoming top Olympic lifter. He progressed beyond any expectation and with little training. He advanced in training during his study for elementary school diploma. He dreamed and worked hard to advance his education, yet lost his struggle for better education to his obligation to support his family. His lack of any higher education put unusual financial burden on him and forced him to quit training to seek a sewing job. His poor understanding of nutritional issues contributed to his insatiable appetite. Sitting in his sewing shop, all day long, caused his weight to increase drastically and became diabetic in early thirties. He started complaining of kidney problems soon after. Despite his little education, he was very bright and quick with arithmetic and sense of humor. His loss as a national Olympic lifter exemplifies the role of education and institutional support in sparing the resourceful youth of a nation.

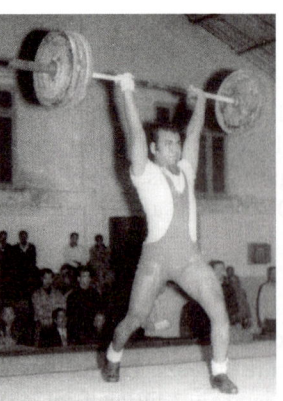 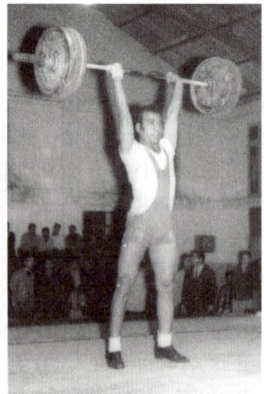 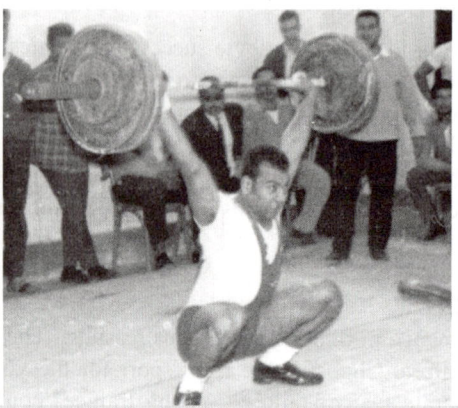 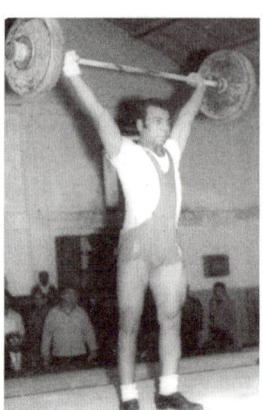

Figure 20.7. The author of this book, started training on Weightlifting in 1967. My coach (seen standing in the third picture from the left) was hoping to see me competing internationally. I attended each training session for twelve years with flawless punctuality. Yet, my medical education and graduate research deprived me from the rest and dedication needed for extensive training. I attended three graduate schools, in the same time, overlapping with Weightlifting training. My main drive stemmed from the fact that I had joined school by mere accident. When I was seven years old, one of my neighbors noticed that my parents did not realize the significance of educating a child. She dragged me to three different schools seeking my admittance to elementary public education, until she found a school manager who agreed to accept me, despite of my old age. From then, education became my obsession and passion.

o   Institutional enforcement in the form of scholarships or other **gains for participation** might suppress unconscious desire to perform different physical activities. Many college athletes quit sport soon after enforcing rewards are removed. Many lead ordinary lifestyle void from any exercise activities. Many elite athletes were driven by individual superiority of physical fitness in certain sports but never comprehend the life-long needs to stay fit. As soon as the excitement of triumph is over, they yield to sedentary lifestyle.

o   Knowledge of the economy of **living healthy** and fit plays crucial role in urging the individual to overcome all difficulties and show up for training. I recall few times when I went shopping for training clothes just because I did not want to miss the opportunity of attending a gym that I accidentally ran across, at remote location during travel or holidays. Paying whatever price to locate a gym and finding my way to training could only be explained by my conviction of the outcome of exercise.

o   Past experience on the sequence of **evolution of gaining strength** and gaining more ability to walk longer, run stronger, and do things with high confidence, eases the anticipation of uncertainties of the outcome of exercise. Enforced belief that fostering health does not lie in the hands of other figures of authority but in our will to acquire knowledge and implement it in everyday activities helps realizing that exercise is a basic, practical duty to maintain and advance health.

o   **Misperceptions** deter some people from exercise. Exercise does not undermine the feminine appearance of a women, it is not man-only playful activity. Exercise does not interfere with scholastic achievements in negative manner, nor does it dull the mind of the young. The negative influence of bad peers in exercise environments could happen in any other environment. Exercise does not cause injuries more than lack of exercise. Despite the high risk of physical activities, they enhance one's skills of managing dangerous affairs. Although younger age is associated with dramatic accomplishments in gaining strength and fitness, exercise never ceases to benefit people from all ages.

20.4.3. PRESENT STRATEGIES

Start with concrete belief that things will change over time as long as efforts are made and gauged to advance your cause. In your personal life, you are the only boss and the executive of all activities, which includes prioritizing deficits according to their significance. The least idea that might skip your attention such as the ill effects of sweetened beverages, for example, might be the best solution to long-term deficit. The most **frustrating exercises** that seem to break your will **might need not be skipped**, but rather performed more frequently, at lower intensity and fewer repetitions. Higher repetitions of exercises only deplete the ATP and CP of the muscle and weaken the muscle, if intensity is not kicked up. The nagging desire to seek swift help from the drug industry to remedy an urge might be suppressed, if you occupy your mind with passionate ideas. Your best strategy to overcome fear of failure and the urge for quick gratification lies in your cognitive realization that you are the boss of your own affairs and that you alone are responsible for making wise decisions that lead to wellness. Your best bid for sound planning is to stick to axial exercises. These will get you where many champions have gone. You will build invincible musculoskeletal frame, with robust cardiopulmonary and neuromuscular systems.

20.4.4. ASSESSING STRATEGIES

If every strategy you have adopted has not got you where you want to be that is perfectly a normal course of affairs. As long as you are breathing, new strategies signify that you are utilizing the gift of creativity. Most probably, you have gotten good things out of the past failures, but not exactly what you originally aimed for. If your aim does not sound totally irrational, you should not settle for humility. A search for the reasons of past failures might not reside in your vicinity. May be you need a change, seeing a movie, visiting the library, traveling abroad, or just asking total aliens if they know of any alternative? The oldest deterrents to strength training were completely preventable, as follows.

o   Strength athletes used to believe that **lifting heavy** everyday makes them strong. In competition, those who used to lift heavy, consistently and for many months, always fail. The wisdom of finding the best load curve for intensity and rest is now well understood from the mistakes of those stubborn predecessors.

o   Athletes used to believe that **repeated lifting** of a light weight enhances circulation and strength. It turns out that repetitive lifting of light weights does not alter the distribution of muscle fibers in the direction of building strength, but rather enhances the aerobic characteristics of muscle to stand endurance. This led to understanding of the relationship between intensity of training and building strength.

o   Athletes used to believe that **waist belts** prevent hernias and Weightlifting might be the cause. Today we know that hernias result from defects in abdominal wall, bearing down with fully loaded guts, or imbalanced strengthening exercises. Strength training helps you feel and sense how to contract your muscles to prevent hernias, dislocation, and fracture, through enhancing muscular balance and motor vigor.

o   **Overtraining** and undertraining were never understood in the past with today's clarity. We still experiment with what is best for healthy activities. We know for sure that hard laborers live longer and healthier than folks sitting in offices for life-long jobs. We know better about the health of muscles and bones than just few decades ago. Muscles were thought to characterize people with low acumen and inferior social status. Today, the presidents of nations take pride in jugging and attending fitness exercises to alleviate public concern about their remoteness from modernity.

o   Nowadays, the overwhelming flood of information and competition for marketing left many people in total loss of what is simple and effective **exercise plan.** The simple fact is that strength training is based on resisting force. That could be any force. You can plan a perfect workout with just running, squatting, push-ups, and few calisthenics exercises, without the need for machines, tools, or memberships, *Figures 20.1* and *20.2.*

20.4.5. WORKOUT ANXIETY

Anxiety is a common component of training psyche that is constantly under suppression of the accomplished athlete. Anxiety increases during stressful times. I recall my worst anxiety after knee surgery when I thought that I might never be able to run again. After few months of mere moving the feet in the air, I was able to gradually control my anxiety. Understanding the course of development of affairs, eases the worried mind than long and tense expectation. The peak of anxiety occurs during or prior to competition, particularly when prior training was not at best compliance with intended planning. The role of a coach is essential in adhering to the sound rules of competition preparation in order to avoid severe incapacitating anxiety. For example, many novice Weightlifters would think that heavy and voluminous leg and arms strengthening prior to contest would promote their performance, while experienced coaches know that relaxed body with adequate recuperation, after proper planning of volume and intensity, would bring best outcome. Convincing novice Weightlifter that the power of lifting originate in the cellular biology, rather than in the external physique of muscles, would require gaining the trust of the trainee over some period of time and being able to establish a rapport with individual athletes, in caring attitude. Without such rapport, novice lifters would err on the side of defiance and trial of impractical ideas that perceived by them to be short cut solution to victory. Regular contact and follow up on development help both athlete and coach understand the proper approach to solve issues that lead to anxiety. The best example is that of lifters who like to skip most of the leg workout assuming that the classical Olympic lifts already accomplish such purpose. Without separate leg strengthening exercises, Olympic lifts become tedious and daunting. The coach might then has to cut down the number of exercises in order to get to the Squat sooner than the trainee becomes bored with the training session. Instilling the habit of prioritizing basic lifts such as legs, back, and shoulders requires persistence trying and convincing until the trainee begins to appreciate its purposeful intent.

20.4.6. WORKOUT COUNSELING

o   Counseling trainees for planning and executing workout is more complex that counseling discrete disciplines such as academic, legal, or health counseling. For the counselor to be effective, he or she must gain the confidence of the trainee by being likable and exhibit interpersonal skills. The trainee might confront an issue that is impervious to the counselor but with some attention and flexibility, the counselor might figure a way to help the trainee out of such troubling situation. The most important principle in counseling is realizing that each trainee has unique and individual identity with specific pros and cons. The effort to understand such traits depends on the ability of the counselor to gather information from various human interactions, directly or indirectly. Some trainees are outspoken and can adequately communicate their mind on time for advice. Others are introvert and require some effort to read their minds in order to understand their concerns. Still, others can offer logical explanation of their problems and appreciate the need for more time to reach solution; while different others put the blame on remote circumstances. The counselor's role in such extremes might vary from direct simple planning to tricky improvisation of workout plan that does not directly confront the illogical thought of the emotional trainee.

o   Also, a compulsive trainee constitutes a challenge to a counselor since deeply seated believes are hard to change. Yet

GUIDELINES FOR OPTIMUM STRENGTH TRAINING

agreeing with the trainee when executing a destructive plan is counterproductive. For example, the trainee who wants to diversify his power training to include Weightlifting, Plyometric, and running might not realize that overtraining and skill acquisition negate against simultaneous cross training. Though engaging is such great activities is commended, yet phasing them out into different sessions of the year would prevent their interference with buildup of power and acquiring motor skill.

o As with other psychiatric counseling, workout counseling relies of listening, talking, remembering, and paying attention to details. The value of verbal communication cannot be overstates. Such art of dialogue serve the purpose of understanding how the trainee perceives his or her world and how he or she acts to accomplishes his or her goals. Effective communication may help the trainee engage in a world of fun and productivity, without interfering thought of apprehension and misperception. The goal of effective communication is to portray to the trainee the value of adhering to strategic planning that distinguishes thoughtful ventures and that will reflect on his or her personality in other fields of life.

o The most invaluable skill the counsel should have is expressing his or her dedication to the art of teaching sport. Even without any educational credentials, a dedicated and passionate coach can produce champions. ***Figures 20.8 thru 20.16***, demonstrate a gratifying campaign by one driven man who taught Weightlifting to his two daughters, his son, in addition to all interested kids in the neighborhood. This champion's maker never attended a school in his life and never competed above and beyond local contests. Yet, his passion for Weightlifting drove him to compete for training with the few educated and renowned coaches with international and Olympic achievements. Most probably, no other man would venture that far, to the extent of transforming his home and street to a training arena, and devoting all his day to watching kids lifting barbells from the floor. Yet, for Ramadan Mohamed, Weightlifting was the only tool to get his voice heard. All his kids got employment offers in companies that permitted and supported them to train and compete.

20.4.7. SKILLFUL WORKOUT

o Engaging in long-term exercise enriches our repertoire of diverse knowledge in the making an athlete. Building up our repertoire starts with learning the roles of our predecessors in making the world the way it is, along with adding our own contributions. We learn how to ration our feeling to endure structured planning, execution of such plans, and expectation of progress. Our skill level depends on the richness of our repertoire of knowledge and encompasses the knowledge of the required expenditure of energy that accomplishes tasks with minimal waste. This involves rationing psychological impulses to exert arousal, when force is needed, and quiet, when building up reserves is needed. Thus, skilled trainees learned to manipulate the mind to master motor harmony, with little interference with sensory or emotional distractions and, reversely, suppress motor activities when replenishments of depleted reserves are needed. Olympic Weightlifters are perfect examples of mastering such sympathetic control. Prior to commencing lifting, Olympic Weightlifters could induce total relaxation of the major lifting muscles, suppress their emotional feeling by relaxing all muscles of the face and hands, and drop their heart rate to lowest level. The muscular deployment of Olympic Weightlifters demonstrates the well-developed **neuromuscular control of the body**. Thus gaining skill modifies the mental, neural, and chemical states of the body in order to channel energy to optimum timely expenditure.

o The level of skill amounts to monitoring every reflex and impulse in the body to time the harmonious activities for certain flawless outcome. High level of skill is needed for multi-joint activities. Freestyle lifting from the floor is an example of activities that require long training to learn how to eliminate extraneous movement and to effectively coordinate muscles to act as a single functional unit. Unskilled lifters, which are the vast majority of the population, do not master the skill of recruiting sequences of muscles that fixate joints prior to setting motion. Skilled lifters are trained heavily, though without analytical explanation, to stabilize joints by hardening postural muscles, before equalizing the resisting weight and inducing the lift. The most common mistake many people make is working out on the **basic elements of movement** assuming that that substitutes for skillful compound exercises. I cannot overemphasize the value of gaining skill through compound exercises. Take for example the skill of riding a bicycle, you can exercise each hand, leg, head, and torso movement separately, but that would not substitutes regular practice on the bicycle in order to enhance your skill in bike riding. The same can be said about mathematics; for example, you can learn the basic operations of addition, subtraction, multiplication, and division, yet you have to go beyond these to become a mathematician. Thus, skill is, basically, a complex mental compilation of motor activities that have to be acquired with constant practice and feedback.

20.4.8. TRAINING NOVICE PERFORMERS

o A novice performer has to manage more information when learning a new motor skill. The perception of a novice performer of the new motor skill directs his or her focus of attention to a specific aspect of the activity that appeals to his mind. This **focus will keep shifting** from one aspect to another until the central aspect of the activity gets maximal attention. A new Weightlifter, for example, might think that performing the Power Clean requires fast and vigorous yanking of the bar from the floor. After few attempts, he may realize that yanking is not the right strategy and may postpone that until the bar gains some momentum. Then afterwards, as the bar gains momentum a new issue arises, regarding whether to yank by Biceps contraction or by trapezius shrugging, and so on until all aspects of the motion get their proper ration of attention. Such dynamic rationing of attention by novice performers causes anxiety during the learning process.

GUIDELINES FOR OPTIMUM STRENGTH TRAINING

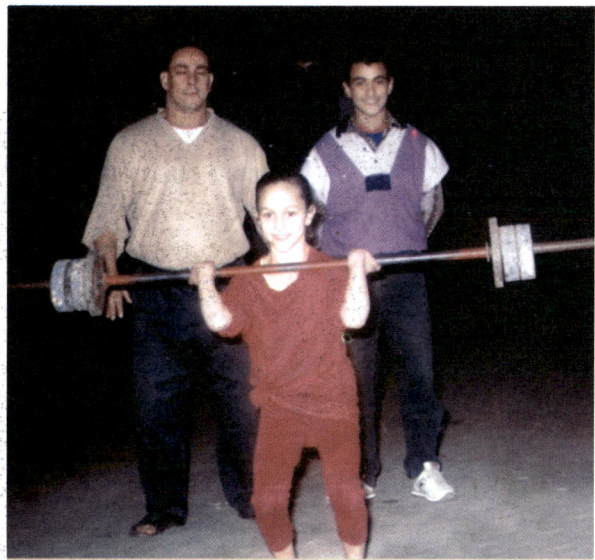

Figure 20.8. Nahla Ramadan Mohamed, 7-year old.

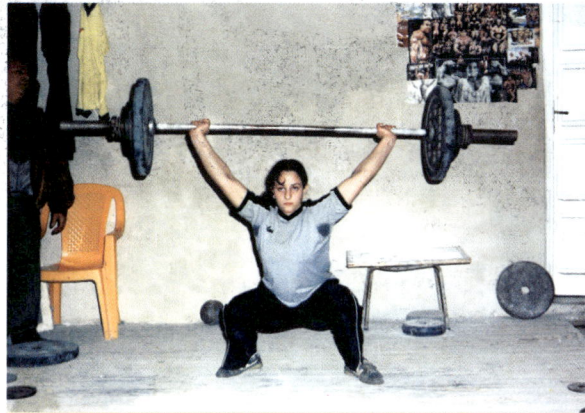

Figure 20.9 Nagham Ramadan Mohamed, the younger sister, 1998.

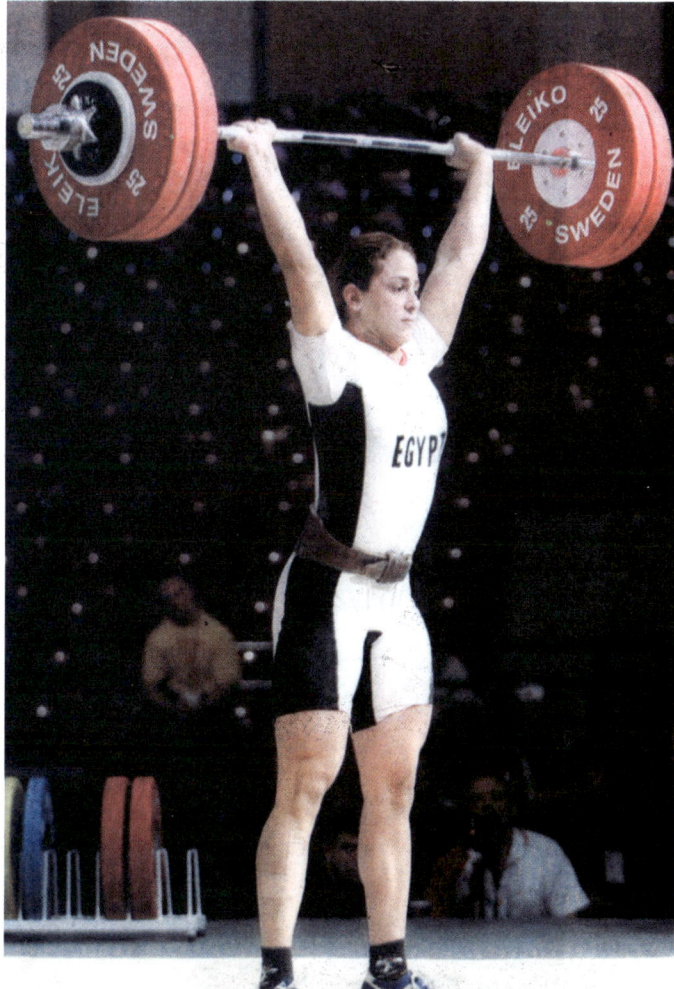

Figure 20.10. Nahla Ramadan Mohamed, 16-year old, 2002.

Figure 20.8. Nahla Ramadan Mohamed, born 1985, Alexandria, Egypt. At the age of seven-year, this girl is learning the Clean lift, under the coaching or her father (standing behind her, bare-footed), in the streets of Alexandria, Egypt. Her father's passion for Weightlifting made him transforms the house and the street into a gymnasium. He started with home-machined barbell and trained his kids and his neighbors' kids on the pavement. When started producing champions, he got this Olympic barbell and wooden platform from the state, *Figure 20.9.*, Nagham is his youngest daughter, among four siblings. The other tow are boys Noor and Nehad. She is training at the front door of her home with her father watching carefully the locking of the elbows in the Snatch lift. Nagham is now old enough to lift more than her father can lift. His oldest sun Noor is shown below, also a Weightlifter. The second daughter, Nagham, is also a World Champion in Weightlifting. His wife abandoned the family because of the blinding passion of her husband for sport. The father of four Weightlifting champions had trained and competed with the author in the 1970's. He can barely read or write. Weightlifting was a morbid affection of his heart and soul. He dreamed every day of his life to make all his kids World Champions. The two daughters were able to climb fast to the top, since few women care about training or have a driven father like Ramadan Mohamed Abdel Mouety. His son made great progress, but not enough to compete in the tough world of men's Weightlifting. Nahla Ramadan Mohamed will become World Champion in the age of seventeen, in 2002, *Figure 20.10.* Her current coach Yerden Ivanov, a Bulgarian national, prohibited her from attending the eighth grade preparatory school, due to the long and gruesome eight hours daily training sessions. In **8th Women's Junior World Weightlifting Championship, Havirov, Czech Republic, 2002,** in weight class 69 kg. She executed the Snatch of 95.0, 100.0, and 102.5 kg and the clean and Jerk of 120.0, 125.0, 127.5 kg. At the World Junior Weightlifting Championship in Budapest, Hungary, May 2003, Nahla Ramadan became the game's top-ranked athlete after collecting three gold medals and breaking two world records in the process, an unprecedented accomplishment for an Egyptian of any sex in the sport. The eighteen-year-old Nahla set a new world record of 145kg in the jerk, two kilograms more than that of Bulgaria's Krenz Geuiguny. Ramadan's second world record was in the total number of kilograms lifted: 260kg, again at Geuiguny's expense and her previous record of 255kg. In the snatch, Ramadan heaved 115kg to clinch her third gold medal but this time failed to break the world record. She picked up $3,500 in prize money for her efforts. In June 6, 2003, in **the Junior World Championships, Hermosillo,** Mexico, Nahla Ramadan, weighing 73.40 kg, made two new world records, 116.5 kg Snatch and 147.5 Kg Clean and Jerk. (From Alexandria, Egypt. Courtesy of Dr. Salah F. El-Hewie and Ramadan and Noor Mohamed Abdel Mouety.)

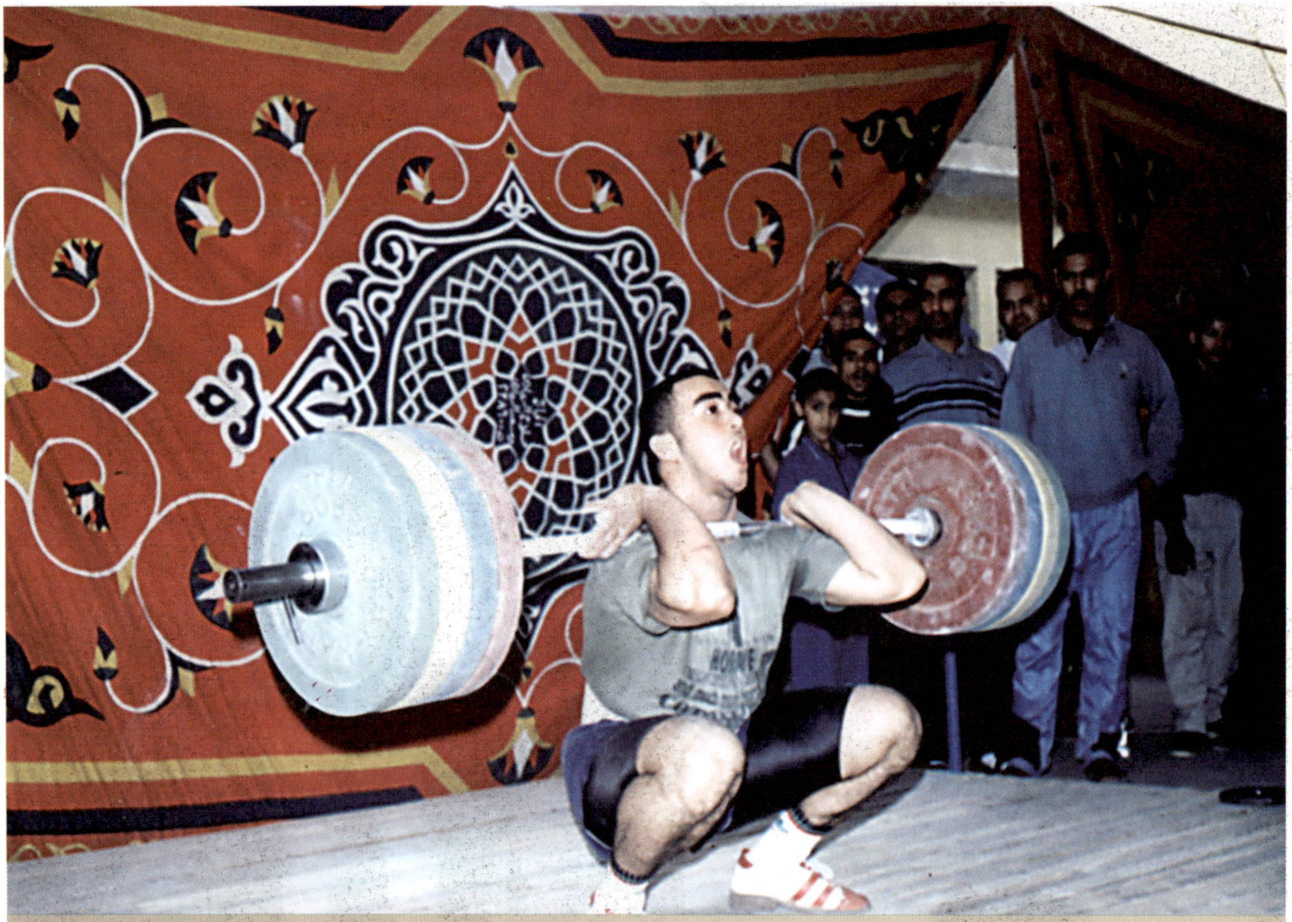

20 GUIDELINES FOR OPTIMUM STRENGTH TRAINING

Figure 20.11 Noor Ramadan Mohamed, born 1981, lifting 165 kg Clean, in 105 kg bodyweight class. Local competition, 1998.

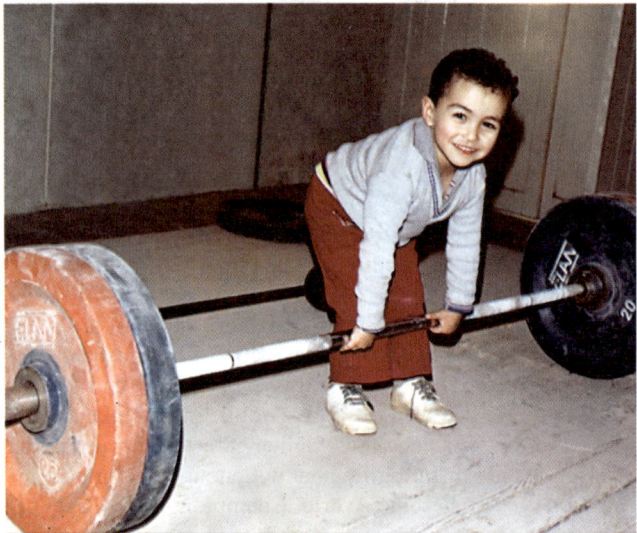

Figure 20.12 Noor Ramadan, 4-year old, 1985, attending his father's street gym.

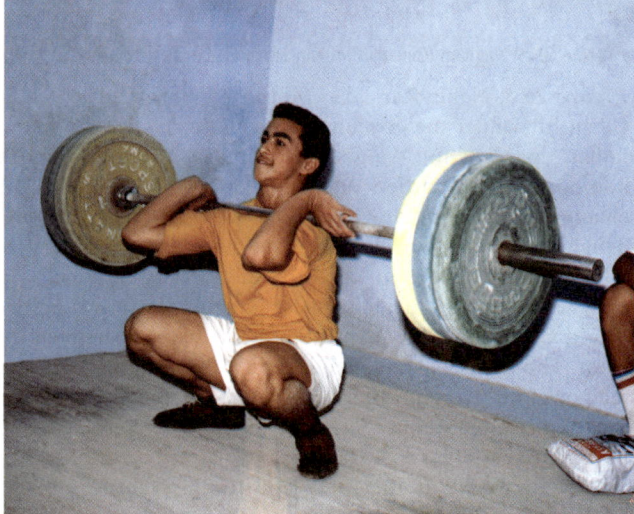

Figure 20.13. Noor Ramadan, 1994, 13-year old, lifting 120 kg Clean, in training.

Figure 20.11. Noor Ramadan Mohamed, born 1981, is the oldest son in the Ramadan's family. Although, his father was morbidly blinded with Weightlifting training and aiming for the gold, despite his family's dire financial blight, Noor never felt bitter about his father's delinquency. In cheerful phone conversation, he explained his dropout from the college of literature by his intend to support his father in refurbishing the street gym. His father used to shout on him relentlessly for his lack of seriousness about lifting, in comparison to the youngest daughter Nahla. He finished a vocational technical school and intends to join the college of engineering. The new and constant records made by the youngest sister, Nahla, provide some financial assistance and a lot of hope to the father and the family that were stigmatized by everyone, for being maniacally obsessed with dead sport and delinquent in securing safe, clean, and healthy home for four growing children. Fortunately, Noor has understood his father's good intention and stood fast behind him in his irrational pursuit for the gold dream of medals. In Figure 20.12, when he was 4-year old, he grew around dumbbells and barbells, and punches of young and old people talking and chatting about Weightlifting techniques. In Figure 20.13, he proved to his father that he is a follower of his doctrine of training. (From Alexandria, Egypt. Courtesy of Dr. Salah F. El-Hewie.)

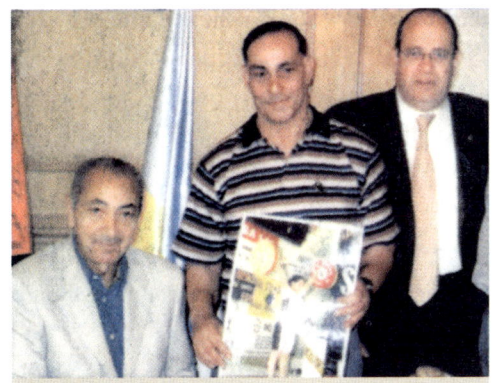
Figure 20.14

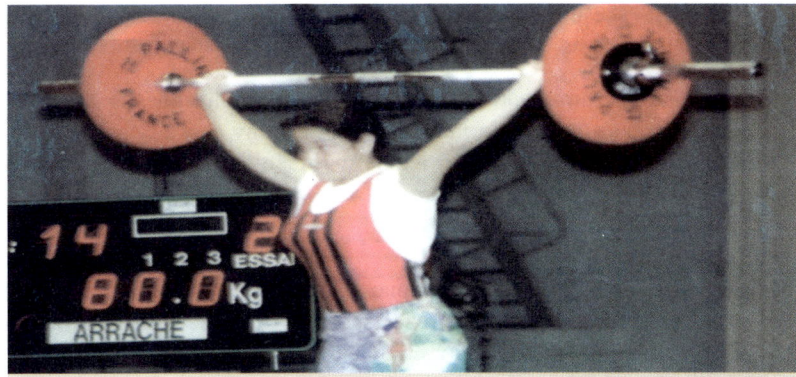
Figure 20.15

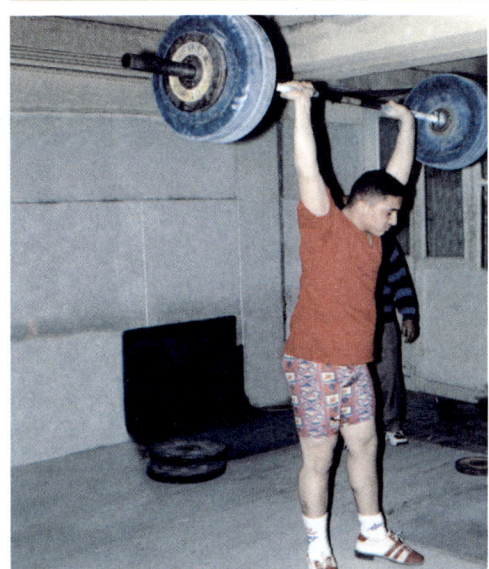
Figure 20.16

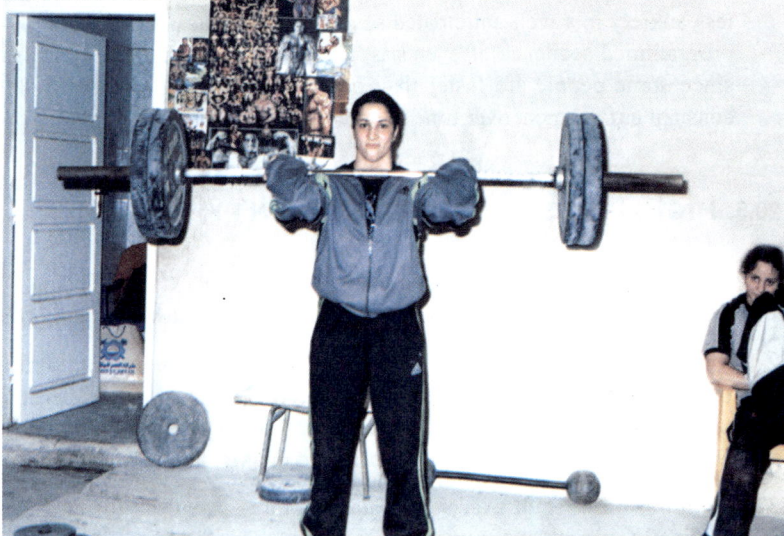
Figure 20.17

Figure 20.14. Ramadan Mohamed Abel Mouety, born 1952, with the governor of the city of Alexandria, in his passionate campaign to promote Weightlifting and support his morbid affection with sport. The governor rewarded the international achievement of his daughter, Nagham Ramadan Mohamed. Nagham was born 1987 and competed in short distance running with a record of 11.08 second on 100-meter race. Her father grabbed her to Weightlifting as soon as women's participation in Weightlifting became real fact. In *Figure 20.15*, she is shown snatching 80 kg in an International Weightlifting Champion. In the In *8th Women's Junior World Weightlifting Championship, Havirov, Czech Republic, 2002,* Nagham weighed 72.93 kg, lifted 97.5, 100.0, and 102.5 kg in the Snatch and 117.5, 122.5, and 125.0 in the Clean and Jerk, thus ranked third in the 75 kg class. Her past competition in short distance running caused her to tear the cruciate ligaments and knee cartilages. She was born with instable knee patellas. Her coach Yerden Ivanov, a Bulgarian national, forced her to freeze her education at senior high school in order to train seriously. In *Figure 20.16,* her younger brother, Nehad, born 1985, is shown lifting in disgust and disinterest in lifting while his father is watching impatiently. This is the only member in the family that got to the college of commerce and resisted the coercion of his father and his coach to train and abandon school. *Figure 20.17,* shows Nahla lifting while her younger sister, Nagham, laughing at her. Nahla and Nagham will have make constant compromises in regard to their weight class. Both weigh 73 kg. In competition, one increases her weight over 69 kg and the other diets harder to stay under 69. Thus, both won medals in many International competitions. (Courtesy of Dr. Salah F. El-Hewie and Noor Ramadan Mohamed).

- o Training constitutes mastering such emotional arousal in order to allow **attention rationing** to proceed with the learning process to fruition. The novice performer will appreciate growing over learning anxiety and managing peripheral stimuli, which distract his attention off the central aspect of motion. As learning proceeds, the long and serious practice of training delegates the acquired knowledge to the unconscious memory. Thus, skills can effectively be performed with less thought to complete the task. This can be facilitated by regular, long, and, planned practice on the motor skill, in addition to supportive enforcement by a trainer in the form of approval of proper performance and disapproval of flaws. Of course, such enforcement has to be gauged in a manner that reduces anxiety; otherwise, it will protract the skill acquisition process.

- o An important aspect of training novice performers is conveying the rationale beyond the motor skill, its dynamics, and role in performance. The novice has to learn to compare his perception of performance to the standards of practice and to feel free to modify and add his individual touches, after learning about the reasonable options of performance. There are always some eloquent phrases that may stick permanently in the mind of novices, when expressed timely an properly. These firing phrases can override many distractions and lend the performer a convenient key to solving their nagging concerns, when and if they arise. The following are examples.

   i. Lifting from the floor is made easy by **breaking the motion down** into three phases. This simple rule can eliminate all the anxiety that faces many novice, as well as expert lifters, when approaching the barbell. Performing one phase at a time will take care of the subsequent phase, without having to worry about the whole process of full lift.
   ii. Brining the bar as **close to the body** as possible eliminates many unnecessary movement and eases lifting by axial muscles.
   iii. Overhead press is better done by pressing the bar backwards and upwards. This eliminates shoulder strain by reducing the torque required to shoulder press the barbell.
   iv. **Thrusting the chest forwards** during lifting will help transmission of forces from the axial muscles to the arms along straight and shorts conduits.

o The now expert performer is more likely able to bring back the old memories of motor skill and execute exercises with less anxiety in a well-anticipated sequence of events. The process of focusing attention by skilled performers on well-programmed sequence of events is, therefore, both acquired by learning and inherited in the instincts of the persons, since some people are faster than others in acquiring new skills. In addition, even long-learned skills also require constant enforcement over time in order to remain viable.

20.5. HIGHLIGHTS OF CHAPTER TWENTY

1. Daily inclusion of **compound exercises** such as the Clean, Snatch, Deadlift, Bent-over row, Squat, Overhead Squat, Jerk, and Standing Shoulder Press will foster strength development of the whole body, if done as core exercises.

2. Muscular strength gained by training diminishes with **inactivity**. After six months intermission more than one third of the gained strength is reduced and up 4/5 reduction by a year intermission. Reclaiming muscular loss does not happen over night with quick and heavy exercise. Training to reclaim loss of muscles alters the cellular strategies of managing energy. Long inactivity diverts excess food intake into fat.

3. **Minimal number of exercise sessions** is three per week for late starters. Longer intervals between sessions lead to decline in strength and increase in injuries.

4. **Exercise should be simplified** in terms of the number of exercise groups, sets per group, and repetitions per set. To overcome boredom changes should be made frequently without undermining the basics of balanced exercise.

5. The reason that many people get easily discouraged, when expected progress does not follow hard work, is the lack of understanding of the **time frame of physical development** and the significance of proper tweaking of efforts in order to foster development. Fast and hard work can cause overtraining and setback in your progress.

6. Exercise alone does not promote health unless you adopt healthy habits in all aspects of your lifestyle. You do not have to know the **caloric contents** of each foodstuff in order to win the slimness contest, but you need to know general ideas about healthy food. The role of thumb is that as little amounts of diverse food intake can maintain steady bodyweight and prevent excess calories and nutritional deficiencies.

7. The principal rule of strength training that applies to all individuals is that, in building maximal strength one should maintain the **number of repetitions below five** with maximal and sub-maximal weights above 60% of maximal, in each particular category of exercises and that the total duration of a session is kept under an hour in order to prevent severe exertion and protracted recovery.

8. **Warm-up should not exceed 15 minutes** if one expects to reach high intensity during session. Full range of motion with progressive weights under 50% 1RM is ideal for warm-up. This prepares the neuromuscular system to stimulate the exact mechanics, which will be performed during the workout. It reduces muscle and joint injury and increases muscular recruitment through enhancing motor skill and breathing.

9. In fact, **without massaging and hot sauna** many Weightlifters would not be able to lift such maximal weight or endure for that many years. Both the Greek lifter Pyrros Dimas and the Turkish lifter Naim Suleymanoglu have hold the Olympic gold medals for 12 consecutive years which is extremely daunting task due to the nature of competition and performance.

10. The truth is that, anybody, even with **past surgical history** of the knees, could advance his or her ability to benefit from aerobic training. Gradual and slow increase of duration and intensity of training are crucial to prevent injuries.

Glossary

1RM	One repetition maximum, is the maximum weight that can be lifted only once in a set.
Acetylation	The addition of an acetyl group (-COCH3) group to a molecule.
Acidic	Having a pH of less than 7.
Acute	Having a short and relatively severe course.
Adjunct	Assisting in the prevention, amelioration, or cure of a disease.
Adrenal glands	A pair of small glands, located above the kidneys, consisting of an outer cortex and inner medulla. The adrenal cortex secretes cortisone-related hormones and the adrenal medulla secretes epinephrine (adrenaline) and norepinephrine (noradrenaline).
AHC	Anterior horn cells of the spinal cord that contain motor neurons that regulate muscular motor function.
AIDS	Acquired immune deficiency syndrome. AIDS is caused by the HIV (Human Immunodeficiency Virus) virus, which attacks the immune system, leaving the infected individual vulnerable to opportunistic infection.
Alkaline	Basic; having a pH of more than 7.
Amino acids	Organic (carbon-containing) molecules that serve as the building blocks of proteins.
Clone	An exact copy of a DNA segment; produced by recombinant DNA technology.
Anaerobic	Refers to the absence of oxygen or the absence of a need for oxygen.
Anemia	The condition of having less than the normal number of red blood cells or hemoglobin in the blood, resulting in diminished oxygen transport. Anemia has many cause, including: iron, vitamin B-12, or folate deficiency, bleeding, abnormal hemoglobin formation (e.g., sickle cell anemia), rupture of red blood cells (hemolytic anemia), and bone marrow diseases.
Angina pectoris	Pain generally experienced in the chest, but sometimes radiating to the arms or jaw, due to a lack of oxygen supply to the heart muscle.
Angiographies (coronary)	A diagnostic test used to identify the exact location and severity of coronary artery disease. During angiography a small tube or catheter is inserted into an artery and guided with the assistance of a fluoroscope (x-ray) to the opening of the coronary arteries, which supply blood to the heart. A dye, visible on x-rays, is then injected into each coronary artery to reveal the extent and severity of blockages. Images produced by angiography are known as angiograms.
Anion	A negatively charged ion.
Antagonist	A substance that counteracts the cellular effects of a natural compound, for example, a nutrient or a hormone. Or a muscle that opposes the action of another muscle.
Antibodies	Also known as immunoglobulins (Ig), antibodies are specialized proteins produced by white blood cells that circulate in the blood recognizing and binding to foreign proteins, microorganisms or toxins in order to neutralize them. They are a critical part of the immune response.
Anticoagulant	A class of compounds that inhibit the formation of blood clots.
Anticonvulsant	A class of medication used to prevent seizures, commonly used in individuals with seizure disorders or epilepsy.
Antigen	A substance that is capable of causing an immune response.
Antihistamine	A chemical that blocks the affect of histamine in a susceptible tissues. Immune cells release histamine during an allergic reaction and also during infection with viruses, which cause the common cold. The interaction of histamine with the mucus membranes of the eyes and nose results in "watery eyes" and the "runny nose" often accompanying allergies and colds. Antihistamines can alleviate such symptoms.
Antioxidant	Any substance that prevents or reduces damage caused by reactive oxygen species (ROS) or reactive nitrogen species (RNS). ROS and RNS are highly reactive chemicals that attack other molecules and modify their chemical structure. Antioxidants are commonly added to foods to prevent or delay their deterioration due to exposure to air.

GLOSSARY

Arrhythmia	An abnormal heart rhythm. The heart rhythm may be too fast (tachycardia), too slow (bradycardia) or irregular. Some arrhythmias, such as ventricular fibrillation, may lead to cardiac arrest if not treated promptly.
Asthma	A respiratory condition characterized by difficulty breathing and reversible narrowing of the airways, known as bronchospasm.
Ataxia	A lack of coordination or unsteadiness usually related to a disturbance in the cerebellum, a part of the brain that regulates coordination and equilibrium.
Atherosclerosis	Also known as arteriosclerosis, atherosclerosis results from the accumulation of cholesterol-laden plaque in artery walls. Plaque accumulation causes a narrowing and a loss of elasticity of the arteries, sometimes referred to as hardening of the arteries.
ATP	Adenosine triphosphate. An important compound for the storage of energy in cells, as well as the synthesis (formation) of nucleic acids.
Atrophic gastritis	A chronic inflammation of the lining of the stomach, which ultimately results in the loss of glands in the stomach (atrophy) and decreased stomach acid production.
Atrophy	Decrease in size or wasting away of a body part or tissue.
Autoimmune disease	Autoimmune diseases occur when the body tissues are mistakenly attacked by its own immune system. The immune system is a complex organization of cells and antibodies designed normally to destroy pathogens, particularly viruses and bacteria that cause infections. Individuals with autoimmune diseases have antibodies in their blood, which target their own body tissues.
Bacteria	Single-celled organisms that can exist independently, symbiotically (in cooperation with another organism) or parasitically (dependent upon another organism, sometimes to the detriment of the other organism). Examples of bacteria include acidophilus (found in yogurt), streptococcus the cause of strap throat, and E. coli (a normal intestinal bacteria, as well as a disease-causing agent).
Bile	A yellow, green fluid made in the liver and stored in the gallbladder. Bile may then pass through the common bile duct into the small intestine where some of its components aid in the digestion of fat.
Bile acids	Components of bile, formed by the metabolism of cholesterol. Bile acid deficiency may lead to the formation of cholesterol gallstones, because bile salts (formed from bile acids) are required to dissolve cholesterol in bile so that it may be eliminated via the intestines.
Bone mineral density (BMD)	A term used in quantifying the mineralization of bone. The mineral component of bone consists largely of calcium and phosphorus. BMD is positively associated with bone strength and resistance to fracture. BMD can be determined through a low radiation X-ray technique known as DEXA.
Bone remodeling	The continuous turnover process of bone that includes bone resorption and bone formation. An imbalance in the regulation of bone remodeling has two contrasting events, bone resorption and bone formation, increases the fragility of bone and may lead to osteoporosis.
Buffer	A chemical used to maintain the pH of a system by absorbing hydrogen ions (which would make it more acidic) or absorbing hydroxyl ions (which would make it more alkaline).
Calcification	The process of deposition of calcium salts. In the formation of bone this is a normal condition. In other organs, this could be an abnormal condition. Calcification of the aortic valve causes narrowing of the passage (aortic stenosis).
Cancer	Also known as malignancy, cancer refers to abnormal cells, which have a tendency to grow uncontrollably and metastasize or spread to other areas of the body. Cancer can involve any tissue of the body and can have many different forms in one tissue. Cancer is a group of more than one hundred different diseases.
Carbohydrate	Considered a macronutrient because carbohydrates provide a significant source of calories (energy) in the diet. Chemically, carbohydrates are neutral compounds composed of carbon, hydrogen and oxygen. Carbohydrates come in simple forms known as sugars and such as starches and fiber.
Carboxylation	The introduction of a carboxyl group (-COOH) or carbon dioxide into a compound.
Carcinogen	A cancer-causing agent; adjective: carcinogenic.
Carcinogenesis	The formation of cancer cells from normal cells.
Cardiomyopathy	Disease of the heart muscle that often leads to abnormal function.
Cardiovascular	Referring to the heart and blood vessels.
Cardiovascular diseases	Diseases affecting the heart and blood vessels. The term has come to encompass a number of conditions that result from atherosclerosis, including myocardial infarction (heart attack), congestive heart failure, and stroke.
Carnitine	A compound that is required to transport long chain fatty acids across the inner membrane of the mitochondria, in the form of acyl-carnitine, where they can be metabolized for energy.

GLOSSARY

Cartilage	A soft, elastic tissue that composes most of the skeleton of vertebrate embryos and except for a small number of structures is replaced by bone during ossification in the higher vertebrates. Cartilage cushions joints, connects muscles with bones, and makes up other parts of the body such as the larynx (voice box) and the outside portion of the ears.
Case reports	Individual observations based on small numbers of subjects. This type of research cannot indicate causality but may indicate areas for further research.
Case-control study	A study in which the risk factors of people who have been diagnosed with a disease are compared with those without the disease. Because the risk factor (e.g., nutrient intake) is generally measured at the time of diagnosis, it is difficult to determine whether the risk factor was present prior to the development of the disease. Another potential draw back is the difficulty in obtaining well-matched control subjects.
Catalyze	Increase the speed of a chemical reaction without being changed in the overall reaction process. See enzyme.
Cataract	Clouding of the lens of the eye. As cataracts progress they can impair vision and may result in blindness.
Catecholamines	Substances with a specific chemical structure (a benzene ring with two adjacent hydroxyl groups and a side chain of ethylamine) that function as hormones or neurotransmitters. Examples include epinephrine, norepinephrine, and dopamine.
Cell membrane	Also called the plasma membrane. The external limiting membrane of a cell. It is composed of lipids (fat molecules) that have a hydrophobic (insoluble in water) end and a hydrophilic (water-soluble) end. Cell membranes are made of lipid bilayers in which the lipids line up in two layers with the hydrophobic ends facing each other and the hydrophilic ends facing the outside and the inside of the cell.
Cell signaling	Communication among individual cells so as to coordinate their behavior to benefit the organism as a whole. Cell-signaling systems elucidated in animal cells include cell-surface and intracellular receptor proteins, protein kinases and protein phosphates (enzymes that phosphorylate and dephosphorylate proteins), and GTP-binding proteins.
Central nervous system (CNS)	The brain, spinal cord, and spinal nerves.
Cerebrospinal fluid	The fluid that bathes the brain and spinal chord.
Cerebrovascular disease	Disease involving the blood vessels supplying the brain, including cerebrovascular accident (CVA), also known as a stroke.
Chelate	The combination of a metal with an organic molecule to form a ring-like structure known as a chelate. Chelation of a metal may inhibit or enhance its bioavailability.
Chemotherapy	Treatment with drugs. Commonly used to describe the systemic use of drugs to kill cancer cells, as a form of cancer treatment.
Cholestatic liver disease	Liver disease resulting in the cessation of bile excretion. Cholestasis may occur in the liver, gall bladder or bile duct (duct connecting the gall bladder to the small intestine).
Cholesterol	A lipid used in the construction of cell membranes and as a precursor in the synthesis of steroid hormones. Dietary cholesterol is obtained from animal sources, but cholesterol is also synthesized by the liver. Cholesterol is carried in the blood by lipoproteins (e.g., LDL and HDL). In atherosclerosis, cholesterol accumulates in plaques on the walls of some arteries.
Cholinergic	Resembling acetylcholine in action, a cholinergic drug for example. Cholinergic nerve fibers liberate or are activated by the neurotransmitter, acetylcholine.
Chorionic villus sampling (CVS)	A procedure for obtaining a small sample of tissue from the placenta (chorionic villi) for the purpose of prenatal diagnosis of genetic disorders. CVS can be performed between 9 to 12 weeks of pregnancy.
Chromosome	Structures composed of a long DNA molecule and associated proteins that carry part of the hereditary information of an organism.
Chronic disease	An illness lasting a long time. By definition of the U.S. Center for Health Statistics, a chronic disease is a disease lasting 3 months or more.
Chronic obstructive pulmonary disease (COPD)	A progressive disease of the lungs, often the result of long-term smoking. COPD is characterized by difficulty breathing, wheezing and a chronic cough.
Cirrhosis	A condition characterized by irreversible scarring of the liver, leading to abnormal liver function. Cirrhosis has a number of different causes, including chronic alcohol use and viral hepatitis B and C.
Classic Clean	Lifting barbell from the floor to shoulders with considerable squatting in order to shorten upward travel.

GLOSSARY

Clean lift	Lifting a barbell from the floor to the shoulders with overhand grip with monotonous motion.
Clinical trial	A research study generally used to evaluate the effectiveness of a new treatment in human participants. Clinical trials are designed to answer specific scientific questions and to determine the efficacy of new treatments for specific diseases.
Coagulation	The process of involved in forming a blood clot.
Coenzyme	A molecule that binds to an enzyme and is essential for its activity, but is not permanently altered by the reaction. Many coenzymes are derived from vitamins.
Cofactor	A compound that is essential for the activity of an enzyme.
Cognitive	An adjective referring to the processes of thinking, learning, perception, awareness, and judgment.
Cohort study	A study that follows a large group of people over a long period of time, often 10 years or more. In cohort studies, dietary information is gathered before disease occurs, rather than relying on recall after disease develops.
Collagen	A fibrous protein that is the basis for the structure of skin, tendon, bone, cartilage and all other connective tissue.
Collagenous matrix (of bone)	The organic (nonmineral) structural element of bone. Collagen is a fibrous protein that provides the organic matrix upon which bone mineralize crystallizes.
Colon	Sometimes called the large bowel or intestine, the colon is a long, coiled, tubelike organ that removes water from digested food after it has passed through the small intestine. The remaining material, solid waste called stool, moves through the colon to the rectum and leaves the body through the anus.
Colorectal adenoma	A tumor of the colon or rectum that arises in glandular tissue. Although not cancer, colorectal adenomas may develop into colorectal cancer over time.
Colorectal cancer	Cancer of the colon (large intestine) or rectum.
Congenital hypothyroidism	Also known as cretinism, congenital hypothyroidism occurs in two forms, although there is considerable overlap. The neurologic form is characterized by mental and physical retardation and deafness. It is the result of maternal iodine deficiency that affects the fetus before its own thyroid is functional. The myxedematous or hypothyroid form is characterized by short stature and mental retardation. In addition to iodine deficiency, the hypothyroid form has been associated with selenium deficiency and the presence of goitrogens in the diet that interfere with thyroid hormone production.
Congestive heart failure (CHF)	A disorder of the heart, resulting in the loss of the ability to pump blood efficiently enough to meet the demands of the body. Symptoms may include swelling, shortness of breath, weakness, and exercise intolerance.
Cornea	The transparent covering of the front of the eye that transmits and focuses light into the eye.
Coronary artery	The vessels that supply oxygenated blood to the heart muscle itself, so named because they encircle the heart in the form of a crown.
Coronary artery bypass graft (CABG)	A surgical procedure used in individuals with significant narrowings and blockages of coronary arteries to create new routes around narrowed and blocked arteries, permitting increased blood flow to the heart muscle. The bypass graft for a CABG can be a vein from the leg or an inner chest wall artery.
Coronary heart disease (CHD)	Also known as coronary artery disease and coronary disease, coronary heart disease is the result of atherosclerosis of the coronary arteries. Atherosclerosis may result in narrowing or blockage of the coronary arteries and is the underlying cause of myocardial infarction (heart attack).
Corticosteroid	Any of the steroid hormones made by the cortex (outer layer) of the adrenal gland. Cortisol is a corticosteroid. A number of medications are analogs of natural corticosteroid hormones.
Creatine phosphate	A high-energy compound found in muscle cells, which is used to convert ADP into ATP by donating phosphate molecules to the ADP. ATP is the molecule, which is converted into ADP with a release of energy that the body then uses.
De novo synthesis	The formation of an essential molecule from simple precursor molecules.
Deadlift	Lifting barbell from the floor to full back extension, the bar moves up to mid-thigh level.
Decarboxylation	A chemical reaction involving the removal of a carboxyl (-COOH) group from a compound.
Dermatitis	Inflammation of the skin. This term is often used to describe a skin rash.
DEXA	Dual energy X-ray absorptiometry. A precise instrument that uses the energy from very small doses of X-rays to determine bone mineral density (BMD) and to diagnose and follow the treatment of osteoporosis.
Diabetes (diabetes mellitus)	A chronic condition associated with abnormally high levels of glucose (sugar) in the blood. The two types of diabetes are referred to as insulin-dependent (type I) and non-insulin dependent (type II). Type I diabetes results from a lack of adequate insulin secretion by the pancreas. Type II diabetes (also known as adult-onset diabetes) is characterized by an insensitivity of the tissues of the body to insulin secreted by the pancreas (insulin resistance).

GLOSSARY

Diabetic ketoacidosis	A potentially life-threatening condition characterized by ketosis (elevated levels of ketone bodies in the blood) and acidosis (increased acidity of the blood). Ketoacidosis occurs when diabetes is not adequately controlled.
Diastolic blood pressure	The lowest arterial blood pressure during the heart beat cycle. The diastolic blood pressure is measured while the heart muscle is filling with blood.
Differentiation	Changes in a cell resulting in its specialization for specific functions, such as those of a nerve cell. In general, differentiation of cells leads to a decrease in proliferation.
Diffusion	A process, which does not require energy expenditure, by which particles in solution move from a region of higher concentration to one of lower concentration.
Diuretic	An agent that increases the formation of urine by the kidneys, resulting in water loss from the individual using the diuretic.
DNA	Deoxyribonucleic acid. A long thread-like molecule made up of large numbers of nucleotides. Nucleotides in DNA are composed of nitrogen containing base, a 5-carbon sugar (deoxyribose), and phosphate groups. The sequence of bases in DNA serves as the carrier of genetic (hereditary) information.
Eccentric contraction (negative contraction)	Contracting muscles while elongation, such as lowering weights to the floor.
Echocardiography	A diagnostic test that uses ultrasound to make images of the heart. It can be used to assess the health of the valves and chambers of the heart, as well as to measure cardiac output.
Edema	Swelling ; accumulation of excessive fluid in subcutaneous tissues (beneath the skin).
Electrocardiogram (ECG)	A recording of the electrical activity of the heart, used to diagnose cardiac arrhythmias, myocardial ischemia and myocardial infarction.
Electroencephalogram (EEG)	A recording of the electrical activity of the brain, used to diagnose neurological conditions such as seizure disorders (epilepsy).
Electrolytes	Ionized (dissociated into positive and negative ions) salts in the body fluids. Major electrolytes in the body include sodium, potassium, magnesium, calcium, chloride, bicarbonate, and phosphate.
Electron	A stable atomic particle with a negative charge.
Electron transport chain	A group of electron carriers in mitochondria that transport electrons to and from each other in a sequence, in order to generate ATP.
Element	One of the 103 chemical substances that cannot be divided into simpler substances by chemical means. For example, hydrogen, magnesium, lead, and uranium are all chemical elements. Trace elements are chemical elements that are required in very small (trace) amounts in the diet to maintain health. For example, copper,
Endocrine system	The glands and parts of glands that secrete hormones that integrate and control the body's metabolic activity. Endocrine glands include the pituitary, thyroid, parathyroid, adrenals, pancreas, ovaries, and testes.
Enzyme	A biological catalyst. That is, a substance that increases the speed of a chemical reaction without being changed in the overall process. Enzymes are vitally important to the regulation of the chemistry of cells and organisms.
Epidemiologic study	A study examining disease occurrence in a human population.
Epididymis	A system of tubules emerging from the testes, which serves as storage site form sperm during their maturation.
Epilepsy	Also known as seizure disorder. Individuals with epilepsy experience seizures, which are the result of uncontrolled electrical activity in the brain. A seizure may cause a physical convulsion, minor physical signs, thought disturbances, or a combination of symptoms.
Erythropoietin	A hormone produced by specialized cells in the kidneys that stimulates the bone marrow to increase the production of red blood cells. Recombinant erythropoietin is used to treat anemia in patients with end stage renal failure.
Esophagus	A soft muscular tube that connects the throat to the stomach. When a person swallows, the muscular walls of the esophagus contract to push food down into the stomach.
Excretion	The elimination of wastes from blood or tissues.
Extracellular fluid (ECF)	The volume of body fluid excluding that in cells. ECF includes the fluid in blood vessels (plasma) and fluid between cells (interstitial fluid).
Fatty acid	An organic acid molecule consisting of a chain of carbon molecules and a carboxylic acid (COOH) group. Fatty acids are found in fats, oils, and as components of a number of essential lipids, such as phospholipids and triglycerides. Fatty acids can be burned by the body for energy
Femoral neck	A portion of the thighbone (femur). The femoral neck is found near the hip, at the base of the head of femur, which makes up the ball of the hip joint. Fractures of the femoral neck sometimes occur in individuals with osteoporosis.

GLOSSARY

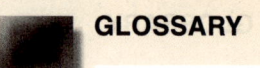

Fracture	A break in a bone or cartilage, often but not always the result of trauma.
Free radical	A very reactive atom or molecule typically possessing a single unpaired electron.
Fructose	A very sweet 6-carbon sugar abundant in plants. Fructose is increasingly common in sweeteners such as high-fructose corn syrup.
Gallbladder	A small pear shaped sac adjacent to the liver. The gallbladder stores bile, which is secreted by the liver and releases bile into the small intestine through the common bile duct.
Gallstones	Pebbles formed by the precipitation (crystallization) of cholesterol (most common in the U.S. and Europe) or bilirubin (most common in Asia) in the gallbladder. Gallstones may be asymptomatic (without symptoms) or they may result in inflammation and infection of the gallbladder.
Gastro esophageal reflux disease (GERD)	A condition in which stomach contents, including acid, back up (reflux) into the esophagus, causing inflammation and damage to the esophagus. GERD can lead to scarring of the esophagus, and may increase the risk of cancer of the esophagus in some patients.
Gastrointestinal	Referring to or affecting the stomach and intestines (small and large bowel).
Gene	A region of DNA that controls a specific hereditary characteristic, usually corresponding to a single protein.
Gene expression	The full use of the information in a gene through transcription and translation leading to production of a protein.
Genome	All of the genetic information (encoded in DNA) possessed by an organism.
Gluconeogenesis	The production of glucose from non-carbohydrate precursors, such as amino acids (the building blocks of proteins).
Glucose	A 6-carbon sugar which plays a major role in the generation of energy for living organisms.
Glutathione	A small peptide consisting of three amino acids (glutamate -cysteine -glycine). It participates in redox reactions and is an important reducing agent inside cells.
Glycogen	A large polymer (repeating units) of glucose molecules, used to store energy in cells, especially muscle and liver cells.
Goiter	Enlargement of the thyroid gland. Goiter is one of the earliest and most visible signs of iodine deficiency. The thyroid enlarges in response to persistent stimulation by TSH (see Function). In mild iodine deficiency, this adaptation response may be enough to provide the body with sufficient thyroid hormone. However, more severe cases of iodine deficiency result in hypothyroidism. Thyroid enlargement may also be caused by factors other than iodine deficiency, especially in iodine sufficient countries, such as the U.S.
Goitrogen	A substance that induces goiter formation by interfering with thyroid hormone production or utilization.
Gout	A condition characterized by abnormally high blood levels of uric acid (urate). Urate crystals may form in joints, resulting in inflammation and pain. Urate crystals may also form in the kidney and urinary tract, resulting in kidney stones. The tendency to develop elevated blood uric acid levels and gout is often inherited.
GTP	Guanosine triposphate. A high-energy molecule, required for a number of biochemical reactions, including nucleic acid and protein synthesis (formation).
Hartnup's disease	A genetic disorder resulting in defective absorption of the amino acid, tryptophan.
HDL	High-density lipoproteins. HDL transport cholesterol from the tissues to the liver where it can be eliminated in bile. HDL-cholesterol is considered good cholesterol, because higher blood levels of HDL-cholesterol are associated with lower risk of heart disease.
Heme	Compounds of iron complexed in a characteristic ring structure known as a porphyrin ring.
Hemoglobin	The oxygen-carrying pigment in red blood cells.
Hemolysis	Rupture of red blood cells.
Hemolytic anemia	Anemia resulting from hemolysis (the rupture of red blood cells).
Hemorrhage	Excessive or uncontrolled bleeding.
Hepatitis	Inflammation of the liver. Hepatitis caused by a virus is known as viral hepatitis. Other causes of hepatitis include toxic chemicals and alcohol abuse.
HIV	Human immunodeficiency virus. The virus that causes AIDS.
Hormone	A chemical, released by a gland or a tissue, which affects or regulates the activity of specific cells or organs. Complex bodily functions, such as growth and sexual development, are regulated by hormones.
Hydroxyapatite	A calcium phosphate salt. Hydroxyapatite is the main mineral component of bone of bone and teeth, and is what gives them their rigidity.
Hydroxylation	A chemical reaction involving the addition of a hydroxyl (-OH) group to a compound.
Hyperparathyroidism	Excess secretion of parathyroid hormone by the parathyroid glands resulting in the disturbance of calcium metabolism. Symptoms may include increased blood levels of calcium (hypercalcemia), decreased blood levels of phosphorus, loss of calcium from bone, and kidney stone formation.

GLOSSARY

Hypertension	High blood pressure, defined as a systolic blood pressure greater than 140 mm Hg and/or diastolic blood pressure greater than 90 mm Hg.
Hyperthyroidism	An excess of thyroid hormone, which may result from an overactive thyroid gland or nodule, or from taking too much thyroid hormone.
Hypoglycemia	An abnormally low blood glucose concentration. Symptoms may include nausea, sweating, weakness, faintness, confusion hallucinations, headache, and loss of consciousness, convulsions, or coma.
Hypoparathyroidism	A deficiency of parathyroid hormone, which may be characterized by low blood calcium levels (hypocalcemia).
Hypothalamus	An area at the base of the brain that regulates bodily functions, such as body temperature, hunger, and thirst.
Hypothesis	An educated guess or proposition that is advanced as a basis for further investigation. A hypothesis must be subjected to an experimental test to determine its validity.
Hypothyroidism	A deficiency of thyroid hormone, which is normally made by the thyroid gland, located in the front of the neck.
Impaired glucose tolerance	A metabolic state between normal glucose regulation and overt diabetes. Generally, blood glucose levels are higher than normal, but lower than those accepted as diagnostic for diabetes.
In vitro	"in glass" referring to a test or research done in the test tube, outside a living organism.
In vivo	inside a living organism. An in vivo assay evaluates a biological process occurring inside the body.
Insoluble	Not dissolvable. With respect to bioavailability, certain substances form insoluble complexes that cannot be dissolved in digestive secretions, and therefore cannot be absorbed by the digestive tract.
Insulin	A peptide hormone secreted by the b-cells of the pancreas required for normal glucose metabolism.
Insulin resistance	Diminished responsiveness to insulin.
Intracellular fluid (ICF)	The volume of fluid inside cells.
Ion	An atom or group of atoms that carries a positive or negative electric charge as a result of having lost or gained one or more electrons.
Ion channel	A protein, embedded in a cell membrane that serves as a crossing point for the regulated transfer of an ion or a group of ions across the membrane.
Ischemia	A low oxygen (hypoxic) state usually related to insufficient blood flow to a tissue.
Isokinetic contraction	Contracting muscles while maintaining constant speed, such as in biking.
Isometric contraction	Muscular contraction without external motion of bones, such as pushing immovable wall.
Isotonic contraction	Muscular contraction with external motion of bones, such as squatting.
Jaundice	A yellowish staining of the skin and whites of the eyes due to increased bilirubin (a bile pigment) levels in the blood. Jaundice can be an indicator of red blood cells rupturing (hemolysis), or disease of the liver or gallbladder.
Jerk	Lifting the bar from shoulders to overhead with leg drive in addition to shoulder drive.
Ketone bodies	Any of three acidic chemicals (acetate, acetoacetate, and beta-hydroxybutyrate). Ketone bodies may accumulate in the blood (ketosis) when the body has inadequate glucose to use for energy, and must increase the use of fat for fuel. Ketone bodies are acidic, and very high levels in the blood are toxic and may result in ketoacidosis.
Kidney stones	Also known as renal calculi, kidney stones are the result of crystallization of certain substances found in urine, including calcium, phosphate, oxalic acid, and uric acid. Stones may form in the urine collecting area (pelvis) of the kidney, as well as the ureters (narrow tubes connecting the kidney to the urinary bladder).
Kyphosis	Abnormal rearward curvature of the spine, resulting in protuberance of the upper back; hunchback
LDL	Low-density lipoprotein. Lipoproteins (particles composed of lipids and protein) are the form in which fats are transported throughout the body, in the bloodstream. LDL transport cholesterol from the liver to the tissues of the body. A high proportion of cholesterol carried in LDL (LDL-cholesterol) is associated with an increased likelihood of developing cardiovascular diseases (heart disease and stroke). Oxidized LDL appears to play an important role in the development of atherosclerosis.
Left ventricular hypertrophy (LVH)	Abnormal thickening of the wall of the left ventricle (lower chamber) of the heart muscle. The ventricles have muscular walls in order to pump blood from the heart through the arteries, but LVH occurs when the ventricle must pump against abnormally high volume or pressure loads. LVH may accompany congestive heart failure (CHF).
Legumes	Members of the large family of plants known as leguminosae. In this context the term refers to the fruits or seeds of leguminous plants (e.g., peas and beans) that are used for food.
Leukemia	An acute or chronic form of cancer that involves the blood-forming organs. Leukemia is characterized by an abnormal increase in the number of white blood cells in the tissues of the body with or without a corresponding increase of those in the circulating blood, and is classified according to the type of white blood cell most prominently involved.

GLOSSARY

Lipid peroxidation	The process by which lipids are oxidatively modified; so named because lipid hydroperoxides are formed in the process.
Lipids	Different types of fat molecules. For example, phospholipids, cholesterol, triglycerides.
Lipoic acid	A cofactor, essential for the oxidation of alpha-keto acids, such as pyruvate, in metabolism.
Lipoproteins	Particles composed of lipids and protein, that allows for transport of fat and cholesterol through the blood. A lipoprotein particle is composed of an outer shell of phospholipid, which renders the particle soluble in water; a core of fats called lipid, including cholesterol and a surface apoprotein molecule that allows tissues to recognize and take up the particle.
Load intensity	Level of difficulty of resistance with respect to maximum resistable force, 1RM.
Load volume	Added intensities of a number of sets over specific intervals. There is session volume for daily session volume, weekly volume, monthly volume, and annual volume.
Lordosis	Arching in the lower back as a "Lord". Exaggerated lordosis is an abnormal forward curvature of the spine in the lumbar region.
Lp(a) lipoprotein	A lipoprotein particle in which the protein (apolipoproteinB-100) is chemically linked to another protein apolipoprotein(a). Increased blood levels of Lp(a) are associated with an increased risk of cardiovascular diseases.
Lumbar spine	The portion of the spine commonly referred to as the small of the back. The lumbar portion of the spine is located between the thorax (chest) and the pelvis.
Lymphocyte	A white blood cell that creates an immune response when activated by a foreign molecule (antigen). T lymphocytes or T-cells develop in an organ called the thymus and are responsible for cell-mediated immunity, while B-lymphocytes develop in the bone marrow and are responsible for the production of antibodies (immunoglobulins).
Macrocytic anemia	Low red blood cell count, characterized by the presence in the blood of larger than normal red blood cells.
Magnetic Resonance Imaging (MRI)	A special imaging technique that uses a powerful magnet and a computer to provide clear images of soft tissues. Tissues that are well-visualized using MRI include the brain and spinal cord, abdomen, and joints.
Malignant	Cancerous
Megaloblastic anemia	Low red blood cell count, characterized by the presence in the blood of large, immature, nucleated cells (megaloblasts) that are forerunners of red blood cells. Red blood cells, when mature, have no nucleus.
Membrane potential	The electrical potential difference across a membrane. The membrane potential is a result of the concentration differences between potassium and sodium across cell membranes, which are maintained by ion pumps. A large proportion of the body's resting energy expenditure is devoted to maintaining the membrane potential, which is critical for nerve impulse transmission, muscle contraction, heart function, and the transport of nutrients and metabolites in and out of cells.
Menstruation	The cyclic loss of blood by a woman, from her uterus (womb) when she is not pregnant. Menstruation generally occurs every 4 weeks after a woman has reached sexual maturity and prior to menopause.
Metabolism	Physical and chemical processes within the body involving energy production and utilization.
Metabolite	A compound derived from the metabolism of another compound is said to be a metabolite of that compound.
Methionine	A sulfur containing amino acid, required for protein synthesis and other vital metabolic processes. It can be obtained through the diet in protein or synthesized from homocysteine.
Methylation	A biochemical reaction resulting in the addition of a methyl group (-CH3) to another molecule.
Migraine headache	A type of headache thought to be related to abnormal sensitivity of blood vessels (arteries) in the brain to various triggers resulting in rapid changes in the artery size due to spasm (constriction). Other arteries in the brain and scalp then open (dilate), and throbbing pain are perceived in the head. The tendency toward migraine appears to involve serotonin, a neurotransmitter that can trigger the release of vasoactive substances in the blood vessels.
Military Clean	It is Clean lift without any knee bending, from the floor to shoulders.
Military Snatch	It is Snatch lift with stiff-legged stand, from the floor to arm stretch overhead.
Minerals	Nutritionally significant elements. Elements are composed of only one kind of atom. Minerals are inorganic, i.e., they do not contain carbon, as do vitamins and other organic compounds.
Mitochondria	Energy-producing structures within cells. Mitochondria possess two sets of membranes, a smooth continuous outer membrane, and an inner membrane arranged in folds. Among other critical functions, mitochondria convert nutrients into energy via the electron transport chain.
Mm Hg	Millimeters of mercury. The unit of measure for blood pressure.

GLOSSARY

Multifactorial	Refers to a disorder or condition that has a number of different causes.
Multiple sclerosis (MS)	An autoimmune disorder, which results in the demyelinization of nerves. In MS, the myelin sheath that allows for efficient transmission of nerve impulses is damaged, resulting in progressive neurological symptoms such as, numbness, tingling, loss of control of certain bodily functions, and paralysis.
Muscular Recruitment	A process by the nervous system to deploy muscular fibers in accordance to feedback from sensors from muscles and ligaments and coordination by the motoneuron of the AHC.
Myelin	The fatty substance that covers myelinated nerves. Myelin is a layered tissue surrounding the axons or nerve fibers. This sheath acts as a conduit in an electrical system, allowing rapid and efficient transmission of nerve impulses. Myelination refers to the process in which nerves acquire a myelin sheath.
Myocardial infarction (MI)	Commonly known as a "heart attack", a myocardial infarction refers to changes that occur in the heart muscle due to an interruption in its blood supply. An MI is often the result of a clot that lodges in a coronary artery, resulting in deprivation of oxygen to a portion of the heart muscle (ischemia), and ultimately the death (necrosis) of a portion of the heart muscle, if the oxygen supply is not restored within a few minutes.
Myocarditis	An inflammation of the heart muscle.
Myoglobin	A heme-containing pigment in muscle cells that binds and stores oxygen.
Myopathy	Any disease of muscle.
Neuropathy	Malfunction or disease pathology of nerves. Peripheral neuropathy refers to a disease or degenerative state of peripheral nerves resulting in pain, numbness, and sometimes muscle weakness.
Neurotoxic	Toxic or damaging to nervous tissue (brain and peripheral nerves).
Neurotransmitter	A chemical that is released from a nerve cell, which transmits an impulse from that nerve cell to another nerve cell, or to another organ (a muscle, for example). Neurotransmitters are chemical messengers that transmit neurological information from one cell to another.
Nucleic acids	DNA (deoxyribonucleic acid) and RNA (ribonucleic acid). Long thread-like molecules made up of large numbers of nucleotides. Nucleotides are composed of nitrogen containing base, a 5-carbon sugar, and one or more phosphate groups. The sequence of bases in DNA or RNA represents the genetic (hereditary) information of a living cell.
Nucleotides	Molecules composed of nitrogen containing base, a 5-carbon sugar, and one or more phosphate groups. Long strands of nucleotides form nucleic acids (see above). The sequence of bases in DNA or RNA represents the genetic (hereditary) information of a living cell.
Nucleus	A membrane-bound cellular organelle, which contains DNA organized into chromosomes.
One-carbon unit	A biochemical term for functional groups containing only one carbon in addition to other atoms. One-carbon units transferred by folate coenzymes include methyl (-CH3), methylene (-CH2-), fomyl (-CH=O), formimino (-CH=NH), and methenyl (-CH=). Many biosynthetic reactions involve the addition of a one-carbon unit to a precursor molecule.
Optimum health	In addition to freedom from disease, the ability of an individual to function physically and mentally at his or her best.
Osteoarthritis	A degenerative joint condition that is characterized by the breakdown of articular cartilage (cartilage within the joint). Symptoms of osteoarthritis include pain and stiffness in the affected joint(s), particularly after activity.
Osteomalacia	A disease of adults that is characterized by softening of the bones due to loss of bone mineral. Osteomalacia is characteristic of vitamin D deficiency in adults, while children with vitamin D deficiency suffer from rickets.
Osteoporosis	A condition of increased bone fragility and susceptibility to bone fracture due to a loss of bone mineral density (BMD)
Oxidant	Reactive oxygen species.
Oxidation	A chemical reaction that removes electrons from an atom or molecule.
Oxidative stress	An organism is said to experience oxidative stress when the effects of prooxidants (e.g. free radicals, reactive oxygen and reactive nitrogen species) exceed the ability of antioxidant systems to neutralize them.
Pancreas	A small organ located behind the stomach. The head of the pancreas is connected to the duodenum (the first section of the small intestine). The pancreas makes enzymes that help digest food in the small intestine and hormones, including insulin, that control the amount of glucose in the blood.

GLOSSARY

Parathyroid glands	Glands located behind the thyroid gland in the neck. The parathyroid glands secrete a hormone called parathormone (PTH) that is critical to calcium and phosphorus metabolism.
Peptide	A chain of amino acids. A protein is made up of one or more peptides.
Peptide hormones	Hormones that are proteins, as opposed to steroid hormones, which are made from cholesterol. Insulin is an example of a peptide hormone.
Peripheral neuropathy	A disease or degenerative state affecting the nerves of the extremities (arms and legs). Symptoms may include numbness, pain, and muscle weakness.
Peripheral vascular diseases	Diseases of the vessels of the extremities such as atherosclerosis, resulting in diminished circulation, pain (claudication), or a blood clot, for example.
Peritoneum	A membrane that lines the walls of the abdominal cavity.
Pernicious anemia	The end stage of an autoimmune inflammation of the stomach, resulting in destruction of stomach cells by one's own antibodies. Progressive destruction of the cells that line the stomach cause decreased secretion of acid and enzymes required to release food bound vitamin B-12. Antibodies to intrinsic factor (IF) bind to IF preventing formation of the IF-B-12 complex, further inhibiting vitamin B-12 absorption.
PH	A measure of acidity or alkalinity.
Pharmacologic dose	The dose or intake level of a nutrient many times the level associated with the prevention of deficiency or the maintenance of health. A pharmacologic dose is generally associated with the treatment of a disease state and considered to be a dose at least 10 times greater than that needed to prevent deficiency.
Phospholipids	Lipids (fat molecules) in which phosphoric acid as well as fatty acids are attached to a glycerol backbone. Phospholipids are found in all living cells and in the bilayers of cell membranes.
Phosphorylation	The creation of a phosphate derivative of an organic molecule. This is usually achieved by transferring a phosphate group (-PO4) from ATP to another molecule.
Physiologic dose	The dose or intake level of a nutrient associated with the prevention of deficiency or the maintenance of health. A physiologic dose of a nutrient is not generally greater than that which could be achieved through a conscientious diet, as opposed to the use of supplements.
Pituitary gland	A small oval gland located at the base of the brain that secretes hormones regulating growth and metabolism. The pituitary gland is divided into two separate glands, the anterior and posterior pituitary glands, which each secrete different hormones.
Plasma	The liquid part of blood (as opposed to blood cells) that makes up about half its volume. Plasma differs from serum in that the blood sample has not clotted. A centrifuge is used to separate plasma from cells in the laboratory.
Platelet	Irregularly shaped cell fragments that assist in blood clotting. During normal blood clotting platelets aggregate (group together) to prevent hemorrhage.
Pneumonia	A disease of the lungs, characterized by inflammation and accumulation of fluid in the lungs. Pneumonia may be caused by infectious agents (e.g., viruses or bacteria) or by inhalation of certain irritants.
Power Clean	Lifting as in the Clean lift without too much dipping with knee bending.
Precursor	A molecule, which is an ingredient, reactant, or intermediate in a synthetic pathway for a particular product.
Prevalence	The proportion of a population with a specific disease or condition at a given point in time.
Prognosis	Predicted outcome based on the course of a disease.
Proliferation	Rapid cell division.
Prooxidant	An atom or molecule that promotes oxidation of another atom or molecule by accepting electrons. Examples of prooxidants include free radicals, reactive oxygen species (ROS) and reactive nitrogen species (RNS).
Protein	A complex organic molecule composed of amino acids in a specific order. The order is determined by the sequence of nucleic acids in a gene coding for the protein. Proteins are required for the structure, function, and regulation of the body's cells, tissues, and organs, and each protein has unique functions.
Pyruvate kinase deficiency	A hereditary deficiency of the enzyme pyruvate kinase. Pyruvate kinase deficiency results in hemolytic anemia.
Radiation therapy	The local use of radiation to destroy cancer cells or stop them from dividing and growing.
RDA	Recommended dietary allowance. Set by the Food and Nutrition Board of the Institute of Medicine, the RDA is the average daily dietary intake level sufficient to meet the nutrient requirements of nearly all (97-98%) healthy individuals in a specific life stage and gender group (e.g., women from 19-50 years of age). It is intended as a goal for daily intake of specific nutrients by individuals.
Receptor	A protein on or protruding from the cell surface to which select chemicals can bind. Binding of a specific molecule (ligand) may result in a cellular signal, or the internalization of the receptor and the ligand.

GLOSSARY

Rectum	The last section of the large intestine (colon). It connects the sigmoid colon (above) to the anus (below).
Reduction	A chemical reaction in which a molecule or atom gains electrons.
Renal	Refers to the kidneys.
Resorption	The process of breaking down or assimilating something. With respect to bone, resorption refers to the breakdown of bone by osteoclasts that result in the release of calcium and phosphate (bone mineral) into the blood.
Retina	The sensory membrane that lines most of the back of the eye. The retina is composed of several layers including one containing the rods and cones. It receives the image formed by the lens and converts it into chemical and nervous signals, which reach the brain by way of the optic nerve.
Rheumatoid arthritis	An autoimmune disease, which causes chronic inflammation of the joints, the tissue around the joints, as well as other organs in the body. Because it can affect multiple other organs of the body, rheumatoid arthritis is a systemic illness and is sometimes called rheumatoid disease.
Riboucelotide	A molecule consisting of a 5-carbon sugar (ribose), a nitrogen containing base, and one or more phosphate groups.
Rickets	Often the result of vitamin D deficiency. Rickets affects children while their bones are still growing. It is characterized by soft and deformed bones, and is the result of an impaired incorporation of calcium and phosphate into the skeleton.
RNA	Ribonucleic acid. A chain of nucleotides, which are composed of nitrogen containing base, a 5-carbon sugar (ribose), and phosphate groups. RNA functions in the translation of the genetic information in DNA to protein synthesis.
Scurvy	A disorder caused by lack of vitamin C. Symptoms includes anemia, bleeding gums, tooth loss, joint pain, and fatigue. Scurvy is treated by supplying foods high in vitamin C as well as with vitamin C supplements.
Seizure	Uncontrolled electrical activity in the brain, which may produce a physical convulsion, minor physical signs, thought disturbances, or a combination of symptoms.
Serotonin	A hormone also known as 5-hydroxytryptamine. Serotonin functions as both a neurotransmitter and a vasoconstrictor (substance that causes blood vessels to narrow).
Serum	The liquid part of blood (as opposed to blood cells) that makes up about half its volume. Serum differs from plasma in that the blood sample has clotted. A centrifuge is used in the laboratory to separate serum from cells after blood has clotted.
Short bowel syndrome	A malabsorption syndrome resulting from the surgical removal of an extensive portion of the small intestine.
Sickle cell anemia	A hereditary disease in which a mutation in the gene for one of the proteins that comprises hemoglobin results in the formation of defective hemoglobin molecules known as hemoglobin S. Individuals who are homozygous for this mutation (possess two genes for hemoglobin S) have red blood cells that change from the normal discoid shape to a sickle shape when the oxygen supply is low. These sickle-shaped cells are easily trapped in capillaries and damaged, resulting in severe anemia. Individuals who are heterozygous for the mutation (possess one gene for hemoglobin S and one normal hemoglobin gene) have increased resistance to malaria.
Sideroblastic anemia	A group of anemias that are all characterized by the accumulation of iron deposits in the mitochondria of immature red blood cells. These abnormal red blood cells do not mature normally, and many are destroyed in the bone marrow before reaching the circulation. Sideroblastic anemias can be hereditary, idiopathic (unknown cause), or caused by such diverse factors as certain drugs, alcohol, or copper deficiency.
Small intestine	The part of the digestive tract that extends from the stomach to the large intestine. The small intestine includes the duodenum (closest to the stomach), the jejunum, and the ileum (closest to the large intestine).
Snatch lift	Lifting barbell from the floor to overhead, with monotonous motion.
Sprue	Also known as celiac sprue and celiac disease, it is an inherited disease in which the intestinal lining is inflamed in response to the ingestion of a protein known as gluten. Treatment of celiac disease involves the avoidance of gluten, which is present in many grains, including rye, oats, and barley. Inflammation and atrophy of the lining of the small intestine leads to impaired nutrient absorption.
Steroid	A molecule related to cholesterol. Many important hormones such as estrogen and testosterone are steroids. See hormone.
Steroid hormone receptor	A protein within a cell, which binds to a specific steroid hormone. Binding of the steroid hormone changes the shape of the receptor protein and activates it, allowing it to activate gene transcription. In this way, a steroid hormone can activate the synthesis of specific proteins.

GLOSSARY

Stress fracture	A hairline or microscopic break in a bone, usually due to repetitive stress rather than trauma. Stress fractures are usually painful, and may be undetectable by X-ray. Though they may occur in almost any bone, common sites of stress fractures are the tibia (lower leg) and metatarsals (foot).
Stroke	The sudden death of some brain cells due to lack of oxygen, when blood flow to the brain is impaired by the blockage (usually due to a blood clot) or rupture of a blood vessel in the brain. A stroke is also called a cerebrovascular accident (CVA).
Subclinical	Without clinical signs or symptoms; sometimes used to describe the early stage of a disease or condition, before symptoms are detectable by clinical examination or laboratory tests.
Substrate	A reactant in an enzyme catalyzed reaction.
Supplement	A nutrient or phytochemical supplied in addition to that which is obtained in the diet.
Syndrome	A combination of symptoms that occur together and is indicative of a specific condition or disease.
Synthesis	The formation of a chemical compound from its elements or precursor compounds.
Systolic blood pressure	The highest arterial pressure measured during the heart beat cycle. It occurs when the heart muscle is contracting (pumping).
Tetany	A condition of prolonged and painful spasms of the voluntary muscles, especially the fingers and toes (carpopedal spasm) as well as the facial musculature.
Threshold	The point at which a physiological effect begins to be produced, for example, the degree of stimulation of a nerve which produces a response or the level of a chemical in the diet that results in a disease.
Thyroid	A butterfly-shaped gland in the neck that secretes thyroid hormones. Thyroid hormones regulate a number of physiologic processes, including growth, development, metabolism, and reproductive function.
Transcription	(DNA transcription); the process by which one strand of DNA is copied into a complementary sequence of RNA.
Transient ischemic attack (TIA)	Sometimes called a small or mini stroke. TIAs are caused by a temporary disturbance of blood supply to an area of the brain; resulting in a sudden, brief (usually less than 1 hour) disruptions in certain brain functions.
Translation	(RNA translation) process by which the sequence of nucleotides in a messenger RNA molecule directs the incorporation of amino acids into a protein.
Trauma	An injury or wound.
Tremor	Trembling or shaking of all or a part of the body.
Triglycerides	A triglyceride consists of three molecules of fatty acid combined with a molecule of the alcohol glycerol. Triglycerides serve as the backbone of many types of lipids (fats). Triglycerides are the major form of fat in our diets and are also produced by the body.
Tuberculosis	An infection caused by bacteria called mycobacteria tuberculosis. Many people infected with tuberculosis have no symptoms because it is dormant. Once active, tuberculosis may cause damage to the lungs and other organs. Active tuberculosis is also contagious and is spread through inhalation. Treatment of tuberculosis involves taking antibiotics and vitamins for at least 6 months.
Typhoid	An infectious disease, spread by the contamination of food or water supplies with the bacteria called salmonella typhi. Food and water can be contaminated directly by sewage or indirectly by flies or poor hygiene. Though rare in the U.S., it is common in some parts of the world. Symptoms include fever, abdominal pain, diarrhea, and a rash. It is treated with antibiotics and intravenous fluids. Vaccination is recommended to those traveling to areas where typhoid is common.
Ultrasonography	A test in which high-frequency sound waves (ultrasound) are bounced off tissues and the echoes are converted into a picture (sonogram).
Vascular dementia	Dementia resulting from cerebrovascular disease, for example a cerebrovascular accident (stroke).
Vascular endothelium	The single cell layer that lines the inner surface of blood vessels. Healthy endothelial function promotes vasodilation and inhibits platelet aggregation (clot formation).
Vasoconstriction	Narrowing of a blood vessel.
Vasodilation	Relaxation or opening of a blood vessel.
Vertebral	Have or pertaining to a vertebra, one of the twenty-three bones that comprise the spine.
Vesicle	A small bag or pouch. Inside a cell, a vesicle is a small organelle surrounded by its own membrane.
Virulent	Marked by a rapid, severe, or damaging course.
Virus	A microorganism smaller than bacteria, which cannot grow or reproduce apart from a living cell. A virus invades living cells and uses their chemical machinery to keep itself alive and to replicate itself.
Vitamin	An organic (carbon-containing) compound necessary for normal physiological function that cannot be synthesized in adequate amounts, and must therefore be obtained in the diet.

Index

A

abdomen, in sit-ups, 471
, in axial back exercises, 466
, in Bent-over Row, 127
, in crunches, 137
, in external abdominal muscles, 487
, in horizontal seated row, 126
, in gymnastics, 266, 267, 269
, in induction of momentum, 180, 190
, in induction of acceleration, 199
, in intestinal muscular contraction, 415
, in leg raises, 138
, in lever rowing, 130
, in lower back deformity, 227
, in oblique leg press, 133
, in one-hand dumbbell curls, 145
, in peripheral training in Weightlifting, 245, 247
, in phase of full squat snatch, 193
, in physiological changes due to exercise, 426
, in Pullover, 160
, in respiration, 427
, in seated leg curls, 134
, in seated trunk twisting, 470
, in Squat, 131
, the role of abdominal muscles, 450
, in torso imbalance, 280
, in unconditioned muscles aerobic component, 275, 392
, in Weightlifting training, 287
abdominal, girth, 486
, circumference, 123
, exercise, 137, 138, 140
, external muscles, 487
, hernias, 55, 491
, major vessels in Squat, 131
, muscles in lateral cable pulldown, 128
, in hip extension, 136
, in shoulder shrugging, 151
, in Pullover, 160
, in Pushups, 162
, in horizontal leg raises, 171
, in inclined sit-ups, 172
, in strengthening the abdominal muscles, 177
, in oblique Bends, 178
, in Jerk lift, 203
, in nervous regulation, 223
, in dynamic forces in running, 226
, in plyometrics exercises, 241
, in local fat deposition, 250
, in hip Flexors, 266, 267, 268, 270, 275, 276
, in Powerlifting training, 294

, in healthy gut, 330
, in trapping of blood inside organs, 365
, in weakness, 392, 393
, in organs in Human development, 423
, in digestion, 427
, in exercises in workout, 445, 446
, in waist belts, 449, 450
, in urinary incontinence, 461
, in Goodmorning exercise, 469
, in seated trunk twisting, 470
, in sit-ups, 470, 471
, in support of organs, 474
, in sprinting, 478
, in fat loss and weight training, 486
, oblique and transverse muscles in trunk twists, 135
abduction, muscular balance, 466
abnormalities, anabolic steroids on menstruation, 124
, antagonists to insulin in circulation, 62
, back pain and vaginal discharge, 46
, body shape curvatures, 120, 243, 245
, coronary arteries and diseased blood vessels, 363
, discomfort in soreness, 398
, female masculinity, 460
, molecules of cancerous tumors, 381
, nerve root syndrome, 45
, overtraining, 293
, spinal cord, 453
, unfit persons, 59
, vitamin B12 deficiency, 340
abortion, family planning, 50
abscess, intravenous injection, 363
, spinal in back pain, 46
absorption, blocking fat, 332
, carbohydrate digestion, 51
, in pernicious anemia, 382
, in bursa fluids, 397
, in digestion, 427
, in seated trunk twisting, 470
, vitamin B12, 340
, vitamin-D and calcium, 248, 338, 460
, waist size, 249, 486
, with alcohol, 371
abstinence from alcohol, 49
, from smoking, 322, 403
, from drugs, 371
, from destructive habits, 253
, from eating fattening food, 62
, from sex, 50
Abu-Khalila (or Kalila), Olympic lifter, 280, 281, 288
abuse, alcohol 371
, arthritis, physical of sport or job, 400

, substance 363, 482
ACC, acetyl-CoA carboxylase enzyme, 430, 431
acceleration, all fingerprints of energy, 407, 408
, ballistic weight training, 213
, basics of physical power, 89
, Hamstrings role, 80
of heart during lifting, 29
, in cable Pulldown, 164
, in the Snatch lift, induction of, 179
, in the Snatch lift, sequence, 183
, in the Snatch, learning with dummy objects, 185
, in the Snatch lift, analysis, 186
, in the Snatch lift, strengthening, 187
, in the Snatch lift, role of shoulder abduction,190, 191
, in the Clean, induction of, 199, 200
, in the Jerk left, 204
, in force, 409
, in inertia, 410
, in gravity, 411
, interpreted as a distortion, 434
, isometric contraction, 217
, load volume of Deadlift, 441
, muscle glycogen, 433
, muscular energy, 418, 477
, Plyometrics, 240
, progressive incremental training, 212
, spinoscopic examination, 47
, timing the pull, 43, 44
, timing energy expenditure, 72
, virtual forces, 270, 287, 446
accessory equipments, distraction of, 16
exercises, to remedy individual deficits, 67
, in session's planning, 69, 77
, in Weightlifting, 73,
, in training on the Snatch lift 182
, in training the clean and jerk lift, 207
, cofactors in biochemistry, 325, 337
muscles of respiration, 223, 225, 241
accident, brain stroke, 381
, fear of liability, 4
, heart attack, 425
, in diabetes, 384
, incurring traumatic, 474
, injuries due to physical activity, 395, 396, 403
, major life threatening, 366
, mobility adaptation in women, 460
, risk of death, 368, 369, 370
, in squatting deep, 448
ACE-inhibitors, in heart disease, 369
acetabular fossa, in hip extension, 167
acetaldehyde, in pyruvate dehydrogenase complex 421
acetoacetyl CoA, in fat metabolism, 415, 416

INDEX

acetone, in ketogenesis, 416
acetyl CoA, in cellular respiration, 63,76,90, 239,253, 339, 340, 418, 421, 476
　, in fatty acid metabolism, 249, 415, 431, 477, 486
　, in cellular metabolism of cholesterol, 331
　, in buildup versus burnout, 333
　, after eating, 432
　, in fasting, 433
　, during muscular contraction, 90, 333, 415, 431, 486
　, fat synthesis, 326, 415, 477
　, and PDH complex, 339-340, 418, 421, 430
　, ketone body formation, 416-419
　, tricarboxylic acid cycle, 419, 476
　, fasting, 433
acetylcholine, in neuromuscular junction, 458
ache, in muscular and fascial pain, 45, 397
　, in muscular imbalance, 108
Achilles tendon, pre-stretching, 39
　, in calf raises, 132
　, in rectifying shoulder imbalance, 283
　, in dealing with long limbed lifters, 286
　, in squatting with raised toes or heels, 452
acidity, in cellular metabolism 220
　, in aerobic enhancement, 237
acidosis, exercise shifts, 235
　, in electronic joggling, 420
acne, in anabolic steroids, 124, 436
acromion process, in shoulder elevation, 151
ACTH, in cortisone Injections, 405,
　, in regulation of hormones, 484
actomyosin, in muscular energy 418, 459, 476
　, see muscle, myoactin
addiction to drugs 5, 11, 50, 371
adductor, hip, 93, 104, 132, 167, 169-173
　, in lifting posture, 29
　, shoulder, 105, 129, 130, 147, 155, 159, 160, 163, 216, 443
adenomas, in anabolic steroids, 124
adenosine mono-phosphate, AMP, 432
adipose tissue, in walking, 331
　, in obesity, 374
　, in fat metabolism, 415
　, after eating, 432
adolescence education, 9
　, back injuries, 423
　, back hunching deformity, 469
　, evolutionary changes, 74
　, maximal growth in strength, 270
　, physical changes, 265, 273
　, Weightlifting training, 286
ADP, during glycolysis, 90
　, high-energy phosphate bonds, 417
　, in mineralization of the skeleton, 248
　, in nitrogen fixing organisms, 416
　, in mitochondria, 420
　, in physical activity, 430
　, in energy consumption, 432
　, in vigorous exercise, 433
　, in cellular chemical decision, 476
　, in muscle fuel, 487
　, respiratory chain of the mitochondria, 418

　, TCA cycle, 419
adrenal gland, aldosterone hormone, 249
　, Hypophyseal-Pituitary-Adrenal axis, 265
　, managing body fat, 327
　, cortisone, 405
　, testosterone, 440
　, in cardiovascular dynamics, 458
　, in women's physiology, 462
　, in fat cells to hormonal regulation, 486
adulthood, peak level of strength, 371,
advertisement, Bodybuilding, 117
　, deceptive marketing, 49
　, Powerlifters, 111
　, training planning, 264
aerobic, adaptation to exercise, 485
　, age variation, 274
　, body fat content, 120, 242
　, Bodybuilders, 117
　　fat burning, 60, 437
　, cardiac muscle, 234,
　, cardiac power output, 251
　, cardiovascular exercises, 465
　, crunches, 136
　, dynamics of circulation, 59
　, energy production, 90, 237, 239, 417-418
　, enhancing endurance, 84, 253, 459
　, in fatigue, 238
　, for mobility gain, 140
　, fuel utilization, 224, 487
　, in knee injuries, 56
　, in running, 81, 173, 225
　, in resting, 277
　, load volume, 114, 292
　, plausibility of training, 336
　, returning from lay-off, 139
　, strength training, 231
　, wasting of major muscles, 110
　, weight training, 60, 475-476
aerobics, group exercise, 20, 332-333, 487
aftereffects, in Weightlifters, 9
　, in squatting, 80, 230
　, in endurance training, 274
　, in strength training, 277, 292
　, in repetitive lifting, 439
　, normal course, 35
age,　and alcohol, 370-371
　, in anabolic steroid, 123
　, in autoimmune decline, 380
　, in axial training, 251
　, in back injury, 31
　, in caloric intake, 335
　, in cardiac output, 234
　, in cardiac arrhythmia, 366-367
　, in compliance of ligaments, 37, 401
　, in cystic fibrosis, 413
　, in degenerative conditions, 334
　, in front Squat, 170
　, in heredity, 371
　, in high blood pressure, 373
　, in human limitations, 4, 11, 59, 238-239, 264, 457, 480
　, in Lumbar deformities, 229

　, in managing body fat, 327, 375-376
　, in mechanics of ventilation, 223
　, in primary spinal tumors, 46
　, in muscle pain and stiffness, 330
　, in overtraining, 488
　, in risk factors for cardiovascular diseases, 364, 369-370, 460
　, in setting goals, 261
　, in sexual function, 471
　, in spasticity and inflexibility, 439
　, in starting training, 6, 60, 74, 195, 265- 266, 477
　, in starting in late adolescence, 270, 280, 444
　, in starting in the twenties, 272
　, in starting in the thirties, 274
　, in strength plateaus, 194, 450
　, in strength training prior to the age of 16, 276
　, in training benefits, 3, 328, 428, 490
　, in urinary incontinence, 461, 470
　, in vitamin B12 over age 50, 338
　, in weak Supraspinatus, 155
　, in weight increase, 65
　, in yanking habit, 34
　, in yoga-style stretching, 485
agility, drawbacks of Powerlifting, 455
　, dynamics of innervation, 60
　, intensity of exercise, 367
　, knee extension, 174, 176
　, little athletes, 17
　, maximal oxygen consumption, 236
　, mobility adaptation, 460, 474
　, partial overloading, 56
　, power and strength, 264
　, Snatch lift, 197
AHC (anterior horn cells), 71, 273
AIDS, immune suppression, 381
　, role of behavior, 363, 368, 370
albumin, free fatty acids transport, 432
alcohol, consumption, 23, 482
　, hypertension, 385
　, in menial occupations, 5
　, lower back pain, 403
　, MAO inhibitors, 435
　, marketing and health ethics, 49-50
　, moderation in drinking, 385
　, neuromuscular integrity, 22
　, planning of Weightlifting program, 9, 15, 76, 257
　, preventable causes of death, 363, 371
　, tumors, 381
　, weight gain, 376
alcoholic beverage, wine, 385, 435
　, whiskey, 341
alcoholism, 11
　, heart causes failure, 366
　, neurological disturbances, 333
almond, niacin content, 355
　, phosphorus contents, 348
　, protein contents, 337, 345
　, riboflavin contents, 357
　, thiamin contents, 356
　, vitamin B6, 351
alveoli, during peak exercise, 251, 424, 465
　, gas exchange, 222

INDEX

, surface tension, 392
amino acid, alanine release during activity, 432
, glycine, 51
, body synthesis, 63, 124, 339, 431
, anabolic androgens, 125
, conversion into acetyl coenzyme-A, 239
, food intake of proteins, 250, 337, 411, 432
, muscle fuel, 253, 475
, colon cancer, 330
, production of ammonia, 330
, dietary supplements, 338
, synthesis by bacteria and animals, 412
, secret for life, 414
, gluconeogenesis, 416, 486
, nitrogen content, 420, 429
, tyramine, 435
, liver deamination, 477
, genetic expression of enzymes, 485
, arginine, 244, 250, 326, 331, 339
, threonine, 339
, creatinine, 238, 425
, globin, 224, 442
, transcription, 125, 325, 392, 406, 415
, tryptophan, 250, 339
, tyramine, 435
, glutamine, 326, 416
, glycine, 339
, hydroxproline, 398
, tyrosine, 339
ammonia, amino acid metabolism, 330
, glutamic acid to glutamine, 326
, in production and growth, 333
, nitrogen fixing organisms, 416
, toxic load, 337
AMP, activity demand signal, 432
, after vigorous work, 433
, chemical energy carries, 248, 430
amphetamines, stimulants, 363
, with MAO inhibitors, 435
amyotrophic lateral sclerosis, ALS, 391
anabolic state, nutritional requirements, 14, 59
, peaking of volume, 81
steroids, 1, 75, 123-125, 336, 435-436
, overtraining, 293
, anabolin-I, 123
, anadrol, 123, 435
, anavar, 123
, androgens, 123-125, 415, 436
, baldness, 124
, cholestasis, 124
, on clitoris, 124
, hepatocellular hyperplasia and adenomas, 124
anadrol, receptor affinity, 435
anaerobic oxidation, 224, 292, 326, 397, 418
analgesic, drugs (NSAIDs), 47
, in muscular and fascial pain, 45, 395, 396, 401, 403, 404
anemia, aplastic, 123, 382, 435
, blood donation, 442
, diseased kidneys, 428
, iron deficiency, 224
, megaloblastic, 340, 391
, over training, 114

, vitamin B6 deficiency, 339
aneurysm, in workup for back pain, 46
, in myocardial infarction, 367
, in high blood pressure, 373
angiogenesis, in obesity, 381
, in strength exercise, 485-486
, L-arginine-nitric oxide pathway, 331
angioplasty, 364
ankle flexion (dorsal flexion), 176
extension (plantar flexion), 176
antibiotic oral administration, 339
, discovery, 3, 87
, infectious arthritis, 401
, intestinal microorganisms, 339
, intravenous drug injection, 363
, rheumatic fever, 366
antibodies, and anabolic androgens, 125
, immune system 381, 382
, in rheumatoid arthritis, 401, 461
anticoagulants, bleeding or hematoma, 46
anticoagulants, hypersensitivity to aspirin or NSAIDs, 47
antidepressant, 332
antidiuretic, 62, 249
antihistaminic, 15
anti-inflammatory, rheumatoid arthritis, 401
, rotator cuff tear, 402
, Synthetic cortisones, 405
antineoplastic, anabolic androgenic steroids, 123
antioxidant, Scientific fallacies, 49, 336
, vitamin-E, 339
anxiety, and night sleep 11
, and ambition, 14
, and performance, 257
, and insight, 483
, exercise, 484, 491
, gym environment, 454
, heart attacks, 366
, in weight-reduction plan, 376
, in brain stress, 391
, MAO inhibitors, 435
, overtraining, 293, 488
, size of the testicles, 436
appearance, athletic muscular, 5, 6, 7, 19, 112, 119, 165-166, 225, 263
, axial strengthening, 118, 264
, body fat content, 120, 429
, change, 327-333, 426
, feminine appearance, 457, 490
, imbalance of muscular, 41, 80, 455
, in runners, 228
, skeletal posture, 248, 475
, of Weightlifter, 115, 485
appendicitis, differential diagnosis of back pain 46
appetite, in high carbohydrate diet, 62
, in fat intake, 436
, in overweight, 489
, overtraining, 293
Archimedes, on natural laws 261
arousal, alcohol in sexual, 436
, brain stem signals, 72
, cortisol level, 405
, drug doping, 113

, during the approach phase, 38
, in unfit body, 395
, neural adaptation, 225, 238
arrhythmia, ambient temperature, 465
, during resistance training, 456, 458
, heart conduction, 239
, heart diseases, 364, 367
, prerequisites to exercise, 380
, sympathetic regulation, 251
arteriolar valve, in muscular contraction, 244, 251
network, in axial training, 248
arteriosclerosis, blood pressure sensors, 234
, cultural differences, 368
, daily activities, 13, 249
, in exercise, 425, 427
, overweight, 376
, perfusion and ventilation, 465
arteritis, temporal, 405
artery, Causes of Morbidity 364
, coronary artery disease, 1, 62, 265, 267, 269
, vasa vasora, 428
artherosclerosis, aging, 399
, in dislocation, 402
arthritis, adhesion, 403
, blood supply, 111
, chondro-osteo-arthritis, 334
, cortisone Injections, 405
, dislocation, 402
, in Deadlift wide stance, 104
, in muscular imbalance, 107, 108
, magnetic mattresses, 51
, osteoarthritis, 399
, preventable maladies in women, 460, 461, 474
, rheumatoid, 382, 402
, strengthening, 393
, variants, 400-401
, walking exercise, 331
articulation, feet stance, 216
, in Weightlifting, 58
, in hips, 166
, in knees 174
, in ankle, 176
, internal acceleration, 434
, lifting from the floor, 409
aspirin, cause of deaths, 363
, cortisone Injections, 405
, heart diseases, 369
, injuries of soft tissues, 396
, rheumatic heart Disease, 368
, treatment of back pain, 47
asthma, administration of corticosteroids, 405
, daily training routine, 68
, respiratory adaptation, 459, 474
atherosclerosis, 5, 223, 248-249, 260, 367, 428
ATP, biological energy, 416, 487
, changes due to exercise, 425
, chemical energy, 248, 419-421, 428, 476
, developing strength, 478, 485
, in glycolysis, 431
, in activity, 432
, in fasting, 433
, in warm-up, 433
, in shakiness during resistance training, 456

511

INDEX

, in chronic fatigue, 253
, in TCA cycle, 383
, in soreness, 397
ATP-CP, creatine phosphate and adenosine triphosphate shuttle, 56, 392, 419, 475, 477
attitude, fitness trainers, 185
, in Weightlifters, 321
, mental rituals, 37
, towards physical training, 8
, workout anxiety, 491
autoimmune system, in cancer 7, 380
, soft tissue pain, 45, 331, 391
, gastrointestinal tract disorders, 330
, heart valves, 367
, alcohol, 371, 381
, autoimmune intolerance, 382
, arthritis, 400, 401, 402
, corticosteroids, 405

B

back extension, see "exercise,, Goodmorning"
back Squat, knee injuries, 56, 445
, descending during lifting, 65-66
, exercise sequence, 70, 262
, accessory Weightlifting exercises, 73, 77-79, 82-83, 215, 259
, maximal records, 80-81
, in Powerlifting, 90, 106-107, 294
, full description, 91-94, 130-131, 169-170, 174, 470-471
, muscular imbalance, 107
, power boosting modalities, 109, 451
, Weightlifting style, 112, 247, 441
, monthly exercise-differentials, 295-316
backache, 449
bacteria, electron transport, 420
, epidemics of the past, 7
, fertilization of the soil, 484
, food borne illness, 378, 379, 389
, gastrointestinal health, 329-330, 337, 427, 460, 470
, infection, 51
, nitrate-fixing, 412, 416
, rheumatic heart disease, 367
, tooth decay, 384
basketball layer Magic Johnson, 381
beginner trainee, personal training, 2, 11, 68, 184, 195, 454
, basic training, 12, 16, 30, 194, 235, 277
, injury, 18, 37, 42
, yanking, 34
, scientific sport, 58
, bodyweight increase, 66
, starting age, 74
, teaching the Snatch, 79
, Powerlifting training, 90, 106
, full squatting, 94
, Front Squat adaptation, 95-96, 283
, military style of lifting, 99
, stiff-legged Deadlift, 104, 126, 442
, avoiding overtraining, 114, 488
, Bodybuilding, 115
, weekly training frequency, 138

, shoulder elevation, 151
, learning the Clean lift, 208, 212
, load volume and training intensity, 232, 451
, adult beginners adjustment, 244
, bar shelving technique, 318
, development, 457
Bench Press, and back extension, 12
, whole range lifting, 35, 80, 90, 118, 139, 294
, and squatting, 36, 451
, individualized exercises, 68, 482
, number of repetitions per sets, 69
, exercise sequence, 70, 197
, contraction mode, 71, 252
, records of Weightlifters, 81
, hindrance effect in Weightlifting, 84
, description, 104-110, 160-161, 163, 472-473
, load volume, 114-115
, forced repetitions, 140
, wrist and finger flexion, 147
, shoulder rotation, 152, 155
, enhancing the Snatch, 187
, axial training, 247
, permanent physical changes, 273
, Powerlifting periodization, 294
, structuring workout sessions, 443-445
, and dumbbell Press, 454
Bend-over rows (BOR), description, 126-127, 153 468
, balance the shoulder muscles, 105
, supersets, 110
, shoulder extension, 166, 191
, enhancing the Clean lift, 207
, axial training, 244, 247
, workout at home, 445
, T-Bar, 154
Bent-over lateral arm raises, 152-153
Beriberi, thiamin deficiency, 339, 421
beverages, alcoholic, 49, 371, 385
, carbohydrate density, 341, 383-384, 490
, dental health, 390
biking, endurance versus weight training, 444
, rehabilitating physical therapy, 399
bile, in fat diet, 63, 415, 432
, in anabolic steroids, 124
, in sclerosing cholangitis, 382
bladder, abdominal muscles and immobility, 474
, bladder cancer, 381
, during lifting, 92
, dysfunction in disk herniation, 45, 46
, urinary incontinence, 461
bleeding, anticoagulants, 46
, myocardial infarction, 367
, older athletes and external pressure, 267
, spinal cord venous congestion, 453
, sudden ankle inversion, 396
, testicles support during training, 112
, vitamin-C deficiency, 339
blindness, deficiency of vitamins, 337, 338
, in diabetes mellitus, 384
blood pressure, baroreceptors, 425, 427
, perfusion, 159, 161, 216, 220, 222, 236, 244, 247, 440, 465
, platelets, 435, 442
, prothrombin, 339

, turbulence, 59, 275, 373, 412
bodyweight issues, 277
bodyweight-to-height relation, 86
bone, clavicle, 28, 156, 158, 160, 184, 275, 403
, coccyx, 173
, coracoid, 143, 144, 145, 158, 160
, cuneiform, 176
, demineralization, in lower back pain 46
, demineralization, in corticosteroids therapy, 405
, epicondyle, 146, 170, 400
, femur, 134, 167, 170, 173, 175, 193, 447
, fibula, 27, 40, 176, 442
, glenoid cavity, 144, 147, 150, 152, 164, 191
, humerus, 142, 144, 145-147, 149-150, 152, 155, 158, 160-163, 283
, iliac, 167
, ilium, 41, 166, 177
, ischial, 26, 39, 167, 175, 442, 447
, Ischium, 150, 167, 173
, olecranon, 147
, ossification, 248, 265
, sacrum, 41, 71, 166, 172
, supra-glenoid, 144
, tuberosities, 26, 144, 173, 442, 447
, ulna, 142, 145, 146, 147
bowel, abdominal hernias, 56
, and diet, 14, 370, 377-378
, and leg raises, 137
, and exercise, 470
, dysfunction, 45, 46
bowlegs, body shape, 120
brain, neural control, 90, 458
breathing, abdominal hernias, 55
, abdominal support, 108, 131, 177, 225, 257, 470
, and gut contents, 14, 29
, chemoreceptors, 425
, during exercise, 59, 223, 380, 418, 426-427
, in back hunching, 18
, in runner, 228
, in untrained people, 251
, in aerobic activities, 328
, in heart attack, 366
, in Squats, 451
, in Bend-over row, 468
, in warm-up, 484
, maximal oxygen consumption, 236
, nervous regulation, 223
, restriction by belt, 449
, strong upper body, 92
, thrusting the chest, 442, 448
, voluntary control, 38
butter, 4, 335, 337, 338, 377, 386, 387, 437

C

caffeine, 363, 465
calcium, coronary artery disease, 367, 373, 461
, hormonal control, 90, 458-459
, Immobility induces bone loss, 474
, in muscle fuel usage, 76, 225, 235, 253, 326, 391, 418, 433
, kidney filtering, 428
, mineralization of the skeleton, 248, 325, 334,

INDEX

338, 426, 428
, osteoporosis, 276
, recommended daily allowance, 121, 336, 377
, soreness, 397, 485
, source, 247, 338-339, 346
, with cortisone, 405
Calisthenics, 276, 442, 491
cancer, annual rate of death, 369
, as preventable diseases, 11, 117, 363, 370, 427
, causes and prevention, 380-381
, chemotherapy, 381
, folic acid enriched grains, 378
, high fat diet, 62, 330
, in autoimmune decline, 7, 327
, testosterone treatment, 123
, with alcohol drinking, 371
carbohydrate, caloric density of, 341, 353
, daily intake 120-121, 436
, density in various food, 341
, diet high, 62-63
, fuel source, 110, 224, 235, 237-238, 383-384, 412, 416, 429, 433, 459, 475, 487
, in fat mobilization, 249, 274, 375, 486
, in overweight, 376-377
, liver role, 325
, metabolism, 326, 391, 431-432
, source, 247, 335, 337, 378
carbon monoxide, affinity to hemoglobin, 371
cardiac arrest, 364, 366, 367
cardiovascular exercises, 465, 474
Carnitine, 419, 433, 476
cartilage, deformity, 227
, function, 226, 414
, in full Squat, 470
, injury during lifting, 36, 72, 112, 334, 398-400, 485
, over training, 293, 488
, Structural changes, 252
, vitamin-C role, 339
, wear and tear, 21, 31, 56-57, 69, 107, 231, 394, 401, 403, 445
cell ribosomes, 383, 416
, cytochrome, 235, 339, 420
, cytoplasm (cytosol), 224, 235, 237, 242, 250, 325, 326, 339, 383, 414, 415, 416, 418, 419, 420, 422, 433, 476, 485, 487
, mitochondria, 56, 124, 213, 220, 225, 232-237, 239, 242, 249, 253, 338-339, 367, 397, 416, 418-421, 433, 456, 459, 475-476, 486-487
cellular furnace of chemical fuel, 419
cellulite, 51
championship, 1999 World, 239, 240
, 2002 World, 290
, 2002 Junior World, 464, 493, 495
, 2003 Junior World, 323
, International, 321
childhood, back injuries, 423
, development and growth, 8, 457
, participation in sport, 377
children, alcoholic beverages, 371
, back pain, 45
, becoming champions, 322, 423

, early start, 265-266, 268, 269, 276
, education and physical training, 8, 9, 380, 461
, food borne illness, 390
, genetic predisposition, 372
, heart problems, 366, 368
, iron requirement, 338
, lordotic versus kyphotic postures, 27
, managing body fat, 327-329, 374, 376-377, 384, 388
, passing habits between generations, 5
, resistance training and strength, 8, 9
, sodium intake, 374
chiropractors, aggressive manipulation, 109
, improper lifting, 32
cholesterol structure, 63
, and alcohol, 371
, blood level, 363-364, 365, 369, 370, 387
, contents of food, 340, 344
, food source, 61, 63, 337, 386
, high blood pressure, 373
, hypercholesterolemia, 223, 364, 373
, managing body fat, 327, 375-376
, myocardial infarction, 367
, Percentage daily value, 336
, plaques deposit in blood vessels, 223, 380, 413, 428
, role in health and disease, 374-375
, synthesis in liver, 326, 332, 333, 415-416, 429
cigarette (see smoking)
cities, Cairo, 87, 277, 321
, Alexandria, Egypt, 254, 255, 257, 258, 265, 272, 288
, Paris, 272
Clean lift, ascent from Squat, 202
clothes, supportive clothing, 112
coaching, Bodybuilding, 7, 117
, children, 268-270, 368, 423, 481, 493, 495
, East German, 263
, in full squatting, 94
, lack of, 85, 114, 257
, learning and objectivity, 184
, mastering the rituals of lifting, 32
, on the mechanics of the vertebral column, 42, 266
, Plyometrics training, 240
, Powerlifting, 90
, relaxation and sequential execution, 258, 283
, stretching, 227
, teaching the Snatch, 194, 195
, training and contests, 319-322, 490, 491-492
, zealous trend, 14, 113
cofactor, NAD, 237, 253, 339, 418, 419, 420, 421, 430, 432, 485
, NADH, 339, 417, 418, 419, 420, 421, 430, 432, 433, 485
, NADP, 339, 420, 430, 431
, NADPH, 415, 417, 431, 432
coffee, 341, 342, 350
colon, abdominal muscles, 461
, cancer, 62, 329, 381
, putrefaction, 330, 486
, toxicity, 393, 486
, transit time, 14, 427

colonoscopy, 381
competition, 120, 138, 182, 205, 206, 218, 254, 261, 272, 273, 276, 287, 295, 311, 436, 449, 485, 491, 545
consciousness, alcohol consumption, 23
, in whiplash, 404
, loss of during maximum lifting, 28
, neural control, 458, 484
, physical activity, 15
constipation, 460, 482
and indigestion, 330
Contest rules of the Clean and Jerk lift, 206
rules of the Snatch lift, 182
, pre-contest-month, 312
corticosteroid, 265, 401, 405, 415, 431
administration, 405
cortisone structure, 405
country, Bulgaria, 80, 81, 84, 542
, Egypt, 254, 255, 257, 258, 265, 271, 272, 277, 288, 424
, France, 65, 66, 84, 272
, Germany, 65, 84, 261, 262, 317
, Italy, 439
, Japan, 65, 84, 367, 368, 369, 382
, Koreas, 84
, Poland, 84, 290
, Sweden, 424
CP (creatine phosphate), 18, 56, 76, 392, 418, 419, 428, 431, 475, 477, 487, 490
CP-ATP, 18, 56, 418, 419, 431, 475, 477
cruciate ligaments, PCL, in leg curls, 133, 134
, strengthening the knees, 174
, knee extension, 175
, ligament sprain, 396
, in arthroscopic photographs, 400
, in leg extensions and shear stresses, 447, 448
, in leg extension and flexion, 471
, in history of tear, 495
crunches, 106, 107, 136, 294, 393, 443, 445, 487
cyanide poisoning, 420
cybernetics, 49
cytochrome, ferric form, 420

D

daily activities, 334, 374
Deadlift, axial training versus peripheral training, 243, 247, 273
, description of, 103-104, 169, 174, 438-439, 468
, exercise-differentials, 315
, fallacies on deadlift, 52
, intensity of resistance, 440
, knee injuries, 56
, limitations of, 52
, load volume, 114, 440
, lordotic back, 53
, muscular imbalance, 108
, pelvic circulation, 440
, power drive, 54, 80
, Powerlifting, 90, 106-107, 294
, range of motion rules, 139
, role of the scapulas, 33, 286
, role in the Snatch lift, 182, 186-187, 190

INDEX

, role in the Clean lift, 210, 215
, role in the Squat, 450
, sequence in session, 18, 439
, shoulder shrugging, 151
, stiff-legged Deadlift, 125-126, 169, 446
, superheavy Weightlifters records, 81, 83-84
, Weightlifting training, 66, 73, 77, 235, 254, 272, 287, 440-441, 475
debility, clinical manifestation, 384
, overcoming by resistance training, 5, 13, 276, 426
, with weight reduction, 12
defecation, abdominal weakness, 392, 471
, in herniated disc, 404
deformities, axial vs. peripheral training, 247
, documentation, 482
, due to daily work, 12, 256
, feminine contours, 460
, impact on choosing sport, 14, 261
, in isolated training, 12, 57, 117-119, 243, 473, 485
, in runners, 17, 226-229, 234, 465
, in the Deadlift, 54, 104
, in planning load volume, 60, 291
, in explosive lifting, 73
, in Powerlifting training, 106
, in muscular imbalance, 107-109, 243, 461
, in shoulder Press, 156, 252
, knee cartilages, 57, 461
, late manifestation, 12
, lordotic versus kyphotic postures, 27, 42, 45, 142, 165, 469
, shoulder dislocation, 402
, special exercises, 159, 164, 173
, scoliosis, 120
, swayback, 108
degeneration, active muscle fibers, 238
, arthritis, 400
, chondro-osteo-arthritis, 334
, degenerative changes of aging, 402, 406
, herniated spinal discs, 45, 404
, in atherosclerosis of the arterial walls, 261, 428
dehydration, Bodybuilding diet, 120
, cramps, 398
, heart attack, 365
, in dizzy spells, 234
dementia, in Wernicke-Korsakoff syndrome, 421
deprivation, circulatory in shaking, 456
, in Discipline, 12, 475
, of oxygen in limited cardiac output, 236, 238, 242, 365
, of oxygen in smoking, 372
, of glucose fuel in diabetes, 383
diabetes mellitus, amputation, 395
, epidemiology of, 382
, adult-onset, 4, 383
dietary habits, 120
dieting, and muscle mass, 437-438
, body and mind, 477
, Bodybuilding diet, 120, 123
, boost of energy, 407
, in resistance training, 12
, with aging, 369
digestion, 49, 51, 61, 249, 250, 384, 413, 415, 427, 458, 460, 470, 487

discipline, 12, 231, 475
disease, cardiac arrhythmia, 367
, cardiomyopathies, 364
, cholangitis, autoimmune intolerance sclerosing 382
, cholera, 7, 88, 424
, chondro-osteo-arthritis, 334
, claudication, 45
, colitis, 405
, compartment syndrome, 397
, diabetes, 1, 7, 11, 50, 62, 117, 276, 278, 285, 328, 333, 363, 364, 367, 368, 370, 376, 382, 383, 384, 426, 431, 461
, fibromyalgia, 45
, gynecomastia, 124
, lupus erythromatosus, 382
, malaria, 7
, manic-depressive, 483
, megaloblastic anemia, 340
, meningitis, 45
, mitral valve stenosis, 367
, myositis, 330, 402
, nerve root syndrome, 45
, osteoarthritis, 399, 401, 405
, osteochondritis, 170, 471
, osteomalacia, 151
, pellagra, 339
, pellagra, 339
, Pneumonia, 368, 370, 392
, Pneumothorax, 392
, polymyalgia, 330
, polymyalgia rheumatica, 330
, polymyositis, 330
, prostatitis, 46
, pseudoclaudication, 45
, pseudo-spondylolisthesis, 45
, rheumatoid arthritis, 382, 401, 402, 461
, sacroiliitis, 46
, sarcoidosis, 405
, schizophrenia, 483
, sciatica, 24, 45, 47, 394
, scurvy, 339
, septicemia, 363
, sinusitis, 403
, spinal stenosis, 45
, syncope, 459
, syphilis, 7, 401
, tendonitis, 18, 108, 396, 401, 402, 403, 447
, tuberculosis, 7, 88, 401, 424
, typhoid, 7, 88, 424
, Wernicke-Korsakoff, 421
dislocation, asymmetrical movements, 20
, in yanking, 37, 395
, in start position, 38
, of hip, 44
, of shoulder, 107, 192, 402
, of knees, 400
, spinal discs, 130, 404, 491
diuretic, in Bodybuilding, 123
dizziness, 25, 28, 51, 95, 244, 247, 251, 380, 381, 404, 435, 442, 465, 484
DNA, 250, 325, 327, 340, 412, 414, 416, 484
DOMS (delayed-onset muscle soreness), 397, 406, 451
drive and the psyche, 489

drowsiness, 435
drug use, 435
, cocaine, 363, 435
, codeine, 47
, cortisone, 401, 402, 403, 405
, Cyclobenzaprine (Flexeril), skeletal muscle relaxant, 47
, D-Bol, 435
, Deca-Durabolin, 123
, Depo-testosterone, 123
, Dianabol, 435
, Ethylestrenol, 123
, Fluoxetine, 435
, Ibuprin, 47
, Ibuprofen, 401
, illicit, 2, 74, 113, 123-125, 363
, Isocarboxazid, 435
, Isocitrate, 419
, Ketoprofen, 47
, MAO-inhibitor, 435
, Marplan (MAO-Inhibitor), 435
, Methandrostenol, 435
, Motrin (Ibuprofen), 47
, Nandrolone Decanoate, 123
, Nandrolone, 123
, Naprelan, 47
, Naprosyn, 47
, Nardil, 435
, Oxandrolone, 123
, Oxymetholone, 123, 435
, Panadol(Acetaminophen), 47
, Phenelzine, 435
, Progestin, 371
, Prozac, 435
, Stanozolol, 123
, Tranylcypromine, 435
, Tylenol, 47
, Vicodin (acetaminophen), 47
, Winstrol, 123
, Cannabis, 363
, clot-busters, 369
, contraceptives, 371
, laxatives, 123
dynamics of moving mass, 258
dysuria, 46

E

ego, 455, 483
EKG, electrocardiography, 365
elbow, applied anatomy, 141
electric charges, 333, 407, 411, 412, 426, 434
electrical stimulators, 333, 336
electrocution, 366
electron, 339, 412, 417, 419, 420, 432, 476
electronic joggling, 420
embryo, 124, 422
emergency, 365, 366, 375
emotion, 185, 257, 258, 325, 425, 484
endocrine system, excess bodyweight, 8, 57, 376, 425, 475
, physical power, 90
, Plyometric exercises, 111
, drug doping, 113, 124-125

INDEX

, in exercise, 121, 414
, and Cholesterol, 374
, women's health, 458, 462
, fat loss and weight training, 486
endurance, aiming for higher optimum, 221
    , cellular energy production, 110, 219-220, 236, 268, 459, 480
    , deceptive information, 51
    ,   muscle mass, 222, 234-235, 240
    ,   metabolism, 222, 234
    ,   cardiovascular system, 222, 225, 233, 275
    ,   ventilation, 222, 225, 275
    , fat burning, 237
    , in starting training in adolescence, 9
    , in free lifting, 15
    , in daily living, 22
    , in highly repetitive lifting, 56, 69, 483
    , in fitness enhancement, 58, 66, 274, 413, 485
    , in aerobics, 60, 84, 131, 418
    , in muscular imbalance, 107
    , in running, 122, 173, 225, 230, 437
    , in heavy lifting, 213, 241, 444, 475
    , in overtraining, 293
    , in physical therapy, 399
    , in strength and flexibility, 462
    , inherence and nurture, 219
    , kinetics, 253
    , load volume and training intensity, 232, 292, 491
    , mitochondrial density, 224
    , muscle fiber type, 268
    , preventing anemias, 224
    vs. weight training, 444
energy disguises, 407
    of combustion, 7, 223, 235, 412
    , managing by live organisms, 429
    flow of in human body, 425
enzyme ACC, 431
    TGL, 433
    , oxidase, 435
    cyclase, 432
    dehydrogenase, 237, 242, 253, 339, 416, 418, 419, 420, 421, 422, 430, 431
    lipase, 61, 250, 419, 432, 433, 476, 486
    , arginase, 326
    , ATPase, 225
    , carboxykinase, 430
    , carboxylase, 415, 430, 431
    , CK(creatine kinase), 392, 398, 406, 430
    , FBPase, 430
    , GS, glycogen synthase, 326, 430, 431, 433, 477
    , hexokinase, 326, 418, 422, 430, 431, 432
    , isomerase, 418
    , kinase, 421, 430, 431, 433
    . lactate-dehydrogenase, 418
    . LDH (lactate-dehydrogenase), 237, 242, 418, 420
    . lyase, 415
    . nitrogenase, 416
    . PDH-complex, 237, 242, 339, 340, 418, 419, 421, 430, 433
    , PDH-kinase, 430
    , PDH-phosphatase, 430
    , PFK(phosphofructokinase), 418, 421, 430, 432, 433

, phosphatase, 326, 421, 430, 431, 433
, phosphatase, 326, 421, 430, 431, 433
, phosphodiesterase, 431, 432
, phosphodiesterase, 431, 432
, phosphofructokinase, 418
, phosphofructokinase, 418
, phosphorylase, 326, 430, 431, 433
, reductase, 339, 415
, synthase, 430, 477
, synthetase, 239
, TGL (triglyceride lipase), 433
, thiolase, 415
, translocase, 419, 420
ephedrine, 332, 435
essence of Bodybuilding, 117
    of physical of strength, 475
esthetics, 120
exercise adaptation, 233, 325, 459, 484
    intensity, 75, 233, 292
    sequence, 18, 70, 297, 484
    intensity, 75, 233, 292
    sequence, 18, 70, 297, 484
    isolation, 19, 59, 82, 101, 146, 152, 440, 443, 446, 447, 475, 479
    , auxiliary variants, 294, 470
    , axial back, 189, 274-275, 465, 466
    ,   versus peripheral, 243, 247
    , back extension, 12, 29, 67, 71, 101, 103, 110, 135-137, 167-168, 193, 268, 466, 470
    , back Squat, exercise sequence, 70
    ,   , in Weightlifting, 73, 112, 441
    ,   , maximal records, 80
    ,   , developing leg strength, 81-82
    ,   , description, 91-97, 174
    ,   , in Powerlifting, 106-107, 294
    ,   , supersets, 109, 130
    ,   , hip extension, 167, 169
    ,   , Jerk leg drive, 215
    ,   , axial training and peripheral training, 247, 259
    ,   , essential component, 262
    ,   , monthly exercise-differentials, 295-316
    ,   , knee pain, 445
    ,   and Bench Press synergy, 451
    ,   , Pelvic girdle exercises, 470
    , cellular adaptation, 325
    , chin-ups, 127, 128, 163, 164, 166, 269, 274, 276, 442, 466, 473, 481
    , Deadlift assisting to Weightlifting, 441
    , Deck flyes, 155, 159
    , dumbbell concentration curls, 142, 143
    ,   flyes, 155, 158
    ,   front raises, 155, 157
    ,   Squat, 167, 168
    ,   rowing, 129, 152
    , elbow extension, 148
    , essential, 17, 18, 19, 465
    , examples of improper sequence, 18
    , exercise, upright barbell arm rows, 165
    , fat burning with diet, 436
    , floor abdominal crunches, 177
    , floor and machine hip abduction, 173

, forearm kickback, 148, 149
, frog-squatting, 191
, Goodmorning, 36, 41, 52, 53, 140, 168, 186, 188, 213, 252, 465, 468, 469
, Goodmorning (back extension), 167, 168, 172, 186, 187, 188, 189, 190, 213, 214, 215, 231, 235, 243, 247, 252, 260, 273, 286, 295, 313, 315, 444, 446, 450, 451, 465, 466, 468, 469, 482
, growing need for good living, 6
, Hack Squat, 133
, Hammer dumbbell curls, 145
, Hang Clean, 21, 80, 101, 207, 208, 214, 247, 281, 295, 296, 297, 298, 299, 300, 301-316, 445, 453
, Hang Pull, 80, 208, 214
, high Pull, 80, 202, 208, 209, 214
, hip abduction, 173
,   adduction, 173
,   extension, 135, 167
,   extension from a bench, 135
,   flexion, 170, 171
, horizontal back extension, 167, 168
,   leg raises, 171
,   seated row, 126
, Incline dumbbell flyes, 155, 158
,   sit-up, 137, 294
,   bench press, 155, 161
,   dumbbell press, 155, 158, 159
,   leg press, 167, 168, 169
,   sit-ups, 171, 172, 471
, Isolation versus compound, 446
,   versus compound, 446
, kickback, 148, 149
, knee flexion, 175
, Ladder vertical leg raises, 171
,   arm raises, 165
,   cable pulldown, 128
,   deck raises, 165
,   push and pull, 473
,   trunk bends, 135
, leg extension and flexion, 471
,   and shear stresses, 447
,   lunges, 73, 216, 470, 471
,   Press, 133, 167, 168, 169, 187, 294, 318, 398, 453, 470, 471
, leg-raising, 45, 137, 138, 487
, lever Bent-over Row, 127
, lever rowing, 129
, low back, 134
, lying leg curls, 133, 175
, military Snatch, 73, 102, 103, 106, 107, 247
, monthly differentials, 295
, Natural versus equipment-aided, 14
, number session, 69, 105
, oblique bends, 177, 178
, oblique leg press, 132
, of back, 31, 63, 78, 125, 134, 294-295, 297, 445, 465-466, 469, 470
, of axial extensors, 268
, one-hand cable curls, 142, 143
,   dumbbell curls, 144, 145
,   elbow extension, 148
,   rows, 152
,   side bends, 151, 152

INDEX

, shoulder dumbbell press, 155, 156
, one-legged hip extension, 167
, parallel bar dip, 155, 162
, parallel bar vertical leg raises, 171
, permanent physical changes, 273
, pulldown, 128, 437, 443
, Pullover, 155, 160, 166, 444
, Push Press, 80, 209, 212
, pushdown, 148, 149
, Push-up, 148, 152, 152, 155, 162, 442, 445, 466, 481, 491
, regenerate new neural dendrites, 333
, reverse barbell curls, 144, 145
, wrist curls, 146
, seated shoulder press, 155, 156, 466, 472
, trunk twisting, 466, 469
, back pushing, 466, 469
, cable rows, 152, 154
, knee extension, 175
, leg curls, 134, 175
, sit-ups, 136-137, 171-172, 176, 186, 231, 268, 294, 446, 450, 470-471
, SLDL, stiff-legged Deadlifts, 441-442, 445
, T-bar bent-over row, 152, 154
, Triceps dips, 148, 149, 150
, trunk rotation, 178
, trunk twists, 134, 135
, upright elbow extension, 148
, vertical sit-ups, 171, 172
exercise-differentials, 295, 296, 438, 439
, 295, 296, 438, 439
, eighth-week daily, 306
, eleventh-week daily, 310
, fifteenth-week daily, 315
, fifth-week daily, 302
, fourteenth-week daily, 314
, fourth week daily, 300
, ninth-week daily, 308
, pre-contest-month daily, 312
, sixteenth-week daily, 316
, sixth-week daily, 304
, tenth-week daily, 309
, twelfth-week daily, 311
exercises, cable curls, 142, 143
, flyes, 155, 159
, front raises, 155, 157
, Pulldown, 164, 166, 247
, pushdown, 148, 149
, rowing, 148, 247, 286, 473
, calf raises, 131, 176, 177, 190
, hip adduction, 132, 173
exhaustion, ambient temperature, 465
, cramps, 398
, electrical stimulators, 333
, in progressive weight training, 3, 65, 73, 76, 132, 172, 485
, in menial occupations, 5
, in overtraining, 293, 488
, in heart attack, 365
, in muscular weakness, 392
, in Deadlift, 440
, in shakiness during resistance training, 456
, lactate accumulation, 419

F
FAD (cofactor), 237, 253, 339, 417, 419, 420, 421, 430
fallacy, on Goodmorning and abdominal muscles, 83
, on monopoly in Weightlifting, 84
, on electrical stimulators, 333
, on commercial promotion, 336
, on high blood pressure, 373
, on masculine look, 460
, on back as a weak link, 468
, on squatting as demanding exercise, 470
fasting, and exercise, 76, 475
, fuel utilization, 90, 421, 433
, gluconeogenesis, 418, 421
, ketone synthesis (ketosis), 416
, loss of voluntary control, 257, 391
fat loss and weight training, 485, 486
, chylomicrons, 432
, linoleic acid, 343
and protein diet, 62
, triglycerides, 121, 124, 327, 371, 375, 432-433, 476, 486
, unsaturated fatty acids, 63, 335, 337, 339, 340, 343, 345, 365, 373-374, 386
fatigue (see also exhaustion), 117, 126, 133, 135, 149, 177, 181, 220, 225, 228, 232, 235, 237, 238, 241, 251, 253, 293, 324, 329, 330, 338, 366, 380, 419, 424, 442, 449, 462, 465, 468, 469, 483, 484, 485, 487, 488
fatty acid oxidation, decarboxylation, 419
, dihydroacetone, 326
fava beans, 347, 435
feet stance, in proprioreceptors, 40
, in back Squat, 92-93, 108, 112, 130-131, 170
, in Powerlifting Deadlift, 104, 108
, in Bent-over Row, 127
, in oblique leg press, 132
, in lateral trunk bends, 135
, in standard snatch, 179, 282, 284
, in standard clean, 199, 208, 216, 282
, in the Jerk, 215
, in enhancing the technique, 263
, in muscular imbalance, 281, 286, 287
, in inclined leg Press, 169
, in hip adduction, 173
ferrous sulfate, iron supplements, 442
fever, 46, 52, 94, 114, 116, 236, 317, 366, 368, 382, 391, 421, 424, 483, 488
fish, 63, 121, 247, 327, 335, 337, 338, 339, 365, 374, 378, 379, 386, 387, 390, 435, 437
, salmon, 339, 386, 437
, whitefish, 345
fitness consideration, 274
, pearls of, 331
flags of alarm, 329
flexibility, after puberty, 9, 481
, during systemic training, 15
, effect of training, 254-256, 398, 485
, in military performance, 13
, in shoulder flexion, 36, 252, 263-265, 278, 281-289
, in Deadlift, 52, 438-441, 445
, in spinal disc herniation, 55-56, 403-404
, in Clean and Snatch, 67, 79, 182, 193, 195, 202, 207, 214, 467
, in Squat, 80, 92-97, 170, 174, 317
, in Bodybuilders, 85, 117, 245, 278, 455
, in muscular imbalance, 107
, in Powerlifting, 111, 113, 284, 455
, in oblique leg press, 133
, in Bench Press, 140
, in one-hand exercises, 148, 156
, in Bent-over Rows, 153
, in Deck Flyes, 160
, in inclined leg Press, 169, 187
, in runners, 227-232
, in women's participation, 462
, in overtraining, 488
, prior to competition, 110
, proper planning of Weightlifting, 9, 30, 60, 66, 221, 271, 274
, range of motion rules, 139
, with mobility, 328
food, asparagus, 349
, avocados, 365, 386, 435
, babassu, 342
, babyfood, 341, 345, 346, 348, 351, 352, 355, 356, 357, 358, 359
, bagels, 327, 488, 437
, balsam-pear, 352
, bread, counts of servings, 335
, bread, whole grain, 338, 378, 389
, bread, nutritional value, 341, 343, 347, 350, 354-355, 360-362, 377, 384
, bread, obesity and overweight In Children, 377, 429
, bread, salt intake, 386
, bread, saturated fat content of different foods, 388
, broadbeans, 347
, brownies, 341
, bulk nutrients, 337
, burger, 356
, butterfish, 345
, buttermilk, 346, 348
, butternuts, 343
, cake, 121, 341, 342, 344
, candies, 337, 384
, caviar, 344, 354, 362
, cereals, 337, 339, 340, 437, 374
, chestnuts, 341
, chickpeas, 347, 353
, chocolate, 121, 340, 341, 355, 359, 384, 435
, clam, 349, 354, 359, 362
, coconut, 342, 347
, cookies, 341, 351, 356, 357
, cottonseed, 345, 348, 350, 360
, crab, 344
, crackers, 341, 347, 351, 362
, dessert, 342
, egg, 121, 335, 374, 378, 386, 387
, garlic, 351
, gelatin, 345, 349, 352
, gingerbread, 341
, Granola, 341
, honey, 341, 346, 348, 351, 353, 355, 356, 357, 359, 362

, jelly, 341
, jellybeans, 341
, lard, 121, 342
, lecithin, 343
, lemon, 341, 348, 350, 352
, lemonade, 341, 346, 348, 352
, lentils, 347
, macaroni, 341, 362
, margarine, 342, 343
, marjoram, 346, 347, 350, 359
, mushroom, 349
, mustard, 343, 348, 362
, nacho, 342, 349
, noodle, 349
, nut, 341
, nutmeg, 435
, oat, 343, 348, 351
, oatmeal, 346, 348, 351, 355, 356, 357, 359
, octopus, 354, 362
, oleic acid, 337
, olive oil, 365, 437
, omega-3 fatty acids, 335, 337, 365, 386
, oyster, 349, 354, 360, 361, 362
, pancakes, 348
, parmesan, 345, 346, 348
, parsley, 346, 347, 350, 352, 353, 358, 359
, pasilla, 347, 350, 351, 357, 358
, pastry, 343
, peanuts, 355
, pectin, 341
, Potato, 429
, potatoes, 350
, pretzels, 121, 341
, pumpkin, 343, 346, 348, 358, 359, 360
, roughage, 120, 337
, safflower, 342, 343, 345
, salt, 123, 335, 336, 338, 339, 373, 374, 385, 386
, saltines, 341
, sardine, 342, 343, 344, 362
, shrimp, 338, 435
, soybeans, 345, 347, 350, 353
, soybn, 340, 342, 343
, spaghetti, 341, 349, 362
, spices, 365, 386
, squid, 344, 361
, sugar, 288, 337, 341-360, 378, 383, 384, 390, 462
, sunflower, 343, 345, 348, 356, 361, 362
, sweet, 377, 378, 384, 482
, sweetpotato, 358
, teriyaki, 349
, tuna, 121, 386, 437
, walnut, 343
, whelk, 345, 354, 361, 362
, whole-wheat, 341, 348, 362
foodstuff contents of protein, fat, carbohydrates, and vitamins, 340
fracture, chronic steroids, 46
, exercise protects women, 460-461
, in osteoporotic people, 372
, injuries to the shoulder, 403
, muscle mass and activity, 327-328, 415, 474, 484, 491

, pinched neck nerves, 405
, role of diet, 373
, start position, 38
, X-ray diagnosis, 396, 399, 402, 404
, yanking injuries, 36
Front Squat, description of, 95
, insidious deformities of shoulders, 57, 161
, exercise sequence in training, 70
, as an accessory Weightlifting exercise, 73, 139
, in enhancing the Clean and Jerk, 78, 114
, records of superheavy Weightlifters, 80
, shoulder muscles, Deltoids role, 82, 166, 167, 252, 264
, description of technique, 94-96
, difference over other variants of Squat, 97
, after military Clean, 100
, in plans of Powerlifting training, 106, 107
, muscular balance in Powerlifting, 108, 286
, power boosting modalities, 109
, as a leg exercise, 130-131, 170, 174, 270-271
, strong wrist and forearm flexors, 147
, in full Squat Clean, 202, 210, 215
, in axial training, 247, 283
, flexibility, 254, 271, 272, 274, 275
, monthly leg differential, 295-316
, in split day workout, 445
, Squat and Deadlift rotation, 251
, and knee pain, 445
fructose, 390, 422, 430
fruit, grape, 349, 358, 361
, grapefruit, 352
, grapes, 247
, grapeseed, 343
, prunes, 341
, strawberry, 341, 351, 355, 360
, apple, 335, 341, 351, 352, 435
, apricot, 341, 343, 350, 352, 358, 389
, banana, 335, 341, 342, 346, 348, 351, 356, 357, 377, 389, 429, 435, 437
fait, 227, 465, 470, 472, 481

G

gallbladder, 415
gas exchange in rest and exercise, 222
gastrointestinal health, 329
gender, 6, 17, 276, 364, 370, 373, 462
consideration, 276
gene expression, 1, 2, 118, 250, 331, 372, 415
mutation, 420, 431, 433
mutation, 420, 431, 433
genitalia, in abdominal sit-ups, 471
, steroid use, 436
, testosterone secretion, 439
gland, parathyroid, 248, 253, 338, 458, 460
, thymus, 344
, thyroid, 366
glenoid cavity, 144, 150, 152
gluconeogenesis, 237, 249, 250, 326, 397, 416, 418, 419, 422, 431, 433, 485, 486
glucose, added sugars on food labels, 390
, alternative source, gluconeogenesis, 250, 416-417, 432
, anabolic steroids and liver, 123-124

, as nervous system fuel, 293, 325, 329
, blood level, 327, 371, 433, 476
, breakdown, glycolysis, 224, 234, 326, 418-419, 424, 431
, constituents of, 337
, digestion inhibition, 51
, disturbance in metabolism, 124
, glucose uptake, 326
, glycogen storage, 330
, hypoglycemia, 234
, in high carbohydrate diet, 62
in energy production, 233, 237, 332, 397, 421, 485-486
, in diabetes mellitus, 383-384
, insulin and transport, 121, 326, 383, 430, 431
, on state of mind, 475
, transport proteins, 422
GLUT-1, affinity to glucose, 421
glycerol, 224, 249, 325, 326, 327, 337, 416, 417, 419, 432, 433, 476, 486
glycogen, 121, 224, 225, 237, 238, 253, 326, 330, 416, 419, 422, 430, 431, 432, 433, 456, 476, 477
glycogenolysis, 430glycerol, 224, 249, 325, 326, 327, 337, 416, 417, 419, 432, 433, 476, 486
Golgi, cellular apparatus, 422
, tendon organs, 455
grains, bean, 327, 335, 338, 340-341, 345, 347-350, 353, 356, 374, 377-378, 386-389, 435
groin, 180, 190, 216, 285, 471
growth hormone administration, 336
GTP, 416, 417, 419, 428

H

handgrip, overhand, 127, 128, 144, 146, 148, 149, 179, 199, 208, 210, 211, 438
, thumb-hook grip, 99
, thumb-hook, 99
, overhand and underhand, 55
HDL, 331-332, 365, 370, 376, 432
headache, 329, 366
health advocacies, 376
, flags of alarm, 329
trends of modern american society, 363
health-care, 487
healthy diet, 14, 335, 337
heart adaptation, right atrium, 233
attack, dyspneic (breathless), 366
adaptation, 233
attack, 364, 365, 366
failure, 366
, cardiac after-load, 234
, coronary occlusion stints, 364
, diastole, 239
and lung racing, 250
, myocardial infarction, atheroma, 367
, out-of-rhythm, 367
, preload, 232, 234
, revascularization, 372
, sinoatrial node, 233, 242
, systoles, 239
heartbeat, 220, 222, 233, 468
heart-size, 59
heat, cellular production, 222-226, 232-233, 235, 237-238

INDEX

, feeling of warmth, 51, 220, 410
, food content, 429
, in therapy, 109, 396-399, 402-404, 449
, in physical activity, 122-123, 424, 475, 487
, in dehydration, 365, 461
, in injury, 478
, on the principle of conservation, 333, 429
, radiation, 407-408, 411-412
, regulation, 375, 462
, strong inter-particular forces, 43, 410
, vitamin destruction by, 339-340
hematocrit, 442
hematoma, 46
hemoglobin, 23, 222, 224, 251, 339, 372, 427, 442
hemolysis, 339
hemorrhage, 339, 373, 381, 391
hepatis, 124
herbivores, 374, 416
herbs, 382, 386
Hercules, Naim Suleymanoglu, 441
, Sudanese, 76
heredity, 364, 371
hernia, abdominal cavity, 29, 55-56, 177, 393, 450
, abdominal cavity, 29, 55-56, 177, 393, 450
, spinal discs, 21, 23, 27, 37, 42, 45-47, 54, 154, 167, 266, 268, 404-406, 410, 452-453
, spinal discs, 21, 23, 27, 37, 42, 45-47, 54, 154, 167, 266, 268, 404-406, 410, 452-453
, using waist belts during, 111, 449
, using waist belts during, 111, 449
heroin, 363
high blood pressure, gangrene, 333
, hypertension, preventable diseases, 11, 328, 369, 385
, epidemic of, 1, 7, 50, 117, 376
, over training, 293
, hormonal control, 327
, cholesterol buildup, 333
, prevalence of cardiovascular Diseases, 363-364
, in women, 276, 371
, smoking, 372
, cause, effect, prevalence, and role of diet, 372-373
, prerequisites to exercise, 380
, impact on public health, 382
, cortisone Injections, 405
, arteriosclerosis, 427-428
, MAO-Inhibitors, 435
, on heart disease, 367-368
, in body overweight, 376
high-risk, diseases, 368
, exercise, 158, 453, 487
hip exercise abduction, 173, 174
Hitler, adolf, 243
HIV, 369, 381
HMG-CoA, 415, 416
homeostasis, 234, 235, 238, 253
homosexuality, 50, 64
hormone, adrenalin, 90, 121, 250, 326, 327, 430, 432, 433, 462, 486
, cortisol, 90, 397, 405, 406, 486
, epinephrine, 430
, erythropoietin, 123
, estrogen, 370, 397, 406, 460

, glucagon, 90, 121 326, 328, 418, 422, 430, 433, 486
, glucocorticoids, 405
, gonadotropin, 124, 239, 436
, HCG, 123
, insulin, 62, 90, 326, 382, 383, 415, 418, 422, 431, 486
, mineralocorticosteroids, 327
, norepinephrine, 435
, parathormone, 397, 406
, progesterone, 276, 397, 406, 415
, prolactin, 397, 406
, renin, 428
, testosterone, 124, 265, 328, 435, 439, 440, 479
, thyrotropin, 397, 406
, thyroxin, 431, 486
, TSH, 124
HRT, hormone replacement therapy, 370
HSCoA, 421
human development, 5, 424
organism, 413, 426, 434
humidification, 424
humidity, 233
hunching, (hunchback) 17, 21, 26-27, 33, 42, 53-55, 95, 135, 142, 145, 151, 157, 164, 226, 248, 334, 465, 469, 474
hunger, 61, 487
hydration, 23, 370
hydrogen, (proton), in Lactate affects on muscle, 220
, aerobic exercise, 487
, in combustion energy, 223, 236, 241, 420
, in Carbohydrates, 337
, in fat synthesis, 415-416
, stored body depots, 225
, transport coenzyme, 339, 419, 485
hydrolysis, 328, 416, 417, 418, 419, 430, 432, 433, 486
hygiene, 120, 384
hyperextension, 79, 83, 255, 272, 449
hyperinsulinism, 124
hyperlipidemia, 374, 415
hyperplasia, 124, 235, 414, 476
hypertension, see high blood pressure
hypertrophy, 134, 143, 213, 225-226, 232-234, 239-240, 282, 414, 475, 476-478, 483
hyperventilation, 223, 251, 257, 459, 474
Hypophyseal-Pituitary-Adrenal axis (HPA), 265
hypothalamus, 125, 239, 458
hypothermia, 123

I

ice in therapy, 109, 395, 396, 398, 400, 402, 449
idiosyncrasy, 123
illicit drug use, aggression, 125
imbalance due to body disproportion, 280
weak arms and shoulders, 281
weak scapular muscles, 282
immobility, 278, 325, 376
improper occupational activities, 21
lifting of a child from the floor, 22
a grocery bag, 22
bending on a sink, 22
inactivity, as cause of deformities, 132, 285, 402

, autoimmune decline, 380, 428
, back injuries, 25, 111, 398, 404, 474
, effects on enzymes, 325, 327
, fuel switching, 330, 375, 383, 393, 414, 418, 430
, in arteriosclerosis, 425
, in alcoholism, 371
, muscle wasting, 41, 119, 129, 166, 238, 250, 384, 392, 440
, muscular balance, 395
, retraining after, 69, 139, 244
, returning from lay-off, 139
, risk to disease, 8-Jul, 11, 13, 50, 234, 364, 383, 426, 483
, with age, 369
indigestion, 330, 461, 482, 488
individualization, 65, 482
inertia, 185, 189, 190, 200, 245, 270, 274, 407, 409, 410, 434
infarction, 333, 364, 366, 367, 369, 370, 371, 372
infection, 293, 328, 363, 367, 428, 461
inflammation, 145, 147, 249, 271, 274, 331, 334, 337, 339, 372, 382, 428, 446, 461
, bursitis, 396, 402
, epicondylitis, 405
inflexibility, 174, 229, 230, 245, 256, 274, 278, 285, 286, 440, 480, 488
information, lack of access to, 10
ingestion, 121, 459
inherence, 219
injuries, alleviating physical injuries of soft tissues, 395
, and warm-up, 20, 258, 276, 484
, and improper lifting, 41-42, 52, 54, 57, 70, 93, 99, 143, 195, 334, 395
, avulsion, 36, 94, 115, 132, 400-401
, back injuries, 403, 448-449, 466, 474
, bursitis, 396
, compartment syndrome, 397
, cortisone injections, 405
, due to inactivity and weakness, 15, 31, 366, 392, 415
, due to shyness, fear, or overconfidence, 37
, entertaining sports, 85
, fallacies, 55, 245, 460, 487, 490
, Hamstrings weakness, 393
, improper sequence of exercises, 18, 66, 197
, in physical activity, 395
, in lifting weights, 25
, in exercise, 11, 18, 25, 89, 212-213, 395, 413, 478, 485
, in modern living, 13, 21-23, 32
, in yanking, 36
, in Calisthenics, 111
, knee injuries, 399-401, 446-447, 471
, knees and back injury, 31, 45, 47, 56, 101, 135, 152, 168, 226, 229-231, 245, 423
, ligament sprain, 396
, load volume and overtraining, 73, 174, 293, 481, 488
, lordotic versus kyphotic postures, 27, 29, 439, 442, 452
, motor recruitment skill, 39, 458

INDEX

, muscular balance, 235, 273
, of back, 403
, of Meniscus, 399
, of tendons, 396, 401
, overweight and knee, 5, 264
, pinched nerves, 118, 404
, Powerlifting, 294
, rehabilitation training, 106, 268, 398-399
, rotator cuff tear, 402, 469
, Safety rules of proper progressive resistance, 16, 35
, soreness, 397-398
, spinal disc herniation, 54, 404
, Supraspinatus weakness, 393
, to knees, 56, 460
, sprain, 20, 57, 132, 170, 212, 252, 395, 396, 442, 445, 452, 488
, whiplash, 404
insomnia, 257, 293, 404, 435, 488
insulin role, 383
, anabolic effect, 62, 431
insulin-resistance, 62
intensity of resistance, 291, 316, 480
intermittent physical work, 232
intestine, 177, 224, 248, 250, 329, 330, 331, 338, 340, 365, 372, 380, 415, 422, 423, 427, 461, 485, 486, 487
involuntary control, 257
iron, 6, 32, 35, 86, 224, 264, 285, 336, 338, 378, 420, 442
. requirement, childbearing, 338 442
iron-deficiency, 442
Isaac Newton, 261
ischemia, 220, 368, 461

J

jackass, 422
jacuzzi, 398
jaundice, 124
Jerk lift, faults, causes and corrections, 215
jogging, 1, 31, 110, 111, 399
joint sublaxation, 396
    stability, with exercise sequence, 10, 18, 56
, alcohol, 23
, knees and back muscles, 31, 111, 202, 229, 241, 399, 447
, in start-position, 40
, in injury, 45, 461
, muscular balance, 63, 70, 109, 185, 192, 257, 391, 426, 468, 478
, in Squat, 93, 94, 96, 174, 181, 394, 470
, in Deadlift, 125, 394, 470
, in shoulder Press, 156, 161, 402, 472
, abdominal muscles, 177, 470
, axial strengthening, 268, 458, 470
    stiffness, in daily work, 4, 254, 485
, in Bodybuilding, 8, 13, 57, 66, 83, 104, 164, 252, 254, 438-439, 445, 481, 485
, managing, 15, 32, 60, 99, 208, 256, 461, 487
, and exercises sequence, 18
, and posture, 19, 29, 289, 484
, causes, 21, 31, 45, 52-54, 69, 111-112, 139, 170, 201, 207, 252, 271, 330, 396-400, 402, 404, 406, 413, 438, 449, 451, 462, 467, 473, 484

, Powerlifting, 469,
, effects, 264, 396-400
, muscles of the knees, 41, 56, 108, 175, 286, 473
, muscular imbalance, 161, 280-281, 330, 473
, in runners, 226, 230-231
, Claviculomandibular, 283
, sternoclavicular, 210
, sternomadibular, 155

K

ketoacids, 326, 416, 432
ketogenesis, 416, 486
ketone bodies, 326, 339, 416, 421, 433, 486
ketosis, 68, 416, 433
kidney, effect of exercise, 428, 485
    , effects of age on training, 238
    , in metabolism, 224, 248, 338, 416, 420, 485
    , in Long recovery, 334
    , in high blood pressure, 372-373
    , juxtaglomerular, 428
    , overweight, 376
    , parathyroid regulation of calcium and potassium, 458, 460
    , risk of death from disease, 368-369, 489
    , water retention, 62, 366, 372
knee-jerk, 46
Krebs' cycle, see tricarboxylic acid cycle
kyphosis, 27, 103, 108, 114, 116, 128, 130, 145, 159, 215, 244

L

lactate threshold, 237
    , activity and oxygen delivery, 395
    , adaptation in the type of muscle fiber, 235
    , anaerobic burning, 224, 234, 326, 421, 485
    , cardiopulmonary limitation, 251
    , gluconeogenesis, 416
    , high intensity training, 233, 242, 424, 456
    , in endurance, 253, 419, 478, 487
    , in soreness, 397
    , in fasting, 433, 485
    , lactic acidosis, 420
    , Low power output exercises, 237-238
    , maximum accumulation, 219-220, 225, 232, 235, 237, 241, 293, 449
    , over training, 488
    , training peripheral muscles, 248
landmarks of progress in the Snatch, 196
LDL (low-density lipoproteins), 331, 332, 365, 371, 376, 415, 432, 476
LDL-receptors, 476
learning the Snatch lift, 184
leg lunge, during lifting, 66-67, 74, 191, 204-205, 209, 211, 216, 218, 283
    lunge, in running, 226
    lunge, in accessory exercise, 73, 445, 450-451, 470-471, 262-263
legume, peanut, 437
leverage at the shoulder joints, 42
    of torque, 39
libido, 124
lifter, Anatoly Pisarenko, 80
    , Andrei Mustrikov, 81

, Andrei Mustrikov, 81
, Andrew Kerr, 81
, Antonio Krastev, 80, 81
, Antonio Krastev, 80, 81
, Aslanbek Yenaldiev, 80
, Aslanbek Yenaldiev, 80
, Bill Kazamaier, 81
, Bruce Wilhelm, 81
, Evgeni Popov, 81
, Ibrahim Abu Kalila, 246, 255, 256, 281, 321
, Ibrahim Shams, 480
, Ibrahim Safa, 489
, Kareem, 288
, Leonid Taranenko, 80
, Mahmoud Fayad, 88, 317, 320, 322
, Naim Suleymanoglu, 441, 485
, Paul Anderson, 80
, Paul Anderson, 80
, Paul Wrenn, 81
, Paul Wrenn, 81
, Pyrros Dimas, 485
, Pyrros Dimas, 485
, Sergei Alexeev, 81
, Viktor Naleiken, 81
, Viktor Naleiken, 81
lifting instincts, 30
    posture, 29
, backward fall and bruises, 96
, bailing out, 9, 23, 36, 42, 96, 115, 213, 216, 258
, bar trajectory, 216, 214
, essence of proper, 31
, forced repetitions, 139
, heavy versus fine movements, 195
, hesitation during, 32, 35, 37, 39, 58, 96, 98, 101, 138, 158, 168, 197, 198
, induction of momentum, 180, 200
, induction of speed, 179, 200
, induction of weightlessness, 180, 201
, insufficient full body extension, 215
, insufficient leg drive, 215
, insufficient shoulder flexion, 215
, insufficient torso torque, 214
, mastering the rituals of, 32
, off-loading, 131
, origin of forces, 184
, plateauing, 76, 441
, premature hip elevation, 214
    speed timing of the, 35
ligament sprain, 396
    , calcification, 135, 264, 401
    , collateral to knees, 400
lignoceric acid, 337
linolenic acid, 337
lipogenesis, 326, 422
lipoic acid, 253, 421, 488
lipolysis, 433
lipoprotein, 124, 326, 332, 376, 432, 476
liver, alcohol effect, 371
    , anabolic steroids effects, 124, 436
    , as abdominal organ, 92, 223, 249
    , autoimmune intolerance, 382
    , cholesterol or ketone metabolism, 339, 364, 374, 387

519

INDEX

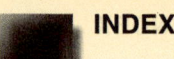

, disease effects, 62, 123, 124, 368-369, 413, 423
, exercise effect, 6, 330, 414, 423, 442, 482
, fat metabolism, 249, 250, 375, 386, 415-416, 425, 431, 486
, glucose metabolism, 237, 325-326, 416-419, 421-422, 430-433, 476-477
, glycerol metabolism, 61, 224, 486
, insulin effect on, 121, 383, 422
, lactates metabolism, 397, 485
, synthesis of clotting factors, 124
, vitamin-D metabolism, 248, 337-338, 460
load volume and intensity training, 232
logical inference and progress in sciences, 2
longevity, 19, 57, 66, 114, 263, 325, 370, 395, 448, 466
lordosis, 38, 48, 91, 108, 130, 135, 156, 181, 186, 192, 200, 205, 210, 211, 215, 229, 273, 282
lung, during warm-up, 52
, during activity, 220, 223, 465, 480
, in axial training, 247, 250-251, 468
, in smoking, 363, 459, 474
, in disease, 365, 368-370, 413, 415, 428
, neural regulation, 29, 223
, scapular muscles role, 82
lupus erythromatosus, 382, 405

M

magazine, Al Lataif Al Musawara, 87
magnesium, 188, 419
making the best out of your rest time, 15
malabsorption, 339, 382, 427
malignancy, 46, 428
malnutrition, 62, 76, 333, 371, 404, 413
mammography, 381
masculinity, 460, 474
massage, 45, 213, 214, 286, 290, 399, 401, 403, 485
meat, and cancer, 63, 381
, and cholesterol, 415
, and MAO inhibitors, 435
, beef, 121, 337, 338, 340, 342, 344, 345, 349, 351, 354-355, 357-362, 388, 416, 429, 437
, chick, 349, 355
, chicken, 121, 247, 342-462 411, 429, 437
, daily servings, 388
, duck, 121, 342, 344, 353, 354, 358, 359, 361
, food borne illness, 390
, goat, 346
, goose, 342, 344, 353, 354, 358, 359, 361
, in diet, 4, 121, 335, 338, 377-379, 386
, lamb, 337, 342, 344-345, 353-355, 357-362
, managing body fat, 327, 337, 365, 374
, nutritional contents, 342, 345, 347, 350, 355, 360
, pork, 121, 342, 344, 345, 349, 354, 355, 357, 358, 359, 362
, poultry, 327, 335, 337, 338, 374, 378, 379, 386, 387, 390
, sausage, 121, 354, 355, 357, 358, 362
, turkey, 121, 377, 437
, veal, 337
mechanics of ventilation, 223
meniscus injuries, arthroscopic trimming, 399-402
, function, 31, 112
, injury, 21, 57, 93, 108, 170, 231, 394-395, 399-401, 406
menopause, 370, 403

menstruation, anabolic steroids, 124
, loss of minerals, 276, 462, 442
, lower back pain, 46
, weight reduction, 332
messenger RNA, 250
milk, and cholesterol, 374, 387
, calcium source, 247, 338-339
, food borne illness, 378-379, 390
, managing body fat, 327, 335, 377, 386, 388
, nutritional contents, 340-360
, preventive diet, 384
, whey, 340-361, 437
mineral depot, 248
modern men's back, 230
momentum of head bouncing, 184
monoamine oxidase Inhibitors, agitation, 435
mood, 124, 239, 435, 481, 483, 484, 489
morbidity, 6, 45, 364, 405, 468
mortality, 6, 363, 364, 372-373, 382
motoneurons, 71, 72, 80, 90, 119, 188, 256, 391, 455, 475, 476
MRI (magnetic resonance imaging), 46, 396, 399, 400, 401, 402, 404, 412
mRNA, 325, 383, 416
muscle protein, actin and myosin, 18, 76, 234, 235, 397, 414, 418
recruitment, 148, 154
recruitment, 118-119, 140, 148, 154, 164, 170, 174, 183, 213, 214, 216, 220, 235-240, 242, 244, 247, 252, 256-257, 260, 267-268, 277, 294, 410, 446, 448, 471, 475-476, 478, 484-485, 487
fuel, 487
, A-band, 418
, adaptation, 235, 240
, anconeus, 147
mass and disproportion in runners, 226, 227
mass and flexibility issues in runners, 227
pain and stiffness, 330
, atrophy, 76, 414
, autoimmune reaction, 331
, axial back exercises, 466
, Biceps, in proper lifting, 25, 32, 35, 39, 466
, , exercise fallacy, 63
, , contraction, mode, 71
, , in Front Squat, 95
, , in overhead Squat, 97
, , in military Clean, 99
, , supersets, 109
, , in horizontal seated row, 126
, , in chin-ups, 128, 163
, , barbell curls, 142
, , one-hand cable curls, 143
, , dumbbell Concentration curls, 143
, , cable curls, 143
, , anatomy and exercises, 144-145
, , role in the Snatch lift, 186-187, 189
, , in full Squat Clean, 202
, , Hang Clean, 207, 453
, , peripheral training, 243, 247
, , structuring workout sessions, 443
, Brachial, 128, 142, 143, 145, 473
, Brachioradialis, 142, 144, 145

, brain control, 3, 71
, burning fuel during activity, 225
, Coracobrachialis, 150, 163, 166, 202, 207, 215, 216, 402
, cramps, 398
, eccentric contraction, 67, 71, 73, 92, 94, 97, 101, 105, 110, 111, 115, 129, 134, 136, 141, 142, 143, 148, 150, 163, 164, 166, 168, 207, 208, 240, 252, 266, 267, 272, 397, 439, 471, 478
, gastrocnemius, 131, 175, 447
, Gemellus, 167, 173
, glutei (glutes, and glueus), 125, 130, 133, 136, 153, 173, 184, 185, 187, 190, 193, 197, 198, 227, 268, 278, 421, 438-440, 444, 446-447, 449, 450-452, 465, 466, 467, 470, 471
, gracilis, 167, 173, 175
, Hamstrings (Hams), 153, 167, 168, 169, 174, 175, 186-189, 193, 197, 200, 204, 210-211, 214, 241, 243, 247, 260, 285, 287, 441
, I-band, 418
, Iliopsoas, 136, 137, 148, 167, 171, 227, 452
, latissimus dorsi, 126, 127, 128, 129, 130, 139, 193, 247, 269, 438, 443, 473
, leg extensions, 447
, Levator scapulae, 93, 99, 108, 151, 164, 170, 197-198, 279
, myoactin, 76, 225, 234, 235, 397, 414, 418, 459, 476
, myoglobin, 235, 398, 406
, Pectineus, 171, 173
, pectoralis, 158, 159, 160, 269, 270, 443
, Peroneus, 176
, pinnation, 147, 183, 191-192, 247, 250, 268
, Piriformis, 167, 173
, Plantaris, 176
, Popliteus, 175
, Quadratus lumborum, 152
, Quadratus lumborum, 152
, Quadriceps (Quad), 130, 133-134, 184-185, 193, 241, 273, 283, 286, 438, 439, 444, 446-447, 449, 466, 471, 482, 484
mass reduction with age, 238
, sarcoplasmic reticulum, 225, 235
, sartorius, 167, 171, 175
, scalene, 405, 406
, Semimembranosus, 167, 175
, Semitendiunosus, 167
, serratus anterior, 118, 160, 161, 164, 193, 270, 469, 472
, soles, 131, 190, 446, 451, 471
, spasm, 22, 37, 38, 40, 82, 213, 398, 403, 449, 478
, spasticity, 216, 391, 439
, Sternomastoid, 151
, subscapularis, 157, 158, 159, 473
, supinator, 144, 145
, Supraspinatus, 143, 144, 150, 155, 156, 159, 164, 180-181, 190-191, 193, 197-198, 201, 207-211, 215, 217, 252, 279, 282, 451
, tenderness, 45, 331, 396, 398, 399
and tendon strain, 396
, teres, 126, 127, 155, 443, 473
, tertius, 176

INDEX

, toning, 135, 155, 165, 228, 231, 445
, transversospinal, 29, 47
, Trapezius, 126, 127, 193, 269, 270, 273, 279, 280, 282, 438, 451, 453, 467, 473, 541
, Triceps, 118, 126, 128, 129, 139, 149, 183, 276, 437, 443, 444, 446, 451, 473
, troponin, 225
, twitching, 119, 125, 212, 213, 214, 216, 235, 238, 241, 259, 267, 331, 414, 433, 435, 476
muscles, agonist, 475
, hip flexors and abdominal, 266
, rotator cuff, 108, 139, 152, 155, 156, 157, 158, 195, 209, 215, 252, 273, 393-394, 402, 443, 451, 454, 472
, wasting of knees and back, 31
muscular imbalance, in weight reduction, 12
, flexibility problems, 13, 174, 256, 441
, in Strenuous work duties, 13
, reliance on equipments, 16, 89
, during inactivity, 30, 456
, body appearance, 41, 107
, in herniated spinal discs, 45
, and pyramidal neural tract, 53
, abdominal hernias, 55-56, 450
, Scapular balance, 63, 244
, in Bodybuilding training, 66, 118, 246, 447, 478
, pelvic, 94, 449
, and military style of lifting, 99
, description, diagnosis, prevention, 107-109, 278-283, 285
, one-hand dumbbell exercises, 148, 153
, reversing shoulder, 160, 161
, in hip adduction, 173
, in the Snatch, 179, 197, 255
, in runners, 227-229, 478
, in axial and peripheral training, 245
, in leg spring, 263
, in Weightlifting, 291, 441
, in Powerlifting, 294, 469
, walking exercise, 331
, heads of the Quadriceps, 394, 451
laxity, 98, 179, 193, 197, 198, 199, 209, 215, 229, 462
weakness, lower neural causes of, 391
definition, 119, 127
effects, 259
imbalance, 12, 13, 89, 99, 107, 108, 109, 148, 264, 278, 281, 291, 294, 331, 441, 445, 448, 449, 451
proportion, 119
and fascial pain, 45
imbalance in runner, 228
myelography, 46
myocardial infarction, 367, 369
myosin, see muscle, myoactin
mystical thinking among athletes, 1
thinking among common people, 2

N

N-acetylglutamate, 416
narcolepsy, 333
narcotics, 47, 363
nature of physical strength, 475, 478
nausea, 465

necessity of ballistic weight training, 213
necrosis, 405
need for community-volunteer work by athletes, 11
nerve, impingement, 45, 46
, afferent of muscle spindle, 71
, afferent of motor unit, 236
, ganglia, 63, 72-73, 174, 236
, Phrenic, 223
, tingling, 404, 406
, vagus, 223
nervous system, cerebellum, 72, 90, 458
, cerebrum, 18, 72, 90, 236, 253
neurons, 236, 273, 293, 407, 410, 422, 458
neurotransmitters, 238, 391, 435, 488
neutrinos, 412
new trends, 118, 457
challenges of urbanization, 363
tools of fitness, 117
niacin administration, 339
, aerobic oxidation, 339
nicotine, 23, 372, 403, 427
NSAIDs, non-steroid anti-inflammatory drugs, 47
nucleic acid, 124, 330, 337, 340, 412, 416, 420, 431, 432
, pyrimidine, 416
nucleus, 235, 250, 383, 412, 414, 416, 417, 420, 452
number of repetitions per sets, 69, 105
nutrition, 117, 120-121, 123, 139, 194, 213, 222, 224, 251, 253, 271-272, 281, 293, 331, 333, 363, 365, 373, 415, 420, 429, 438, 441, 450, 455, 459, 460, 469, 477, 481, 488
and coronary artery diseases, 62

O

obesity, 1, 49, 50, 61, 62, 223, 230, 243, 276, 328, 364, 372, 375, 376, 383, 438, 460, 461, 474
and overweight in Children, 376
Ohm, 251
oil of oregano, 51
old eating habits, 61
Olympic games, Atlanta 1996, 86, 221
, Barcelona 1988, 6, 246, 489
Olympic lifts, Clean, safety rules, 16
, Clean, mobility versus stability, 18
, Clean, lifting rituals, 37
, Clean, synchronizing the Pull, 44
, Clean, insidious deformities, 57
, Clean, chronological evolution, 65
, Clean, strength exercises, 66, 73, 90, 106, 107, 110
, Clean, technique assisting exercises, 67
, Clean, exercise sequence, 70
, Clean, contraction mode, 71
, Clean, core Weightlifting exercises, 73
, Clean, Standard Weightlifting training Sessions, 77-79
, Clean, leg drive, 80
, Clean, "military" style of lifting, 99
, Clean, muscular imbalance issues, 161
, Clean, standard technique of the clean, 199-203, 210, 280-281, 285-287
, Clean, contest rules, 206
, Clean, dissecting the motion, 207, 212

, Clean, errors in the Clean and Jerk, 214
, Clean, relative and absolute strength, 221, 239
, Clean, skeletal muscle adaptation, 234
, Clean, axial training and peripheral, 247, 466
, Clean, at 9-year old, 266
, Clean, imbalance due to weak scapular muscles, 282
, Clean, Powerlifting periodization, 294
, Clean, monthly exercise-differentials, 295-320
, Clean, plateauing in Squat, 450
, Clean, learning the Hang Clean, 453
, Clean, style variants, 466-467
, Snatch, mistakes, 195
, Snatch, final ascent, 181
, Clean finalizing, 203
, Jerk, flawed leg split, 216
, Snatch phase of acceleration, 186
, Snatch phase of descent, 191
, Snatch phase of full ascent, 193
, Snatch phase of full squat, 192
, Snatch phase of initiating momentum, 187
, Snatch phase of maximal momentum, 189
, Snatch phase of maximal speed, 188
, Snatch phase of shoulder abduction, 190
, full Squat Clean, 199, 202, 217, 254, 259, 317
, general tips on technique, 216
, Snatch, specific features of the mechanism, 183
, Clean faults, causes and corrections, 214
, proper Clean and Jerk technique, 210
, framework of training for the snatch, 194
, initiating the Jerk lift, 204
, Jerk, 147, 203, 206, 207, 216, 265, 271, 285, 441, 466, 469
, military Clean, 73, 98, 99, 100, 102, 106, 107, 199, 207, 214, 217, 245, 247, 466, 467
, Clean lift, 466
omentum, 188, 189, 200, 249, 407
optimization of energy expenditure, 219, 220, 234
in Weightlifters, 220
orchestrated central delivery, 251
overhead Squat, attentive posture, 28, 258
, future of Weightlifting, 80, 209, 451, 475
, full description, 96-97, 181-182
, muscular imbalance, 107, 161, 274, 296
, axial strengthening, 118, 167, 193-194, 197, 247
, flexibility, 254
overtraining, causes, 58, 69, 76, 89, 114, 117, 233, 236, 291-293, 439, 488
, circadian disturbance, 293
, clinical signs, 293, 488
, consequences, 94, 138, 216, 257, 264, 270, 366, 398, 456, 488, 491
, managing, 45, 78-79, 81-82, 149, 168, 293, 450, 471
, prevention, 110, 232, 441, 450, 481, 488
, recuperation and load, 488
overweight, 93, 228, 363, 375, 376, 383, 396, 438
, and obesity, 375
, back extension, 470
, body mass index, 375

521

INDEX

, cardiovascular exercises, 465
and decline in health, 376
, definition, 376
, epidemic, 50, 117, 363
, in runners, 228-229
, in children, 327, 376
, in heart failure, 366
, in diabetes mellitus, 382
, in ligament sprain, 396, 401
, in women, 460-461
, knees and back injury, 31, 399-401
, lifters, 92-93, 277
and obesity, 375, 376, 438
, one-legged hip extension, 167
, risk factor for chronic diseases, 332, 364, 369
and weakness in runners, 228
oxygen administration, 366

P

pain, of joint, 334
palmitic acid, 337
pancreas, 92, 121, 249, 250, 371, 383, 422, 462
passing habits between generations, 5
peliosis, 124
pelvic girdle exercises, 465, 470
penis size, 436
perception, 120, 125, 195, 212, 238, 245, 254, 261, 329, 335, 407, 427, 428, 482, 541, 544
perfecting lifting skills, 36
peripheral exercises, 465, 473
peripheral exercises, 465, 473
peristalsis, 330
perspiration, 36, 249, 251, 257, 485
phosphate, 247, 248, 253, 325, 326, 336, 338, 416, 418, 419, 425, 426, 428, 430, 431, 432, 433, 459, 485
phosphate-ATP, 326, 456
phospholipids, 326, 415, 432
phosphorus in food, 340, 348
phosphorylation, 338, 339, 415, 418, 420, 430, 432, 433
photons, 409, 427
physical appearance, 327
physiological consideration, 265
physiotherapy, 22
physique, 7, 14, 17, 20, 23, 39, 117, 120, 140, 246, 276, 444, 491
plankton, 337
planning load volume, 60
plateau in Squat, 450
Plyometric exercises, 139, 240, 492
Plyometrics, 236, 240, 245, 257, 258, 260
exercises, zig zags, 241
polysaturated fatty acids, 340, 342
polyunsaturated, 337, 343, 373
popularity of peripheral training, 245
potassium, 235, 378, 384, 385, 389, 413, 421, 458, 459, 486
administration, 459
potassium-sodium, 476
power Clean, as assisting exercises, 67, 199
, description, 100-102, 258, 265
, in Powerlifting training, 106-107, 294, 455
, muscular imbalance, 108, 281

, high intensity training, 110, 212, 479
, axial strengthening, 118, 247, 271, 275, 443-445, 467
, elevation of hips, 214
, maintaining flexibility, 254
, execution by children, 266
, monthly exercise-differentials, 295-316
Snatch, description, 102-103
, in powerlifting training, 106-107, 455
, in muscular imbalance, 107-108
, in axial strengthening, 118, 247, 254
, as assisting exercise, 189, 271, 455
, monthly exercise-differentials, 295-316
, structuring workout sessions, 443
, elements of physical, 90
and strength, 264
Powerlifting, 134, 277, 287, 294, 324, 439, 440, 455
periodization, 294
practical tricks of proper lifting, 25
pre-contest, exercise-differentials, 312-316
, load volume, 74, 233
, training trends, 235
pregnancy, alcohol consumption in, 371
, folic acid in, 378
, milk requirements, 388
, recreational drugs in, 363
, thiamin need in, 421
preparation for the Jerk lift, 203
prestretch, and yanking, 164
, in start position, 39, 200
, in shoulder Press, 156
, in the Clean lift, 216
, in learning the Hang Clean, 453
, leg drive, 80, 215
prestretch, muscle spindle reflex, 29, 127, 151, 273
problems with illicit drug use, 125
proliferation of the sport of general weight training, 8
proper eating, 61
technique for the Clean, 210
technique for the Jerk, 210
caloric intake, 61
sequence of the Snatch in training sessions, 197
resistance training leads to strength, 8
proprioception, 216, 410, 455, 476
prostaglandin, 47
prostate, 46, 327
protein synthesis, 76, 90, 113, 124, 219, 234, 235, 242, 250, 253, 325, 337, 392, 397, 398, 406, 416, 424
protein-balance, 429
psyche, 12, 123, 264, 482, 483, 489, 491
puberty, 9, 265, 423
pure strength exercises, 66
pyruvates (pyruvic acid), 234, 237, 253, 326, 332, 338, 339, 340, 416, 417, 418, 419, 421, 430, 432, 433, 456, 476, 485, 487, 488

Q

quadriceps weakness, 394

R

radiography, 399
rationing demands, 248
rationing your emotion, 257

RDA, recommended daily allowance, 121
real living emulation, 98
recovering from the Jerk motion, 205
rectifying shoulder imbalance, 282
recuperation, 45, 74, 106, 110, 113-114, 139, 182, 207, 212-213, 217, 220, 237, 241, 270, 282, 284, 291, 293, 478, 488-489, 491
recuperative intervals, 292, 324
reflex, cologastric, 487
regurgitation, 59
rehabilitation, 69, 151, 173, 175, 336, 395, 405, 447
resistance training a new experiment, 6
respiration, 122, 139, 142, 173, 202, 218, 220, 222-223, 225, 232, 239, 250, 251, 266, 270, 274, 329, 330-331, 338, 372, 375, 383, 423, 427, 456, 472, 484, 487
retracting the scapulae, 29
rheumatic heart Disease, 367
ribonucleic acid, 250, 325, 416
role of exercise, 398
rotator cuff tear, 402
rounded back during squatting, 452
runner, marathon, 122, 253
, lumbar deformities in, 229
, wasted leg muscles in, 230
running, accessibility of, 225
, dynamic forces in, 226
for endurance and strength, 225

S

saccharin, 350
satiety, 61, 487
sauna, 45, 214, 281, 398, 403, 478, 485
scapular balance, 63
sclerosis, blood vessels, 327
sclerosis, disease, multiple, 382, 391
sclerosis, soft tissue, 396
search for ultimate role models, 14
sequential hardening of muscles, 40, 438
serotonin, 435
sets, repetition, intensity, and volume, 291
setting goals, 261
setting priorities in a wise manner, 15
sexuality, 50, 51, 120, 374
shedding calories by physical activities, 122
shoes, 94, 100, 379, 396, 399, 446
shoulder abduction, synchronizing the pull, 44
, Deltoids and Suprapinatus, 83
, military Clean, 99, 100, 101
, muscular imbalance, 108
, transverse abduction, 153
, Bent-over Row, 154
, basic exercises, 164, 165
, induction of weightlessness, 180
, arm usage in transfer of forces, 183
, in Snatch, 190, 191, 196
, induction of weightlessness in the Clean, 201
, in the Clean and Jerk, 207
, in the Hang Clean, 208
, proper technique for the Clean, 210
, Suprapinatus weakness, 393
, in Hang Clean, 453
shoulder Press, lower back shearing, 21
, muscles of the scapulas, 67

INDEX

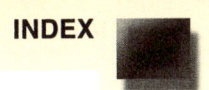

, core Weightlifting exercises, 73, 77-78, 296-315
, exercise intensity, 75
, front Squat enhancement, 96
, overhead Squat enhancement, 97
, military Clean enhancement, 100
, Bench Press enhancement, 105
, Powerlifting training, 107-109, 294
, enhancing the Snatch, 179, 182, 192, 194, 197
, enhancing the Jerk, 203, 205, 469
, slow motion training, 110
, mobility, 114
, range of motion rules, 139
, forced repetitions, 140
, shoulder internal rotation, 155-159, 161
, defaulted Jerk, 206
, Push Press, 209-210
, peripheral training, 245
, description, 252
, permanent physical changes, 273
, weak arms and shoulders, 281
, rotator cuff tear, 402, 450
, in split day workout, 445
, axial back exercises, 466, 472, 475
, individualization, 482
shoulder elevation, 151
    extension, 166, 201, 207
    flexion, 36, 98, 166, 282
    shrug, 83, 98, 102, 151, 152, 208, 230, 473
    abduction, 164
    drive and leg lunging, 204
    press and jerk, 469
    adduction and extension, 163
    abduction by Deltoid muscle, 33
    girdle exercises, 465, 472
    strengthening in children, 269
    and pelvis imbalance, 278
    external rotation, 152
    internal rotation, 155
    elevation and chest thrusting, 28
    , drooping, 107, 465, 474
similarities in health and physical sciences, 3
sitting in couch, 23
skeletal pain, 45
    muscle adaptation, 234
skiing, 40, 60, 396, 400
skill acquisition, 59, 70, 185, 238, 492
    transferability, 117, 140
    acquisition in the Snatch 196
skillful workout, 492, 541
skills, enhancing the Clean and Jerk, 78
    , enhancing the Snatch, 79
sleep, and diet, 370, 427
    , and pain, 398-399, 402-403, 405, 485
    , destructives habits, 9, 74
    , distribution of body fat, 120, 327
    , exercise role, 10, 11, 22, 43, 58, 77, 230, 236, 257, 465
    , exercising axial extensors, 268, 469, 488
    , Hot applications, 398
    , impact of modern times, 15, 276, 462
    , in unconditioned states, 22, 450, 456, 462, 469, 486

, modifying, 7, 422, 465, 481
, narcolepsy, 333
, recuperation of vital organs, 76, 293, 366, 450, 482, 486
, weekly training frequency, 138, 437-438
, yoga exercises, 214, 236, 256
smoking, alcohol and, 49, 257, 325, 371, 403, 470
, bodyweight control, 332, 376
, cultural views, 1, 321
, in cardiovascular diseases, 363-364, 366-367
, inorganic ashes, 427
, risks to health, 2, 5, 9, 12, 22, 41, 76, 224, 293, 383, 456, 486
, serious habits, 23-24, 372
Snatch technique, emphasis on, 77
Snatch lift, synchronizing the pull, 44
Snatch lift, deep Squat, 66
    , assisting exercises, 67, 77-79, 147, 152, 165-166, 197
    , maximum speed, 73, 272
    , and farmer's lifting, 98
    , role of the arms, 101, 102
    , description, 179
    , contest rules, 182, 195
    , learning, 184-185, 190-191, 197
    , teaching, 194
    , tweaking, 196
    , maintaining flexibility, 254-256
    , monthly exercise-differentials, 295
    , axial back exercises, 466-468
sodium, 120, 235, 335-336, 340, 366, 373-374, 378, 385-386, 391, 413, 421, 459, 486
soreness, 35, 139, 244, 247, 397, 398, 485
    , after-exercise, 139
speed of lifting, 72
speed-of-light, 408
spinal disk, nucleus pulposus, 452
    herniation, 54
spinoscopic examination, 47
split Jerk, 80, 209, 210, 211
split-session, 106, 294
sport versus exercise, 57
Squat, flat-footed, 452
    , leaning over during, 448
    and shoulder pain, 450
squatting with raised toes or heels, 452
stabilizing the Jerk motion, 205
stamina, 15, 51, 84, 235, 253, 274, 334, 479
standard training, 77
    technique of the Clean, 199
    technique of the Jerk, 203
    Snatch technique, 179
standards that achieve noticeable improvement, 17
standing very close to the object, 26, 438
start position, 38, 91, 95, 98, 102, 103, 125, 126, 127, 128, 129, 130, 131, 132, 133, 134, 135, 136, 137, 183, 186, 207, 217
    of the snatch, 185
starvation, 391, 421, 430
stearic acid, 337
stomach, acid secretion, 420, 427
    , after ingestion, 61
    , and injury, 22, 456

, in abdomen hardening, 92
, intrinsic factor secretion, 340, 382
straight and upright posture, 27
strength buildup, load volume, 73, 138, 304, 425, 480-481
, spastic muscles and yoga, 214
, peripheral training, 252
, and aerobics, 333, 418, 431, 480, 481
strength training and quality of ambulant living, 3
    , essence of resistance and energy, 39
    , Jerk-to-Snatch, 221
strength-development, 109
strength-training, 274, 287, 292, 440, 480
streptococcus bacteria, rheumatic heart disease, 367
stretch, benefit, 45, 159, 215, 230, 254, 328, 395-399, 403, 446, 481, 487
    , during lifting, 39, 41, 80, 82, 94, 200, 449, 476
    , exercises, 73, 100, 106, 130, 131-138, 158, 160, 162, 165, 168, 268, 471
    , muscular balance, 45, 109, 158, 283, 452, 485
    , spinal, 22, 27, 126, 168
submaximal cardiac power output, 251
suicide, 368, 371, 452
supraspinatus weakness, 393
surpassing others in the new sport, 6
swimming, 4, 59, 60, 84, 123, 220, 257, 392, 455, 485
switching muscle fuels, 60
symmetry rules, 139

T

TCA cycle, decarboxylation, 421, 430, 432
teaching the snatch lift, 194
technique assisting exercises, 67
    versus strength, 69
tensor fascia lata, 171, 173, 174, 193
testicles, during vigorous, 112
    , glucose transport, 422
    , in steroid usage, 436
    , metabolism, 417
testosterone ester after its oral administration, 435
therapy, chelation, 62, 336
tissue regeneration, 224, 232, 242, 253, 330, 418, 424, 426, 429
tobacco, 2, 9, 23, 372, 376, 482
torques and forces, 44, 438
torso imbalance, 279
training adherence, 11, 119, 457, 481, 485
    psychology, 488, 489, 490, 491, 492, 541
    frequency, 6, 15, 79, 81, 138, 292, 450, 456, 478, 484
    methods, 89
    load-volume, 172, 292, 294, 324
    habits, procrastination, 7
    , adjustment, 482
    volume and physical decline with age, 238
    , availability of space and equipment, 16
    , issues, 276, 284-285
    , balancing joints and muscles, 3, 17, 19, 30, 54, 485
    , in pyramidal start-position, 38
    Glutei and Iliopsoas, 41
    in Irregular squatting, 56

INDEX

, muscles of the scapulas, 67, 259, 286
, in machine aided training, 89
, in overhead Squat, 97
, in squatting style, 112
, in load volume, 114
, in Jerk motion, 205
, pelvis and lower back, 231
, in starting in the twenties, 272
, extensors and flexors, 275, 343, 446
, Snatch overhead, 279
, shoulder muscles, 283, 287
, core lifts and assisting exercises, 302
, postural training, 424
, in back and the abdomen, 450
, dealing with long limb bones, 285
, difficulties with axial, 244
, early education, 8
, early start, 265, 266
, effects of strength exercise, 222, 485-486
for endurance and strength, 232
, fundamentals of strength, 478, 479, 480, 481, 482, 483
, Fundamentals versus details of workout, 271
, getting involved, 6
, individualized exercises, 68
, intensity-volume, 293, 324, 462
, managing load intensity and volume, 217
, normal course of aftereffects, 35
, of gymnast, 267, 268, 269, 270
, off-season, 70, 120, 233
, on decarboxylation enzymes, 397
practice on the Clean and jerk lift, 207, 212
practice on the Snatch lift, 182
, periodization, 294, 295, 324
, periodization, 84, 213, 292, 294, 295, 324
, periodization, 84, 213, 292, 294, 295, 324
, plain common sense, 16
, scientific planning of resistance, 11
, spinal balancing, 286
, starting in the thirties, 274
, starting in late adolescence, 270
, starting in the twenties, 272
, two-day split workout, 443
, weekly frequency, 138
, workout counseling, 491
, workout anxiety, 491
trauma, 41, 42, 45, 50, 56, 64, 72, 79, 205, 212, 229, 252, 259, 397, 398, 399, 400, 402, 403, 405, 485
treadmill, 17, 236
treatment of back pain, 47
tremors, 92, 193, 205, 391, 435
tricarboxylic acid cycle, TCA, Krebs' cycle, 63, 76, 90, 234, 326, 330, 332, 338, 339, 375, 383, 415, 418, 419, 421, 425, 431, 432, 433, 476, 477, 486, 488
troponin, affinity for calcium, 225
tweaking the Snatch lift, 196

U

ulcers, 172
ultrasound, 109, 364
underweight, 375
urbanization role, 1, 13, 117, 254, 363, 424, 484

urea, 250, 326, 330, 416, 432
urinalysis, 46
urinary incontinence, 460-461, 471, 474
urine, 6-sulphatoxymelatonin, 256
, bladder cancer, 381
, calcium, 325, 373
, creatinine excretion, 238
, myoglobin, 398
, protein loss, 339
, stagnation of, 428
USDA, US Department of Agriculture, 327, 328, 329, 331, 332, 335, 338, 339, 340, 385
use your knees as a probe in lifting, 31
of simple and reliable equipments, 20
using waist belts during Squats, 448
uterus, 327, 461, 471, 474

V

vaccines, 23, 381
vasa vasora, atrophy, 428
vascularity, 69, 424, 466, 478
vasopressin, 397, 406
vegetables, broccoli, 352, 358, 389, 437
, cabbage, 121, 339, 389
, carrots, 338, 389
, cauliflower, 339, 349, 352
, lettuce, 121
, onion, 341, 349-350, 360
, pepper, 347, 350, 351, 358, 359
, tomatoes, 338, 341-361, 377, 389
ventilation, 219, 220, 222, 223, 225, 230, 232, 233, 235, 237, 241, 242, 244, 247, 248, 275, 424, 459, 465, 472
, perfusion, and circulation, 222
vertebral column, articulation, 42
vertebral column, spinal disc herniation, 54, 404
vitality, 39, 365, 367, 415, 425, 471
vitamin, B2, dermatitis, 339
, biotin, 340
, calciferol, 338
, flavoprotein, 330, 420, 488
, Folic acid, 340, 352, 353, 378
, niacin, 330, 336, 339, 378, 421, 488
, pantothenic, 339
, pyridoxine, 339
, riboflavin, 339, 340, 357
, thiamin, 253, 339, 340, 356, 421, 456, 488
, thiamine requirement in breastfeeding, 421
vitamin-A, effect on cornea, 338
vitamin-B12, cyanocobalamin, 340
vitamin-B6 administration, 339
vitamin-C, ascorbic, 339
vitamin-C, collagen, 339
vitamin-C, on dentine, 339
vitamin-E administration, 339
vitamin-E, tocopherol, 339
vitamin-K, 339, 374
vitamin-K, diarrhea, 339
vomiting, 392

W

waist-belt, 394
waistline, 375

water balance, 62
weakness, higher neural causes of muscular, 391
, Infraspinatus, 394
, of peripheral muscles, 392
, of Hamstrings, 393
of spinal erectors, 394
, 293, 324, 366, 488
weight reduction, adrenergic stimulation, 332
training, pros and cons of explosive, 212
Weightlifting training, from start to end, 286
, greatest assets, 283, 284
weight-to-bodyweight, 86, 221
wheezes, 68
whole performance and regional participation, 270
workout, environment auditory signals, 72
at home, 444, 445
workup for back pain, 46
worn cartilage, 400
wrestling, 35, 41, 59, 405
wrist curls, 146, 247
straps, 19, 182, 401
and finger extensors, 146
and finger flexors, 146
wrist-curling, 146
wrist-elbow-shoulder, 144

X

X-ray, 46, 396, 401-404, 412

Y

yanking, in Power Clean, 100
, in Bent-over Row, 127
, in lateral cable pulldown, 128
, in lever rowing, 130
, in cable hip adduction, 132
, in seated leg curls, 134
, in one-hand cable curls, 143
, in cable pulldown, 164
, in lower back pain, 403
, inertia, 410
, pulling versus yanking, 34-37
, speed of lifting, 72
, synchronizing the pull, 44
, training novice performers, 492
yeast, 345, 347, 348, 350, 351, 353, 355, 356, 357, 359, 360, 435
yogurt, low-fat, 327, 387
, saturated fat content, 388
, serving, 335
, source for calcium, 247

Z

zinc, in meat, fish, and poultry, 338
, low basic nutrients, 121